Clinical Chemistry
Fundamentals and Laboratory Techniques

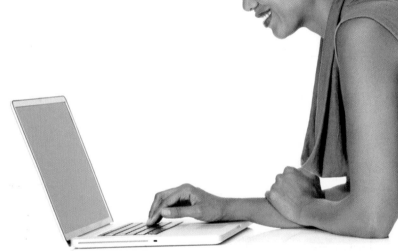

Clinical Chemistry
Fundamentals and Laboratory Techniques

Author

Donna Larson, EdD, MT (ASCP), DLM

Vice President for Academic and Student Affairs
Clatsop Community College
Astoria, Oregon

Consulting Editors

Joshua Hayden, PhD, DABCC

Assistant Professor of Pathology and Laboratory Medicine
Weill Cornell Medical College
Director, Toxicology and Therapeutic Drug Monitoring
Assistant Director, Central Laboratory
New York Presbyterian Hospital—Cornell Campus
New York, New York

Hari Nair, PhD, DABCC

Technical Director
Boston Heart Diagnostics
Framingham, Massachusetts

ELSEVIER

ELSEVIER

3251 Riverport Lane
St. Louis, Missouri 63043

CLINICAL CHEMISTRY: FUNDAMENTALS AND
LABORATORY TECHNIQUES

ISBN: 978-1-4557-4214-1

Notices

Knowledge and best practice in this field are constantly changing. As new research and experience broaden our understanding, changes in research methods, professional practices, or medical treatment may become necessary.

Practitioners and researchers must always rely on their own experience and knowledge in evaluating and using any information, methods, compounds, or experiments described herein. In using such information or methods they should be mindful of their own safety and the safety of others, including parties for whom they have a professional responsibility.

With respect to any drug or pharmaceutical products identified, readers are advised to check the most current information provided (i) on procedures featured or (ii) by the manufacturer of each product to be administered, to verify the recommended dose or formula, the method and duration of administration, and contraindications. It is the responsibility of practitioners, relying on their own experience and knowledge of their patients, to make diagnoses, to determine dosages and the best treatment for each individual patient, and to take all appropriate safety precautions.

To the fullest extent of the law, neither the Publisher nor the authors, contributors, or editors, assume any liability for any injury and/or damage to persons or property as a matter of products liability, negligence or otherwise, or from any use or operation of any methods, products, instructions, or ideas contained in the material herein.

Library of Congress Cataloging-in-Publication Data

Larson, Donna, editor. | Hayden, Joshua (Joshua A.), editor. | Nair, Hari, editor.
Clinical chemistry : fundamentals and laboratory techniques / edited by Donna Larson ; consulting editors,
    Joshua Hayden, Hari Nair.
Clinical chemistry (Larson)
St. Louis, Missouri : Elsevier/Saunders, [2017] |
    Includes bibliographical references and index.
LCCN 2015044074 | ISBN 9781455742141 (paperback : alk. paper)
| MESH: Clinical Chemistry Tests.
LCC RB40 | NLM QY 90 | DDC 616.07/56--dc23 LC record
    available at http://lccn.loc.gov/2015044074

Executive Content Strategist: Kellie White
Content Development Manager: Jean Sims Fornango
Content Development Specialist: Beth LoGiudice, Spring Hollow Press
Publishing Services Manager: Catherine Jackson
Senior Project Manager: Daniel Fitzgerald
Designer: Margaret Reid

Printed in Canada

Last digit is the print number: 9 8 7 6 5 4 3 2 1

Working together
to grow libraries in
developing countries

www.elsevier.com • www.bookaid.org

To my mom and dad, Donald and Barbara Bedard (I wish they could have been here to see this); to my husband, Earl, and my son, Adrian, for their love and support; to my sister and her family for their warmth and love; to the Allards for their support during my clinical year and college years; and to all the friends and colleagues I worked with at Wentworth-Douglass Hospital (NH), 509th Strategic Hospital (NH), RAF Lakenheath Regional Hospital (UK), Winston-Salem State University (NC), Mt Hood Community College (OR), Portland Community College (OR), and Clatsop Community College (OR).

Donna Larson

Acknowledgments

I appreciate the opportunity Elsevier provided for me to write the first edition of this clinical chemistry book for medical laboratory technology students. The process was exciting, exhausting, challenging, and an educational experience like no other. I would like to thank the contributors for their hard work to help make this book possible.

I would like to thank the Elsevier staff for the assistance, guidance, encouragement, and experience that they shared with me throughout the development of the book. Thank you to Ellen Wurm-Cutter, who helped me through the proposal and beginning stages of manuscript development.

A big thank you to Kellie White, Jean Sims Fornango, and Beth LoGiudice for joining the team and seeing this project through to completion. The final product has been a long time coming. My Thursday mornings will never be the same! Thanks also to Dan Fitzgerald and his team for putting everything together in a beautiful full-color book. Everyone was understanding, patient, compassionate, empathetic, and truly amazing.

Donna Larson

Contributors

Sheryl Berman, PhD
Division Dean of Health Professions
Lane Community College
Eugene, Oregon

Jimmy L. Boyd, CLS (NCA), MS/MHS
Assistant Professor, Department Head
Medical Laboratory Technology
Arkansas State University, Beebe
Beebe, Arkansas

Craig Foreback, PhD
Senior Consultant
Clear Medical Solutions, LLC
Bradenton, Florida
Senior Lecturer Emeritus
University of Wisconsin School of Medicine
    and Public Health
Madison, Wisconsin

Danielle Fortuna, MD
Department of Pathology, Anatomy, and
    Cell Biology
Sidney Kimmel Medical College
Thomas Jefferson University
Philadelphia, Pennsylvania

Thomas Kampfrath, PhD, DABCC
Clinical Biochemist
Santa Clara Valley Medical Center
Department of Pathology and Laboratory Medicine
San Jose, California

Laura J. McCloskey, PhD
Department of Pathology, Anatomy, and Cell Biology
Sidney Kimmel Medical College
Thomas Jefferson University
Philadelphia, Pennsylvania

M. Laura Parnas, PhD, DABCC, FACB
Director of Clinical Science
Sutter Health Shared Laboratory
Livermore, California

John W. Ridley, PhD, RN, MT (ASCP)
Formerly, Director of Medical Laboratory Technology
West Central Technical College
Waco, Georgia

Laird C. Sheldahl, PhD
Instructor, Anatomy and Physiology, Biology
Mount Hood Community College
Gresham, Oregon

Douglas F. Stickle, PhD, DABCC, FACB
Department of Pathology, Anatomy, and Cell Biology
Sidney Kimmel Medical College
Thomas Jefferson University
Philadelphia, Pennsylvania

Zi-Xuan Wang, PhD
Department of Pathology, Anatomy, and Cell Biology
Sidney Kimmel Medical College
Thomas Jefferson University
Philadelphia, Pennsylvania

Reviewers

Keith Bellinger, PBT (ASCP)
Medical Technologist
The United States Department of Veterans Affairs New
   Jersey Health Care System
East Orange, New Jersey
Assistant Professor, Phlebotomy
Rutgers—The State University of New Jersey
Newark, New Jersey

Stephanie Bielas, PhD
Assistant Professor of Human Genetics
University of Michigan
Ann Arbor, Michigan

Jimmy L. Boyd, CLS (NCA), MS/MHS
Assistant Professor, Department Head
Medical Laboratory Technology
Arkansas State University, Beebe
Beebe, Arkansas

Russell Cheadle, MS, MLS (ASCP)
Professor, Clinical Laboratory Technology
Macomb Community College
Warren, Michigan

Cathy Crawford, BS, MT (ASCP)
Clinical Courses Instructor and MLT Teaching Assistant
Mount Aloysius College
Cresson, Pennsylvania

Karen M. Escolas, EdD, MT (ASCP)
Chair, Department of Medical Laboratory Technology
Farmingdale State College, State University of New York
Farmingdale, New York

Roger Fortin, MS, MBA, MLS (ASCP)
Program Director
Bunker Hill Community College
Charlestown, Massachusetts

Trent Freeman, MA, BS, MLS (ASCP)
Education Coordinator
Medical Education and Training Campus
The George Washington University
Fort Sam Houston, Texas

Amy Gatautis, MBA, MT (ASCP), SC
Program Director, Medical Laboratory Technology
Cuyahoga Community College
Cleveland, Ohio

Kristine Hayes, MAT, MLS (ASCP)
MLT and Phlebotomy Program Coordinator
Moberly Area Community College
Moberly, Missouri

Candy Hill, MEd, MT (ASCP)
CLT Program Coordinator
Jefferson State Community College
Birmingham, Alabama

Lorri Huffard, PhD, MT (ASCP), SBB
Dean, Science & Health Programs
Wytheville Community College
Wytheville, Virginia

Phyllis Ingham, EdD, MEd, MT (ASCP)
Director Clinical Laboratory Technology Program
West Georgia Technical College
Waco, Georgia

Stephen M. Johnson, MS, MT (ASCP)
Program Director
Saint Vincent Health Center School of Medical
   Technology
Erie, Pennsylvania

Haywood Joiner Jr., EdD, MT (ASCP)
Chair, Department of Allied Health
Louisiana State University at Alexandria
Alexandria, Louisiana

Stephanie Jordan, BS, MLS (ASCP), CM
Assistant Professor
Pierpont Community and Technical College
Fairmont, West Virginia

Jeffrey Josifek, MS, MLS (ASCP), CLS (NCA)
Department of Medical Laboratory Technology
Portland Community College
Portland, Oregon

Minh Kosfeld, PhD, MLT (ASCP)
Assistant Professor
Department of Biomedical Laboratory Science
Doisy College of Health Sciences
St. Louis University
St. Louis, Missouri

Marc L. Meyers, MBA, MT (ASCP)
PM Laboratory Coordinator
Centegra Clinical Laboratories
McHenry, Illinois

Constance Moore, MS, MT (ASCP)
Program Director, Laboratory Sciences
Eastern Gateway Community College
Steubenville, Ohio

Richard C. Mroz Jr., DA, MS, BSMT, MT (ASCP)
MLT Program Director
Fortis Institute
Fort Lauderdale, Florida

Dawn Nelson, MA, MT (ASCP)
MLT Program Director
Florence-Darlington Technical College
Florence, South Carolina

Kathleen C. Perlmutter, MBA, MT (ASCP)
Phlebotomy Coordinator, MLT Faculty
Montgomery County Community College
Blue Bell, Pennsylvania

Jennifer D. Perry, MS, BSMT (ASCP)
Associate Professor and Chairperson
Clinical Laboratory Sciences Department
Marshall University
Huntington, West Virginia

Ellen F. Romani, AAS (MLT), MS
Department Chair
Medical Laboratory Technology/Phlebotomy/Therapeutic
    Massage
Spartanburg Community College
Spartanburg, South Carolina

Ryan Rowe, MLS (ASCP)
Weber State University
Ogden, Utah

Mary Sadlowski, MT (ASCP)
Medical Technologist
Greater Baltimore Medical Center and Community
    College of Baltimore County
Towson, Maryland

Cheryl Selvage, MS, MT (ASCP)
Associate Professor
Lorain County Community College
Elyria, Ohio

Anita Marie Smith, MT (AMT), MBA
Laboratory Administrative Director
Moberly Regional Medical Center
Moberly, Missouri

Angela Sparkman, MEd, MT (ASCP)
Program Director, Assistant Professor of the Medical
    Laboratory Technology Program
Ivy Tech Community College
Sellersburg, Indiana

Andrea Thompson, BS, MLT (ASCP)
MLT Instructor
Barton Community College
Great Bend, Kansas

Dionne M. Thompson, MSE, MT (ASCP)
MLT Program Director/Instructor
Three Rivers College
Poplar Bluff, Missouri

Preface

Clinical Chemistry: Fundamentals and Laboratory Techniques is a comprehensive, readable, and student-friendly text for 2-year medical laboratory technology programs. The textbook has a full-color design along with detailed illustrations and diagrams to help students with complex chemistry concepts. Pathophysiologic concepts are included to help students understand the clinical relevance of clinical chemistry assays.

Purpose and Organization

As I look back at my journey in clinical laboratory science, I cannot help but marvel at how laboratory test methods rapidly changed over the course of the 20th century and into the 21st century. While researching my dissertation, *The Structure of Knowledge in Clinical Laboratory Science,* I was amazed to read articles in laboratory journals (1940s) concerning how to build a better cage for laboratory animals. (Pregnancy tests during that time used rabbits to determine whether a woman was pregnant.) The radioimmunoassays that were popular in the 1970s and into the 1980s were largely replaced by colorimetric immunoassays in the late 1980s and 1990s. Looking back, there was always new information in the expanding discipline of clinical laboratory science. The more the knowledge base expands, the more the students are asked to learn. This is especially true of medical laboratory technology (MLT) students.

MLT students have a mere 2 years to learn all the clinical laboratory science (CLS) knowledge (with few prerequisite and general education courses) on which to build a solid knowledge foundation. Pieces from various disciplines are incorporated or embedded in their CLS. When writing this book, I envisioned a clinical chemistry book that would incorporate just-in-time learning concepts for which the material would be fortified with additional material when needed. Building on this approach, Part 1, Laboratory Principles, covers laboratory principles, safety, quality assurance, and other fundamentals of laboratory techniques. The concepts are essential for anyone working in a clinical laboratory, and this section provides a good reference for beginning MLT students. For example, the students do not take a statistics course, but statistical concepts and calculations are included in Chapter 7, Laboratory Quality Management Systems. Quality management methods,

including the applications of Westgard rules for control charts and the calculation of the mean, mode, and standard deviation, are explained and practiced in that chapter.

Part 2, Pathophysiology and Analytes, covers the diseases, broken down by body system, that are commonly diagnosed through chemical tests. Each chapter in this section contains information about anatomy and physiology of a specific body system, disease mechanisms of common conditions that require clinical chemistry testing, and how laboratory results correlate with clinical disorders. This is a key section of the book because MLT students usually do not have room in their program for a separate pathophysiology class, unlike other health science students, for whom it is part of the program paradigm.

Pathophysiologic mechanisms of diseases and the resultant effects on clinical chemistry tests are discussed in each of the chapters. For example, it is easier to remember test results that are elevated after an acute myocardial infarction (MI) if it is known that the muscle is damaged and that the dying cells release specific chemicals into the blood. If blood is drawn at timed intervals after the MI, the person who understands the pathophysiologic mechanism behind the infarct will know what types of clinical chemistry results to expect from each specimen.

When diseases are discussed that do not use laboratory tests for diagnoses or when laboratory tests are used to rule out other disorders, this information is given so that students can understand the laboratory test ordering patterns of health care providers. This information also helps students better understand reflex testing and how the algorithms are developed.

Part 3, Other Aspects of Clinical Chemistry, covers therapeutic drug monitoring, toxicology, transplantation, and emergency preparedness. The clinical laboratory has a critical role in these areas, providing ongoing testing and assistance.

To complement the organization, the book is written in the active voice to help students better understand the material. Although this may be unconventional for a textbook at this level, I believe it helps students to better understand complex clinical chemistry concepts and master the material.

Most individuals are visual learners. To that end, many figures, photographs, tables, and flowcharts are included to help students better understand concepts. Many figures summarize complex and complicated processes or pathways to provide better comprehension of the material by students.

Key Features

Chapter Outline

Each chapter starts with a chapter outline that shows the main topics that are covered. It provides students and instructors with a roadmap to the chapter and can be easily referenced at any time.

Objectives

The textbook format facilitates the learning process by providing students and educators with detailed objectives that address the knowledge required to master each chapter's content. The learning objectives are listed at the beginning of each chapter, giving students and instructors definitive evaluation tools to use as the chapter's content is covered. Objectives are provided at various cognitive mastery levels: comprehension, application, analysis, synthesis, and evaluation.

Key Terms

Key terms are identified at the beginning of each chapter and highlighted in the chapter, putting valuable terminology at students' fingertips. The key terms are also included in the Glossary at the back of the book.

Case in Point

A key clinical case study is provided at the beginning of every appropriate chapter. The Case in Point feature provides application of the student's knowledge for correlating the clinical side of test results. Students are asked to think about important questions related to each scenario and to use fundamental information from the chapter to determine the answers.

Points to Remember

A bulleted list of important concepts is included in the first part of the chapter, providing an overview of the chapter content. This list gives students a simple study tool for easy reference.

Summary

A short summary at the end of the chapter highlights key information from the chapter. Students can revisit the various chapter topics in short form for review and reinforcement.

Review Questions

Multiple-choice review questions at the end of every chapter provide students with a unique tool as they prepare for classroom examinations and certification examinations. The review questions give students a chance to quiz themselves on the chapter content, assess their knowledge of important chapter topics, and evaluate which topics need follow-up review.

Critical Thinking Questions

The Critical Thinking Questions allow students and instructors to discuss the chapter topics in a broader way. Although these questions have correct answers, they require more in-depth thinking, analysis, evaluation, and reflection than other questions in the chapter.

Case Studies

Additional Case Studies round out each most chapters, giving students another opportunity to apply the knowledge gained from the chapter. The scenarios are meant to stimulate interest and critical thinking and to encourage discussion of chapter topics with other students.

Evolve Companion Website

Clinical Chemistry comes with a companion website, found on Evolve (evolve.elsevier.com/Larson). This website contains helpful ancillaries for instructors and additional materials for students.

For the Instructor

The Evolve website has multiple features for the instructor:
- A test bank with multiple-choice questions and rationales.
- PowerPoint presentations for every chapter that can be used as is or as a template to prepare lectures.
- A detailed Answer Key with rationales for all in-text questions.
- The Image Collection that provides electronic files of all the chapter figures that can be downloaded into PowerPoint presentations.

For the Student

Additional content is available for the student:
- High-definition animations to illustrate key physiologic and pathophysiologic processes.
- Extra Case Studies for certain chapters for more practical application of textbook content.

Contents

1

Laboratory Essentials

DONNA LARSON

CHAPTER OUTLINE

OBJECTIVES

At the completion of this chapter, the reader will be able to:

1. Describe the history of the clinical laboratory.
2. List the typical departments of a clinical laboratory.
3. List the personnel employed in a clinical laboratory.
4. List the characteristics of reference, federal, and military laboratories.
5. Briefly describe The Joint Commission and the College of American Pathologists and their roles in clinical laboratory oversight.
6. Describe the types of water and the uses for each.
7. Compare and contrast the types of glassware and plasticware.
8. Describe the types of centrifuges used in the laboratory.
9. Describe the operating instructions and precautions for centrifuges.
10. Describe the types of balances and their use in the laboratory.
11. Compare and contrast serologic and volumetric pipettes.
12. Describe the various methods used to calibrate pipettes.
13. Define molarity and mole and perform the calculations needed for preparing and working with molar solutions.
14. Define molality and perform the calculations needed for preparing and working with molal solutions.
15. Define normality, equivalent weight, and milliequivalent weight and perform the calculations needed for preparing and working with normal solutions.
16. Define g/dL and mg/dL units and perform calculations necessary to prepare solutions of a desired g/dL and mg/dL concentration.

17. Solve dilution problems for final volume and concentration given the initial volumes and concentrations.
18. Describe how serial dilutions are prepared.

19. Convert metric units from one unit to another, the three temperature scales (i.e., Fahrenheit, Celsius, and Kelvin), between SI units and conventional units, absorbance to transmittance and transmittance to absorbance, and absorbance values to concentration of the unknown.

KEY TERMS

Accrediting Bureau of Health Education Schools
Acid
Alcohols
Aldehyde
American Society for Clinical Pathologists
Amines
Anatomic pathology
Anion
Aromatic ring
Atomic theory
Automated pipettes
Balances
Base
Beer's law
Biochemistry
Blood bank
Bloodborne pathogens
Board of Registry
Carbohydrates
Cations
Centers for Disease Control and Prevention
Centrifuge
Chemical symbols
Clinical chemistry

Clinical Laboratory Improvement Act
Clinical laboratory scientists
Clinical laboratory technicians
Clinical pathology
College of American Pathologists
Commission on Accreditation of Allied Health Education Programs
Covalent bond
Ester
Governing board
Gram per deciliter concentration
Hazard communication
Hazardous chemicals
Hematology
Hydrocarbons
International units
Ionic bond
Ions
Ketone
Laboratory manager
Lipids
Medical laboratory assistants
Medical staff
Medical technologist
Microbiology department
Molality
Molarity

Mole
Nalgene
Needlestick Safety and Prevention Act of 2000
Neutralization reaction
Normality
Nucleic acids
Outpatient clinic
Pathologist
pH
Phenol
Phlebotomists
Physicians' office laboratories
Pipettes
Proficiency testing
Protein
Pyrex
Reagent-grade water
Reagents
Reference laboratories
Serial dilution
Serologic glass pipette
Standard curve
Sterols
The Joint Commission
Volumetric pipette
Valence

Points to Remember

- The American Society for Clinical Pathologists (ASCP) was formed in 1922 to meet the needs of the growing pathology profession.
- The ASCP created the Board of Registry in 1928 to certify laboratory technicians and then the Board of Schools to accredit laboratory training schools.
- In 1933, clinical laboratory technicians formed a professional society, the American Society for Clinical Laboratory Technicians, to provide autonomy and a voice for the growing profession of clinical laboratory science.
- Laboratories produce 80% of the objective data that health care providers use to diagnose and rule out diseases, and they provide blood for transfusion and determine the susceptibility of pathogenic bacteria to antibiotics.
- Clinical laboratories began as part of a hospital in the early 20th century and remain a critical part of hospitals today.

- Hospitals have an organizational structure consisting of a governing board, medical staff, and management.
- Anatomic pathology comprises surgical pathology, histology, and cytology.
- Clinical pathology is the largest portion of the clinical laboratory, and it is composed of hematology, clinical chemistry, microbiology, immunohematology, toxicology, immunology and serology, urinalysis, specimen collection, and customer service.
- Pathologists are medical doctors who oversee laboratory testing.
- A laboratory manager is responsible for the daily activities of the laboratory.
- Clinical laboratory scientists possess a bachelor's degree in clinical, medical, or laboratory science; 3 years of academic course work; and 6 months to 1 year of clinical experience.
- Clinical laboratory technicians or medical laboratory technicians have a 2-year associate degree, and they perform all the routine testing in the laboratory.

- Medical laboratory assistants are trained to perform or assist in performing routine laboratory testing allowed by law and administrative tasks.
- Phlebotomists draw blood from patients.
- An outpatient clinic or a physician's office is a location where patients receive medical care.
- Public health laboratories are responsible for health reference tests; disease prevention, control, and surveillance; population-based interventions; and emergency response efforts.
- The Department of Defense operates many clinical laboratories across the world.
- Federal regulations that affect clinical laboratories include the Clinical Laboratory Improvement Act (CLIA) of 1967 and 1988, the Needlestick Safety and Prevention Act of 2000, and regulations for bloodborne pathogens, hazardous chemicals, and hazard communication.
- The Health Insurance Portability and Accountability Act affects the laboratory as it relates to patient privacy.
- Accreditation is a voluntary process with which laboratories maintain standards of quality.
- The Joint Commission accredits hospitals and many other health care organizations.
- The College of American Pathologists is an internationally known agency that accredits clinical laboratories.
- Competency testing involves testing the ability of the laboratory professionals that perform the diagnostic tests.
- Characteristics of glassware include thermal durability; alkali, zinc, or heavy metal content; chemical stability; electrical conduction; optical qualities; and color.
- Plasticware can be made from polystyrene, polypropylene, polycarbonate, Teflon, and nylon.
- The four basic types of centrifuges are horizontal head or swinging bucket, angle-head or fixed angle, axial, and ultracentrifuge.
- Pipettes are classified as manual, semiautomated, and automated.
- The volumetric pipette is a long glass tube with a bubble in the middle.
- There are two types of serologic pipettes—those used to deliver and to contain.
- Reagents must be monitored for reliability and reproducibility.
- To ensure high-quality laboratory results, high-quality chemicals and high-quality water must be used.
- The term *gram molecular weight* is often used as a definition of *mole*.
- Molarity = (grams of compound/gram molecular weight)/liters of solution.
- The molal concentration of a solution is equal to the number of moles of solute per 1000 g of solvent.
- The definition of *normality* is 1 gram equivalent weight of a compound dissolved in a liter of solution.
- The g/dL concentration is defined as the number of grams of a compound dissolved in 100 mL of water.
- A percent (%) solution can be written as g/dL or g%.

- $volume_1 \times concentration_1 = volume_2 \times concentration_2$.
- Remember:

  grams → milligrams, multiply by 1000
  decigrams → milligrams, multiply by 100
  centigrams → milligrams, multiply by 10
  mm^3 → mL (cc), divide by 1000
  milligrams → grams, divide by 1000

- Conversion of Celsius to Fahrenheit: $C = 5/9 \times (F - 32)$
- Conversion of Fahrenheit to Celsius: $F = (9/5 \times C) + 32$
- Conversion of Celsius to Kelvin: $K = C + 273$.
- The amount of dissociation that occurs and the number of hydrogen ions (H^+) in the solution correlate with the strength of the acid and the pH of the solution.
- Beer's law: $A = 2 - \log \%T$
- $A_{unknown}/A_{standard} = C_{unknown}/C_{standard}$
- Standard curves are constructed by plotting points for at least three standards for a test procedure.

Introduction

This chapter provides a short history of the clinical laboratory, various practice sites for laboratories and their organizational structures, levels of laboratory personnel, laboratory departments, and accreditation agencies. Chemistry principles and essential laboratory mathematics are also reviewed.

History of Clinical Laboratories

The first clinical laboratory in the United States opened in 1896 at Johns Hopkins Hospital. Laboratories were small rooms with very little equipment where pathologists performed tests on patients' specimens. After the discovery of causative agents of tuberculosis, diphtheria, and cholera, laboratories became more important in medicine. As the volume of laboratory tests increased, pathologists trained young women to perform some of the simpler laboratory tests to free the pathologist to do more complex testing.

The American Society for Clinical Pathologists (ASCP) was formed in 1922 to meet the needs of the growing pathology profession. In 1926, the accrediting body for hospitals, the American College of Surgeons, mandated hospitals to have a pathologist on staff. During World War I, hospitals experienced a critical shortage of laboratory assistants. Pathologists viewed this as an opportunity to standardize educational programs for laboratory assistants, now called technologists or scientists. To meet this need, the ASCP created the Board of Registry in 1928 to certify laboratory workers and the Board of Schools to accredit laboratory training schools. When an individual completed an accredited program, she could take the Board of Registry examination. Successful completion of the examination conferred the ASCP title of medical technologist (MT).

The ASCP played a major role in the formation of the clinical laboratory science profession by approving education programs and certifying laboratory workers. The National Credentialing Agency (NCA) was an independent certification agency created by laboratory professionals in the 1970s to credential laboratory professionals. The ASCP Board of Registry and the NCA merged in 2009 to create the ASCP Board of Certification.

Another organization that certifies laboratory professionals and other medical professionals is the American Medical Technologists (AMT). The AMT was founded in 1939 and is a nationally and internationally recognized certification and membership society for medical technologists, medical laboratory technicians, phlebotomy technicians, medical laboratory assistants, clinical laboratory consultants, medical assistants, medical administrative specialists, dental assistants, and allied health instructors.

In 1933, clinical laboratory technicians formed a professional society, the American Society for Clinical Laboratory Technicians, to provide autonomy and a voice for the growing profession of clinical laboratory science. Years later, the organization changed its name to the American Society for Medical Technology and then to the American Society for Clinical Laboratory Science (ASCLS).

In the 1940s and 1950s, clinical laboratory testing analyzed specimens such as blood and urine. Laboratories also housed and used animals in the test procedures. An example is the pregnancy test where urine from a woman suspected of being pregnant was injected into a rabbit. After a specific time period, the rabbit's ovaries were examined for ovulation. If the ovaries were swollen and ovulating, the woman was pregnant. In the 1960s, laboratories used frogs to detect pregnancy in women. By the 1970s, more reliable and valid test procedures were introduced into the clinical laboratory for pregnancy testing. More sensitive test procedures were introduced in the 1970s (e.g., radioimmunoassay) and 1980s (e.g., enzyme immunoassays). Bioluminescence assays attained widespread use in the 1990s. As more sensitive test procedures were introduced in the clinical laboratory, more test analyses were added.

Types of Clinical Laboratories

Clinical laboratories are a dynamic area in health care. Laboratories produce 80% of the objective data that health care providers use to diagnose and rule out diseases, to provide blood for transfusion, and to determine the susceptibility of pathogenic bacteria to antibiotics. Clinical laboratories are found in hospitals, outpatient clinics, and physicians' offices and as stand-alone reference laboratories. Laboratories are constantly integrating new technology and instruments to better meet the needs of health care providers and patients. The following sections describe the types of clinical laboratories, structures of organizations and laboratories, laboratory personnel, and laboratory departments.

Inpatient Laboratories

Clinical laboratories began as part of a hospital in the early 20th century and remain a critical part of hospitals today. Although the clinical laboratory may be located in the hospital, work from outpatient clinics, nursing homes, and other settings may be sent to the hospital's clinical laboratory for analysis. Clinical laboratory workers are hospital employees, and they are an important part of the health care team.

Organizational Structure

Hospitals are an invention of the 20th century. Hospitals were known as almshouses before the 20th century. Almshouses were places where poor people or people without family members to care for them would go to receive care. These facilities provided food, shelter, and rest. Before the 20th century, the best medical care was received at home; even operations were performed in the home. As medical procedures and equipment became more advanced, the patient went to see the doctor instead of the doctor coming to see the patient.

Hospital

There are approximately 6500 hospitals in the United States. They are classified as public, private, specialty, community, federal, military, or other types.

Hospitals are organized in three distinct parts: governing board, medical staff, and management. The **governing board** is the body responsible for the financial health of the organization and for setting institutional policies and goals. The governing board appoints the medical staff as the party responsible for quality patient care.

The **medical staff** members of the hospital are not usually considered to be employees; however, more hospitals and hospital systems are employing health care providers. In the traditional structure, the medical staff is granted the right to admit patients and perform procedures in the hospital.

The management portion of the hospital consists of the hospital administrator as the chief executive officer who is responsible for managing all hospital departments. Figure 1-1 shows the relationships among the three parts of the hospital and shows where the laboratory fits into the organizational structure.

Clinical Laboratory

Clinical laboratories are composed of many different departments. The laboratory services department is usually separated into anatomic and clinical pathology. The **anatomic pathology** department examines all tissues, fluids, organs, and limbs removed from the body. This discipline comprises surgical pathology, histology, and cytology. Personnel in the anatomic pathology department include pathologists, pathologists' assistants, histology technicians, and cytology technicians. In the anatomic pathology department, tissues are described by pathologists, cut into sections, fixed with chemicals, sliced very thin, placed on glass slides, and stained with special chemicals. After the slides are stained and cover slipped, the pathologist examines the tissue for abnormalities.

Clinical pathology is the largest portion of the clinical laboratory. This section is composed of hematology, clinical chemistry, microbiology, immunohematology, toxicology,

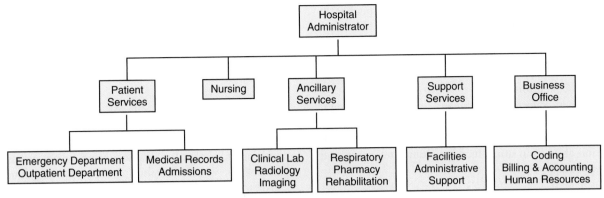

• **Figure 1-1** Hospital organizational chart.

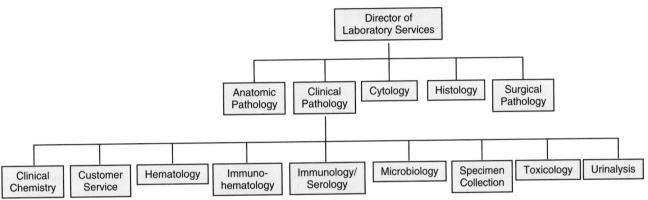

• **Figure 1-2** Clinical laboratory organizational chart.

immunology and serology, urinalysis, specimen collection, and customer service. The individual laboratory sections are described later (Fig. 1-2).

Departments and Their Functions

Clinical Chemistry

Clinical chemistry is the medical discipline that uses various methods of analysis and instrumentation to determine values for chemical components in normal and diseased states, types and concentrations of blood toxins, and therapeutic drug levels. Routine tests run by the clinical chemistry section analyze levels of glucose, blood urea nitrogen (BUN), electrolytes, calcium, phosphorus, magnesium, lipids, liver function values, alkaline phosphatase, creatinine kinase, creatinine, protein, albumin, and hemoglobin A_{1C}. The clinical chemistry department also runs hepatitis panels, tests for rubella and human immunodeficiency virus (HIV), and determines levels of antibodies in the blood. Hormone levels (e.g., thyroid-stimulating hormone, prolactin, follicle-stimulating hormone) are tested in another section of this laboratory.

The routine tests are usually run in the main clinical chemistry department. The antibody and hormone levels are usually considered subspecialties. Other subspecialty departments include the toxicology, therapeutic drug monitoring, molecular diagnostics, and fecal analysis. Some clinical chemistry laboratories have a section that analyzes blood gases.

Hematology

Hematology is the study of blood cells. Blood cells include erythrocytes (i.e., red blood cells), leukocytes (i.e., white blood cells), and thrombocytes (i.e., platelets). The most common test performed in this department is the complete blood count (CBC), which is a summary of cell counts (i.e., red, white, and platelet), total hemoglobin level, red blood cell size, and hematocrit. A CBC usually includes a differential count, which reports the percentage of each type of white blood cell in the blood sample. Cell counts for body fluids are also performed in this department. Other tests include reticulocyte counts and erythrocyte sedimentation rates.

In many laboratories, coagulation testing is performed in the hematology department. Routine coagulation tests include the prothrombin time (PT) and the activated partial thromboplastin time (aPTT). These tests assess the two major clotting pathways in the body.

Microbiology

The microbiology department identifies microorganisms that cause disease and determine the most effective antibiotic to destroy bacterial pathogens. This department grows cultures from major body systems such as the throat, urine, stool, wound, blood, eyes, ears, body fluids, nasal, abscesses, vagina, urethra, and tissues. Surgeons often perform a culture after they drain or débride an infected area.

Routine cultures include aerobic and anaerobic incubation environments. This department also performs identification or presumptive identification of fungi, parasites, and bacteria.

Specimen Collection

The specimen collection department collects tissue, blood, and urine samples from patients. In the outpatient area of the laboratory, phlebotomists also educate patients about collection of 24-hour urine, fecal fat, clean-catch urine, and other specimens.

Urinalysis

The urinalysis department performs chemical tests on urine specimens and analyzes formed elements that may be present in specimens. Urine is tested for color, clarity, specific gravity, glucose, protein, ketones, occult blood, and pH. These tests are used to monitor metabolic diseases such as diabetes.

Blood Bank

The blood bank or immunohematology department tests red blood cells from donors for antigens and serum from recipients for antibodies. Testing ensures that people receive compatible units of blood during a transfusion. The blood bank also transfuses other blood components such as platelets, fresh frozen plasma, and specific clotting factors.

Immunology and Serology

When invaded by microorganisms or other foreign bodies, the human body produces antibodies to protect itself from the threat. The immunology and serology department tests blood for antibodies produced against pathogenic microorganisms. Detection of antibodies against a particular pathogen affects the diagnosis and treatment of the disease, such as hepatitis B virus and HIV infections. The department also tests for abnormal configurations of antibodies.

Much testing is performed across laboratory departments. For example, molecular diagnostics can be performed in a microbiology laboratory to test for specific viruses and other microorganisms. Serology and immunology testing may be performed in the chemistry department. To increase laboratory efficiency, many large laboratories have a core laboratory. The composition of a core laboratory varies according to the needs of the institution and its clients. One possible configuration uses a menu of testing services for general chemistries, hematology, coagulation, blood gases, therapeutic drugs, endocrine profiles, emergency toxicology, and drugs of abuse. It usually includes automated analytic systems and specialized information management for critical care testing on a 24-hour basis.

Technical Personnel

Laboratory workers include pathologists, laboratory managers, clinical laboratory scientists, clinical laboratory technicians, medical laboratory assistants, and phlebotomists. The educational requirements and duties of each type of worker are discussed in the following sections.

Pathologist

A pathologist is a medical doctor who examines tissues and oversees the quality of laboratory test results from a clinical laboratory. Pathologists must complete medical school, an accredited student resident program, and an approved residency.

Pathologists are responsible for analyzing tissue samples (e.g., looking for cancer cells) and interpreting the meaning of laboratory test results. They consult with treating physicians to determine diagnostic and follow-up tests for patients. They are also responsible for performing autopsies.

Anatomic pathologists assist surgeons by examining biopsies during surgery to produce an immediate diagnosis. This helps the surgeon to determine whether additional tissue must be removed from the patient's body to eradicate disease. Clinical pathologists oversee testing of body fluids and confirm cellular identification in the hematology laboratory. The clinical pathologist also consults with physicians about blood transfusions and antibiotic treatment of bacterial and other infections. Forensic pathologists examine evidence to provide information for criminal and civil law cases.

Laboratory Manager

A laboratory manager is responsible for the daily activities of the laboratory. He or she has at least a bachelor's degree and is a clinical laboratory scientist. The person is responsible for the laboratory workers conducting tests and reporting test results.

Clinical Laboratory Scientists

Clinical laboratory scientists (CLSs) are also known as medical laboratory scientists (MLSs) or medical technologists (MTs). They perform routine and specialized laboratory tests. They also troubleshoot problems with specimens, procedures, and instruments to ensure quality test results. They examine blood and body fluids under the microscope for microorganisms and possibly even cancer. These workers communicate laboratory results to physicians and pathologists. Clinical laboratory scientists train new employees, perform quality control procedures on analytic test runs, and evaluate instruments and new procedures. These individuals may also advance to department supervisors, technical supervisors, or the laboratory manager. They can also choose to specialize in disciplines such as clinical chemistry, immunology, molecular pathology, microbiology, and blood bank services.

CLSs possess a bachelor's degree in clinical or medical laboratory science, 3 years of academic course work, and 6 months to 1 year of clinical experience. This is the most common route to certification. Several other routes combine education with experience that can be used to become certified. Most employers require CLSs to obtain a certification from the ASCP Board of Certification (BOC) or the AMT.

Clinical Laboratory Technicians

Clinical laboratory technicians (CLTs) or medical laboratory technicians (MLTs) possess a 2-year associate degree, and they perform all the routine testing in the laboratory. CLTs who graduate from accredited programs are able to sit for the national certification examination offered through the BOC. CLTs use microscopes and all of the instrumentation in a clinical laboratory. CLTs also specialize in the same disciplines as the CLSs.

Medical Laboratory Assistants

Medical laboratory assistants (MLAs) are trained to perform or assist in performing routine laboratory testing as allowed by law and to perform administrative tasks. Some MLAs also have duties involving patient contact. Most of these professionals receive on-the-job training, but some graduate from short-term educational programs accredited by the Commission on Accreditation of Allied Health Education Programs (CAAHEP) or the Accrediting Bureau of Health Education Schools (ABHES).

Phlebotomists

Phlebotomists draw blood from patients. Usually, CLSs and CLTs are also trained to draw blood as part of their education. It is more cost effective to hire phlebotomists to draw blood and have the CLSs and CLTs perform laboratory tests. Phlebotomists are high school graduates with specific training in phlebotomy. The ASCP BOC offers a certification examination for phlebotomy technicians (Table 1-1).

Outpatient Clinics and Physicians' Office Laboratories

An outpatient clinic or a doctor's office is a location where patients receive medical care. Clinics usually have small laboratories that perform routine tests as allowed by law. Physicians' office laboratories (POLs) range from a small laboratory (for one to five physicians) that performs a few tests to laboratories with a large volume (500,000 tests per year) that serve up to 200 physicians. The large POL is usually the exception. POLs are defined as a laboratory that performs tests in a physician office setting, provides results to be used during the office visit, and performs tests to be used for screening, diagnosis, and monitoring.

Reference Laboratories

Reference laboratories are independent, commercial, large laboratories that perform routine and specialty testing. POLs, nursing homes, and hospital laboratories send laboratory testing to these facilities. Reference laboratories have specialized equipment and perform low-volume specialized tests. Reference laboratories usually have drawing stations located in convenient locations for patients.

State and Federal Laboratories

The Centers for Disease Control and Prevention (CDC) operates one of two biosafety level 4 laboratories in the United States. It is an example of a federal laboratory. Many public health laboratories are operated at a state level. The network of public health laboratories plays a vital role in keeping Americans healthy. Public health laboratories are responsible for performing public health reference tests; disease prevention, control, and surveillance; population-based interventions; and emergency responses.

TABLE 1-1 Laboratory Professionals' Profiles

Laboratory Professionals	What They Do	Where They Work	Special Skills	Education Required
Laboratory director	Directs laboratory operations and consults with physicians	Hospitals, reference laboratories, pharmaceutical companies	Attention to detail, big picture; good communicator, planner, leader	PhD or MD
Clinical laboratory scientist (CLS)	Performs routine and complex tests Performs quality control	Hospitals, reference laboratories, clinics	Problem solver, troubleshooting skills, attention to detail, organized, good time management	Bachelor's degree Licensure or certification
Clinical laboratory technician (CLT)	Performs routine tests Performs quality control with supervision	Hospitals, reference laboratories, clinics	Good coordination, ability to manipulate small objects, attention to detail, computer literate	Associate degree Licensure or certification
Clinical laboratory assistant (CLA)	Performs or assists with routine laboratory tests as allowed by law	Hospitals, reference laboratories, clinics	Good coordination, ability to manipulate small objects, attention to detail, computer literate	On-the-job training or completion of a short-term program
Phlebotomist	Collects blood specimens from patients	Hospitals, reference laboratories, clinics	Good coordination, ability to manipulate small objects, attention to detail, computer literate	On-the-job training or completion of a short-term program

Military Laboratories

The Department of Defense operates many clinical laboratories across the world. Military hospitals perform routine laboratory testing and are accredited by the College of American Pathologists (CAP). The very large military hospitals perform routine tests for the physicians assigned to that hospital and specialized tests for other military hospitals around the world.

Military hospitals operate American hospitals to treat military members and their dependents. Military hospitals have laboratory officers and medical laboratory technicians staffing the clinical laboratory. Laboratory officers have at least a bachelor's degree and CLS certification, and the enlisted members serve as medical laboratory technicians and are graduates of the service's medical laboratory technician school.

Regulation and Accreditation of Clinical Laboratories

Federal regulations and accreditation agencies govern the operation of clinical laboratories. Federal regulations that affect clinical laboratories include the Clinical Laboratory Improvement Act (CLIA) of 1967 and the Clinical Laboratory Improvement Amendments of 1988, the Needlestick Safety and Prevention Act of 2000, and those for bloodborne pathogens, hazardous chemicals, and hazard communications. The regulations concerning safety are discussed in Chapter 2, and CLIA is discussed in the next section. The Health Insurance Portability and Accountability Act affects the laboratory as it relates to patient privacy.

Regulation

Congress first passed the CLIA in 1967. The purpose of this Act was to regulate clinical laboratories involved in interstate commerce. Hospital and reference laboratories were the only clinical laboratories affected by the Act. In 1988, Congress passed regulatory amendments to the Act in response to public concern about the quality of Pap smears. The provisions of CLIA 1988 govern the activities of all laboratories. It was designed to enhance the quality of laboratory services provided to all patients by mandating quality control, quality assurance, and proficiency testing. Trained personnel were required to perform particular levels or complexities of tests. The more complex tests a laboratory performs, the higher the standards required for the personnel working in that laboratory. If a laboratory performs only simple tests, the laboratory can obtain a certificate of waiver. Laboratories performing "waived" tests are exempt from proficiency testing requirements under CLIA.

Accreditation

Accreditation is a voluntary process by which laboratories maintain certain standards of quality. Two accrediting agencies have been given "deemed status" by the federal government's Centers for Medicare and Medicaid Services (CMS). If laboratories are accredited by either agency, the laboratory does not need to be inspected by the Department of Health and Human Services. The two accrediting agencies are The Joint Commission and the College of American Pathologists (CAP).

The Joint Commission

The Joint Commission (formerly known as the Joint Commission for the Accreditation of Healthcare Organizations [JCAHO]) accredits hospitals and many other health care organizations, such as ambulatory care facilities, stand-alone surgery centers, long-term care facilities, behavioral health centers, and laboratories. A team of individuals from peer institutions that are accredited by The Joint Commission visits an institution seeking accreditation or reaccreditation. These site visitors examine each standard and the evidence compiled by the institution for compliance with the standard. Institutions must also collect data on core measures (ORYX) and must comply with the National Patient Safety Goals annually issued by The Joint Commission. The Joint Commission accepts accreditation by the CAP as evidence of compliance with a good portion of laboratory standards.

College of American Pathologists

The CAP is an internationally known agency that accredits clinical laboratories. Clinical laboratory professionals perform inspections at clinical laboratories using accreditation checklists developed by CAP. CAP strives for excellence well beyond regulatory compliance to assist physicians in providing the best patient care possible. The foundation of CAP accreditation is rigorous accreditation standards that are molded into specific, comprehensive checklists. The inspection team uses the checklists to analyze laboratory operations.

Proficiency Testing

Proficiency testing is required by CAP, The Joint Commission, and the federal government through CLIA 1988. Proficiency testing is a process in which a laboratory is provided samples to analyze with a regular run. These samples are provided for every department in the laboratory that performs diagnostic tests. The laboratory analyzes the samples and then sends the results back to the agency that provided the samples. The agency analyzes the laboratory's results and provides the analysis to the laboratory. This process tests the accuracy of laboratory results being produced in that laboratory. Excellent clinical laboratories must produce accurate and reliable laboratory test results.

Competency Testing

Competency testing involves testing the ability of the laboratory professionals who perform the diagnostic tests. This must occur yearly to ensure that individuals performing diagnostic tests are well trained and competent.

Laboratory Materials

Laboratory professionals use many types of equipment and chemicals in the laboratory. The following sections describe common, nonautomated equipment and chemicals used in the laboratory.

Glassware and Plasticware

All glassware is not made the same and has different characteristics for different purposes. Characteristics of glassware include thermal durability; alkali, zinc, or heavy metal content; chemical stability; electrical conduction; optical qualities; and color. Pyrex can be used in high-temperature experiments, and it is heat shock resistant. Other qualities of Pyrex include acid resistance and a low alkali content, which is good for high-purity laboratory work. The name probably looks familiar because Pyrex glassware is used for home baking.

Many types of plasticware are sold for laboratory use. Nalgene is a leader in providing high-quality plasticware to laboratories. Plasticware can be made from polystyrene, polypropylene, polycarbonate, Teflon, and nylon. Many types of plasticware are biologically inert, chemically resistant, break resistant, and durable. Because breakage is less of an issue than when working with glassware, plasticware makes good laboratory equipment.

Cleanliness of laboratory equipment is extremely critical because contaminants residing in a piece of glass or plasticware can severely disrupt the next analysis performed. All glass and plasticware should be rinsed thoroughly after use with water and a mild detergent solution. After using the detergent, the item should be rinsed thoroughly with water. If using a dishwasher to clean glass and plasticware, follow manufacturer's guidelines for the best results.

Centrifuges

A centrifuge is a piece of motorized equipment that uses centrifugal force to separate a mixture such as clotted blood. There are four basic types of centrifuges: horizontal head or swinging bucket, angle-head or fixed angle, axial, and ultracentrifuge. Centrifuges can be small enough to set on a bench top or large enough to stand alone on the floor. They can be refrigerated or nonrefrigerated. They can have small openings for placing test tubes or large openings for placing a unit of blood.

Uses for Centrifuges

There are many uses for centrifuges in a clinical laboratory. Blood specimens are spun down in a centrifuge to separate the red blood cells from the serum or plasma. Urine specimens can be poured into a disposable plastic tube and spun down in a centrifuge to concentrate the nonliquid material that may be present in the urine specimen. Antibodies and antigens can be separated through centrifugation.

Periodic Maintenance

New centrifuges should be calibrated before they are put into service in the laboratory and after repair. Centrifuges should spin at the speed recommended by the manufacturer because spinning too fast can lyse or break apart red blood cells, and spinning too slowly can fail to adequately concentrate materials in a urine or other specimen. The speed should be checked approximately every 3 to 6 months using an external tachometer.

The timer should also be checked for accuracy periodically. If the centrifuge is refrigerated, the temperature should be checked and recorded monthly. The temperature should fall within the manufacturer's guidelines.

Balances
Types of Balances

Balances are devices used to accurately weigh substances. There are two designs for balances: double pan and single pan. The double pan balance has a single beam with two arms of equal length. The single pan balance has arms of unequal length. Both types of balances can be mechanical or electronic. Balances should be placed in a vibration-free and airflow-free area away from centrifuges.

Analytical balances are used in laboratories for precision measuring in weighing substances requiring 0.1-mg to 10-μg readability. Analytical balances can be electronic or manual. Types of electronic balances are the electromagnetic balancing or electrical resistance wire. Although they are based on different principles, neither type of balance directly measures mass. Instead, they measure the force that pushes the pan downward. This force is converted to an electrical signal, and the signal on the digital display is interpreted as the mass of the object on the pan. The electromagnetic balancing principle uses a magnet and a coil to generate an electromagnetic force that is converted to an electronic signal and interpreted as mass. The electrical resistance wire uses the change in resistance of a wire that is attached to a piece of metal that bends when a force is applied. Balances use reference weights to calibrate the output, which correlates force to a particular number of grams.

Periodic Maintenance

Analytical standard weights are used to verify the accuracy of balances. The National Institute of Standards and Technology (NIST) recognizes five different classes of analytical weights: M, S, S-1, P, and J. Class M weights are designated as primary standard quality and are used to calibrate other weights. Usually laboratories use class S weights to verify the accuracy of balances for weights between 100 g and 1 mg.

Pipettes

Pipettes are devices used to transfer a specific amount of a liquid to another container. Pipettes are classified as manual, semiautomated, and automated. The two types of manual pipettes are volumetric (i.e., transfer) and serologic (i.e., measuring). Semiautomated pipettes can have a fixed volume or variable volume. These pipettes use plastic, disposable pipette tips to draw up and dispense the liquid. Semiautomatic pipettes are especially useful for transferring extremely small volumes of liquids, such as 10 µL, 5 µL, 100 µL, or 200 µL.

Automated pipettes are usually electronic, computerized pipettes that control the amount of liquid aspirated and the amount of time allowed for aspirating and dispensing liquids. All types of pipettes used in the laboratory must be routinely calibrated to ensure accuracy. The manufacturer's instructions provide details on calibration.

Volumetric Pipettes

The volumetric pipette is a long glass tube with a bubble in the middle. The liquid being transferred is drawn up in the pipette until it reaches an etched mark on the pipette. This mark indicates the exact volume for the pipette. Volumetric pipettes come in different sizes, and each pipette has only one volume.

Serologic Pipettes

The serologic glass pipette is etched with gradations so that different amounts can be delivered with the same pipette. There are two types of serologic pipettes: "to deliver" and "to contain." "To deliver" pipettes retain some liquid in the tip after the specified amount of liquid has been delivered. The "to contain" pipettes require the liquid that remains in the tip after delivery to be pushed out of the pipette for accurate delivery.

Reagents

Reagents are chemical solutions that are used in diagnostic tests. They are usually liquid, lyophilized, or frozen. Reagents come in various purity states. Because there is no agreement about the purity of a reagent, the standards put forth by the American Chemical Society (ACS) are used to determine reagent or analytical reagent grade. ACS chemicals are considered to have very high purity and to be suitable for quantitative analyses.

Reagents must be monitored for reliability and reproducibility. The U.S. Food and Drug Administration Department of Biologics enforces tough federal regulations to ensure quality. Laboratories must be vigilant and verify the integrity of purchased reagents. When changing lots of reagents, the laboratory must perform parallel testing to ensure reliable results. Laboratories develop operating instructions for performing this function.

Water

Water is a common substance with many laboratory uses. Drinking water contains many impurities that can affect laboratory test results. To ensure high-quality laboratory results, high-quality chemicals and high-quality water must be used.

Several methods are used to produce water that is free of impurities and suitable for laboratory use. The methods

are discussed in great detail in the Clinical Laboratory Standards Institute (CLSI) guideline, *Preparation and Testing of Reagent Water in the Clinical Laboratory: Approved Guideline,* 4th edition.

The most common purification processes used in clinical laboratories include distillation, deionization, reverse osmosis, and ultrafiltration. Distillation is a good process for removing particulates and some dissolved contaminants. It is less effective at removing dissolved ions. Deionization involves passing water through cation- and anion-exchange resins. This is an excellent method for removing ions, and when coupled with a carbon filter, most dissolved organic compounds can be removed. This process is less effective at removing particulate matter. Reverse osmosis involves forcing water under pressure through a semipermeable membrane. The semipermeable membrane filters out dissolved organic, ionic, and particulate impurities. This method is less effective at removing dissolved gases. Ultrafiltration involves passing water through semipermeable membranes (i.e., pores less than 0.2 mm) to remove most particulates from the water. It does not do a good job of removing dissolved solids and gases. Most laboratories choose water filtration systems that produce the best water possible for its use.

There are three types of reagent-grade water. Type I reagent-grade water is the highest quality water, and it is used in test methods requiring minimal interference and maximum sensitivity. Type II water is used for general laboratory testing. Type III water is used for the initial rinsing and washing of glassware. The CLSI standard bases the purity of reagent-grade water on microbiology content (colony forming units per ml), pH, resistivity, silicates, organics, and particulate matter. Water used for most routine clinical laboratory testing is defined as clinical laboratory reagent water by CLSI and has a resistivity of at least 10 mΩ · cm at 25° C.

Chemistry Review

A clinical laboratory analyzes specimens from the human body and other living animals. Clinical chemistry deals with the concentrations of chemicals and ions in the body and the changes that occur to these chemicals and ions in normal and disease states of the body. The following sections review the chemical principles needed to understand clinical chemistry.

Atomic Theory

Atomic theory states that all matter is made up of atoms. Atoms have protons (i.e., positively charged particles [1+]) and neutrons (i.e., neutral particles) in the center or nucleus and electrons (i.e., negatively charged particles [1–]) that circle around the nucleus. Electrons are located in specific areas around the nucleus called *electron shells*. The shells are located a specific distance from the nucleus. Smaller shells are located closer to the nucleus of the atom, and larger shells are located farther away from the nucleus. Scientists think there are up to seven electron shells surrounding the nucleus. In most cases, electrons fill or partially fill the lower energy level electron shells before filling the higher energy level shells.

Various atoms have different numbers of protons, neutrons, and electrons. The outermost shell containing electrons is called the *valence shell*. Electrons located in the valence shell are usually involved in bonding with other atoms to produce chemical compounds.

The valence of an atom is the number of electrons that can be lost, gained, or shared by an atom when forming a compound. If the atom gains electrons (–1 charge), the atom's valence is negative. If the atom loses electrons, the atom's valence is positive. As a rule, when 2 atoms combine to form a molecule, the sum of the valences of the atoms is zero. The resulting molecule is considered to be neutral. For example, hydrogen and oxygen combine to make water. The valence of hydrogen is +1, and the valence of oxygen is –2. The result of combining 1 hydrogen atom and 1 oxygen atom is a molecule with a valence of –1. Another hydrogen atom is needed to form the neutral molecule of water (H_2O). When an atom loses or gains electrons, it becomes an ion.

Ions are charged atoms. If a hydrogen atom loses its electron, it becomes a positively charged (+1) ion, also known as a *cation*. If the oxygen atom adds 2 electrons, it becomes a negatively charged (–2) ion, also known as an *anion*. Oppositely charged atoms attract each other, and this force holds the resulting molecule together. The force that holds atoms together to form molecules is called a *bond*.

Chemical Bonds

Atoms combine through ionic, covalent, coordinate covalent, nonpolar covalent, and polar covalent bonds. In an ionic bond, one atom transfers its electrons to another atom. The atoms in this molecule each have their valence shells completed. These atoms are held together with an electrovalent bond. In a covalent bond, each atom donates one or more electrons that are subsequently shared between the two atoms. A coordinate covalent bond is a special case of a covalent bond in which one atom donates all the electrons to be shared. A nonpolar covalent bond occurs when both atoms sharing electrons have similar characteristics. A polar covalent bond occurs when one atom in a molecule is more electronegative than the other atom. Chemical bonds play a role in chemical reactions.

Factors Affecting Chemical Reactions

Many factors affect chemical reactions. Some chemical reactions are reversible, and others are irreversible. Some chemical reactions go much faster than other chemical reactions. By understanding the factors that affect chemical reactions, it is easier to predict the outcome or troubleshoot a problem. Factors affecting a chemical reaction include temperature, light, pressure, concentration, and catalysts.

An increase in temperature causes an increase in the rate of a chemical reaction. A higher temperature provides energy for the molecules to move faster and collide more frequently. Due to the increased collisions, the chemical reaction rate increases. Conversely, lowering the temperature slows the chemical reaction rate and the collisions between the molecules. Light is another form of energy that can increase the rate of a chemical reaction. When working with gases, increased pressure adds energy to the chemical reaction and forces more molecular collisions, resulting in an increased chemical reaction rate. The concentrations of the reactants may also influence the reaction rate.

Important factors affecting a chemical reaction rate are catalysts. Many biological reactions are extremely slow by nature and require a catalyst to increase the reaction rate. Some catalysts are organic and are called *enzymes*. Enzymes are a clinically important group of compounds for diagnosing diseases. Chemical reactions are also affected by the concentration of the reacting compounds.

Acid, Bases, and Salts

Acids, bases, and salts are important compounds in the body. Acids and bases are produced and used in urine formation and respiration. Salt is the basis for the blood that runs through our veins. Understanding the properties of these substances helps to explain and troubleshoot test principles.

An acid is a substance that donates hydrogen atoms in a water solution. Acids occur as liquids, solids, and gases. When a strong acid is mixed with water, the acid completely dissociates or ionizes. When a weak acid is mixed with water, the acid partially dissociates or ionizes. Weak acids are used as buffers to minimize large pH changes with the addition of strong acids or bases to a system such as blood.

A base is a substance that donates hydroxide (OH^-) ions in a water solution. Acids donate protons, and bases accept the protons. Most bases have an –*ide* suffix: sodium hydroxide ($NaOH$), potassium hydroxide (KOH), or lithium hydroxide ($LiOH$).

A neutralization reaction consists of combining an acid and a base to produce a salt and water as products. The hydrogen donated by the acid and the hydroxide ion donated by the base combine to form water. The other atoms in the acid and base compounds combine to form the salt.

Organic Chemistry

Organic chemistry is the study of carbon-based compounds. Carbon is a special compound that can have a valence of +4 or –4, meaning that it can donate all four of its electrons or take on four electrons. Examples of other atoms that are found in organic molecules include hydrogen, nitrogen, sulfur, chlorine, bromine, and iodine. The versatility of the carbon atom's bonding creates more than 5 million known organic compounds. Most organic compounds are held together by covalent bonds.

Covalent bonds in organic compounds create lower melting and boiling points than in inorganic compounds.

Hydrocarbons

Hydrocarbons are compounds made of hydrogen and carbon atoms. The atoms can be arranged as straight chains, branched chains, or rings.

The two main types of hydrocarbons are aliphatic and aromatic. Aromatic hydrocarbons contain one or more benzene rings, and aliphatic hydrocarbons do not contain benzene rings. Organic molecules can contain a special group of atoms called a *functional group.* Five functional groups are important in clinical chemistry: alcohols, aldehydes and ketones, esters, sterols and phenols, and amines and amides.

Alcohols

Alcohols are compounds that contain a hydrocarbon chain (R) and one or more hydroxyl (OH^-) groups. Alcohols are extensively used in the clinical laboratory as preservatives or solvents, and they may be a component of stains and reagents. Examples of alcohols are ethyl alcohol, isopropyl alcohol, isopropanol, and glycerol.

$$R-O-H$$

Aldehydes and Ketones

The aldehyde functional group consists of an oxygen atom that is double bonded to a carbon atom, which also has a hydrogen atom attached. This group is attached to a hydrocarbon chain.

$$R-\overset{O}{\overset{\|}{C}}-H$$

The ketone functional group consists of an oxygen atom that is double bonded to a carbon atom that is bonded to two other carbon atoms.

$$C-\overset{O}{\overset{\|}{C}}-C$$

Aldehydes usually have a detectable odor. Some smell very bad, and others smell good. Examples of aldehydes include formaldehyde and paraldehyde. An example of a ketone is acetone.

Esters

An ester is an alcohol derivative of carboxylic acids. Carboxylic acids are organic acids. Esters occur in plants and produce the fragrance in fruits. Esters may be found in reagents used in chemical tests.

Sterols and Phenols

Sterols are high-molecular-weight cyclic alcohols produced from fat metabolism. A cyclic structure has three or more carbons joined together in a closed ring. If one of the carbons is attached to an alcohol functional group, the cyclic structure is a cyclic alcohol. Examples of cyclic sterols are benzene, toluene, and xylene. The benzene molecule (C_6H_6) is the smallest example of an aromatic ring. Benzene contains

six carbon atoms with alternating double bonds and single bonds in the ring.

An aromatic ring that contains a hydroxyl group (OH^-) is a phenol. Phenol is a carbolic acid and is highly poisonous. Phenols are toxic to most organisms, especially microorganisms. Phenol is an ingredient in many antiseptics and disinfectants. Examples of phenols include vanillin (i.e., found in vanilla beans), eugenol (i.e., oil of cloves), and thymol (i.e., oil of thyme, a member of the mint family).

OH

Amines and Amides

Amines are derivatives of ammonia (NH_3), and amides are compounds in which a nitrogen atom is attached to a carbon chain. Amines and amides are found in alkaloids, antihistamines, sulfa drugs, and barbiturates. A well-known amine is amphetamine, which is a powerful stimulant. A well-known amide is acetaminophen, which is a nonprescription pain reliever.

$$R-\overset{H}{\underset{H}{N}}$$
amine

$$R-\overset{O}{\overset{\|}{C}}-NH_2$$
amide

Biochemistry

Biochemistry, also called physiologic chemistry, is the study of the chemistry of living organisms. A sample of the biological processes that are studied in biochemistry includes the study of digestion, urine formation, reproduction, metabolism, and respiration. The four classes of functional molecules in biochemistry are carbohydrates, lipids, proteins, and nucleic acids.

Carbohydrates

Carbohydrates are polyhydroxy aldehydes or polyhydroxy ketones. This means that the functional groups are aldehydes or ketones and that there are several hydroxyl groups on each compound. When carbohydrates are hydrolyzed, the resulting compounds are aldehydes or ketones.

Carbohydrates are the main food source for humans; the body uses carbohydrates for energy. Carbohydrates are also found in connective tissue and nucleic acids (i.e., ribose in RNA and deoxyribose in DNA).

Carbohydrates have a general molecular formula of CH_2O. They exist as sugars, starches, and cellulose. Simple sugars are called saccharides and have names ending in *–ose.* Examples include glucose, sucrose, fructose, and maltose. Carbohydrates are classified by the number of saccharide units in the molecule: monosaccharides, disaccharides, oligosaccharide, and polysaccharides. Glucose is a monosaccharide, sucrose is a disaccharide, and starch is a polysaccharide.

Lipids

Lipids, mainly fats and oils, are insoluble in water and found in living organisms. As a general rule, fats, which are solid at room temperature, come from animals, and oils, which are liquid at room temperature, come from vegetable sources. Fats are part of messenger systems (e.g., hormones), are structural components of membranes, and provide energy storage in animals.

Fats and oils share a similar structure; each has three ester functional groups. These compounds are esters of trialcohol, or glycerol. The common name is triglycerides, and the more scientific name is triacylglycerol.

The popular media often discuss the good qualities of polyunsaturated fats and the bad qualities of saturated fats. Polyunsaturated fats have double bonds in the ester chains, and saturated fats have single bonds in the ester chains.

A *trans* fat has a double bond in a specific type of isomer (see figure below).

Other classes of lipids include phospholipids, glycolipids, and steroids. Phospholipids are found in the brain, spinal cord, and liver. Glycolipids (i.e., cerebrosides) are mainly found in the brain and at nerve synapses. Fats are the building blocks of steroids. Cholesterol is the major steroid in the body.

Proteins

Protein is considered by many to be the most important compound in the body. Proteins are found in every tissue of the body. Proteins are responsible for structure; they are the main component in hair, skin, and nails. Proteins are responsible for movement; muscles are made of protein. Proteins are responsible for catalyzing chemical reactions in the body; catalytic enzymes are proteins. Proteins are responsible for transport; proteins transport molecules across cell membranes and carry oxygen and carbon dioxide in blood. Proteins are part of hormones that regulate many body processes, including growth. Proteins are responsible for protection; specialized white blood cells (i.e., lymphocytes) produce antibodies (i.e., immunoglobulins) to destroy foreign invaders that enter the body. Proteins facilitate storage; specialty proteins store materials, such as iron in the liver by ferritin.

Proteins are made of linear chains of amino acids (Fig. 1-3). Twenty amino acids make up the proteins in the body. Protein synthesis plays a large part in producing proteins to replace those that wear out. Protein synthesis is controlled by genes.

Nucleic Acids

There are two types of nucleic acids in the body: deoxyribonucleic acid (DNA) and ribonucleic acid (RNA) (Fig. 1-4). Genes are composed of chromosomes, which are composed of nucleic acids and DNA-bound proteins. DNA controls the hereditary traits that are expressed in an individual, and RNA plays an important role in protein synthesis. Many inherited conditions, such as hemophilia and sickle cell anemia, are caused by the absence of a protein or presence of an abnormal protein.

Butyric acid–saturated fatty acid

Oleic acid–monounsaturated fatty acid

Linoleic acid–polyunsaturated fatty acid

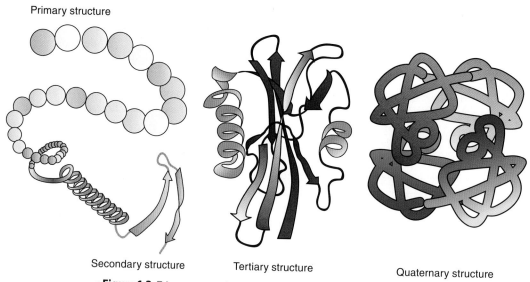

Primary structure

Secondary structure   Tertiary structure   Quaternary structure

• **Figure 1-3** Primary, secondary, tertiary, and quaternary protein structures.

Laboratory Mathematics

Everyone who works in the clinical laboratory needs to know the basic concepts of mathematics for technical procedures. Computers perform most of the calculations, but laboratory workers must verify the results. It is important to understand how to do mathematical calculations and to understand the concepts behind a formula. Understanding the basis of a formula allows a laboratory worker to modify the formula to better suit a particular situation.

When performing mathematical calculations, follow the procedure below to efficiently solve problems and reduce errors:

1. Read the problem carefully.
2. Determine the principles and relationships involved.
3. Determine exactly what the problem is asking and the results required.
4. Think about all possible methods to solve the problem.
5. Write the intermediate stages of the calculations clearly in a sequential format. Avoid writing one number on top of another as a method of correction. Make each digit legible.
6. Recognize different forms of the same value, such as: ½, 0.5, and 50%.
7. Position the decimal point carefully.
8. Mentally estimate an answer before working the problem; compare the calculated result with the estimated answer. If the two figures disagree drastically, determine which is wrong.

Molarity

Definition

Atoms and molecules combine or separate during chemical reactions. In other words, chemical reactions take place at the level of the atoms and molecules of the reactants. Because atoms and molecules are not visible in a solution, some way to know the relative number of reactant particles involved in a chemical reaction would be useful. The mole and molarity measurements are useful methods for this purpose.

A **mole** of a substance is the number of grams equal to the atomic or molecular weight of the substance. Laboratory professionals work mostly with compounds, and use the molecular weight of a molecule more often than that of a single element. An easier way to determine the molecular weight of a compound is to add the atomic weights of the atoms comprising the molecule.

Examine the periodic chart of the elements on the inside back cover. In the center of each block, there is a capital letter or a capital letter and a small letter. These letters are the **chemical symbols** for the elements. Beneath the chemical symbol is a number (e.g., 52.01) that represents the atomic mass (*mass* and *weight* are used synonymously throughout this chapter). This number is the sum of the number of protons and neutrons in the nucleus of the element.

To find the molecular weight of NaCl, first find the atomic weight of Na (23 g). Next find the atomic weight of Cl (35.5 g). The total of 23 + 35.5 equals the molecular weight, or 58.5 g. All atomic weights for elements are rounded to the nearest whole number, except for Cl. The atomic weight for Cl is always 35.5. The 58.5 g also represents 1 mole of NaCl. The term *gram molecular weight* is often used as a definition of *mole*.

Find the molecular weight of H_2SO_4. The atomic weight for hydrogen (H) is 1 g. Because there are 2 hydrogen atoms, multiply the atomic weight by 2: 2 H = 1 g × 2 = 2 g. The atomic weight of sulfur (S) is 32 g, and because there is only 1 sulfur atom, there is no need to multiply the atomic weight: S = 32 g. The last element needed in this problem is oxygen (O). Because there are 4 atoms of oxygen in the chemical formula, the atomic weight of oxygen (16 g) must be multiplied by 4 to derive the weight. 16 g/atom × 4 atoms = 64 g. To calculate the

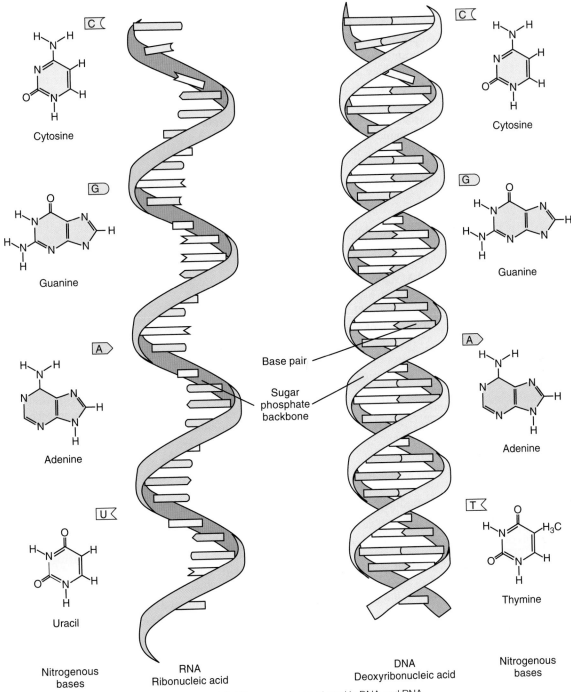

Cytosine

Guanine

Adenine

Uracil

Nitrogenous
bases

RNA
Ribonucleic acid

Base pair

Sugar
phosphate
backbone

DNA
Deoxyribonucleic acid

Cytosine

Guanine

Adenine

Thymine

Nitrogenous
bases

• **Figure 1-4** Nitrogenous bases found in DNA and RNA.

molecular weight of H_2SO_4, sum the molecular weights of the individual atoms:

$$2 \text{ g (hydrogen)} + 32 \text{ g (sulfur)} + 64 \text{ g (oxygen)} = 98 \text{ g} (H_2SO_4)$$

● Practice Problems

1. Review the process and then calculate the molecular weights of the following compounds: KBr, H_2O, $AgNO_3$, $Fe_2(SO_4)_3$.

Calculations

One way to calculate the concentration of a solution is to use **molarity.** Because one mole of a substance is equal to the gram molecular weight of a compound, mixing 1 mole or gram molecular weight of a compound with 1 L of water produces a 1 molar solution. In the previous example, we found that 1 gram molecular weight of H_2SO_4 (i.e., sulfuric acid) equals 1 mole of H_2SO_4 or 98 g. If we measure 98 g of H_2SO_4 (i.e., 1 mole of H_2SO_4) and dissolve it in 1 L of water, the concentration of the resulting solution is *1 molar*. **When 1 gram molecular weight (or mole) of a compound is dissolved in**

1 L of water, the concentration of the resulting solution is 1 molar. The molar concentration is also called *molarity*.

If two times the molecular weight of a compound is dissolved in 1 L of solution, the concentration is 2 molar and molarity = 2. Given this information, how is a 5 molar (5 M) solution of NaCl made? Unless the volume is specified, always use the standard 1 L solution. To make a 5 M solution of NaCl, first calculate the gram molecular weight of NaCl. The atomic weight of Na is 23, and the atomic weight of Cl is 35.5. Add these two atomic weights together to find the gram molecular weight of NaCl (58.5 g). To make a 5 M solution, 5 × 58.5 g of NaCl must be dissolved in 1 L of solution.

Practice Problems

2. If 5 moles of NaCl are dissolved in 5 L of solution, what is the molarity of the resulting solution?

Consider also how to make 1 L of 3 M sodium hydroxide (NaOH) solution. The molecular weight of NaOH is 40 (23 + 16 + 1). To make a 3 M solution of NaOH, dissolve 3 moles × 40 g/mole = 120 g of NaOH in 1 L of water. This is a 3 M solution.

Molarity (M) is a number that expresses the number of moles of substance in 1 L of solution. This is stated in mathematical terms as

$$\text{molarity} = \frac{\text{moles}}{\text{liter}}$$

$$1 \text{ mole} = \frac{\text{grams of compound}}{\text{gram molecular weight}}$$

By substituting grams of compound/gram molecular weight the formula becomes

$$\text{molarity} = \frac{(\text{grams of compound/gram molecular weight})}{\text{liters of solution}}$$

Using algebra, the equation can be simplified:

$$\text{molecular weight} \times \text{molarity} = \text{grams/liter}$$

This formula is based on the fact that molarity is equal to the number of moles per liter. For example, a 2 M solution contains 2 moles/L, and a 0.5 M solution contains 0.5 moles/L. Use the formula to make 1000 mL of 0.5M NaCl (molecular weight of NaCl is 58.5 g):

$$\text{molecular weight} \times \text{molarity} = \text{grams/liter}$$
$$58.5 \times 0.5 = 29.25 \text{ g/L}$$

Weigh 29.25 g/L of NaCl, and make 1000 mL (1 L) of solution.

Practice Problems

3. How much $CaCl_2$ would you weigh out to make a liter of a 2 M solution?
4. How much KOH would it take to make 3.5 L of a 1.5 M solution?

If you know how a solution is made, you can calculate the concentration. For example, an NaOH solution was made by dissolving 100 g of NaOH in enough water to make 1 L. To find out the molar concentration, find out how many gram molecular weights the 100 g represent. NaOH has a molecular weight of 23 + 16 + 1 = 40, and 40 g represents 1 gram molecular weight. Therefore, 100 g is 100/40 = 2.5 gram molecular weights. This makes the solution 2.5 M.

When faced with a volume other than 1 L, the same process applies. Suppose you have a solution made by dissolving 3 g of NaOH in 100 mL of solution. Because molarity is based on grams per liter, the first step is to find out how much NaOH was used to make a liter of the same concentration. This is done with a simple proportion equation. If there are 3 g in 100 mL, there would be x grams in 1000 mL:

$$\frac{3 \text{ g}}{100 \text{ mL}} = \frac{x \text{ g}}{1000 \text{ mL}}$$

$$100x = 3000 \text{ g/mL}$$

$$x = 30 \text{ g/mL}$$

The numerators and denominators must be in the same units—grams to grams or milligrams to milligrams, not grams to milligrams; and liters to liters or milliliters to milliliters, not milliliters to liters. The 1 gram molecular weight is 40, and there are 40 g in 1 L of water in a 1 M solution. Because there are only 30 g in 1 L of water, the molar concentration is 30/40 = 0.75 M.

Practice Problems

5. A solution of NaCl is made by dissolving 9 g in enough water to make a liter. What is the molarity?
6. A solution of NaCl is made by dissolving 100 g in 2 L of solution. What is the molarity?
7. How would you make (a) 1 L of 3 M NaOH, (b) 3 L of 1 M KCL, and (c) 2.5 L of 2 M $CaCl_2$?
8. What is the concentration of a KCl solution made by dissolving 200 g of KCL in 900 mL of water?

Molality

Definition

Molality is a system of expressing concentration and is similar to molarity. The *molal concentration of a solution is equal to the number of moles of solute per 1000 g of solvent.* It is a more accurate method of measuring concentration than molarity, but it is usually much less convenient than molarity and is infrequently used in the clinical laboratory.

The molal solution volume varies with temperature, the density of the materials used, and the pattern of the interaction of molecules of solutes and solvent. However, the relative masses of the constituents of the solution remain constant.

Calculations

A one molal solution could be made by placing 1 mole (1 gram molecular weight) in 1000 g of solvent. The resulting solution's volume may be greater or less than the volume of the separate parts of the mixture. Why? A molal solution does not use volume as a method of measure, only mass.

Place 58.5 g of NaCl into 1000 g of water. The volume of the solution is 1000 mL. Why? The salt dissolves into the water and does not add a measurable amount of volume to the solution.

Practice Problems

9. Make a 3 molal solution of NaCl and water. NaCl is the solute and water is the solvent.
10. What is the molality of a solution of 35 g of LiOH (solute) in 750 g of $NaC_2H_3O_2$?
11. How many grams of NH_4OH (solvent) must 44 g of NaCl be dissolved in to make a 2.75 molal solution?
12. How many grams of $CaCl_2$ must be dissolved in 475 g of H_2SO_4 to produce a 1.4 molal solution?

Normality

Definition

Laboratory testing requires an understanding of normality and normal solutions. The concentration of solutions often is expressed in normality, and many of the concepts learned about molarity can be applied to normality. The main difference is equivalent weights are used rather than gram molecular weights.

Equivalent weight is the gram molecular weight of a compound divided by the total positive valence in the compound. For example, the gram molecular weight of NaCl is 58.5, and the total positive valence is 1. Therefore, the equivalent weight of NaCl is 58.5/1 or 58.5. When the total positive valence is 1, the equivalent weight is equal to the gram molecular weight.

What if the total positive valence is different from 1? The gram molecular weight of $MgCl_2$ is 95.3, and the total positive valence is 2. The equivalent weight is 95.3/2 or 47.7. The gram molecular weight of $FeCl_3$ is 162.5, and the total positive valence is 3. The equivalent weight is 162.5/3 or 54.2. The molecular weight of Na_2CO_3 is 106. The total positive valence is 2, and the equivalent weight is 106/2 or 53 (notice the radical (CO_3^{-2}).)

What is the equivalent weight of K, $MgSO_4$, and $Ca_3(PO_4)_2$? The answers are 39 for K, 60.2 for $MgSO_4$, and 51.7 for $Ca_3(PO_4)_2$. It is important to use a periodic table to obtain the elemental gram weights.

When determining the total positive valence, some basic chemistry is applied. An atom has a positive nucleus that contains neutrons and protons. Surrounding this positive nucleus are electrons arranged in specified and ordered orbits. Because the number of electrons is equal to the number of protons in the nucleus, an atom has no net charge. When an atom reacts to form a compound, it tries to give up or accept electrons to form a completed outer orbit. The first orbit can only hold 2 electrons. When it contains one electron (as in hydrogen), it can give up the electron, as it does in most instances, forming

a hydrogen ion having a charge of +1. The valence is equal to the charge on the ion and is therefore +1, meaning that each atom can give up one electron. In special cases, hydrogen can accept another electron, giving it a valence of –1.

The second orbit can contain 8 electrons. The periodic chart shows the 8 major families of elemental atoms, labeled IA to VIIIA. Each atom under IA contains one electron in its outer orbit; and each atom under IIA contains 2 electrons in the outer orbit, continuing in that pattern until group VIIIA, which has 8 electrons in the outer orbit. Atoms in group IA can obtain a completed outer orbit by giving up the 1 electron each atom has in its outer shell or accepting 7 electrons into the outer shell. These atoms give up the 1 electron, giving them a valence of +1.

Atoms in group IIA have 2 electrons in the outer orbit. They could get to a completed outer orbit by giving up these electrons or by accepting 6 electrons. Similar to the previous example, the atom gives up the 2 electrons.

The atoms in group VIIIA have 8 electrons in their outer orbit, making it completely filled. These atoms are *inert*. They neither give up nor accept additional electrons because the outer orbit is already completed. Group VIIA, which has 7 electrons in the outer orbit, can get a completed outer orbit by accepting 1 additional electron, producing a valence of –1. Atoms in group VIA accept 2 electrons into the outer orbit to make it complete, giving them a valence of –2. The other possibility is to give up 6 electrons. Groups IIIA, IVA, and VA have 3, 4, and 5 electrons, respectively, in their outer orbits. Some of these elements, especially C and Si, develop covalent bonds in which they share electrons rather than give up or accept electrons.

Practice Problems

13. Indicate the number of electrons in the outer orbit of the following elements and the most likely valence.

Element	Electrons in Outer Orbit	Valence
K	_____	_____
Ca	_____	_____
Br	_____	_____
Fe	_____	_____
O	_____	_____

Calculations

If you can determine the equivalent weight, you can determine normality. Normality is the gram equivalent weight of a compound per liter. We need to know two things: the equivalent weight and the actual number of grams per liter. If you dissolve 1 gram equivalent weight of a compound in a liter of water, the resulting solution is 1 normal (1 N). If 2 times the gram equivalent weight of a compound is dissolved in a liter of water, the normality is 2 N.

Consider how to prepare a 3 N solution of a compound with an equivalent weight of 35. A 1 N solution by definition contains 35 g in a liter of water, and a 3 N solution contains 3 × 35 or 105 g of the compound in a liter of water; 3 N is the normality of the solution.

To determine the normality of a solution of NaCl containing 117 g of NaCl in 2 L of water, start with the equivalent weight. The molecular weight of NaCl is 23 + 35.5 = 58.5, and the total positive valence is 1; the equivalent weight of NaCl is therefore 58.5/1 or 58.5. A simple proportion problem shows how many grams there are per liter.

$$\frac{117\text{ g}}{2\text{ L}} = \frac{x}{1\text{ L}}$$

$$x = 58.5\text{ g}$$

The solution contains 58.5 g/L, and the gram equivalent weight is 58.5 g. The normality of the solution therefore equals 58.5/58.5 (actual g/L per gram equivalent weight) = 1.

To determine the normality of a solution containing 20 g of NaOH per 800 mL, we need to know the equivalent weight and the grams per liter. The gram molecular weight is 23 + 16 + 1 = 40 g, and the total positive valence is 1; the gram equivalent weight is also 40. Set up the proportion equation:

$$\frac{20\text{ g}}{0.8\text{ L}} = \frac{x}{1\text{ L}}$$

$$x = 25\text{ g/L}$$

The normality is equal to 25 g/40 g/equivalent weight or 0.625 N.

Practice Problems

14. Calculate the normal concentration of the following solutions:
    a. 10 g of NaOH dissolved in 500 mL water
    b. 90 g of $MgCl_2$ dissolved in 1500 mL of water
15. How would you prepare the following?
    a. 1 L of a 3 N solution of KOH
    b. 5 L of a 1 N solution of $CaCl_2$

Concentrations often are expressed in milliequivalents per liter (mEq/L). This represents the equivalent weight in milligrams per liter. A milliequivalent is $\frac{1}{1000}$ of an equivalent weight. All calculations are identical to those used in normality problems. The only difference is that you are working with milligrams rather than grams.

Dilutions

Weight/Volume Dilutions

The concepts of grams per deciliter (g/dL) and milligrams per deciliter (mg/dL) are easy compared with normality and molarity. The gram per deciliter concentration is defined as the number of grams of a compound dissolved in 100 mL of water. The prefix *deci* means one tenth, and a deciliter is one tenth of a liter or 100 mL. The most common determination reported in g/dL units is that for serum protein. A normal serum protein concentration is 6 to 8 g/dL, which is 6 to 8 g of protein per 100 mL of serum.

In g% solutions, the molecular or equivalent weight does not enter into the calculations, and a 10 g/dL solution

of any compound contains 10 g of that compound per 100 mL. For example, a 10 g/dL solution of glucose contains 10 g of glucose per 100 mL of water, and a 10 g/dL solution of NaCl contains 10 g of NaCl per 100 mL of water.

How many grams of NaCl do you need to prepare 600 mL of a 0.9 g/dL solution? By definition, a 0.9 g/dL solution contains 0.9 g per 100 mL, and a simple proportion completes this problem:

$$\frac{0.9\text{ g}}{100\text{ mL}} = \frac{x\text{ (grams)}}{600\text{ mL}}$$

$$x = \frac{(0.9 \times 600)}{100}$$

$$x = 5.4\text{ g of NaCl per 100 mL}$$

Prepare 1 L of a 1 g/dL solution of glucose. By definition, a 1 g/dL solution contains 1 g per 100 mL, and

$$\frac{1\text{ g}}{100\text{ mL}} = \frac{x}{1000\text{ mL}}$$

$$x = 10\text{ g/L}$$

Notice that the volume is expressed the same way on both sides of the equation. The liter is expressed as 1000 mL. It would also be correct to express the 100 mL as 0.1 L.

Practice Problems

16. How would you make the following solutions?
    a. 3 L of 1.5 g/dL KOH
    b. 600 mL of 4 g/dL $MgCl_2$
    c. 50 mL of 10g/dL NaOH

The concentration of many clinically important compounds such as glucose, blood urea nitrogen (BUN), and cholesterol is reported in units of mg/dL. *Mg/dL* is defined as the number of milligrams per 100 mL. A blood glucose level that is reported as 100 mg/dL contains 100 mg of glucose per 100 mL of blood, and a BUN value reported as 20 mg/dL contains 20 mg of the solute per 100 mL of solution. To make a liter of a glucose standard containing 200 mg/dL, the solution must contain 200 mg of the solute per 100 mL of solution:

$$\frac{200\text{ mg}}{100\text{ mL}} = \frac{x}{1000\text{ mL}}$$

$$x = 2000\text{ mg} = \frac{2\text{ g}}{1\text{ L}}$$

The liter was converted to 1000 mL so that both volumes are in the same units (there are 1000 mg in 1 g, and 2000 mg = 2 g). All calculations involving mg/dL units are done exactly like the g/dL calculations.

Although g/dL and mg/dL are the scientifically preferred terms, in many instances, g% is used instead of g/dL and mg% or mg/100 mL instead of mg/dL. Sometimes, a solution's concentration is indicated only as a percentage, such as 10% NaCl. This percent solution is a shorthand way of writing g/dL or g%. A 10% NaCl solution contains 10 g of NaCl per 100 mL of water.

Practice Problems

17. For these problems, recall the information on normality and molarity.
    a. What is the molarity of 10% NaOH?
    b. How would you prepare 20 L of 0.9% NaCl?
    c. What is the concentration in mg/dL of a 0.1 N KOH solution?

Volume/Volume Dilutions

Being able to correctly dilute concentrated solutions to a desired concentration is an important time-saving skill. It is much easier to make a simple dilution than it is to weigh out and dissolve the raw material. This topic can be condensed into one equation:

$$\text{volume}_1 \times \text{concentration}_1 = \text{volume}_2 \times \text{concentration}_2$$

Use of this equation is necessary to become proficient in making dilutions. For example, you have a 4 N solution of NaOH, and you need 1 L of 1 N solution. Solution one has a concentration of 4 N and a volume of x (i.e., the required volume). We want to make 1 L of 1 N, so solution 2 has a concentration of 1 N and a volume of 1000 mL. The equation then reads as follows:

$$4x = (1)(1000)$$

$$x = \frac{1000}{4} = 250 \text{ mL}$$

The units of volume and concentration must be the same on both sides of the equation. If the volume of the desired solution is expressed as 1000 mL, the volume of the initial solution is 250 mL, and if the volume of the desired solution is expressed as 1 L, the required volume of the initial solution is 0.25 L (0.25 L = 250 mL). Because the initial and final concentrations are expressed in normality, this is not an issue.

You want to make 500 mL of 1 N NaOH from the 10% NaOH solution available. Because one concentration is expressed in normality and the other in percent, the first step is to convert both to the same units. Since it does not make a difference which one you convert to the other, convert the 10% to normality. By definition, the solution contains 10 g per 100 mL:

$$\frac{10 \text{ g}}{100 \text{ mL}} = \frac{x}{1000 \text{ g}}$$

$$x = \frac{1000 \text{ g}}{10} = 100 \text{ g}$$

There are 100 g per liter. The equivalent weight of NaOH is 40, so the normality is 100/40 or 2.5. That can be substituted into the dilution equation:

$$2.5x = 500 (1) \text{ mL}$$

$$x = \frac{500}{2.5} = 200 \text{ mL}$$

Solve the same problem by converting the concentration of the desired solution to a percentage (%).

A 1 N solution contains 40 g/L. If there are 40 g/L, the equation is

$$\frac{40 \text{ g}}{1000 \text{ mL}} = \frac{x}{100 \text{ mL}}$$

$$x = \frac{4 \text{ g}}{100 \text{ mL}} = 4\%$$

Substitute this information in the dilution equation:

$$10x = (500 \text{ mL})(4)$$

$$x = \frac{2000}{10} = 200 \text{ mL}$$

The result shows that 200 mL of 10% NaOH diluted to 500 mL produces a 1 N solution.

Practice Problems

18. Concentrated sulfuric acid is 36 N. How much concentrated sulfuric acid is needed to prepare 5 L of 2 N H_2SO_4?
19. You have a 1 M solution of NaCl. How much do you need to dilute to make 10 L of isotonic saline (0.9%)? Remember that the units of volume and concentration must be the same on both sides of the equation.

Serial Dilutions

Many procedures call for a dilution series in which all dilutions after the first one are the same. This type of dilution series is referred to as a **serial dilution.** The methods and calculations discussed for any type of dilution series apply to serial dilutions. This procedure is used in producing a series of solutions having equal increments of concentration.

For example, a serum sample is diluted 1:2 with buffer. A series of five dilutions is made of this first dilution by diluting it 1:10 and then three times more, with each resulting solution being a 1:10 dilution of the previous one in the series. The concentration of serum in each solution is as follows: 1:2, 1:20, 1:200, 1:2000, 1:20,000, 1:200,000.

The instructions indicate that a 1:10,000 dilution of a substance is to be made. This means 1 part of solute in a total volume of 10,000 parts. A 1:10,000 dilution of serum in saline is made by taking 1 mL of serum and diluting it up to a total volume of 10,000 mL. However, this quantity of a solution is rarely needed. If the approximate volume needed is known, a dilution problem procedure may be used to determine how to make a smaller quantity or volume of the desired concentration. The preceding dilution of serum can be made in several ways:

- Make a 1:10 dilution of serum, redilute 1:10, redilute 1:10, and redilute 1:10.

$$\frac{1}{10} \times \frac{1}{10} \times \frac{1}{10} \times \frac{1}{10} = \frac{1}{10,000}$$

This produces 10 mL of a 1:10,000 dilution of serum in saline.

- Make a 1:10 dilution of serum, redilute 1:10, and redilute 1:100.

$$\frac{1}{10} \times \frac{1}{10} \times \frac{1}{100} = \frac{1}{10,000}$$

This yields 100 mL of a 1:10,000 dilution of serum in saline.
- Make a 1:100 dilution of serum and redilute 1:100.

$$\frac{1}{100} \times \frac{1}{100} = \frac{1}{10,000}$$

This procedure gives 100 mL of a 1:10,000 dilution of serum in saline (Fig. 1-5). Any combination of dilutions that yields a final concentration of 1:10,000 may be used. The combination is determined in part by the glassware available and the volume needed.

Several factors affect the decision about what dilutions to use:
- Original concentration of the substance being diluted
- Final volume desired
- Final concentration desired
- Number of dilutions to be made (sometimes)

For example, a 1:200 stock solution of boric acid is on hand. The patient requires 50 oz of a 1:500 solution. Follow the process to make the necessary amount without making an excess amount.
- Recall the general rule for determining the concentration of a dilution series:

$$\text{original concentration} \times \text{dilution 1}$$
$$\times \text{dilution 2} \cdots = \text{final concentration}$$

- Fill in the known parts:

$$\text{original concentration} \times \text{dilution 1} = \text{final concentration}$$

$$1/200 \; x \,(\text{unknown}) = 1/500$$

- Recall that the volume of the last dilution in a dilution series is the volume of the final solution. Fifty ounces of the 1:500 solution are needed. If 50 is inserted for the total volume of the dilution to be made, it will leave the amount to be diluted as the unknown *(x)*.

$$1/200 \times x/50 \text{ oz} = 1/500$$

$$x/10,000 = 1/500$$

$$500x = 10,000$$

$$x = 20 \text{ oz}$$

In 20 oz of the stock 1:200 solution diluted up to 50 oz, 50 oz of the desired 1:500 solution are present.

Conversions
Unit Conversions

When converting a larger unit (g) to a smaller unit (mg), multiply by the appropriate factor (in this case, 1000). When converting a smaller unit to a larger unit, divide by the appropriate factor (Table 1-2).

grams → milligrams, multiply by 1000
decigrams → milligrams, multiply by 100
centigrams → milligrams, multiply by 10
mm^3 → mL (cc), divide by 1000
milligrams → grams, divide by 1000

● Practice Problems

20. How many milliliters in 1 L?
21. How many milliliters in 20 L?
22. How many milligrams in 3 dg?
23. How many milliliters in 1 dL?
24. How many grams in 1 kg?
25. How many kilograms in 1 g?

TABLE 1-2	Prefixes for Unit Conversions	
Prefix	**Prefix Symbol**	**Numeric Equivalent**
kilo	K	10^3
centi	c	10^{-2}
deci	d	10^{-1}
milli	m	10^{-3}
micro	μ	10^{-6}
nano	n	10^{-9}
pico	p	10^{-9}

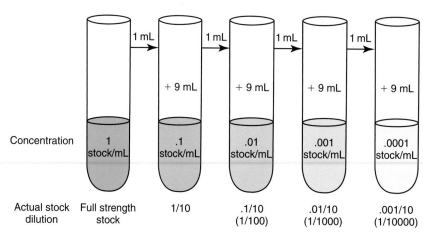

	1 mL	1 mL	1 mL	1 mL
	+ 9 mL	+ 9 mL	+ 9 mL	+ 9 mL
Concentration	1 stock/mL	.1 stock/mL	.01 stock/mL	.001 stock/mL	.0001 stock/mL
Actual stock dilution	Full strength stock	1/10	.1/10 (1/100)	.01/10 (1/1000)	.001/10 (1/10000)

• **Figure 1-5** Serial dilution.

26. How many liters in 1 mL?
27. How many milligrams in 1 cg?
28. How many grams in 1 cg?

Temperature Conversions

It is often necessary to convert Fahrenheit temperatures to Celsius and Celsius temperatures to Fahrenheit. It may also be necessary to convert temperatures from Celsius to Kelvin. Three formulas are used for conversions:

$$\text{Celsius to Fahrenheit: } C = 5/9 \times (F - 32)$$

$$\text{Fahrenheit to Celsius: } F = (9/5 \times C) + 32$$

$$\text{Celsius to Kelvin: } K = C + 273.$$

In the Kelvin system, zero represents absolute zero. Absolute zero is the point at which there is no heat in an element.

● Practice Problems

29. Convert 39° F to C.
30. Convert 50° C to F.
31. Convert 67° F to C.
32. Convert 33° C to F.
33. Convert 98° F to C.
34. Convert 45° C to F.
35. Convert 53° F to C.
36. Convert 53° F to K.
37. Convert 100° C to K.
38. Convert –50° F to K.

Conversion Between SI Units and Conventional Units

Results may be received from external laboratories with test results in international units (Système International [SI]). Every laboratory may not report test results in SI units, and hospital and clinic personnel may ask for assistance in converting SI units to the units used for reporting.

This formula is used to change mass concentrations (mass units/dL to mass unit/L):

$$\frac{\text{numeric value in mass units}}{dL} \times 10 = \text{mass units/L}$$

Use the formula to change the protein value of 7.5 g/dL to g/L:

$$7.5 \text{ g/dL} \times 10 = 75 \text{ g/L}$$

This formula is used to change mass concentration to substance concentration:

$$\frac{(\text{numeric value in mass concentration/dL} \times 10)}{\text{molecular mass}} = \text{substance units/L}$$

Use the formula to change the serum albumin value of 7.5 g/dL to μmol/L:

$$7.5 \times \frac{10}{69000} = 1087 \text{ μmol/L}$$

This formula is used to calculate the mass amount to amount of substance:

$$\frac{\text{numeric value in mass units}}{\text{molecular mass}} = \text{amount of substance}$$

Use the formula to calculate urine albumin:

$$300 \text{ mg/dL} = \frac{300 \text{ mmol/dL}}{69000} = 4.4 \text{ μmol/dL}$$

Use the formula to calculate urine urate:

$$300 \text{ mg/dL} = \frac{300}{168} = 1.8 \text{ mmol/dL}$$

pH

Many chemical reactions result from an interaction of charged particles. Ions are atoms or molecules in which the total number of protons does not equal the number of electrons. Ions with more protons than electrons carry a net positive charge and are called cations. Ions with more electrons than protons carry a negative charge and are called anions. Cations are attracted to anions by the electromagnetic forces associated with atoms and molecules. Cations and anions are attracted to one another and bond together to form a molecule. The bonds between ions are called ionic bonds. If the positive charges equal the negative charges, a neutral compound is formed. When such compounds are not in solution, the molecules remain intact. NaCl is an example of this type of a compound. When these compounds are added to an ionic solvent such as water, the compound dissociates into its ionic molecules.

Acids are ionic compounds that dissociate when dissolved in water. Dissociation releases H^+ ions into the solution. The amount of dissociation that occurs and the number of H^+ ions in the solution correlate with the strength of the acid and the pH of the solution. The pH is an expression of the acidity or alkalinity of a solution on a logarithmic scale (1 to 10) on which 7 is neutral, values lower than 7 are more acid, and values higher than 7 are more alkaline. This can be defined mathematically as pH = –log[H^+], with the hydrogen ion concentration given in moles per liter. More hydrogen ions in solution indicate a strong acid. Fewer hydrogen ions in solution indicate a weak acid. A strong acid may have a pH of 1 or 2, and a weak acid may have a pH of 5 or 6. Any pH value above 7 is basic (i.e., alkaline).

The acidity or alkalinity has a profound effect on the kinds and speed of chemical reactions that occur in a solution. Because of this, it is important to know the relative concentrations of the hydrogen and hydroxyl ions or pH in a solution.

Beer's Law

The optical density (OD) or absorbance (A) of a substance is proportional to the amount of light of a wavelength that it absorbs. The greater the absorbance, the more light it absorbs and the less it transmits. The relationship between absorbance and percent transmission (%T) is

$$A = 2 - \log \% T$$

If the %T of a solution is 100, the absorbance is 0:

$$A = 2 - \log \% T$$

$$A = 2 - \log 100$$

$$A = 2 - 2 = 0$$

In the clinical laboratory, absorbance is used to calculate concentration of an unknown component of serum or plasma. When the test reaction follows Beer's law, absorbance is directly related to concentration. The law says that the absorbance (A) of a colored solution is equal to the product of the concentration of the color-producing substance (C) times the depth of the solution through which the light must travel (L) times a constant (K):

$$A = C \times L \times K$$

This one formula can refer to the standard and to the unknown.

$$\text{Standard: } A_s = C_s \times L_s \times K$$

$$\text{Unknown: } A_u = C_u \times L_u \times K$$

Using algebraic manipulations of these equations and canceling out the K, the equation becomes

$$A_{unknown}/A_{standard} = C_{unknown}/C_{standard}$$

$$C_{unknown} = A_{unknown} \times C_{standard}/A_{standard}$$

Practice Problems

39. Absorbance of the unknown = 0.16; absorbance of the standard = 0.14; and concentration of the standard = 100 mg%. What is the concentration of the unknown?

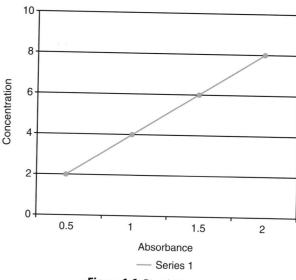

• **Figure 1-6** Standard curve.

Standard Curves

Constructing a standard curve involves running at least three standards for a test procedure. The three points are plotted on regular graph paper with concentration on the *y* axis and absorbance on the *x* axis (Fig. 1-6). Treat the standards and controls as you treat a specimen.

Never draw the lines of the curve past the last point on the curve. What happens to the relationship between the readings and the concentration is not known beyond the extremes of the curve.

Summary

Clinical laboratories were created in the early 20th century. They were usually located in closet-sized rooms and staffed with one pathologist. They progressed to larger rooms with animal cages and laboratory assistants. As laboratories grew, tests were logically grouped into sections or departments. Modern departments commonly include clinical chemistry, hematology, microbiology, specimen collection, blood bank, urinalysis, and immunology and serology. Clinical laboratories evolved into one of the most important aspects of medicine, employing physicians and a variety of academically credentialed professionals.

Clinical laboratories can be located in hospitals, physicians' offices, and stand-alone reference laboratories. All laboratories are governed by federal regulations and accrediting organizations, which include The Joint Commission and the CAP.

Laboratories are unique workplaces that use specialized equipment. Specially prepared water is a mainstay of any laboratory. Reagent-grade water, the purest water available, is used for reagents prepared for analyses. Special types of glassware and plasticware are routinely used in the laboratory. One specialized piece of equipment in every laboratory is a centrifuge. Centrifuges are used to spin down or separate blood cells and clots from the liquid portion of the blood. Balances are also a basic piece of equipment found in most laboratories. All laboratories make extensive use of pipettes. Pipettes can be manual or serologic, volumetric, semiautomatic, or automatic. Pipettes are used to transfer chemicals and patient specimens.

Atomic theory states that chemicals are made of atoms that contain protons (positively charged) and neutrons (no charge) in the center or nucleus, with electrons (negatively charged) revolving around the nucleus. Valence electrons inhabit the outer electron shell of a chemical.

Organic chemistry focuses on the characteristics and combining properties of hydrocarbons. Several functional groups are important in clinical chemistry: aldehydes, ketones, amines, alcohols, and esters. Biochemistry is often referred to as the chemistry of life, and important biochemical compounds include proteins, carbohydrates, lipids, and nucleic acids.

Laboratory math is important. Laboratory professionals must understand the processes for calculating molarity, molality, normality, volume/volume dilutions, weight/volume dilutions, serial dilutions, conversions, pH, Beer's law, and standard curves (Table 1-3).

TABLE 1-3	Useful Laboratory Formulas	

Function	Equations
Molarity	M = (grams/molecular weight)/liters of solution
Molality	m = (grams/molecular weight)/kg of solution
Normality	N = [(grams/molecular weight)/(valence)]/liters of solution
Weight/volume dilutions	g/dL (i.e., g%) = grams of solute/deciliters of solution
Volume/volume dilutions	$\dfrac{C_1}{V_1} = \dfrac{C_2}{V_2}$
F to C conversion	$F = (9/5 \times C) + 32$
C to F conversion	$C = 5/9 \times (F - 32)$
C to K conversion	$K = C + 273$

C, Celsius; *F*, Fahrenheit; *K*, Kelvin.

Review Questions

1. A pathologist is
   a. A medical doctor specializing in pathology
   b. A person with a bachelor's degree who is able to perform complex tests
   c. A person with an associate degree who is able to perform routine laboratory tests
   d. A medical doctor specializing in laboratory medicine

2. The agency that accredits laboratories only and has "deemed status" from the Centers for Medicare and Medicaid is
   a. The Joint Commission
   b. The National Agency for Accreditation of Clinical Laboratory Science
   c. The College of American Pathologists
   d. The National Certifying Agency

3. All of the following are departments in a clinical laboratory EXCEPT
   a. Microbiology
   b. Hematology
   c. Paleontology
   d. Urinalysis

4. One type of pipette used in the laboratory is
   a. Glass
   b. Routine
   c. Calibrated
   d. Volumetric

5. The most common type of centrifuge used in the laboratory is the
   a. Refrigerated
   b. Bench top
   c. Fixed angle
   d. Floor model

6. Determine how to make each solution:
   a. Make 1 L of a 1 M solution of H_2SO_4.
   b. Make 300 mL of a 0.45 M solution of $Cu(NO_3)_2$.
   c. Make 250 mL of a 0.1M solution of KBr.
   d. Make 700 mL of a 7.0 M solution of $CaCO_3$.
   e. Make 500 mL of a 3.2 M solution of H_2O_2.
   f. Make 3 L of 1 M NaBr.
   g. Make 2.5 L of 2 M Na_3PO_4.
   h. Make 450 mL of 3.33 M $NaC_2H_3O_2$.
   i. Make 200 mL of a 4 M solution of $Ni_2(S_2O_3)_3$.

7. What is the molarity of the following solutions?
   a. 100 g of $NaHSO_4$ in 3 L of solution
   b. 250 g of KNO_3 in 250 mL of solution
   c. 75 mg of NH_4OH in 100 mL of solution
   d. 99 g of $NaBO_3$ in 1 L of solution
   e. 30 g of Na_3PO_4 in 1 L of solution
   f. 3.0 g of Na_3PO_4 dissolved in 100 mL of solution
   g. 44 g of $Mg(OH)_2$ dissolved in 800 mL of solution
   h. 1 kg of KNO_3 dissolved in 2.75 L of solution
   i. 55 dg of SnF_2 in 1.11 L of solution
   j. 75 g of Co_2O_3 in 4.25 L of solution
   k. 44 g of $Li_2Fe(CN)_6$ in 3.5 L of solution

8. Determine the normality of the following solutions:
   a. 100 g of $NaHSO_4$ in 3 L of solution
   b. 250 g of KNO_3 in 250 mL of solution
   c. 75 mg of NH_4OH in 100 mL of solution
   d. 99 g of $NaBO_3$ in 1 L of solution
   e. 30 g of Na_3PO_4 in 1 L of solution
   f. 3 g of Na_3PO_4 dissolved in 100 mL of solution
   g. 44 g of $Mg(OH)_2$ dissolved in 800 mL of solution
   h. 1 kg of KNO_3 dissolved in 2.75 L of solution
   i. 55 dg of SnF_2 in 1.11 L of solution
   j. 75 g of Co_2O_3 in 4.25 L of solution
   k. 44 g of $Li_2Fe(CN)_6$ in 3.5 L of solution

9. Calculate the normality or the molarity of the following solutions:
   a. Normality of a 125 mg% solution of $Na_2Cr_2O_7$.
   b. Molarity of a 29.5 mg% solution of $Cs_2C_2O_4$.
   c. Normality of an 18 mg% solution of $Ba_3(BO_3)_2$

   d. Molarity of a 0.9g% solution of NaCl

   e. Normality of a 21 mg% solution of $CaCO_3$

   f. Molarity of a 15 mg% solution of NH_3

   g. Normality of a 24 mg% solution of $HgCl_2$

   h. Molarity of a 17.5 mg% solution of HCl

   i. Normality of a 30 mg% solution of $FeCl_3$

   j. Molarity of a 41 mg% solution of ZnO

10. Determine the mg% concentration of the following solutions:

   a. 0.25 N solution of NaOH

   b. 1.2 M solution of $Na_2Cr_2O_7$

   c. 1.8 N solution of $Ba_3(BO_3)_2$

   d. 0.9 M solution of NaCl

   e. 2.1 N solution of $CaCO_3$

   f. 1.5 M solution of NH_3

   g. 2.4 N solution of $HgCl_2$

   h. 1.75 M solution of HCl

   i. 3.0 N solution of $FeCl_3$

   j. 4.1 M solution of ZnO

11. Answer the following questions:

   a. A solution of 100 mg% of ammonia nitrogen has an A = 0.15. The A of an unknown blood sample is 0.11. What is the ammonia concentration of the sample?

   b. A solution of 50 mg% has an A = 0.2. The A of an unknown blood sample is 0.48. What is the glucose concentration of the blood sample?

   c. A solution of 500 mg/dL glucose has an A = 0.63, and the A of an unknown sample is 0.80. What is the glucose concentration of the sample?

   d. A solution of 350 mg/dL cholesterol has an A = 0.44, and the A of an unknown sample is 0.30. What is the cholesterol concentration of the sample?

   e. A solution of 9.0 mg/dL calcium has an A = 0.5, and the A of an unknown sample is 0.15. What is the calcium concentration of the sample?

   f. A solution of 1000 mg/dL triglyceride has an A = 0.968, and the A of an unknown sample is 0.550. What is the triglyceride concentration of the sample?

   g. A solution of 6.0 mg/dL uric acid has an A = 0.25, and the A of an unknown sample is 0.70. What is the uric acid concentration of the sample?

   h. A solution of 4.5 g/dL albumin has an A = 0.48, and the A of an unknown sample is 0.32. What is the albumin concentration of the sample?

Bibliography

American Medical Technologists. *Get Certified: Medical Lab Assistant.* <http://www.americanmedtech.org/GetCertified/CMLAEligibility.aspx> Accessed 08.05.15.

American Society for Clinical Pathology, Board of Certification. *Phlebotomist Technician, PBT (ASCP) and International Phlebotomy Technician, PBT (ASCP^i) Examination Content Guideline.* <http://www.ascp.org/PDF/BOC-PDFs/Guidelines/ExaminationContentGuidelinePBT.aspx> Accessed 08.05.15.

Austin A, Wetle V. *The United States Health Care System: Combining Business, Health, and Delivery.* Upper Saddle River, NJ: Pearson Prentice Hall; 2008.

Burke MD. Laboratory medicine in the 21st century. *Am J Clin Pathol.* 2000;114:841–846. <http://ajcp.ascpjournals.org/content/114/6/841.full.pdf> Accessed 08.05.15.

Burtis CA, Ashwood ER, Bruns DE. *Tietz Textbook of Clinical Chemistry and Molecular Diagnostics.* 4th ed St. Louis: Saunders; 2006. 4–5.

Carlson B. Physician office lab diagnostic market. *Genetic Engineering & Biotechnology News.* 2010;30(21). <http://www.genengnews.com/gen-articles/physician-office-lab-diagnostic-market/3493/> Accessed 08.05.15.

College of American Pathologists. *About the CAP Accreditation Program.* Updated July 1, 2014. <http://www.cap.org/apps/cap.portal?_nfpb=true&cntvwrPtlt_actionOverride=%2Fportlets%2FcontentViewer%2Fshow&_windowLabel=cntvwrPtlt&cntvwrPtlt{actionForm.contentReference}=laboratory_accreditation%2Faboutlap.html&_state=maximized&_pageLabel=cntvwr> Accessed 08.05.15.

Corning Incorporated, Life Sciences. *Characteristics of Corning Plasticware.* <http://csmedia2.corning.com/LifeSciences//media/pdf/CLS_AN_10> Accessed 08.05.15.

Delwiche FA. Mapping the literature of clinical laboratory science. *J Med Libr Assoc.* 2003;91(3):303–310. <http://www.ncbi.nlm.nih.gov/pmc/articles/PMC164393/> Accessed 08.05.15.

Lab Tests Online. *Where Lab Tests Are Performed.* Last modified October 2012. <http://labtestsonline.org/lab/labtypes/start/2> Accessed 08.05.15.

Lab Tests Online. *Who's Who in the Lab: A Look at Laboratory Professionals.* <http://labtestsonline.org/lab/who/start/1> Accessed 08.05.15.

Lee J. *Basic Biolumeniscence.* Updated March 2014. <http://www.photobiology.info/LeeBasicBiolum.html> Accessed 08.05.15.

Moran LA, Horton RA, Scrimgeour G, Perry M. *Principles of Biochemistry.* 5th ed Upper Saddle River, NJ: Prentice Hall; 2011.

The Joint Commission. *Accreditation Guide for Hospitals.* March 2013. <http://www.jointcommission.org/assets/1/6/Accreditation_Guide_Hospitals_2011.pdf> Accessed 08.05.15.

Tro NJ. *Introductory Chemistry Essentials Plus Mastering Chemistry with eText—Access Card Package.* 4th ed. Upper Saddle River, NJ; 2012.

Valley Design Corp. *Properties of 7740 (Pyrex).* <http://www.valleydesign.com/pyrex.htm> Accessed 08.05.15.

2

Practical Laboratory Safety

DONNA LARSON

CHAPTER OUTLINE

OBJECTIVES

At the completion of this chapter, the reader will be able to:

1. Discuss the Occupational Exposure to Hazardous Chemicals in Laboratories standard, the Hazardous Communication standard, the Bloodborne Pathogens standard, and the Needlestick Safety and Prevention Act.
2. Compare and contrast the four biosafety levels and their meaning for a clinical laboratory.
3. Describe the risks posed by sharp objects, centrifuges, refrigerators and freezers, fires, electricity, compressed gases, and biohazardous waste in the laboratory.
4. Describe how each of the following can reduce hazards: standard operating procedures, warning signs and labels, fire prevention, electrical safety, and procedure for disposal of hazardous waste.
5. Compare and contrast seven pieces of laboratory safety equipment.
6. Describe how immunizations can protect laboratory workers.
7. Describe six practices that can help keep laboratory workers safe in the laboratory.
8. Describe the correct method for washing your hands.

KEY TERMS

Biohazard
Biohazardous waste
Biological safety cabinet
Biosafety level 1
Biosafety level 2
Biosafety level 3
Biosafety level 4
Bloodborne pathogens
Centrifuge
Chemical hazard
Chemical hygiene plan

Decontamination
Dry chemical extinguisher
Engineering controls
Ergonomic hazards
Exposure Control Plan
Flammable
Fume hood
Halotron
Hazard communication
National Fire Protection Association (NFPA) label

Other potentially infectious materials (OPIM)
Occupational Safety and Health Administration (OSHA)
Personal protective equipment (PPE)
Safety Data Sheet (SDS)
Sharps
Standard operating procedures (SOPs)
Standard precautions
Sterilization
Universal precautions

◆ Case in Point

A laboratory worker drops a volumetric flask onto the floor, breaking the flask and sending glass shards off in many directions. The worker is embarrassed and begins picking up the pieces of glass with her bare hands. What is the correct way for this worker to pick up the glass? Why should the worker not use her hand to pick up the glass pieces of the flask?

Points to Remember

- Four federal regulations address laboratory safety: the Occupational Exposure to Hazardous Chemicals in Laboratories standard, the Hazard Communication standard, the Bloodborne Pathogens standard, and the Needlestick Safety and Prevention Act.
- The federal agency that oversees interpretation and enforces federal safety regulations is the Occupational Safety and Health Administration (OSHA).
- One way to increase needlestick safety is through engineering controls and worker training.
- A laboratory safety program minimizes the risk of injury by assuring that employees have training, information, support, and equipment needed to work safely.
- There are four biosafety levels for clinical laboratories. Level 1, the lowest level, is for organisms that are not known to cause human disease. Level 2 is the level assigned to a regular laboratory in which human disease-producing bacteria are handled. Level 3 is assigned to a specialty laboratory in which organisms that cause severe or potentially lethal diseases are handled. Level 4, the highest level, is where organisms that are transmitted through an aerosol route and cause fatal or incurable diseases are housed.
- Risks in the laboratory include sharp objects, potential infectious materials, centrifuges, refrigerators and freezers, fires, electrical devices, compressed gases, and biohazardous waste disposal.
- Laboratory safety equipment includes the biological safety cabinet, fume hood, needlestick engineering controls, fire suppression system, pipetting aids, eye wash stations, and emergency showers.
- Other ways employers keep laboratory workers safe is through immunizations, standard operating procedures, biohazard signage, training, personal protective equipment, dress codes, and hand washing procedures.

Introduction

This chapter covers laboratory safety from a practical viewpoint. It begins with an overview of the federal regulations that govern laboratory safety practices, continues with a description of the typical laboratory safety program, biohazards, chemical hazards, laboratory safety equipment, and employee health and concludes with employee safety. Laboratory safety is critical for a healthy workforce and workplace.

Safety Regulations

The major federal regulations affecting laboratory safety are the Occupational Safety and Health Act of 1970 (OSH Act), the Occupational Exposure to Hazardous Chemicals in Laboratories standard (29 CFR 1910.1450), the Hazard Communication standard (29 CFR 1910.1200), the Bloodborne Pathogens standard (29 CFR 1910.1030), and the Needlestick Safety and Prevention Act of 2000. A short summary of each of these regulations follows.

Occupational Safety and Health Act

In 1970, the U.S. Congress passed the OSH Act, which created the Occupational Safety and Health Administration (OSHA) within the Department of Labor. Its mission is to help employers and employees reduce on-the-job injuries, illnesses, and deaths by maintaining a safe and healthy workplace. This approach leads to lower workers' compensation insurance costs and medical expenses for employers and greater productivity from healthier workers. OSHA focuses on enforcement of regulations, outreach and training for employers and employees, and partnerships through voluntary programs (Box 2-1).

The Occupational Exposure to Hazardous Chemicals in Laboratories Standard

In 1990, OSHA issued the Occupational Exposure to Hazardous Chemicals in Laboratories standard to protect laboratory workers from small amounts of hazardous chemicals used in laboratories. It was most recently updated in 2012. This standard applies to clinical laboratories; however, because there is a low potential for exposure when a laboratory uses a test kit, the chemicals in the kit are not covered by this standard. The provisions in the Occupational Exposure to Hazardous Chemicals in Laboratories standard cover the routes of exposure, chemical inventory, storage of chemicals, chemical spills, and compressed gases.

• BOX 2-1	Methods Used by the Occupational Safety and Health Administration (OSHA) to Promote a Safe and Healthy Workplace

1. Implement new or improved health and safety systems.
2. Perform work site inspections.
3. Promote cooperative programs.
4. Establish rights and responsibilities of both employers and employees.
5. Support innovations in workplace safety.
6. Implement recordkeeping and reporting requirements for employers.
7. Establish training programs for employers and employees.
8. Partner with state occupational safety and health programs.
9. Provide consulting.

From Occupational Health and Safety Administration.

Routes of Exposure

There are several ways that a hazardous chemical can enter the body. Hazardous chemicals can enter through the mouth or a cut on the hand, but also through the lungs or eyes. Some hazardous chemicals can enter the body through intact skin.

Chemical Inventory

Laboratories keep an inventory of all chemicals used for testing and other procedures. A chemical inventory is valuable and is required by law for employers, but an inventory is also useful in other ways. For example, laboratories share their chemical inventory with the local fire department, so that fire department personnel can come prepared to resolve a hazardous chemical spill, an explosion, or another type of chemical emergency. The local law enforcement or appropriate county officials may also need to know the chemical inventory of a laboratory.

Storage of Chemicals

Storage of chemicals is important to ensure not only the safety of the individuals working in a laboratory but also the safety of others in the same building. Even if chemicals are stored in proper containers, vapors may escape from the storage vessel and interact with vapors from other chemicals. This interaction could cause corrosion in the storage cabinet, explosions when released from the storage cabinet, or hazardous conditions for employees working with the chemicals. Two classes of chemicals that are notorious for causing problems with off-gassing are acids and bases. Specially developed cabinets are widely available for storing acids and bases separately. Some storage cabinets for organic materials contain a flame-retardant covering over the shelf.

Store similar chemicals together to minimize interactions between chemicals—do not store chemicals alphabetically. Keep flammable chemicals together in an approved, dedicated, flammable-storage cabinet. Store hazardous chemicals separately from nonhazardous chemicals. Store liquid chemicals in unbreakable containers or in double packaging; the containers, packaging, and cabinet for storing liquid chemicals should be able to contain the chemical in case a container breaks or spills. Do not store chemicals on the floor, on the very top shelf of a cabinet, or higher than eye level. The shelves on chemical storage cabinets should have anti-roll lips.

Always be alert when opening chemical storage cabinets. Check for improperly stored chemicals, leaking containers, spilled chemicals, unusual temperature (too hot or too cold), poor lighting, open flames (cigarettes or matches), absence of warning signs in area, and lack of security in the chemical storage area. Correct the deficiencies or notify the appropriate individual so that the deficiencies can be corrected. Keeping yourself and others safe in the laboratory is everyone's responsibility.

Chemical Spills

Although most individuals are extremely careful when handling chemicals, chemical spills are inevitable. The person spilling the chemical should take responsibility for cleaning it up. Notify the supervisor and report the spilled chemical and location.

The nature of the spilled chemical will dictate the personal protective equipment (PPE) necessary for the person cleaning up the spill and whether the area must be evacuated.

Chemical Hygiene Plan

OSHA mandates that each laboratory creates a chemical hygiene plan (CHP) for good laboratory practices and standard operating procedures (SOPs) guiding chemical usage. This plan must specify procedures, equipment, personal protective equipment (PPE), and laboratory practices to protect workers from chemical health hazards. Required elements of the CHP include:

- SOPs
- Criteria for exposure control measures
- Adequacy and proper functioning of fume hoods and other protective equipment
- Information and training
- Requirement of prior approval of laboratory procedures
- Medical consultations and examinations
- Chemical hygiene officer designation
- Particularly hazardous substances

See Table 2-1 for a suggested CHP format.

The Hazard Communication Standard

Another federal regulation pertaining to protecting workers from adverse health effects due to chemical exposure is the Hazard Communication standard, which was issued in 1983 and most recently updated in 2012. The purpose of the Hazard Communication standard is to protect workers from illnesses and injuries due to chemical exposure through information and training about chemical hazards and protective measures. This standard mandates employers to implement at least four steps to educate and train employees (Box 2-2).

Once the laboratory identifies all of its hazardous chemicals, the chemicals must be documented and a Safety Data Sheet (SDS) must be obtained for each chemical. SDS is provided by chemical suppliers and manufacturers. An SDS will contain information about physical hazards; health hazards; routes of entry; exposure limits; precautions for safe handling and use; spill cleanup procedures; PPE to be worn when handling the chemical; emergency first aid; and name, address, and phone number of the manufacturer. The SDS must be written in English and readily available to workers close to the location of the chemical.

The Bloodborne Pathogens Standard

The Bloodborne Pathogens standard was issued in 1991 and most recently updated in 2012. Its purpose is to protect workers from microbiological pathogens that are carried in blood and body fluids. This standard covers workers who are "reasonably anticipated" to become exposed to blood and other potentially infectious materials (OPIM) when performing job duties. OPIM include body fluids—semen, vaginal secretions, cerebrospinal fluid, synovial

TABLE 2-1	Information Contained in a Chemical Hygiene Plan

Heading	Content
Purpose	This section states why this document was created.
Scope	This section states the employees and other types of workers that will be covered by the plan's provisions.
Responsibilities of Employer and Employees	This section states the responsibilities of employers and employees as dictated by law.

Classification of Chemical Hazards
    Corrosive chemicals
    Sensitizing/irritant chemicals
    Flammable/combustible liquids
    Flammable solids
    Highly reactive/unstable chemicals
    Acute toxicity chemicals
    Explosive chemicals
    Organic peroxide
    Pyrophoric
    Select carcinogenic chemicals
    Reproductive/developmental toxins
    Respiratory system–damaging chemicals
    Restricted chemicals
    Cryogenic liquids
    Solid dry ice
    Compressed gases
	This section discusses the various types of chemical hazards that are present in the specific laboratory.

Routes of Exposure	This section explains the different routes of exposure for hazardous chemicals.
Laboratory Standard Operating Procedures	The laboratory's standard operating procedures for handling hazardous chemicals in the laboratory are compiled in this section.
Chemical Exposure and Medical Examination	This section explains what employees need to do after exposure to a hazardous chemical and whether the employee needs to have a medical examination.
Hazardous Waste Disposal	This section addresses the procedures used at the laboratory for disposing of hazardous waste.

Employee Information and Safety Training
    Content of OSHA standard and appendices
    Location and explanation of chemical hygiene plan
    Location of SDS and reference materials
	This section contains much information about the hazardous chemicals in the laboratory and the required safety training for all laboratory workers. It also discusses the content of the OSHA standard and appendices, the location and purpose of the chemical hygiene plan, and the locations of the SDS for all the hazardous chemicals in the laboratory as well as reference materials for chemicals.

• BOX 2-2 Requirements of the Hazard Communication Standard

1. Create a written plan to educate and train employees about the chemical hazards in the workplace, including lists of chemicals present in the laboratory.
2. Label all chemicals in the laboratory and chemicals that are shipped to others with National Fire Protection Association (NFPA) labels.
3. Assemble Safety Data Sheets (SDS) of chemicals that workers may be exposed to and store them in an area accessible to employees.
4. Create training programs to inform workers about the chemical hazards they may be exposed to and mandatory methods for protecting themselves during use of these chemicals.

---

fluid, pleural fluid, pericardial fluid, peritoneal fluid, amniotic fluid, saliva, and other body fluids contaminated with visible blood. Requirements of the standard are listed in Box 2-3 and in Figure 2-1.

Exposure Control Plan

Every employer is required to have an **Exposure Control Plan** to protect employees from exposure to blood, body fluids, and OPIM (see Fig. 2-1). The Exposure Control Plan includes listing jobs and associated tasks that may expose employees to potentially infectious materials; implementing exposure control through **universal precautions,** engineering and work practice controls, good housekeeping, and PPE; documenting hepatitis B vaccination or declination, evaluating employees after exposure, and following up with

1. Train workers before they are exposed to blood and OPIM and annually thereafter.
2. Offer each employee the hepatitis B vaccination series. Each worker has the right to decline the hepatitis B vaccination series.
3. Provide appropriate PPE such as gloves, laboratory coats, face shields, and goggles, and instruct personnel on when and how to use this equipment.
4. Develop an Exposure Control Plan so that potential exposure situations for each job category are identified and engineering and work practice controls are implemented to lessen or remove the potential exposure.
5. Follow the practice of universal precautions, standard precautions, or transmission-based precautions.
   a. Universal precautions is an infection control practice in which blood and other body fluids from all patients are handled as if they contained human immunodeficiency virus (HIV), hepatitis B virus, or other bloodborne pathogens.
   b. Standard precautions is a system of minimizing the transmission of pathogens in a hospital setting. Standard precautions apply to blood, fluids produced by the body (except sweat), non-intact skin, and mucous membranes and include hand hygiene and wearing PPE whenever touching a patient's body fluids.
   c. Place all specimens of blood and body fluids in a well-constructed container with a secure lid to prevent leakage during transport.
   d. Be careful when collecting each specimen to avoid contaminating the outside of the container or the laboratory form accompanying the specimen.
   e. If there is potential for or actual contamination, use an outer container such as a biohazard transport bag.
   f. Label specimens with biohazard insignia.
   g. All persons processing blood and body fluid specimens (e.g., removing tops from vacuum tubes) should wear gloves.
   h. Personnel should wear facial barrier protection if splashes or sprays of blood or body fluids may occur.
   i. Use mechanical pipetting devices for manipulating all liquids in the laboratory.
   j. After use, place all sharps in a clearly labeled, puncture-resistant container for transport to disposal sites.
   k. Place sharps containers as close to the work site as practical.
   l. To prevent overfilling and resultant accidental skin punctures, remove sharps containers when they are two-thirds to three-quarters full.
   m. Decontaminate work benches with a fresh 1:10 solution of chlorine bleach after blood or body fluids have been spilled on the bench and at the end of each work shift. Leave the bleach on the bench for at least 15 minutes to ensure that all microorganisms are killed.
   n. Dispose of all contaminated materials used in the laboratory in biohazard bags and treat them as regulated medical waste.
   o. Decontaminate and clean contaminated laboratory equipment before the equipment is repaired in the laboratory or transported to the manufacturer for repair.

From Occupational Safety and Health Administration.

employees; keeping files and records; communicating and training employees about hazards; and analyzing exposures to prevent similar exposures in the future.

Needlestick Safety and Prevention Act

The Needlestick Safety and Prevention Act was signed into law on November 6, 2000, marking the first time in American history that the federal government became involved with the safety of health care workers. This Act requires employers to distribute safer medical devices to employees after identifying and evaluating several different devices; to record sharps injuries in a log; to let health care workers assist in selecting devices; to use engineering controls for sharps disposal containers, self-sheathing needles, and other systems that will eliminate or lessen exposure of employees to bloodborne pathogens; and to train employees to properly use engineering devices and work practice controls to improve employee safety. About a year after this Act was approved, OSHA modified its Bloodborne Pathogens standard to include language pertaining to sharps and sharps injuries.

The Laboratory Safety Program

Laboratory-associated infections occur infrequently in the medical laboratory. In most cases, no one specific incident can be traced as the source of the infection (Box 2-4). The medical laboratory is a hazardous place to work; however, good hygiene practices, appropriate training, and proper use of PPE can reduce the risk of laboratory-associated infections for laboratory personnel.

The goal of any laboratory safety program is to minimize the risk of injury or illness to employees by ensuring that they have the training, information, support, and equipment needed to work safely in the laboratory. The guidelines and standards set forth by regulatory agencies such as OSHA and accrediting bodies such as the College of American Pathologists assist laboratories in ensuring that this goal is met. This section discusses the concept of biosafety levels, SOPs, and specific good laboratory practices. Laboratory safety equipment, employee health, and employee safety are also discussed.

Clinical Laboratories and Biosafety Levels

Clinical laboratories represent a unique working environment because not only hazardous chemicals but also biological hazards are part of the environment. The Centers for Disease Control and Prevention (CDC) developed a system for rating the safety level in a clinical laboratory. Biosafety levels are used to describe the potential biological hazard and the function of the laboratory. There are four biosafety levels, with 1 being the safest environment and 4 being the most hazardous environment (see Fig. 2-4).

Biosafety Level 1

A biosafety level 1 laboratory contains equipment, practices, and facilities that will be used with organisms that do

Requirements of Employers: OSHA Bloodborne Pathogens Standard

EXPOSURE CONTROL PLAN

Each medical office must develop a written Exposure Control Plan (ECP). The purpose of an ECP is to identify tasks where there is the potential for exposure to blood and other potentially infectious materials.

- A timetable must be published indicating when and how communication of potential hazards will occur.
- The employer must offer employees the hepatitis B vaccine within 10 working days of employment (at no cost to the employee). If employees sign a form to refuse the vaccine, they can change their mind at no cost to the employee.
- The employer must document the steps that should be taken in case of an exposure incident, including a postexposure evaluation and follow-up, strict record keeping, implementation of engineering controls, provision for personal protective equipment, and general housekeeping standards. This plan must be posted in the medical office.
- There must also be written procedures for evaluating the circumstances of an exposure incident.
- Training records must be kept for 3 years.

ENGINEERING CONTROLS AND WORK PRACTICES

The employer must provide engineering controls, or equipment and facilities that minimize the possibility of exposure. Examples of engineering controls include the following:

- Providing puncture-resistant containers for used sharps.
- Providing handwashing facilities that are readily accessible.
- Equipment for sanitizing, decontaminating, and sterilizing.

The employer must also enforce work practice controls. Work practice controls also minimize the possibility of exposure by making sure employees are using the proper techniques while working. Examples include the following:

- Enforcing proper handwashing or sanitizing procedures.
- Enforcing proper technique for using and handling needles to prevent needle sticks.
- Enforcing proper techniques to minimize the splashing of blood.

PERSONAL PROTECTIVE EQUIPMENT

Employers must provide, and employees must use, personal protective equipment (PPE) when the possibility exists of exposure to blood or contaminated body fluids. This equipment must not allow blood or potentially infectious material to pass through to the employee's clothes, skin, eyes, or mouth. Examples of PPE include the following:

- Gowns
- Face shields
- Goggles
- Gloves

If an employee has an allergy to powder or latex, the employer must provide hypoallergenic or powderless gloves. The employee cannot be charged for PPEs.

EXPOSURE INCIDENT MANAGEMENT

An exposure incident is contact with blood or biohazard infectious material that occurs when doing one's job. When an exposure incident is reported, the employer must arrange for an immediate and confidential medical evaluation. The information and actions required are as follows:

- Documenting how the exposure occurred.
- Identifying and testing the "source" individual, if possible.
- Testing the employee's blood, if consent is granted.
- Providing counseling.
- Evaluating, treating, and following up on any reported illness.

Medical records must be kept for each employee with occupational exposure for the duration of employment plus 30 years.

COMMUNICATION OF POTENTIAL HAZARDS TO EMPLOYEESS

A medical assistant will be exposed to hazardous chemicals on the job. Most chemicals handled by assistants are not any more dangerous than those used in the home. In the workplace, however, exposure is likely to be greater, concentrations higher, and exposure time longer.

The "right to know" law, OSHA's hazard communication standard, states that each employee has a right to know what chemicals he or she is working with in the workplace. The right-to-know law is intended to make the workplace safer by making certain that all information regarding chemical hazards is known to the employee. This information is supplied in the material safety data sheet (SDS), a fact sheet about a chemical that includes the following information:

- Identification of the chemical
- Listing of the physical and health hazards
- Precautions for handling
- Identification of the chemical as a carcinogen
- First-aid procedures
- Name, address, and telephone number of manufacturer

Many SDS information sheets can be obtained in repositories on the Internet. An SDS should be updated at least every 3 years. Employers must ensure that all products have an up-to-date SDS when they enter the workplace.

Potential hazards are also communicated with labels and color. Any containers with biohazard waste must be orange (or reddish orange) and must display the biohazard symbol. These labels and colors alert employees to the risk of possible exposure.

• **Figure 2-1** Requirements of employers: OSHA's Bloodborne Pathogens standard. (From Occupational Safety and Health Administration. <http://www.osha.gov> Accessed 08.05.15.)

• **BOX 2-4** **Origin of Rocky Mountain Spotted Fever**

One famous laboratory-associated infection involved Dr. Howard Taylor Ricketts. Dr. Ricketts discovered the causative agent of Rocky Mountain spotted fever, which was named after him—*Rickettsia*. Dr. Ricketts also isolated the causative agent of scrub typhus, then died from that disease a few days later.

not consistently cause disease in healthy adults. This type of laboratory is suitable for high school and undergraduate students. Commonly known strains of *Bacillus subtilis*, *Staphylococcus epidermidis*, *Serratia marcensens*, and *Streptococcus bovis* are examples of organisms used in these laboratories. Although they are not known to cause disease in healthy adults, immunocompromised individuals such as the very young and the very old may become infected with these opportunists.

Biosafety Level 2

A biosafety level 2 laboratory contains equipment, practices, and facilities used to identify and characterize moderate-risk agents derived from the community that cause disease in immunocompromised and immunocompetent people. The biosafety level 2 laboratory differs from a biosafety level 1 laboratory in that laboratory personnel receive training for handling pathogenic organisms, access to the laboratory is restricted when work is in progress, and procedures that produce aerosols are conducted in a biological safety cabinet. Organisms encountered in a biosafety level 2 laboratory may include *Salmonella* spp., *Staphylcoccus aureus*, *Streptococcus pyogenes*, and *Escherichia coli*.

Biosafety Level 3

A biosafety level 3 laboratory contains equipment, practices, and facilities used to identify and characterize organisms that cause severe or potentially lethal infections transmitted through inhalation. Personnel working in a biosafety level 3 laboratory receive training for handling specific pathogenic and lethal organisms. In addition, all procedures involving organisms are performed in a class II or class III biological safety cabinet. Organisms encountered in a biosafety level 3 laboratory may include *Bacillus anthracis*, *Yersinia pestis*, and the smallpox virus.

Biosafety Level 4

A biosafety level 4 laboratory contains equipment, practices, and facilities used to identify and characterize extremely hazardous infectious organisms, usually transmitted through aerosols, that frequently cause fatal diseases, diseases with no cure or treatment, or diseases with an unknown transmission mechanism. Personnel must receive training not only in handling extremely dangerous organisms but also in containment procedures. An accidental release of these organisms into the atmosphere could have catastrophic results. A biosafety level 4 laboratory is characterized by decontamination units (which include showers) at every entry point, positive-pressure suits worn by laboratory personnel, and biological safety cabinets. Organisms in this category include viruses that cause Ebola hemorrhagic fever, Lassa fever, Marburg hemorrhagic fever, and Hantavirus pulmonary syndrome.

Management of Risks

Laboratory personnel work in a hazardous environment. The hazards are presented by the many pathogenic organisms that are present in medical laboratories. These organisms include not only those present in a microbiology laboratory but also those present in blood, body fluids, and tissues. Infection control is a laboratory safety practice that assesses the risks to laboratory personnel by examining the chain of infection. The chain of infection includes infectious agents as well as the routes of transmission of an organism in the laboratory (e.g., injection from a contaminated sharp), the amount of the organism necessary to produce an infection (e.g., 1 drop vs. 1 mL), the stability of the organism in the environment (e.g., how long it is infective while traveling in the air), the types of hosts that the organism will infect (e.g., children vs. adults), the immunocompetency of its hosts (e.g., presence of antibodies to the hepatitis B organism), and the pathogenicity of the host (the likelihood that the organism will produce disease). As a result, employers proactively use many approaches to minimize the risk to laboratory workers.

The first step in managing the risks to laboratory workers is to determine what risks exist in each particular laboratory. Infectious agents can be transmitted to laboratory workers through five main routes:

1. Skin puncture with a contaminated needle or other sharp object
2. Spills and splashes of contaminated material onto mucous membranes or cuts in the skin
3. Ingestion, usually through mouth pipetting
4. Animal bites and scratches
5. Inhalation of infectious aerosols

According to the CDC, the first four routes of exposure account for only a minimal amount of laboratory associated infections (about 20%). The remaining 80% of exposures cannot be traced back to one particular incident, and experts assume that the greatest route of exposure for laboratory workers is through inhalation of infectious aerosols. This assumption makes sense because aerosols cannot be seen, so workers are unaware that they are being infected. This is only the microbiological hazard; laboratories will use a multifaceted approach to keep workers safe from this and other hazards.

As observed earlier, training plays a big part in keeping workers safe. Workers need training in the characteristics of the hazards, good laboratory techniques, SOPs, PPE and its use (Fig. 2-2), attentiveness to details at all times, safety policies and procedures, and awareness of surroundings.

Standard Operating Procedures

Standard operating procedures (SOPs) are one way that a laboratory can help reduce the exposure of workers to hazards. SOPs for clinical chemistry vary slightly from those of other departments. The usual headings for a written clinical chemistry SOP include the following:

- Introduction
- Principle of method
- Specimen types—collection and storage
- Reagents, standards, and controls—preparation and storage
- Equipment, glassware, and other accessories
- Detailed procedure
- Calculations and calibration curve
- Analytical reliabilities (quality control and statistical assessments)
- Hazardous reagents
- Reference range and clinical interpretation

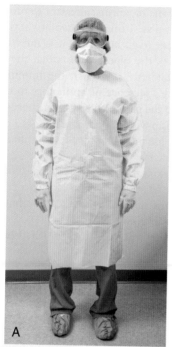

1. Discard broken or chipped glassware.
2. Dispose of broken or discarded pieces in a specially marked, separate, puncture-resistant container.
3. Handle contaminated broken glassware with puncture-resistant gloves or mechanical devices.
4. When using sharp objects, observe the following precautions:
   a. Extreme caution will be used when handling sharp objects, including needles and broken glass.
   b. All sharp objects will be handled with mechanical devices or one-handed techniques.
   c. Used needles will not be sheared, bent, broken, or recapped by hand.
   d. Used needles will not be removed from disposable syringes.
   e. Sharp objects will be placed immediately into the puncture-resistant red sharps containers located throughout the laboratory.
   f. Sharps containers will be sealed and disposed of when three-quarters full.

From Occupational Health and Safety Administration.

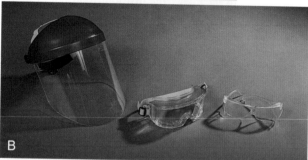

• **Figure 2-2 A,** Personal protective equipment (PPE). Not all parts of PPE are required for all situations. **B,** Eye protection: face mask, goggles, and glasses. (**A,** from Proctor DB, Adams AP. *Kinn's The Medical Assistant: An Applied Learning Approach.* 12th ed. St. Louis: Saunders; 2014. **B,** from Bonewit-West K. *Clinical Procedures for Medical Assistants.* 9th ed. St. Louis: Saunders; 2015.)

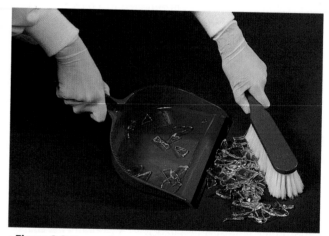

• **Figure 2-3** Proper cleanup of broken glassware is a very important part of laboratory safety. (From Bonewit-West K. *Clinical Procedures for Medical Assistants.* 9th ed. St. Louis: Saunders, 2015.)

- Limitations of method (e.g., interfering substances, troubleshooting)
- References
- Dates and signature of authorization
- Effective date and schedule for review

Sharp Objects

Use of laboratory glassware and sharp objects in a laboratory requires a certain amount of care and awareness (Box 2-5). Glassware in good condition represents a small hazard to laboratory workers; broken or damaged glassware becomes a larger hazard.

When laboratory workers use extreme caution handling glassware and sharp objects, the number of puncture incidents in the laboratory can be minimized (Fig. 2-3).

Centrifuges

The **centrifuge** is the workhorse of the laboratory, and the dangers created by this piece of equipment can be forgotten or minimized. Centrifuges spin at thousands of revolutions per minute and can hurl objects at incredible speeds. When a tube breaks in the centrifuge, glass shards and infectious particles can be spread over a large area in a short time.

Centrifuges can produce mechanical and biological hazards. Follow centrifugation procedures to minimize the possibility of aerosolization of infectious particles. Ensure that all specimen tubes are capped before starting the centrifuge. Close centrifuge covers, and keep hair, clothing, and dangling items away from the centrifuge. Such items may get caught in the centrifuge as it spins, resulting in injuries to the scalp, damage to clothing, or other types of damage.

Flammable liquids require much care during centrifugation. Centrifugation creates a vacuum and causes liquids to

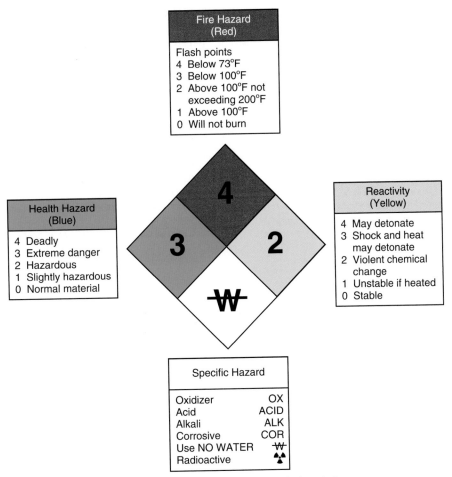

• **Figure 2-4** NFPA hazardous chemical symbol.

become volatile and flammable liquids to become bombs. Use caps or parafilm to cover tubes, and centrifuge at low speeds only.

Disinfect centrifuges periodically with a 1:10 dilution of bleach. Balance centrifuges properly before operation. Imbalance of the rotor causes vibration; as a result, tubes break more frequently, and the centrifuge wears out more rapidly.

Centrifuges are potentially dangerous weapons. Load imbalances may launch projectiles that can injure laboratory workers; broken glass tubes will liberate tiny glass particles and infectious agents into the air; and flammable liquids may become bombs and cause damage to the laboratory.

Refrigerators and Freezers

Refrigerators and freezers used in a laboratory setting may be commercial or household models. Observe the following precautions with laboratory refrigerators: Do not store flammable liquids in household refrigerators or freezers, because there are numerous ignition sources that could ignite vapors from the flammable liquids. To minimize the risk of fire or explosion, store flammable liquids in specially designed flammable-storage refrigerators or freezers. Store food in specially designated refrigerators. Food should not be stored in refrigerators containing reagents, media, specimens, or chemicals.

Warning Signs and Labels

Most laboratories use the National Fire Protection Association's (NFPA) 704 standard for labeling chemicals in the laboratory. This chemical labeling system allows laboratory and emergency response personnel to determine the characteristics of a chemical quickly and accurately during an emergency such as a fire or a chemical spill. Containers of hazardous chemicals must be labeled (Fig. 2-4), tagged, or marked with the specific information (Box 2-6).

Signage

Several areas and equipment require specific signage in the laboratory. Label refrigerators that are approved for storage of food as "For Food Only." Place biohazard stickers on all instruments and equipment in the laboratory. Place biohazard and "Authorized Personnel Only" signs on each external entrance to the laboratory. Post radiation hazard signs in areas where radioactive materials are handled. Post "Eye Wash Station" signs above the eye washing equipment. Post "Emergency Shower" signs close to the shower. Ensure that emergency exits are clearly marked. Post "Lab Coats Must Be Worn in This Area" signs in the working areas in the laboratory. Place "Spill Kit Station" signs at each spill kit location.

- State the identity or contents of the container
- Include appropriate warnings for health hazards (blue), flammability (red), instability (yellow), and specific hazards (white), such as oxidizer or reactive with water on the label.
- Include numbers on the label to indicate the severity of the hazard (1 stands for low severity, and 4 stands for high severity).
- Include the name and address of the chemical manufacturer, or other responsible party, as well as the emergency telephone number.
- Label secondary containers into which hazardous chemicals are transferred from labeled containers with the chemical identity of the contents and any precautionary handling hazards, including specific effects of the chemical and target organs affected.
- Do not remove or deface existing labels on containers carrying hazardous chemicals.
- Labels must be legible, in English, and prominently displayed on the container.
- Label all chemicals and reagents with date of receipt, date of preparation and/or date placed in service, and where appropriate, date of expiration.
- Return unlabeled containers of chemicals to the supplier unopened.

Emergency Evacuation

When an emergency arises in a laboratory or hospital, employees may be required to evacuate the laboratory and possibly the building. If this should occur, follow the emergency evacuation procedures in the laboratory's emergency response plan.

Fire Safety

Fire Prevention

Fire prevention is a very important aspect of any laboratory safety program. Assess and inventory the type, nature, and quantity of fuel sources in the laboratory. To keep the laboratory safe and efficient, use the smallest amounts possible of flammable and combustible liquids. Keep less than 2 gallons per 100 square feet in approved storage cabinets or safety cans (or less than 1 gallon if kept on an open shelf). Use fire safety cabinets and safety cans for storing chemicals. Keep open flames, heating elements, and electrical sparks (light switches, electric motors, friction, and static electricity) away from flammable and combustible chemicals.

Fire Classes

Regardless of prevention methods, a fire can occur in the laboratory (Box 2-7). There are four classes of fires:

- Class A fire—involves ordinary combustible materials such as wood, paper, and plastic
- Class B fire—involves flammable or combustible liquids such as kerosene, gasoline, grease, and oil
- Class C fire—involves laboratory instruments, wiring, circuits, and outlets

1. Pull the fire box to get help and to initiate evacuation of the area or building. Small fires can rapidly become large fires.
2. Immediately notify all persons in the area.
3. Call the fire department (911) and give them the following information: the building, your name, and the location within the building. Stay on the phone until the fire department arrives or terminates the call.
4. Contain the fire by closing all doors to the area and by placing wet towels or sheets at the base of the doors.
5. Evacuate all personnel from the premises.
6. Remember the acronym RACE: Rescue, Alarm, Contain, and Evacuate.
7. When evacuating the building, help patients and other visitors to the exits.
8. Close all doors and windows as personnel exit the building.

- Class D fire—involves combustible metals such as potassium, sodium, and magnesium

Different types of fire extinguishers are available to extinguish different types of fires.

Use water extinguishers on Class A fires only. Never use a water extinguisher on an oil fire, because it will spread the oil, thus expanding the fire to a wider area and increasing the danger from the fire. Dry chemical extinguishers can be used on Class A, B, or C fires because they are filled with dry chemicals such as bicarbonate or monoammonium phosphate. The chemical left on the fire is noncombustible; this reduces the chance of re-ignition of the fire.

Carbon dioxide extinguishers are used on Class B or C fires. This extinguisher contains highly pressurized CO_2 that can effectively stop the flow of oxygen to the fire. It does not leave a harmful residue on computers or other electrical devices and is a good choice for extinguishing sensitive electrical device fires.

Halotron is a clean fire-extinguishing agent that is found in handheld extinguishers and larger fire-extinguishing systems. Halotron is noncorrosive and will not damage equipment after discharge. It is approved for fighting fires in marine and aviation areas.

Fire blankets are used for clothing fires, and personnel are trained to "stop, drop, and roll" immediately after clothing catches on fire.

Electrical Safety

Repairs to electrical equipment and electrical systems are made only by qualified persons—biomedical technicians or manufacturer's technical service representatives. Unplug any instrument before attempting electrical repairs. Use approved extension cords that are appropriately rated for the equipment. Do not use electrical devices on wet surfaces. When unplugging a piece of equipment, always grasp the plug of the electrical cord between forefinger and thumb, then pull the plug from the socket. Do not pull on the cord. Do not use equipment with frayed or damaged

1. Secure cylinders (usually with wall mounts) in an upright position at all times to prevent them from falling.
2. Do not store cylinders with or near flammable materials.
3. Leave valve safety covers on the cylinder until pressure regulators are attached.
4. Clearly mark gas cylinders with the name of the contents.
5. Use hand trucks or dollies to move cylinders; do not roll or drag cylinders.
6. Do not attempt to repair damaged cylinders or to force frozen cylinder valves.

• **BOX 2-9** **Guidelines for Pressure Regulators and Needle Valves**

1. Use needle valves and regulators with the properly designated fittings.
2. Threads and surfaces must be clean and tightly fitted with no lubricants used on valves.
3. Use the proper size wrench to tighten regulators and valves.
4. Completely open the diaphragm control knob to release diaphragm pressure before opening the control valve; this prevents damage to the diaphragm.
5. Slowly open valves and stand to the side of the gauges in case the gauge face blows out; do not force sticking valves.
6. Check connections for leaks resulting from damaged faces at connections or from improper fittings.
7. Leave valve handles attached to the cylinders.
8. Set the maximum rate of flow by the high-pressure valve on the cylinder; then fine tune the flow using the needle valve.

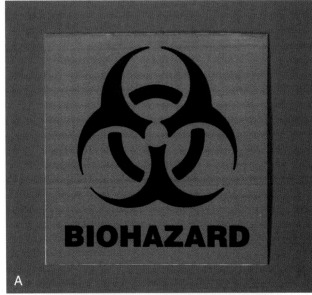

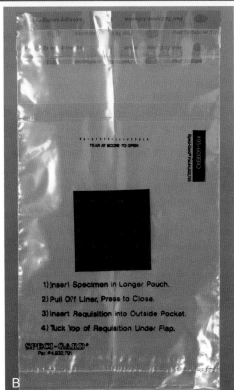

• **Figure 2-5 A,** Biohazard warning label. **B,** Biohazard bag used to hold and transport blood or other potentially infectious materials (OPIM). (From Bonewit-West K. *Clinical Procedures for Medical Assistants.* 9th ed. St. Louis: Saunders; 2015.)

cords. Plug only one piece of equipment into each electrical outlet. Do not plug one power strip into another power strip to increase the number of available outlets.

Compressed Gases

Compressed gases pose a unique hazard (Box 2-8 and Box 2-9). The cylinders themselves are heavy and can fall on someone, causing injury, or the cylinder itself can be propelled by the gas inside, making it a projectile and causing damage to anything in its path. The gas leaking out of the cylinder also constitutes a hazard because it may be poisonous, inert, explosive, flammable, or corrosive.

Biohazardous Waste Disposal

Biohazardous waste is waste that contains infectious or possibly infectious materials. No Federal regulations cover the disposal of medical waste. Responsibilities of laboratories generating biohazardous waste include properly sterilizing and disposing of the waste; properly packaging the waste to prevent puncture wounds; having the waste transported to a site where it will be sterilized or incinerated; and properly labeling the containers of biohazardous waste with the generator's name and date generated (Fig. 2-5).

Biohazardous waste includes several categories of waste.
- *Human blood and blood components:* Liquid or semiliquid blood or blood components are considered biohazardous. Contaminated items that release liquids when compressed and items with caked-on blood or blood products that release flakes when handled are also considered biohazardous.
- *Body fluids:* Certain specific body fluids are considered to be contaminated, including semen, vaginal fluids,

cerebral spinal fluid, synovial fluid, amniotic fluid, pericardial fluid, peritoneal fluid, and saliva from dental procedures. Any body fluid that is normally considered not biohazardous can become a biohazard if it is contaminated with visible blood.

- *Microbiological waste:* Any waste coming from a microbiology laboratory in which pathogenic organisms are concentrated is considered biohazardous, including culture plates, stock organism strains, and supplies used to transfer, inoculate, and mix infectious organisms.
- *Pathological waste:* Any human tissues, organs, or body parts are considered pathological waste.
- *Sharps waste:* Sharps include anything that can puncture a person's skin. Examples are needles, broken glass, glass pipets, razor blades, and scalpels. Contaminated sharps are considered biohazardous waste, but sharps must first be placed in a puncture-proof container that can be sealed before discarding.

Shipping of Biohazardous Materials

Shipping of biohazardous materials is governed by the International Air Transport Association (IATA). IATA leads air transport efforts to provide the safest handling of dangerous goods being transported through the air. This association publishes guidelines for documentation, packaging, handling, and transporting dangerous goods including biohazardous materials. IATA also publishes Dangerous Goods regulations with training requirements for personnel handling dangerous goods.

Laboratory Safety Equipment

Biological Safety Cabinet

A biological safety cabinet or biosafety cabinet is used to provide primary containment and to keep laboratory workers safe from potentially infectious materials. There are three types of biological cabinets: class I, class II, and class III. A class I biological safety cabinet is an open-front, negative-pressure cabinet. The exhaust air from this cabinet is filtered through a high-efficiency particulate air filter (HEPA filter). This type of cabinet will protect the worker and the environment from contamination.

A class II biological safety cabinet is an open-front, ventilated cabinet with vertical laminar flow. The air inside the cabinet is vented through a HEPA filter and recirculated through the cabinet. The exhaust from the cabinet is filtered through a HEPA filter. This cabinet will provide worker, environment, and product protection from exposure to potential infectious material.

A class III biological safety cabinet is a totally enclosed, ventilated cabinet. Laboratory workers manipulate items in the cabinet through attached rubber gloves that are accessible from outside the cabinet. When in use, the cabinet maintains a negative-pressure atmosphere. The intake air is filtered through HEPA filters, and the exhaust air is filtered through two HEPA filters, arranged in a series, before being discharged outside of the building.

Fume Hood

A fume hood is an enclosed area, similar to a cabinet, with an exhaust fan that directs harmful vapors away from the bench top and out through a vent, usually at the top of the fume hood. Laboratory workers can handle and store chemicals with harmful vapors by using a fume hood.

Needlestick Prevention Engineering Control

Needlestick prevention engineering controls are devices that remove, eliminate, or isolate the sharps hazard. These include retractable syringe needles, self-sheathing needles, needless devices, and sharps containers.

Fire Suppression Systems

All clinical laboratories must be equipped with a fire suppression system. This system is set off when heat or smoke triggers sensors to release a fire suppression agent throughout that area of the laboratory. Many buildings have sprinkler systems installed in the ceilings. Water might damage sensitive laboratory equipment, so an alternative system with a clean fire suppression agent is preferred for use in a laboratory setting.

Pipetting Aids

Pipetting aids are small pieces of equipment that allow the laboratory worker to draw liquid up into a pipet to a precise level and then discharge the liquid into a container. Pipetting aids come in several different shapes and sizes so that they fit onto volumetric and transfer pipets. Very small amounts of liquids, such as 10 µL, 50 µL, or 200 µL, can be pipetted with the use of micropipettes.

Eye Wash Stations

Eye wash stations are located at the sink of each technical area (Fig. 2-6). Eye washing devices are tested weekly to ensure proper functioning and to flush out stagnant water. When a laboratory worker gets chemicals into his or her eyes, it is imperative to rinse the chemicals out immediately.

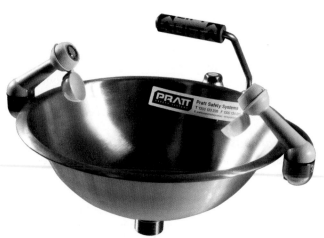

• **Figure 2-6** Eye wash station. (From Proctor DB, Adams AP. *Kinn's The Medical Assistant: An Applied Learning Approach.* 12th ed. St. Louis: Saunders; 2014.)

If the person is wearing contacts, the contacts must be removed before the eyes are rinsed.

Wash the eyes from outside to inside, ensuring that the water source is positioned at an angle toward the eyes. Rinse the eyes for a minimum of 15 minutes. Have the person roll the eyes and look up and down to ensure that the entire eye is rinsed. The stream of water should not be damaging to the person's eyes. Instead, have a steady stream of water with enough pressure to rinse the eyes thoroughly. Have someone else call 911 while the worker is rinsing his or her eyes.

Emergency Showers

Emergency showers are located in laboratories and are designed to douse a person with water after contamination with a chemical that is highly corrosive, irritating, or toxic to humans. The purpose of the shower is to rinse away as much of the chemical as possible. The first few seconds after exposure to a hazardous chemical is important, because the longer the chemical remains in contact with the skin, the more tissue damage will result.

Employee Health

Most hospitals have an employee health department. The employee health department is there to help workers with immunizations, workers' compensation claims, and incident reports related to health and safety issues such as needlesticks. Immunizations are the best protection for laboratory workers against many communicable diseases. Employers are required to offer workers the hepatitis B vaccination series or a booster. Antibodies are good protection against many infectious diseases. Employers may also offer employees free flu shots to keep them healthy during influenza season.

Needlestick Follow-up Procedures

Every employer mandates specific actions after an employee is stuck by a dirty sharp. The general procedure involves reporting to the employee health nurse for HIV and hepatitis B tests. If the employee knows which patient the dirty sharp was from, then the patient will also be asked to be tested for HIV and hepatitis B.

Incident Reports

When situations occur in a laboratory environment, an incident report must be filled out to protect both the worker and the employer. The incident report is a record of facts about the occurrence of a particular situation. Incident reports are filled out, for example, after a needlestick injury, a slip on a wet floor, or drawing blood from the wrong patient.

Employee Safety
Food and Drink

Food and drink are prohibited in all areas except the break room. Do not store food and drink items in technical refrigerators. The refrigerator to be used exclusively for food and drink items is located in the office and is marked accordingly. Do not store food and specimens in the same refrigerator.

Cosmetics

Do not apply cosmetics in the technical work area. Use of hand creams is allowed, but the cream must be stored in a drawer or cabinet. Do not store it on the workbench.

Eye and Face Protection

Safety glasses, facial shields, or other eye and face protectors (see Fig. 2-2, *B*) are worn when handling body fluids, infectious materials, or caustic or toxic materials. Contact lenses (especially soft lenses) absorb solvent and therefore constitute a hazard during splashes or spills. Contact lenses offer no protection from splashes, and they may concentrate caustic material against the cornea or prevent tears from washing a caustic substance away. Do not wear contact lenses in hazardous areas of a laboratory unless protective goggles or face shields are also worn. Face shields, masks with goggles, or other eye-protective devices are worn for splash protection when working with agents that can infect through mucous membranes or skin or when splashing is likely.

Clothing and Personal Protective Equipment

Wear appropriate attire, such as scrubs, when working in a laboratory. Sturdy, close-toed shoes are worn in the laboratory. PPE is appropriate only if it does not permit blood or OPIM to pass through to or reach the employee's work clothes, undergarments, skin, eyes, mouth, or other mucous membranes under normal conditions of use. Personnel working in technical areas need to wear water-impermeable laboratory coats that are long-sleeved with cuffs and worn with a closed front. Other PPE, such as gloves or goggles, may also be required in certain situations (see Fig. 2-2, *A*). Remove laboratory coats before leaving contaminated areas in the laboratory. Wear disposable gloves when handling infectious substances. Gloves are also worn when drawing blood from patients and are changed between patients. Gauze or another engineering device is used when removing tube stoppers to minimize spatter, and an appropriate shield is also worn.

Hair and Jewelry

Wear hair secured back and off the shoulders in such a manner as to prevent it from contacting contaminated materials or surfaces and also to prevent shedding of organisms into the work area. Do not wear jewelry that can become caught in equipment or hang into infectious materials.

Hand Washing

Hand washing is the best way to break the chain for spreading infections. Hand washing is the single best way to make sure workers in a clinical laboratory stay healthy. Hands should be washed before and after touching a patient; after working with infectious agents; before leaving the laboratory; before eating; after using the toilet; after blowing your nose, coughing, or sneezing; and after removing gloves. It is easy to do and everyone does it, but not everyone washes their hands correctly. Proper hand washing procedure is covered in Box 2-10.

Good Housekeeping

All technical areas of the laboratory, including the drawing room, are considered "contaminated" areas. All telephones, computer terminals, microscopes, and other surfaces are considered contaminated. Persons entering these areas with ungloved hands to use telephones, computer terminals, or other equipment are responsible for gloving and for thorough hand washing after touching equipment.

All office areas are considered "clean" areas. Gloves are removed before using the telephone, computer terminals, and other equipment to prevent contamination. Laboratory coats are not worn in office areas.

Work areas are kept neat and uncluttered. Bench tops are cleaned at least daily using a 1:10 dilution of bleach, which is prepared fresh weekly, or another disinfectant that will kill the tuberculosis bacterium. All spills are cleaned using a spill kit. Gloves and appropriate PPE are worn when dealing with sample spills and grossly contaminated work surfaces.

Refrigerators, freezers, and centrifuges are cleaned and disinfected weekly and when gross contamination occurs. Gloves, gown, and appropriate PPE are worn during cleaning. Outer clothing, such as laboratory coats, are properly hung up away from radiators, steam pipes, and heating instruments. Use of compressed gas cylinders or fire extinguishers as coat hooks is not appropriate. Do not obstruct the view through glass partitions in doors by hanging clothing over the glass. Store contaminated and uncontaminated PPE separately.

Trash should not be allowed to accumulate. Housekeeping staff should dispose of trash at least daily.

Festive decorations on lights, light fixtures, or instruments are not permitted. Electrical decorations, wax candles, dried arrangements, live Christmas trees, and other decorations that present potential fire hazards are not to be used.

Do not store personal belongings, such as purses, coats, boots, coffee mugs, sweaters, prepackaged foods, or medications in the technical work area. Storage of large amounts of disposables in the workplace should be avoided.

Hazardous liquids such as acids or alkalis should be stored below eye level. Large containers are stored down low and smaller containers higher up. Items should be stored no less than 36 inches from the ceiling in nonsprinkled areas and no less than 18 inches in sprinkled areas.

Exits and aisles must not be obstructed in any way. No trash, supplies, equipment, or furniture should be permitted in exit routes or aisles. Exit doors must not be obstructed, bolted, or blocked in any way. Do not cover or block access to fire extinguishers, fire alarm boxes, emergency blankets, safety showers, or exits at any time for any reason.

Decontamination and Sterilization

Decontamination is defined as the removal of contaminating substances from an object. It is just as important to physically scrub away the microorganisms as it is for the antimicrobial chemicals in the agent to kill the microorganisms. Some debris may actually inactivate antimicrobial agents, thus protecting the microbial agents.

Sterilization is defined as destruction of all microorganisms to create an aseptic environment. Many different agents can be used to disinfect or sterilize bench tops and other objects. The most effective disinfectants contain iodophors, chlorine, alcohol, phenols, or quaternary ammonium compounds. These compounds effectively kill the tuberculosis bacterium. With its thick, waxy outer cell wall, the tuberculosis bacterium is one of the most difficult microorganisms to kill with a disinfectant. By choosing a disinfectant that kills the tuberculosis bacterium, one can safely assume that other bacteria are also destroyed.

The amount of time needed to disinfect an area depends on the surface structure of the area. If there are many cracks, crevices, or joints, the disinfectant must be left in contact with the surface for an extended period to ensure that the microorganisms are killed. Workers who are using disinfectants must always wear appropriate PPE—fluid-resistant laboratory coat, gloves, and safety glasses—if splashes are expected. Always follow the manufacturer's instructions for use of the disinfectant.

Ergonomic Hazards

Ergonomic hazards are inherent in tasks that involve prolonged repetitive motion. Workers need to make themselves aware of the potential risks associated with all tasks. Adjustments can be made to chairs and workstations to minimize the risk of developing an injury. Workers can also help prevent prolonged repetitive motion injuries by taking frequent short breaks and using alternative activities. Also, practicing proper body posture while working on a computer can help prevent injuries.

• BOX 2-10   Hand Washing Technique

1. Wet your hands with hot or cold water.
2. Dispense soap into one of your hands.
3. Rub hands together to produce lather.
4. Scrub your hands well, including the backs and palms of the hands, between the fingers, and around and under the nails.
5. Scrub your hands for at least 20 seconds. (Sing the "Happy Birthday" song twice to equal 20 seconds.)
6. Rinse your hands well, then dry them with a clean paper towel or air.
7. If a sink, soap, and running water are not available, then use an alcohol-based hand sanitizer. Squirt a small amount of the sanitizer into one palm and rub both hands together, including between the fingers, until the hands are dry.

Summary

There are many hazards facing laboratory workers. As a result, the federal government has passed at least four laws that dictate the type of safety precautions that must exist in clinical laboratories: the Occupational Exposure to Hazardous Chemicals in Laboratories standard, the Hazard Communication standard, the Bloodborne Pathogens standard, and the Needlestick Safety and Prevention Act. Some hazards are physical hazards, such as sharp objects, and some are biohazards, such as blood and body fluids.

There are several different ways to be exposed to biohazards, including by aerosol, ingestion, mucous membranes and eyes, and direct inoculation. The severity of the biohazard is reflected in the biosafety level assigned to the laboratory—biosafety level 1, 2, 3, or 4. Biosafety level 1 has lower-level biohazards, whereas biosafety level 4 contains microorganisms that can cause fatal diseases. There are also fire hazards and electrical hazards in the laboratory.

Many hazards can be prevented through good housekeeping, fire prevention, electrical safety, and a good laboratory safety program. Immunizations can also help prevent infections if laboratory workers are exposed to biohazards. Every laboratory has a laboratory safety program to keep its workers as safe as possible.

Review Questions

1. The laboratory safety program is mainly dictated by all of the following federal regulations EXCEPT
   a. OSH Act of 1970
   b. Needlestick and Safety Act of 2000
   c. Hazard Communication standard
   d. Bloodborne Pathogens standard

2. Which of the following is *not* part of a chemical hygiene plan?
   a. SDS
   b. Procedures
   c. Equipment
   d. PPE

3. Which of the following is part of an Exposure Control Plan?
   a. Documenting Hepatitis B immunization or declination
   b. Biohazard spill cleanup procedures
   c. N-95 respirator instructions for use
   d. SDS

4. The Hazard Communication standard mandates employers to
   a. Label all chemicals in the laboratory with NFPA labels
   b. Lock away all hazardous chemicals
   c. Not store hazardous chemicals on the laboratory floor
   d. Register all hazardous chemicals with the fire department

5. Compressed gases hazards for the clinical laboratory professional include all the following EXCEPT
   a. The cylinders can present a projectile hazard if the compressor breaks off of the cylinder.
   b. The gas contained in the cylinder can be hazardous.
   c. The cylinders are very heavy.
   d. Cylinders can present a chemical hazard due to the composition of the cylinder.

6. A worker can take all of the following actions to help prevent exposure to potentially infectious materials EXCEPT
   a. Get vaccinated.
   b. Wear appropriate PPE.
   c. Do not eat or drink in the laboratory.
   d. Practice good hand washing techniques.

7. The Needlestick Safety and Prevention Act requires employers to do all of the following EXCEPT
   a. Choose all the devices used for invasive procedures.
   b. Use self-sheathing needles.
   c. Use engineering controls for sharps disposal containers.
   d. Record sharps injuries in a log.

8. Which of the following statements concerning biosafety levels for clinical laboratories is true?
   a. A biosafety level 2 laboratory identifies moderate-risk agents such as *Salmonella* spp., *Staphylococcus aureus*, *Streptococcus pyogenes*, and *Escherichia coli*.
   b. A biosafety level 1 laboratory identifies viruses that cause Ebola hemorrhagic fever, Lassa fever, Marburg hemorrhagic fever, and Hantavirus pulmonary syndrome.
   c. A biosafety level 3 laboratory identifies *Bacillus subtilis, Staphylococcus epidermidis, Serratia marcensens,* and *Streptococcus bovis.*
   d. A biosafety level 4 laboratory identifies *Bacillus anthracis, Yersinia pestis,* and the smallpox virus.

9. Shipping procedures for biohazardous substances are regulated by
   a. The International Air Transport Association (IATA)
   b. OSHA
   c. The Federal Department of Transportation
   d. The Federal Aviation Administration (FAA)

10. The goal of a laboratory safety program is to
    a. Minimize the risk of injury or illness to employees
    b. Reduce the number of needlesticks involving laboratory personnel in 1 year
    c. Decrease the amount of biological waste generated by the laboratory
    d. Make sure all OSHA regulations are met

Critical Thinking Questions

1. How does a laboratory safety program minimize the risk of exposure for clinical laboratory workers?
2. Describe three pieces of PPE and why each is effective at preventing exposure.
3. Explain the acronym RACE. Why is it important?

CASE STUDY

Eddie was working in the microbiology department, and one of the incubators was getting low on carbon dioxide. He had another CO_2 cylinder delivered to the department. The maintenance man left the cylinder at the door instead of bringing it to the incubator. Rather than calling maintenance back, Eddie decided to move the cylinder himself. He rolled it on its bottom headed toward the incubator with the low tank. As he was dragging the cylinder, he took his eyes off of it, and the cylinder slipped out of his hands. It crashed down on the floor and, because the tank cover was removed, the regulator popped out of the cylinder. The gas cylinder, with pressurized gas streaming out of it, was transformed into a torpedo, penetrating the wall. The wall was thick enough to stop the momentum of the cylinder. No one was hurt as the cylinder went shooting across the floor and became impaled in the wall.

Bibliography

American National Standards Institute. *ANSI Eyewash Z358.1-2009 In-Depth Compliance Guide.* <http://www.eyewashdirect.com/v/vspfiles/assets/images/ANSI%20Eyewash%20Z358.1-2009%20In-Depth%20Compliance%20Guide.pdf> Accessed 08.05.15.

Centers for Disease Control and Prevention. *CDC Features: Wash Your Hands.* December 2013. <http://www.cdc.gov/features/handwashing/> Accessed 08.05.15.

Clinical and Laboratory Standards Institute. *Clinical Laboratory Safety: Approved Guideline.* 2nd ed. Wayne, PA: NCCLS; 2004. NCCLS document GP17–A2 (ISBN 1-56238-530-5).

Kanagasabapathy AS, Kumari S: *Guidelines on Standard Operating Procedures for Clinical Chemistry.* World Health Organization, Regional Office for Southeast Asia (last updated 2006). <http://www.searo.who.int/entity/bloodsafety/documents/en/> Accessed 08.05.15.

International Air Transport Association. *Dangerous Goods Regulations.* 52nd ed. Effective January 2011. <http://dgitraining.com/content/pdf/iataaddendumjan2011.pdf> Accessed 08.05.15.

National Institutes of Health. NIH Office of Research Services. *Decontamination and Sterilization.* <http://www.ors.od.nih.gov/sr/dohs/BioSafety/decon/Pages/decontamination.aspx> Accessed 08.05.15.

Occupational Safety and Health Administration. *Healthcare Wide Hazards: (Lack of) Universal Precautions.* <http://www.osha.gov/SLTC/etools/hospital/hazards/univprec/univ.html> Accessed 08.05.15.

Occupational Safety and Health Administration. *Healthcare Wide Hazards: Needlestick/Sharps Injuries.* <http://www.osha.gov/SLTC/etools/hospital/hazards/sharps/sharps.html> Accessed 08.05.15.

Occupational Safety and Health Administration. *Laboratory Safety Guidance.* OSHA; 3404–11R 2011. <http://www.osha.gov/Publications/laboratory/OSHA3404laboratory-safety-guidance.pdf> Accessed 08.05.15.

Occupational Safety and Health Administration. *Model Plans and Programs for the OSHA: Bloodborne Pathogens and Hazard Communications Standards.* OSHA; 3186–06N 2003. <http://www.osha.gov/Publications/osha3186.pdf> Accessed 08.05.15.

SAFENEEDLE.org. *Needlestick Safety Facts and Figures, 2010.* <http://safeneedle.org/us-needlesticks/the-needlestick-safety-and-prevention-act/> Accessed 08.05.15.

U.S. Department of Health and Human Services. Section IV: Laboratory biosafety level criteria. In: *Biosafety in Microbiological and Biomedical Laboratories.* 5th ed. DHHS/PHS/CDC/NIH/HHS publication no. (CDC)21-112. Revised December 2009. <http://www.cdc.gov/biosafety/publications/bmbl5/bmbl5_sect_iv.pdf> Accessed 08.05.15.

U.S. Department of Health and Human Services. *Biosafety in Microbiological and Biomedical Laboratories.* 5th ed. DHHS/PHS/CDC/NIH/HHS publication no. (CDC)21-112. Revised December 2009. <http://www.cdc.gov/biosafety/publications/bmbl5/> Accessed 08.05.15.

3

Principles of Laboratory Instrumentation

CRAIG FOREBACK AND DONNA LARSON

CHAPTER OUTLINE

OBJECTIVES

After completion of this chapter, the reader will be able to:

1. Describe the relationships among wavelength, frequency, energy, and color of the ultraviolet and visible spectra.
2. Describe the relationship between percent transmittance (%T) and absorbance (A).
3. Discuss the Beer-Lambert law and its limitations.
4. Describe how the instrumentation and basic principles of photometry are modified with the applications of turbidimetry, nephelometry, or fluorometry.
5. State the applications for fluorescence, chemiluminescence, and bioluminescence.
6. Compare and contrast the principles of absorption and emission spectroscopy.

7. Differentiate between potentiometric and voltammetric techniques.
8. State the general principles of chromatography and describe their application to the divisions and subdivisions of chromatography, supporting each description with an illustration of mechanism.
9. Describe the separation processes involved with the following types of chromatography and list the class of molecules that can be separated by each type: absorption, partition, ion exchange, and gel permeation.
10. State the requirements for internal standard selection and use.

OBJECTIVES—cont'd

11. Diagram and describe the basic column liquid chromatographic system.
12. Diagram and describe the basic components of a gas chromatographic system.
13. Name four common carrier gases and state the function of a carrier gas.
14. Diagram and describe the basic components of a mass spectrometer.
15. Discuss the principles of using a mass-fragmentation pattern to identify unknown molecules.
16. Describe the common support media for electrophoresis.
17. Compare and contrast freezing-point depression and vapor-pressure depression for osmolality determinations.
18. Compare and contrast the technology used in point-of-care testing devices, including reagents and instruments, with routine laboratory instruments.
19. Discuss the method of measurement for flow cytometers.
20. Describe resolution in a flow cytometer and one way to improve the resolution.
21. Discuss hydrodynamic focusing in flow cytometry.
22. Discuss how fluorescent light and refraction are used in flow cytometry.
23. Discuss six clinical applications for flow cytometry.

KEY TERMS

Adsorption chromatography
Affinity chromatography
Agarose
Amperometry
Anodic stripping voltammetry
Beer's law
Bioluminescence
Capillary electrophoresis
Capillary gel electrophoresis
Capillary isoelectric focusing
Capillary zone electrophoresis
Chemical ionization
Chemiluminescence
Chromatography
Chromogen
Clark electrode
Colligative properties
Column chromatography
Conductometry
Coulometry
Cuvette
Diffraction grating
Electrochemiluminescence
Electron ionization
Electrophoresis
Electrospray ionization
Fiberoptics

Filters
Flow cytometry
Fluorescence
Fluorescence polarization
Fluorometer
Fluorometry
Fluorophore
Gas chromatography
High-performance liquid
 chromatography
Incandescent lamp
Interference filter
Ion exchange chromatography
Ion-selective electrode
Isocratic procedure
Isoelectric focusing
Isotachophoresis
Linear ion trap
Liquid chromatography
Luminometer
Mass spectrometer
Mobile phase
Monochromatic
Monochromator
Nephelometry
Osmolality
Osmotic pressure

Partition chromatography
Photodetectors
Photodiodes
Photomultiplier
Planar chromatography
Point-of-care testing
Polyacrylamide
Potentiometric sensor
Prism
Quadrupole mass spectrometer
Redox electrode
Reflectance density
Reflection
Refraction
Resolution
Size-exclusion chromatography
Spectral bandwidth
Spectral purity
Spectrophotometry
Specular reflectance
Stationary phase
Tandem mass spectrometry
Time-of-flight mass spectrometer
Turbidimetry
Vapor pressure
Voltammetry

Points to Remember

- Beer's law (A = abc) is the relationship among the absorbance (a) of light by a solution, the path length of light (b), and the concentration of the solution (c).
- A spectrophotometer contains a light source, spectral isolation device, fiberoptics, cuvette holders, photodetector, readout device, recorder, and microprocessor.
- A cuvette is a small vessel used to hold a liquid sample to be read in the light path of the spectrophotometer.
- Fluorometry is the measurement of emitted fluorescence, and it is used for medically important analyses.

- A fluorometer contains a light source, sample cells, photodetectors, and detectors.
- Luminometry is a technique that employs chemiluminescence, bioluminescence, and electroluminescence to detect medically important analytes.
- Basic components of a luminometer are a light-tight sample chamber, an injection system, and a detector.
- Turbidimetry and nephelometry are used to measure proteins and antibody-antigen complexes.
- Potentiometric electrodes are used to measure pH, partial pressure of carbon dioxide (P_{CO_2}), and Na^+, K^+, Cl^-, Ca^{2+}, Mg^{2+}, and Li^+ ions.

- The silver–silver chloride electrode is an example of a redox electrode.
- Ion-selective electrodes are used extensively in clinical chemistry to measure pH, P_{CO_2}, and Na^+, K^+, Ca^{2+}, Mg^{2+}, and Li^+ ions.
- The valinomycin membrane on a potentiometric electrode makes it highly selective for K^+ measurement.
- Voltammetry uses the Clark electrode to measure oxygen.
- Conductometry is used to measure the number of red blood cells and uses the Coulter principle.
- Several chloride analyzers work on the principle of coulometry.
- Ion exchange chromatography is performed in columns and is used to separate anions, cations, amino acids, peptides, and proteins.
- Affinity chromatography was the earliest method used to measure glycohemoglobin
- Size-exclusion chromatography is useful for determining the tertiary and quaternary structures of purified proteins.
- Gas chromatography is used to measure volatile analytes such as alcohols.
- Liquid chromatography is more useful than gas chromatography because more analytes are nonvolatile than volatile.
- Applications of mass spectrometry include analysis of therapeutic drugs, drugs of abuse, trace metals, and vitamins. It is also used in proteomics to identify and quantify proteins.
- Mass spectrometer components include an ionizer, analyzer, and detector system.
- Mass spectrometers are used to analyze glycans, lipids, proteins, peptides, and oligonucleotides.
- A basic electrophoresis system consists of a buffer tray, electrophoretic medium, and power supply.
- Isoelectric focusing is used to separate proteins.
- Blotting techniques are used to detect RNA (i.e., Northern blotting), DNA (i.e., Southern blotting), and proteins (i.e., Western blotting).
- Capillary electrophoresis is used for separating serum proteins, immunotyping, separation of abnormal hemoglobins, and purity analysis of oligonucleotides and RNA.
- Freezing point depression osmometers are used to quantitate ethanol, methanol, isopropane, and osmolar gaps in acid-base disturbances.
- Point-of-care testing instruments have transformed health care by running laboratory tests and getting results at the patient's bedside.
- Flow cytometers are used to measure cell size, stage of the cell cycle, DNA content of the cell, presence or absence of cell markers, and other cellular characteristics.
- A flow cytometer contains fluidics systems, optic electronics, and a data analyzer.

Introduction

Analytical chemistry techniques and instrumentation provide the basis for most measurements in the clinical laboratory. Applications include spectrometry, spectrophotometry, refractometry, reflectance photometry, atomic absorption, mass spectrometry, fluorescence, chemiluminescence, nephelometry or turbidimetry, electrophoresis, potentiometry, voltammetry or amperometry, conductometry, coulometry, and gas, liquid, and thin-layer chromatography. Flow cytometry is an application of several analytical principles, including light scattering, fluorescence, and immunochemical methods.

With improvements in optics, electronics, and computerization, instrumentation has become miniaturized and more powerful. Benefits include smaller sample requirements, smaller physical size, and reduced cost. Current mass spectrometers are a fraction the size of their predecessors, electrodes for multiple analytes are available on a single chip, and many point-of-care tests are now available on handheld, portable devices.

Properties of Light

Light is electromagnetic radiation that has wavelike properties and particle-like properties (i.e., photons). Electromagnetic radiation includes a spectrum of energy from short-wavelength gamma rays (0.01 to 10 nm) to long-wavelength radiofrequencies (1 to 100 cm). The relationship between wavelength and energy, E, is described by Plank's equation:

$$E = h\nu$$

In the equation, h is Plank's constant (6.62×10^{-27} erg-sec) and ν is frequency.

Because the frequency of a wave is inversely proportional to the wavelength, it follows that the energy of electromagnetic radiation is inversely proportional to wavelength. This relationship is described in the following equations:

$$\nu = \frac{c}{\lambda}$$

$$E = \frac{hc}{\lambda}$$

In these equations, c is the speed of light and λ is the wavelength.

Beer's Law

The relationship between the absorption of light by a solution and the concentration of the solution has been described by August Beer and others including Johann Heinrich Lambert and Pierre Bouguer. Beer's law states that the amount of light absorbed by a solution is directly proportional to the concentration of a solution. Conversely, the logarithm of the transmitted light of a substance is inversely proportional to its concentration. The amount of light absorbed or transmitted is mathematically related to the concentration of the analyte in question. The amount of light absorbed (A) by a sample is defined in the following equation:

$$A = -\log\frac{I_s}{I_r} = -\log T$$

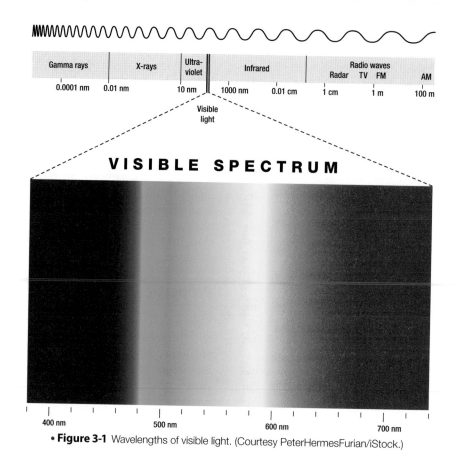

• Figure 3-1 Wavelengths of visible light. (Courtesy PeterHermesFurian/iStock.)

where I_s is the intensity of the light transmitted through the sample, I_r is the intensity of light transmitted through a reference cell, and T is transmittance. Beer's law is expressed as follows:

$$A = \varepsilon bc$$

In this equation, A is absorbance, ε is absorptivity (a characteristic of the absorbing compound), b is the light path in centimeters, and c is concentration.

Spectrophotometry

Photometry is the measurement of light without specifying a wavelength. Spectrophotometry is the measurement of light at selected wavelengths (Figs. 3-1 and 3-2), typically in the ranges of ultraviolet (UV), visible, and infrared light (Table 3-1). The technique depends on the light-absorbing properties of the analyte of interest or a derivative of the analyte. The intensity of transmitted light passing through a solution that contains an absorbing substance, or chromogen, is decreased by the absorbed fraction. This fraction is detected, measured, and used to relate the light transmitted or absorbed to the concentration of the analyte of interest. Beer's law is valid only under the following conditions:

- Incident radiation on the solution is monochromatic (i.e., single wavelength).
- The solvent absorption is insignificant compared with the solute absorbance.

- The solute concentration is within given limits.
- There is no optical interference.
- A chemical reaction does not take place between the molecule of interest and another solute or solvent molecule.

Components

Modern instruments isolate a narrow range of wavelengths for optical measurements. Those that use filters are called *photometers,* and those that use prisms or gratings are referred to as *spectrophotometers.* The basic components of a single-beam photometer or spectrophotometer are a light source, a spectral isolation device, fiberoptics in automated instruments, cuvettes, a photodetector, a readout device, a recorder, and a microprocessor (Fig. 3-3). In many modern instruments, the last three components are replaced by a personal computer with printer.

Light Sources

Light sources include incandescent lamps, hydrogen or deuterium lamps, and lasers. Incandescent lamps use a tungsten filament housed in a fused-silica envelope around a low-pressure iodine or bromine vapor in the lamp. This greatly increases the lifetime of the filament. Because a tungsten lamp does not supply sufficient radiant energy below 320 nm, hydrogen or deuterium lamps must be used for measurements in the UV region.

Absorbance

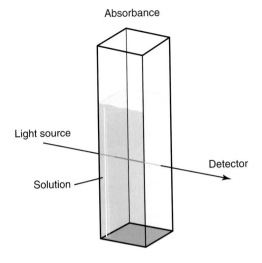

Fluorescence

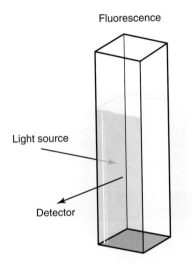

• **Figure 3-2** The amount of light that exits the cuvette after passing through a solution depends on the amount of light that is absorbed by the sample. In the case of fluorescence, light is absorbed and then emitted by the sample.

TABLE 3-1	Ultraviolet, Visible, and Short Infrared Spectrum Characteristics Colors	
Wavelength (nm)*	Region Name	Characteristics
<380	Ultraviolet†	Invisible
380-440	Visible	Violet
440-500	Visible	Blue
500-580	Visible	Green
580-600	Visible	Yellow
600-620	Visible	Orange
620-750	Visible	Red
800-2500	Near-infrared	Not visible
2500-15,000	Mid-infrared	Not visible
15,000-1,000,000	Far-infrared	Not visible

*Because of the subjective nature of color, the wavelength intervals shown are only approximations.
†The ultraviolet (UV) portion of the spectrum is sometimes further divided into near UV (220 to 380 nm) and far UV (<220 nm). This distinction has a practical basis because cuvettes made from silica transmit light effectively at wavelengths of 220 nm or greater.
From Burtis CA, Bruns DE. *Tietz Fundamentals of Clinical Chemistry and Molecular Diagnostics*. 7th ed. Elsevier: St. Louis; 2015.

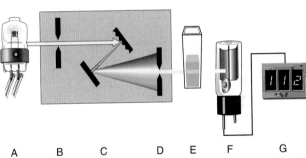

A   B   C   D   E   F   G

• **Figure 3-3** Major components of a single-beam spectrophotometer. **A,** Exciter lamp. **B,** Entrance slit. **C,** Monochromator. **D,** Exit slit. **E,** Cuvette. **F,** Photodetector. **G,** Light-emitting diode (LED) display. (From McPherson RA, Pincus MR. *Henry's Clinical Diagnosis and Management by Laboratory Methods*. 22nd ed. Philadelphia: Elsevier; 2012.)

Laser Sources

The term *laser* is an acronym for "light amplification by stimulated emission of radiation." Lasers are different from regular light sources because they emit collimated light. They are used as light sources in many instruments that measure the interactions of light and matter, including spectrophotometers, nephelometers, and flow cytometers, because they provide intense radiation of a narrow wavelength. These devices are based on the capacity of certain materials to absorb energy and store all or part of it remaining in an excited state. If the excited material has yet more energy pumped into it, a rapid decay to a lower energy state may occur with the emission of highly quantified light. Because of the kinetic mechanisms of decay to a lower energy state, a highly collimated beam of light is produced that is almost monochromatic and has minimum scatter (Fig. 3-4).

Spectral Isolation

A system for isolating radiant energy of a desired wavelength and excluding that of other wavelengths is called a **monochromator**. The term is somewhat of misnomer because most monochromators that are described in this chapter do not isolate a single wavelength.

Devices used for spectral isolation include filters, prisms, and diffraction gratings. Combinations of lenses and slits are usually employed before or after the monochromatic device to render light rays parallel or to isolate narrow portions of the light beam. Various slits may be used to allow adjustments in the radiant energy reaching the photodetector.

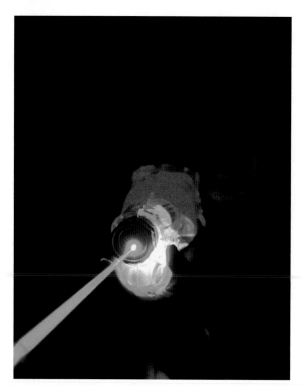

• **Figure 3-4** Lasers provide intense, highly collimated beams of monochromatic light. (©Rich Legg/iStock)

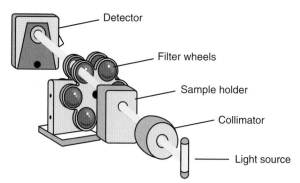

• **Figure 3-5** Filter wheels contain many filters to ensure only light of a particular wavelength enters the sample holder.

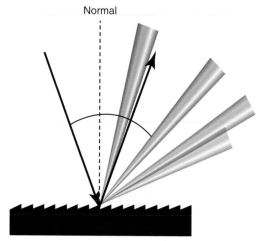

• **Figure 3-6** Diffraction grating.

Filters

The simplest filters are thin layers of colored glass. The spectral purity of a filter or other monochromator is described in terms of its spectral bandwidth, which is defined as the width, in nanometers, of the spectral transmittance curve at a point equal to one half of the peak transmittance. Commonly used glass filters have spectral bandwidths of approximately 50 nm. These wide band-pass filters are not used in most spectrophotometric applications.

Interference filters are often used as monochromators. They have narrow spectral bandwidths in the range of 5 to 15 nm. Interference filters are commonly used in automated multichannel instruments (Fig. 3-5).

Prisms and Gratings

Prisms and gratings are widely used as monochromators. A prism separates white light into a continuous spectrum by refraction: Shorter wavelengths are bent or refracted more than longer wavelengths as they pass through the prism. A diffraction grating is prepared by depositing a thin layer of an aluminum–copper alloy onto the surface of a flat glass plate and then ruling many small parallel grooves into the metal coating. Diffraction gratings can be mass produced using a laser in high-precision machining mode (Fig. 3-6). Because gratings cost less to produce than high-quality quartz prisms, are highly accurate, and have low light scatter, they have replaced prisms in most UV-visible spectrophotometers and infrared spectrophotometers. UV high-performance liquid chromatography (HPLC) detectors frequently use concave holographic gratings in their optical systems. High-quality spectrophotometers may have bandwidths of less than 0.5 nm.

Fiberoptics

In traditional single-beam or double-beam spectrophotometers, the positions of individual components dictate the path the light beam must travel from the source to the detector. This places restrictions on design, size, and cost of the instrument. To overcome these restrictions, fiberoptics are integrated into the optical design. Fiberoptics, also known as flexible light pipes, are bundles of thin, transparent fibers of glass, quartz, or plastic that are enclosed by a material with a lower index of refraction. They transmit light through internal reflections. Fiberoptics improve directional control of the light beam within the confines of the instrument, allowing the design and manufacture of miniature, inexpensive optical subsystems for use in automated devices. A single light source can be multiplexed with many optical channels using fiberoptics. Disadvantages of fiberoptics include greater amounts of stray light, refractive index changes, and the loss of transmitted energy when exposed to UV light.

Cuvettes

A cuvette is a small vessel used to hold a liquid sample in the light path of a spectrophotometer for measurement. Square or rectangular cuvettes are preferable to round cuvettes because

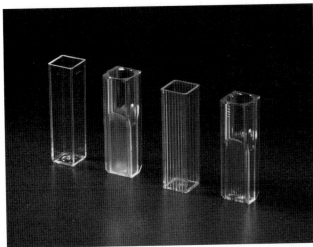

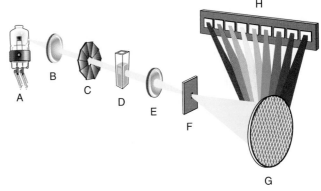

• **Figure 3-8** Diode array in a spectrophotometer. **A,** Lamp. **B,** Lens. **C,** Shutter. **D,** Cell. **E,** Lens. **F,** Slit. **G,** Grating. **H,** Photodiode array. (From McPherson RA, Pincus MR. *Henry's Clinical Diagnosis and Management by Laboratory Methods.* 22nd ed. Philadelphia: Elsevier; 2012.)

they have plane-parallel optical surfaces and a constant light path. They can be constructed of glass, quartz, or plastic. Borosilicate glass cuvettes are suitable for the visible portion of the spectrum, but for readings below 340 nm, quartz cuvettes are usually required. Plastic cuvettes are available that have good clarity in the UV region (Fig. 3-7). Many of the plastic cuvettes are designed for disposable, single-use applications, eliminating issues with cleaning and drying. In the case of plastic UV cuvettes, the expense may justify washing, but care must be taken to avoid scratching. Other issues include etching by organic solvents and temperature deformations.

Photodetectors

Photodetectors are devices that convert light into an electrical signal by detecting photons that strike a photosensitive or photoemissive surface. The detector surface releases electrons in proportion to the number of photons striking it. The two main types of detectors used are photomultiplier tubes (PMTs) and photodiodes. A **photomultiplier** is an electron tube that contains a cathode, a light-sensitive metal, and a series of dynodes (up to 16) enclosed in a glass enclosure, as well as an anode that collects the amplified electrons. When photons strike the cathode, emitted primary electrons are attracted to the first dynode, causing the emission of three to six secondary electrons. This sets up a chain reaction that results in an amplified current up to 10^6 times the initial energy. The resultant measured current is directly proportional to the light intensity striking the PMT.

Photodiodes or light-sensing diodes are semiconductor photodetectors; they have begun to replace PMTs in many clinical laboratory instruments. Photodiodes are popular detectors because they can measure light simultaneously at many wavelengths with speed and accuracy. They can be arranged in a linear array of hundreds of diodes, each calibrated to respond to a specific wavelength by its placement in the array. As shown in Figure 3-8, the diffraction grating is positioned after the sample cell when a diode array is employed in a spectrophotometer.

Readout Devices and Computers

The signal processing or readout device amplifies and mathematically manipulates the electrical signal produced by the photodetector and converts it to a convenient format. The use of computers for readout has largely supplanted that of all other devices for that purpose. Computers can plot and store standard curves, control instrument functions, and automate trouble-shooting functions. In every type of instrumentation discussed in this chapter, the computer has become an essential component for collecting, converting, and storing analytical data.

Performance Parameters

Wavelength accuracy, linearity of detector response, stray light, and absorbance accuracy are important quality control measures that should be checked according to manufacturers' instructions to certify that the spectrophotometer is functioning within specifications. Optical test methods use particular wavelengths to quantitate analytes. If the wavelength is not accurate, the test result is not accurate.

Wavelength Accuracy

A spectrophotometer must be calibrated to ensure that the exact desired wavelength is passing through the specimen. Three common methods are used to calibrate wavelength. The first involves using a light source with strong emission lines at specific wavelengths. Mercury vapor or hydrogen lamps are often used for calibrating spectrophotometers. The second method uses rare earth glass filters such as holmium oxide and didymium. These filters have strong absorption bands. The third method uses a solution of chromogen. This method is usually a secondary wavelength calibration standard. Spectrophotometers using gratings require calibration at two wavelengths, and spectrophotometers using prisms require calibration at three wavelengths.

Linearity

For analytical and spectrophotometric accuracy, there must be a linear relationship between the amount of light absorbed by a sample and the corresponding instrument readout. Two methods are used to determine linearity: solid glass filters and liquid solutions. Solid glass filters are inserted into the spectrophotometer, and the linearity is measured at particular wavelengths. Liquid solutions are made from stable chromogens at various concentrations. The absorbance of the solution is read, and the data are analyzed for linearity.

Stray Light

Stray light can cause erroneous results and can be detected at the far ends of the spectral range. It is detected with the use of filters or solutions that are opaque at a particular wavelength. If the filter or solution does not transmit light at the appropriate wavelength but light is detected, then stray light is getting into the spectrophotometer. If the amount of stray light detected is greater than 1%, the instrument is malfunctioning and needs to be fixed.

Absorbance Accuracy

Standards are used to confirm absorbance accuracy. Absorbance standards have a stable absorbance at a suitable wavelength. The National Institute of Standards and Technology (NIST) offers a set of three neutral-density glass filters to determine the absorbance accuracy of a spectrophotometer.

Reflectance Photometry

Reflection occurs when light (i.e., incident ray) is deflected by the surface of a substance. The reflected light is in the same plane as the incident ray and is perpendicular to the reflecting plane. Specular reflectance occurs when light is reflected from a smooth or mirror-like surface; this contrasts with diffuse reflectance, which occurs when light is reflected from an irregular surface.

Specular reflectance is used as an analytical technique to measure sample concentrations in reflectometry instruments (i.e., reflectometers). A reflectometer measures the amount of light reflected by a colored reaction product on a reflective surface composed of paper or plastic. The term reflectance density describes the amount of light absorbed by the colored reaction product on the smooth surface; it is inversely proportional to the light intensity reflected by the sample. As sample concentration increases, the intensity of the color increases and the amount of light reflected decreases. The reflectance is inversely proportional to the concentration of the analyte of interest and is nonlinear, requiring the use of a mathematical algorithm to linearize the data and determine the sample concentration.

Reflectance techniques are used in many point-of-care applications and in analysis of macroscopic urine test strips. They also are used in many of the measurements performed on the Vitros (Ortho Clinical Diagnostics) series of analyzers.

Refractive Index Measurements

Refraction is the change in direction as light passes from one medium to a second medium. A common example is a prism, which disperses white light into its constituents. The use of prisms as monochromators has been discussed. Refractometry is an analytical method that is routinely used to measure specific gravity in urine. It has been incorporated into some automated instruments. Refractive index detectors have been employed in HPLC systems, and for many years, they were the only universal detectors available for HPLC. However, their poor limit of detection and inability to be interfaced with gradient HPLC separations limit their utility.

Fluorometry

Fluorescence occurs when a molecule absorbs light at one wavelength and reemits light at a longer wavelength. An atom or molecule that fluoresces is called a fluorophore. Fluorophores are frequently used as labels in immunoassays and flow cytometry.

Fluorometry is the measurement of the emitted fluorescence. Fluorometric analysis is a widely used technique that is more sensitive and specific than absorption spectrophotometry. The increased sensitivity results from the fact that the emitted fluorescent signal comes directly from the sample.

Instrumentation

Fluorescence intensity is measured with the use of a fluorometer or a spectrofluorometer. This instrument contains the same components found in an absorbance photometer or spectrophotometer, but there are some important differences in each component. A fluorometer uses filter monochromators to isolate excitation and emission light, whereas a spectrofluorometer uses a diffraction grating, similar to a spectrophotometer (Fig. 3-9).

Light Source

The excitation source needs to be a high-intensity lamp or laser producing intense light in the UV and short-wavelength visible spectra. Xenon lamps are ideal because they provide intense, full-spectrum light. They are also ideally suited as light sources for pumping atoms in a laser to excited states so that they can be stimulated to emit collimated, monochromatic light. Laser sources are especially useful in flow cytometry applications.

Sample Cells

Rectangular sample cells are preferred over round cells to minimize excitation light scatter interference, and they must be composed of UV light–transmitting material such as quartz or fused silica. The sample cell is placed at the 90-degree angle intersection point between the excitation light path and the emission light path. The front surface geometry is useful in measuring front surface fluorescence

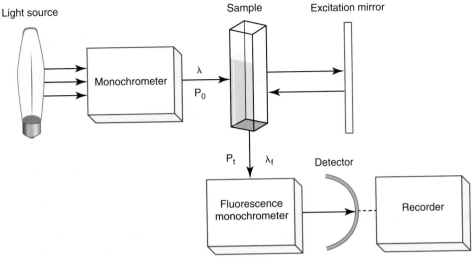

• **Figure 3-9** Diagram of a fluorometer. (Adapted from schematic by Delmar Larsen, University of California-Davis.)

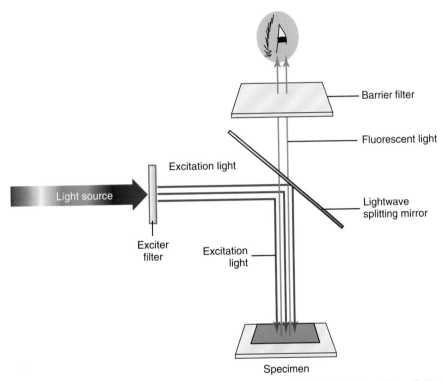

• **Figure 3-10** Geometry of excitation and emission in a photomultiplier. (Adapted from Tille P. *Bailey and Scott's Diagnostic Microbiology*. 13th ed. Philadelphia: Mosby; 2014.)

of a turbid solution or solid support matrix. Front surface geometry is commonly used in heterogeneous, solid-phase fluorescent immunoassay systems.

Detectors

Sensitive photodetectors are required because sample fluorescent emission is typically weak. A PMT is often used to amplify and measure light. The detector is positioned at 90 degrees to the excitation light source to minimize stray light interference from the excitation light source. Excitation and emission geometries are shown in Figure 3-10.

Fluorescence Polarization

Fluorophores absorb light most effectively in the plane of their electronic energy levels. If the rotational relaxation is slower than the fluorescence decay time (e.g., with large fluorescent-labeled molecules), the emitted fluorescence becomes polarized. Small molecules have rotational relaxation times that are much shorter than their fluorescence decay time, and their emitted fluorescence is depolarized. However, when a small fluorescent molecule is attached to a macromolecule such as an antibody, the small molecule emits polarized light. Application of this technique to immunoassays minimizes the background noise typically associated with fluorescent labels. **Fluorescence polarization**, P, is defined by the following equation:

$$P = \frac{(I_v - I_h)}{(I_v + I_h)}$$

where I_v is the intensity of the emitted fluorescence light in the vertical plane and I_h is the intensity of light in the horizontal plane. Fluorescent polarization is measured by placing an electrically driven polarizer between the sample and the detector, as shown in Figure 3-11.

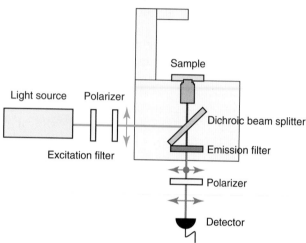

• **Figure 3-11** Schematic diagram of a fluorescence polarization instrument. (From Erdogan T, Prabhat P. *Fluorescence Polarization in Life Sciences.* Courtesy Semrock, Inc., a unit of IDEX Corporation.)

The polarization analyzer is first positioned to measure the emitted fluorescence in the vertical plane and then rotated 90 degrees to measure the emitted fluorescence in the horizontal plane. The fluorescence polarization is calculated from the equation, and a standard curve is created. Fluorescence polarization is used to quantitate analytes according to the change in the polarization of fluorescent light after an immunologic reaction (see Chapter 4).

Quantitation is accomplished by adding a known quantity of fluorescent-labeled analyte molecules to a reaction mixture containing an antibody specific to the analyte. The labeled analyte binds to the antibody, which causes a change in its rotational relaxation time that results in fluorescence polarization. Addition of an unlabeled analyte from a standard sample results in competition with the fluorescent-labeled analyte for binding to the antibody. For example, the presence of an unknown quantity of a therapeutic drug in a urine or serum specimen results in competition with the fluorescent-labeled analyte for binding to the antibody. The change in binding of the fluorophore-labeled analyte causes a change in fluorescence polarization that is inversely proportional to the concentration of the analyte in the sample. Because the change in fluorescence polarization is a direct response to the reaction mixture, the bound fluorophore does not have to be separated from the free fluorophore. Fluorescence polarization is applicable to homogeneous assays of low-molecular-weight molecules such as therapeutic drugs or small peptides (Fig. 3-12).

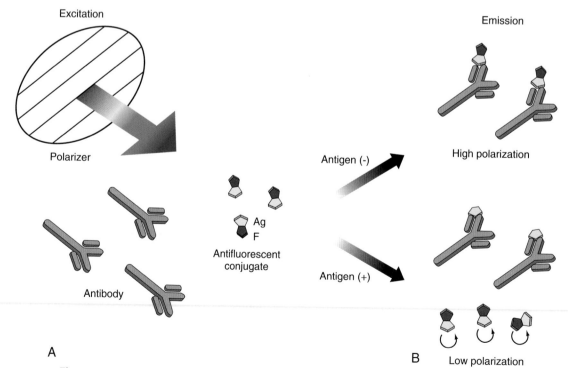

• **Figure 3-12** Diagram of the fluorescence polarization immunoassay (FPIA). (From McPherson RA, Pincus MR. *Henry's Clinical Diagnosis and Management by Laboratory Methods.* 22nd ed. Philadelphia: Elsevier; 2012.)

Luminometry

Chemiluminescence, bioluminescence, and electrochemiluminescence are types of luminescence in which the excitation event is caused by a chemical, biochemical, or electrochemical reaction rather than by photoillumination. Instruments that measure this type of light emission are called **luminometers.**

Chemiluminescence is a reaction that produces light without producing heat. In chemiluminescence, the excitation process is caused by an oxidant such hydrogen peroxide, hypochlorite, or oxygen and involves the oxidation of an organic compound such as luminol, luciferin, or an acridinium ester. The reaction occurs in the presence of a catalyst such as an enzyme (e.g., alkaline phosphatase, horseradish peroxidase, microperoxidase), metal ions, or metal complexes.

Bioluminescence is a special form of chemiluminescence found in biological systems. The glow from a firefly on a warm summer evening is a commonly observed example of bioluminescence. In bioluminescence, an enzyme or photoprotein increases the efficiency of the reaction. Bioluminescence assays have attomole to zeptomole detection limits with a wide dynamic range. Luciferase and aequorin are two examples of biological catalysts. They are used as components of detection in automated immunoassay and DNA probe assay systems (see Chapter 4).

Electrochemiluminescence differs from chemiluminescence in that the oxidative species is generated from a stable precursor at the surface of an electrode. A ruthenium chelate is commonly used as an electrochemiluminescence label. The advantage of this process is improved reagent stability, simple reagent preparation, and enhanced sensitivity. The detector is usually a PMT, and photons are counted in a manner similar to a radioimmunoassay. The basic components of a luminometer are a light-tight chamber housing the sample cell, an injection system to add reagents to the sample cell, and a detector.

Nephelometry and Turbidimetry

Turbidimetry and nephelometry are analytical methods used to measure light scatter by particles in solution (Fig. 3-13). **Turbidimetry** measures the reduction of light transmitted through a colloidal solution. It is in many aspects analogous to absorption spectrophotometry. It is used to assay smaller particles at higher concentrations. The reduction in source light results from light scattering, reflectance, and absorption.

Nephelometry is based on detection of the portion of light scattered or reflected by the particles in a solution toward a detector not in the direct path of the transmitted light. It is the method of choice for assaying larger particles at lower concentrations.

Figure 4-30 illustrates the basic components of an instrument used to measure light scattering, including a light source, collimating optics, a sample cell, and collection optics, which include light-scattering optics, a detector optical filter, and a detector.

Light Sources and Wavelength Selection

High-intensity light sources such as lasers, tungsten–halogen lamps, and xenon lamps are used for nephelometry. Lasers are particularly well suited for this purpose because they provide highly collimated, intense beams of monochromatic light. Laser sources provide dramatic improvements in sensitivity compared with conventional high-intensity lamps. Wavelength selection is typically in the 320- to 380-nm or the 500- to 650-nm range to avoid absorption by protein and by some serum chromogens (e.g., porphyrins). When conventional light sources are employed, wavelength selection can be accomplished with the use of interference filters. Lasers provide monochromatic light and do not require a mechanism for wavelength selection.

Because turbidimetry has the same spatial arrangement as spectrophotometry, turbidimetric assays are usually performed along with color development assays using a standard automated spectrophotometer-based analyzer. Theoretically, nephelometry is more sensitive than turbidimetry, but with currently available instruments and techniques, nephelometric methods are only slightly more sensitive for low-level antigen–antibody complex reactions and almost equally sensitive for specific protein quantitation. Assay sensitivity for both techniques depends primarily on the absence of stray light scatter.

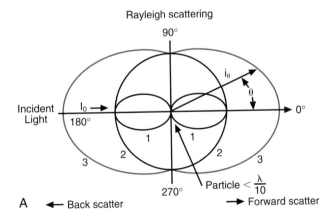

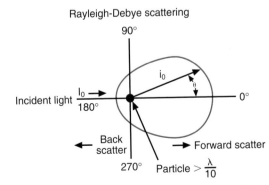

• **Figure 3-13** The angular dependence of light-scattering intensity with nonpolarized and polarized incident light for small particles **(A)** and the angular dependence of light scattering with nonpolarized light for larger particles **(B)**. (From Burtis CA, Bruns DE. *Tietz Fundamentals of Clinical Chemistry and Molecular Diagnostics.* 7th ed. St. Louis: Saunders; 2015.)

Electrochemistry and Chemical Sensors

Many analytical methods used in the clinical laboratory are based on electrochemical interactions. The fundamental electrochemical principles of potentiometry, amperometry, conductometry, and coulometry are discussed along with clinical applications in the following sections.

Potentiometry

Potentiometric sensors are widely used in clinical applications for the measurement of an electrical potential difference between two electrodes or half-cells in an electrochemical cell. Applications include pH; partial pressure of carbon dioxide (pCO_2); electrolytes (e.g., Na^+, K^+, Cl^-, Ca^{2+}, Mg^{2+}, Li^+) in whole blood, serum, plasma, and urine; and as transducers for developing biosensors (Fig. 3-14).

Basic Concepts

Potentiometry is the measurement of an electrical potential between two electrodes, called half-cells, in an electrochemical cell. The two electrodes in the half-cell are connected by an electrolyte solution such as sodium chloride (NaCl), which ionizes when dissolved in water. Electrolyte solutions typically can conduct an electric current because the charged ions are mobile in solution. An electrode consists of a single metallic conductor that is in contact with the electrolyte solution.

The two half-cells either are in direct contact with each other or are separated by membranes permeable to specific anions or cations. One of the half-cells (i.e., the indicator electrode) consists of the sample or a reference solution for calibration purposes, and the other half-cell is the reference electrode and reference solution. In this system, only the potential difference between the two electrodes is measured, because the absolute potential of each individual half-cell is unknown and cannot be routinely measured. The measured potential is related to the activity of a specific ion in sample (e.g., H^+, Na^+).

Types of Electrodes

Redox Electrodes

Redox electrodes consist of inert metal electrodes immersed in solutions containing redox couples or electrodes whose metal functions as a member of a redox couple. Gold and platinum are examples of inert metals that are used to record the redox potential of a redox couple dissolved in an electrolyte solution.

The silver–silver chloride electrode is an example of a metal electrode that participates as a member of a redox couple. The electrode consists of a silver (Ag) wire or rod, coated with silver chloride (AgCl), that is immersed in a chloride solution of constant activity that sets the half-cell activity. The Ag-AgCl electrode by itself is considered a potentiometric electrode because its boundary potential is fixed by an oxidation-reduction electron transfer equilibrium reaction that occurs at the surface of the silver:

$$AgCl + e^- \rightarrow Ag^0 \,(a\ solid) + Cl^-$$

This electrode can be used as an internal reference element in **ion-selective electrodes** (ISEs) or as an external reference electrode of constant potential to complete a potentiometric cell (Fig. 3-15). In either case, the electrode must be in equilibrium with a solution of constant chloride ion activity. In the application as an external reference electrode half-cell, it is commonly in contact with saturated potassium chloride (KCl) that is separated from the sample by a porous membrane or glass frit. The calomel electrode consists of mercury covered by a layer of calomel (Hg_2Cl_2), which is in contact with an electrolyte solution containing chloride ions. The calomel electrode is widely used as a reference electrode, especially for pH measurements.

Ion-Selective Electrodes

Membrane potentials are caused by the permeability of certain types of membranes to selected anions or cations. Membranes are constructed to selectively interact with a single ionic species. The potential produced at the membrane-sample interface is a function of the logarithm of the ionic activity or concentration. The glass membrane electrode was the first ISE and is still the most commonly used ISE for measuring hydrogen ion activity (Fig. 3-16). It is also used as an internal transducer for pCO_2 sensors. By varying the composition of the glass, ion-selective measurement of sodium ions is possible.

Polymer membrane ISEs have been constructed to measure K^+, Ca^{2+}, Na^+, Mg^{2+}, and Li^+ ions. They are the most prominent class of potentiometric ISEs used in modern clinical analyzers. Polyvinyl chloride (PVC) membranes incorporate various sequestering agents to measure specific ions. For example, valinomycin incorporated into a PVC membrane results

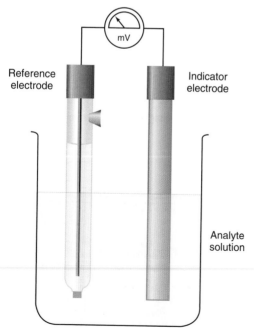

• **Figure 3-14** Diagram of a potentiometric electrode. (From Chemistry Glossary. *Indicator Electrode.* <http://glossary.periodni.com/glossary.php?en=indicator+electrode> Accessed 15.07.15.)

in a sensor with a high selectivity for potassium. The Ca^{2+}-selective ion exchange or complexation properties of 2-ethyl-hexyl phosphoric acid dissolved in dioctyl phenyl phosphate have been cast into a PVC membrane to produce a rugged and convenient electrode. Dissociated anion exchanger–based electrodes employing lipophilic quaternary ammonium salts as active membrane components are used for the determination of Cl^- ions in whole blood, serum, or plasma.

A pH electrode is used as an internal element in a potentiometric cell for measurement of pCO_2 in blood. A thin membrane that is permeable only to gases and water is in contact with the sample. The membrane can be made of silicone rubber, Teflon, or another polymeric material. On the other side of the membrane is a thin layer of a dilute bicarbonate salt and a chloride salt. A pH electrode is in contact with this solution. Carbon dioxide from the sample or calibration matrix diffuses through the membrane and dissolves in the internal electrolyte layer, shifting its pH. The amount of shift in pH is indirectly related to the Pco_2 concentration.

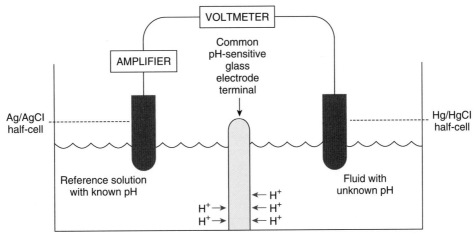

• **Figure 3-15** Schematic diagram of an ion-selective membrane electrode-based potentiometric cell. (From Malley WJ. *Clinical Blood Gases: Assessment and Intervention.* 2nd ed. St. Louis: Saunders; 2005.)

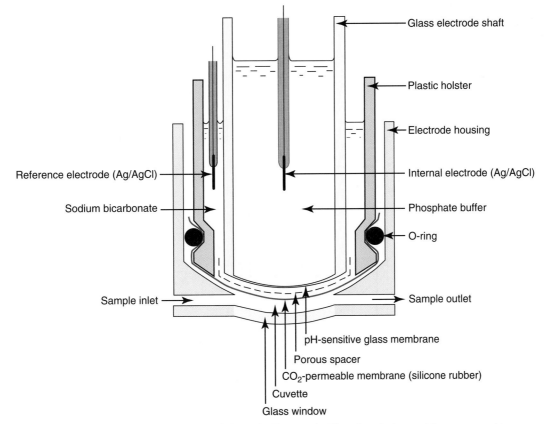

• **Figure 3-16** Ion-selective electrode. Schematic diagram of a Stow-Severinghaus–style sensor used to monitor carbon dioxide concentrations in blood samples. (Adapted from Burtis CA, Bruns DE. *Tietz Fundamentals of Clinical Chemistry and Molecular Diagnostics.* 7th ed. St. Louis: Saunders; 2015.)

Direct Potentiometry: Comparison With Diluted or Indirect Sampling

Classic analytical methods for measurement of electrolytes provide the total concentration of a given ion in the sample. Many instruments use direct potentiometry (undiluted) by ISEs for measurement of electrolytes. A primary advantage is that the technique is sensitive to molality and is therefore not affected by variations in the concentrations of proteins or lipids in the sample.

Methods requiring sample dilution (e.g., high-volume chemistry analyzers) underestimate the concentration of electrolytes because of the volume contribution of proteins and lipids. In these methods, only the water phase of the sample is diluted. There is a risk of reporting a falsely low sodium concentration (i.e., pseudohyponatremia) in cases of significantly elevated protein and lipid concentrations. This is known as the volume exclusion effect.

Direct potentiometry enables the measurement of activity (a), which is the concentration of free, unbound ions in solution. In contrast to methods sensitive to ion concentration, ISEs do not sense the presence of bound or electrostatically hindered ions in the sample. This allows measurement of ionized calcium and ionized magnesium. In the body, activity of ions is more relevant than concentration of ions.

Voltammetry is used to measure current flowing into or out of an electrode in a solution. It is the study of current as a function of applied potential. Amperometry is based on the measurement of the current flowing through an electrochemical cell and the electrochemical potential between the two electrodes while a constant external voltage is applied.

Measurement of the partial pressure of oxygen (pO_2) is based on an amperometric principle. When electricity passes from a metal such as platinum to an electrolyte solution or from the electrolyte to the metal, oxidation or reduction takes place. In the case of oxygen in solution, oxygen is reduced with the release of electrons, and the current increases. The increase in current is directly proportional to the oxygen in the solution:

$$O_2 + 2\,H_2O + 4^- \rightarrow 4\,OH^-$$

The pO_2 electrode, often referred to as a Clark electrode, consists of a platinum cathode surrounded by a tubular silver anode. The two electrodes are separated from each other and make contact through a drop of electrolyte at the electrode tip. A gas-permeable membrane holds the drop at the tip of the electrode and separates it from the blood sample to be measured. Oxygen in the blood diffuses across the membrane into the electrolyte, where it is reduced and quantitated by the change in current.

Enzyme biosensors are primarily based on the Clark electrode (Fig. 3-17). The first amperometric sensor, developed by Clark and Lyons, was used for measuring glucose and was based on immobilizing glucose oxidase (GO) on the surface of an immobilized pO_2 electrode. A solution of glucose oxidase is trapped between the gas-permeable membrane of the electrode and an outer semipermeable membrane. The outer membrane has a low-molecular-weight cutoff, allowing glucose (i.e., substrate) and oxygen from the sample to pass while restricting proteins and other macromolecules. Oxidation of glucose proceeds according to the following equation:

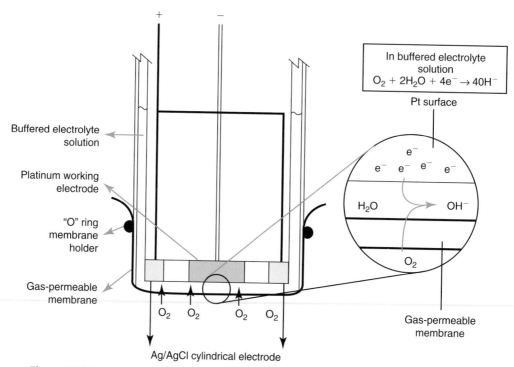

• **Figure 3-17** Design of Clark-style amperometric oxygen sensor used to monitor oxygen concentrations in blood. (Adapted from Burtis CA, Bruns DE. *Tietz Fundamentals of Clinical Chemistry and Molecular Diagnostics.* 7th ed. St. Louis: Saunders; 2015.)

$$Glucose + O_2 \xrightarrow{GO} Gluconic\ acid + H_2O_2$$

This reaction consumes oxygen near the surface of the sensor. The rate of decrease in pO_2 is a function of the glucose concentration of the substrate. The measured current decreases as a function of increased glucose concentration. Alternatively, reversing the polarizing voltage of the electrode and replacing the gas-permeable membrane with a hydrophilic membrane containing the immobilized enzyme allows oxidization of the H_2O_2 produced by the GO:

$$H_2O_2 \rightarrow 2\,e^- + 2\,H^+$$

The steady-state current is directly proportional to the glucose concentration in the sample. Substitution of other oxoreductase enzymes for GO allows other amperometric biosensors to be constructed. Examples include lactate, cholesterol, pyruvate, and even creatinine.

A method for detecting trace levels of toxic metals in clinical samples is **anodic stripping voltammetry** (ASV). ASV uses a carbon electrode that is sometimes coated with a film of mercury metal. The applied electric current is first fixed at a very negative potential so that all of the metal ions in solution are reduced to elemental metals within the mercury film or on the surface of the carbon electrode. The electrode is then made more positive, and the reduced metals are rapidly reoxidized, yielding a large anodic current proportional to the concentration of the metal ions in the original sample (Fig. 3-18).

In the clinical laboratory, the ASV technique is limited to the analysis of lead in whole blood. A small benchtop analyzer (Lead Care II, Magellan Diagnostics, North Billerica, MA) can perform an analysis of lead in whole blood on a fingerstick specimen. The instrument is used in clinics, local health departments, and industrial sites where exposure to lead must be monitored. The small sample size makes it a useful instrument in pediatric settings.

Conductometry

Conductometry is measurement of electrolytic conductivity to monitor the progress of a chemical reaction (Fig. 3-19). The technique makes use of the ability of electrolytes in a solution to carry an electrical current by migration of ions. The current is proportional to the concentrations of the ions. An increase in conductivity represents a decrease in resistance because they are reciprocal functions. Red blood cells act as electrical insulators because of their lipid-based membranes. This property was first used in the 1940s to measure the volume fraction of erythrocytes in whole blood (i.e., hematocrit), and it is used now to measure hematocrit on multianalyte instruments such as blood gas analyzers.

These measurements have limitations. For instance, abnormal protein levels are a source of error. Determination of hemoglobin is a much better marker for monitoring of blood loss and the need for transfusion because of trauma or surgery. Despite the limitations, the electrical measurement of hematocrit in conjunction with blood gases and electrolytes by conductometry continues because of its simplicity and convenience.

Another clinical application of conductometry is for electronic counting of blood cells in suspension. Based on the Coulter principle, this method relies on the fact that the conductivity of blood cells is lower than that of the salt solution used as a suspension medium. The cell suspension is forced to flow through a tiny orifice. A constant current is established between two electrodes placed on either side of the orifice.

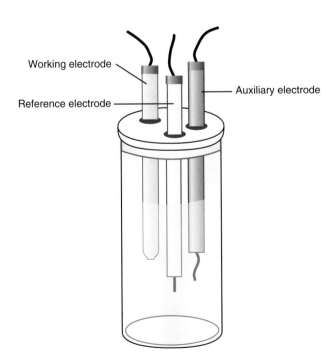

• **Figure 3-18** Voltammetry electrode.

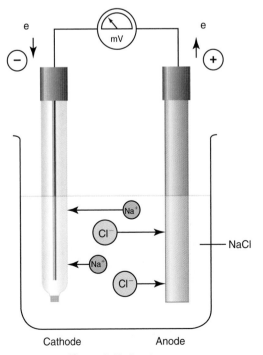

• **Figure 3-19** Conductometry.

Each time a cell passes through the orifice, the resistance increases, causing a spike in the potential difference between the electrodes. These pulses can be amplified and counted to determine the number of cells in a prescribed volume.

Coulometry

Coulometry, which is based on amperometry, measures the amount of charge (in coulombs) passing between two electrodes at a fixed potential (Fig. 3-20). The number of coulombs is a direct measurement of the quantitative oxidation or reduction of an electroactive species at one of the electrodes. Several chloride analyzers work on the principle of coulometry. When a carefully controlled current is passed between two electrodes, silver ions are produced by oxidation at one of the electrodes. Chloride ions in the solution combine with the released silver ions to produce insoluble silver chloride:

$$\text{Anode electrode reaction}: Ag^0 \rightarrow Ag^+ + e^-$$

$$\text{Solution reaction}: Ag^+ + Cl^- \rightarrow AgCl \text{ (a solid)}$$

The Buchler-Cotlove titrator is based on this principle. A silver-detecting electrode and a reference half-cell are included in the system to sense the excess of free silver ions. When silver is detected, the current to the silver-releasing electrode is stopped. If the amperage of the oxidizing current and the time during which it was flowing are known, the coulombs that passed can be calculated. Faraday's law states that a set amount of electricity produces more moles of analyte with lower oxidation numbers and fewer moles of analyte with higher oxidation numbers. The silver ions released by the oxidation of the silver metal therefore exactly equal the number of chloride ions that were in the solution.

In the clinical laboratory, a constant-current coulometric assay is used for the determination of chloride in fluids in a fixed volume of sample. The concentration of chloride in the unknown (in mmol/L) is calculated from the concentration (in mmol/L) of the standard (STD) and the titration times for the blank (T_{blk}), the standard (T_{std}), and the unknown (T_{unk}):

$$[Cl] = \frac{(T_{unk} - T_{blk})}{(T_{std} - T_{blk})} \times [STD]$$

This method was employed in the Beckman Astra 8 and Astra 4 systems, but it has been replaced by ISEs for the determination of chloride because the response of the method was unable to keep pace with the higher throughput of modern automated chemistry analyzers. However, small benchtop analyzers employing coulometry are currently used for sweat chloride analysis. Sweat chloride analysis continues to be the gold standard for the diagnosis of cystic fibrosis.

Chromatography

Chromatography is used in the clinical laboratory to separate and quantify a variety of clinically important analytes. The basic concepts, separation mechanisms, types of chromatography, and resolution are discussed in the following sections.

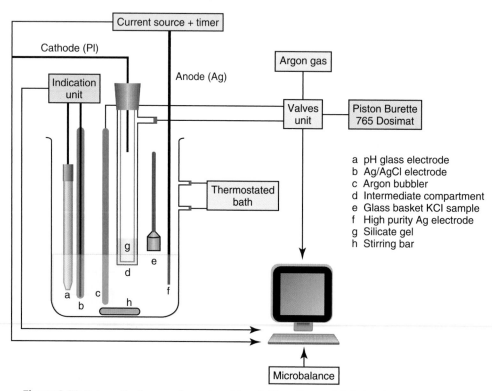

• **Figure 3-20** Schematic diagram of a coulometric cell. (From Borges PP, Sobral SP, da Silva L, Araújo TO, Silva RS. Constant-current coulometry and ion chromatography bromide determination to characterize the purity of the potassium chloride. *J Braz Chem Soc.* 2011;22(10), 1931–1938.)

Basic Concepts

Chromatography is the collective term for a set of laboratory techniques used for the physical separation of mixtures. The sample containing solute is dissolved in a fluid called the mobile phase, which carries it through a bed, layer, or column containing another material called the stationary phase. As the mobile phase flows past the stationary phase, the solutes with higher affinity for the stationary phase reside in the stationary phase and migrate more slowly than those with less affinity. Those with less affinity reside primarily in the mobile phase and migrate faster.

Chromatography was first employed by Russian scientist Mikhail Tsvet in 1900. He continued to work with chromatography in the first decade of the 20th century, primarily for the separation of plant pigments such as chlorophyll, carotenes, and xanthophylls. These components had different colors (green, orange, and yellow, respectively), and the technique was named *chromatography,* meaning "color writing."

Types of Chromatography
Separation Mechanisms

Ion Exchange Chromatography

Ion exchange chromatography, also called ion chromatography, uses an ion exchange mechanism to separate analytes based on their charge (Fig. 3-21). It is usually performed in columns but can also be useful in planar mode. Ion exchange chromatography uses a charged stationary phase to separate charged and amphoteric species such as anions, cations, amino acids, peptides, and proteins. In conventional methods, the stationary phase is an ion exchange resin that contains charged functional groups that interact with the oppositely charged groups of the analyte in the compound, resulting in retention.

Partition Chromatography

Partition chromatography is based on the differential distribution of solutes between two immiscible liquids, as in liquid chromatography or gas chromatography (Fig. 3-22).

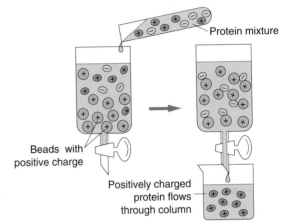

• **Figure 3-21** Ion exchange chromatography. This figure depicts an anion exchange column. Negatively charged protein binds to positively charged beads, and positively charged protein flows through the column. (From Baynes JW, Dominiczak MH. *Medical Biochemistry.* 4th ed. Edinburgh: Saunders/Elsevier Limited; 2015.)

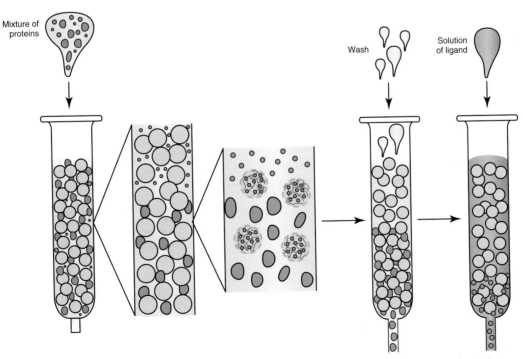

• **Figure 3-22** Partition chromatography. The smaller proteins will be attracted to the matrix and actually enter pores in the matrix. The larger proteins are too large to enter the pores and stay within the matrix. A wash step is performed to wash away the unwanted large proteins. A ligand solution at a particular pH elutes the smaller molecules in the pores of the matrix.

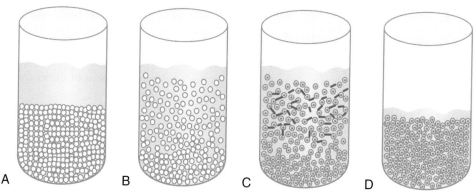

• **Figure 3-23** Adsorption chromatography. In adsorption chromatography, the reaction of the matrix and the analyte occur on the surface of the molecule. Different solutes are used to separate the unwanted analytes from the analyte of interest.

In liquid chromatography, one of the immiscible liquids serves as the stationary phase by adsorbing or chemically bonding a thin film of the liquid onto the surface. In gas chromatography, a nonvolatile liquid is coated or chemically bonded onto particles of column packing or directly onto a capillary wall. In normal-phase liquid chromatography, a polar medium is used as the stationary phase, and a relatively nonpolar solvent or solvent mixture is used as the mobile phase. In reverse-phase partition liquid chromatography, the stationary phase is nonpolar, and the mobile phase is polar. Ion suppression and ion pair chromatography are two forms of reverse-phase chromatography that employ an acid-base modifier to allow separation of ionic solutes. Although there is a wide selection of mobile phases and stationary phases, the basis of most separations is partitioning.

Adsorption Chromatography

In **adsorption chromatography,** analytes are separated by the adsorption and desorption of solutes at the surface of a solid particle (Fig. 3-23). Adsorption chromatography uses electrostatic hydrogen bonding, and dispersive interactions are the physical forces that facilitate this technique. In gas chromatography, this technique is used to separate and quantitate volatile compounds such as methanol, ethanol, and isopropanol or any compounds that can be converted to gases. Support particles such alumina or styrene divinylbenzene act as molecular sieves. In liquid chromatography, nonpolar, acidic polar, and basic polar adsorbents are used.

Affinity Chromatography

Affinity chromatography is a liquid chromatographic technique that makes use of a biological interaction for the separation and analysis of analytes in a sample (Fig. 3-24). Examples of these interactions include binding of an enzyme with a substrate, of a hormone with its receptor, or of an antibody with an antigen.

In affinity chromatography, a binding agent *(affinity ligand)* that selectivity interacts with the desired analyte is obtained and placed into a solid support in a column. After the immobilized ligand has been prepared, it can be used

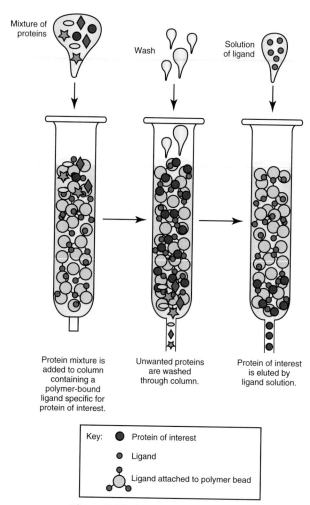

• **Figure 3-24** Affinity chromatography.

for isolation or quantification of the analyte. Adjustments of pH and ionic strength are required to achieve optimal binding of the analyte to the ligand.

Affinity methods that use boronic acid or boronates as ligands are one group of chromatographic techniques that have been used successfully with clinical samples. These methods, known collectively as *boronate affinity chromatography,* include one of the earliest reported quantitative

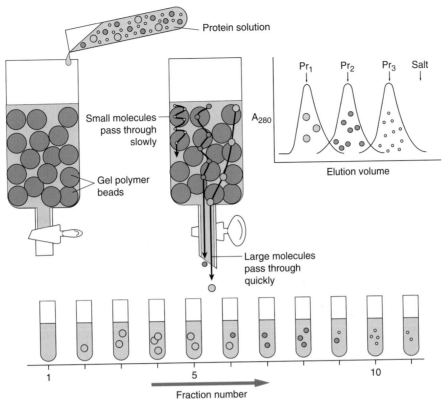

• **Figure 3-25** Size exclusion chromatography. (From Baynes JW, Dominiczak MH. *Medical Biochemistry.* 4th ed. Edinburgh: Saunders/Elsevier Limited; 2015.)

applications of affinity chromatography in the clinical laboratory, the determination of glycohemoglobin (i.e., glycated hemoglobin) for assessment of long-term diabetes management. At pH values greater than 8, most boronate derivatives form covalent bonds with compounds that contain *cis*-diol groups in their structure. Because sugars such as glucose possess *cis*-diol groups, boronates are valuable for distinguishing glycoproteins (e.g., glycohemoglobin) from nonglycoproteins (e.g., normal hemoglobin).

Size-Exclusion Chromatography

Size-exclusion chromatography, also known as gel permeation chromatography or gel filtration chromatography, separates molecules according to their size (i.e., hydrodynamic diameter or hydrodynamic volume) (Fig. 3-25). Smaller molecules can enter the pores of the medium, and the molecules are trapped and removed from the flow of the mobile phase. The average residence time in the pores depends on the effective size of the analyte molecules. However, molecules that are larger than the average pore size of the packing are excluded and have essentially no retention; these species are the first to be eluted.

Size-exclusion chromatography is a low-resolution chromatography technique. It is often reserved for the final polishing step of purification. It is also useful for determining the tertiary structure and quaternary structure of purified proteins, especially because it can be carried out under native solution conditions.

Forms of Chromatography

There are two other chromatography techniques: planar chromatography, which includes paper and thin-layer chromatography, and column chromatography, which includes gas and liquid forms of chromatography. Methods can be classified by their form and separation mechanism. For example, the separation mechanism of a gas chromatography method can be partition or adsorption.

Planar Chromatography

Planar chromatography is a separation technique in which the stationary phase exists on a plane (Fig. 3-26). The plane can be a paper impregnated by a substance that serves as the stationary bed (i.e., paper chromatography), or a layer of solid particles can be spread on a support such as a glass plate (i.e., thin-layer chromatography). Different compounds in the sample mixture travel different distances according to how strongly they partition between the stationary phase and mobile phase. The specific retention factor (R_f) aids in the identification of an unknown analyte.

The use of paper chromatography in the clinical laboratory has largely been discontinued. Thin-layer chromatography has been used in tandem with immunoassay for screening purposes. Positive immunoassay screens can be followed up with a thin-layer chromatography assay such as the Toxi-Lab System before confirmation with gas chromatography or liquid chromatography and mass spectrometry. Most laboratories find it more efficient to go directly to

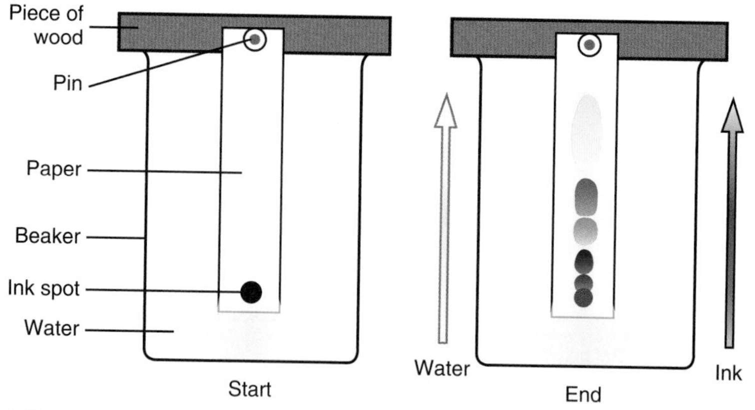

• **Figure 3-26** Planar chromatography. (From MicroMountain. Simple time lapse chromatography animation. <www.micromountain.com> Accessed 15.07.15.)

confirmatory methods, and some may bypass immunoassay screens, depending on the circumstances.

Column Chromatography

In column chromatography, the stationary phase is coated onto or chemically bonded to support particles that are then packed into a tube or capillary. Alternatively, the stationary phase may be coated onto the inner surface of the tube.

Gas Chromatography

In gas chromatography, a gaseous mobile phase is used to carry a mixture of volatile solutes through a column containing the stationary phase, and it cannot be reused. The mobile phase is typically an inert gas such as helium, hydrogen, or nitrogen, referred to as the *carrier gas.* Solutes separate based on their relative differences in vapor pressure and their interactions with the stationary phase. A more volatile substance elutes from the column before a less volatile one, and a solute that selectively interacts with the stationary phase elutes from the column after one that has less interaction with the stationary phase. The carrier gas moves separated solutes to a detector in the order of their elution. Solutes are identified by their retention time and quantitated by comparing peak area or height to a known standard.

Packed or capillary columns are used. Packed columns are filled with support materials that are used uncoated in gas-solid chromatography (GSC). In gas-liquid chromatography (GLC), a nonvolatile liquid is coated or chemically bonded with the support particles or directly onto the wall of a capillary column.

In gas chromatography, an extraction of the sample is often necessary. The sample may have to be acidified, such as to convert the compound of interest to a form that is soluble in an organic solvent. This allows the desired analyte to be separated from interferences such as proteins. Solvent extraction can be used to preconcentrate the analyte before chromatographic analysis. Many clinically relevant compounds are nonvolatile and are difficult to separate by gas chromatography. Chemical modification or derivatization increases the volatility for gas chromatographic analysis.

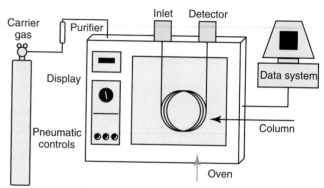

• **Figure 3-27** Schematic diagram of a gas chromatograph. (Adapted from Burtis CA, Bruns DE. *Tietz Fundamentals of Clinical Chemistry and Molecular Diagnostics.* 7th ed. St. Louis: Saunders; 2015.)

Components of gas chromatography include a carrier gas supply and flow control, injector, temperature control, detector, and computer or controller (Fig. 3-27). The injector provides the means to introduce a sample into a continuous flow of carrier gas. The injector is a piece of hardware attached to the column head. One commonly used injector type is the split/splitless injector. A sample is introduced into a heated small chamber with a syringe through a *septum.* The heat facilitates volatilization of the sample and sample matrix. The carrier gas then sweeps all (i.e., splitless mode) or a portion (i.e., split mode) of the sample into the column. In split mode, a part of the sample and carrier gas mixture in the injection chamber is exhausted through the split vent. Split injection is preferred when working with samples with high analyte concentrations (>0.1%), whereas splitless injection is best suited for trace analysis of low amounts of analytes (<0.01%).

In splitless mode, the split valve opens after a preset time to purge heavier elements that would otherwise contaminate the system. This preset (splitless) time should be optimized. The shorter time (e.g., 0.2 minutes) ensures less tailing but causes a loss in response; a longer time (e.g., 2 minutes) increases tailing but also the signal.

Temperature-programmable injection ports are used in the split or splitless mode. This allows injection of larger volumes of sample compared with a standard injector, increasing the

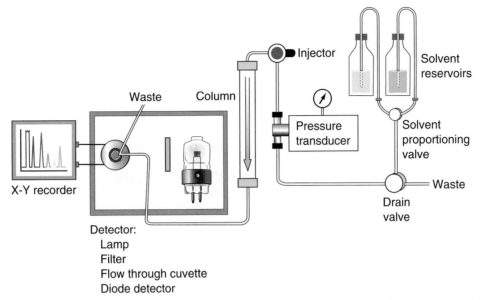

• **Figure 3-28** Liquid chromatography instrument. (From McPherson RA, Pincus MR. *Henry's Clinical Diagnosis and Management by Laboratory Methods.* 22nd ed. Philadelphia: Elsevier; 2012.)

sensitivity. Typically, the sample is injected at a temperature slightly higher than the boiling point of the solvent.

Gas chromatography columns are contained in an oven, the temperature of which must be precisely controlled. The rate at which a sample passes through the column is directly proportional to the temperature of the column. The higher the column temperature, the faster the sample moves through the column. However, the faster a sample moves through the column, the less it interacts with the stationary phase, and the less the analytes are separated. The column temperature selected is usually a compromise between the length of the analysis and the level of separation.

A method that holds the column at the same temperature for the entire analysis is called *isothermal.* Most methods, however, increase the column temperature during the analysis. The initial temperature, rate of temperature increase (i.e., temperature ramp), and final temperature are called the *temperature program.* A temperature program allows analytes that elute early in the analysis to separate adequately while shortening the time it takes for late-eluting analytes to pass through the column.

Resolution. Resolution is a measure of how well analytes are separated by chromatography. The resolution, *R,* between two peaks in a chromatogram is given by the following equation:

$$R = \frac{(t_{r2} - t_{r1})}{1/2\,(w_1 + w_2)}$$

In the equation, t_{r1} and t_{r2} and w_1 and w_2 are the retention times and widths, respectively, of the two immediately adjacent peaks. In chromatography, the retention time is the time at which the center, or maximum, of a symmetric peak occurs in a chromatogram.

Detectors. Before advances in mass spectrometry, a flame ionization detector was the most commonly used detector for gas chromatography. It is reliable, versatile, and easy to

use. It is still widely used for the identification and detection of volatile analytes such as alcohols. The mass spectrometer is a detector that provides structural information and positive identification of a wide variety of substances.

Liquid Chromatography

Liquid chromatography is a separation technique in which the mobile phase is a liquid (Fig. 3-28). Modern liquid chromatography that uses very small stationary-phase particles and a relatively high performance is called high-performance liquid chromatography. Most HPLC applications are partition separations, but ion exchange columns, affinity columns, and size-exclusion columns are often used.

Components for liquid chromatography are somewhat different from gas chromatography components. Both techniques include a column, an injector, a detector, and a computer. Liquid chromatography also includes a solvent reservoir and a pump for solvent delivery.

Columns. The internal diameter (ID) of an HPLC column is an important parameter that influences the detection sensitivity and separation selectivity in gradient elution (Fig. 3-29). It also determines the quantity of analyte that can be loaded onto the column. Analytical scale columns (4.6 mm) have been the most common type of columns, although smaller columns are rapidly gaining in popularity. They are used in traditional quantitative analysis of samples and often use a UV-visible absorbance detector.

Narrow-bore columns (1 to 2 mm) are used for applications when more sensitivity is desired with special UV-visible detectors, fluorescence detection, or other detection methods such as liquid chromatography with mass spectrometry. Capillary columns (<0.3 mm) are used almost exclusively with alternative detection means such as mass spectrometry. They are usually made from fused silica capillaries rather than the stainless steel tubing that larger columns employ.

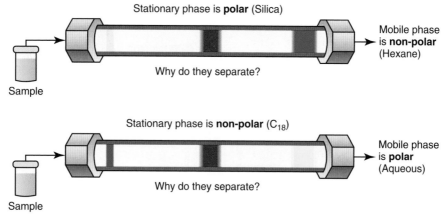

Stationary phase is **polar** (Silica)

Why do they separate?

Sample

Mobile phase is **non-polar** (Hexane)

Stationary phase is **non-polar** (C$_{18}$)

Why do they separate?

Sample

Mobile phase is **polar** (Aqueous)

• **Figure 3-29** High-performance liquid chromatography (HPLC) columns. (Courtesy Waters Corporation, Milford, MA.)

Most traditional HPLC is performed with the stationary phase attached to the outside of small spherical silica particles (i.e., very small beads). These particles come in a variety of sizes, but 5-μm beads are the most common. Smaller particles provide more surface area and better separations, but the pressure required for optimal linear velocity increases as the inverse of the particle diameter squared. This means that changing to particles that are one half as big while keeping the size of the column the same doubles the performance but increases the required pressure by a factor of four.

Pumps vary in pressure capacity, but their performance is measured by their ability to yield a consistent and reproducible flow rate. Pressure may reach as high as 40 MPa (6000 lbf/in^2), or about 400 atm. Modern HPLC systems can work at much higher pressures than earlier models and can use much smaller particle sizes (<2 μm) in the columns. These ultrahigh-resolution systems (i.e., RSLCs or UHPLCs) can work at up to 100 MPa (15,000 lbf/in^2) or about 1000 atm.

In an isocratic procedure, the mobile-phase composition remains constant throughout the separation; *isocratic* means "constant composition." In isocratic elution, the peak width increases with retention time linearly according to the equation for N, the number of theoretical plates. This leads to flattening and broadening of the peaks. Gradient elution decreases the retention of the later-eluting components so that they elute faster, giving narrower (and taller) peaks for most components. This also improves the peak shape for tailed peaks because the increasing concentration of the organic eluent (in reverse-phase mode) pushes the tailing part of a peak forward. This approach also increases the peak height (i.e., peak looks sharper). The gradient program may include sudden step increases in the percentage of the organic component or different slopes at different times according to the desire for optimal separation in a minimum time.

Detectors may be UV-visible spectrophotometers, fluorometers, and electrochemical. Sample concentration, purification, or derivatization may be required. In preparing the mobile phase, dissolved gasses must be removed from the solvents, and they must be free of particulate.

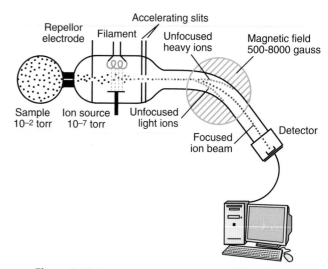

• **Figure 3-30** Mass spectrometer. (Courtesy William Reusch.)

Mass Spectrometry

Mass spectrometry (MS) is a powerful qualitative and quantitative analytical technique that is used to measure a wide variety of clinically relevant analytes (Fig. 3-30). It has become the detector of choice for gas chromatography and liquid chromatography. Applications include monitoring therapeutic drugs, drugs of abuse, trace metals, and vitamins. Liquid chromatography with tandem MS has become the method of choice for drugs used for suppression of the immune system after organ transplantation (i.e., immunosuppressants) and for vitamin D$_3$ analysis. It is a key tool in the emerging field of proteomics because of its ability to identify and quantify proteins.

The development of soft ionization techniques such as matrix-assisted laser desorption ionization (MALDI) have facilitated the use of time-of-flight mass spectrometers (TOF-MS) in microbiology. A mass spectrometer is an analytical instrument that is coupled with an ionization source that ionizes a target molecule and then separates and measures the mass of the molecule or its fragments. Mass analysis provides the concentration for a given ion or ions. All MS methods require an ionization step in which an ion is produced from a neutral atom or molecule. The mass spectrum is represented by the relative abundance of each ion plotted as a function of its mass-to-charge (m/z) ratio.

Ionization Techniques

Electron Impact Ionization

Electron impact ionization (EI) is an ionization method in which energetic electrons emitted from a heated filament are attracted to a collector electrode. The electrons interact with gas-phase atoms or molecules to produce ions (Fig. 3-31). This process must occur in a vacuum to prevent filament oxidation. The technique is widely used in mass spectrometry, particularly for gases and volatile organic molecules.

Matrix-Assisted Laser Desorption/Ionization

MALDI is a soft ionization technique, which produces mass spectra with little or no fragment ion content. MALDI is used in mass spectrometry to analyze biomolecules (e.g., DNA, proteins, peptides, and sugars) and large organic molecules (e.g., polymers, dendrimers, and other macromolecules), which tend to be fragile when ionized by more conventional ionization methods. It is similar to electrospray ionization (ESI) in relative softness and the ions produced; ESI produces multiple charged ions for larger molecules such as proteins and peptides.

MALDI is a two-step process (Fig. 3-32). First, desorption is triggered by a UV laser beam. Matrix material heavily absorbs UV laser light, which ablates the upper layer (≈1 μm) of the matrix material. Gas phase produced during ablation contains many species: neutral and ionized matrix molecules, protonated and deprotonated matrix molecules, matrix clusters, and nanodroplets. The second step is ionization by gaining or losing a proton from or to the UV-absorbable matrix molecules. Protonation or deprotonation of analyte molecules takes place in the gas phase. The matrix is a low-molecular-weight, UV-absorbing material, and this solution is placed on a target that can be introduced into the mass spectrometer. Identification of suitable matrix compounds is determined to some extent by trial and error, but they are based on some nonspecific molecular design considerations.

MALDI-TOF spectra are used for the identification of microorganisms such as bacteria or fungi. A colony of the microbe in question is smeared directly on the sample target and overlaid with matrix. The mass spectra generated are analyzed by dedicated software and compared with stored profiles. Species diagnosis by this procedure is much faster, more accurate, and cheaper than other procedures based on immunologic or biochemical tests. MALDI-TOF may become the standard method for species identification in medical microbiological laboratories over the next few years.

Inductively Coupled Plasma Mass Spectrometry

Inductively coupled plasma mass spectrometry (ICP-MS) is a type of mass spectrometry that can detect metals and several nonmetals at concentrations as low as one part per

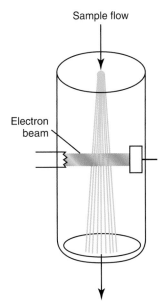

• **Figure 3-31** Electron impact ionization.

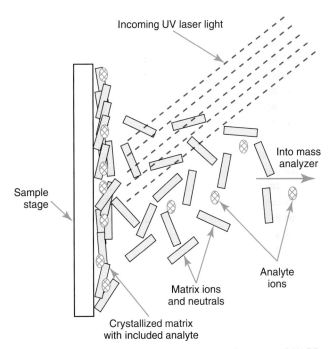

• **Figure 3-32** Matrix-assisted laser desorption/ionization (MALDI). Co-crystallized matrix and analyte molecules are irradiated with an ultraviolet (UV) laser. The laser vaporizes the matrix, producing a plume of matrix ions, analyte ions, and neutral molecules. Gas phase ions are directed into a mass analyzer. (Adapted from Burtis CA, Bruns DE. *Tietz Fundamentals of Clinical Chemistry and Molecular Diagnostics.* 7th ed. St. Louis: Saunders; 2015.)

trillion (10^{12}) (Fig. 3-33). This is achieved by ionizing the sample with inductively coupled plasma and then using a mass spectrometer to separate and quantify the ions.

Compared with atomic absorption techniques, ICP-MS has greater speed, precision, and sensitivity. However, analysis by ICP-MS is also more susceptible to trace contaminants from glassware and reagents. Some ions can interfere with the detection of other ions.

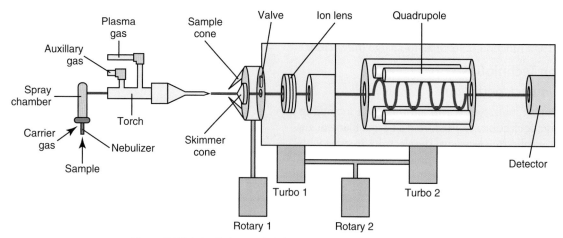

• **Figure 3-33** Inductively coupled plasma mass spectrometry (ICP-MS).

The ICP-MS allows determination of elements with atomic mass ranges between 7 and 250 (i.e., elements Li to U). Some masses are prohibited, such as 40 due to the abundance of argon in the sample. Other blocked regions may include a mass 80 (due to the argon dimer) and mass 56 (due to argon oxide), which greatly hinders iron (Fe) analysis unless the instrumentation is fitted with a reaction chamber. Detection limits of a typical ICP-MS are in the region of nanograms per liter to 10 or 100 mg/mL, or about eight orders of magnitude in concentration units.

Unlike atomic absorption spectroscopy, which can measure only a single element at a time, ICP-MS can scan for all elements simultaneously, allowing rapid sample processing. A growing trend in elemental analysis involves the speciation of certain metals such as chromium and arsenic. One of the primary techniques uses an ICP-MS in combination with HPLC or field-flow fractionation (FFF). From a clinical standpoint, there are advantages in knowing the specific species in a patient's body. For example, one species of chromium, known as trivalent chromium (Cr III), is needed by the body and causes no ill effects, but hexavalent chromium (Cr VI), is very toxic. Chromium VI can cause mutations that may lead to cancer if not repaired by the body. Another concern is arsenic in shellfish. Frequent consumption of shellfish can lead to elevated levels of arsenic in blood, but the arsenic is usually in the organic form, which is less toxic. Analysis of arsenic in humans must include the identification of the specific species.

One of the largest uses for ICP-MS is in the medical and forensic field of toxicology. A physician may order a metal assay for a number of reasons, such as suspicion of heavy metal poisoning, metabolic concerns, or hepatologic issues. Depending on the specific parameters of each patient's diagnostic plan, samples collected for analysis may be whole blood, urine, plasma, serum, or packed red blood cells. This instrument is also used in the environmental field. Applications include water testing for municipalities or private individuals and soil, water, and other material analysis for industrial purposes.

Industrial and biological monitoring require metal analysis that is done with ICP-MS. Individuals working in plants where exposure to metals is likely and unavoidable, such as a battery factory, are required by their employer to have their blood or urine analyzed for metal toxicity on a regular basis. Monitoring has become a mandatory practice implemented by the Occupational Safety and Health Administration (OSHA) to protect workers from their work environment and ensure proper rotation of work duties.

Clinicians use speciation analysis for preventative medicine. Many patients who have elevated levels of certain metals do not know when or where the exposure occurred. By identifying the exact species, a physician can better narrow the search for possible exposure sites, helping the patient to avoid certain areas in the future. ICP-MS has replaced atomic absorption for the routine determination of trace metals. It is superior for the analysis of samples when the composition is unknown, it has better sensitivity, and it can analyze multiple elements simultaneously.

Chemical Ionization

Chemical ionization (CI) is a technique that is rarely used in mass spectrometry. Chemical ionization is a lower-energy process than electron ionization. The lower energy yields less fragmentation and usually a simpler spectrum. A typical CI spectrum has an easily identifiable molecular ion. In a CI experiment, ions are produced through the collision of the analyte with a reagent gas with easily exchangeable protons or other ionizable functional groups that are present in the ion source.

Electrospray Ionization

Electrospray ionization (ESI) is the ion source of choice to couple liquid chromatography with mass spectrometry. Samples for injection into the electrospray ionization mass spectrometer work the best if they are first purified. Purity in a sample is important because this technique does not work well when mixtures are used as the analyte. A means of purification is often employed to inject a homogeneous sample into the capillary needle. HPLC, capillary electrophoresis, and liquid-solid column chromatography are preferred methods for this purpose.

The chosen purification method is attached to a capillary needle to which a 3- to 5-kV charge is applied. The sample

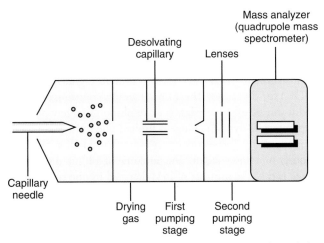

• **Figure 3-34** Electrospray ionization. (Adapted from schematic by Delmar Larsen, University of California-Davis.)

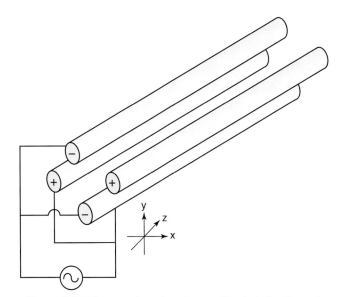

• **Figure 3-35** Diagram of quadrupole mass filter, including the radio-frequency (RF) part of the voltages applied to the quadrupole rods. (Adapted from Burtis CA, Bruns DE. *Tietz Fundamentals of Clinical Chemistry and Molecular Diagnostics*. 7th ed. St. Louis: Saunders; 2015.)

can be introduced directly. ESI belongs to methodologies known as *atmospheric pressure ionization* techniques, in which ions or molecules in solution are transferred to the gas phase before sampling into a mass analyzer as ionized species (Fig. 3-34). ESI interfaces are available from all manufacturers of mass spectrometry detectors.

Atmospheric pressure chemical ionization (APCI) is similar to ESI, but it has no voltage applied to the inlet capillary. Instead, a separate corona discharge needle, located perpendicular to the capillary, is used to emit a cloud of electrons that ionize compounds after they are converted to the gas phase. This technique yields very little fragmentation.

Vacuum Requirements

Almost every step in mass spectrometry requires a vacuum. The vacuum lowers the probability of an ion colliding with an ambient molecule before hitting the detector. The ion signal is reduced by collisions with ambient gas molecules, and the filament used to generate the electron beam for ionization rapidly oxidizes in air.

Some instruments use electrostatic lenses, which focus the ion beam, using sufficiently high-voltage electric fields that can discharge through ambient gas. The electron multiplier detector is essentially a capacitor carrying 1000 to 3000 volts, and a discharge would destroy it. The electron multiplier can detect neutral collisions, and its operational life depends on the number of collisions it detects; the density of gas molecules at ambient pressure is sufficiently large that the detector lifetime is rapidly exceeded.

High vacuum pressures are approximately 10^{-8} to 10^{-3} torr, although the lower limit may vary. To achieve a high vacuum pressure, an oil diffusion or turbomolecular pump is used in series with a mechanical pump. The mechanical pump is called a foreline or backing pump. Pressures below 10^{-8} torr are called an ultra-high vacuum. To achieve pressures this low, cyropumps or ion pumps are used in series with mechanical pumps. However, the system must be pumped to a low to moderate vacuum pressure before the pumps can be operated, and their pumping speed is comparatively low. An ultra-high vacuum requires other specialized techniques, such as metal-metal connections and high-temperature baking of system components to eliminate adsorbed residual gas.

Classes of Mass Spectrometers

Beam-Type Designs

Quadrupole Mass Spectrometer

The quadrupole mass analyzer is used in mass spectrometry. In a **quadrupole mass spectrometer** (QMS), the quadrupole is the component of the instrument that is responsible for filtering sample ions based on their m/z ratio. Ions are separated in a quadrupole based on the stability of their trajectories in the oscillating electric fields that are applied to the rods. The quadrupole consists of four parallel metal rods. Each opposing pair of rods is connected electrically, and a radiofrequency (RF) voltage is applied between one pair of rods and the other. A direct current voltage is then superimposed on the RF voltage. Ions travel down the quadrupole between the rods. For a given ratio of voltages, only ions with a certain m/z value have stable trajectories and reach the detector. Other ions have unstable trajectories and collide with the rods. This allows selection of an ion with a particular m/z value or allows the operator to scan for a range of m/z values by continuously varying the applied voltage.

Ideally, the rods are hyperbolic. Circular rods with a specific ratio of rod diameter to spacing provide an adequate approximation to hyperbolas that are easier to manufacture. Small variations in the ratio have large effects on resolution and peak shape. Different manufacturers choose slightly different ratios to fine-tune operating characteristics for anticipated application requirements. Some manufacturers have produced quadrupole mass spectrometers with true hyperbolic rods. A diagram of a quadrupole mass filter is shown in Figure 3-35.

Time-of-Flight Mass Spectrometry

TOF-MS is a method in which an ion's m/z ratio, which determines its velocity, is determined by a time measurement. Ions are accelerated by an electric field of known strength. An ion has the same kinetic energy as any other ion with the same charge. The time required for the particle to reach a detector at a known distance is measured; heavier particles reach lower speeds. From this time and the known experimental parameters, the m/z ratio of the ion can be calculated.

Continuous ion sources (most commonly ESI) are interfaced with the TOF mass analyzer by orthogonal extraction, in which ions introduced into the TOF mass analyzer are accelerated along the axis perpendicular to their initial direction of motion.

The combination of ion collisional cooling and orthogonal acceleration has significantly increased the resolution of modern TOF-MS without compromising the sensitivity. Orthogonal acceleration combined with collisional ion cooling allows separation of ion production in the ion source and mass analysis. Very high resolution can be achieved for ions produced in MALDI or ESI sources. Before entering the orthogonal acceleration region (i.e., pulser), the ions produced in continuous (ESI) or pulsed (MALDI) sources are focused (i.e., cooled) into a beam of 1 to 2 mm in diameter by collisions with a residual gas in RF multipole guides. A system of electrostatic lenses mounted in a high-vacuum region before the pulser makes the beam parallel to minimize its divergence in the direction of acceleration.

The kinetic energy distribution in the direction of ion flight can be corrected with a reflectron. The reflectron uses a constant electrostatic field to reflect the ion beam toward the detector. The more energetic ions penetrate deeper into the reflectron and take a slightly longer path to the detector. Less energetic ions of the same mass-to-charge ratio penetrate a shorter distance into the reflectron and take a shorter path to the detector. The flat surface of the ion detector (typically a microchannel plate) is placed at the point where ions with different energies reflected by the reflectron hit a surface of the detector at the same time and are counted with respect to the onset of the extraction pulse in the ion source. A point of simultaneous arrival of ions of the same mass and charge but with different energies is referred to as a TOF focus.

An additional advantage to the reflectron-TOF arrangement is that twice the flight path is achieved in a given length of instrument. TOF-MS uses a time-to-digital converter (TDC) for detection. The TDC is an ion-counting detector, and it can be extremely fast (i.e., resolution of a few picoseconds), but its dynamic range is limited due to its inability to properly count the events when more than one ion simultaneously hits the detector. The outcome of a limited dynamic range is that the number of ions detected in one spectrum is somewhat small. This problem of limited dynamic range can be alleviated by using multichannel detector designs.

Trapping Mass Spectrometers

Quadrupole Ion Trap

A quadrupole ion trap is designed to trap ions in three dimensions rather than allowing the ions to pass through as in a quadrupole mass filter, which confines ions to two dimensions. It is commonly used as a component of a mass spectrometer for structural identification and sample identification.

Linear Ion Trap

The linear ion trap is based on a modification of the quadrupole mass filter and uses a set of quadrupole rods to confine ions radially and a static electrical potential on end electrodes to confine the ions axially. The linear form of the trap can be used as a selective mass filter or as an actual trap by creating a potential well for the ions along the axis of the electrodes. Advantages of the linear trap design are increased ion storage capacity, faster scan times, and simplicity of construction, although quadrupole rod alignment is critical, adding a quality control constraint to their production. This constraint also affects the machining requirements of the three-dimensional trap.

Tandem Mass Spectrometry

Tandem mass spectrometry (MS/MS) is rapidly becoming important in clinical laboratories, where it is used for the quantitative analysis of routine samples (Fig. 3-36). MS/MS has very high selectivity and good sensitivity.

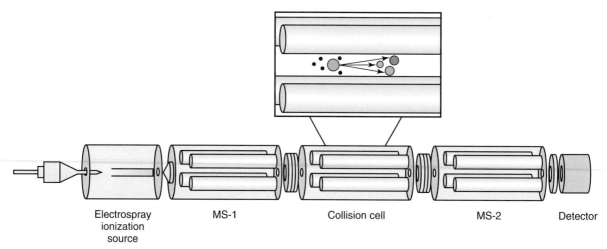

Electrospray ionization source   MS-1   Collision cell   MS-2   Detector

• **Figure 3-36** Tandem mass spectrometer. *MS,* Mass spectrometer.

Two mass spectrometers are arranged in sequence with a collision cell between the two instruments. The first instrument is used to select ions of a particular m/z called the *parent ion*. The parent ions are directed into the collision cell, where they are broken into fragment ions. The second MS acquires the mass of the fragment ions. The key to the high selectivity of MS/MS is that it characterizes a compound by two structural properties. If combined with a chromatographic separation, the retention time adds a third property. Another development in MS/MS is the combination of two TOF mass spectrometers. These instruments are especially useful in proteomics research.

Detectors

Most mass spectrometers use electron multipliers for ion detection. The three main classes of detectors work on the same physical principle. When an ion strikes the first dynode in the multiplier, one or more electrons are ejected from the dynode surface. On striking the second dynode, two or three more electrons are ejected. This process is repeated through a chain of dynodes numbering between 12 and 24. This cascade process typically produces a gain of 10^4 to 10^8.

Computer and Software

As with most modern laboratory instruments, sophisticated computers and software programs are required to control instrument parameters and acquire and analyze data. In toxicology laboratories, another important function is the data system library used to assist in compound identification. Identification is accomplished by matching the mass spectrum generated from the unknown specimen with an in-house database that may contain hundreds or thousands of spectra. This process depends on the use of a computer. Software packages exist or can be custom designed that aid in characterizing spectral data to identify intact protein mass, amino acid subsequences, and posttranslational modifications.

Electrophoresis

Electrophoresis is the separation of analytes on a medium using an electrical current. The most popular technique is zone electrophoresis, which involves a porous supporting medium such as a film of agarose gel or a slab gel using polyacrylamide. Charged particles migrate as zones on a porous medium such as agarose gel after the sample is mixed with a buffer. The process generates an electropherogram or display of protein zones that are usually sharply separated from neighboring zones on the supporting medium. The zones are stained with a protein stain specific for the protein class of interest. The medium is then dried, and the zones are visually examined or quantified by scanning with a densitometer. The dried support medium is stable almost indefinitely and is retained as a permanent record.

In an electrophoresis system, chemical species such as proteins take on an electrical charge dictated by the p*Ka* of the functional groups and the pH of the buffer, and they become ionized. Ions then move toward the positive electrode (i.e., anode) or the negative electrode (i.e., cathode) according to the charge they carry. An *ampholyte* is a molecule that contains both acidic and basic groups. Because proteins contain many ionizable amino (basic) and carboxyl groups (acidic), they behave as ampholytes in solutions. In a solution that is more alkaline than its isoelectric point (pI) (i.e., pH at which a particular molecule or surface carries no net electrical charge), ions migrate toward the anode. In a solution that is more acidic than its pI, they migrate toward the cathode.

The rate of migration depends on factors such as the net charge of the molecule, its size and shape, electric field strength, properties of the supporting media, and the temperature of the operation. Electrophoretic mobility is directly proportional to net charge on the ion and inversely proportional to molecular size and viscosity of the electrophoresis medium.

Other factors that affect mobility include endosmotic flow (discussed later) and wick flow. Wick flow results from the heat generated by the electrophoretic process, causing evaporation of solvent from the electrophoretic support. The drying effect causes buffer from both buffer compartments to flow into the supporting media to replace the lost solvent. This wick flow affects protein migration and mobility.

Instrumentation and Reagents

A diagram of a typical electrophoresis system is shown in Figure 3-37. Two buffer boxes with baffle plates contain the buffer used in the process. Each buffer box contains an electrode made of carbon. The polarity of the electrodes is determined by the manner in which the connection is made to the power supply. The electrophoresis support on which the separation takes place contacts the buffer directly. The entire apparatus is covered to minimize evaporation. Power is supplied by a direct current power supply.

Commercially available power supplies allow operation using constant voltage, current, or power. The flow of current through a medium offering electrical resistance produces heat (measured in joules). The heat produced during the procedure increases the conductance of the system. In a constant-voltage system, the current rises, increasing the migration rate of the proteins and the rate of evaporation. To minimize these effects, a constant-current power supply is recommended. In isoelectric focusing, constant power is recommended. Capillary electrophoresis uses a power supply that can provide voltages in the kilovolt range.

Pulsed-power or pulsed-field techniques change the orientation of the applied field relative to the direction of migration by alternately applying power to different pairs of electrodes. During each cycle, the molecules must be reoriented to the new field direction to fit through the pores in the gel before migration can continue. Because reorientation time is related to molecular size, net migration is a function of the frequency of the field alteration, permitting the separation of large

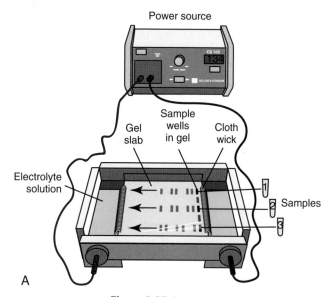

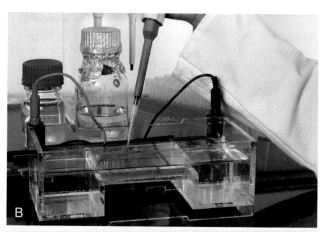

• **Figure 3-37** Gel electrophoresis. **A,** Schematic. **B,** Actual equipment. (**B,** Courtesy eROMAZe/iStock.)

molecules such as DNA fragments that cannot be resolved by the relatively small pores in agarose or polyacrylamide gels.

Buffers

The buffer serves several purposes in an electrophoretic separation. It carries the current and establishes the pH at which the electrophoresis is performed, which determines the charge of the solute. The ionic strength of the buffer affects the conductance of the support, the thickness of the ionic cloud surrounding a charged molecule (buffer and nonbuffer ions), the rate of the solute's migration, and sharpness of the electrophoretic zones. Buffers of high ionic strengths yield sharper band separations but produce more heating, which can denature heat-labile proteins.

Support Media

Various types of support media are used in electrophoresis. Pure buffer solutions can be used inside a capillary. Insoluble gels in sheets, slabs, or columns of agarose or polyacrylamide have been used as support media. Gels are cast in the same buffer that is used in the procedure.

Agarose

Agarose is the neutral fraction of agar obtained by separating it from agaropectin. It is used in agarose gel electrophoresis (AGE). AGE has many applications, including separation of proteins in serum, urine, and cerebrospinal fluid; hemoglobin variants; lipoproteins; and many other substances.

Because the pore size of agarose is large, it allows all proteins to pass through unimpeded. Separation is based solely on the charge of the proteins. It has a lower affinity for proteins, and its native clarity after drying permits superb densitometric examination. It is free of ionizable groups and therefore exhibits little endosmosis. *Endosmosis* is the preferential movement of buffer in one direction through an electrophoretic medium due to selective binding of one type of charge on the surface of the medium. Macromolecules in solution that would normally move in the opposite direction to this flow may remain immobile or are swept back toward the opposite pole if they are insufficiently charged.

Disadvantages of cellulose acetate membranes include endosmosis and the need to be softened before use and cleared before densitometric scanning. As a result, cellulose acetate is seldom used in clinical laboratories.

Polyacrylamide

Polyacrylamide is a polymer prepared by heating acrylamide with a variety of catalysts with or without crosslinking. The advantages of polyacrylamide gel (PAG) include thermostability, transparency, and durability. It is relatively inert chemically, and unlike agarose, the gels are relatively uncharged, limiting endosmosis.

PAGs are prepared in a variety of pore sizes. The average pore size in a typical 7.5% PAG is about 5 nm, which allows most serum proteins to migrate unimpeded. However, some proteins with larger radial dimensions, such as fibrinogen, α_1-lipoprotein, α_1-macroglobulin, and $\alpha\beta$-globulins, are impeded in their migration. With PAGs, proteins are separated on the basis of charge and molecular size (i.e., molecular sieving). When used for the separation of nucleic acids, polyacrylamide is capable of resolving DNA molecules that differ by as little as 2% in length. It accommodates a larger sample than agarose, and the DNA recovered is extremely pure.

Automated Systems

Because of the increased volume of testing (mostly serum proteins), most clinical laboratories that perform electrophoresis for clinical purposes have automated the process to reduce labor, increase throughput, and reduce turnaround. It also reflects the reality that most manufacturers no longer market manual systems. Systems such as the Helena SPIFE

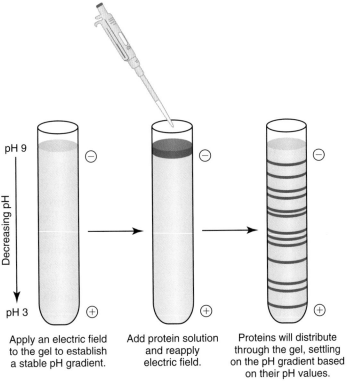

pH 9

Decreasing pH

pH 3

Apply an electric field
to the gel to establish
a stable pH gradient.

Add protein solution
and reapply
electric field.

Proteins will distribute
through the gel, settling
on the pH gradient based
on their pH values.

• **Figure 3-38** Isoelectric focusing.

4000 and Sebia Hydrasys 2 have automated the entire process from sample and reagent application to staining and drying.

Sebia's second-generation instrument, the Hydrasys 2, is a semiautomated agarose gel electrophoresis system that automatically performs the many tedious steps involved in traditional electrophoresis and immunofixation testing. The Hydrasys 2 system can carry out all phases of electrophoresis, including application, migration, incubation, staining, destaining, and drying. The scan option allows for high-resolution image capture and quantification of a gel in less than 1 minute. The system has a throughput of 162 proteins, 45 hemoglobins, or 18 immunofixations in 1 hour.

The SPIFE 4000 is the most recent innovation in automated electrophoresis from Helena Laboratories. It eliminates all manual steps, including sample application, addition of stains and antisera, gel transfers, dilutions, removal of gel blocks, and scanning. In a single 8-hour shift, the SPIFE 4000 can process 80 immunofixation electrophoresis or 560 serum protein electrophoresis samples.

Most capillary electrophoresis systems have autosampling capabilities. Throughput is enhanced by using multiple capillaries.

Procedure

General operations performed in conventional electrophoresis include separation, staining, and quantitation. Several blotting techniques also have been developed. Common types of electrophoretic methods used in clinical laboratories are zone electrophoresis, isoelectric focusing, and capillary electrophoresis.

Specific procedures are not described in this chapter; the technician should follow the procedure provided in the manufacturer's kit insert.

Zone Electrophoresis

In zone electrophoresis, separation is determined by charge differences of the solutes in a single continuous buffer. Zone electrophoresis most commonly uses agarose gels.

Isoelectric Focusing

In **isoelectric focusing** (IEF), proteins are applied to polyacrylamide gels (i.e., IEF gels) or immobilized pH gradient (IPG) strips containing a fixed pH gradient (Fig. 3-38). An electrical field is applied, and the protein sample containing a mixture of proteins migrates through the pH gradient. Individual proteins are immobilized in the pH gradient as they approach their specific neutral pH.

Two-dimensional electrophoresis provides superior resolving ability for the separation of complex mixtures of proteins. Using two high-resolution techniques, it can resolve hundreds of proteins on a single gel. The first step uses IEF. The second step uses sodium dodecyl sulfate–polyacrylamide gel electrophoresis (SDS-PAGE), which eliminates differences in the charge on the protein. In this step, the protein profile is determined by size of the molecule instead of charge. The result is a gel with proteins spread out on its surface.

The separated proteins can be detected by a variety of means, but the most common protocols employ silver or Coomassie Brilliant Blue staining. In the former case, a silver colloid is applied to the gel. The silver binds to cysteine groups within the protein. The silver is darkened by exposure to UV light. The amount of silver correlates with the degree of darkness and therefore the amount of protein at a given location on the gel. This process provides an approximate measurement, but it is adequate for most purposes.

Molecules other than proteins can be separated by two-dimensional electrophoresis. In supercoiling assays, coiled DNA is separated in the first dimension and denatured by a DNA intercalator such as ethidium bromide or the less carcinogenic chloroquine in the second. Two-dimensional electrophoresis is not well suited for routine clinical analysis but is primarily employed in research applications.

Blotting techniques are widely used to detect DNA or RNA fragments (see Fig. 5-25 in Chapter 5). Southern blotting requires an electrophoretic separation of DNA or DNA fragments by agarose gel electrophoresis. A strip of nitrocellulose is then laid over the agarose gel, and the fragments are blotted onto it. They are then detected by hybridization with a labeled, complementary nucleic acid probe. Northern blotting is identical to Southern blotting except that a labeled RNA probe is used for hybridization. Western blotting is used to identify one or more proteins in a complex mixture. It involves separation of the proteins by PAGE and their transfer onto a nitrocellulose strip by electroblotting. The strip is reacted with a reagent that contains an antibody raised against the protein of interest.

Capillary Electrophoresis

Capillary electrophoresis (CE) encompasses a family of separation techniques that use narrow-bore, fused-silica capillaries to separate a complex array of large and small molecules (Fig. 3-39). High electric field strengths are used to separate molecules based on differences in charge, size, and hydrophobicity. Sample introduction is accomplished by immersing the end of the capillary into a sample vial and applying pressure, vacuum, or voltage.

CE separation techniques depend on the types of capillaries and electrolytes used:

- Capillary zone electrophoresis (CZE), also known as free-solution CE (FSCE), is the simplest form of CE. The separation mechanism is based on differences in the charge of the analytes. Fundamental to CZE are homogeneity of the buffer solution and constant field strength throughout the length of the capillary. The separation relies principally on the pH-controlled dissociation of acidic groups on the solute or the protonation of basic functional groups on the solute.

- Capillary gel electrophoresis (CGE) is an adaptation of traditional gel electrophoresis for the capillary using polymers in solution to create a molecular sieve, also known as a replaceable physical gel. It allows analytes having similar charges to be resolved by size. This technique is commonly employed in SDS-PAGE analysis of the molecular weights of proteins and in applications of DNA sequencing and genotyping.

- Capillary isoelectric focusing (CIEF) allows amphoteric molecules such as proteins to be separated by electrophoresis in a pH gradient generated between the cathode and anode. A solute migrates to a point where its net charge is zero (isoelectric point). At the solute's isoelectric point (pI), migration stops, and the sample is focused into a tight zone. After a solute has focused at its pI, the zone is mobilized past the detector by pressure or chemical means. This technique is commonly employed in protein characterization to determine a protein's pI.

- Isotachophoresis (ITP) is a focusing technique based on the migration of the sample components between leading and terminating electrolytes. Solutes having mobilities intermediate to those of the leading and terminating electrolytes stack into sharp, focused zones. Although it is used as a mode of separation, transient ITP has been used primarily as a sample concentration technique.

- Electrokinetic chromatography (EKC) is a family of electrophoresis techniques. EKC derives its name from electrokinetic phenomena that include electroosmosis, electrophoresis, and chromatography. An example is cyclodextrin-mediated EKC, in which differential interaction of enantiomers with cyclodextrins allows separation of chiral compounds. This approach to enantiomer analysis has had a significant impact on the pharmaceutical industry's approach to assessing drugs containing enantiomers.

- Micellar electrokinetic capillary chromatography (MECC or MEKC) is a mode of electrokinetic chromatography in which surfactants are added to the buffer solution at concentrations that form micelles. Separation with MEKC is based on a differential partition between the micelle and the solvent. This principle can be employed with charged or neutral solutes and can involve stationary or mobile micelles. MEKC has great utility in separating mixtures that contain both ionic and neutral species, and it has

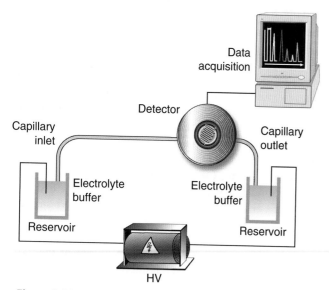

• **Figure 3-39** Schematic diagram of capillary electrophoresis instrumentation. *HV,* High voltage. (From Ward KM, Lehmann CA, Leiken AM. *Clinical Laboratory Instrumentation and Automation; Principles, Applications, and Selection.* Philadelphia: WB Saunders; 1994, with permission.)

become valuable in the separation of very hydrophobic pharmaceuticals from their very polar metabolites.

- Microemulsion electrokinetic chromatography (MEEKC) is a CE technique in which solutes partition with moving oil droplets in a buffer. The microemulsion droplets are usually formed by sonicating immiscible heptane or octane with water. SDS is added at relatively high concentrations to stabilize the emulsion. This technique allows separation of aqueous and water-insoluble compounds, and it is used effectively by the pharmaceutical industry as a general method to analyze a broad spectrum of pharmaceuticals.

- Nonaqueous capillary electrophoresis (NACE) involves the separation of analytes in a medium composed of organic solvents. The viscosity and dielectric constants of organic solvents affect sample ion mobility and the level of electroosmotic flow. The use of nonaqueous medium allows additional selectivity options in method development and is valuable for the separation of water-insoluble compounds.

- Capillary electrochromatography (CEC) is a hybrid separation method that couples the high separation efficiency of CZE with HPLC and uses an electric field rather than hydraulic pressure to propel the mobile phase through a packed bed. Because there is minimal backpressure, it is possible to use small-diameter packing and achieve very high efficiencies. Its most useful application appears to be online analyte concentration before separation by CZE.

In CE, the most common techniques of zone electrophoresis, IEF, and gel electrophoresis are carried out in a small-bore (10 to 100 μL), fused-silica capillary tube 20 to 200 cm long. CE has two advantages over traditional electrophoresis: the ability to apply much higher voltages and the ease of automation. CE has a much wider range of applications, including inorganic ions, amino acids, organic acids, proteins, drugs, vitamins, oligonucleotides, and DNA fragments. CE has the highest resolution of any liquid separation technique.

Two forces are dominant in CE: the electrophoretic mobility of the solutes and the electroosmotic flow (EOF) of the liquid. EOF refers to the flow resulting from interactions of the charged ions on the capillary walls. The capillary has a large surface, and the negative charge effect of EOF plays a major role in the separation of solute constituents in a mixture. All solutes ultimately move toward the cathode because the EOF is usually sufficient to force the movement in one direction.

CE systems are available from several manufacturers. They provide more consistent and standardized results with less time and effort (i.e., rapid and robust) than gel electrophoresis. Using CE, DNA fragments are rapidly separated with a high-voltage gradient because the capillary dissipates heat quickly. One CE run can take 30 minutes or less, and with current systems equipped with 16 capillaries that are run simultaneously, the process is shorter than the 3 to 4 hours required for standard electrophoresis. CE systems can separate up to 80 serum protein samples per hour.

Other applications include immunotyping, an alternative to immunofixation, and separation of abnormal hemoglobins.

Genetic Analysis

Since the publication about DNA's double-helix structure by Watson and Crick in 1953, electrophoresis has been a standard among the analytical tools used in modern biochemistry. CE's automation and quantitation capabilities made it a natural successor to the slab-gel format for genetic analysis. By introducing replaceable physical gels (i.e., polymers in solution) into a capillary, a molecular sieve is created that resolves molecules of DNA and RNA by size. Automation of this format has enabled significant advances in genetic analysis, accelerating the discovery of new genomic information.

CE technology is routinely used for purity analysis of oligonucleotides and siRNAs. If not pure, synthesized oligonucleotides can cause problems in hybridization reactions, and good quality assurance can save significant time and money. Rigorous characterization is particularly essential in the development of nucleic acid–based therapeutics.

Colligative Properties

Colligative properties of solutions depend on the ratio of the number of solute particles to the number of solvent molecules in a solution. They are independent of the nature of the solute particles and result from dilution of the solvent by the solute. Colligative properties include relative lowering of vapor pressure, elevation of boiling point, depression of freezing point, and osmotic pressure.

The term *colligative* is derived from the Latin *colligatus,* meaning "bound together." The properties are bound together because they all depend on the number of solute particles and not on the type of chemical species.

Vapor pressure, which is the pressure of the evaporated solvent, decreases as the concentration of solute particles increases. The solute particles take up a portion of the surface area between the solvent and the gas it is evaporating into. Because the solvent has fewer opportunities to evaporate, there are fewer evaporated or vaporized solvent particles, decreasing the vapor pressure.

Addition of solute to form a solution stabilizes the solvent in the liquid phase and lowers the solvent chemical potential so that solvent molecules have less tendency to move to the gas or solid phases. As a result, liquid solutions slightly above the solvent boiling point at a given pressure become stable, which results in an increased boiling point. Similarly, liquid solutions slightly below the solvent freezing point become stable, resulting in a decreased freezing point. The boiling point elevation and freezing point depression are proportional to the lower vapor pressure in a dilute solution. Adding 1 mole of solute particles to 1 kg of water raises the boiling point of water by 0.52° C, lowers the freezing point by 1.86° C, lowers the vapor pressure by 0.3 mm Hg, and raises the vapor pressure by 17,000 mm Hg (22.4 atm).

Osmometry is a technique for measuring the concentration of solute particles that contribute to the osmotic pressure of a solution. Osmotic pressure governs the movement of a solvent across a membrane that separates two solutions. In physiologic conditions, the solute is water. Examples of biologically important membranes are those enclosing glomerular and capillary vessels that are permeable to water, ions, and small molecules but not to large protein molecules. Differences in the concentrations of osmotically active molecules that cannot cross a membrane cause molecules that can cross the membrane to move for the purpose of establishing an osmotic equilibrium. The movement of solute and permeable ions or molecules exerts an osmotic pressure. Osmosis is the movement of a solvent across a membrane in response to differences in osmotic pressure across the membrane to the side containing a higher concentration of solute. The number of particles in a solution per given mass of solvent determines the total osmotic pressure of the solution.

Osmolality expresses concentrations relative to the mass of the solvent. A 1 molal solution contains 1 mole of solute per 1 kg of water. Osmolarity expresses concentration per volume of solvent. Osmolality is thermodynamically a more accurate expression because solutions expressed on a weight/weight basis are temperature independent. Although the term *osmolarity* is often used by medical staff and in medical literature, osmolality is what the laboratory measures.

Osmolality is the number of moles of solute particles per kilogram of pure solvent. Because most ionic species do not completely dissociate, osmolality is a unit of concentration, which takes into account the dissociative effect. Measured osmolality is usually expressed in mOsm/kg of water. One milliosmol (mOsm) is 10^{-3} osmols. Technically, any of the colligative properties could be used as a basis for osmolality, but freezing point depression is most commonly measured in the clinical laboratory. Some analyzers rely on the relationship between vapor pressure and osmolality. However, it is less precise than the freezing point depression method. Unlike vapor pressure, freezing point depression is independent of ambient temperature. The vapor pressure measures the dew point temperature, which has a much lower slope of increase compared with freezing point depression. Freezing point depression osmometers are reliable (Fig. 3-40).

Substances such as ethanol, methanol, and isopropanol escape from the sample, which increases the vapor pressure of the solvent rather than lowering it. This makes the use of vapor pressure osmometers impractical for identifying osmolar gaps in acid-base disturbances. This is a particular problem for the physician in an emergency room. Advanced Instruments, the major manufacturer of freezing point osmometers, produces instruments with multisampling capability by employing a sample turntable, enabling analysis with less labor and attention.

Point-of-Care Testing

Point-of-care testing (POCT) is a mode of testing performed at or near the site of patient care. Some definitions

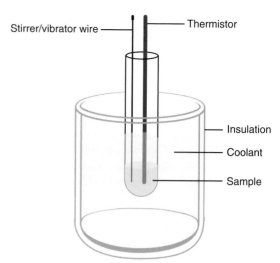

• **Figure 3-40** Freezing point depression osmometer.

include satellite testing or other types of decentralized testing. POCT is usually performed by the caregiver rather than the central laboratory personnel. Another variant of POCT is arterial blood gas (ABG) analysis done by respiratory therapists in satellite laboratories (i.e., satellite testing), usually near an intensive care unit but not at the bedside. POCT can be performed in physician's offices, workplace clinics, paramedical support vehicles, pharmacies, emergency rooms, hospital-based critical care units, and satellite clinics. Advantages of POCT include quicker test results by eliminating the time required for transportation to a central laboratory, reduction of the delays associated with a central testing facility, and time saved by the immediate reporting of results.

POCT has expanded because of the long-term trend of miniaturization in clinical diagnostics instrumentation. An early report described the advantages of using electrochemical sensors for bedside monitoring in critical care units. Small, handheld or benchtop devices can measure electrolytes, blood gases, cardiac markers, glucose levels, and coagulation markers. Although the throughput for the devices is low, the time required for an individual result is usually short. Because these devices are often small enough to be portable, they can be taken directly to the patient. Many devices use the same analytical technologies as those found on analyzers in central laboratories (Table 3-2).

Most POCT analyzers are single-use strips or cartridges with a monitoring device capable of measuring reflectance, light scattering, electrochemical changes, absorbance, or fluorescence. Many POCT devices can read bar codes and identify test packages, or they incorporate factory calibration data. Some devices use a magnetic strip to store similar information. Other important bar-code functions include identifying the operator and the patient sample, providing traceability to the person who performed the test and linking the results to the correct patient.

Because most POCT devices are usually single use only, reproducibility in manufacturing is required to ensure that consistent performance extends across an entire lot of strips

TABLE 3-2   Classification of Point-of-Care Testing Instruments or Devices

Type of Technology	Analytical Principle	Analytes
Single-use, qualitative or semiquantitative cartridge or strip tests	Reflectance	Urine and blood chemistry
	Lateral-flow or flow-through immunoassays	Infectious disease agents, cardiac markers, hCG
Single-use quantitative cartridge or strip tests with a reader device	Reflectance	Glucose
	Electrochemistry	Glucose
	Reflectance	Blood chemistry
	Light scattering or optical motion	Coagulation
	Lateral-flow, flow-through, or solid-phase immunoassays	Cardiac markers, drugs, CRP, allergy and fertility tests
	Immunoturbidimetry	HbA$_{1C}$, urine albumin
	Spectrophotometry	Blood chemistry
	Electrochemistry Fluorescence, electrochemistry with PCR	pH, blood gases, electrolytes, metabolites Infectious agents
Multiple-use quantitative cartridge or benchtop devices	Electrochemistry	pH, blood gases, electrolytes, metabolites
	Fluorescence	pH, blood gases, electrolytes, metabolites
	Multiwavelength spectrophotometry	Hemoglobin species, bilirubin
	Time-resolved fluorescence	Cardiac markers, drugs, CRP
	Electrical impedance	Complete blood count

CRP, C-reactive protein; HbA$_{1C}$, glycosylated hemoglobin; hCG, human chorionic gonadotropin; PCR, polymerase chain reaction.
From Burtis CA, Bruns DE. *Tietz Fundamentals of Clinical Chemistry and Molecular Diagnostics.* 7th ed. Elsevier: St. Louis; 2015.

or devices. The manufacturing process includes steps to ensure the devices provide reproducible results and remain stable for the stated period of time.

POCT is most often used to measure glucose levels. Several approaches are used to measure glucose levels, but all devices are called biosensors because they use an enzyme as the recognition agent. Enzymes such as GO, hexokinase, and glucose dehydrogenase have been used with reflectance or electrochemical detection. All modern glucose strips are some variation of thick-film technology. The film is composed of several layers, with each having a unique function. When blood is added to the strip, water and glucose pass into the analytical layer. For some photometric (reflectance-based) systems, red blood cells must be excluded. This can be achieved by a separating layer that may contain glass fibers, fleeces, membranes, or special latex formulations. Photometric systems require a spreading layer for fast, homogeneous distribution of the sample. Electrochemical strips use capillary fill systems. The support layer usually consists of a thin plastic material. In reflectance-based systems, the support layer may also have reflective properties, which can be achieved through inclusion of titanium oxide, barium sulfate, or zinc oxide.

Since the introduction of glucometers, it is easier for patients to obtain test results quickly. Manufacturers make meters that are small and easy to use; have a low risk of error; and reduce interference from substances such as ascorbic acid and maltose, low oxygen tension, and hematocrit extremes. One meter that overcomes these interferences is the Nova StatStrip. A major step in solving the problem was the use of ferrocene or its derivatives as immobilized mediators in the construction of electrochemical strips. The introduction of electrochemical technology has facilitated the production of smaller meters and nonwipe strips, eliminated instrument optics, and produced faster results. Other applications of the thick-film technology include immunosensor-based POCT devices capable of measuring a panel of analytes such as cardiac markers, allergens, fertility indicators, and drugs of abuse.

In contrast to the thick-film technology, single-use sensors have been constructed using thin-film technology. The most common commercial device is the i-STAT analyzer (Abbott Laboratories). The Epoc Blood Analysis System (Alere) is a more recent introduction to the field. Both are handheld devices with wireless capability. The i-STAT can measure electrolytes, blood gases, glucose, coagulation markers, cardiac markers, and creatinine. The epoc can measure blood gases, electrolytes, and lactate. In thin-film applications, electrodes are wafer structures constructed of thin metal oxide films using microfabrication techniques. The small, single-use cartridges contain an array of electrochemical sensors that operate in conjunction with a handheld portable analyzer.

Connectivity

POCT and critical care device connectivity continues to be a matter of high priority for hospitals, point-of-care coordinators, respiratory care managers, and caregivers. At a time when mainstream laboratory-based instrumentation is automatically interfaceable to a laboratory information system (LIS) or hospital information system (HIS), it seems unimaginable that almost 70% of all POCT results never make it into the patient's electronic medical record. The benefits of POCT can be optimized only if rapid and high-quality test results are consistently available.

Many factors such as user certifications, on-time quality control testing, and up-to-date reagent control must be managed effectively. Several considerations and questions must be addressed to properly manage an institution's POCT program.

Implementation and Management Considerations

A POCT coordinating committee must be in place to organize and manage all aspects of POCT, including
- Need for POCT
- Development of a POCT policy
- Training and certification
- Equipment procurement and evaluation
- Quality control and quality assurance
- Auditing
- Maintenance and inventory control

Several sources can be consulted about the implementation and management of a POCT program.

Flow Cytometry

Cytometry is the measurement of cells or cellular particles. Cytometric methods can determine cell size, cell cycle stage, DNA content, cell surface and cytoplasmic proteins, and other indicators of the internal cellular complexity.

In *flow cytometry*, measurements are performed while the cells or particles pass through the measuring device in a single file in a fluid stream. Some regard flow cytometry as an esoteric and expensive technology for producing data that can be obtained by traditional and less expensive methods. Flow cytometry is valuable for diagnosing and staging leukemias, lymphomas, and other cancers involving deviant T and B cells; it often provides the diagnosis when other methods fail. Advances in flow methods combined with novel monoclonal antibodies have allowed it to replace many established clinical tests used to diagnose chronic granulomatous disease and paroxysmal nocturnal hemoglobinuria.

Although flow cytometers can be classified as analyzers or sorters, the most common instrument in a clinical laboratory is the analyzer. Sorters, which can physically separate different cell populations, are more expensive and find few applications in a diagnostic laboratory. Sorters are primarily applied in research.

Instrument Components

Fluidics, optics, and electronics are the three main systems that make up a flow cytometer (Fig. 3-41). Operation of a flow cytometer involves the following steps. A tube or other

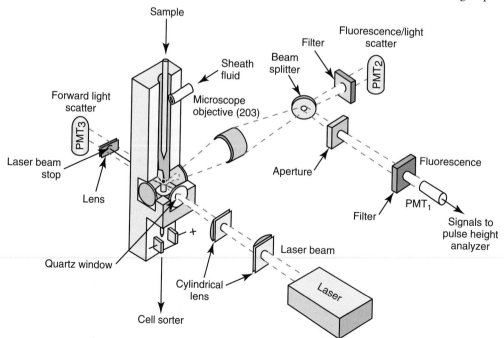

• **Figure 3-41** Schematic diagram of a flow cytometer. *PMT,* Photomultiplier tube. (From Burtis CA, Bruns DE. *Tietz Fundamentals of Clinical Chemistry and Molecular Diagnostics.* 7th ed. St. Louis: Saunders; 2015.)

type of sample vessel containing the prepared cells under investigation is placed in the flow cytometer. The sample is drawn up from the sample vessel and pumped into the flow chamber (i.e., flow cell) through tubing. Cells flow through the flow chamber one at a time very quickly and are presented to one or more light sources (i.e., lasers). The laser beam impacts the cells as they pass through the flow chamber. Light scatter (fluorescence if fluorescent molecules are on the particle), is captured, spectrally filtered, and directed to appropriate photodetectors for conversion to electrical signals. The detected light that bounces off each cell gives information about the cell's physical characteristics.

Flow cytometers interrogate one cell at a time and collect data at a high rate. The cytometer's flow cell prepares the sample for presentation to the laser light source in a single-cell fluid stream. The sample in an isotonic fluid is forced through the flow cell surrounded by a sheath fluid (also isotonic) to produce a laminar flow. The laminar flow creates an optimal differential pressure for cells to enter a conical nozzle assembly and exit the orifice of the nozzle for intersection by the laser. The sample is then collected as waste or sorted if the instrument is designed for sorting.

Optics

Many cytometers come with two lasers. The laser sources generate parallel waves of monochromatic (single-wavelength) light. Inert gas ion lasers (e.g., argon, krypton, helium-neon), diode lasers, and tunable dye lasers have been used. Signals from the scatter of the laser light and the fluorescent emission are separated and directed into individual PMTs through a series of beam splitters, dichroic mirrors, and wavelength-selective filters. With the development of newer fluorescent dyes, four-color analysis is easily performed with two lasers.

Electronics

Most modern laboratory instruments are controlled by a personal computer, and electrical signals from a detector (e.g., PMT, photodiode, electrochemical cell, GLC-MS detector) are converted to digital signals. Light signals collected by the cytometer's PMT detectors are digitalized and stored in the instrument's computer, where the data can be retrieved and analyzed. Specimen types that can be analyzed by flow cytometry include those that can be processed into single-cell suspensions, including ascites fluid, bone cores and marrow, cerebrospinal fluid, lymph nodes, fine-needle aspirates, peripheral blood, pleural fluid, products of conception, spleen, solid tumors, and paraffin blocks.

Flow cytometry has increased in popularity among physicians because it has several advantages over histology and histochemistry. Results are quantitative or semiquantitative, and most instruments can detect and analyze rare cells with a high level of confidence not possible with other methods. Expense and the requirement for highly trained personnel to operate the instrument and interpret the results are limitations of this technology. Tissue morphology can be lost during specimen preparation, and there is the potential to lose highly fragile cells during preparation and analysis. Flow cytometry is not a replacement for standard histologic and immunohistologic procedures but is a secondary procedure.

Data Analysis

Initially, data from the cytometer are analyzed to determine light-scattering properties of the cells, which define the populations to be subjected to further examination. Although light from the laser source is scattered in all directions, it is collected at 90 degrees and a low forward angle, usually 10 to 30 degrees. The right-angle scatter indicates internal cellular complexity or granularity related to the density of the cell. The forward-angle scatter is directly related to the size of the cell. By plotting both light-scattering profiles along two axes results in a characteristic pattern for each cell type. Mature lymphocytes, monocytes, and granulocytes can be easily identified by light scatter alone (Fig. 3-42). Abnormal cells can often be identified in terms of size or density.

After the desired populations of leukocytes are identified, fluorescent-labeled monoclonal antibodies are added, and the fluorescent properties of the chosen cells are examined. As many as four markers can be examined on a single cell at the same time using four monoclonal antibodies labeled with four different fluorochromes.

In addition to measuring cell size and granularity, flow cytometers can measure DNA and RNA content, DNA nucleotide ratios (A+T/G+C), chromatin structure, antigens, total protein content, cell receptors, membrane potential, and intracellular calcium ion concentration as a function of pH. These parameters can be used in hematology, immunology (i.e., T-cell subsets, tissue typing, lymphocyte stimulation, and antigen–antibody reactions), oncology (i.e., diagnosis, prognosis, and monitoring of treatment), microbiology (i.e., bacterial identification and antibiotic sensitivity), virology, genetics (i.e., karyotyping and carrier state detection), parasitology, reproduction, and fertility studies.

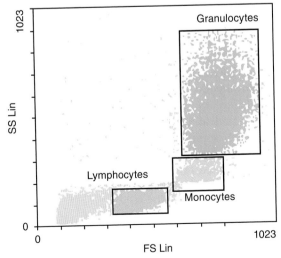

• **Figure 3-42** Data from the flow cytometer.

Flow cytometric bead arrays and multiplexed, solid-phase, particle-based immunoassays or techniques have been used to measure cytokines or their receptors, antibodies, and genes. This technology has also been approved for transplantation studies. Other clinical applications include the diagnosis of chronic lymphocytic leukemia, chronic granulomatous disease (e.g., leukocyte adhesion deficiency), paroxysmal nocturnal hemoglobinuria, and the presence of fetal cells in circulation.

Summary

Laboratory tests are performed on many different types of instruments. Routine chemistry tests are performed on instruments that measure the concentration of an analyte by the amount of light a solution with an analyte and reagent absorbs. Beer's law allows a curve to be constructed from standards. Unknown concentrations can be calculated from the standard curves. This type of analysis is called *spectrophotometry,* and it uses a spectrophotometer.

Fluorometry is a method for identifying and characterizing analytes. The analyte is complexed with a compound that fluoresces when stimulated by a light source. Detectors measure the amount of fluorescent light emitted at the characteristic wavelength.

Nephelometry and turbidimetry measure the scattering of the light transmitted through a sample. Detectors are placed at 180, 90, and 45 degrees with respect to the analysis cuvette. The amount of light scattered is proportional to the concentration of the analyte.

Analytes with ionic characteristics such as electrolytes can be measured using electrochemical techniques. There is usually a reference electrode and a sample electrode. The ions at the sample electrode are measured by potentiometric, conductometric, and coulometric methods.

Organic compounds can be separated based on their physical characteristics through chromatography. Chromatography separation methods include ion exchange, partition, adsorption, affinity, and size exclusion. Planar and columnar supports are used for gas and liquid chromatography. A mass spectrometer separates substances, which are ionized and moved through magnetic fields. This instrument is used as a confirmatory test for drugs and toxic substances.

Electrophoresis separates proteins and DNA in body fluids by running an electrical current through a slab of semisolid material such as agarose. The semisolid matrix allows the organic materials to separate when a current is applied.

Colligative properties can be used to quantify chemical compounds in body fluids. The most common applications include freezing point depression, osmometry, and colloidal osmotic pressure.

Flow cytometry is used to differentiate cell types. Different types of cells scatter light in characteristic ways. The amount of light scattered in a particular pattern identifies the cell and the number of cells in a sample.

Researchers are constantly improving methods for detecting analytes. As computers become more powerful, the opportunities increase for detecting analytes more quickly and precisely. Better laboratory results benefit patients and providers.

Review Questions

1. Beer's law states that the amount of light absorbed is directly proportional to the concentration of a substance. This is expressed by which of the following formulas?
   a. $A = \varepsilon bc$
   b. $A = \lambda bc$
   c. $A = \varepsilon/bc$
   d. $A = b/\lambda c$

2. Light sources for spectrophotometers include all of the following EXCEPT
   a. Lasers
   b. Incandescent lights
   c. Fluorescent lights
   d. Hydrogen lamps

3. Devices used for spectral isolation include all of the following EXCEPT
   a. Filters
   b. Lenses
   c. Prisms
   d. Diffraction gratings

4. Which of the following components of a spectrophotometer converts light into an electrical signal by detecting photons that strike a photosensitive surface?
   a. Photodetector
   b. Monochromator
   c. Cuvette
   d. Interference filter

5. Which of the following light sources is used in fluorometry?
   a. Incandescent
   b. Halon
   c. Halogen
   d. Xenon

6. Potentiometric sensors are used to measure all of the following EXCEPT
   a. pH
   b. Oxygen
   c. P_{CO_2}
   d. Potassium

7. Which of the following types of chromatography was first used to quantitate hemoglobin A_{1C}?
   a. Ion exchange
   b. Gas
   c. Affinity
   d. Partition
8. Which of the following is the method of choice for immunosuppressive drugs used to prevent transplant rejection?
   a. Gas chromatography
   b. HPLC
   c. Liquid chromatography with tandem mass spectrometry
   d. Amperometry

9. In which of the following techniques are proteins applied to polyacrylamide gels containing a fixed pH gradient, after which an electrical field is applied and the protein sample containing a mixture of proteins migrates through the pH gradient?
   a. Nonaqueous capillary electrophoresis
   b. Capillary electrophoresis
   c. Isotachophoresis
   d. Isoelectric focusing
10. Colligative properties include all of the following EXCEPT
   a. Osmolality
   b. Vapor pressure
   c. Freezing point
   d. Osmotic pressure

Critical Thinking Questions

1. Diagram a spectrophotometer and label the parts.
2. Draw a diagram of a tandem mass spectrometer.
3. Explain the principle of electrophoresis.

Bibliography

Bosserhoff A, Hellerbrand C. Capillary electrophoresis. In: Patrinos G, Ansorge W, eds. *Molecular Diagnostics*. Burlington, MA: Academic Press; 2005.

Burtis CA, Ashwood ER, Bruns DE, eds. *Tietz Textbook of Clinical Chemistry*. 5th ed. St. Louis: Elsevier; 2012.

Chew D, Cameron A, Goodwin D, et al. Considerations for primary vacuum pumping in mass spectrometry systems. *Spectroscopy*. 2005;20(1):44–51.

Clark L, Lyons C. Electrode systems for continuous monitoring in cardiovascular surgery. *Ann N Y Acad Sci*. 1962;102:29–45.

Collison M, Meyerhoff M. Chemical sensors for bedside monitoring of critically ill patients. *Anal Chem*. 1990;62:425A–437A.

Croxatto A, Prod'hom G, Greub G. Applications of MALDI-TOF mass spectrometry in clinical diagnostic microbiology. *FEMS Microbiol Rev*. 2012;36:380–407.

Eleventh Annual Symposium on Advanced Analytical Concepts for the Clinical Laboratory. Oak Ridge, TN; *Clin Chem*. 1979;25(9): 1622–1661.

Holtzinger C, Szelag E, DuBois J, et al. Evaluation of a new POCT bedside glucose meter and strip with hematocrit and interference corrections. *Point of Care*. 2008;7(1):1–6.

Lyon M, DuBois J, Fick G, Lyon A. Estimates of total analytical error in consumer and hospital glucose meters contributed by hematocrit, maltose, and ascorbate. *J Diabetes Sci Technol*. 2010;4(6):1479–1494.

Mercier D, Feld R, Witte D. Comparison of dew point and freezing point osmometry. *Am J Med Technol*. 1978;44:1066–1069.

Price C, St. John A, Kricka L. *Point-of-Care Testing: Needs, Opportunity, and Innovation*. 3rd ed. Washington, DC: AACC Press; 2010.

Ward-Cook K, Lehmann C, Schoeff L, Williams R, eds. *Clinical Diagnostic Technology: The Total Testing Process*. The Analytical Phase; Vol. 2. Washington DC: AACC Press; 2005.

4

Immunoassays

DONNA LARSON

CHAPTER OUTLINE

OBJECTIVES

After completion of this chapter, the reader will be able to:

1. Discuss the structure of an antibody.
2. Compare and contrast affinity and avidity, and discuss the importance of both concepts.
3. Define and discuss the term cross-reactivity.
4. Differentiate polyclonal and monoclonal antisera.
5. Describe the principles of solid-phase sandwich assays, distinguishing between those that measure antigen and those that measure antibody.
6. List the labels used for sandwich assays, comparing their sensitivities, advantages, and disadvantages.
7. Differentiate between homogenous and heterogeneous immunoassays.
8. Compare and contrast competitive and noncompetitive immunoassays.
9. Describe the interactions of polyclonal and monoclonal antibodies in the formation of antibody–antigen complexes.
10. Name the two researchers who introduced the radioimmunoassay (RIA) technique in 1957.
11. List the principles, labels, and enzyme for the following techniques: RIA, enzyme immunoassay (EIA), enzyme-linked immunosorbent assay (ELISA), enzyme-multiplied immunoassay technique (EMIT), cloned enzyme donor immunoassay (CEDIA), fluorescence polarization immunoassay (FPIA), microparticle enzyme immunoassay (MEIA), and chemiluminescent microparticle immunoassay (CMIA).
12. Compare and contrast radial immunodiffusion (RID), Ouchterlony double immunodiffusion, Laurell technique, immunoelectrophoresis (IEP), counterimmunoelectrophoresis (CIE), and Western blot.
13. Differentiate turbidimetry and nephelometry
14. Describe five factors that affect immunoassay analytical performance.

KEY TERMS

Affinity
Antibodies
Antigens
Avidity
Cloned enzyme donor immunoassay
Chemiluminescent microparticle
   immunoassay
Competitive immunoassay
Counterimmunoelectrophoresis
Cross-reactivity
Dose-response curve
Enzyme-linked immunosorbent assay
Enzyme-multiplied immunoassay
   technique
Epitope

Fluorophores
Fluorescence polarization immunoassay
Hapten
Heterogeneous immunoassays
High-dose hook effect
Homogenous immunoassays
Hybridomas
Immunodiffusion
Immunoelectrophoresis
Labels
Laurell technique
Liquid-phase adsorption
Luminophors
Microparticle enzyme immunoassay
Monoclonal antibodies

Nephelometry
Noncompetitive immunoassay
One-step format
Ouchterlony double immunodiffusion
Polyclonal antibodies
Precipitation
Radial immunodiffusion
Radioimmunoassay
Solid-phase adsorption
Traceability
Turbidimetry
Two-step format
Western blot

 Case in Point

Technicians in a hospital laboratory used an enzyme-linked immunosorbent assay (ELISA) to measure rubella antibody titers. They noticed that over the past 3 weeks their control values were consistently above the mean and all values for patients were high. There was also poor within-assay precision. They double-checked the lot numbers of the kits, and they were the same lot numbers that had been used for the past 3 months. All kits had been properly stored. What is the likely explanation for the consistently high values? Hint: Look at the type of immunoassay used.

Points to Remember

- Antibodies are produced by the body against antigens.
- The underlying principle of immunochemical techniques is that antibodies combine with an antigen or analyte of interest and react with an indicator that allows the lab technician to determine the amount of antigen or analyte in the sample.
- The equilibrium reached between antibody (Ab) and antigen (Ag) in the reaction Ab + Ag ⇌ Ab-Ag can be expressed as an equilibrium constant (K_a) defined by the following formula:

$$K_a = \frac{[Ab - Ag]}{[Ab][Ag]}$$

- In the binding reaction, avidity is based on affinity of the antibody for the antigen, number of binding sites in the antibody and antigen, and the way the two molecules combine.
- Polyclonal antibodies are produced by many B-cell lineages against a specific antigen; each binds a different epitope on the antigen.
- Monoclonal antibodies are produced by a single B-cell clone and target a specific epitope of an antigen.

- A major disadvantage of using polyclonal antibodies in diagnostic assays is that they can cross-react with unrelated molecules.
- Because monoclonal antibodies are produced from cell culture instead of live animals, an unlimited amount of antibody can be produced.
- Heterogeneous immunoassays require separation through a wash step of the free labeled antigen from the bound labeled antigen in the solution.
- Homogenous immunoassays do not require separation of bound and free labeled antibody or antigen (i.e., no wash step).
- A competitive immunoassay is based on the competition between the unlabeled analyte in the sample and the labeled antigen in the immunoassay. Concentration of the analyte is inversely proportional to the absorbance of the solution.
- Noncompetitive immunoassays, which have the highest levels of sensitivity and specificity, are used to measure cardiac markers and hepatitis markers.
- Labels, including enzymes, fluorophores, luminophors, chemiluminescent compounds, and radioisotopes, are used to detect free antigen or antigen–antibody complexes, but labels cannot distinguish between free and bound antigens.
- In an enzyme-linked immunosorbent assay (ELISA) absorbance of the sample wells is measured; sample absorbance is inversely proportional to the analyte concentration.
- Enzyme-multiplied immunoassay technique (EMIT) is used primarily for quantitating therapeutic drugs and drugs of abuse.
- Fluorescence polarization immunoassay (FPIA) is a homogeneous, competitive, fluorescence immunoassay used to measure hormones, therapeutic drugs, abused drugs, toxic substances, and hormones.
- FPIA combines three principles to increase sensitivity and accuracy: fluorescence, rotation of molecules in solution, and polarized light.

- The microparticle enzyme immunoassay (MEIA) measures large molecules such as cardiac markers, fertility hormones, tumor markers, hepatitis antigens, thyroid hormones, and metabolic markers in an automated instrument.
- The chemiluminescent microparticle immunoassay (CMIA) is one of the most sensitive immunoassays.
- The cloned enzyme donor immunoassay (CEDIA) is a homogenous enzyme immunoassay (EIA), and it was the first EIA designed using genetic engineering techniques.
- Radial immunodiffusion (RID) is used to determine the concentration of an antigen.
- The Ouchterlony double immunodiffusion technique is used to test the similarity between antigens.
- The Laurell technique is one-dimensional electroimmunodiffusion.
- Immunoelectrophoresis (IEP) uses electricity to enhance the double immunodiffusion technique by increasing the speed and specificity of the reaction.
- In counterimmunoelectrophoresis, antigens and antibodies migrate toward one another using electrophoresis, which moves charged particles under the influence of an electric field.
- The Western blot method can detect antigens with concentrations 10-100 times smaller than those detected with immunodiffusion methods.
- Turbidimetry and nephelometry are common laboratory methods that measure antibody–antigen complexes in solution.
- For immunoassays, a dose-response curve is established to correlate certain values of signals with known analyte concentrations.
- The high-dose hook effect is usually seen when performing sandwich immunoassays. Very high antigen concentrations in the sample bind to all available antibody binding sites in the antibody–solid phase and the antibody-labeled conjugate, which prevents formation of the sandwich and falsely decreases the test result.

Introduction

Immunochemistry offers rapid, sensitive, and easily automated methods for routine analyses in clinical laboratories. Immunochemical methods involve principles of antibody–antigen interactions; determinations of hormones, pharmaceuticals, and disease biomarkers; in serum, urine, plasma, saliva, and blood samples. Immunochemistry can be used in conjunction with histochemistry to visualize specific cells. This chapter reviews the principles of antibody–antigen reactions, production of polyclonal and monoclonal antibodies, and technical aspects of particle, light-scattering, and label immunochemical methods.

Antibodies, Antigens, and Analytes

Antibodies are produced by the body against antigens. An epitope is the part of the antigen recognized by the antibody. Each antibody has an affinity and avidity for a specific epitope. These characteristics determine the sensitivity and specificity of the antibodies and antigens used in laboratory assays. Antibody–antigen interactions are used for qualitative and quantitative assays. The underlying principle of immunochemical techniques is that antibodies combine with an antigen or analyte of interest and react with an indicator, allowing determination of the amount of antigen or analyte in a sample. These immunochemical techniques are used to diagnose and monitor the progression of disorders such as autoimmune diseases. The following sections examine antibody structure and behavior, the chemical basis for antibody–antigen binding, and the production of polyclonal and monoclonal antibodies.

Antibody Classification

The presence of antibodies was first proposed by Paul Ehrlich (1854-1915). His work provided the basis for the genetic theory of antibody specificity. Karl Landsteiner discovered the ABO system of blood group antigens. Landsteiner proposed the template theory of antibody formation and coined the term hapten. A hapten is small molecule that cannot elicit an immune response unless it is attached to a large carrier molecule. The template theory of antibody formation recognized that antibodies are produced in response to an antigen. Antigens can be proteins, lipids, carbohydrates, or polysaccharides. B lymphocytes are the cells responsible for producing antibodies. B lymphocytes are preprogrammed to recognize specific epitopes on nonself molecules (i.e., antigens). Clonal expansion of each preprogrammed B lymphocyte produces a line of cells with the independent capacity to make antibodies in response to encountering a specific antigen (Figs. 4-1 and 4-2)

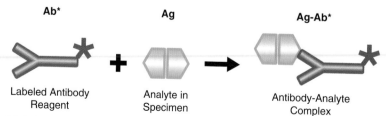

• **Figure 4-1** Labeled antibody (Ab*) binds with antigen (Ag), allowing detection of labeled antigen–antibody (Ag-Ab*) complexes in immunoassays. (Used with permission of Abbott Laboratories. All rights reserved.)

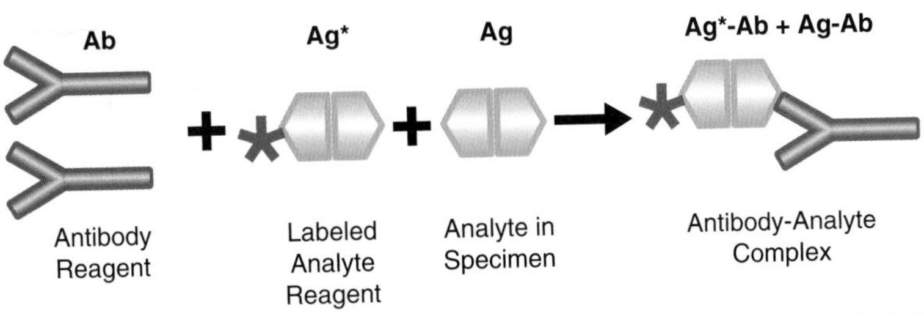

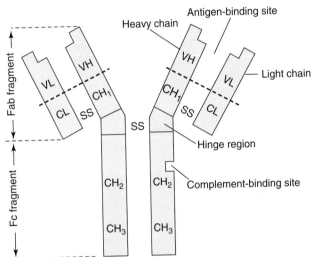

• **Figure 4-2** Antibody binds with both labeled antigen *(Ag*)* and unlabeled antigen *(Ag)*; the labeled antigen–antibody complexes can be separated and detected in immunoassays. (Used with permission of Abbott Laboratories. All rights reserved.)

Antibodies are immunoglobulins (Ig). The five classes of antibodies are IgG, IgA, IgM, IgD, and IgE. The antibody molecule is made up of a constant region and a variable region. The variable region binds to the antigen, and the constant region is responsible for biological activity by initiating the immune response. The structure resembles a Y, as seen in Figure 4-3. The heavy chains are located in the constant area of the antibody, and the light chains are located in the variable region of the antibody.

Affinity and Avidity

Antigen binds antibody through weak, reversible chemical interactions, and bonding is essentially noncovalent. Electrostatic interactions, hydrogen bonds, hydrophobic interactions, and Van der Waals forces are involved. **Affinity** refers to the strength of the bond between the antigen and the antibody. This interaction can be expressed as a reversible reaction, $[Ab] + [Ag] \rightleftharpoons [Ab\text{-}Ag]$, in which $[Ab]$ is the molar concentration of unoccupied binding sites on the antibody, $[Ag]$ is the molar concentration of unoccupied binding sites on the antigen, and $[Ab\text{-}Ag]$ is the molar concentration of the antibody–antigen complex. The affinity (association) constant, K_a, is expressed by the following formula:

$$K_a = \frac{[Ab - Ag]}{[Ab][Ag]}$$

K_a describes the amount of antigen–antibody complex that exists when there is equilibrium between association (i.e., binding) and dissociation (i.e., release). High-affinity antibodies can bind with more antigen than low-affinity antibodies can during a specified time. The affinity of an antibody for an antigen can be affected by environmental conditions such as pH and temperature.

Avidity describes the overall stability of an antibody–antigen complex. Avidity is based on affinity of the antibody for the antigen, the number of binding sites available, and the way the two molecules combine—factors that influence the binding reaction.

Polyclonal and Monoclonal Antibodies

Polyclonal antibodies are antibodies produced by different B-cell lineages against a specific antigen, with each

• **Figure 4-3** Structure of an antibody shows two light *(L)* and two heavy *(H)* polypeptide chains held together by disulfide bonds *(SS)*. The molecules have a variable *(V)* portion, a constant *(C)* portion, and flexible hinge region, which can be cleaved at this site by the enzyme papain in experimental studies. The variable portion or antibody-binding *(Fab)* region of the molecule binds with the antigen epitope. The fragment crystallizable *(Fc)* region interacts with cell surface receptors and complement. (From Price SA, Wilson LM. *Pathophysiology: Clinical Concepts of Disease Processes.* 6th ed. St. Louis: Mosby; 2003.)

antibody identifying a different epitope. The antibodies attach to different epitope sites on the same antigen (Fig. 4-4).

Monoclonal antibodies are antibodies that come from a single B-cell clone and are produced against one specific epitope of an antigen. Monoclonal antibodies usually do not cross-react to form large antibody–antigen complexes. One antibody usually attaches to one antigen epitope (Fig. 4-5).

The first generation of immunoassays used polyclonal antibodies to measure specific analytes. When producing antibodies for an immunoassay, a standard procedure is followed to produce an antiserum that allows an immunoassay to perform at a particular specificity and sensitivity level, although these levels often vary. After the antigen is prepared, it is purified so that only antibodies to the targeted antigen are produced. The purified antigen is then injected into a rabbit to produce a population of antibodies to the antigen. This population consists of heterogeneous subpopulations

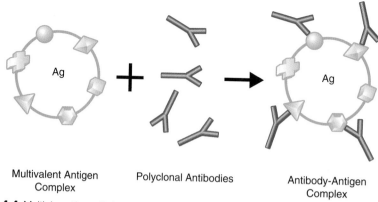

Multivalent Antigen Complex   Polyclonal Antibodies   Antibody-Antigen Complex

• **Figure 4-4** Multiple antigen *(Ag)* specificities of polyclonal antibodies. The shapes on the multivalent antigen represent different antigens on the multivalent antigen. Note that different polyclonal antibodies attach to different antigens. (Used with permission of Abbott Laboratories. All rights reserved.)

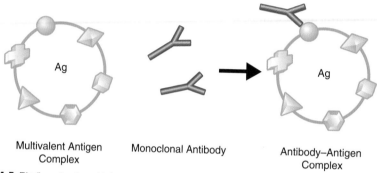

Multivalent Antigen Complex   Monoclonal Antibody   Antibody–Antigen Complex

• **Figure 4-5** Binding of antigen *(Ag)* to monoclonal antibodies. The different shapes on the multivalent antigen represent different antigens. Monoclonal antibodies are exactly the same; therefore, only one antibody attaches to one antigen on the multivalent antigen. (Used with permission of Abbott Laboratories. All rights reserved.)

of antibodies directed at individual epitopes on the antigens. After a specified time, the animal is checked for antibodies in its blood against the injected antibody. After antibodies are detected, the animal is bled. The serum is separated from the cells, and the generated antiserum is stored.

The antiserum varies from bleeding to bleeding and from animal to animal because the immune response in a particular animal at a particular time can modify the concentration, affinity, or specificity of the antibodies. A major disadvantage of using polyclonal antibodies in diagnostic assays is that cross-reactivity with unrelated molecules can occur.

In 1975, Cesar Milstein and George Kohler developed the monoclonal antibody technique. A monoclonal antibody is one that has been produced by a single B-cell clone. Antibody-producing B cells from mice sensitized to a particular antigen are fused with myeloma cells to form hybridomas (i.e., hybrid cell lines). The hybridoma is placed in a selective medium and grown in vitro. The clones that produce a large quantity of antibodies are grown in tissue culture. They are recloned as soon as possible to increase the amount of monoclonal antibodies produced. Hybridomas can be frozen for future use. This procedure produces homogenous antibodies that all recognize a single antigen epitope and with the same affinity. Because monoclonal antibodies are produced from a cell culture instead of live animals, an unlimited amount of near-identical antibodies is available (Fig. 4-6).

Immunochemical Methods

Heterogeneous Immunoassays

The distinguishing feature of heterogeneous immunoassays is that they require separation of the free labeled antigen from the bound labeled antigen in the solution (i.e., they involve a wash step) (Fig. 4-7). Widely used separation techniques include chemical or immunologic precipitation, liquid-phase adsorption, and solid-phase adsorption.

Chemical precipitation consists of adding a protein-precipitating chemical to the solution to precipitate the free labeled antigen. Immunologic precipitation consists of adding a second precipitating antibody to the solution. In liquid-phase adsorption, the free antigen is adsorbed onto charcoal added to the solution. All of these separation methods include centrifuging the specimen to remove the precipitin (i.e., antibody that forms a precipitate when it unites with its antigen) or the charcoal.

In the solid-phase adsorption, antibody binding to an analyte takes place on the surface of a solid support, such as the inner surface of plastic tubes or microtiter wells or the outer surface of cellulose beads, latex beads, or magnetic particles.

Homogenous Immunoassays

Homogenous immunoassays do not require separation of bound and free forms of labeled antibody or antigen (i.e., no wash step). The activity of the label is controlled by antibody binding to the analyte. These methods are used to quantitate drugs of abuse and therapeutic drugs. Because the antibody–antigen complexes do not need to be separated from the test solution, these assays are usually easier and faster to perform (Fig. 4-8).

Competitive Immunoassays

A competitive immunoassay is based on competition between the unlabeled analyte in the sample and the labeled antigen in the immunoassay. The analyte concentration is inversely proportional to the absorbance of the solution (Fig. 4-9). Less label measured in the assay means that more of the unlabeled antigen (i.e., test sample) is present. The radioimmunoassay was the prototype for the competitive immunoassay.

The competitive assay is performed in a one-step format or a two-step format. One-step competitive assays

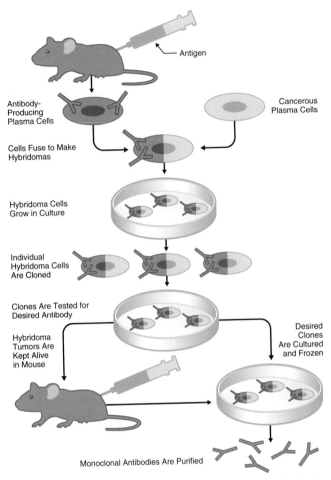

• **Figure 4-6** Monoclonal antibody production using cloned antibody-producing mouse hybridoma cells. (Used with permission of Abbott Laboratories. All rights reserved.)

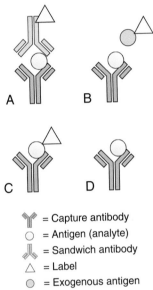

• **Figure 4-7** Various types of immunochemical methods. **A,** Sandwich method. **B,** Competitive method. **C,** Direct-label method. **D,** Label-free method.

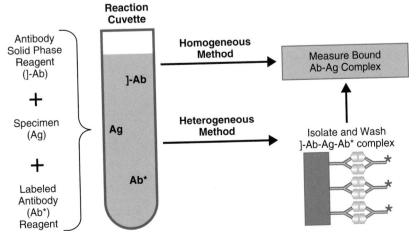

• **Figure 4-8** Schematic diagram of homogenous and heterogeneous competitive immunoassays. (Used with permission of Abbott Laboratories. All rights reserved.)

allow labeled antigen and the unlabeled sample to compete for a limited amount of antibody (Fig. 4-10). In two-step competitive assays, excess antibody is incubated with the sample in step 1, in which antibodies bind antigens in the sample. In step 2, labeled antigen is added to the solution from step 1. Any open antibody binding sites bind with the labeled antigen. Less bound labeled antigen indicates that there is a higher amount of antigen in the sample (Fig. 4-11).

Noncompetitive Immunoassays

Noncompetitive immunoassays have the highest level of sensitivity and specificity. These assays are used to measure cardiac markers and hepatitis markers. Similar to the competitive assays, the noncompetitive assays are performed in one- and two-step formats. The two-step format includes wash steps in which the sandwich binding complex (i.e., bound antibody and antigen) is isolated and washed to remove unbound labeled reagent (Fig. 4-12). After a labeled antibody specific for the antigen is added, the resulting complex of antigen sandwiched between antibodies can be detected by fluorescence microscopy. Measurement of the labeled antibody is directly proportional to the amount of antigen in the sample (Fig. 4-13). These tests are referred to as sandwich assays (Fig. 4-14).

Label Methods

The current field of immunochemistry can be divided into label methods, particle methods, and light-scattering methods. Labels are used in immunochemical assays to detect or quantify small quantities of clinically important substances. Labels are applied to antibodies or antigens (see Figs. 4-1 and 4-2). Types of labels include enzymes, fluorophores, luminophors, chemiluminescent compounds, and radio-isotopes. Labels are used to detect free antigen and antigen–antibody complexes, but labels cannot distinguish between free and bound antigens. The substance used for labeling must be easy to attach, easy to measure, noninterfering, inexpensive, and nontoxic. Table 4-1 lists the advantages and disadvantages of each type of label.

Early Methods: Radioimmunoassay and Enzyme Immunoassay

In the 1950s, Rosalyn Yalow and Solomon Berson developed radioimmunoassay (RIA) detection of insulin, and in 1977, they were award the Nobel Prize for their discovery. In the 1960s, radioisotopes were replaced with enzymes and

Inverse Relationship

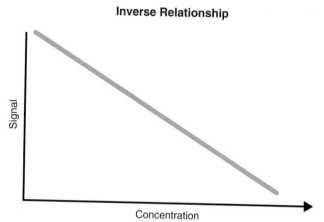

• **Figure 4-9** Signal versus concentration graph for a competitive immunoassay. (Used with permission of Abbott Laboratories. All rights reserved.)

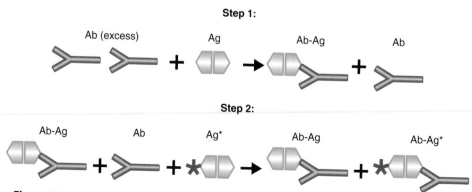

• **Figure 4-10** One-step competitive assay. *Ab,* Antibody; *Ag,* antigen; *Ag*,* labeled antigen. (Used with permission of Abbott Laboratories. All rights reserved.)

Step 1:

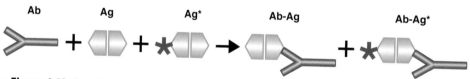

Step 2:

• **Figure 4-11** Two-step competitive assay. *Ab,* Antibody; *Ag,* antigen; *Ag*,* labeled antigen. (Used with permission of Abbott Laboratories. All rights reserved.)

Sandwich Assays: Antibodies bind to two sites on analyte

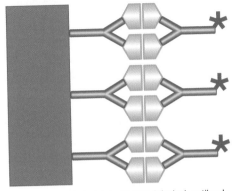

Solid Support:
microparticles
beads
microtiter plates

• **Figure 4-12** Sandwich assay. *Asterisk* indicates labeled antibody. (Used with permission of Abbott Laboratories. All rights reserved.)

Direct Relationship

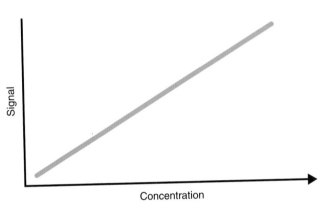

• **Figure 4-13** Signal versus concentration graph for noncompetitive immunoassays. (Used with permission of Abbott Laboratories. All rights reserved.)

color generation and were used as the detection method as opposed to radiation. This new method was called enzyme immunoassay (EIA). This method had faster reaction times and longer shelf lives of components than RIA. The technique was not applied in clinical laboratories for another 10 years, when personal computers became available for analyzing data. The use of enzyme immunoassays (EIAs) to quantitate hormones, drugs, and other analytes has grown dramatically since the 1970s.

Enzyme-Linked Immunosorbent Assay

In the enzyme-linked immunosorbent assay (ELISA) (Fig. 4-15), antibodies are absorbed to the surface of a solid phase, usually a microtiter plate well. Samples and standard solutions containing the antigen are added to the wells and then incubated. After incubation, the wells are washed, leaving the antibody–antigen complexes in the well. Enzymes are added, the wells are washed again, and a substrate is added. Absorbance of the wells is measured. Sample absorbance is inversely proportional to the analyte concentration. This technique is used to measure cytotoxins, hormones, antibodies, drugs, tumor markers, cardiac markers, and toxic substances.

Enzyme-Multiplied Immunoassay Technique

The enzyme-multiplied immunoassay technique (EMIT) (Fig. 4-16) is used primarily for quantitating therapeutic drugs and drugs of abuse. Drug in a sample (if any) competes with drug labeled with glucose-6-phosphate dehydrogenase (G6PD) for antibody binding sites. Binding of antibody to antigen inhibits enzyme activity, and

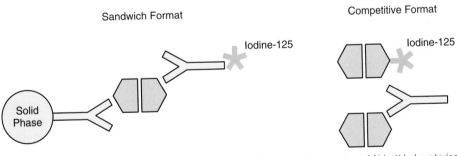

Sandwich Format

Competitive Format

Iodine-125

Iodine-125

Solid Phase

• **Figure 4-14** Sandwich format versus competitive format. (Used with permission of Abbott Laboratories. All rights reserved.)

TABLE 4-1 Test Advantages and Disadvantages

Label	Advantages	Disadvantages
Enzymes	Diversity, amplification, versatility	Lability, size, heterogenicity
Fluorophores	Size, specificity, sensitivity	Hardware, limited selection, background
Luminophors	Size, sensitivity	Hardware
Radioisotopes	Flexible, sensitive, size	Toxicity, shelf-life, disposal costs

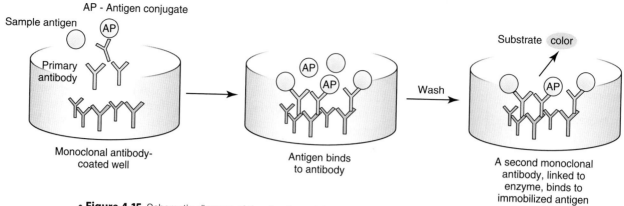

• **Figure 4-15** Schematic diagram of the direct sandwich method in an enzyme-linked immunosorbent assay (ELISA).

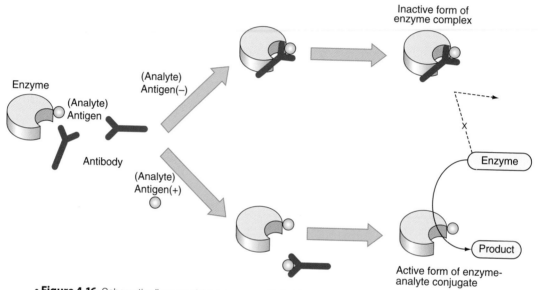

• **Figure 4-16** Schematic diagram of the enzyme-multiplied immunoassay technique (EMIT). (From Nakamura RM, Kasahara Y, Rechnitz GA, eds. *Immunochemical Assay and Biosensor Technology for the 1990s.* Washington, DC: American Society for Microbiology; 1992.)

higher concentrations of drug in the sample lead to higher concentrations of free enzyme. Only the free enzyme can convert the substrate to the product, and enzyme activity is directly proportional to the drug concentration in the sample.

Fluorescence Polarization Immunoassay

Fluorescence polarization immunoassay (FPIA) is a homogeneous, competitive immunoassay (Fig. 4-17). Labeled, antibody-bound antigen in the sample competes with labeled, free antigen for antibody binding sites. This method provides accurate and sensitive measurement of therapeutic drugs, abused drugs, toxic substances, and hormones. It was one of the first fully automated methods used to detect these analytes.

FPIA combines three principles to increase sensitivity and accuracy: fluorescence, rotation of molecules in solution, and polarized light (Fig. 4-18). Fluorescein is the label

of choice for this method; when the molecule is activated, it produces fluorescent light at a wavelength of 520 nm. The antibody–antigen–fluorescein molecules are large and rotate slowly in solution when excited by polarized light, whereas the smaller antigen–fluorescein molecules in the solution rotate rapidly. When the solution is exposed to polarized light, the smaller antigen–fluorescein molecules emit light in a different plane (520 nm) from that which was absorbed (490 nm). When the larger antibody–antigen–fluorescein molecule is exposed to polarized light, it emits light in the same plane as the absorbed light energy. There is an inverse relationship between the signal (i.e., light emission) and the concentration of analyte in the sample (Fig. 4-19). This technique is used in fetal lung maturity tests.

Microparticle Enzyme Immunoassay

The **microparticle enzyme immunoassay** (MEIA) uses the surface of small beads called microparticles to isolate

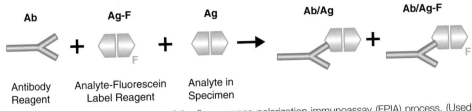

• **Figure 4-17** Schematic diagram of the fluorescence polarization immunoassay (FPIA) process. (Used with permission of Abbott Laboratories. All rights reserved.)

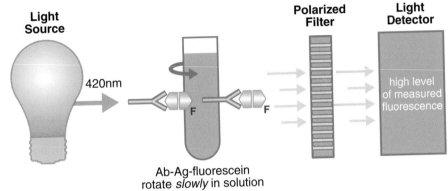

• **Figure 4-18** Detection schematic for fluorescence polarization immunoassay (FPIA). *Ab–Ag–fluorescein,* Fluorescein-labeled antibody–antigen complex. (Used with permission of Abbott Laboratories. All rights reserved.)

Chemiluminescent Microparticle Immunoassay

The **chemiluminescent microparticle immunoassay** (CMIA) uses a chemiluminescent compound to detect analytes. Chemiluminescent labels produce light when combined with a trigger reagent. The CMIA is similar to the MEIA in that both techniques use a noncompetitive sandwich assay to measure analytes. In this type of assay, the amount of analyte present in the sample is directly proportional to the intensity of the measured signal. In MEIA, the solid phase is latex microparticles, the separation step uses a glass fiber matrix, the label is alkaline phosphatase enzyme, and the detector is a fluorescence detector. In CMIA, the solid phase is a magnetic microparticle, separation is achieved with a magnet, the label is a chemiluminescent compound, and the detector is a chemiluminescence photomultiplier tube (Fig. 4-22).

CMIA is one of the most sensitive immunoassays. It measures antibodies and is useful for measuring antibodies to the human immunodeficiency virus (HIV).

Cloned Enzyme Donor Immunoassay

Cloned enzyme donor immunoassay (CEDIA) is a homogenous EIA. It was the first EIA designed with the use of genetic engineering techniques (Fig. 4-23). Inactive fragments of enzyme (β-galactosidase) and analyte are prepared using *Escherichia coli*. These two molecules automatically bind to form

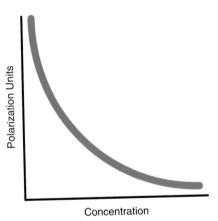

• **Figure 4-19** Signal dose-response curve for fluorescence polarization immunoassay (FPIA). (Used with permission of Abbott Laboratories. All rights reserved.)

antibody–antigen complexes (Fig. 4-20). The solid phase consists of latex particles coated with antibodies to the analyte being measured. The antibody–enzyme molecule consists of an antibody with alkaline phosphatase attached. The enzyme substrate is fluorescent 4-methylumbelliferone phosphate (4-MUP) (Fig. 4-21). This method is used to measure large molecules such as cardiac markers, fertility hormones, tumor markers, hepatitis antigens, thyroid hormones, and metabolic markers in an automated instrument.

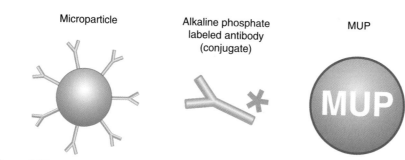

Microparticle   Alkaline phosphate labeled antibody (conjugate)   MUP

• **Figure 4-20** Components of the microparticle enzyme immunoassay (MEIA). *MUP,* 4-Methyl umbelliferone phosphate fluorescent substrate. (Used with permission of Abbott Laboratories. All rights reserved.)

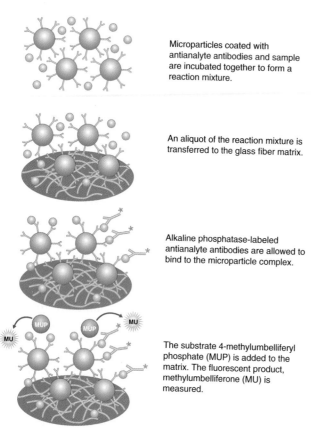

Microparticles coated with antianalyte antibodies and sample are incubated together to form a reaction mixture.

An aliquot of the reaction mixture is transferred to the glass fiber matrix.

Alkaline phosphatase-labeled antianalyte antibodies are allowed to bind to the microparticle complex.

The substrate 4-methylumbelliferyl phosphate (MUP) is added to the matrix. The fluorescent product, methylumbelliferone (MU) is measured.

• **Figure 4-21** Microparticle enzyme immunoassay (MEIA) method. (Used with permission of Abbott Laboratories. All rights reserved.)

an active enzyme. An antibody to the enzyme–donor antigen complex inhibits binding and renders the enzyme inactive. As with other immunoassays, a high antigen concentration produces a high-level signal, and low antigen concentration produces a low-level signal. This technique is used to measure therapeutic drugs and drugs of abuse (Table 4-2).

Particle Methods

Characteristics of particle methods include precipitation of an antigen–antibody complex, no labels, and qualitative and quantitative applications. Antibodies precipitate antigens through multivalent bonding, and a single antibody can bind more than one antigen. This results in a matrix of antigen–antibody complexes that precipitates from the solution.

The solubility of an antigen–antibody complex depends on particle size, charge, temperature, and ionic strength of the solvent. The solubility of the antigen–antibody complex follows a curve that has antibody excess on one end, antigen excess on the other end, and a zone of equivalence in which the precipitate is formed in the center (Fig. 4-24). In the area with excess antibodies, there is not enough cross-reactivity occurring to create an antigen–antibody complex. In the area with excess antigens, antigens attach to both binding sites in the antibody, preventing cross-reactivity and formation of the antigen–antibody complex. These concepts are applied in immunodiffusion techniques, immunoelectrophoresis (IEP), counterimmunoelectrophoresis, and Western blotting.

Immunodiffusion

Immunodiffusion is a laboratory technique that allows antigens and antibodies to diffuse through agar or agarose. It is used to determine relative concentrations, compare antigens, or determine the purity of a preparation. The technique does not use electricity to speed the reaction. The immunochemical concepts for immunodiffusion are the same as for antibody–antigen precipitation reactions that occur in the liquid state. Immunodiffusion techniques are more sensitive than liquid assays and therefore more widely used.

Methods that use passive diffusion include radial immunodiffusion, Ouchterlony double immunodiffusion, and the Laurell technique. The Western blot test uses electrophoresis to separate antibodies and labels to visualize them.

Radial Immunodiffusion

Radial immunodiffusion (RID) is used to determine the concentration of an antigen. An antibody is suspended in agar or agarose, a small well is punched in the medium, and a measured amount of antigen is added to the well (Fig. 4-25). The antigen diffuses into the medium from the well, after which the antibody–antigen complex precipitates, forming precipitin lines or circles that mark the zone of equivalence between the antibody and the antigen. The clarity and density of the precipitin lines or circles increase with time. The antigen's concentration is directly proportional to the area

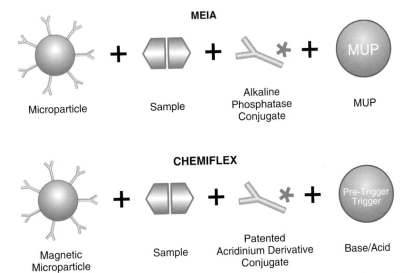

• **Figure 4-22** Microparticle enzyme immunoassay (MEIA) versus chemiluminescent microparticle immunoassay (CMIA). *MUP*, 4-Methyl umbelliferone phosphate fluorescent substrate. (Used with permission of Abbott Laboratories. All rights reserved.)

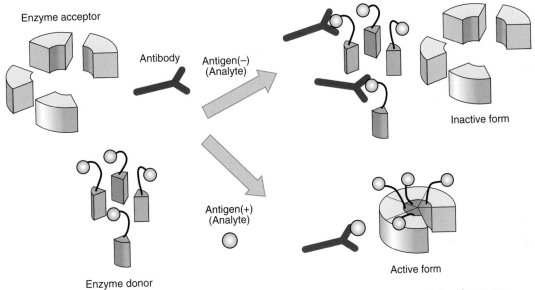

• **Figure 4-23** Cloned enzyme donor immunoassay (CEDIA). Enzyme acceptors associate with enzyme donors to form an active β-galactosidase tetramer. The antibody inhibits association of the enzyme acceptor with the enzyme donor–antigen conjugate. (With permission from Nakamura RM, Kasahara Y, Rechnitz GA, eds. *Immunochemical Assay and Biosensor Technology for the 1990s.* Washington, DC: American Society for Microbiology; 1992.)

TABLE 4-2	Labels	
Label Name	**Type of Label**	
Iodine-125 (^{125}I)	Radioactive	
Horseradish peroxidase	Colorimetric	
Alkaline phosphatase	Colorimetric	
β-Galactosidase	Colorimetric	
Fluorescein isothiocyanate	Fluorescent	
Isoluminal	Chemiluminescent	
Acridinium esters	Chemiluminescent	

of the circle and the square of the circle's diameter, whereas the antibody's concentration is inversely proportional to the measurement. Temperature affects only the speed of the diffusion, not the size of the circle at the end point.

Ouchterlony Double Immunodiffusion

Double diffusion is also called **Ouchterlony double immunodiffusion.** This technique was developed by Orjan Ouchterlony in 1948. The test is rarely used in current practice.

In the technique, the antigen and antibody are allowed to diffuse into the gel medium. This technique is used to test the similarity between antigens. Two separate samples

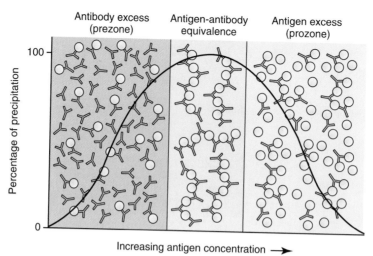

• **Figure 4-24** Antibody precipitation curve shows prezone (antibody excess) and prozone (antigen excess) regions. (Modified from Kaplan LA, Pesce AJ. *Clinical Chemistry: Theory, Analysis, Correlation.* 5th ed. St. Louis: Mosby; 2010.)

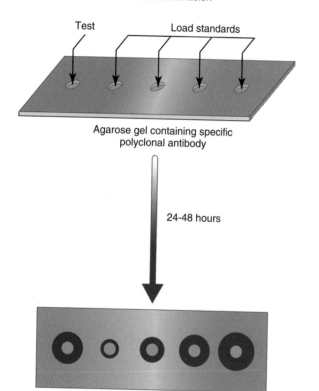

• **Figure 4-25** Measurement of immune-relate proteins by a radial immunodiffusion (RID). (From Peakman M, Vergani D. *Basic and Clinical Immunology.* 2nd ed. Edinburgh: Churchill Livingstone; 2009.)

containing antigens are loaded into the wells, and the known antibody is loaded into a third well located between and slightly below the antigen wells; the arrangement forms a triangle. The three possible results are identity, partial identity, and nonidentity (Fig. 4-26).

Laurell Technique

The Laurell technique, also called *rocket electroimmunodiffusion,* was developed by Carl-Bertil Laurell at Lund University in Sweden in 1966. It is a type of one-dimensional electro-immunodiffusion. This technique is an adaptation of radial immunodiffusion in which electrophoresis is used to move antigens out of the well and into the antibody-containing agar. As the antigen migrates out of the well, precipitin lines form and disappear until equilibrium is reached (Fig. 4-27). The resulting pattern is a precipitin spike that resembles the shape of a rocket. The height of the rocket is measured and is directly proportional to the amount of antigen in the sample.

This technique is used when the protein concentration is too low to be detected by nephelometry and too high to be measured by RID. Analytes commonly measured by this technique include α-fetoprotein, immunoglobulins in spinal fluid and urine, and complement in body fluids.

Immunoelectrophoresis

Immunoelectrophoresis was introduced by Graber and Williams in 1953. The technique uses electricity to enhance the double immunodiffusion technique by increasing the speed and specificity of the reaction. This technique is used for semiquantitation of antigens and is considered a qualitative technique. The method is a two-step process. First, antigens in the sample are separated by electrophoresis. Next, a trough is cut in the medium that is parallel to the electrophoresed antigens. Antisera are placed in the trough, and the medium is incubated for a day. The precipitin lines form at right angles to the separated antigens, developing where antigens and antibodies react (Fig. 4-28). These reactions are compared with control sera. Immunoelectrophoresis is commonly used to detect immunodeficiencies, complement deficiencies, and excess protein production; to identify monoclonal antibodies and urine proteins; and to assess antigen purity.

Counterimmunoelectrophoresis

Counterimmunoelectrophoresis (CIE) is used to evaluate antibody–antigen binding. An electrical field is applied across the diffusion medium, causing antigens and antibodies to rapidly migrate toward one another. When the two meet, a precipitin line forms. This technique can be used only when the antigens and antibodies have opposite charges. The qualitative technique typically is used to identify antinuclear ribonucleoproteins, although this is often done by fluorescence microscopy.

Western Blot

Most immunodiffusion techniques use immunoprecipitation to identify and determine the concentration of an analyte. Some media, such as polyacrylamide, do not allow precipitation of antibody–antigen complexes, and in some cases, the amount of antigen in a sample is so small that there are not enough antibody–antigen complexes to cause a visible precipitation line in the medium. The Western blot technique allows quantitation of antigen in both cases (Fig. 4-29).

The analyte first undergoes electrophoresis, and the separated proteins are transferred to a nitrocellulose strip or nylon membrane. The transfer process is called *electroblotting*.

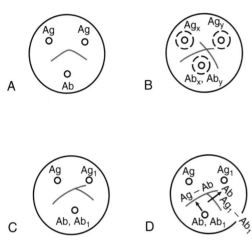

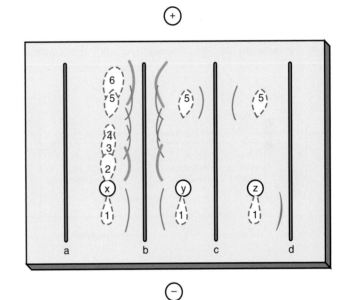

• **Figure 4-26** Ouchterlony double immunodiffusion result. A sample is placed in each antigen (Ag) circular well. Antibodies or serum is placed in each antibody (Ab) circular well. At the completion of the reaction, the Ag-Ab complex is visualized as a precipitated line. **A,** Reaction of identity. A single continuous line of precipitation is seen. The two samples have the same antigen (or antigens) recognized by the antibody placed in the Ab circular well; the samples are antigenically identical. **B,** Reaction of nonidentity. Two lines briefly overlap but appear to be independent. The two samples, Ag_x and Ag_y, are different antigens that react with their respective antibodies, Ab_x and Ab_y; no cross-reaction is seen. **C,** Reaction of partial identity. Two lines partially join and a spur is formed; the two samples (Ag and Ag_1) have some epitopes that overlap, but complete identity does not occur. **D,** Direct and cross-reactions with the antibodies Ab and Ab lead to spur formation. (From Burtis CA, Bruns DE. *Tietz Fundamentals of Clinical Chemistry and Molecular Diagnostics.* 7th ed. St. Louis: Saunders; 2015.)

• **Figure 4-28** Configuration for immunoelectrophoresis (IEP). Sample wells (*x, y,* and *z*) are punched in the agar/agarose medium, the sample is applied, and electrophoresis is carried out to separate the proteins in the sample. Antisera are loaded into the troughs (*a* through *d*), and the gel is incubated in a moist chamber at 4° C for 24 to 72 hours. Track *x* represents the shape of the six protein zones after electrophoresis; antiserum against proteins 1 through 6 is present in trough *b*. Tracks *y* and *z* show the reactions of proteins 5 and 1 with their specific antisera in troughs *c* and *d*, respectively. (From Burtis CA, Bruns DE. *Tietz Fundamentals of Clinical Chemistry and Molecular Diagnostics.* 7th ed. St. Louis: Saunders; 2015.)

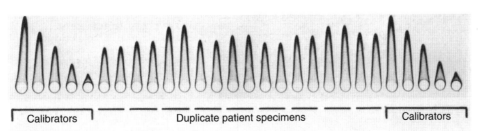

• **Figure 4-27** Laurell technique or rocket immunoelectrophoresis of human serum albumin. Patient samples were applied in duplicate. Calibrators were placed at opposite ends of the plate. (From Burtis CA, Bruns DE. *Tietz Fundamentals of Clinical Chemistry and Molecular Diagnostics.* 7th ed. St. Louis: Saunders; 2015.)

The proteins are then fixed to the membranes, and radioactive isotope or enzyme probes are used to detect the proteins. Concentrations that are 10 to 100 times smaller than those measured by immunodiffusion methods can be detected with this method.

Light-Scattering Methods

When antibody–antigen complexes are created in a liquid solution, the solution becomes cloudy. The light may be absorbed by the particles, transmitted unimpeded through the solution, or scattered in many directions. Turbidimetry and nephelometry are common laboratory methods that measure this light.

Turbidimetry

Turbidimetry techniques use spectrophotometers to measure the amount of light transmitted and the amount absorbed by suspended particles in a solution; these values are used to determine the amount of a substance in the sample. The amount of transmitted light that is absorbed depends on the number of particles in the solution and their size. Most often, absorbance of the solution is measured. Clinical applications for turbidimetry include protein determinations in urine or cerebrospinal fluid using trichloracetic acid and lipase determinations using triglycerides as the substrate.

Nephelometry

Nephelometry measures light scattered by particles in a solution to determine the amount of a substance in a sample. Nephelometry is less susceptible to interference from bilirubin and hemoglobin than similar approaches.

The components for a nephelometer are the same as for a spectrophotometer, except that the light detector is placed at a specific angle (90, 70, or 37 degrees) in relation to the solution (Fig. 4-30). The light detector is a photomultiplier

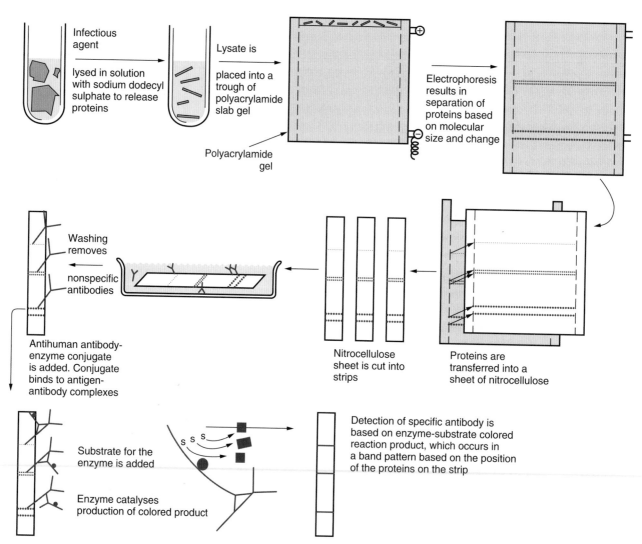

• **Figure 4-29** Western blot immunoassay. (From Turgeon ML. *Immunology and Serology in Laboratory Medicine.* 5th ed. St. Louis: Mosby; 2014. [Modified from Tille PM. *Bailey and Scott's Diagnostic Microbiology.* 13th ed. St. Louis: Mosby; 2014.])

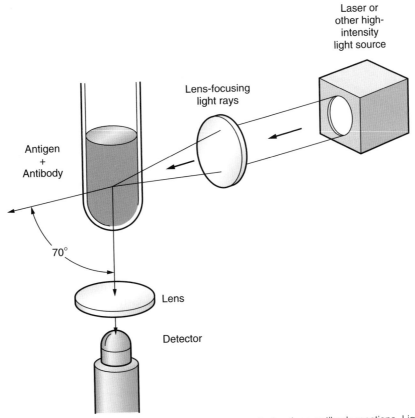

• Figure 4-30 Principle of nephelometry for the measurement of antigen–antibody reactions. Light rays are collected in a focusing lens and can ultimately be related to the antigen or antibody concentration in the sample. (From Turgeon ML. *Immunology and Serology in Laboratory Medicine.* 5th ed. St. Louis: Mosby; 2014.)

tube that detects forward light scatter, and its placement angle depends on the angle with the most scattered light. Nephelometry is more sensitive than turbidimetry because a cloudy solution scatters more light than it transmits.

The amount of light scattered by the particles in a solution depends on the size and number of particles in the solution. Laser light nephelometers can be used for higher sensitivity or in applications that determine the size and number of particles in solution. Clinical applications of nephelometry include quantitating serum proteins (e.g., haptoglobin, transferrin, C-reactive protein, α_1-antitrypsin) and immunoglobulins.

Factors Affecting Immunoassay Analytical Performance

Many factors can affect the outcome of immunoassays, including calibrators, controls, interfering substances, and other phenomena. These factors may also affect the outcome of chemical assays.

Calibrators

Calibrators contain known amounts of an analyte, and they establish the absorbance (in chemical tests) or the amount of signal produced (in immunoassays) for specific analyte concentrations. In chemical reactions, a calibration curve is generated using calibrators with known concentrations, and the curve is then used to determine concentrations in patient samples (unknowns) according to their absorbance (Fig. 4-31). In immunoassays, a dose-response curve is established to correlate certain values of signals to known analyte concentrations. The sample signal level is compared with the dose-response curve, and the amount of analyte in the sample is determined from this curve. If the dose-response curve is incorrect, the sample and control results will also be incorrect.

Calibrators must be handled according to the manufacturer's instructions, or an incorrect dose-response curve may result. Calibration is automated on modern immunoassay analyzers, and most are liquid, ready-to-use calibrators.

Immunoassays differ from manufacturer to manufacturer. Patient samples tested on one immunoassay may yield different results when tested for the same analyte on an immunoassay analyzer made by a different manufacturer. This can cause much confusion for physicians, especially if the medical decision levels (i.e., cutoffs) for the two immunoassays are different.

Discrepancies in test results can be caused by different antibody specificities of the two immunoassays or lack of calibration traceability. Manufacturers seldom use identical antibodies for their immunoassays, but they are increasingly

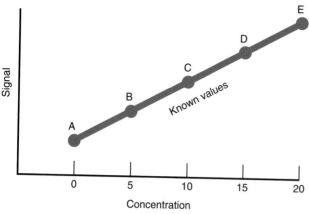

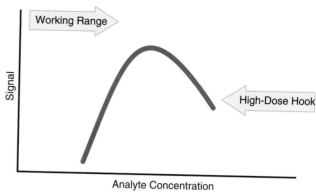

using reference materials recommended by the Joint Committee for Traceability in Laboratory Medicine (JCTLM). This international consortium identifies reference materials and methods that are suitable for calibration traceability purposes. If all manufacturers used these materials and methods, the variations in test results for different manufacturers' kits would decrease.

Controls

Controls are solutions of known concentration used to measure the accuracy and precision of an assay and analyzer. Controls are usually run periodically according to the manufacturer's instructions. Control values are plotted on a Levy-Jennings control chart, and Westgard control rules are used to analyze the results for outliers, trends, or shifts. Controls should be made of high-quality materials using a base matrix that mimics patient specimens. Controls should also follow the same traceability guidelines as calibrators.

Assay Interference

One-step immunoassays are more likely to experience interference with antigen–antibody binding due to agents that block binding. Heterophile antibodies are produced against poorly defined antigens, and they are generally weak. They can interfere with immunoassays by binding to antibodies used in the immunoassay, causing falsely elevated or falsely reduced results. Two-step assays are less prone to this type of interference because the free antigen or antibody and endogenous proteins are removed during the wash step. Two-step assays are used when there is a concern about heterophile antibodies being present in a patient sample.

High-Dose Hook Effect

The high-dose hook effect is usually seen when sandwich immunoassays are performed. Very high antigen concentrations in the patient sample bind to all available antibody binding sites, in both the antibody solid phase and the antibody-labeled conjugate. This prevents formation of the sandwich complex and causes a falsely decreased test result. This phenomenon gets its name from the shape of the dose-response curve when the data are plotted as signal versus analyte concentration (Fig. 4-32). In serology, this is referred to as a *prozone effect*.

Summary

Antibodies are produced by the body in reaction to antigens, but they can also be used to detect analytes in immunochemical assays. Polyclonal and monoclonal antibody production allows many types of assays to be used for detection. Antibodies are ideally suited for immunochemical techniques because they are specific and sensitive, allowing small amounts of antigen to be detected. Immunochemical techniques include particle methods, light-scattering techniques, and labeling methods. Specific assays include RID, Ouchterlony double immunodiffusion, Laurell technique, IEP, CIE, Western blot, turbidimetry, nephelometry, ELISA, MEIA, CMIA, RIA, EIA, EMIT, CEDIA, and FPIA (Table 4-3). Factors affecting immunoassay analytical performance include calibrators, controls, and interfering substances.

TABLE 4-3 Immunoassay Techniques

Name of Technique	Analyte Measured
Radioimmunoassay (RIA) (older, rarely used)	Hormones, drugs, proteins
Enzyme immunoassay (EIA) (older, rarely used)	Hormones, drugs, proteins
Enzyme-linked immunosorbent assay (ELISA)	Cytokines, hormones, antibodies, drugs, tumor markers, cardiac markers, toxins
Enzyme multiplied immunoassay technique (EMIT)	Therapeutic drugs, drugs of abuse
Cloned enzyme donor immunoassay (CEDIA)	Drugs
Fluorescence polarization immunoassay (FPIA)	Therapeutic drugs, drugs of abuse, toxic substances, hormones
Microparticle enzyme immunoassay (MEIA)	Cardiac markers, fertility hormones, tumor markers, hepatitis antigens, thyroid hormones, metabolic markers
Chemiluminescent microparticle immunoassay (CMIA)	Antibodies
Radial immunodiffusion (RID)	Concentration of antigens
Ouchterlony double immunodiffusion	Tests similarities of antigens
Laurell technique (rocket electroimmunoassay)	Antigens
Immunoelectrophoresis (IEP)	Semiquantitation of antigens
Counterimmunoelectrophoresis (CIE)	Identify antinuclear ribonuclear protein
Western blot	Antibodies and specific proteins
Nephelometry	Plasma proteins
Turbidimetry	Plasma proteins

Review Questions

1. All immunoassays require
   a. A chemiluminescent label
   b. The use of labeled material to detect the amount of antibody or antigen
   c. A wash cycle
   d. Monoclonal antibodies
2. In the two-step noncompetitive assay format, the wash step isolates
   a. The labeled antibody
   b. The labeled antigen
   c. The binding proteins
   d. The sandwich complex
3. Which of the following is the format that offers the highest specificity and sensitivity?
   a. One-step noncompetitive
   b. Two-step noncompetitive
   c. One-step homogenous
   d. Two-step competitive
4. Typical labels for ELISA tests include all of the following EXCEPT
   a. β-Galactosidase
   b. Alkaline peroxidase
   c. Alkaline phosphatase
   d. Horseradish peroxidase
5. Which of the following immunoassay types uses fluorescence, rotation of molecules in solution, and polarized light to quantitate analytes?
   a. CEDIA
   b. ELISA
   c. CMIA
   d. FPIA
6. Which of the following solid phase types is used by MEIA?
   a. Latex microparticles
   b. Magnetic microparticles
   c. Microtiter plates
   d. Inside wall of polystyrene tubes
7. Which of the following factors may interfere with the results of immunoassays?
   a. Cloned antibodies
   b. Heterophile antibodies
   c. Exogenous antigen
   d. Antibody–antigen complexes
8. What is the difference between a spectrophotometer and a nephelometer?
   a. There is no difference.
   b. The detector is placed at a 90-degree angle, and there is a forward scatter angle in the spectrophotometer.

c. The detector is placed at a 180-degree angle in the spectrophotometer.

d. The detector is placed at a 90-degree angle, and there is a forward scatter angle in the nephelometer.

9. Which of the following methods can detect analytes at concentrations 10 to 100 times smaller than those detected by immunodiffusion?
   a. Counterimmunoelectrophoresis
   b. Ouchterlony technique
   c. Western blot
   d. Laurell technique

10. Which of the following techniques is used when the protein concentration is too low to be detected by nephelometry and too high to be measured by radial immunodiffusion?
    a. Counterimmunoelectrophoresis
    b. Immunoelectrophoresis
    c. Laurell technique
    d. Western blot

Critical Thinking Questions

1. Explain the processes used to create polyclonal and monoclonal antibodies.

2. What is the high-dose hook effect, and why is it important?

CASE STUDY

An MLT was running adrenocorticotropic hormone tests. This test is an immunoassay that uses the sandwich methodology. A nurse called on the phone inquiring about one of the patient samples in the run. She said that they were testing a particular patient to see if they had an ectopic tumor. Normally, in individuals with ectopic tumors, the ACTH levels are very high.

The technician decided to run the patient sample straight and also a 1 to 10 dilution. At the end of the run, the technician checked the patient's results and found that the straight sample was 650 ng/mL, while the diuted sample was 975 ng/ml. Why is there such a large difference between the two results?

Bibliography

Abbott Laboratories. Learning guide: immunoassay. <http://www.drtanandpartners.com/wp-content/uploads/2014/05/learning_immunoassay.pdf> 2008 Accessed 28.06.15.

Bailey GS. Ouchterlony double immunodiffusion. In: *The Protein Protocols Handbook*. New York: Humana Press; 1996:749–752.

Burtis CA, Ashwood ER, Bruns DE. *Tietz Textbook of Clinical Chemistry and Molecular Diagnostics*. 5th ed. St. Louis: Elsevier Health Sciences; 2012.

Mancini G, Vaerman JP, Carbonara AO, Heremans JF, Peeters H. Protides of the biological fluids. In: *Proceedings of the 11th Colloquium*. Bruges, The Netherlands: Elsevier; 1963:370.

Ouchterlony O, Nilsson LA. In: Weir DM, ed. *Handbook of Experimental Immunology, vol 1: Immunochemistry*. 4th ed. Oxford, England: Blackwell Scientific; 1986:32.1–32.50.

Wild D, ed. *The Immunoassay Handbook: Theory and Applications of Ligand Binding, ELISA and Related Techniques*. 4th ed. Oxford: Newnes; 2013.

Wild G. Immunofluorescent techniques. In: *Bancroft's Theory and Practice of Histological Techniques*. New York: Churchill Livingstone; 2012:427.

Williams C, ed. *Methods in Immunology and Immunochemistry*. Vol. 1. St. Louis: Elsevier; 2012.

Wu AH. A selected history and future of immunoassay development and applications in clinical chemistry. *Clin Chim Acta*. 2006;369:119–124.

5

Molecular Diagnostics

DONNA LARSON

CHAPTER OUTLINE

OBJECTIVES

At the completion of this chapter, the reader will be able to:

1. Define the key terms.
2. State who discovered the double helix form of DNA and in what year.
3. Describe how information is transferred within the cell.
4. Describe the three components of the nucleotide.
5. Name the two types of nitrogenous heterocyclic bases and give two examples of each type.
6. Draw the structures for the five nitrogenous heterocyclic bases.
7. Describe how nucleotides bond in DNA structure.
8. Describe the rule for pairing of bases in DNA.
9. Describe the position of the hydrogen bonds in the DNA molecule.
10. Describe the two external helical grooves.
11. Draw the structures for DNA, mRNA, tRNA, and rRNA.
12. Describe the DNA in a chromosome.
13. Describe DNA replication.
14. Describe two substances needed for DNA replication.
15. Describe antiparallel DNA.
16. Explain DNA transcription and translation.
17. Describe the process of restriction fragment length polymorphism (RFLP) analysis.
18. Describe the process of polymerase chain reaction (PCR).
19. Explain the use of DNA probes, cloning, DNA microchips, and DNA microassays.
20. Describe the Southern blot test methodology and what it tests for.
21. Review the application of molecular diagnostics for testing and treatment of genetic and infectious diseases.

KEY TERMS

Anneal
Denaturation
DNA probe
Endonuclease

Enzyme
Helicase
Nucleotide
Polymerase chain reaction (PCR)

Polynucleotide
Primer
Restriction
Southern blot

Points to Remember

- DNA and RNA are composed of building blocks called nucleic acids.
- Nucleotides are composed of a sugar, a phosphate group, and a heterocyclic nitrogenous base.
- Adenine and guanine are classified as purines, whereas thymine, cytosine, and uracil are classified as pyrimidines.
- The covalent bonds between the phosphate group and the 3′ and 5′ carbons of the heterocyclic base form the "backbone" of the DNA and RNA molecules.
- Complementary bonding occurs when a free 3′ carbon at the end of one chain associates itself with a free 5′ carbon at the end of the other chain.
- Adenine and thymine bond together, and guanine and cytosine bond together; adenine will not bond with guanine or cytosine, and neither will thymine.
- RNA has three distinct forms: ribosomal RNA (rRNA), messenger RNA (mRNA), and transfer RNA (tRNA).
- The bases found in RNA are adenine, guanine, cytosine, and uracil.
- rRNA is an integral part of the ribosome.
- mRNA is produced at the DNA and migrates to the ribosome, where it serves as the template for synthesis of a specific protein.
- tRNA carries the amino acid to the codon on the mRNA molecule to synthesize a protein.
- Chromosomes contain all of the DNA for an organism, but the basic unit of inheritance is the gene.
- A gene is a sequence of DNA bases that occurs at a particular location on a chromosome.
- DNA produces an exact copy of itself through replication: The DNA separates at several locations, and replication occurs at all sites simultaneously, proceeding until the replication forks meet.
- The "central dogma" for life is DNA → RNA → protein.
- Transcription is the process of producing RNA from DNA to create proteins via protein synthesis.
- Transcription is not as complicated as DNA replication because the RNA molecule separates from the DNA after production and migrates to the ribosome to act as a template for protein synthesis.
- Translation or protein synthesis occurs when an mRNA molecule migrates to a ribosome and tRNA brings amino acids (dictated by the mRNA) to the ribosome so that they can be connected to each other by peptide bonds to form a protein molecule.
- The restriction fragment length polymorphism (RFLP) technique enables scientists to analyze DNA for definitive identification of an individual.
- Polymerase chain reaction (PCR) is a technique that uses thermal cycling to amplify or produce many copies of DNA in vitro.
- DNA probe assays are among the most sensitive and specific techniques to identify genes or specific DNA sequences in samples.
- Cloning is making an identical copy of a living being.
- DNA microarrays are single microscope slides that arrange tiny amounts (hundreds or thousands) of gene sequences on their surface to determine whether a gene is expressed more in a tumor than in tissue from a normal person, more in normal tissue than in a tumor, or equally in both samples.
- A Southern blot test is used to detect specific DNA sequences in samples.
- Structural abnormalities in chromosomes include deletions, duplications, translocations, inversions, and rings.
- One of the biggest diagnostic applications for molecular diagnostics is in the realm of infectious diseases.

Introduction

Molecular diagnostics is one of the newer areas in the clinical laboratory, and it is rapidly becoming an integral part of laboratory work. In 1953, Francis Crick and James Watson published a groundbreaking article on the double helix structure of deoxyribonucleic acid (DNA). This model was the culmination of the work of many scientists over many years. Some scientists studied how characteristics are passed from one generation to the next (heredity). Others worked on isolating chemical matter from the nucleus of cells. Still others exposed the chemical matter from the nucleus of cells to x-rays to investigate the structures of the nucleic chemicals. Little by little, scientists chipped away at the puzzle of how a chemical material encodes the instructions to produce a living organism. This chapter discusses the basic chemistry of nucleic acids, DNA, and ribonucleic acid (RNA); chromosomes; transcription; and the chemistry of life. This section also discusses clinical laboratory techniques that are used in molecular diagnostics and clinical applications for these techniques.

Nucleic Acid Structure and Function

Genetic information for each living organism is encoded within its DNA. This information is passed from the organism's DNA to its RNA to its proteins. DNA is passed from one organism to its offspring through DNA replication. RNA is also found in the nucleus of cells and plays an important role in DNA expression.

DNA and RNA are composed of building blocks called nucleic acids. Nucleic acids are found exclusively in the nucleus of cells. However, viruses—which do not have a nucleus, only a capsid—can contain either DNA or RNA. Nucleic acids have a specific structure and functions.

Nucleic Acid Structure

Nucleic acids are called **polynucleotides,** meaning that they are composed of a linear arrangement of many **nucleotides.** Each nucleotide is composed of a sugar, a phosphate group, and a heterocyclic nitrogenous base (Fig. 5-1). The sugar moiety differs in DNA and RNA molecules; it consists of deoxyribose in DNA and ribose in RNA. The five

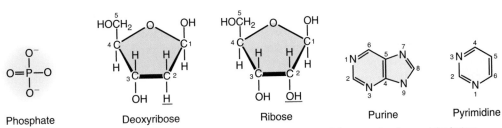

• **Figure 5-1** Atomic structures of a phosphate group, deoxyribose and ribose molecules, and the heterocyclic nitrogenous bases purine and pyrimidine.

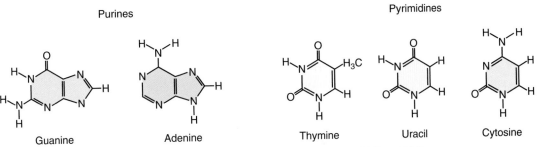

• **Figure 5-2** Structures of the five nucleotides found in DNA and RNA.

nucleotides found in DNA and RNA are adenine, guanine, thymine, cytosine, and uracil; adenine and guanine are classified as purines, whereas thymine, cytosine, and uracil are classified as pyrimidines. (See chemical structures in Figure 5-2.)

DNA and RNA Structure

Nucleotides are the building blocks of DNA and RNA. The chain of covalent bonds between the phosphate groups and the 3′ and 5′ carbons of the heterocyclic bases forms the backbone of DNA and RNA molecules (Fig. 5-3). This is considered the primary structure of DNA.

The secondary structure of DNA follows the Watson and Crick model in which two of these chains are wound together in helical fashion. The two chains are configured in an opposite manner—that is, the free 3′ carbon at the end of one chain associates itself with the end of the other chain containing a free 5′ carbon. This type of association is called complementary. In essence, the strands are running in opposite directions. When the strands associate themselves in this manner, the bases in the strand are turned toward the inside of the molecule and the backbone is on the outside. The bases that are paired on the inside form hydrogen bonds between the strands.

In DNA, the bases adenine and thymine bond together, and the bases guanine and cytosine bond together (Fig. 5-4). These are the only possible combinations: Adenine will not bond with guanine or cytosine, and neither will thymine. This order of pairing is important to note because, if the order of the bases in one strand of DNA is known, the order of bases in the "complementary" strand of DNA can be constructed from that information.

The base pairs in DNA and RNA are "stacked" one above the other on the inside of the molecule and are oriented perpendicular to the molecule's backbone.

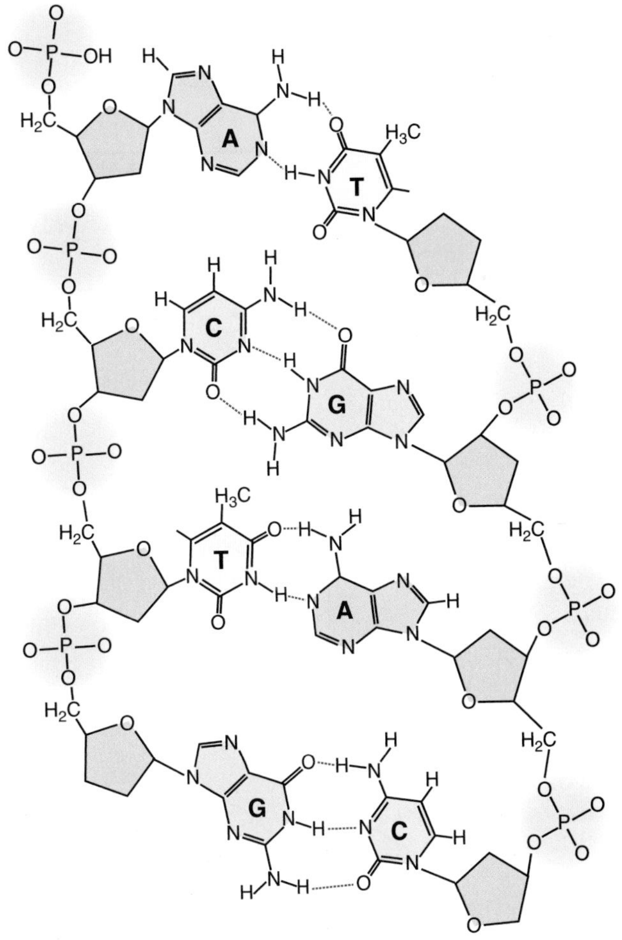

• **Figure 5-3** The chemical structure of DNA, showing the "sugar backbone." The nucleotides are adenine (A), thymine (T), guanine (G), and cystosine (C).

This is important because the backbone is polar and interacts with the liquid portion of the cell, whereas the bases on the interior of the molecule are hydrophobic and are not soluble in polar solvents. Therefore, the external backbone is the portion of the molecule that reacts with the solvent.

The DNA structure does not form a perfectly symmetric molecule (Fig. 5-5). Instead, the twists are elongated and skewed. The reason is that a combination of two purines would be too big, and a combination of two pyrimidines would allow large gaps in the helix.

Therefore, pairing of one purine with one pyrimidine is the most effective and efficient way for the helix to maintain an intact molecule.

Ribonucleic Acid

RNA plays an important role in biological functions and has three distinct forms: ribosomal RNA (rRNA), messenger RNA (mRNA), and transfer RNA (tRNA). The chemical makeup of RNA is similar to that of DNA and consists of a heterocyclic base, a ribose sugar molecule, and a phosphate group. As in DNA, the sugar establishes the

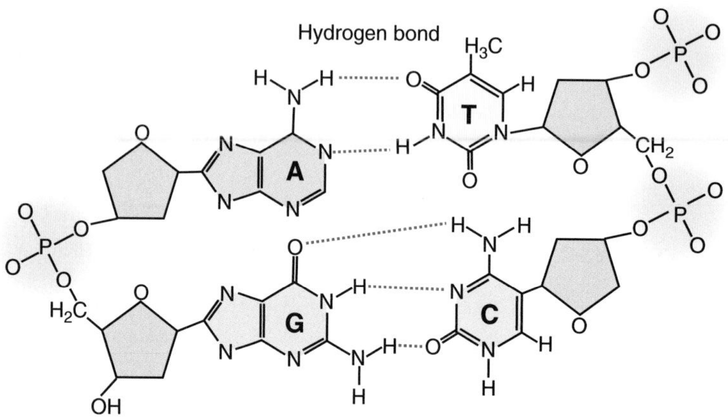

• **Figure 5-4** In DNA, hydrogen bonds are formed between thymine (T) and adenine (A) and between guanine (G) and cytosine (C).

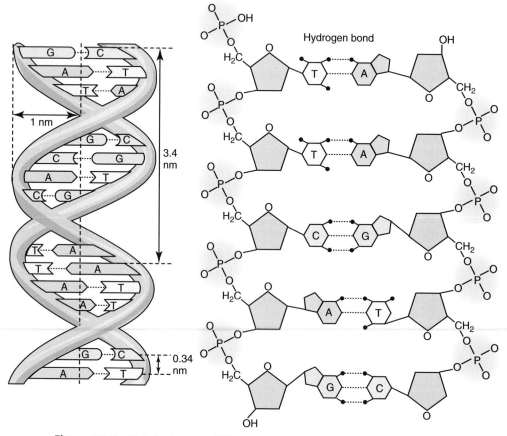

• **Figure 5-5** Double helix structure of DNA. *A*, Adenine; *C*, cystosine; *G*, guanine; *T*, thymine.

backbone of the molecule, forming phosphoester bonds between 3′ and 5′ carbons. The bases found in RNA are adenine, guanine, cytosine, and uracil.

Ribosomal RNA

rRNA is the type of RNA that is found in the ribosome, an organelle in the cytoplasm that serves as the site where protein synthesis occurs. A cell contains approximately 80% rRNA, 5% mRNA, and 15% tRNA.

Messenger RNA

mRNA plays an integral role in protein synthesis (Box 5-1). It is produced at the DNA and migrates to the ribosome, where it serves as the template for synthesis of a specific protein (Fig. 5-6). A different mRNA molecule is needed for synthesis of each protein. After a protein is synthesized, the mRNA is broken down and its nucleotides are reused.

Transfer RNA

tRNA functions as a transporter for amino acids during protein synthesis. tRNA carries to the codon on the mRNA molecule the appropriate amino acid that is needed at that point to synthesize a protein (Fig. 5-7).

• BOX 5-1	Components Necessary for Protein Synthesis

mRNA
tRNA
Large ribosomal unit
Small ribosomal unit
Codons

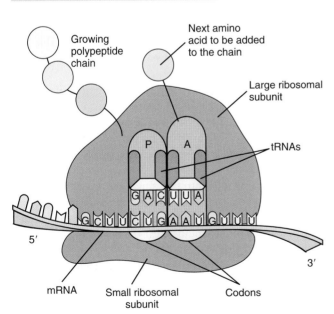

• **Figure 5-6** Protein synthesis at the ribosome. The P-site holds growing polypeptide chain. The A-site is where new amino acids enter. *A,* Adenine; *C,* cytosine; *G,* guanine; *mRNA,* messenger RNA; *tRNA,* transfer RNA; *U,* uracil.

Chromosomes

Chromosomes are the structures that contain all of the DNA in a cell. A chromosome is made by supercoiling of the long DNA helix. It twists and twists until coils start to form. Once the DNA is supercoiled, it wraps around proteins called histones. These DNA-wrapped proteins (nucleosomes) are densely compacted together into the structure called a chromosome (Fig. 5-8).

Chromosomes are not visible in the cell's nucleus until the cell begins to divide. A chromosome has two sides that are joined together by a centromere. The chromosome resembles an asymmetric letter X with two sets of arms—on each side there is a shorter *p arm* and a longer *q arm*. The centromere (center area of attachment) can also be used as a marker to locate specific genes on a chromosome.

Humans have 23 pairs of chromosomes for a total of 46 chromosomes. Twenty-two of the chromosomes are autosomes and look the same in males and females. The twenty-third pair is the sex chromosome, which looks different in males and females (Fig. 5-9).

Chromosomes contain all of the DNA for an organism, but the basic unit of inheritance is the gene. Genes are those DNA sequences that control the inheritance of specific characteristics of a species. The genes are designated as specific portions of the DNA contained in a chromosome. Humans have approximately 23,000 genes, and each gene is

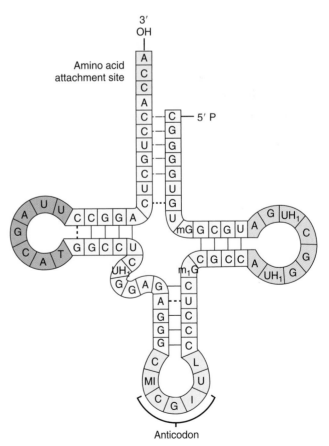

• **Figure 5-7** A transfer RNA molecule. *A,* Adenine; *C,* cytosine; *G,* guanine; *U,* uracil.

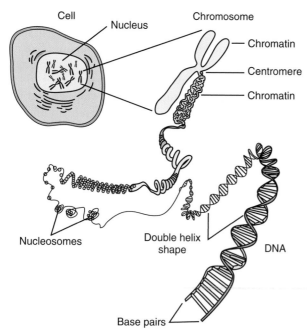

• **Figure 5-8** A chromosome: DNA begins as a double helix and it supercoils into a strand that then wraps around histones. DNA wrapped around a histone is called a *nucelosome*. The nucleosomes continue to coil into thicker coils. The thicker coils form a chromosome.

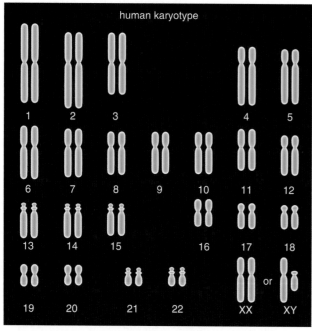

• **Figure 5-9** Normal human karyotype. Note that the pair of sex chromosomes is usually *XX* or *XY*. (© isomersault18:24/iStock.)

a sequence of DNA bases that occurs at a particular place in a chromosome. The National Human Genome Project has sequenced the DNA in each human chromosome.

Sequencing all the DNA in the human chromosomes was no small task. There are 3 billion bases in human DNA. To put this into perspective, if each base were identified by a letter (A, G, U, or T) and printed on one piece of paper, the stack of paper for 3 billion bases would be as tall as

the Washington Monument! Now, scientists are working to identify genes and diseases that can be linked to gene mutations. Mutations can occur when DNA replicates itself before a cell divides and at other times.

DNA Replication and Repair

DNA Replication

DNA provides everything an organism needs to carry its species and individual characteristics to its offspring. Every time a cell divides, identical copies of the cell's DNA are synthesized and passed on to its daughter cells.

DNA produces an exact copy of itself through *replication*. Replication is a complex and incompletely understood process. For DNA to replicate, the chromosome must unwind, and each strand must serve as a template for a new complementary strand. However, an entire strand of DNA cannot completely unwind and separate during cell division. Instead, the DNA separates from its opposite strand at several locations, and replication occurs at all of these sites simultaneously, proceeding until the replication forks meet (Fig. 5-10). The final product is two new double-stranded DNA molecules—each of which contains one strand of the old DNA. This is called semiconservative replication.

Factors in the replication of DNA include the following:
- Energy is required to unwind the helix.
- Single-stranded DNA tends to form intrastructure base pairs.
- DNA has an antiparallel or complementary structure.
- Systems are in place to help minimize errors during the replication process.
- The DNA molecule is very long compared to the size of a cell.
- Unwinding of DNA presents a mechanical problem.

The two helixes of a DNA molecule are wound together and must revolve around each other at the unwinding fork. The unwinding must be compensated for somewhere down the molecule, and the result is supercoiling. This step requires energy because the hydrogen bonds between the bases must be broken for it to occur.

DNA replication proceeds through a number of steps:
1. An **enzyme** called a DNA gyrase enters a small area in the DNA helix and separates the two strands a bit.
2. An enzyme called a DNA **helicase** begins to unwind the molecule where it was separated by the DNA gyrase (Fig. 5-11).
3. The helix unwinds into two single strands of DNA for a small distance along the DNA molecule. To keep the two strands separated, single strand–binding proteins attach to each side of the strands, near the beginning of the replication fork (Fig. 5-12).
4. Short pieces of RNA called **primers** attach to the leading and the lagging DNA strands.
5. DNA polymerase elongates the primers by adding new nucleotides to the 3′ end of the strand (see Fig. 5-12). Nucleotides pair with complementary nucleotides: adenine with thymine and guanine with cytosine.

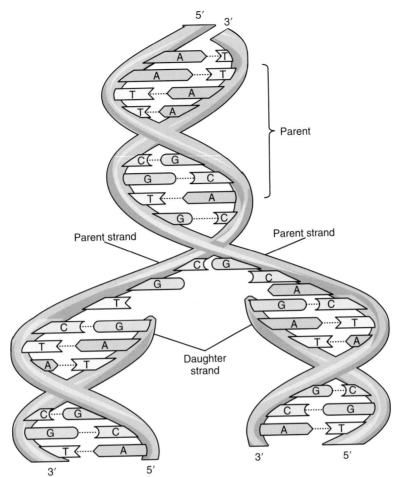

5′ 3′

A ⋯⋯ T
A ⋯⋯ T
T ⋯⋯ A
T ⋯⋯ A

Parent

C ⋯⋯ G
G ⋯⋯ C
T ⋯⋯ A
G ⋯⋯ C

Parent strand   Parent strand

C ⋯⋯ G
G   C
                                          A
T   G ⋯⋯ C
C ⋯⋯ G   A ⋯⋯ T
T ⋯⋯ A   T ⋯⋯ A
A ⋯⋯ T

Daughter
strand

C ⋯⋯ G
G ⋯⋯ C   G ⋯⋯ C
T ⋯⋯ A   C ⋯⋯ G
                                          A ⋯⋯ T

3′   5′   3′   5′

• **Figure 5-10** The products of replication are two daughter molecules.

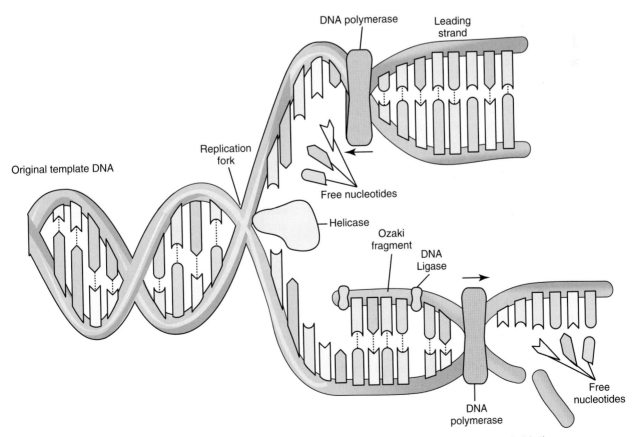

DNA polymerase   Leading
                                     strand

Replication
fork

Original template DNA

Free nucleotides

Helicase

Ozaki
fragment   DNA
                    Ligase

DNA
polymerase   Free
                     nucleotides

• **Figure 5-11** Initiation of DNA replication. DNA must separate in order to replicate. Helicase holds the strand open as the DNA polymerase carries out replication.

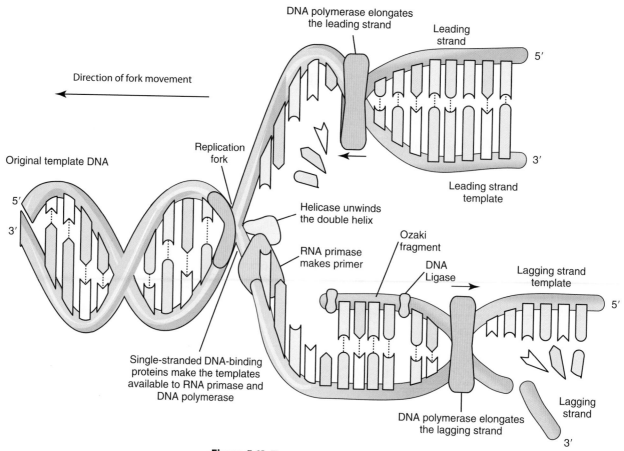

Direction of fork movement

DNA polymerase elongates
the leading strand

Leading
strand

5′

3′

Leading strand
template

Replication
fork

Original template DNA

5′

3′

Helicase unwinds
the double helix

Ozaki
fragment

RNA primase
makes primer

DNA
Ligase

Lagging strand
template

5′

Single-stranded DNA-binding
proteins make the templates
available to RNA primase and
DNA polymerase

Lagging
strand

3′

DNA polymerase elongates
the lagging strand

• **Figure 5-12** The process of DNA replication.

6. When the DNA polymerase has completed a small portion of the DNA replication, it removes the RNA primer and replaces it with DNA.
7. Ligase joins the short DNA fragments on the newly replicated DNA molecule together until the new molecule is an exact copy of the parent DNA strand.
8. The new strands automatically wind back up.

This process, in which the DNA in a cell is replicated in such a way that daughter cells are produced with the same exact complement of DNA, is important for life. In addition, RNA and proteins must be produced. Because most of the body is composed of proteins put together in a particular way, creation of proteins is very important. The "central dogma" for life is DNA → RNA → protein.

Transcription

Transcription is the process of producing RNA from DNA for the purpose of synthesizing proteins (Fig. 5-13). As discussed earlier, rRNA is found in the ribosomes of the endoplasmic reticulum. The ribosomes are the site for protein synthesis. mRNA molecules migrate to the ribosomes and act as a coded template for the production of proteins. rRNA is an integral piece of the ribosome and is part of that tissue. rRNA is an enzyme that catalyzes the production of peptide bonds.

DNA is used as the template for transcription. Transcription is not as complicated as DNA replication because the

RNA molecule (i.e., mRNA) separates from the DNA after production and migrates to the ribosome to act as a template for protein synthesis (Fig. 5-14).

The steps for transcription include the following:
1. Helicase enzymes separate the DNA strands in a particular area of the helix to expose unpaired DNA nucleotides. (Recall that particular areas of the DNA helix, called genes, encode for specific proteins.)
2. RNA polymerase attaches to the unpaired DNA nucleotides on one strand and adds matching RNA nucleotides to produce a complementary strand of RNA. (Recall that DNA bases include guanine, cytosine, adenine, and thymine, whereas RNA bases include guanine, cytosine, adenine, and uracil.) The RNA polymerase will add a uracil, instead of adenine, when it encounters a thymine base on the DNA strand.
3. RNA polymerase also aids in the formation of the RNA sugar-phosphate backbone while the mRNA molecule is being created.
4. The hydrogen bonds holding the RNA and the DNA strand together during the process break after production of the mRNA molecule is complete. This allows the newly synthesized mRNA strand to migrate.
5. The mRNA is slightly modified as it moves through the nucleus and enters the cytoplasm on its way to the endoplasmic reticulum and ribosome. The resulting mRNA includes the code for the protein as well as other regulatory codes at the beginning and end of the molecule.

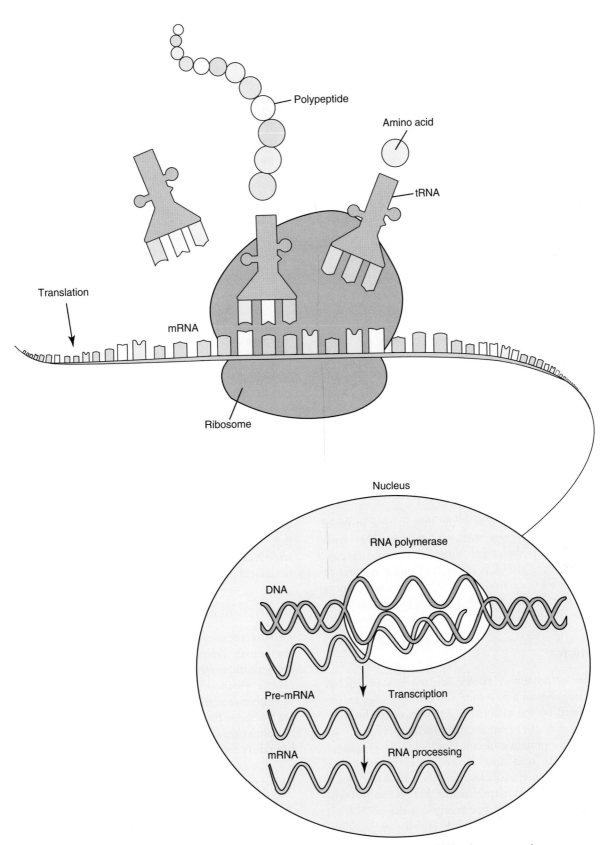

• **Figure 5-13** Production of messenger RNA: transcription and translation. The RNA polymerase creates pre-mRNA strands from the DNA template. The pre-mRNA molecule is processed into the usable mRNA molecule. The mRNA molecule travels out of the nucleus to the ribosome where it is the template for protein synthesis (translation).

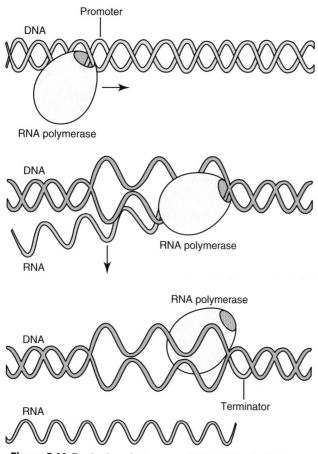

• **Figure 5-14** Production of messenger RNA: initiation (top), elongation (middle), and termination (bottom).

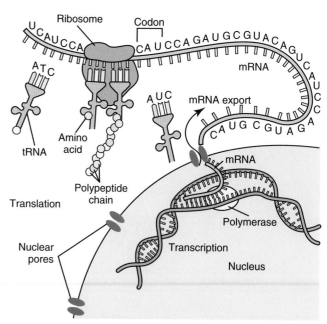

• **Figure 5-15** Relationship between transcription and translation. Transcription takes place in the nucleus, after which the mRNA is transported from the nucleus to the ribosome, where translation occurs. *A,* Adenine; *C,* cytosine; *G,* guanine; *mRNA,* messenger RNA; *tRNA,* transfer RNA; *U,* uracil.

tRNA is another RNA molecule that is used to make proteins. tRNA molecules transport specific amino acids to the ribosome in the correct order to allow a polypeptide chain to form. tRNA is made in a similar manner to mRNA, but after transcription the tRNA folds into a more compact molecule than mRNA. RNA molecules are at the heart of the process of making a protein or translation.

Translation

Translation, or protein synthesis, occurs when an mRNA molecule migrates to a ribosome and tRNA brings amino acids (dictated by the mRNA base sequence) to the ribosome so that they can be connected to each other by peptide bonds to form a protein molecule (Fig. 5-15). The sequence on the mRNA is "read" in groups of three nucleotides, or codons, each of which codes for a specific amino acid. Each tRNA has a codon sequence that matches (is complementary to) that of the mRNA. For example, if the mRNA has the three bases guanine, cytosine, and guanine in its codon, then the matching tRNA will have cytosine, guanine, and cytosine in its codon. Also, any adenine nucleotide sequence on the mRNA will be matched with uracil (rather than thymine) on the tRNA.

As the tRNA molecules read the mRNA and work along the mRNA chain, specific amino acids are added to the growing polypeptide chain in a specific order that determines the particular protein that is created. Because RNA contains 4 nucleotide bases, there are 64 possible codons. Three of those 64 codons are termination or stop codons, which end protein synthesis, and 61 codons code for 20 different amino acids. When the end of the mRNA chain is reached, the mRNA is disconnected from the ribosome, and so is the protein. The mRNA moves to another ribosome to complete another protein chain, and the protein is folded and assembled into a functional protein at other cell organelles.

Restriction Enzymes and Nucleases

Restriction enzymes are enzymes found in bacteria that cut human DNA at specific locations (Fig. 5-16). They are very important in recombinant DNA technology and genetic engineering. These enzymes break the hydrogen bonds between the bases and the phosphoester bonds holding the sugar backbones together. The fragments produced by restriction enzymes can be identified by many different laboratory methods.

Laboratory Methods

There are many laboratory methods to identify DNA. This section covers the more prevalent techniques. Some methods are a combination of several different techniques.

Restriction Fragment Length Polymorphism

The restriction fragment length polymorphism (RFLP) technique (Fig. 5-17) enables scientists to analyze DNA to

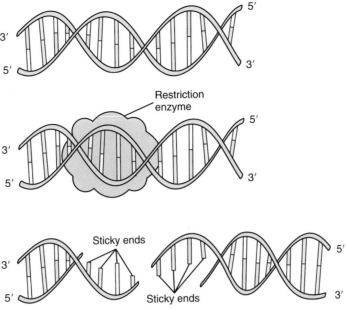

• **Figure 5-16** Action of a restriction enzyme.

make a definitive identification of an individual. For this method, the sample DNA is cut into small fragments by endonucleases. The procedure calls for use of more than one type of endonuclease so that DNA fragments of different lengths are produced. It is important to note that each set of fragments is unique to the individual. These DNA fragments are separated by gel electrophoresis to reveal the characteristic pattern for that individual.

Polymerase Chain Reaction

Kary Mullins created the polymerase chain reaction (PCR) technique in 1983 (Fig. 5-18). This method uses thermal cycling to amplify or produce many copies of DNA. The following materials are needed to amplify DNA by the PCR technique: DNA to be amplified, two primers (3′ and 5′), polymerases, nucleotides, buffer, and magnesium and potassium ions. The PCR procedure is straightforward:

1. Denaturation step—Heat the solution containing DNA to 94° C to 98°C for 20 to 30 seconds. This separates the double-stranded DNA by breaking the hydrogen bonds between the nucleotides.
2. Annealing step—Lower the reaction temperature to 50° C to 65°C for 20 to 40 seconds. This allows the primers to anneal to the single-stranded DNA template. Once the primers anneal, the polymerase begins DNA formation.
3. Extension/elongation step—The optimum temperature is that at which the polymerase is most active. For most procedures, this temperature is 72°C. The time required for this step depends on the polymerase and the length of the DNA template. A good estimate is that the DNA polymerase will polymerize 1000 bases per minute. Theoretically, if there were no limiting

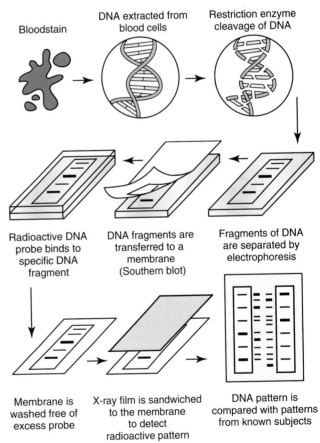

• **Figure 5-17** Steps in restriction fragment length polymorphism analysis.

factors (such as bases or polymerases), the amount of the target DNA in the solution would be doubled by each PCR cycle.

The cycle described in steps 1 through 3 is repeated to produce the amount of DNA needed.

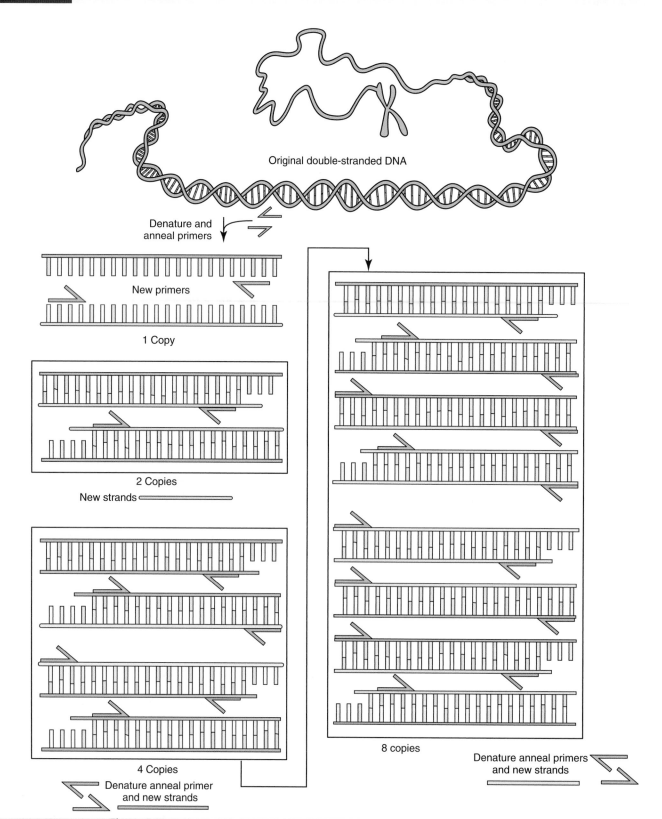

• **Figure 5-18** Polymerase chain reaction. The number of copies increases exponentially; after 20 to 30 cycles, many millions of copies will have been produced.

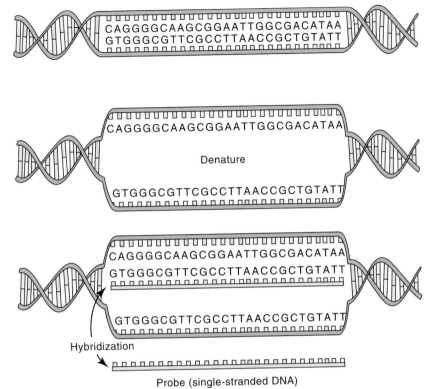

• **Figure 5-19** Hybridization. The single-stranded DNA probe bonds to a complementary segment in the DNA being tested. *A*, Adenine; *C*, cytosine; *G*, guanine; *T*, thymine.

4. Final elongation—To ensure that all of the single-stranded DNA has been amplified, the solution remains at 70° C to 74°C for 5 to 15 minutes after the last PCR cycle.

5. Final hold—To preserve the DNA produced through PCR, hold the solution at 4° C to 15° C for an indefinite period (short-term storage).

Great quantities of DNA can be produced by following this simple method. It is usually performed on equipment that can maintain the timing and temperature within small tolerances. These devices can be small enough to sit on a benchtop.

DNA Probes

DNA probes are small segments of DNA that are designed to attract other complementary pieces of DNA in a biological system (Fig. 5-19). These assays are among the most sensitive and specific techniques to identify genes or specific DNA sequences. The small segment of DNA is usually attached to a mounting structure. The single-stranded DNA probe attaches to the structure on one end, leaving the other end free to bond to complementary strands of DNA in the solution.

The general procedure for DNA probes includes the following steps:

1. Treat the sample to be tested with detergents and enzymes to remove non-DNA materials.

2. Denature the DNA using acid solutions.

3. Place the solution containing the denatured DNA onto the probe structure. The exposed probe DNA will hybridize with a complementary strand of single-stranded DNA in the solution.

4. The unbound DNA is detected by various methods such as fluorescence.

Cloning

The term *cloning* refers to making an identical copy of a living being. Cloning uses the DNA from a living being, copies it, and makes an identical living being from the copied DNA. There are three different types of cloning: gene cloning, reproductive cloning, and therapeutic cloning (Figs. 5-20 and 5-21). Gene cloning creates clones of genes or DNA segments; reproductive cloning creates clones of whole animals; and therapeutic cloning creates clones of embryonic stem cells. All types of cloning are ethically and socially controversial.

DNA Microchip

DNA microchip techniques are new tools used to identify mutations in genes. The chip consists of a small glass plate encased in plastic that resembles a microchip. The surface of the chip contains thousands of short single-stranded DNA pieces that, when added together, compose the normal gene in question. This is currently only a research tool.

A sample is drawn from an individual who may possess a gene mutation. The sample is run in tandem with a sample

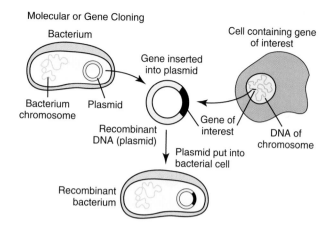

Molecular or Gene Cloning

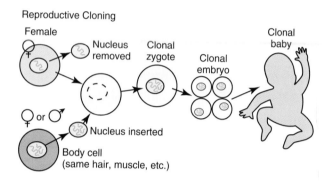

Reproductive Cloning

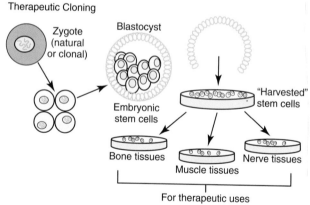

Therapeutic Cloning

• **Figure 5-20** Types of cloning: molecular or gene cloning, reproductive cloning, and therapeutic cloning.

that does not have the mutation. The DNA is denatured into single-stranded molecules. The long DNA molecules are cut into smaller fragments by restriction enzymes, and then each small fragment is labeled with a fluorescent dye. Usually, the patient's DNA is labeled with one color (e.g., red) and the normal control with another color (e.g., green). Both sets of DNA are inserted into the chip and allowed to hybridize. If the patient does not have a mutation, both the red and green samples will bind to the DNA on the chip. If the patient does have a mutation, the patient's DNA will not bind properly where the mutation is located. Further examination is then needed to confirm the presence of a mutation.

DNA Microarray

DNA microarrays are single microscope slides that arrange tiny amounts of hundreds or thousands of gene sequences on their surface (Figs. 5-22 and 5-23). Sanger sequencing uses different colored fluorescent labels and capillary electrophoresis to determine a DNA sequence. Scientists attach different colored fluorescent nucleotides to samples from the patient's tumor. If a gene is very active, there will be a very bright fluorescence in the area of that gene. Some genes are not quite as active and produce a dimmer fluorescent area. Sometimes there is no fluorescence because the gene is inactive. Scientists combine the tumor and normal (control) samples together to determine whether a gene is expressed more in the tumor than in normal tissue, expressed more in normal than in tumor tissue, or equally expressed in both samples.

Southern Blot

A Southern blot test is used to detect specific DNA sequences in samples (Fig. 5-24). DNA fragments are separated by electrophoresis, then transferred to a filter membrane where the fragments are detected by DNA probes.

The Southern blot procedure includes the following steps:

1. Restriction endonucleases cut DNA strands into fragments.
2. Electrophoresis on agarose gel separates the fragments by size.
3. A sheet of nitrocellulose membrane is placed onto the agarose gel containing the DNA fragments. Capillary action moves the DNA to the membrane, and ionic interactions allows the DNA to bind to the membrane. (DNA is negatively charged, and the membrane is positively charged.)
4. The membrane is baked in an 80° C oven for 2 hours to permanently attach the DNA to the membrane.
5. The membrane is exposed to a DNA probe.
6. The excess probe is washed from the membrane, and the pattern of hybridization is examined.
7. The pattern reveals the sequence of the DNA fragments present in the original sample.

Diagnostic Applications

Genetic Disease

Genetic diseases can be produced by an abnormal number of chromosomes or by an abnormality in a chromosome's structure. Abnormal number may occur if one of a specific pair of chromosomes in an individual is missing (monosomy) or if one of a pair is present in duplicate (trisomy). An example of monosomy is Turner syndrome, in which a female is born with only one X chromosome instead of two. Trisomy 21 is known as Down syndrome: The individual is born with three copies of chromosome 21 rather than two.

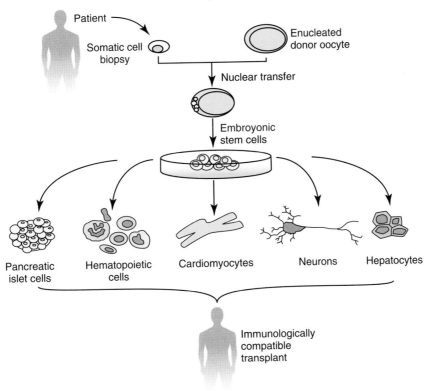

Human Therapeutic Cloning

Patient

Somatic cell biopsy

Enucleated donor oocyte

Nuclear transfer

Embryonic stem cells

Pancreatic islet cells

Hematopoietic cells

Cardiomyocytes

Neurons

Hepatocytes

Immunologically compatible transplant

• **Figure 5-21** Therapeutic cloning can be used to treat a variety of conditions in humans.

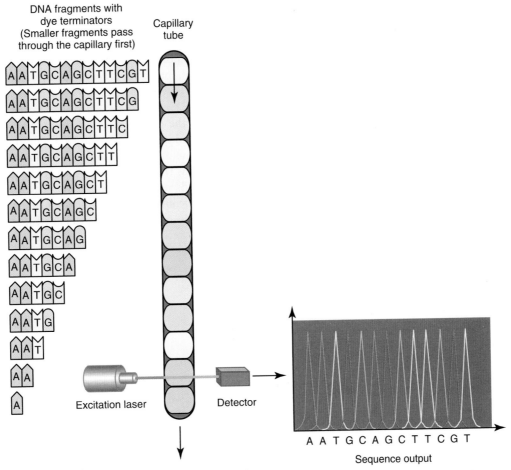

DNA fragments with dye terminators (Smaller fragments pass through the capillary first)

Capillary tube

AATGCAGCTTCGT
AATGCAGCTTCG
AATGCAGCTTC
AATGCAGCTT
AATGCAGCT
AATGCAGC
AATGCAG
AATGCA
AATGC
AATG
AAT
AA
A

Excitation laser

Detector

AATGCAGCTTCGT

Sequence output

• **Figure 5-22** Sanger sequencing. As each band of color (caused by collections of dye-terminated fragments of the same length) moves past the detector, a peak signal for the terminal nucleotide is produced on a graph. *A*, Adenine; *C*, cytosine; *G*, guanine; *T*, thymine.

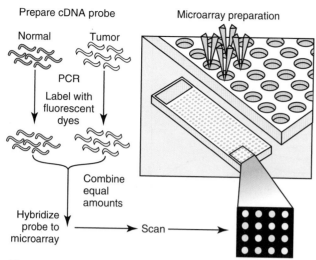

• **Figure 5-23** Microarray preparation. *cDNA,* Complementary probe; *PCR,* polymerase chain reaction.

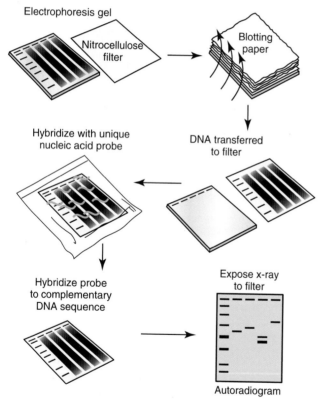

• **Figure 5-24** Southern blot test.

There are many more variations of structural abnormalities of chromosomes, including deletions, duplications, translocations, inversions, and rings. In *deletions,* part of the chromosome is deleted. In *duplications,* there are extra portions of chromosomes. In *translocations,* a portion of one chromosome is transferred to another chromosome. Translocations are produced primarily by reciprocal translocation, in which segments from two different chromosomes are exchanged, and Robertsonian translocation, in which two chromosomes are attached at one central point. There are also *inversions,* in which a piece of a chromosome breaks off and reattaches at the same location but upside down. *Rings* are pieces of chromosomes that break free; the two ends join to form rings that are outside the main chromosome.

Many times, a mutation or abnormality occurs in the egg or in the sperm cell before conception. Other mutations or abnormalities are inherited from a parent or are new to the individual. Environmental influences may play a large part in causing new mutations.

Infectious Diseases

One of the biggest diagnostic applications for molecular diagnostics is in the field of infectious diseases. Molecular techniques to identify bacteria and genotype bacteria and viruses have revolutionized microbiology. For example, microbiological molecular diagnostic assays are used to identify viruses such as influenza, respiratory syncytial virus, Epstein-Barr virus, and herpes simplex virus. Many fastidious species of bacteria are also identified by molecular techniques, including *Chlamydia trachomatis, Neisseria gonorrhoeae, Bordetella pertussis, Mycobacterium tuberculosis,* and *Mycoplasma pneumoniae. Aspergillus* species are also identified with the use of molecular techniques. Other uses for these techniques include viral load monitoring in Epstein-Barr disease, hepatitis B and C, and human immunodeficiency virus (HIV) infection; viral genotyping of HIV and hepatitis B and C viruses; bacterial resistance detection for methicillin-resistant *Staphylococcus aureus* (MRSA), vancomycin-resistant enterococci (VRE), and *M. tuberculosis;* and bacterial genotyping of *M. tuberculosis* and *Neisseria meningitides.*

Summary

DNA exists in double strands in human chromosomes. DNA contains all the genetic information for an organism and is located in the nucleus of every cell in the body. Watson and Crick uncovered the double helix formation of DNA, and this discovery led to the sequencing of the human genome in the 1990s. More powerful computers are enabling scientists to identify genes on chromosomes as well as genes associated with diseases. Several techniques have speeded up these discoveries, including PCR, DNA probes, DNA microarrays, DNA chips, and the Southern blot test.

Review Questions

1. What type of bonding occurs to twist the DNA backbones?
   a. Hydrogen bonding between the nucleotides located on separate strands
   b. Intrastrand bonding of the DNA strand
   c. Phosphodiester bonding
   d. Organoester bonding
2. Which of the following is *not* a DNA nucleotide?
   a. Adenine
   b. Uracil
   c. Guanine
   d. Cytosine
3. All of the following are types of cloning EXCEPT
   a. Therapeutic cloning
   b. Reproductive cloning
   c. Organ cloning
   d. Gene cloning
4. Which of the following contain the correct steps for a PCR technique?
   a. Mix sample with detergent, heat solution to 95° C, mix solution with primers, cool solution.
   b. Heat solution to 95° C, mix sample with detergent, mix solution with primers, mix solution with endonucleases, cool solution.
   c. Cool solution, add primers, denature, elongate, anneal.
   d. Denature by heating solution, anneal solution, and elongate.
5. Which of the following bacteria are identified with the use of molecular techniques?
   a. *Escherichia coli*
   b. *Lactobacillus*
   c. *Mycobacterium tuberculosis*
   d. *Haemophilus influenzae*

6. Which technique uses thermal cycling to produce many copies of DNA?
   a. PCR
   b. RFLP
   c. DNA microarray
   d. Southern blot
7. Which technique enables scientists to analyze DNA so as to make a definitive identification of an individual?
   a. PCR
   b. DNA probe
   c. Southern blot
   d. RFLP
8. What technique is the most sensitive and specific to identify genes in samples?
   a. RFLP
   b. PCR
   c. DNA probe assays
   d. Southern blot
9. Transcription is
   a. Producing DNA from DNA
   b. Producing proteins from RNA
   c. Creating chromosomes from DNA and histone proteins
   d. Producing RNA from DNA
10. All of the following are needed for translation EXCEPT
   a. Amino acids
   b. Heterocyclic bases
   c. tRNA
   d. mRNA

Critical Thinking Questions

1. Draw a diagram that describes the complex steps in replication.
2. Discuss the bonding structure in DNA and draw diagrams to illustrate the bonds.
3. Compare and contrast RNA and DNA.

Bibliography

Apps DK, Cohen BB, Steel CM. *Biochemistry: A Concise Text for Medical Students.* 5th ed. London: Baillaiere Tindall; 1992.

Berk A, Zipursky SL. *Molecular Cell Biology.* Vol. 4. New York: WH Freeman; 2000.

Burtis CA, Ashwood ER, Bruns DE. *Tietz Textbook of Clinical Chemistry and Molecular Diagnostics.* 5th ed. St. Louis: Elsevier Health Sciences; 2012.

Burtis CA, Bruns DE. *Tietz Fundamentals of Clinical Chemistry and Molecular Diagnostics.* 7th ed. St. Louis: Saunders; 2015.

Genetics Home Reference. *What Is a Chromosome?* <http://ghr.nlm.nih.gov/handbook/basics/chromosome> Accessed 12.05.15.

National Human Genome Research Institute. *Fact Sheets on Science, Research, Ethics and the Institute.* <http://www.genome.gov/10000202> Accessed 12.05.15.

Piper MA, Unger ER. *Nucleic Acid Probes: A Primer for Pathologists.* Chicago, IL: American Society for Clinical Pathologists; 1989.

Speers DJ. Clinical applications of molecular biology for infectious diseases. *Clin Biochem Rev.* 2006;27(1):39–51.

6

Automation in the Laboratory

DONNA LARSON

CHAPTER OUTLINE

OBJECTIVES

After completion of this chapter, the reader will be able to:

1. Discuss the goals of automating clinical chemistry tests.
2. Compare and contrast continuous flow, centrifugal, discrete, random access, and batch analyzers.
3. Discuss fluidics in automation.
4. Explain optics and testing in automation.
5. Discuss detection in automation.
6. Discuss data management.
7. Describe total laboratory management and why it is an important part of large laboratories.

KEY TERMS

Analyte
Analytic run
Aspiration
Assays
Batch analyzers
Bioluminescence
Cap piercer
Centrifugal analyzer
Chemiluminescence
Continuous flow analyzer

Cuvette
Data management
Detection
Detector
Discrete analyzers
Fluidics
Laboratory information systems
Monochromator
Optics
Peristaltic pumps

Photodiode
Photomultiplier tube
Pneumatic tubes
Probe assembly
Random access analyzer
Random sampling
Reagents
Rotor
Test profile
Throughput

Points to Remember

- The first automated chemistry analyzer was the Technicon AutoAnalyzer, which was a continuous flow analyzer.
- A centrifugal analyzer uses centrifugal force to mix reagents and specimens.

- In discrete analyzers, each specimen is contained in a separate reaction vessel, and the analyzer can run multiple tests on one sample or multiple samples one test at a time.
- The principle behind the use of dry slides is reflectance photometry.
- Fluidics, optics, testing, detection, and data management allow automated instruments to perform clinical

chemistry tests faster and more accurately than manual testing.

- The fluidics system of an analyzer controls the movement of fluids with pumps.
- Specimen integrity is based on preanalytical handling, and proper handling ensures a good specimen for testing.
- Each specimen must be positively identified before, during, and after an analytic run.
- The pumps attached to a probe assembly are programmed to aspirate a particular amount of sample for each test.
- Most probes are washed with water or a washing solution between aspirating specimens.
- Reagents must be prepared and handled according to manufacturers' instructions to produce accurate and reliable test results.
- Probe assemblies are washed between dispensing different specimens and reagents.
- Temperature regulation when performing tests is important for accurate test results.
- Test methods are based on principles for quantitating analytes.
- Laboratory information system (LIS) software packages help laboratorians report patient results and manage data.
- Total laboratory automation integrates preanalytical, analytical, and postanalytical functions with software interfaces, bar codes, and status indicators.

Introduction

Automation has revolutionized clinical laboratory science. Improved technology has led to the development of automated instruments that perform tests quicker, cheaper, and with more precision and accuracy than ever before. Large reference laboratories perform a million or more tests each day. This huge volume dictates that they use total laboratory automation to keep pace with the number of tests ordered by physicians. This chapter provides a short history of automated clinical chemistry analyzers, a discussion of various types of automation, and a description of total laboratory automation.

Goal of Automation

Physicians depend on laboratory results to confirm or rule out a diagnosis. In addition to producing more results more quickly and with better precision and accuracy, automation has decreased the laboratory worker's exposure to hazardous chemicals. Automated instruments have reduced the exposure of laboratory professionals to hazardous chemicals through the use of smaller amounts of these chemicals and the decreased amount of manual pipetting required.

Automation enables a clinical laboratory to handle more tests. In the mid-1960s, physicians were ordering more laboratory tests than ever, and the laboratory professional could not perform the manual tests fast enough to keep up with the orders. Adding more technicians was not an option because not enough trained laboratory professionals were

available. Automation allowed the laboratory to operate with fewer technicians.

The Medicare program was established in 1965, and the law provided people 65 years of age or older with hospital and medical insurance that paid for tests ordered by a physician. Clinical laboratories were then able to generate revenue for hospitals by performing laboratory tests.

History of Automated Analyzers

Automated analyzers have evolved over the past 50 years. The first automated analyzer was based on the principle of continuous flow. Other categories of automated clinical chemistry analyzers include centrifugal, random access, discrete, and batch analyzers.

Continuous Flow Analyzers

The first automated chemistry analyzer was the Technicon AutoAnalyzer, which made its debut in 1957. The Technicon AutoAnalyzer used large amounts of plastic tubing to move the specimens and reagents (i.e., substances or mixtures used in chemical analysis) through the instrument (Fig. 6-1). A continuous flow analyzer pumped reagent nonstop while injecting samples into the system at regular intervals. The analyzer used peristaltic pumps for pumping the fluids and bubbles to separate samples and reagents in the tubing. The bubbles also scrubbed the plastic tubes to ensure that there was no carryover from previous samples or reagents. However, the bubbles were found to be less than effective, and carryover from one sample to the next could be very large.

Advantages of this type of instrument include cost-effectiveness when running one test or one test profile

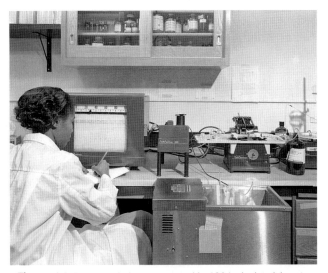

• **Figure 6-1** This historic image, created in 1964, depicts laboratory technician Dorothy Roland at work in one of the Centers for Disease Control's laboratories. Ms. Roland was in the process of recording data captured by an AutoAnalyzer machine while seated at her workbench. (Public Health Image Library/Dorothy Roland, courtesy Centers for Disease Control, Atlanta, GA.)

(i.e., array of laboratory tests run on many specimens). One disadvantage is that all tests are run on all samples, not just the tests ordered by a physician. Another disadvantage is that a test run cannot easily be interrupted to analyze stat samples.

Later-generation clinical chemistry automated instruments used similar technology. The machines evolved from bench-top analyzers to stand-alone floor models. Examples of continuous flow analyzers include the Technicon AutoAnalyzer, SMA 6/60, SMA 12/60, Technicon Chem-1, and Technicon RA.

Centrifugal Analyzers

As automated analyzers evolved, different automation strategies were used. Some analyzers used centrifugation to mix the sample and reagents, and others packaged the reagents separately and used various methods to mix samples and reagents. Some analyzers used bulk reagents, and others used individually packaged reagents. In 1969, Norman Anderson from the National Aeronautics and Space Administration developed the first clinical chemistry centrifugal analyzer, and Electro-Nucleonics marketed the first commercially available centrifugal analyzer, GEMSAEC, in 1970.

In a centrifugal clinical chemistry analyzer, the specimen and reagent are pipetted into rotor compartments, which are clear areas or cuvettes located at one end of the rotor. As the rotor spins, the centrifugal force pushes the specimen and reagent into the cuvette, where they mix and react. Light passed through the resulting solution is used to determine the concentration of an analyte. A disadvantage of this instrument is that it must run one test at a time for many specimens. It takes a long time to run many tests on many samples using this instrument. Examples of a centrifugal analyzer are the Cobas Bio and the IL Monarch.

Discrete Analyzers

Discrete analyzers allowed laboratorians to select individual tests to be run on samples. In 1971, DuPont released the Automated Clinical Analyzer (ACA). The ACA changed clinical laboratory testing because the reagents were self-contained in packets. The original ACA was a stand-alone floor model analyzer. In 1983, DuPont introduced a smaller analyzer, the ACA IV, which could fit on a bench top and meet the needs of small hospitals, clinics, and emergency departments. The specimen was placed in an elongated cup in the ACA, and a reagent packet was added for each test to be run on that specimen.

In 1976, Kodak introduced the Ektachem, which used dry slide technology to test specimens. This was innovative because all of the reagents for a particular test, including electrolytes, were contained on a small slide (Fig. 6-2). When the sample was applied to the slide, it moved through the spreading layer, enabling chemical reactions that led to quantitation of the analyte (e.g., creatinine, glucose). The principle behind the dry slides is reflectance photometry.

Most modern analyzers are discrete analyzers, in which each specimen is contained in a separate reaction vessel. The analyzer can run multiple tests on one sample or multiple

samples one test at a time (Fig. 6-3). This ability is called random sampling. Modern analyzers can be configured to perform batch analysis or random access testing. Modern analyzers use many test methods (e.g., immunoassays, hormone analysis), unlike the original analyzers that used only spectrophotometric test methods.

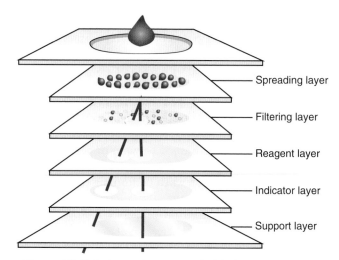

• **Figure 6-2** Reflectance photometry principle for the dry slide used in the Ektachem analyzer.

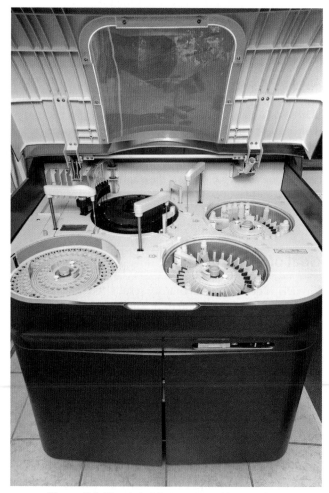

• **Figure 6-3** Blood chemistry analyzer. (© Iculig/iStock)

Random Access Analyzers

The random access analyzer allows the laboratory technician to select tests to be performed on each specimen. Each specimen and its reagents are independent of other specimens in the analyzer. This instrument can run many specimens one test at a time or many tests on one sample at a time.

Batch Analyzers

Analyzers that sequentially perform a test on each of a group of specimens are called batch analyzers. They provide an effective means of keeping down costs for performing a particular test. Some specialty tests are more cost-effective when using this method because only a small number of tests are ordered at one time. By accumulating specimens until a batch is formed, one test run contains many samples instead of one, reducing reagent and personnel costs. Continuous flow, centrifugal, and random access analyzers can run in batch mode.

Automating Clinical Chemistry Tests

Automation of instruments includes fluidics, optics, testing, detection, and data management. These components allow automated instruments to perform clinical chemistry tests faster and more accurately than manual tests.

Fluidics

In automated instruments, movement of specific amounts of specimens and reagents to a particular location so that they can react is an important function of the analyzer. The fluid-handling portion of automation is called fluidics. The system encompasses pipetting and dispensing of specimens, reagents, and wash solutions. The fluidics system of an analyzer controls the movement of fluids with pumps.

Specimen Handling

Specimen integrity is based on preanalytical handling, and proper handling ensures a good specimen for testing. Specimen handling varies according to the analyte. Most assays require specimens to be refrigerated, and some (e.g., bilirubin) require specimens to be protected from light. These are important factors in testing specimens.

Preparation

Blood specimens drawn for chemical analysis must have time to clot and to be centrifuged before a test can be performed. This process takes time, and methods are being developed to shorten or eliminate some of these steps. For example, anticoagulants that do not interfere with laboratory tests are employed so that centrifuged whole blood can be used for analysis, eliminating the time needed for a specimen to clot.

Specimen Identification and Loading

The link between a specimen and a patient is a critical aspect of clinical testing. Each specimen must be positively identified before, during, and after an analytic run. This process can be started at a nursing station or in the laboratory by using the laboratory information system software (see later discussion). Many systems produce bar codes that can be affixed to the specimen tube to positively identify the specimen (Fig. 6-4). Some instruments can obtain a sample directly from the bar-coded tube. Other instruments require aliquots of specimens be placed in secondary containers, which must also be labeled with the bar code before testing is performed. Smaller instruments may not be linked to a laboratory information system, and the identification and sequencing of specimens on the analyzer must be performed manually.

Many analyzers use circular trays, a rack, or a series of racks to introduce specimens to the analyzer. Specimen tubes or secondary containers (i.e., cups) are placed in the circular tray or rack in a particular order with controls and calibrators before the test is run. The sampling mechanisms for patient specimens and reagents are usually robotic arms that enter a specimen and aspirate exactly the correct amount of specimen and reagent needed for the test.

Aspiration

Aspiration is accomplished with a peristaltic pump system. When an instrument accesses capped sample tubes, the probe assembly usually includes a cap piercer and a liquid sensor. The

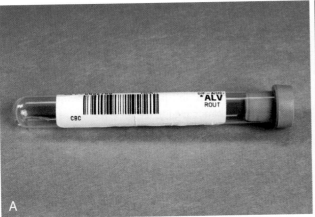
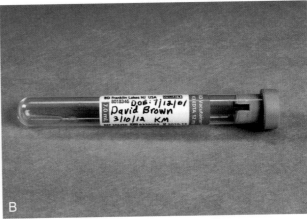

• **Figure 6-4 A,** Computerized bar code label. **B,** Hand-labeled blood tube. (From Bonewit-West K. *Clinical Procedures for Medical Assistants.* 9th ed. St. Louis: Elsevier; 2015.)

cap piercer is a sturdy piece of metal with a sharp end that can easily pierce rubber caps on specimen tubes. The liquid sensor allows the probe to detect liquid at a particular level and aspirate a sample. The liquid sensor can also detect a clot in the specimen. The pumps attached to the probe assembly are programmed to aspirate a specific amount of sample for each test.

Delivery

After the sample is aspirated, the probe moves to the cuvette or mixing chamber and dispenses the sample. Because carryover or contamination of another specimen with a prior specimen is a problem, most probes are washed with water or a washing solution between aspirating specimens.

Reagent Handling

Reagents for different tests have different requirements. Reagents must be prepared and handled according to the manufacturer's instructions. If the instructions are not followed, tests will not produce correct results for quality control and patient specimens. Attention to detail in this area is important for valid and accurate test results.

Reagent Storage

Reagents are stored on the analyzer in temperature-controlled compartments. Some reagents are heated, and others are refrigerated before and during analysis. The reagent containers are covered to prevent evaporation during the storage and analysis phases.

Reagent Aspiration

Reagents are aspirated with a probe assembly, similar to patient specimens. Probe assemblies usually contain a probe tube that aspirates the reagent and a level sensor to detect the liquid level in the reagent container. Typically, a peristaltic pump is used to aspirate specific amounts of reagent during the testing process.

Reagent Delivery

After the reagent is aspirated, the probe moves to the cuvette or mixing chamber and dispenses the reagent. Because carryover or contamination of a reagent with a prior reagent is a problem, most probes are washed with water or a washing solution between aspirating reagents.

Optics

The term optics refers to the properties of transmission and deflection of light. All routine chemistry analyzers have an optical system. The optical system consists of a light source, a monochromator or other device that can separate light into distinctive wavelengths, a light path, and a detector.

Mixing

The optical path includes an area for mixing the reagent and the specimen. In some analyzers, reagent and specimen are mixed in the cuvette; other analyzers mix the two in a mixing chamber made of a transparent material such as plastic, glass, or quartz.

The light from the light source must be able to shine through this area so that changes in intensity can be picked up by a detector.

Timing

Timing of chemical reactions is critical in testing. Routine photometric chemistry tests require a specific amount of time for the chemical reaction between reagents and samples to reach equilibrium. The characteristics of the solution should be measured at this point. For enzyme tests, the reagent or sample solution is read at more than one time because the concentration of the enzyme is determined by the change in absorbance of the solution over a specified period.

Temperature Regulation

All chemical reactions are performed at specified temperatures. Test results depend on the temperature at which the reaction occurs. The instrument must be able to maintain the correct temperature in the testing area. The temperature at which tests are performed also affects the reference ranges established by the laboratory.

Cuvettes

Routine and enzymatic chemistry tests require a transparent testing vessel, often called a cuvette. The reagents and specimens are usually mixed in the cuvette or transferred into the cuvette after mixing so that the characteristics of the solution can be measured. In routine chemistry tests, absorbance is usually measured, but other characteristics of the solution can be measured. The light shines through the cuvette from one side, and changes in the light characteristics are detected on the other side by a component called a detector.

Detection Methods

The detector used for a particular test depends on the test method. Instruments use time sharing to accommodate many test methods that are performed in parallel. While one test is incubating, another may reach equilibrium and is ready to be read. Using every millisecond of time in an efficient and effective manner increases the throughput of an analyzer. Throughput is the number of tests performed per hour.

Spectrophotometry

In a spectrophotometric test method, absorbance of the resulting mixed solution is measured. A single photodiode or an array of photodiodes is used to measure transmittance in routine chemistry tests (see Fig. 3-8 in Chapter 3). Software programs in the instruments convert transmittance to absorbance measurements.

Reflectance Photometry

Reflectance photometry measures diffuse, reflected light. The cuvette or reaction vessel holding the test solution is illuminated by diffuse light, which is reflected by the solution and measured. The intensity of the light from the reaction vessel is measured and compared with the intensity of a reference. This type of detection method is used primarily with dry

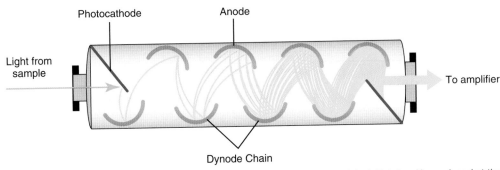

- **Figure 6-5** Schematic diagram of a photomultiplier tube. A tenfold amplification of the initial signal is produced at the anode.

slide technology and in unit-dose reagent systems. Unit-dose reagent systems perform a test on one specimen at a time, and the specimen is added to a self-contained reagent cartridge.

Fluorometry

In fluorometry, the reaction vessel is illuminated by an exciter light; the products from the reagent and specimen interaction absorb the exciter light and then reemit light. Light reemission is measured by a photomultiplier tube (Fig. 6-5). Photomultiplier tubes are extremely sensitive and can detect very small amounts of light. The concentration of product is directly proportional to the amount of light reemitted.

Polarization Fluorometry

Polarization fluorometry is a modification of the fluorometry method. The exciter light is polarized, and the change in the degree of polarization of the emitted light is measured. This method uses a photomultiplier tube, as in fluorometry. Polarization fluorometry is used to measure low-molecular-weight compounds such as therapeutic and abused drugs, hormones, tumor markers, and antibodies.

Turbidimetry and Nephelometry

The interaction of reagents and specimen forms a precipitate, which makes the solution cloudy. If a beam of light is passed through a cloudy sample, its intensity is reduced by scattering, and the amount of light scattered or transmitted depends on the concentration and size of the particles.

In nephelometry, the intensity of light is measured as the forward scatter created by particles in solution, usually at 90-degree angles to the incident light beam, depending on placement of the photomultiplier tubes. Turbidimetry measures the intensity of light transmitted through the sample. The precipitate suspended in the solution reduces the amount of transmitted light. These methods are used to measure the concentrations of therapeutic drugs and proteins.

Chemiluminescence and Bioluminescence

Chemiluminescence and bioluminescence are often confused with fluorescence. Fluorescence involves absorption of an exciter light, which is then reemitted. In chemiluminescence (i.e., emission of light during a chemical reaction) and bioluminescence (i.e., biochemical emission of light by living organisms), exciter light is absorbed, which

produces a chemical or biochemical reaction that emits light at a lower wavelength. This method uses photomultiplier tubes to detect very small amounts of light (Fig. 6-6) and is used in immunoassays.

Electrochemical Method

Ion-specific electrodes (ISEs) are used to measure electrolytes, including sodium and potassium. Peristaltic pumps transfer the specimen into ISE vessels, which house the tips of a reference electrode and an ISE. The specimen comes into contact with both electrodes and remains in contact until a steady state is reached. The ion is measured at this point. ISEs with immobilized enzymes can also be used to measure analytes such as glucose.

Data Management

For many years, laboratory results were transcribed from instruments onto laboratory request slips, and some small laboratories continue to use this technique for data management. This method of reporting patient results can yield many transcription errors.

As automated instruments evolved, software packages called laboratory information systems (LISs) were developed to report patient results and manage quality control data. The computerized reports greatly reduced transcription errors, which were further reduced as laboratory instruments interfaced with the LIS and directly downloaded patient results into the system.

Automated analyzers use computers and sophisticated software to process data; control the fluidic, optic, and mechanical systems of the analyzer; and respond to the commands of the operator. Several computer chips in many locations in the analyzer control actions for particular areas. Automated analyzers can be linked through interfaces to other analyzers. Analyzers are also linked to the LIS that stores patient results.

Total Laboratory Automation

Total laboratory automation begins after a specimen is drawn and continues until the test results are sent to the physician. Components of total laboratory automation include centrifugation, specimen integrity, decapping, aliquotting, instrument interfaces, sorting, recapping, storage, and retrieval.

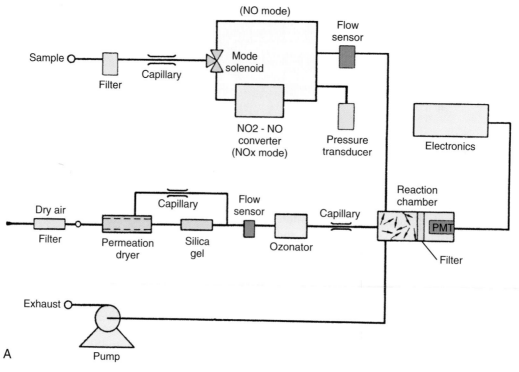

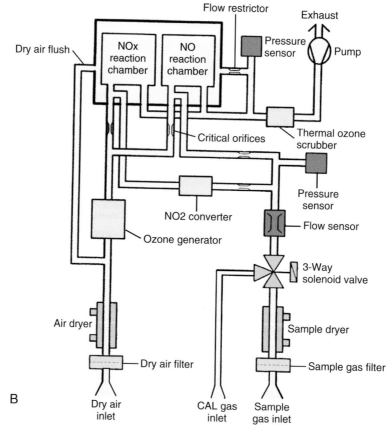

• **Figure 6-6** Schematic diagrams of a single-reaction **(A)** and a dual-reaction **(B)** chamber chemilumi-nescence analyzer. *PMT,* Photomultiplier tube. (Modified from Kacmarek RM, Dimas S. *The Essentials of Respiratory Care.* 4th ed. St. Louis: Mosby; 2005.)

Total laboratory automation is becoming a necessity for large reference clinical laboratories. It involves the integration of preanalytical, analytical, and postanalytical functions in a laboratory using communication software, electromechanical interfaces, specimen containers and racks, specimen identification bar codes, and status indicators.

Automated Specimen Delivery

Laboratory professionals and other hospital personnel are still required to collect specimens and transport them to the laboratory. Common ways to transport specimens to the laboratory include couriers, pneumatic tubes, and robots.

Couriers

Human couriers, once the only way to transport laboratory specimens, are still a common method for transporting specimens to the laboratory and between laboratories. This method works well for routine specimens, but if there is a stat test, an additional charge is incurred if the courier must make a dedicated trip from a laboratory or collection center. Another disadvantage is that specimens can be broken or lost in transit.

Pneumatic Tubes

Pneumatic tubes work well when the system is installed so that the tubes travel from the collection point to the laboratory (Fig. 6-7). If the tube needs to be redirected during its travel to the laboratory, delays in reporting and lost specimens can occur. Another concern is that acceleration and deceleration can damage specimen containers.

Robots

In some large hospitals, mobile robots have been effective for transportation of specimens between various departments and the laboratory. Robots can be dispatched from a department to the laboratory or from the laboratory to the department. Personnel load the properly packaged specimen into the robot and then set its destination. The robot navigates the hallways and the elevators to make its way to the laboratory (Fig. 6-8).

Automated Specimen Processing

The preanalytical phase, in which specimens are processed, centrifuged, sorted, and aliquotted, is one of the most important and error-prone parts of specimen handling. The U.S. Food and Drug Administration has approved systems that perform these non–value-added processes. Some systems can process up to 300 specimens per hour. The system design features a single point of entry for all specimens, automated centrifugation, and automated cap removal. In the postanalytical phase, the patient results are downloaded into the LIS.

Transport to Analyzers

During the analytical phase, automated chemistry instruments perform appropriate tests on each specimen. Specimens must be transported from the specimen processing

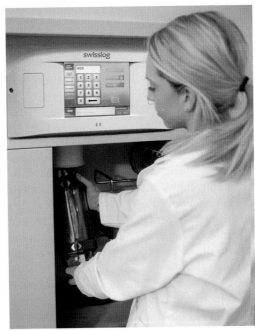

• **Figure 6-7** Pneumatic tube system in use. A pneumatic tube system can be used to transport samples to different areas of the hospital. (Courtesy of Swisslog Healthcare Solutions, Buchs/Aarau, Switzerland.)

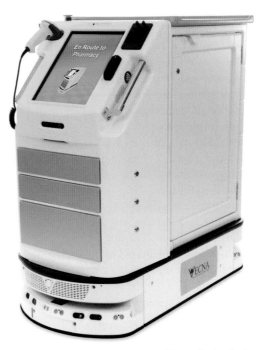

• **Figure 6-8** Vecna QC Bot. (Courtesy Vecna Technologies, Cambridge, MA.)

area to the analyzers. Conveyor belt systems and robotic arms successfully transport specimens in large laboratories. The automated analyzer identifies the specimen through a bar code and then performs appropriate tests by using fluidics, optics, and mechanical systems to route the specimen through the appropriate stations. After the specimens are tested, data are sent to the postanalytical portion of the system to transform the data into patient results. The patient reports are generated and sent to the ordering physician.

Storage and Retrieval

After testing is completed on a specimen, the specimen is stored. Many of the automated specimen processing units include automated storage and retrieval. These units have refrigerators that can store approximately 5400 samples. Automated retrieval is a good idea when the refrigerator stores 5400 specimens! This process saves time and money by having the instrument instead of the laboratory professionals locate specimens. The location of a specimen is maintained in a database of the specimen delivery system. When a request is sent to retrieve a specimen, the location in the database is obtained, and the specimen is retrieved.

Summary

The automated chemistry analyzers introduced in 1957 were continuous-flow analyzers. Four distinct categories of analyzers were developed over the next 20 years: continuous flow analyzers, centrifugal analyzers, discrete analyzers, and random access analyzers. Batch analyzers run tests on all specimens in the sampling area. All analyzers can run in batch mode.

Automated analyzers use fluidics, optics, and robotic systems to test patient specimens for analytes. Analytes include routine chemical substances, hormones, drugs of abuse, therapeutic drugs, and proteins. Data from testing are analyzed and processed by the computer in the analyzer. The results are sent to the LIS so that reports can be created and sent to the physician.

Total laboratory automation is available but used only by large clinical laboratories. These systems are equipped for automatic centrifugation, specimen integrity verification, decapping, aliquotting, instrument interfaces, sorting, recapping, storage, and retrieval of specimens.

Specimens are delivered to the laboratory for processing by human couriers, pneumatic tubes, and mobile robots. The preanalytical phase, in which specimens are processed, centrifuged, sorted, and aliquotted, is one of the most important and error-prone parts of specimen handling. Some totally automated systems perform these non–value-added functions to shorten the turnaround time for laboratory test results. After test results are reported, the specimens are transported to a refrigerator, where they are stored for a predetermined amount of time.

Review Questions

1. All of the following are detection methods used in automated analyzers EXCEPT
   a. Polarization fluorometry
   b. Reflectance photometry
   c. Spectrophotometry
   d. Polarization nephelometry

2. Hardware process components of total laboratory automation include all the following EXCEPT
   a. Status indicators
   b. Instrument interfaces
   c. Sorting
   d. Retrieval

3. Specimens can be delivered to the laboratory by which of the following methods?
   a. Elevators
   b. Internal mail systems
   c. Pneumatic tubes
   d. Phone calls

4. Which of the following is a software package developed to report patient results and manage quality control data?
   a. Proficiency testing
   b. Instrument interfaces
   c. Laboratory information systems
   d. Audit systems

5. Which of the following principles is used by dry slide analyzers?
   a. Reflectance photometry
   b. Nephelometry
   c. Turbidimetry
   d. Fluorescence polarization

6. Another name for a transparent testing vessel is
   a. Dry slide
   b. Cuvette
   c. Photodiode
   d. Monochromator

7. Reagents are aspirated with a
   a. Peristaltic probe
   b. Level sensor
   c. Mixing chamber
   d. Probe assembly

8. If an instrument accesses capped tubes, which of the following does the probe assembly include?
   a. Mixing chamber
   b. Bar code
   c. Fluidics
   d. Cap piercer

9. The fluidics of an analyzer encompasses pipetting and dispensing of all of the following EXCEPT
   a. Specimens
   b. Reagents
   c. Detector solutions
   d. Wash solutions

10. Coordinated aspects of automated instruments that perform clinical laboratory tests faster and more accurately than ever include all of the following EXCEPT
    a. Proficiency testing
    b. Data management
    c. Fluidics
    d. Optics

Critical Thinking Questions

1. Give an example of a discrete analyzer, and describe how it differs from a continuous flow analyzer.

2. What are some of the disadvantages of batch analyzers?

3. What aspects of reagent handling are important to consider in an analyzer? Why are they important?

Bibliography

Alpert N. Automated instruments for clinical chemistry: review and preview. *Clin Chem*. 1969;15:1198–1209.

American Association Clinical Chemistry. *History Division Analyzer Archive*. <https://www.aacc.org/publications/cln/articles/2013/august/history-analyzer.aspx> Accessed 26.06.15.

Bär H, Hochstrasser R, Papenfub B. SiLA: basic standards for rapid integration in laboratory automation. *J Lab Autom*. 2012;17:86–95.

Boyd JC, Felder RA, Savory J. Robotics and the changing face of the clinical laboratory. *Clin Chem*. 1996;42:1901–1910.

Choder G. Laboratory information systems (LIS) in the 21st century: the challenges and the promises. *DARK Daily Clinical Laboratory and Pathology News and Trends*. White paper, DARK Intelligence Group 2011. <http://leadgen.darkdaily.com/Media.aspx?id=36&recordView=1> Accessed 26.06.15.

Cooper GR, ed. *Standard Methods of Clinical Chemistry: By the American Association of Clinical Chemists*. St. Louis: Elsevier; 2013.

Crissman J. Making the most of clinical laboratory automation: achieving best practices with total laboratory automation in your laboratory. *DARK Daily Clinical Laboratory and Pathology News and Trends*. 2011. White paper, DARK Intelligence Group. <http://leadgen.darkdaily.com/Media.aspx?id=17&recordView=1> Accessed 26.06.15.

Cunningham DD. Fluidics and sample handling in clinical chemistry analysis. *Anal Chim Acta*. 2001;429:1–18.

Felder predicts clinical laboratory automation to become faster, more efficient. *DARK Daily Clinical Laboratory and Pathology News and Trends*. April 7, 2010. DARK Intelligence Group. <http://www.darkdaily.com/felder-predicts-clinical-laboratory-automation-to-become-faster-more-efficient-407#axzz-3St3QgP9j> Accessed 26.06.15.

Mattheakis L. Screening robotics and automation. *J Biomol Screen*. 2015;20:299–301.

Melanson SE, Lindeman NI, Jarolim P. Selecting automation for the clinical chemistry laboratory. *Arch Pathol Lab Med*. 2007;131:1063–1069.

Midyett R. Ten instruments that changed the lab. *MLO*. 2005;37:30–32.

O'Connor C, Fitzgibbon M, Powell J, et al. A commentary on the role of molecular technology and automation in clinical diagnostics. *Bioengineered*. 2014;5:155–160.

Olsen K. The first 110 years of laboratory automation technologies, applications, and the creative scientist. *J Lab Autom*. 2012;17:469–480.

Sarkozi L, Simson E, Ramanathan L. The effects of total laboratory automation on the management of a clinical chemistry laboratory: retrospective analysis of 36 years. *Clin Chim Acta*. 2003;329:89–94.

You WS, Park JJ, Jin SM, Ryew SM, Choi HR. Point-of-care test equipment for flexible laboratory automation. *J Lab Autom*. 2014;19:403–412.

7

Laboratory Quality Management Systems

JOHN W. RIDLEY AND DONNA LARSON

CHAPTER OUTLINE

OBJECTIVES

After completion of this chapter, the reader will be able to:

1. Discuss the questions answered by laboratory tests.
2. Discuss the role played by the Clinical Laboratory Improvement Amendments of 1988 (CLIA 88) in the initiation and maintenance of a quality management program.
3. Discuss the twelve essential elements of a laboratory quality management system (QMS).
4. Describe the roles of assessment, customer service, and facilities and safety in the laboratory's QMS.
5. Discuss the purpose of preventive maintenance.
6. Discuss the purpose of service contracts.
7. Discuss the purpose of troubleshooting.
8. Describe how purchasing and inventory contribute to the laboratory's QMS.
9. Discuss function verification of instruments.
10. Recall eight preanalytical variables.
11. State the purpose of a control specimen.
12. Name the characteristics of a control.
13. Differentiate between an assayed control and an unassayed control.
14. Describe the importance of performing lot-to-lot correlations when changing reagent lot numbers.
15. Differentiate between a calibrator and a control.
16. Differentiate between two different types of quality control (QC).
17. Recall eight analytical variables.
18. Differentiate between precision and accuracy.
19. Describe the purpose of statistical methods in QC.
20. Explain the procedure to be followed if a test is performed and the control values are not within range.

OBJECTIVES—cont'd

21. Give the formula for and calculate the SD from a given set of values.
22. State the percentage of the population represented by the mean ±1 standard deviation (SD), mean ±2 SD, and mean ±3 SD.
23. Give the formula for and calculate the coefficient of variation from a given set of values.
24. Discuss the origins and uses of reference ranges.
25. Discuss the importance of properly constructed reference ranges.
26. Differentiate between diagnostic sensitivity and diagnostic specificity of a laboratory test.
27. Discuss why graphic summaries are used in QC.
28. Describe the main type of graphic summary used in QC in the clinical laboratory.
29. Discuss what is done with QC values that are "out of control."
30. Draw and label a Levey-Jennings graph.
31. Draw and label a Youden graph.
32. Discuss the purpose of the Westgard rules.
33. Define the following Westgard rules: 1_{2s}, 1_{3s}, 2_{2s}, R_{4s}, 4_{1s}, and 10_x.
34. Discuss why corrective actions must be documented.
35. Describe a proficiency survey.
36. Identify two methods for analyzing data from proficiency surveys.
37. Discuss performance verification.
38. Discuss critical values.
39. Explain why at least annual competency testing is required for all laboratory personnel performing tests.
40. Describe occurrence management.
41. Discuss the importance of problem-solving mechanisms in a QMS.
42. Describe the difference between laboratory documents and reports and how these fit into a laboratory QMS.
43. Describe important aspects of information management in a laboratory.

KEY TERMS

Accreditation
Accuracy
Analytical phase
Assayed control
Assessment
Bias
Calibrator
CLIA 88
Clinical and Laboratory Standards Institute
Coefficient of variation
Competency assessment
Competency testing
Confidence interval
Continuous process improvement program
Continuous quality improvement cycle
Control
Control limits
Correlation coefficient (r)
Critical value
Customer service
Delta check
Diagnostic sensitivity
Diagnostic specificity
Diurnal variation

Equipment maintenance program
External audit
Flag
Hemolysis
Internal audit
Inventory management
ISO 15189
ISO/IEC 17025
Key quality concept
Laboratory information system (LIS)
Laboratory quality manuals
Lean
Levey-Jennings chart
Linear regression
Linearity
Lipemia
Lyophilized
Mean
Median
Mode
Normal or gaussian distribution or curve
Occurrence
Occurrence management
Out of control
Policy

Postanalytical phase
Preanalytical phase
Precision
Preventive maintenance program
Procedure
Process
Proficiency testing
Quality control chart
Quality control chart rules
Quality control plan
Quality improvement plan
Quality management system (QMS)
Random error
Record
Reference range
Shift
Six Sigma
Specimen processing
Standard deviation (SD)
Standard operating procedures (SOPs)
Systematic error
Trend
Unassayed control
Validation
Westgard rules
Youden plot

◆ Case in Point

A laboratory technician is processing specimens sent to the laboratory from a doctor's office. The technician notices that one of the chemistry serum-separating tubes (SSTs) is not fully separated. What are the effects of incomplete separation of a specimen on test results? What test results will be affected the most? How should the laboratory technician proceed?

Points to Remember

- Quality in the clinical laboratory is important for accurate test results, efficient laboratory operations, and timely reporting of information to providers.
- Laboratory quality standards are developed by outside agencies such as accreditation agencies, the federal government, and international organizations. Examples include the College of American Pathologists, the

Centers for Medicare and Medicaid, and the Clinical Laboratory Standards Institute.

- Every laboratory should implement a quality management system (QMS) that includes the twelve quality system essentials: facilities and safety, customer service, process improvement, documents and records, occurrence management, assessment, purchasing and inventory, process control, information management, equipment, personnel, and organization.
- Laboratories practice risk management by using safety standards to manage physical hazards, needles and sharps, and chemical and biological hazards.
- Laboratory instruments are the cornerstone of laboratory operations because they perform the tests that provide objective information to health care providers.
- Instruments must have preventive maintenance plans and regular servicing to perform at optimal levels.
- For a laboratory to produce accurate, reliable test results, reagents used in the testing process must have a long shelf life and must be stored properly.
- The workflow in a laboratory consists of a preanalytical phase, which includes physiologic factors and other variables that occur before testing; an analytical phase, which includes all the variables that occur during the testing process; and a postanalytical phase, which includes processes and variables that occur after the test result is released.
- The preanalytical workflow phase includes identification of the patient, specimen collection, specimen handling, and transport of the specimen to the laboratory.
- The analytical or testing phase of laboratory workflow uses quality control (QC) processes to detect errors or problems with the testing system.
- The Clinical Laboratory Improvement Amendments of 1988 (CLIA 88) require at least annual competency testing for all laboratory personnel who perform laboratory tests.
- Control specimens are materials used in QC processes that are made with the same matrix as patient samples and contain specific analytes in measurable quantities. These samples are run along with the patient specimens to help detect errors and instrument malfunctions.
- CLIA 88 established guidelines for the frequency of testing control specimens.
- Calibrators are used to align instrument signals with particular values of analytes.
- QC analysis uses Westgard rules to analyze control charts containing control values for analytes. Six common rules are applied to the analysis: 1_{2s}, 1_{3s}, 2_{2s}, R_{4s}, 4_{1s}, and 10_x.
- Reference ranges are constructed using at least 120 values from people who show no sign of disease at the time of the blood draw. The samples are tested over a period of time. The results are analyzed, and ranges of ±2 standard deviations (SD) are created for each analyte tested in the laboratory.
- Proficiency testing is used to assess the accuracy of test methods in a laboratory. Proficiency testing and

required performance on proficiency tests are mandated by CLIA 88.

- Assessments can help laboratories determine where there are gaps in performance.
- Audits can include site visits from accreditation agencies that compare the laboratory's policies, procedures, and processes with accreditation standards.
- Customer service is defined as meeting the customer's requirements.
- Continuous quality improvement is an integral part of a laboratory's QMS.
- Standard operating procedures are guidelines used by laboratory personnel to help them perform laboratory testing in a standardized way.

Introduction

Because health care providers rely on laboratory tests to diagnose and rule out health conditions, it is important for laboratory findings to be valid and to reflect meaningful, accurate test results. Such findings are also used in monitoring treatment and determining disease prognosis. Federal regulations and accreditation standards require laboratories to implement processes and procedures to ensure quality laboratory test results.

This chapter describes a laboratory's quality management system (QMS), which is comprehensive and includes twelve quality system essentials. It also covers the statistical techniques for measuring variation in laboratory results (i.e., descriptive, inferential, linear regression, correlation, reference ranges, predictive values, and method evaluation), tools used to evaluate statistics (i.e., Levey-Jennings graphs, quality control chart rules, assayed and unassayed control materials, standards, and corrective actions), and systematic processes and procedures that help laboratories continually improve their services, including a continuous quality improvement (CQI) program, standard operating procedures, and accreditation. These terms are defined and discussed later in the chapter.

Introduction to Quality

The term *clinical laboratory quality* comprises clinical laboratory operations that are reliable and test results that are as accurate as possible and are reported in a timely manner so as to be useful to a health care provider. Because of the complexity of clinical laboratory testing, test results will not be exactly the same every time a test is run; there is always some variation due to the limitations of testing systems. Quality systems help to reduce the level of inaccuracy as much as possible and alert technicians when systems are not functioning properly.

An individual's health outcomes depend on the accuracy of the laboratory test results. Inaccurate results can cause unnecessary treatments, treatment complications, failure to provide the proper treatment, delay in correct diagnosis, and additional and unnecessary laboratory testing.

The laboratory's QMS examines all of the processes, procedures, and components that lead to quality laboratory results that are reliable and accurate. This system also includes troubleshooting and adjusting components as needed to maintain clinical laboratory quality.

Laboratory Standards

Quality management emphasizes assessment, in which data are gathered on the various components of the QMS. Assessment measures a laboratory's performance against a standard or benchmark. *ISO standards* are developed by the International Organization for Standardization (ISO) and are known as quality standards for industrial manufacturing. There are two ISO standards that apply to the clinical laboratory: ISO 15189 *(Medical Laboratories—Particular Requirements for Quality and Competence, 2007)* and ISO/IEC 17025 *(General Requirements for the Competence of Testing and Calibration Laboratories, 2005).* These are two international standards that are widely accepted by the clinical laboratory industry.

Another international standards organization that produces many different standards for clinical laboratories is the Clinical and Laboratory Standards Institute (CLSI, formerly known as the National Committee for Clinical Laboratory Standards). CLSI develops standards using a consensus process that involves many stakeholders. Two CLSI standards are important to ensure clinical laboratory quality: CLSI document HSI-A2 *(A QMS Model for Health Care; Approved Guideline—Second Edition)* and CLSI document GP26-A3 *(Application of a QMS Model for Laboratory Services; Approved Guideline—Third Edition).* There are many other standards organizations and laboratory standards, some of which apply only to particular laboratory departments.

The QMS Model

A quality management system (QMS) is defined by ISO and CLSI as "coordinated activities to direct and control an organization with regard to quality." Every aspect of a clinical laboratory is related to the quality of the test results it produces: organization structure, processes and procedures, facilities, purchasing, and even housekeeping. Laboratory processes comprise a workflow and are divided into preanalytical, analytical, and postanalytical phases. A key quality concept is the workflow concept, which must be considered when one is developing quality practices. A QMS takes a systematic approach to quality as it considers all processes used by the laboratory.

There are twelve essential elements of a laboratory QMS: facilities and safety, customer service, process improvement, documents and records, occurrence management, assessment, purchasing and inventory, process control, information management, equipment, personnel, and organization. These essentials serve as the building blocks for QMS because each one must be assessed for overall laboratory quality to occur, as in the following list:

1. A strong organizational structure is required to establish quality policies and procedures and to implement and monitor these policies and procedures.
2. Highly trained and competent personnel are required to achieve CQI and a quality laboratory service.
3. Laboratory tests are performed on various types of equipment, so selection of equipment, proper installation, validation of proper function, and implementation of a robust equipment maintenance program all contribute substantially to a quality laboratory service.
4. The availability of good-quality reagents and supplies, storage procedures that preserve the integrity and reliability of reagents, and cost-effective purchasing all contribute to a quality laboratory service.
5. Sample management, quality control of testing, method verification, and validation play vital roles in ensuring that laboratory tests results are reliable, accurate, and precise.
6. Dissemination of accurate laboratory test results in a secure manner to comply with federal regulations is extremely important. The results will not produce the desired outcomes if they do not reach the provider in a timely manner.
7. One way to build quality laboratory services is to standardize testing for more consistent tests results and maintain records in accordance with accreditation and federal standards.
8. The laboratory's QMS must be able to detect errors before the test results are communicated to providers so that actions can be taken to correct the problems and make sure they do not happen again.
9. The QMS assesses laboratory performance by comparing it (internally and externally) to standards and benchmarks. These standards and benchmarks include laboratory quality standards.
10. The QMS contains CQI processes that allow a laboratory to become a learning organization wherein processes and procedures are constantly updated as the laboratory makes changes to correct errors and adapt to change.
11. Laboratories are organizations that provide services to customers; therefore, customer needs must be understood and customers provided with needed services. A QMS ensures that this function of a laboratory is assessed.
12. Facilities and safety is an integral part of a laboratory QMS. Security, risk assessment, safety, and adherence to all state and federal regulations are important and sometimes overlooked quality indicators.

There is no magic system that will ensure that any laboratory's test results are 100% accurate, precise, and timely. Implementing a QMS will not produce an error-free laboratory, but it will help laboratories become learning organizations that identify errors and prevent the same errors from recurring. Everyone in the laboratory is responsible for quality.

Facilities and Safety Overview

In a quality laboratory, the facilities and work spaces are designed so that a technician can perform essential duties without compromising the quality of the work or the safety of the individual worker, the entire laboratory, and the community. As a laboratory worker, it is important to adhere to the basic safety rules and processes, including donning the appropriate personal protective equipment (PPE) when working with toxic chemicals, biological samples (hazards), and physical hazards. Everyone in the laboratory is responsible for safety. For a complete discussion on laboratory safety, see Chapter 2.

Risk Management

Laboratory technicians are exposed to a significant number of risks when working in a clinical laboratory. The risk categories include physical hazards, needles and sharps, chemical hazards, and biological hazards. Laboratory managers identify the possible risks for technicians, then create appropriate training to teach technicians how to work safely. See Chapter 2 for more information on this topic.

Instruments

Because medical laboratories provide essential services in the diagnosis and treatment of diseases, laboratory staff are responsible for ensuring continuous functioning and adequate performance of instruments. Properly functioning laboratory equipment ensures valid and reliable test results. Ignoring an effective equipment maintenance program eventually leads to equipment failure with extensive downtime and loss of use. This results in increased expenses for the laboratory, dissatisfaction on the part of medical staff, and undue stress on the technical personnel of the laboratory.

Instruments are a key element in the production of quality test results. By implementing a good equipment management program, laboratories can ensure a high level of performance, reduced variation in test results, lower repair costs, longer instrument life expectancy, reduced interruptions in workflow, and greater customer satisfaction. Elements to be considered when planning an equipment management program include selection, installation, calibration, performance evaluation, maintenance, service, repair, and disposal of old equipment. Technicians are usually responsible for the calibration and day-to-day maintenance of every piece of equipment.

Selection

Laboratory managers may be responsible for selecting or providing input into the selection of new equipment, and technicians may be asked for input into the decision as well. Many large chemistry instruments require separate electrical and water supplies, and knowing all instrument specifications from the beginning of the selection process saves time and money during the installation process. These requirements can add to the cost and complexity of installing an instrument.

Preparation for Use

After the instrument is installed, developing processes and procedures for testing; performing maintenance; calibrating, operating, and verifying performance; and establishing a scheduled maintenance program must be accomplished before the instrument can be placed into service. In addition, technicians who will operate the instrument must receive adequate training before the instrument is placed into service.

The initial calibration of an instrument is critical to its proper functioning, and the manufacturer's instructions must be followed carefully. It is prudent to calibrate an instrument with each test run during its initial testing period. The calibration frequency for specific tests and specific instruments is dictated by the manufacturer and by federal regulations published as the Clinical Laboratory Improvement Amendments of 1988 (CLIA 88).

Laboratories must verify the manufacturers' performance claims for all new instruments in the laboratory using the laboratory's own personnel. Many laboratories perform parallel testing using fresh patient specimens: The patient specimens are run on both the old and the new instrument, and the results are compared. In planning a parallel testing study, CLSI standard EP-9A2 (Method Comparison and Bias Estimation Using Patient Samples) recommends using 40 duplicate samples with values distributed over the analytical measurement range. The parallel testing should take place over at least 5 days so that the results do not represent only one analytical run. Statistics are used to evaluate the differences in the test results and determine whether one method can replace the other without a general change in measured concentration. A regression method is used for this analysis (see later discussion).

Implementing an Equipment Maintenance Program

The equipment maintenance program begins when an instrument is purchased and becomes a fixed asset for the organization. The instrument should be added to the laboratory's equipment inventory—even if the organization has a fixed asset inventory. As the instrument is installed and readied for service, all maintenance performed on the instrument and any corrective actions are documented in a log. A preventive maintenance plan guides troubleshooting and repair of the instrument, and these procedures are also included in the equipment maintenance program.

Preventive Maintenance

The proper functioning of equipment requires careful operation and preventive maintenance. Early detection of malfunctions and appropriate corrective measures are needed to prevent inaccurate results due to equipment issues, unexpected costs, delays in reporting results, low productivity, and deterioration of the quality and credibility of the laboratory. In the equipment management plan, all major laboratory instruments have a detailed maintenance program specifically designed for the instrument. The manual that accompanies the instrument is a good resource when setting up a preventive maintenance program geared toward the unique functions of the instrument. The more complex an instrument, the more a user will depend on the support of the manufacturer for its maintenance. Some companies provide periodic checks of the equipment as part of a maintenance plan that can be purchased along with the instrument. In any case, daily maintenance is the responsibility of the laboratory's technicians to ensure that the instrument remains in proper operating condition.

Many instruments provide self-diagnostic functions, but others do not and must be manually checked. Sophisticated instruments may be programmed to perform their own self-checks and to alert the operator, even during operation, when errors are detected. Continuous use of these devices when errors are present, as occurs in many large laboratories, can damage the components and lead to unusually increased wear and tear on the instrument. This can result in functional inaccuracies and erroneous test results.

Systematic and routine cleaning, adjustment of systems, and replacement of parts at specified intervals comprise the preventive maintenance program for laboratory instruments. The manufacturer creates a schedule of tasks to be performed at daily, weekly, monthly, and yearly intervals. If the manufacturer's instructions are followed, a laboratory instrument should perform with maximum efficiency, accuracy, and precision and with an increased lifespan.

Troubleshooting Equipment Problems

When laboratory instruments do not function normally, imprecise or inaccurate laboratory test results will be produced. Sometimes, instrument malfunctions can be observed as shifts or trends in quality control (QC) values (see later discussion) or as drifts in calibrator values. Sometimes the instrument does not function normally (e.g., the carousel does not turn, the probe does not move). Sometimes the instrument fails to power up, makes funny noises, or produces absurd results. Sometimes errors are caused when a technician uses a set of controls with the wrong lot number; at other times, the cause of errors can be as complex as a broken part or a programming glitch, both of which require intervention from the manufacturer through a technical service representative. The manufacturer's instrument guide, the preventive maintenance guide, or the instrument log book should contain troubleshooting guidelines or checklists to assist instrument operators in identifying the source of the issue. See Box 7-1 for common troubleshooting questions to consider.

A valuable function of the well-trained laboratory professional is the ability to quickly recognize errors that signal inaccurate patient test results. Most preanalytical errors can be resolved quickly by validating patient identification and ensuring that the reagents are correct and

---

> **• BOX 7-1** **Common Questions to Consider When Troubleshooting Instrument Function**
>
> Is the problem related to a poor-quality sample?
>   Has the sample been collected and stored properly?
>   Are factors such as turbidity or coagulation affecting instrument performance?
> Is there a problem with the reagents?
>   Have the reagents been stored properly, and are they still in date?
>   Have new lot numbers been introduced without updating instrument calibration?
> Is there a problem with the water or electrical supply?
> Is there a problem with the equipment?

---

in date. After need for recalibration of the instrument, the next greatest source of error is analytical error. Proper maintenance of instruments can eliminate many equipment malfunctions; however, components of the instrument can and will fail as the equipment ages and the components wear down.

When one is troubleshooting an instrument issue, only a single change should be made at a time based on symptoms. This makes it possible to determine whether that particular factor is the cause of the malfunction. If the troubleshooting process does not pinpoint the source of the problem, or if the problem cannot be corrected in house, the use of the instrument must be stopped and an alternative method for producing test results must be used. Alternatives include using a back-up instrument, asking a manufacturer to provide a replacement instrument while the main instrument is being repaired, and sending critical samples to reference laboratories for testing. The supervisor, laboratory manager, and health care providers must be made aware of the problems with the instrument as well as the alternative methods for providing results for patient samples. Under no circumstances should faulty instruments continue to be used. A note should be placed on the instrument so that technicians working other shifts do not use that instrument for testing.

Random Errors

Random errors can make troubleshooting extremely frustrating and difficult. A random error is an unexplainable abnormal test result. These unforeseen and unanticipated errors may occur for a variety of reasons, exacerbating the difficulty in identifying them. Random errors are the most difficult type of error to detect, analyze, and correct. Sometimes a physician may contact the laboratory and complain that the provided test results do not match the patient's clinical condition. In such cases, the result is often categorized as a random error. Quite often (and unfortunately), a random error is not detected unless it involves control values and not a patient sample. The reason for the error may never be identified, and merely repeating the test using both the control sample and the patient sample provides an acceptable value.

Random errors occur more frequently than other types of analytical errors. They may occur in any department of a clinical laboratory. Random errors may result from such innocuous sources as environmental factors, differences in operator function, fatigue of certain components that affect high or low levels, transient interference, or almost any other factor that could be included in laboratory instrument operation.

Theoretically, repeated analysis of a given sample should yield the same results. However, this may be impossible due to limitations of the procedure, sample aspiration, light source variation, and a host of other issues. Because of the large volume of routine chemistry tests typically performed, the chemistry department is the one most often affected by errors. Some common sources for random errors are the following:

- Aging or deterioration of chemicals and reagents
- Fluctuations in electrical power flow to instruments
- Experience of the instrument operator
- Laboratory bias based on instrumentation and test methodology
- Environmental factors during any phase of testing
- Personal habits or methods used by testing personnel
- Recent changes in test methodology
- Physical changes in standards, controls, or new lot numbers for reagents and test materials

Random errors occur without warning and sometimes without detection. Good troubleshooting skills are required to differentiate random errors from systematic errors. Good preventive maintenance and instrument service can help reduce the incidence of random errors.

Instrument Service Contracts

When attempts to resolve problems affecting instrument function and test results exceed the abilities of laboratory personnel, the instrument may need to be repaired. In large medical facilities, a staff of biomedical technicians may be able to perform some repairs on laboratory instruments. Some laboratories use instruments acquired through a reagent rental or lease program that requires the laboratory to purchase a specific amount of reagents and supplies from a particular manufacturer, who then provides the instrument at no additional cost to the laboratory. Other organizations that purchase instruments and do not have a biomedical department to perform repairs may purchase a service contract by which manufacturer representatives or service personnel are contracted to provide service and repair instruments. These contracts are fee based and vary with the number of visits and the amount of time spent by technical service representatives working on the laboratory's instruments. If the time spent by repair technicians exceeds the agreed time limit, the laboratory will have to pay extra for additional service.

Because laboratories provide a service for health care providers, they cannot afford to have instruments with considerable down time. Laboratory personnel are a valuable asset because they assist in ensuring that quality results are continuously produced by the clinical laboratory.

Retiring Equipment

As instruments age, their reliability and dependability decrease. Laboratories maintain policies and procedures to guide decisions for retiring older laboratory equipment. This usually occurs when the instrument is not functioning and not repairable. If the laboratory instrument has been acquired on a temporary basis (e.g., through a reagent rental agreement), it will be removed by the manufacturer or replaced by an updated version according to the contract. If an instrument is to be removed from service and from the laboratory, all safety disposal procedures put forth by the organization must be followed to avoid release of biohazardous materials into the community.

Equipment Maintenance Documentation

An individualized maintenance plan for each piece of equipment, including a log for recording preventive maintenance, service repairs, and corrective actions, is required by accrediting and licensing agencies. These documents are essential components of the laboratory QMS. Each major piece of laboratory equipment has its own, step-by-step operating instructions for performing and documenting preventive maintenance, function checks, calibrations, troubleshooting, and other information. Telephone numbers for contacting technical service providers should also be included in the operating instructions.

There is an old adage in the clinical laboratory: "If it is not documented, it is not done." This is particularly true when it comes to preventive maintenance required to maintain top performance. Because several different technicians will work on an instrument, all preventive maintenance must be documented so that anyone picking up the log book can determine when and what work was performed. The same log book should contain the following:

1. Preventive maintenance schedules and activities
2. Forms for recording function checks and calibrations
3. Paperwork from routine maintenance performed by the manufacturer
4. Complete information on instrument problems, including the date on which the problem occurred, the date and time at which the instrument was removed from service, the reason for breakdown or failure, troubleshooting activities and follow-up information for problem resolution, corrective actions taken (including paperwork from any service provided by the manufacturer), the date on which the instrument was returned to use, and any changes to procedures that resulted from problem resolution.

Purchasing and Inventory

Laboratory quality includes efficient and cost-effective laboratory operations. The major service provided by a clinical laboratory is producing quality laboratory results for health care providers. Laboratory tests are run on instruments using test reagents and supplies. Careful inventory management can prevent waste, ensure that supplies and reagents are available when needed, maximize cost savings, and maximize productivity.

Implementing an Inventory Management Program

Laboratory managers are responsible for developing policies, procedures, purchase agreements, inventory records, and delivery schedules. Laboratory technicians are responsible for following established procedures for receiving, inspecting, testing, storing, and handling all materials used in the laboratory. Record keeping is an important aspect of an inventory management program. Laboratory technicians are responsible for recording the date on which reagents and supplies were received; the lot numbers for all supplies, reagents, and kits; the date on which the lot number was put into service; and the date and method of disposal. Other information that may be recorded includes the name and signature of the person receiving the materials, expiration dates, quantities of reagents or supplies received, minimum stock on hand, and current stock balance. New shipments should be stored behind existing stock so that the oldest reagents and supplies will be used first. Box 7-2 lists good practices for storing reagents and supplies.

Computer-based inventory systems may be used in some laboratories. Some laboratories also use automated systems (e.g., Pyxis) that allow users to track inventory with the use of bar codes. A user who removes an item from inventory swipes the bar code, and the inventory record is automatically updated.

Process Control

Process control analyzes three distinctive phases in the laboratory testing cycle: the preanalytical phase (sample management and interferences), the analytical phase (quality control), and the postanalytical phase (reporting and interpretation). For clinical laboratory test results to be meaningful for health care providers, preanalytical factors such as physiologic states that might influence the test results need to be minimized. Collecting, processing, storing, and transporting of samples can also affect laboratory test results.

> **• BOX 7-2   Good Practices for Storing Reagents and Supplies**
>
> 1. Keep the storeroom clean, organized, and locked to protect the inventory.
> 2. Storage areas should be well ventilated and away from direct sunlight.
> 3. Store reagents and supplies according to the manufacturer's instructions; pay attention to temperature and safety requirements.
> 4. Always organize the storeroom so that older materials are at the front of the storage shelves and will be used first.
> 5. Always label reagents with the date opened and make sure the expiration date is clearly visible.

Analytical factors that may influence test results include instrument function, reagent quality, reagent lot number, calibrator lot number, method performance, personnel competence, and procedures. Postanalytical factors that may affect customer satisfaction include critical value decision limits, reference ranges, diagnostic accuracy, result interpretation, correlation of results, and transmission of results.

Preanalytical Phase

The preanalytical phase contains two types of variables—uncontrollable and controllable. The uncontrollable variables are physiologic factors such as diurnal variation, exercise, fasting, diet, stress, posture, and age. Diurnal variation affects hormone levels, iron concentration, and urinary excretion of sodium, potassium, and phosphorus. Exercise may increase levels of lactate, creatine phosphokinase (CK), aspartate aminotransferase (AST), lactate dehydrogenase (LD), and platelets. The reference ranges for most laboratory tests are based on fasting specimens, and many test results are affected by food absorption (especially glucose); therefore, reliable laboratory test results are obtained by using fasting specimens. Diet also affects laboratory test results: Glucose, alkaline phosphatase, and triglycerides are elevated after eating, and potassium and diets high in meat can increase serum urea and uric acid. Stress increases levels of cortisol and adrenocorticotropic hormone and decreases high-density lipoprotein (HDL) cholesterol. Upright posture during phlebotomy can increase concentrations of protein, albumin, calcium, enzymes, and bilirubin. Laboratory values for infants, children, adults, and elderly individuals are very different.

Precollection Variables

Controllable variables in the preanalytical phase include all the tasks that occur before the sample arrives in the laboratory: proper patient preparation, collection, identification of the sample, storage, and delivery of the sample to the appropriate work unit or department of the laboratory. The quality of laboratory test results is only as good as the specimens used for testing. Errors in this phase of the laboratory workflow can cause unnecessary procedures for patients (redraws) and additional costs for the health care organization. Laboratory personnel should use proper collection techniques to minimize patient injuries such as nerve or arterial damage and subcutaneous hemorrhage, as well as infections and injuries such as needlesticks for the laboratory worker.

Collection

Collection of quality specimens is the laboratory's responsibility, even if specimens are collected by non-laboratory staff. For example, nurses may collect specimens at a patient's bedside in the hospital, or home health nurses may collect specimens at a patient's home. Most laboratories produce manuals that detail specimen collection and handling procedures and provide individuals who collect specimens with necessary tubes, needles, and other equipment.

TABLE 7-1	Ten Common Errors in Specimen Collection and the Impact of the Errors	
Common Errors in Specimen Collection		**Impact of the Errors**
Misidentification of patient		Errant results
Mislabeling of specimen		Errant results
Short draw or wrong anticoagulant/blood ratio		Unable to perform the test
Mixing problems or clots		Unable to perform the test
Wrong tube or wrong anticoagulant		Unable to perform the test
Hemolysis or lipemia		Skewed results
Hemoconcentration from prolonged tourniquet time		Skewed results
Exposure to light or extreme temperatures		Altered chemicals
Improperly timed specimen or delayed delivery to laboratory		Chemical alterations
Processing errors such as incomplete centrifugation, incorrect log-in, or improper storage		Chemical alterations

From McPherson RA, Pincus MR: *Henry's Clinical Diagnosis and Management by Laboratory Methods.* 22nd ed. Philadelphia: Elsevier; 2012. Errors in specimen collection lead to recollection of specimens.

Additional variables are associated with collecting the specimen (Table 7-1). Because of the volume of specimens brought to the laboratory every day for testing, clerical errors account for a large percentage of laboratory errors. Examples of clerical errors are misidentification of the patient and mislabeling of specimens. Every laboratory has an operating procedure for proper identification of patients before samples are collected. Phlebotomists and technicians collecting blood specimens need to follow these instructions to greatly reduce the incidence of misidentified patients. Each sample should include the following information on its label: patient identification, test or tests requested, time and date of sample collection, phlebotomists' initials, and name of requesting health care provider. In 2008, the Joint Commission released National Patient Safety Goals for Laboratories. The number one goal was to improve "the accuracy of patient identification." Misidentifying a patient during sample collection (especially for transfusions) can be a life-threatening medical error. Laboratories use bar-coded labels that are placed on tubes to help reduce labeling errors (see Fig. 6-4, *A,* in Chapter 6).

For blood samples, technical issues such as mixing problems, clots, wrong tube type, wrong anticoagulant, hemoconcentration due to prolonged tourniquet time, and hemolysis can lead to erroneous results. Operating instructions should detail the proper mixing techniques and tubes to use for each test. Lipemia is a condition that occurs in patients with particular medical conditions and can interfere with testing. This condition can be corrected when the specimen is processed.

Hemolysis occurs when the red blood cells are mechanically lysed by the phlebotomy needle. It can result from a slow draw, probing, use of a needle smaller than the red blood cell diameter, pulling back too fast on a syringe plunger, forcefully expelling blood into a tube, hard shaking of the tube to mix, or collecting a sample before the alcohol at the collection site has dried. A hemolyzed specimen's serum appears pink (slight hemolysis) or red (severe hemolysis) after centrifugation. Potassium is one of the most important analytes (products being measured by a laboratory procedure) that is elevated in a hemolyzed specimen. Because potassium is critical for heart function, an elevated or decreased potassium level can be a life-threatening medical issue.

When collecting blood in tubes, it is important to follow the proper order of the draw and to thoroughly mix (by inversion) any tubes that contain additives. If tubes containing anticoagulants are not inverted immediately after collection, chances are good that the blood specimen will clot. Clots may be very small, but they can cause erroneous test results.

Tubes are color coded to help identify the additives in each tube. Table 7-2 provides a list of tube colors and their associated additives.

Processing

Specimen processing is another area in which variables can affect laboratory test results. Once the specimen arrives in the laboratory, the sample is checked for proper labeling, sufficient quantity, good condition, and correct tube, as well as appropriate and complete paperwork. The specimen is then entered into the laboratory information system (LIS) and centrifuged before being delivered to the laboratory department for testing. Information recorded in the LIS includes the date and time of collection, date and time at which the sample arrived in the laboratory, sample type, patient name, tests to be performed, provider name, and laboratory-assigned identification. Samples are tracked from the time they arrive in the laboratory until the time test results are reported to the provider.

If a sample does not meet the criteria described, it will go through a laboratory's specimen rejection procedures, which are established by each laboratory. A poor sample will yield erroneous results. Laboratory personnel are responsible for

TABLE 7-2 Tube Color and Additives

Stopper Color	Anticoagulant/Additive	Specimen Type/Use	Mechanism of Action
Red (plastic/Hemogard)	Clot activator	Serum/chemistry and serology	Silica clot activator
Red (glass)	None	Serum/chemistry and serology	N/A
Lavender (glass)	K_3EDTA in liquid form	Whole blood/hematology	Chelates (binds) calcium
Lavender (plastic)	K_2EDTA/spray-dried	Whole blood/hematology	Chelates (binds) calcium
Pink	Spray-dried K_2EDTA	Whole blood/blood bank and molecular diagnostics	Chelates (binds) calcium
White	EDTA and gel	Plasma/molecular diagnostics	Chelates (binds) calcium
Light blue	Sodium citrate	Plasma/coagulation	Chelates (binds) calcium
Light blue	Thrombin and soybean trypsin inhibitor	Plasma/coagulation	Fibrin degradation products
Black	Sodium citrate	Plasma/sedimentation rates—hematology	Chelates (binds) calcium
Light green/black	Lithium heparin and gel	Plasma/chemistry	Inhibits thrombin formation
Green	Sodium heparin, lithium heparin	Plasma/chemistry	Inhibits thrombin formation
Royal blue	Sodium heparin, K_2EDTA	Plasma/chemistry/toxicology	Heparin inhibits thrombin formation; K_2EDTA binds calcium
Gray	Sodium fluoride/potassium oxalate	Plasma/glucose testing	Inhibits glycolysis
Yellow	Sterile containing sodium poly-anetholesulfonate	Serum/microbiology culture	Aids in bacterial recovery by inhibiting complement, phagocytes, and certain antibiotics
Yellow	Acid citrate dextrose	Plasma/blood bank, HLA phenotyping, and paternity testing	WBC preservative
Tan (glass)	Sodium heparin	Plasma/lead testing	Inhibits thrombin formation
Tan (plastic)	K_2EDTA	Plasma/lead testing	Chelates (binds) calcium
Yellow/gray and orange	Thrombin	Serum/chemistry	Clot activator
Red/gray and gold	Clot activator separation gel	Serum/chemistry	Silica clot activator

From McPherson RA, Pincus MR: *Henry's Clinical Diagnosis and Management by Laboratory Methods*. 22nd ed. Philadelphia: Elsevier; 2012.
EDTA, Ethylenediaminetetraacetic acid; *HLA,* human leukocyte antigen; K_2EDTA, dipotassium EDTA; K_3EDTA, tripotassium EDTA; *N/A,* not applicable; *WBC,* white blood cell.

ensuring that the procedures for specimen rejection are followed. In practice, this may be more difficult than it seems (Box 7-3). If a sample is rejected, the provider must be notified as soon as possible that the sample is not acceptable and why. Next, a request is made for another sample to be collected and resubmitted to the laboratory. The rejected sample must not be thrown away but kept until the provider has been contacted. The provider may decide that testing should proceed on the sample that was rejected. For example, the sample may be a cerebrospinal fluid specimen that was sent to the laboratory without a label. Some specimens cannot be recollected, so testing will proceed with a disclaimer on the report stating the problem with the specimen (e.g., not labeled).

If a sample meets the criteria for acceptance, it will be centrifuged (if not already done) and delivered to the

• BOX 7-3 Reasons for Specimen Rejection

Hemolysis or lipemia
Clots present in an anticoagulated specimen
Nonfasting specimen when test requires fasting
Improper blood collection tube
Short draw or wrong volume
Improper transport conditions (e.g., ice for blood gases)
Discrepancies between test requisition and specimen label
Unlabeled or mislabeled specimen
Contaminated specimen or leaking container

From McPherson RA, Pincus MR. *Henry's Clinical Diagnosis and Management by Laboratory Methods.* 22nd ed. Philadelphia: Elsevier, 2012.

appropriate department for testing. Centrifugation is the accepted method for separating the cells from the liquid in a blood sample. All samples placed in a centrifuge must be in their original container and capped to prevent aerosol development inside the centrifuge. Usually, samples are centrifuged for 10 minutes at a relative centrifugal force of 1000 to 1300 g.

Most chemistry tests require serum for testing, and sometimes a chemistry tube that appears to be clotted arrives in the laboratory and is spun down in the centrifuge. When the tube is removed from the centrifuge, the cells are at the bottom of the tube, but the serum above the cells is clotted. Samples from patients receiving anticoagulant therapy can have an extended clotting period. If the sample is spun before it has fully clotted, the result is clotted serum above the red blood cells. This also happens when normal specimens are not allowed to fully clot before being placed into the centrifuge.

Most automated chemistry analyzers accept bar-coded reports and samples for matching the laboratory results with the proper patient. Identification of samples and their entry into the LIS initially occurs as the specimens arrive at the receiving area of the laboratory and are integrated normally into the computer system used by the entire facility. Although the use of bar codes for sample identification is not infallible, it may help to eliminate a large percentage of errors related to the identification of samples.

Transport, Storage, and Retention

Transporting laboratory specimens to the laboratory is a part of the preanalytical activities. Transportation is important because environmental factors (e.g., light, temperature) can affect laboratory results. When specimens for arterial blood gas analysis are drawn, they must be protected from ambient air and transported to the laboratory on ice for quality test results. Other specimens that must be transported at 4° C include those to be tested for plasma renin and ammonia levels. When specimens are obtained in a physician's office, it is not practical to immediately transport every specimen to the laboratory. Instead, the physician's office will follow laboratory guidelines to preserve the specimens until they are transported to the laboratory. Specimens that arrive in leaking or broken containers are biohazards and must be recollected.

The Occupational Safety and Health Administration (OSHA) Bloodborne Pathogens Standard (OSHA 1910.1030) requires that blood specimens and other potentially infectious materials (OPIM) be housed in a leak-proof container labeled with or color coded according to specific requirements (OSHA 1910.1030[g][1][i]) during collection, handling, processing, storage, transport, and/or shipping. According to the standard, if the outside of the primary container becomes contaminated with the specimen, or if the primary container could be punctured by the specimen, then the primary container must be housed in a leak-proof, color-coded, puncture-resistant secondary container (OSHA 1910.1030[d][2][xiii]). In addition to

the color coding, the outer container and any shipping container must be labeled with the OSHA "BIOHAZARD" label. Acceptable color coding for the "BIOHAZARD" label is fluorescent orange (see Fig. 2-5, *A*, in Chapter 2).

Laboratory specimens are stored in a manner that best preserves the particular analyte. Storage of a sample may cause the analyte concentration to change through adsorption to the glass or plastic tube, denaturing of protein, evaporation of serum or the analyte, or continuing metabolism of red and white blood cells. When blood is collected from a vein, the red blood cells, white blood cells, and platelets do not die. They continue to live and therefore continue to metabolize chemicals in the blood. They also produce acids as a result of metabolism. This causes the pH of serum to drop rapidly if the serum is not separated from the cells. Serum can be preserved, however; for example, serum from specimens used for testing creatinine can be stored at 2° to 8° C for up to 5 days or frozen at –20° C indefinitely. Storage instructions accompany the manufacturer's instructions for any test performed in house, and referral laboratory guides are available for specimens that are sent to reference laboratories.

Laboratory specimens are retained for a specific amount of time, usually 5 to 7 days for blood samples. Specimens are retained for a variety of reasons—most commonly, to be able to repeat the result if it is in question or to perform other tests not originally ordered by the provider.

Analytical Phase

Advances in technology, especially computer technology, are revolutionizing the laboratory testing process. The procedures involved in the analytical phase of testing include sample aspiration and transportation to a cuvette or dilution cup, reagent addition, sample and reagent mixing, incubation, detection, calculations, readout, and report writing. Testing problems that occur during the analytical phase are often mechanical in nature, because the analytical phase of laboratory testing chiefly measures instrument function and the quality of the supplies (e.g., reagents) used for testing. But this phase also includes laboratory technician competence, equipment management, reagents, controls, standards, and statistical analysis.

Technician Competence

To be employed in a clinical laboratory, laboratory personnel must have appropriate postsecondary credentials, certification, and, in some states, licenses. CLIA 88 mandates competency testing for all individuals who perform laboratory tests. Competent technicians are those who apply their skills, knowledge, and experience to correctly perform their laboratory duties. Competency is assessed semiannually for new personnel and annually thereafter, to ensure that laboratory personnel are fulfilling their duties in accordance with federal regulations. Competency testing is required for each test an individual is approved by the laboratory director to perform. The minimal regulatory requirements for competency assessment applied to all personnel performing laboratory tests consist of the six procedures detailed in Box 7-4.

Equipment

In the chemistry laboratory, several different pieces of equipment may be used for specific laboratory tests. Some of these devices are capable of performing only a few special tests, whereas others are complicated devices capable of performing hundreds to thousands of procedures per day. Each instrument must undergo preventive maintenance, cleaning, and function checks according to CLIA 88 and the manufacturer's instructions. This is covered more fully in Chapter 3.

In addition, daily and periodic maintenance is required for smaller pieces of equipment that are used in the laboratory. Required preventive maintenance for water baths and heat blocks, refrigerators and freezers, and centrifuges are summarized in the following sections.

Water Baths and Heat Blocks

Heat blocks and water baths are not used as frequently today as in the past. Water baths provide a complete immersion and consistent warming throughout the mixture. Dry heat blocks are used where specific levels of heat application may not be as critical to the reaction. Water baths require monitoring (e.g., for sufficient water level in the bath) and a thermometer to maintain the optimal temperature. Heat blocks require a tube set into one of the wells, containing a liquid that does not evaporate quickly, and a thermometer in the tube to monitor the temperature. A glycerol solution may last for a considerable period, although there are other solutions that work equally well. In both a water bath and a heat block, too much heat will invalidate the laboratory results, and insufficient heat may not facilitate the reaction desired.

• BOX 7-4 Minimal Regulatory Requirements for Assessing the Competency of All Personnel Performing Laboratory Testing

1. Direct observation of routine patient test performance, including patient preparation if applicable, specimen handling, processing, and testing
2. Monitoring of the recording and reporting of test results
3. Review of intermediate test results or worksheets, quality control records, proficiency testing results, and preventive maintenance records
4. Direct observation of performance of instrument maintenance and function checks
5. Assessment of test performance through testing of previously analyzed specimens, internal blind testing of samples, or proficiency testing of samples
6. Assessment of problem-solving skills

From *What Do I Need to Do to Assess Personnel Competency?* November 2012. <http://www.cms.gov/Regulations-and-Guidance/Legislation/CLIA/Downloads/CLIA_CompBrochure_508.pdf> Accessed 21.07.15.

Thermometers used in heat blocks and water baths require monitoring with properly calibrated temperatures recorded on a daily basis. Frequent cleaning of water baths is necessary to prevent growth of microorganisms. Heat blocks need to be cleaned of spills and debris from the environment because these particles may prevent proper transfer of heat to the reaction tubes. Logs of temperature levels for all cooling or heating devices is necessary to ensure effective practices in laboratory technology and to be open for inspection by site visitors.

Refrigerators and Freezers

Laboratory refrigerators and freezers are most frequently used to cool or freeze samples for preservation. Refrigerators are used to store samples at a temperature between 2° C and 8° C, whereas freezers normally store samples at a temperature between –25° C and –15° C. Laboratory refrigerators and freezers are used for storage of certain specimens that might degrade if exposed to higher temperatures.

Refrigerators and freezers that are insulated for storage of flammable materials are designed to prevent electrical sparking from relays, switches, or thermostats that could ignite flammable vapors. Refrigerators and freezers that contain hazardous biological or other materials must be identified as such. These pieces of equipment require periodic cleaning and daily monitoring of temperatures, which are logged onto a chart for observation. Some units are frost free, whereas others require defrosting as the need arises.

Centrifuges

Centrifuges are used to separate solid matter from liquids. In the case of blood used for laboratory testing, the solid portion includes red and white blood cells along with platelets. The liquid portion is called *serum* when it is obtained from a clotted specimen and *plasma* when an anticoagulant is used to prevent clotting of the blood sample. Centrifuges come as benchtop or floor models. Some are equipped as refrigerated units and run at slower speeds to process samples of serum or plasma that do not contain blood cells to be separated.

Daily care of the centrifuge includes scrupulous cleaning of blood or debris. Periodic maintenance includes checking the revolutions per minute with a tachometer. If a centrifuge is not achieving the proper speed, motor parts (i.e., brushes) may need to be replaced to restore the functions of the instrument.

Operators of a centrifuge should follow standard precautions due to potential exposure to aerosolyzed blood or body fluids. Gloves, facial protection (masks or shields), laboratory coats, and plastic aprons help protect operators from biohazardous material.

Reagents

Most reagents are purchased ready to use or as part of a kit. The reagent containers are placed on temperature-controlled areas of the instruments—some reagents are warmed to 37° C, and others are kept at 4° C while on the instrument.

Reagents vary with the tests performed. Deterioration of reagents can be a source of erroneous test results. The reagent should always be checked as part of troubleshooting an issue with a test.

Laboratory reagents and materials are manufactured under strict precautions to prevent contamination. A product insert will accompany reagents; if certain levels of analytes affect results, the package insert should alert the laboratorian to this possibility.

In some cases, it is necessary to test certain reagents for appropriate reactivity on every day of use. If the results are inadequate, a new lot of reagent must be opened and used after reagent testing. Reagents may provide accurate results to a certain level, after which the relationship between the absorbance of the solution and its concentration is no longer linear. This is called the linearity of the reagent. When a patient sample with an extremely elevated level of a certain analyte is tested, the result may be elevated but not accurate. In these cases (i.e., when a sample result exceeds the upper level of linearity), the sample must be diluted and the test rerun. The test result is then multiplied by the dilution factor to arrive at the accurate test result. The linearity of the reagent is noted in the package insert accompanying each reagent.

Controls

Controls are materials that contain a specific amount of an analyte. Controls are tested in the same manner as patient samples: Whatever is done to patient specimens in performing a test is also done to control specimens. Controls are used to test the validity and reliability of a test measurement system and the operator's competence in a particular environment. The purpose of controls is to ensure that the test measurement system is working as expected.

Control samples (also called quality control specimens) are prepared using the same matrix as the patient samples being tested (e.g., serum, plasma, urine). For example, if a serum glucose concentration is being measured, the control material will also be serum-based. Control samples have a constant value and are placed with patient specimens to monitor the testing process. The values of control samples should include at least the lower and upper ends of the analytical measurement range (the reagent linearity). When the test method begins to become unstable, values at the high and low ends of the measurement range are usually affected first. Having controls in the low and high ranges allows errors to be detected early and corrected to reduce errors in patient test results (Fig. 7-1). In clinical chemistry, a two-level set of controls is considered the absolute minimum, and a three-level set of controls is often used. Such a set may provide low-level, normal level, and high-level values for all the metabolites being assessed.

Most often, control samples are run throughout the day and night as needed to detect errors in a test methodology. As a result, much control material is used over the course of a month. Every time the lot number of the control samples changes, the values for the controls also change. These shifts may make it difficult to detect changes in the measurement

methodology. As a result, clinical laboratories purchase large amounts of control materials to last for months, even up to a year. The amount purchased depends on the stability and the useful life of the control materials. By purchasing large amounts of control materials, the laboratory reduces the amount of work that occurs when control lot numbers change. New control ranges must be established before a new lot number of controls is run.

Control materials come in several forms—frozen, lyophilized, or liquid. The control materials must be handled according to manufacturer's specifications to ensure the longest life for them. If the controls are lyophilized (i.e., freeze-dried), the manufacturer's instructions should be followed for reconstitution. Controls may be reconstituted with reagent-grade water or with special diluents provided by the manufacturer. Because controls are usually serum based, it is important to use universal precautions when handling them.

Manufacturers produce two types of controls—assayed and unassayed. Assayed controls are those that come with a predetermined target value that is established by the manufacturer. Unassayed controls do not come with a predetermined target value.

Assayed Controls

Initially, assayed controls are purchased and ranges for acceptable values are provided through statistics developed by the manufacturer. The package insert for these controls may contain predetermined values for specific instruments. For example, if a laboratory is using a Beckman Coulter AU480 chemistry system, there will be a list of values in the package insert for this instrument. As the program evolves for each test, a meaningful range of acceptable values is developed by the individual laboratory for the assayed controls. This range should be somewhat smaller than the manufacturer's range. The cost for assayed controls is quite high because the manufacturer must expend resources to develop the mean and standard deviation for each analyte in the control. After it is satisfied with the control results over a period of time, a laboratory may switch to using unassayed controls.

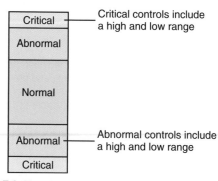

• **Figure 7-1** Choosing appropriate control ranges. Critical control ranges are very high or very low; abnormal control ranges are somewhat high and somewhat low; and normal ranges are the biggest percentage of results, in the middle. This mirrors a normal distribution curve.

Unassayed Controls

Unassayed controls are those that do not have predetermined values. Each laboratory is responsible for determining the mean and standard deviation for each test on its particular instruments. It is considerably less expensive for a laboratory to use unassayed controls. The unassayed controls are of the same quality and come in the same forms (i.e., frozen, lyophilized, and liquid) as the assayed controls.

Lot-to-Lot Correlations

When a change from one lot number of control to another is being made, parallel testing is necessary. Clinical laboratory reagents, as well as control samples, are exposed to environmental factors during transportation and storage that may affect the values obtained in testing. The validation of new reagent kits (i.e., comparing results obtained using the new versus the old kit) ensures that, regardless of the conditions endured by the new lot-numbered kit, there will be no clinically significant differences caused by the switch to the new lot.

Placement of Controls

When large numbers of tests are performed as a batch, it is prudent to intersperse control samples at intervals between the samples. When a control is out of range, the samples measured before the aberrant result (up to the last control that was in range) may be reported. This saves time and resources because the entire batch of samples will not have to be repeated.

Frequency of Analysis

The frequency at which controls need to be assayed is based on the stability of the measurement system—less frequent testing of controls is required with stable systems, more frequent testing with unstable systems. The CLIA 88 regulations (section 493.1256, published by the Department of Health and Human Services in 2003) mandate that controls must be run at least one time every 24 hours or more frequently if recommended by the manufacturer. Laboratories with blood gas instruments must run one set of controls (including both high and low control samples) every 8 hours over a 24-hour period. If the blood gas instrument automatically calibrates itself every 30 minutes, patient samples may be run without running a control; if not, a control must also be run with every patient sample.

Erroneous test results can harm a patient if they influence the medical interventions that may occur after a health care provider receives the laboratory results. QC testing is a way for a laboratory to minimize the risk that erroneous patient results will reach providers. Given the cost of a medical error compared with the cost of repeating patient or control samples, it is certainly worth establishing a more frequent QC sampling schedule so that any error will be caught in a timely manner. The CLSI provides a guideline for clinical laboratories developing a quality control plan that is based on evaluating the risk for patient harm and assessing risk mitigation by referencing the information from manufacturers and local health care conditions.

Calibrators (Standards)

Calibrators are different from controls, so it is important not to confuse them. Calibrators have precisely set concentrations and are used to calibrate an instrument. Some calibrators are traceable to the National Institute for Standards and Technology. Calibrators should not be used as controls because they often contain a different matrix from that used for controls and patient samples.

Calibrators are used to align the signal strength of an instrument to a particular concentration of an analyte. Several calibrators are used to create a linear relationship between signal strength and analyte concentration (Fig. 7-2). (See also the discussion of Beer's law in Chapter 3.)

Most often, calibrators are produced by instrument manufacturers. Many times, such as in point-of-care testing, instruments are calibrated during manufacturing and laboratories merely verify the calibration. The manufacturer's calibrators are designed to produce accurate patient results. Therefore, only calibrators produced by a specific manufacturer for their particular test method should be used.

An instrument should be recalibrated whenever QC results show a shift or a trend (see later discussion). Because trends can be difficult to detect, laboratories usually set up a calibration schedule based on the reliability and stability of a given technology. CLIA requires calibration or calibration verification at least every 6 months or according to the manufacturer's schedule.

Quality Control

QC, also known as statistical process control, is an essential piece of the QMS. The goal of QC processes is to detect, evaluate, and correct errors caused by analytical test system failure, environmental conditions, or operator performance before patient test results are reported. Statistical process control evaluates the accuracy and precision of an analytical system by testing control samples of known values. If the measured control value is within the acceptable range established for that control (i.e., the control limits), then the analytical system is considered to be "in control" (i.e., performing as expected), and patient results are considered to be accurate and precise. If the QC values are not within the control limits, then the analytical system is considered to be "out of control," and the patient results are not reported. Troubleshooting of the analytical system is then required to discover the cause of the error, and corrective actions must be initiated as soon as possible.

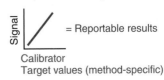

Calibration (or recalibration)

Signal | = Reportable results

Calibrator
Target values (method-specific)

• **Figure 7-2** Steps in calibration or recalibration. (From McPherson RA, Pincus MR. *Henry's Clinical Diagnosis and Management by Laboratory Methods.* 22nd ed. Philadelphia: Elsevier; 2012.)

QC processes discussed in this section deal with producing accurate and precise values from quantitative measurements (Fig. 7-3). QC procedures must be created and established in the laboratory's QMS for qualitative and semi-quantitative methods. The QC plan should contain written policies and procedures (including corrective actions), laboratory staff training information, documentation, and methods for reviewing and analyzing QC data.

Statistics

The QC program lays the groundwork for the calculations to determine accuracy and precision in all quantitative tests performed in the laboratory. **Accuracy** (or validity) is how close a laboratory test result is to its true value. **Precision** (or reproducibility) is how close test results for the same specimen tested several times are to each other. **Bias** is the difference between the average value obtained from a large series of measurements and the true value based on the reference methodology for that test. The goal of laboratory testing is to produce test results that are both **accurate** and **precise.** It is possible for test results to be precise but not accurate, or accurate but not precise (Fig. 7-4).

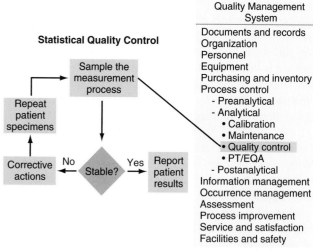

• **Figure 7-3** Statistical quality control. *PT/EQA,* Proficiency testing/external quality assessment. (From McPherson RA, Pincus MR. *Henry's Clinical Diagnosis and Management by Laboratory Methods.* 22nd ed. Philadelphia: Elsevier; 2012.)

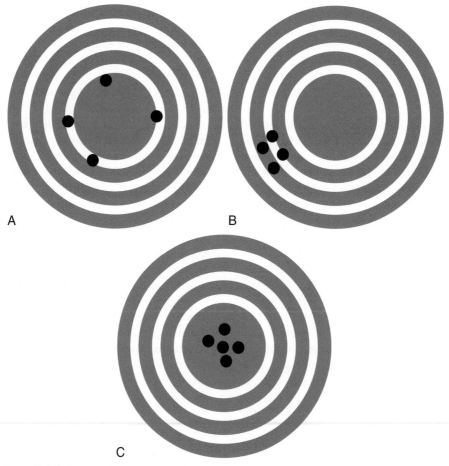

• **Figure 7-4 A,** Repeated measurements are accurate but not precise. They are all close to the bullseye, but they are not close to each other. **B,** Measurements are precise but not accurate. They are precise because they are clustered together, but they are not accurate because they are far from the bullseye. **C,** Measurements are both accurate and precise. They are together in the bullseye of the target. This is the goal for laboratory testing.

Statistical QC is part of the laboratory QMS. This system monitors the accuracy and precision of laboratory test results before patient results are released to the provider. The laboratory QMS combines good laboratory practice with competent personnel and written operating procedures. The operating procedure for statistical QC should cover the sampling frequency for each test methodology and describe method performance using statistical parameters, analysis of statistical parameters, acceptance and rejection of QC results, correction of problems, documentation of all activities, and review of all processes by a supervisor. The operating procedure should also indicate which individuals are authorized to establish acceptable control limits, release results, review performance parameters, or allow exceptions to a policy or procedure.

Laboratory professionals use QC statistics to determine whether the data are in control or out of control. Controls must be repeatedly analyzed over a period of time—with at least 20 data points collected over a 20- to 30-day period for initial analysis. If possible, more points should be used to provide better statistics, and multiple laboratory workers should perform the analysis to discover any procedural variation. The use of at least 20 data points to calculate statistics allows normal variation in test measurement. The 20 data points should not contain any extremely high or extremely low values (outliers). If such points are in the data set, they should not be included in the statistical calculations.

When many measurements are made of a particular sample, the test results will show normal variation. If the results are plotted on a graph, with the data points on the x-axis and the frequency of each value on the y-axis, they should form a bell-shaped curve around the mean. This is called a **normal or gaussian distribution or curve** (Fig. 7-5). In a normal distribution, the mean is the center of the curve and shape of the curve is similar on both sides of the mean. The gaussian distribution curve is one of the most widely used mathematical models in existence. Most biological systems follow this model. Statistics used in the laboratory include mean, mode, median, standard deviation, confidence intervals, and coefficient of variation.

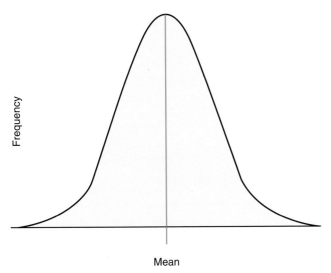

• **Figure 7-5** Normal distribution curve.

The **mean** for a set of data is the same as its average: The data are summed, then divided by the number of individual data points:

$$\bar{x} = \frac{\sum x}{n}$$

The symbol, $\bar{x}$, stands for the mean, and x represents the individual data items in the data set. The large symbol, $\sum$, is a function (i.e., an instruction to sum the values that follow, in this case all the values of x). The number of unique data items in the data set is represented by n. As an example calculation, consider the following data set: 5, 2, 7, 8, 3, 4, 2, 6, 4, 5. To calculate the mean, sum (add) all of the data elements (giving a total of 47), then divide the sum by the number of data elements (10) to arrive at the mean (4.7).

$$\bar{x} = \frac{5+2+7+8+3+4+3+6+4+5}{10} = \frac{47}{10} = 4.7$$

The **median** is the midpoint value—half of the data points (sample values) lie above the median, and half lie below it. The **mode** is the sample value that appears with the greatest frequency.

One of the most useful calculations in the clinical laboratory is the **standard deviation (SD)**. The mathematical symbol for SD is s. The SD measures the amount of variation in a set of data. It is calculated by the following formula:

$$s = \sqrt{\sum_{i=1}^{n} \frac{(x_i - \bar{x})^2}{n-1}}$$

This calculation is more complex than that for the mean, but it uses many of the same symbols. As before, the symbol $\sum$ denotes a summation function. This time, the symbol contains additional notation that indicates exactly which values are to be summed. The notation "$i = 1$" means that the sum function begins with the value calculated from the first number in the data set; the "n" notation means that the function ends with that from "nth" (last) item in the data set. Therefore, all n elements in the data set are to be used. The actual values to be summed are represented by $(x_i - \bar{x})^2 / n - 1$. To perform this function, the mean value $(\bar{x})$ is subtracted from each of the values (x_i) to be included; the resulting number is squared and then divided by the number of data elements (n) minus 1. Dividing by $n-1$ reduces bias because calculating the mean reduces the number of data points by 1. This process is repeated for each value of x between 1 and n. The final calculated values are then summed, and the square root of the result is taken to complete the calculation of s.

In the example, there are ten data elements, so $n - 1 = 9$. The mean for this data set is $\bar{x} = 4.7$. The first calculation to be performed is $(x_i - \bar{x})^2$. This done for each of the data elements:

$$(5-4.7)^2 = 0.09$$
$$(2-4.7)^2 = 7.29$$
$$(7-4.7)^2 = 5.29$$
$$(8-4.7)^2 = 10.89$$
$$(3-4.7)^2 = 2.89$$
$$(4-4.7)^2 = 0.49$$
$$(2-4.7)^2 = 7.29$$
$$(6-4.7)^2 = 1.69$$
$$(4-4.7)^2 = 0.49$$
$$(5-4.7)^2 = 0.09$$

Next, each number is divided by n–1, as in the formula:

$$n-1\left((x_i-\bar{x})^2/n-1\right)$$
$$0.09/9 = 0.01$$
$$7.29/9 = 0.88$$
$$5.29/9 = 0.66$$
$$10.89/9 = 1.21$$
$$2.89/9 = 0.32$$
$$0.49/9 = 0.05$$
$$7.29/9 = 0.88$$
$$1.69/9 = 0.19$$
$$0.49/9 = 0.05$$
$$0.09/9 = 0.01$$

Next, the numbers are summed:

$$0.01 + 0.88 + 0.66 + 1.21 + 0.32 + 0.05 +$$
$$0.88 + 0.19 + 0.05 + 0.01 = 4.35$$

Finally, the square root of the sum (4.35) is determined:

$$\sqrt{4.35} = 2.09$$

Therefore, the SD for this data set is

$$s = 2.09$$

The SD is helpful in analyzing QC data. Mathematically, 68.2% of the data points on a gaussian curve fall between +1 SD and –1 SD from the mean value. If the range is increased to between +2 SD and –2 SD, 95.4% of the data points will be included, and 99% of all values will fall between +3 SD and –3 SD from the mean (Fig. 7-6). When SD ranges are calculated (e.g., from repeated measurements of a control sample) and set up on a curve, they are called **confidence intervals.** For example, there is reasonable confidence that 95% of individual test values will fall within ±2 SD of the true mean of the data set; this is the 95% confidence interval. Values that fall outside the desired confidence interval may require further investigation. (Of course, the larger the data set, the closer the curve will be to a normal distribution.)

To set up such a curve for the small data set used in the example, the SD (2.09) is multiplied by –3, –2, –1, 1, 2, and 3, and those values are placed on the graph, with the mean (4.7)

at the center (Fig. 7-7). In this case, the 95% confidence interval (i.e., the range between +2 SD and –2 SD) is 0.52 to 8.88.

The **coefficient of variation** (CV) is used to monitor precision in the laboratory. Whereas the SD represents the average distance of data points from the mean value, the CV represents the degree of variability or dispersion of the data points relative to the mean. The coefficient of variation is calculated using the following equation:

$$CV(\%) = (s/\bar{x}) \times 100$$

For the example data set,

$$CV(\%) = (2.09/4.7) \times 100 = 4.44\%$$

The CV can be used to determine precision of the methods when a laboratory changes from one test method to another. Precise methods have a CV of less than 5%.

Statistical methods are useful for analyzing QC data, enabling laboratory personnel to produce accurate and precise laboratory test results. Laboratories also use statistical methods to construct reference ranges, create predictive values, and evaluate alternative test methods.

Reference Ranges

When statistical processes are used, the terms *population* and *sample* have distinct meanings. Each laboratory serves

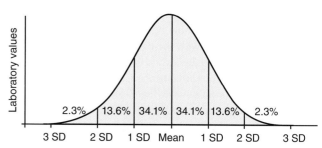

• **Figure 7-6** Standard deviations (SD) on a normal distribution curve, showing the expected percentage of data points falling within each interval.

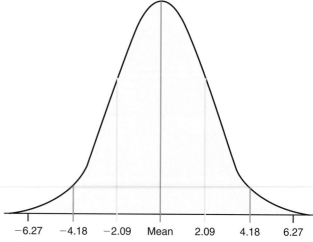

• **Figure 7-7** Example of confidence intervals on a normal distribution curve, using the sample data set provided in the text. The mean of the measured values is 4.7, and the standard deviation (SD) is 2.09 (see text).

a particular population consisting of all the people who use its services, regardless of age, income, and other factors. A sample is a portion of the original population. For example, if the population is a town, a sample would be a neighborhood in that town. A patient specimen is also referred to as a sample: The small amount of blood taken from a person is a sample of the entire amount of blood in that person's body. This distinction is particularly important when discussing reference ranges.

Reference ranges (also called normal ranges) for individual laboratory test results are very important in medical decision making. A reference range is defined as the range within which 95% of normal (non-diseased) persons' test results will fall. (In therapeutic drug testing and toxicology, results are usually reported in relation to *therapeutic ranges* rather than reference ranges.) Reference ranges are developed by each clinical laboratory because ethnic, genetic, cultural, and lifestyle differences and population norms may vary slightly in different geographic locations. Laboratory test values for an entire ethnic or geographic group constitute a generic range that is broad enough to include individuals with slight differences based on inherited physical traits.

According to CLSI standard EP28-A3c (*Defining, Establishing, and Verifying Reference Intervals in the Clinical Laboratory,* October 2010), the reference range (or interval) for an individual test is determined by testing a large group of at least 120 healthy individuals. The mean and SD are calculated for the data set, and then a range from –2 SD to 2 SD is calculated; this is the laboratory's reference range for that test. Laboratories can also verify a reference range used for a different method by showing that the new method produces identical results to the old method. Another option for a laboratory is to verify the manufacturer's reference range for a test.

The initial assumption when establishing reference ranges is that all persons who do not demonstrate clinical symptoms or signs of any disease will have normal laboratory test results. But this is not always true. An individual may be determined to be physically free of disease even if one or more test results fall outside the reference range; therefore, not all persons will fall within an established range even when free from disease. For some diagnostic laboratory tests, *normal* is defined as the absence of clinical evidence associated with a particular disease or medical condition.

A second assumption is also made: Test results from those persons considered normal will have a random distribution. Certain factors other than disease in a given geographic population may place a significant group of test values toward either the low or the high side of the previously normal range. The higher the number of subjects used in establishing reference ranges, the less the effect of a small number of individual results.

A patient whose results are outside the reference range may actually be free of disease, at least in relation to the test results. And because 99.7% of all individual test results fall into the range of ±3 SD in a normal distribution, it is obvious that 0.3% of individuals may have results that fall outside this range but still be of good health. There are several reasons for this. Genetic variations within a specific group (e.g., ethnicity in the population) may be found, with no clinical reason or outward manifestation accounting for the abnormal value of an analyte. Ranges have been established for indigenous population groups from specific areas over the entire globe.

Additional Limits for Control Values

Medical Decision Limit. In addition to reference ranges, a second set of limits for control values provides a wider span of medically acceptable results. These limits relate to the *medical usefulness* requirement, which ensures that the laboratory tests used will identify results that are medically significant (i.e., would alter a physician's diagnosis, treatment, or assessment of the patient).

Clinical Decision Limit. Physicians mentally adopt another set of acceptable values, with limits that are more subjective based on underlying conditions the patient may possess. These limits may represent a wider set of medically acceptable values for laboratory procedures on which the medical diagnosis is based.

Method Evaluation

Laboratory procedures change frequently, and many methods are available for measurement of different compounds in the body. Therefore, it is often necessary to consider new or different methods for producing quality laboratory results. Usually, experienced laboratory professionals are tasked with choosing the best test method for a specific laboratory. The accuracy of the method is of prime importance, but a number of other factors are also involved. Some test methods yield a considerable number of false-positive or false-negative results, so this is also an important consideration. Other factors that may be considered include cost of testing, amount of time required for the test, quality of test results, efficiency of testing, specificity, sensitivity, and satisfaction of those using laboratory services.

Two important criteria that should be considered when selecting a new method are diagnostic specificity and sensitivity. These parameters reflect the ability of a laboratory test to correctly identify the presence or absence of a disease based on a particular cutoff value. Diagnostic sensitivity refers to a test's ability to detect a disease in an individual who actually has the disease. It is reported as the percentage of people with the disease whose test result will be positive. For example, a test with 90% diagnostic sensitivity will yield a positive result in 90% of those patients with the disease (true positive) and a negative result in 10% of those people with the disease (false negative). Diagnostic specificity refers to the ability of a test to detect the absence of disease. It is reported as the percentage of people without the disease whose test result will be negative. For example, a test with a 90% diagnostic specificity will yield a negative result in 90% of those people without the disease (true negative) and a positive result in 10% of those people without the disease

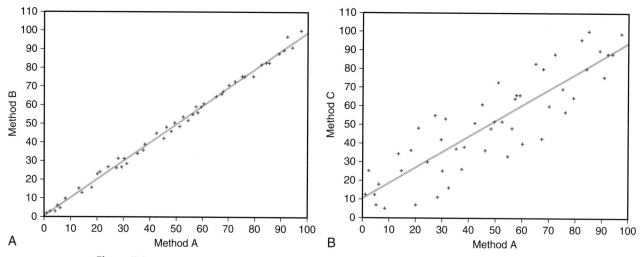

• **Figure 7-8** Examples of linear regression analysis with strong correlation **(A)** and weaker correlation **(B)**. (From McPherson RA, Pincus MR. *Henry's Clinical Diagnosis and Management by Laboratory Methods.* 22nd ed. Philadelphia: Elsevier; 2012.)

(false positive). No diagnostic test is both 100% sensitive and 100% specific.

Once a decision is made to change test methods and the new method is selected, the new method should be evaluated to ensure that it meets the needs and expectations of the laboratory. First, the linear range for the method is confirmed by analyzing a number of standards. This procedure verifies the method's linearity and demonstrates the precision of the method. In addition, because precision is an important attribute of a test method, all levels of control samples are run several times using the new method.

Linear Regression

When two methods are being evaluated for measurement of the same clinical material (e.g., glucose), there should be agreement between the values obtained with each method. When plotted against each other on a graph, the values of test samples measured by the two methods should approximate a straight line. Random errors in testing of the sample are represented by the distance of the values from that line. The statistical technique used for comparing the methods is called linear regression (Fig. 7-8).

The strength of the correlation between two different methods is described by the correlation coefficient (r), which can range from –1 to +1. A correlation of zero indicates that there is no relationship between the two values, whereas a value of 1 indicates a perfect relationship and –1 indicates an inverse relationship. Values between –1 and +1 indicate varying degree of relationship.

Analysis of Quality Control Data

Quality control charts are an essential method for observing the validity of test results from run to run. (A run is a batch of samples tested together or as part of a battery of tests that are performed concurrently.) These charts graphically demonstrate values of control samples over a period of time and provide information used to construct a range of

acceptable values or to determine whether a run has produced valid results that can be reported.

When control values fall outside the acceptable ranges established by the laboratory or the manufacturer's suggested ranges, warning signals indicate that problems associated with testing may be developing. The suspect areas may lie in the condition of the control samples, environmental factors affecting the samples or the equipment, or failure of components of the equipment used for testing. Control values are a marker of precision (reproducibility) and allow laboratory technical personnel to isolate the problem causing the error. In years past, manually prepared charts were displayed in the clinical chemistry department of the laboratory and could be observed by management as well as site visitors from accreditation agencies. Now, computerized pieces of equipment compile data from control values for automated tests, and the results may be viewed or printed for review. Use of control charts allows detection of errors to occur sooner rather than later. An example of a blank control chart is shown in Figure 7-9. The mean is represented by a line across the center of the charting area, and additional lines are drawn to represent –3 SD, –2 SD, +2 SD, and +3 SD. These precharted lines make it easier for laboratory personnel to identify an error.

Errors are broken down into two categories. An errant result can be random in nature, and no cause may be discovered, or it can be a systematic error. Random errors do occur infrequently and may be positive or negative in their effects on the value obtained through testing. Systematic errors consistently shift values in one direction (positive or negative). Common errors relate to variations in technique, inaccurately reconstituted control samples, and dirty sampling components of the testing equipment.

Systematic errors include trends and shifts. A trend is identified when six consecutive control results gradually move in either a positive or a negative direction on the

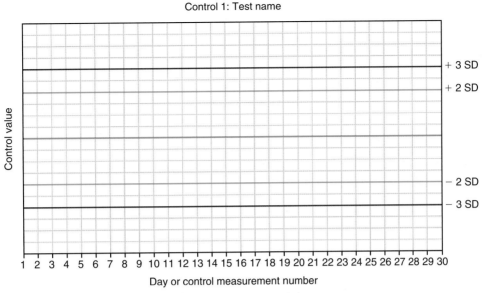

Control 1: Test name

• **Figure 7-9** Blank control chart.

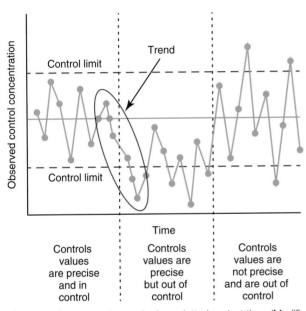

• **Figure 7-10** Display of control values plotted against time. (Modified from Burtis CA, Bruns DE. *Tietz Fundamentals of Clinical Chemistry and Molecular Diagnostics.* 7th ed. St. Louis: Saunders; 2015.)

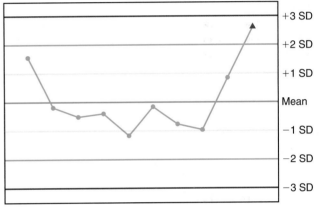

• **Figure 7-11** Levey-Jennings chart.

control chart (Fig. 7-10). When trends occur, they may signal a gradual deterioration of the equipment used for testing and may suggest eminent equipment failure without any further warning. A **shift** occurs when there is a sudden change in control results and at least six consecutive results lie on either the positive or the negative side of the mean value. A shift may announce an impending equipment malfunction, or it may indicate that a new lot number of controls is being used and the QC charts have not been updated.

Levey-Jennings Chart

The **Levey-Jennings chart** is representative of the data used to complete the normal or gaussian (bell-shaped) curve. A Levey-Jennings chart shows daily values in a graph form.

The mean is represented by a line drawn across the middle of the chart; for a given test, both negative and positive values (i.e., above and below the mean) should be seen over a given period of time, such as 1 month.

Levey-Jennings charts are included in the computerized system of the large and sophisticated automated analyzers. These reports are stored in the LIS and can be retrieved for review by site visitors from licensing and accreditation agencies.

Figure 7-11 depicts a Levey-Jennings chart with eleven control values plotted. Ten of the values are within the limit of ±2 SD from the mean and are considered to be in control; the eleventh value exceeds mean +2 SD and is considered out of control. The interpretation rules for these charts are discussed later.

Youden Plot

A **Youden plot** is another method for analyzing QC data. It is a graphic depiction for analyzing data variability from two levels of control materials within a laboratory or between two different laboratories. This technique is used with both

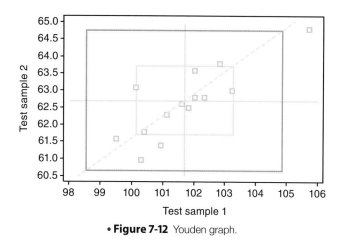

• **Figure 7-12** Youden graph.

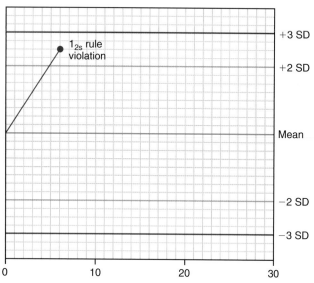

• **Figure 7-13** Levey-Jennings chart showing a 1_{2s} rule violation. The control measurement has exceeded the control limit of mean +2 SD.

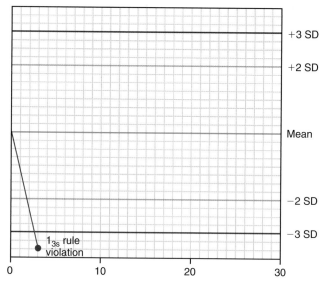

• **Figure 7-14** Levey-Jennings chart showing a 1_{3s} rule violation. A single control measurement has exceeded the control limit of mean −3 SD.

normal and abnormal control results and can differentiate between systematic and random errors. When control results are plotted on a Youden chart, there should be little or no difference between the spread of data for the two samples or two laboratories. On the graph, the center box represents 1 SD; the second box, 2 SD; and the third box, 3 SD; this makes it easy to visualize and understand the data presented (Fig. 7-12). The box is usually divided by lines parallel to the X and Y axes that bisect each other. A 45-degree reference line is drawn from the lower left to the upper right corner. As in the Levey-Jennings chart, control values that fall within the 2 SD box indicate that acceptable patient results are being generated. Points lying far from the line are random errors; results that lie along the 45-degree line but outside the 2 SD box represent systematic errors (see Fig. 7-12).

Quality Control Chart Rules

Quality control chart rules for interpretation of control results should enable a laboratory to detect an analytical error

quickly with a small false-positive alert rate. A laboratory needs to establish performance characteristics before selecting QC rules. The QC interpretive rules established by Westgard have been adopted by clinical laboratories to determine whether a test method is producing out-of-control results. Safeguards based on this system help to demonstrate quality of results and to develop practices for preventing errors; potential problem areas can be identified even before test results are distributed to the offices of medical practitioners and to medical records. Statistical process control verifies that test results are producing expected variability from a properly calibrated and stable operating system.

A laboratory chooses rules in order to detect calibration and precision changes that require corrective action before reporting patient results. The most common Westgard rules used in clinical laboratories are the following:

- 1_{2s} A control value that exceeds the established mean by ±2 SD is considered a warning to carefully inspect the control data (Fig. 7-13).
- 1_{3s} When a control value exceeds the established mean by ±3 SD, a random error is suspected (Fig. 7-14).
- 2_{2s} When two control values on two consecutive runs exceeds the same mean + 2 SD (or mean −2 SD) limit, a systematic error is probable (Fig. 7-15).
- R_{4s} When one control measurement exceeds the mean + 2 SD limit and another exceeds the mean −2 SD limit, a random error is indicated (Fig. 7-16).
- 4_{1s} When four consecutive control values exceed the same mean +1 SD (or mean −1 SD) limit, a systematic error is indicated (Fig. 7-17).
- 10_x When ten consecutive control values fall on the upper or lower side of the mean (without regard to distance from the mean), a systematic error is indicated (Fig. 7-18).

When a laboratory's control results violate the rules formulated by Westgard, patient test results may not be

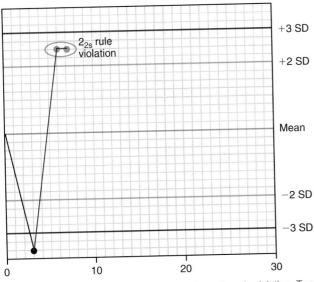

• **Figure 7-15** Levey-Jennings chart showing a 2$_{2s}$ rule violation. Two consecutive measurements have exceeded the same control limit (mean +2 SD).

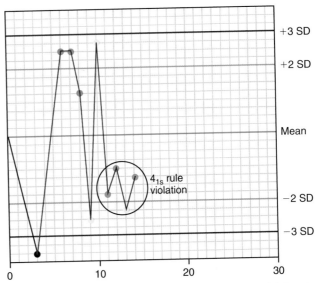

• **Figure 7-17** Levey-Jennings chart showing a 4$_{1s}$ rule violation. In this case, four consecutive control measurements have exceeded the same mean −1 SD limit.

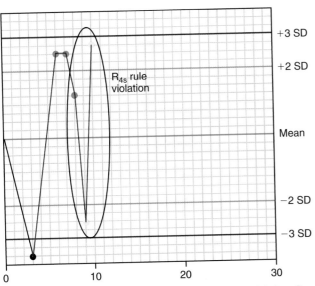

• **Figure 7-16** Levey-Jennings chart showing a R$_{4s}$ rule violation. One control measurement in a group has exceeded the limit of mean +2 SD, and another has exceeded mean −2 SD.

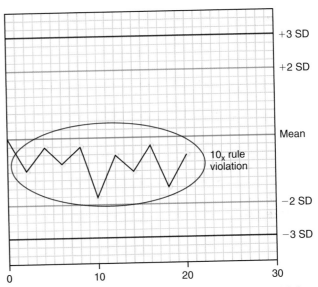

• **Figure 7-18** Levey-Jennings chart showing a 10$_x$ rule violation. Ten consecutive control measurements have fallen on one side of the mean.

acceptable for reporting. The typical definition of acceptable QC results is that all three control levels are within 2 SD of their true value, but this definition may vary by medical facility. None of Westgard's rules has a 100% error detection rate until the error is large. The 1$_{2s}$ rule detects 90% of all errors, but it also has many false alarms. The 1$_{3s}$ rule does not have a high rate of false alarms, but it also does not detect many errors (55%). For better results, laboratories should use more than one rule to evaluate QC data. For example, the 1$_{3s}$ and 2$_{2s}$ rules can be used together (i.e., a 1$_{3s}$/2$_{2s}$ rule violation would occur when one control exceeds ±3 SD or two controls exceed ±2 SD in the same direction from the mean).

This combination has a low false alarm rate but an improved ability to detect an error.

Corrective Actions

When QC results lead to violation of a Westgard rule, a problem may exist with the analytical system, and patient results cannot be reported until the issue is resolved. Any violation of the Westgard rules requires further investigation. A general schema for troubleshooting is presented in Figure 7-19.

Performance of proper and regular preventive maintenance and replacement of worn or defective parts lead to fewer out-of-control results. The following steps should rule out the occasional random error that invariably occurs in a small percentage of laboratory tests.

- Step 1: Analyze the control sample that is out of control. Obvious human error may be evident rather quickly. Ensure that the correct control was chosen and that the lot number of the control correlates with the QC chart.
- Step 2: Reconstitute (if applicable, because some controls come in a liquid form) a new vial of control specimen, and allow adequate time for complete dissolution of the mixture.
- Step 3: Repeat the test using a new control vial; if acceptable control values are obtained, the problem was most likely with the original control sample.
- Step 4: If the control value is still out of range, perform basic daily maintenance. A number of components should be checked as outlined in the operational manual for the instrument.

- Step 5: Unacceptable control values may also indicate that the instrument needs to be recalibrated, a step that may be required periodically.
- Step 6: In the event that recalibration does not return the control results to the acceptable range, another laboratory professional with more technical experience may be able to help. The last step in this series of corrective actions should be to obtain help from an expert, usually a manufacturer's technical representative.

After the technical issue has been resolved, the control samples must be repeated with the patient run. The test results from the repeated run must meet laboratory criteria to determine whether results from both runs have adequate agreement so that the patient test results from the original run can be reported. If the test results from the two runs are very different, a corrected report should be released.

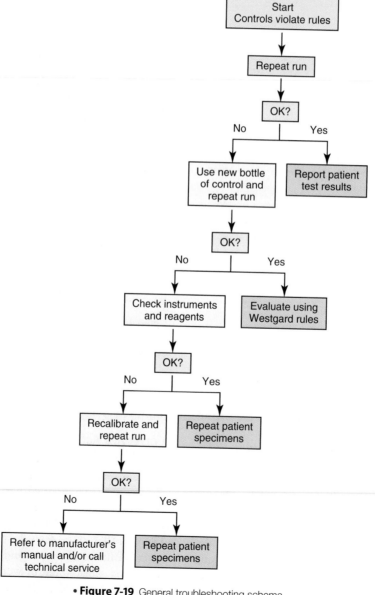

• **Figure 7-19** General troubleshooting schema.

External Quality Control (Proficiency Testing)

Proficiency testing is a form of external QC in which external organizations send unknown samples to laboratories for testing. Whereas QC procedures are useful in providing precision, proficiency testing measures accuracy. Laboratory technical personnel need to understand the differences between routine QC testing and proficiency sample testing. The majority of clinical laboratories use the proficiency testing program provided by the College of American Pathologists, but a number of others are approved by the Centers for Medicare and Medicaid Services. Acceptable proficiency testing performance is required for a laboratory to maintain accreditation. CLIA 88 mandates specific performance results in proficiency testing; otherwise, a laboratory will be unable to report patient test results for tests that do not meet the performance criteria.

A laboratory subscribes to a proficiency testing service offered by an external organization. This organization sends unknown samples to the laboratory on a prearranged schedule. The schedule usually matches or exceeds the schedule set forth by CLIA. These unknown specimens, or proficiency test materials, are tested as routine samples along with patient samples. Proficiency testing samples may be purchased from a number of providers and can be tailored to meet the specific needs of a particular laboratory. The test results from the proficiency test samples are documented by the laboratory and returned to the testing agency, where they are compared with results submitted from all laboratories using similar instrumentation for a particular test. Test results can differ depending on which instrument and reagents are used to perform the testing. The test results from a laboratory must fall within an established range in order to document accurate test performance. Repeated failure to achieve acceptable results for a particular test will lead to prohibitions against reporting patient results for that test until corrective action is taken and acceptable results are validated by future proficiency testing. In extreme cases and for repeated failures on multiple tests, the laboratory may be forced to close.

During testing of proficiency samples, laboratories are expected to adhere to the following practices:

1. Each laboratory performs its own analyses without consultation with other laboratories.
2. Tests are performed by the technical personnel who normally perform patient testing for the various analytes by inserting these samples into the normal workflow without placing special attention on the proficiency samples.
3. Tests are performed within the same time frame as is routinely used for patient tests (some tests are performed only when a sufficient number of tests have been ordered) so that, within reason, proficiency testing is performed along with routine testing.

Postanalytical Phase

The final phase of process control, the postanalytical phase, involves interpreting test results and reporting them in a systematic fashion. This phase requires proper reporting of results and delivery of the reports to the appropriate provider. Automation has improved this task, and errors in transcribing and reporting results are diminished with the use of computerized systems. The LIS prevents many report transmission issues when properly programmed.

Test results produced by a clinical laboratory undergo two postanalytical evaluations. First, the laboratory ensures that the results are reviewed for analytical reliability by flagging results that are outside the reference range, checking the linearity of the test methods, and using delta checks. The health care provider performs the second analysis when clinical data are combined with laboratory data to diagnose and treat patients.

Automated instruments are programmed to flag specimens that require additional review before results are released to the LIS. Flagged test results can indicate a problem with the specimen itself. For example, instrument sample probes are programmed to detect the amount of sample in the tube, and a flag is generated if there is not enough sample to run the test. Instruments also flag specimens with high concentrations of interfering substances (e.g., lipemia, hemolysis).

Instruments can also generate flags when a test result exceeds the linearity of the test method. Sometimes, the instrument automatically dilutes the specimen and reruns it; in other cases, the specimen must be manually diluted and rerun to get a valid test result.

In addition to QC rules, comparison of a patient's current test result for a particular analyte against a previous result for the same analyte (delta check) can be used to identify laboratory errors. Test results are chosen from a specific time interval in the past when a physiologic change in the patient's status was not likely. Not all tests can be monitored with a delta check. The main purpose of a delta check is to detect mislabeled samples and possibly samples that are diluted with intravenous fluid. A suitable threshold level must be selected so that excessive false alerts are avoided. Samples chosen for delta checks must identified, and follow-up investigations must ensue if there is a discrepancy.

When laboratory technicians review test results before releasing them to the LIS, they always check for critical values (also called panic values). A critical value is a test value that indicates a life-threatening condition. Critical values require an immediate call to the clinician so that the clinician can provide necessary medical interventions for the patient. The rapid communication of critical values to the provider is required by accreditation organizations and is one of the national Patient Safety Goals of The Joint Commission. Federal regulations require laboratory technicians to call the clinician and then have the clinician repeat the test result and the patient's name back to the technician to verify the communication. The laboratory technician must then document the communication of this value to the clinician, including the name and title of the person receiving the information, the time and date of the conversation, and the readback by the clinician. Critical values are set by each laboratory, as is the policy for contacting clinicians (i.e., registered nurse, nurse practitioner, physician assistant, or medical doctor). As a result, procedures for reporting critical values vary at each institution.

Using Reference Ranges

Difficulties occur when reference ranges are followed so closely by providers that normal (healthy) patients may be required to undergo the expense and discomfort of further testing simply because one test result was outside the reference range by a small amount. All living organisms have differences in their metabolic processes, and slight differences in a population may be of a genetic or environmental nature, rather than indicating the existence of a disease condition. Chemistry tests in the laboratory are not often ordered as a single procedure; usually, they are performed as a batch of tests that measure many aspects of the metabolism of one or more body systems. When all of the results of a battery of chemistry tests are within normal ranges except for one or two, this may merely reflect individual differences and may not be indicative of a medical abnormality.

Moreover, a supposedly normal population used to establish a reference range of values may contain a small but definite group of clinically normal persons with subclinical manifestations of disease. Some who report themselves as "normal" may have an undetected disease but nevertheless be included in the data used to establish the values.

References ranges obtained by one analytical method may be inappropriately used with another method. The reference ranges for most procedures vary depending on the methodology used for the test as well as the selected instrumentation.

Assessment

Assessment is an important quality system essential because it helps a laboratory determine the effectiveness of its QMS by evaluating performance. Assessment is defined as a systematic examination of the policies, processes, and procedures contained in a laboratory's QMS. The assessment function demonstrates that a laboratory is meeting regulatory, accreditation, and customer requirements. Usually, accreditation standards form the basis for laboratory assessment. Some questions answered through assessment practices are the following:

- What procedures and processes are being followed in the laboratory?
- Are there written policies and procedures?
- Do the current procedures and processes align with written policies and procedures?
- Do written policies and procedures comply with standards, regulations, and requirements?

There are many different ways to conduct assessments. The ISO standards detail specific assessment requirements. ISO standards also refer to assessments as *audits*. Assessments or audits provide data for managers to understand the laboratory's performance compared with a standard or benchmark. Gaps in performance can reveal areas where

policies, procedures, or processes may need to be revised. Gaps can also reveal that existing policies, procedures, or processes are not being followed. The audits provide good information for CQI in laboratory operations.

Audits

There are two types of audits that laboratories may use to gather information: internal and external. Internal audits may consist of individuals from different departments conducting assessments in the laboratory. External audits may be conducted by external groups such as accrediting agencies, CMS, or state agencies. Audits need to examine all processes in the laboratory—preanalytical, analytical, and postanalytical. Well-designed audits can help find the performance gaps. Information is usually gathered about processes and operating procedures, staff competence and training, equipment, environment, handling of samples, QC practices, and recording and reporting practices. This information is then compared with the laboratory's internal policies, procedures, and processes and with an external benchmark.

Accreditation organizations are external groups that visit laboratories to assess adherence to accreditation standards. Accrediting bodies audit a laboratory when the laboratory first applies for accreditation to ensure compliance with standards. Once the laboratory is accredited, the accreditation organization periodically returns to the laboratory to ensure that it is still compliant with the accreditation standards.

When a laboratory is notified of an external audit, it will prepare by organizing documents and records ahead of time and informing staff as well as scheduling meetings of appropriate staff with auditors. At times, external auditors do not provide prior notification for a site visit or give only a very short notification time frame. In any case, laboratories should always ensure that they are in compliance with accreditation standards.

The auditors usually provide a verbal summary of their findings and recommendations before they leave the laboratory, and they always follow up with a written report. A laboratory should use the information and recommendations generated by the audit to identify gaps where standards were not fully met, plan to correct the gaps, record the actions taken to correct the gaps, and document the CQI cycle.

Laboratories are familiar with external audits, but internal auditing may be a new idea. Internal audits allow laboratories to look at their policies, procedures, and processes as frequently as needed. If a new policy is implemented, an internal audit can be a way to gather information and determine whether the policy is working. Internal audits can also help a laboratory prepare for an external audit, increase staff awareness of quality system requirements, identify gaps in performance, understand areas where preventive or corrective action is needed, identify areas for further training, and determine whether the laboratory is meeting its own quality standards.

Continuous monitoring is the key to a successful **continuous quality improvement cycle** (CQI). It starts with a **quality improvement plan,** which is followed by corrective actions and finally by monitoring and evaluation. Audits can help a laboratory monitor and evaluate its policies, procedures, and processes.

Proficiency testing is an external quality assessment method used by laboratories to determine the accuracy of their test results (see earlier discussion).

Personnel

Personnel are the most valuable resource in any laboratory. People who possess integrity, recognize the importance of their work, and participate in the CQI process are important partners in any health care system. It is important for laboratory technicians employed by a clinical laboratory to participate in training and educational opportunities, request training that may be needed to perform a job well, and maintain records of personal professional development. A laboratory will thrive or fail based on the knowledge, skills, commitment, and motivation of its employees.

Competency and Competency Assessment

Laboratory technicians are considered competent when they are able to apply knowledge, skills, and behavior to the performance of specific job tasks. Laboratory technicians should be competent in performing a wide variety of procedures that occur throughout the testing process. CLIA 88 requires laboratories to implement competency testing for all employees performing laboratory tests. A **competency assessment** is a system for measuring and documenting the competency of laboratory personnel. Competency assessment is important because issues with employee performance need to be corrected before patient test results are affected. Competency assessments are performed when a laboratory technician is first hired and periodically throughout his or her employment. If issues with a technician's performance are recognized during competency testing, training can be provided for the technician.

There are a few ways that competency assessment can be accomplished: direct observation (using checklists), monitoring of laboratory records, review and analysis of QC records and results of proficiency testing performed by the employee, retesting or rechecking of results for comparison, and use of case studies to assess knowledge or problem-solving skills. Competency assessments must be documented, showing the date and results, and they should also remain confidential. These records are part of the laboratory's QMS documentation and should be considered as part of the laboratory's CQI activities.

Customer Service

Customer service is part of a QMS because if the customer is not well served, the laboratory is not fulfilling its mission.

Philip Crosby, one of the founding fathers of the quality movement, defined quality **customer service** as meeting the customer's requirements. The same is true for clinical laboratories. The clinical laboratory should know its clients and their expectations, needs, and requirements. Customer service is extremely important for laboratories, and laboratory technicians should always treat clients respectfully and courteously.

The laboratory's clients are customers. However, even though the laboratory requisition identifies a health care provider or physician and this person is considered the primary customer, there are many other individuals who are also considered customers. Other customers include nurses, medical assistants, phlebotomists, secretaries, clerks, patients, family members, public health officials, companies, and the community. In the United States, only licensed health care providers are authorized to order laboratory tests. Laboratories know they are providing good customer service when they deliver valuable information for the best patient care, valuable information for public health organizations, and an image as a professional, quality, reliable laboratory.

Assessing customer satisfaction is an important process in the laboratory's CQI program. Information about customer satisfaction can be gathered through reporting customer complaints, assessing quality indicators, administering satisfaction surveys, and conducting interviews and focus groups. Information gathering can lead to changes in laboratory policy, procedures, or processes.

Occurrence Management

Occurrence management is a central tenet in laboratory CQI. It is a process by which the laboratory identifies and handles errors and near misses. It is a proactive process that leads to changes in policies, procedures, processes, or communication to prevent errors from occurring.

An **occurrence** is an event with a negative impact on an organization, its personnel, or the organization's product, equipment, or environment. If the laboratory fails, significant effects can include inadequate or inappropriate health care, inappropriate public health actions, undetected infectious disease outbreaks, and even patient death.

Process Improvement

The **continuous process improvement program** of a laboratory is based on W. Edward Deming's fourteen quality points. Two of these points—"Create constancy of purpose for improvement" and "Improve constantly and forever"—are the mainstay of laboratory programs. There is always room for improvement, and this process is never finished. As in other aspects of today's world, change is the only constant.

Concepts

The basis for Deming's CQI cycle is his Plan–Do–Check–Act cycle (Fig. 7-20). The laboratory first identifies issues

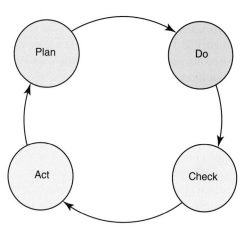

• **Figure 7-20** Plan–Do–Check–Act method for continuous improvement.

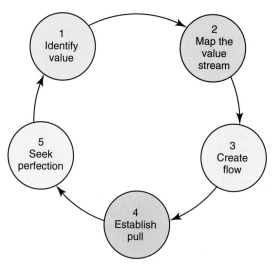

• **Figure 7-21** Lean processes.

and system weaknesses and then gathers the related information. A plan is developed with stakeholders for improvement. Next, the plan is implemented, and data about policies, processes, and procedures are gathered. The data are assessed for effectiveness of the action taken to improve the process. The plan is then updated to ensure that the identified improvements occur. Finally, corrective action is taken to ensure that the plan is effective. Then the process begins again—it is a cycle.

Tools

Several tools are used in the CQI process. Internal audits, external audits, and proficiency testing are all tools that can pinpoint weaknesses and problem areas in laboratory policies, processes, and procedures. The information gained from these tools can be used to identify opportunities for improvement as long as they align with a laboratory goal or standard.

Two newer processes that originated in the manufacturing industry are now also being used in the laboratory: Lean and Six Sigma. Lean optimizes space, time, and activity to improve physical paths of workflow. A lean analysis can lead to improved processes and changes in laboratory floor plans (Fig. 7-21). Six Sigma uses a formal project planning structure that moves the process of reducing error to the lowest levels in the organization. Six Sigma uses a five-step cycle: Define, Measure, Analyze, Improve, and Control (Fig. 7-22).

Quality Indicators and Their Selection

Standardized international quality indicators are described in the ISO 9001 and ISO 15189 regulations. ISO 9001 requires a laboratory to create measurable objectives that can be assessed to determine the success of the quality system. Required indicators include customer satisfaction, conformity to customer requirements, a count of preventive

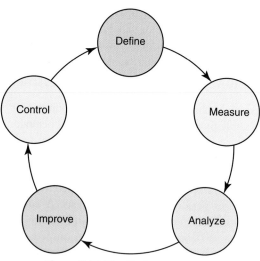

• **Figure 7-22** The Six Sigma sequence.

actions addressed, and quality materials provided by suppliers. ISO 15189 requires a laboratory to implement quality indicators to systematically monitor and evaluate the laboratory's contribution to patient care. This indicator also requires the laboratory to engage laboratory personnel at all levels in this work.

Implementation

Implementing a CQI process requires the participation of managers as well as all other laboratory personnel. All levels of laboratory staff must commit to this process for it to work well. The analysis of information by management should lead to careful planning so that goals can be achieved. Even though all personnel must participate in CQI for it to be successful, top management must be engaged and supportive.

Planning of quality improvement activities involves establishing a timeline, using a team approach, using appropriate tools, implementing actions, and reporting activities and findings to everyone in the laboratory.

Documents and Records

A major goal in keeping documents and records is to be able to find information whenever it is needed. Laboratory *documents* include policies, processes, and procedures. A quality manual and a standard operating procedure notebook are considered documents. A **policy** is a written statement of intentions and directions defined by a laboratory and endorsed by management. Each laboratory develops policies for its own operations. A **process** is a set of interrelated activities that convert inputs (test requisitions) into outputs (test results). A **procedure** is a step-by-step guideline for performing a test. Documents are important in a laboratory because they guide all laboratory operations.

Laboratory *records* include information produced during performance and reporting of laboratory tests. Examples include forms, charts, sample logs, QC charts, and patient reports.

Standard Operating Procedures

Accreditation organizations and licensure agencies require that a procedure manual for the clinical laboratory be produced and used for reference by laboratory staff who perform laboratory procedures. These manuals may be in a written format, or they may be stored on a computer. Examples are available from a number of Internet sites and are quite lengthy. CLSI provides a template for creating a procedure for each test offered on the laboratory menu; it requires, at a minimum, the following pieces of information:

- *Heading, Number, Title:* Necessary for identifying tests in an unmistakable format
- *Procedure Prepared by:* Responsible person to whom questions may be addressed
- *Approved by:* Procedures approved by the laboratory manager and/or a pathologist
- *Effective Date:* When the particular methodology was employed
- *Supersedes:* The methodology used before the current procedure method was adopted
- *Laboratory Section:* Laboratory department in which the procedure is performed
- *Procedure:* Narrative name of procedure identified as a number previously
- *Purpose of Procedure:* What is being tested for (e.g., glucose in urine)
- *Principle of Procedure:* The basis for how the procedure works (e.g., a certain molecule binds to a chemical, producing a color reaction)
- *Specimen:* The required type of specimen; this is needed because many body fluids may be used for testing (e.g., urine, blood serum and plasma, whole blood)

- *Patient Preparation:* For many laboratory procedures, the patient needs to be fasting before the test; some procedures require extensive preparation of the patient
- *Handling Conditions:* Biosafety precautions, proper storage of samples
- *Equipment and Materials:* Items needed for performing the test (must be obtained before testing begins)
- *Equipment:* Instruments used for testing
- *Preparation:* Preparatory steps needed (e.g., proper preparation of the sample, rehydration of standards or controls)
- *Performance Parameters:* Limitations of the procedure, such as inability to measure very large or very small levels of a metabolite; the linearity limits of the procedure are available from the manufacturer's package insert accompanying test reagents
- *Storage Requirements:* Precautions for storing specimens and reagents
- *Calibration Procedure:* When and how measuring instruments are calibrated
- *Quality Control:* Control specimens to be used and recorded to validate test results
- *Procedural Steps:* Numbered steps required to perform the procedure; must be written in an understandable fashion
- *Calculations:* An outline of any calculations that are required to obtain meaningful results
- *Reporting Results:* Any special instructions regarding the reporting of results that must be annotated; test values are chiefly reported electronically to medical offices requesting the procedures
- *Reference Ranges:* These are usually printed on report forms
- *Reporting Abnormal Results:* Values above and below established values to be reported promptly and often verbally to the treating physician
- *Reporting Format:* Results are primarily reported electronically in a standardized format
- *Procedure Notes:* Any unusual finding or anything not reported on a standard report form
- *Limitations of Procedure:* These data may be obtained from the manufacturer's package insert
- *References:* Sources researched in writing the procedure; manufacturer's references are found on the package insert
- *Signature/Date Information:* Signature of the employee who completed the annual review

Standard operating procedures (SOPs) are step-by-step instructions for performing tests and operating equipment in the laboratory. Laboratory staff follow these procedures when performing laboratory tests. SOPs improve consistency because everyone performing a test does so according to the procedures. SOPs can also improve accuracy because laboratory staff do not need to rely on memory to perform the tests. Finally, SOPs produce quality laboratory results through consistent and accurate test performance.

A good SOP is detailed, clear, concise, easily understood, up-to-date, and reviewed and approved by laboratory management. New personnel, students, and staff normally not performing tests should be able to follow the SOP if performing the test. Manufacturers' product inserts should not be substituted for the SOPs; the information from the product insert should be used to develop the SOP.

The Quality Manual

Laboratory quality manuals are used to clearly communicate information and to serve as a framework for achieving a QMS. The manual should contain policies addressing all twelve essential elements of a quality system, a reference to policies and procedures, and a table of contents. Like SOPs, the quality manual needs to be signed and dated by the laboratory manager. The manual should be updated regularly, and a schedule should be prepared for this purpose. Any change to the manual requires approval of those individuals with authority to make the changes. Laboratory personnel should know how to use the manual and must understand and follow the policies in the manual.

Quality is a way of thinking, and time invested in a QMS today will help accomplish quality goals. All laboratory personnel are responsible for quality. Leaders and managers must commit to meeting quality needs, and personnel must commit to following all policies, processes, and procedures.

Overview of Records

Records contain laboratory information and are permanent, with no revisions or modifications allowed. Records can be used for continuous monitoring, sample tracking, evaluating problems, and managing the laboratory. Records must not be changed. If an addition is required, the information should be added, then signed (or initialed), and the date recorded. If a deletion is necessary, a line should be drawn through the information, then signed (or initialed), and dated.

Examples of records include logbooks, worksheets, instrument printouts, QC data, proficiency testing records and reports, patient test reports, continuous improvement projects, incident reports, user surveys, customer feedback, and letters from regulatory or accreditation organizations. Records that need to be maintained include specimen rejection logs with reasons for rejection, information about adverse occurrences and investigations, inventory and storage records, and equipment records.

Reports of patient test results should contain the name of the test, the name of the laboratory, a unique patient identification number, patient location, name and address of provider requesting the test, date and time of collection, date and time received in the laboratory, date and time of report, sample type, results reported in units, reference intervals, comments such as sample quality or sample adequacy, and identification and signature of the patient authorizing release of the report. Some laboratory reports may also include the patient's gender and age.

Storage of Documents and Records

Documents and records must be stored so that the information can be easily retrieved. During accreditation visits, documents and records are often requested to be reviewed. Laboratories must retain documents and records for specific periods of time according to government requirements or standards, accreditation standards, or best practices.

Information Management

The LIS incorporates all the processes needed to effectively manage incoming and outgoing patient information. Unique identifiers for patient samples are important to eliminate confusion and mix-up of samples. The records of patient results must be kept confidential and protected from loss of data.

Organization

The management and supporting structure of a laboratory play a part in the quality of the test results produced by the laboratory. Managerial commitment is a principal element for a successful laboratory QMS. Managers must support and participate in quality system activities. Staff should receive support when needed to reinforce the importance of the QMS in the laboratory. Because the QMS requires policies and resources, management must support this system for it to be successful.

Organizational requirements for a successful QMS include the following:

1. Leadership—Laboratory leaders must commit to the laboratory QMS through good communication and wise use of resources.
2. Organizational structure—The laboratory's functional organizational chart should have clear lines of responsibility.
3. Planning process—A plan should be drafted for the QMS that includes a time frame for implementation, responsibility for conducting activities, use of human resources, workflow management, and financial resource allocation.
4. Implementation—Implementation of the laboratory's QMS requires project management, allocation of resources as needed, adherence to the time line, and goal achievement.
5. Monitoring—Processes for monitoring the QMS need to be developed to ensure that monitoring of the system occurs, benchmarks and standards are being met, and improvements are continually being implemented as the organization learns through errors and error correction.

Responsibilities of managers in a QMS include the following:

1. Establish policies and processes.
2. Document all policies, processes, procedures, and instructions.

3. Ensure that personnel understand documents, instructions, and their duties and responsibilities.
4. Provide personnel with authority and resources to implement the QMS.

Laboratory personnel are responsible for understanding where the authority and responsibility for quality management are assigned. Personnel are responsible for following the quality policies in their daily work. A laboratory QMS must have a laboratory quality manager. Typical responsibilities for this individual include monitoring the QMS, checking staff compliance with quality policies and procedures, reviewing all records, coordinating internal and external audits, investigating deficiencies identified in audits, and communicating observations on the CQI activities.

Summary

The laboratory QMS includes the twelve key quality essentials: facilities and safety, customer service, process improvement, documents and records, occurrence management, assessment, purchasing and inventory, process control, information management, equipment, personnel, and organization.

Process control includes the preanalytical, analytical, and postanalytical phases of laboratory testing. The preanalytical phase consists of physiologic variables, specimen collection and handling, and transport. The analytical phase consists of the test measurement process and includes statistical process control (QC). Descriptive statistics are used to interpret control values and assist in analysis. Control values are monitored using Westgard rules to ensure that reliable and accurate test results are produced. The postanalytical phase includes releasing test results and reporting test results to providers.

The laboratory generates many documents and reports that must be maintained and retained according to accreditation and federal regulations. Information management is vitally important to the laboratory. The laboratory's product is information, and this information must be kept safe, secure, and confidential. The information should be stored so that it is secure but easily retrievable.

At the heart of the QMS is the CQI cycle. This cycle ensures that the laboratory is constantly reviewing and correcting errors and always looking for ways to increase efficiency and effective operation. Internal and external audits help identify gaps in performance where improvement can be made.

Review Questions

1. Preanalytical variables include all the following EXCEPT
   a. Freezing
   b. Handling
   c. Collection
   d. Transportation

2. Which of the following indicates *accuracy*?
   a. When consecutive laboratory test results yield the same number
   b. When a laboratory test result is close to its known value
   c. When two consecutive test results from the same specimen have exactly the value
   d. When consecutive laboratory test results are within ±2 SD

3. Which of the following is a sample of known concentration used to monitor the testing process?
   a. Assayed control
   b. Unassayed control
   c. Liquid control
   d. Standard

4. Which of the following statements about reference intervals is true?
   a. They are drawn from the first 20 patients of the day.
   b. They are not useful for medical decision limits.
   c. They are calculated by each laboratory for every test they run.
   d. They include only specific groups of people.

5. When automated instruments are used, what must be done before patient results are released?
   a. Repeat high values
   b. Count workload data
   c. Assign numbers to patients
   d. Analyze QC and patient values

6. Levey-Jennings charts
   a. Are constructed using ±2 SD
   b. Are constructed using ±3 SD
   c. Do not contain useful information
   d. Are an old concept not used in laboratories today

7. Which of the following is an ISO standard that applies to the clinical laboratory?
   a. ISO 9000
   b. ISO 7000
   c. ISO 15789
   d. ISO 15436

8. A preventive maintenance program includes which of the following?
   a. Free technical support
   b. Systematic and routine cleaning, adjustment of the system, and replacement of parts
   c. A plan that prevents testing when maintenance is performed
   d. Replacement of parts when the instrument is malfunctioning

9. Which of the following is the most common cause of a shift in a control chart?
   a. Not refrigerating controls
   b. Different control lot number used
   c. Poor placement in the run
   d. Outdated reagent

10. All of the following are common errors encountered in specimen collection EXCEPT
    a. Specimen mislabeling
    b. Hemoconcentration
    c. Short draws
    d. Complete centrifugation

Critical Thinking Questions

1. Why is a laboratory quality management system important?
2. Why are Westgard rules used to analyze quality control values?
3. Describe the continuous quality improvement process in a laboratory.

CASE STUDIES

1. A technician is running one of the large automated analyzers in the chemistry department. The control values are shown in the graph. What Westgard rule is broken, and what should the technician do next?

2. The next day, the technician runs the same test and has the results shown in the graph. What Westgard rule is broken, and what should the technician do now?

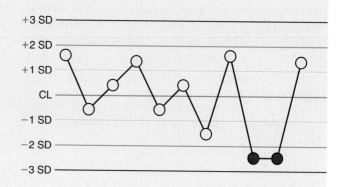

Bibliography

Bachner P. Quality assurance in hematology. In: Howanitz JF, Howanits JH, eds. *Laboratory Quality Assurance.* New York: McGraw-Hill; 1987:214–243.

Centers for Disease Control and Prevention. Centers for Medicare and Medicaid Services, Department of Health and Human Services. Medicare, Medicaid, and CLIA programs; Laboratory requirements relating to quality systems and certain personnel qualifications. Final rule. *Fed Reg.* 2003;68:3639–3714.

Clinical and Laboratory Standards Institute. *Statistical Quality Control for Quantitative Measurements: Principles and Definitions.* Wayne, PA: CLSI; 2006.

Dux J. *Handbook of Quality Assurance for the Analytical Chemistry Laboratory.* New York: Springer Science & Business Media; 2012.

International Committee for Standardization in Haematology. Standardization of blood specimen collection procedures for reference values. *Clin Lab Haematol.* 1982;4:83–86.

Westgard JO, Klee GG. Quality management. In: Burtis CA, Ashwood ER, eds. *Fundamentals of Clinical Chemistry.* 4th ed. Philadelphia: Saunders; 1996:211–223.

Kearney HM, Thorland EC, Brown KK, et al. American College of Medical Genetics standards and guidelines for interpretation and reporting of postnatal constitutional copy number variants. *Genet Med.* 2011;13(7):680–685.

Konieczka P, Namiesnik J. *Quality Assurance and Quality Control in the Analytical Chemical Laboratory: A Practical Approach.* Boca Raton, FL: CRC Press; 2009.

Krouwer JS, Rabinowitz R. How to improve estimates of imprecision. *Clin Chem.* 1984;30:290–292.

Levey S, Jennings ER. The use of control charts in the clinical laboratory. *Am J Clin Pathol.* 1950;20:1059–1066.

National Committee for Clinical Laboratory Standards. *Proposed Guideline for Evaluation of Linearity of Quantitative Analytical Methods* Document no. EP6–P2. Villanova, PA: NCCLS; 2001.

Ryder KW, Glick MR. Erroneous laboratory results from hemolyzed, icteric, and lipemic specimens. *Clin Chem.* 1993;39:175–176.

Statland BE, Westgard JO. Quality management. In: Henry JB, ed. *Clinical Diagnosis and Management by Laboratory Methods.* 18th ed. Philadelphia: Saunders; 1991:81–100.

8

Enzymes

M. LAURA PARNAS AND THOMAS KAMPFRATH

CHAPTER OUTLINE

OBJECTIVES

At the completion of this chapter, the reader will be able to:

1. Describe the four levels of an enzyme.
2. Name two ways to increase the reaction rate of a chemical equation.
3. Describe the first two laws of thermodynamics.
4. Explain why a state of equilibrium is dynamic.
5. Draw an energy diagram for a thermodynamically favorable forward chemical reaction and an energy diagram for a thermodynamically unfavorable forward chemical reaction.
6. Compare and contrast zero-order and first-order kinetics.
7. Describe the specificity of enzymes.
8. Describe how an enzyme works.
9. Name six major classes of enzymes and state their functions.
10. Demonstrate the naming convention for enzymes.
11. Explain the properties of enzymes.
12. Explain how the free energy of activation is involved in enzyme-catalyzed reactions.
13. Discuss the alternate reaction pathway used in enzymatically catalyzed reactions.
14. Discuss the Michaelis-Menten model for enzyme-catalyzed reactions.

15. Write the Michaelis-Menten equation and discuss the assumptions on which the equation is based.
16. Describe a Lineweaver-Burk plot and its use.
17. Discuss competitive inhibition of enzyme-catalyzed reactions.
18. Describe the effect of competitive inhibition on the maximum velocity (V_{max}) of a reaction, Michaelis constant (K_m), and Lineweaver-Burk plot.
19. Discuss noncompetitive inhibition of enzyme-catalyzed reactions.
20. Describe the effect of noncompetitive inhibition on V_{max}, K_m, and the Lineweaver-Burk plot.
21. Describe when a primary reaction is a rate-limiting step.
22. Describe the effect of temperature on the reaction rate.
23. Describe the effect of enzyme concentration on reaction rate.
24. Describe the effect of substrate concentration on reaction rate.
25. Describe the mechanism for drugs to act as enzyme inhibitors.
26. Compare and contrast reversible and irreversible inhibition.

OBJECTIVES—cont'd

27. Define isoenzymes and give three examples of isoenzymes.
28. Discuss how serum or plasma enzymes can be used as diagnostic tools.
29. Discuss the correlation of isoenzymes with diseases.
30. Describe enzyme activators.
31. Describe coenzymes and prosthetic groups and how they work.
32. Describe how chemical changes are measured in a diagnostic test that uses an enzymatic reaction.
33. Describe why enzyme reactions do not require standards or use a standard curve to determine concentrations of unknowns.
34. Compare and contrast four methods used to differentiate isoenzymes in the clinical laboratory.
35. Summarize the physiology, clinical significance, and laboratory procedures and limitations of transaminases, alkaline phosphatase, γ-glutamyl transferase, creatine kinase, lactate dehydrogenase, amylase, and lipase.

KEY TERMS

Activation energy
Activators
Active site
Allosteric sites
Coenzymes
Cofactors
Competitive inhibition
End-point or one-point method
Enzyme
Enzyme kinetics

Enzyme–substrate complex
Hydrolase
International unit
Isoenzyme
Isomerase
Kinetic or multipoint fixed time method
Ligase
Lyase
Michaelis-Menten kinetics
Noncompetitive inhibition

Oxidoreductase
Product
Product formation
Prosthetic groups
Substrate
Transferase
Transition state
Uncompetitive inhibition
Zero-order kinetics

Case in Point

A 57-year-old man is admitted to the emergency department with complaints of acute onset of intense abdominal pain. On physical examination, the pain appears to be localized to the upper abdomen near the epigastric area and radiating to the back. While being examined, the patient experiences nausea and vomiting. The patient denies recent alcohol consumption and states that he has not been feeling well during the past few days. What diagnoses should be considered for the patient? What laboratory tests can aid in making a definitive diagnosis?

Points to Remember

- Enzymes are the biological catalysts that make chemical reactions in living organisms possible.
- Enzymes are highly efficient, allowing a limited number of enzyme molecules to quickly transform large amounts of substrates into products.
- Enzymes are classified according to a system developed by the Nomenclature Committee of the International Union of Biochemistry and Molecular Biology (NC-IUBMB) and published in 1961. Each enzyme is given a four-digit code, known as the Enzyme Commission (EC) number. New recommendations and periodic updates are readily available.
- The rate of a chemical reaction is described by enzyme kinetics and specific reaction conditions. The rate of product formation is affected by enzyme concentration, pH, temperature, cofactors, and inhibitors.

- Enzymes accelerate reactions by lowering the activation energy needed to overcome the transition state on the way to product formation.
- Nonprotein substances that are essential for enzyme activity and must bind to the enzyme before the reaction takes place are known as cofactors; they include activators, coenzymes, and prosthetic groups.
- Isoenzymes are enzymes that catalyze the same reaction but have different structural and biochemical properties derived from genetically distinct variations in primary structure.
- Enzymes are commonly measured in serum, plasma, and other body fluids to detect tissue damage and altered enzyme production. They can also be measured in a tissue to identify abnormalities that may cause disease.
- Enzyme concentration is measured by determining catalytic activity. The international unit (IU) is the amount of enzyme needed to convert 1 μmol of substrate to product per minute. Enzyme concentration is expressed in IU/L units.
- Clinical applications of aminotransferases are exclusively related to the evaluation of liver disease. Alanine aminotransferase (ALT) activity usually is higher than aspartate aminotransferase (AST) activity in most forms of liver disease.
- Clinically significant increases in alkaline phosphatase (ALP) activity are seen in obstructive hepatobiliary disease and osteoblast-mediated bone disease. ALP isoenzymes are commonly separated and quantitated.
- Increases in γ-glutamyl transferase (GGT) are not specific and occur in most individuals with liver disease. However, elevated GGT activity is a useful finding in the context of alcoholic hepatitis and chronic alcohol

drinking. Determination of GGT activity can distinguish the source of elevated ALP activity because GGT activity is normal during pregnancy and in bone disorders, conditions that exhibit elevated ALP activity.

- Increases in total creatine kinase (CK) activity are common in pathological conditions involving skeletal and cardiac tissue and are commonly seen when direct muscle injury occurs (e.g., intense physical activity, severe falls, surgery). Separation and quantitation of CK isoenzymes provide information relevant to specific disorders that exhibit elevated total CK activity.
- The greatest increases in serum amylase activity are seen in acute pancreatitis and salivary gland inflammation.
- Lipase activity determinations are used to diagnose acute pancreatitis and are more specific for this purpose than amylase activity.

Introduction

The physiologic properties and principles of enzymes and enzymatic mechanisms are discussed in this chapter. Assay methods for clinically relevant enzymes also are described.

Enzymes are biological catalysts that increase biochemical reaction rates without undergoing permanent changes or being consumed. They alter the rate but not the chemical equilibrium point of the reaction. Enzymes catalyze the conversion of substrate molecules to products. The catalyzed reactions are specific and essential to physiologic functions that include DNA synthesis, nerve conduction, cell growth, and energy generation.

Enzyme concentrations in body fluids are measured to detect cellular injury or altered enzyme production in a particular tissue that produces the enzyme. Enzymes are measured in a specific tissue to identify abnormalities that cause disease.

The Nature of Enzymes

Enzyme Structure and Properties

A catalyst is defined as a substance that accelerates (catalyzes) the rate of a chemical reaction without becoming modified itself. Biochemical and biological reactions necessary for all living processes require the involvement of catalysts. Enzymes are the biological catalysts that make chemical reactions in living organisms possible. Each enzyme catalyzes a specific physiologic reaction, which is facilitated by the enzyme's three-dimensional structure and other factors.

Although a few enzymes are catalytic RNA molecules (e.g., ribozymes), most are proteins or conjugated proteins with molecular masses ranging from 10 to 500 kD and the structural characteristics of proteins. The linear sequence of the amino acids (i.e., polypeptide) of the enzyme determines its *primary* structure. Three-dimensionally coiled polypeptides generate *secondary* structures, and subsequent folding creates *tertiary* structures. In some cases, assemblies of two or more folded polypeptide chains (i.e., subunits) are further arranged in a *quaternary* structure to provide catalytic activity. The structural characteristics of specific enzyme molecules give them unique properties, and the structural integrity of the enzyme molecule is essential for optimal biological activity.

Cells contain a variety of enzymes in different quantities. Enzymes are part of the cell membrane, reside in subcellular organelles (e.g., mitochondria, microsomes), are part of the cytoplasm, and also exist free (unbound) in plasma. Enzymes largely occur in cells as part of a metabolic pathway, but some tissues (e.g., liver) also generate enzymes in response to specific stimuli.

Enzymes contain an active site, where the substance that is acted on (i.e., substrate) interacts and binds. In the folded enzyme, the active site is usually a cleft or crevice with specific amino acid residues that determine substrate specificity. The enzyme–substrate complex, known as the *adduct*, is formed by noncovalent binding forces between the enzyme molecule and the substrate molecule. The specificity of the bond correlates with the alignment of atoms in the enzyme active site with the atoms in the substrate molecule. Regulator molecules may bind to alternative sites on the enzyme molecules known as allosteric sites, causing conformational changes that affect the active site and therefore the reaction rate. Enzymes are highly efficient due to their extraordinary catalytic properties, which allow for a limited number of enzyme molecules to quickly transform large amounts of substrate into product.

Enzyme Nomenclature

Names of enzymes historically included the name of the substrate or group acted on by the enzyme followed by the suffix –*ase*. For example, the enzyme that hydrolyzes urea was called *urease.* In some cases, the name indicated the reaction catalyzed by the enzyme, such as glucose oxidase. Other enzymes were given empirical names, such as trypsin and pepsin.

Because of the rapid increase in enzyme discovery, the common or trivial and semisystematic naming conventions were considered inadequate, and in 1956, the International Union of Biochemistry (now called the International Union of Biochemistry and Molecular Biology, or IUBMB) established an international commission on enzymes to address the issues of enzyme classification and nomenclature. The enzyme classification system was developed by the Nomenclature Committee of the IUBMB (NC-IUBMB) into the NC-IUBMB Enzyme List, which was published in 1961 and updated in 1965, 1972, 1978, 1984, and 1992. Recommendations and periodic updates are available (http://www.chem.qmw.ac.uk/iubmb/enzyme/).

The NC-IUBMB system assigns a common or trivial name (i.e., accepted name) and a systematic name to each enzyme. The accepted name typically is the most commonly used name for the enzyme and is suitable for everyday use. The systematic name delineates the reaction catalyzed by the enzyme and is associated with a unique numeric code. Each enzyme is given a code called the Enzyme Commission (EC) number, which consists of four digits separated by periods. The first digit classifies the enzymes into six groups, which are characterized by the type of reaction they catalyze:

TABLE 8-1 Classification of Clinically Relevant Enzymes

Enzyme Class and EC Number	Other Name (Accepted Name)	Systematic Name	Standard Abbreviation[†]	Alternative Name (Abbreviation)
Oxidoreductases				
1.1.1.27	Lactate dehydrogenase (L-lactate dehydrogenase)	(S)-Lactate:NAD+ oxidoreductase	LD	LDH
Transferases				
2.6.1.2	Alanine aminotransferase (alanine transaminase)	L-Alanine:2-oxoglutarate aminotransferase	ALT	Glutamate-pyruvate transaminase (GPT)
2.6.1.1	Aspartate aminotransferase (aspartate transaminase)	L-aspartate:2-oxoglutarate aminotransferase	AST	Glutamate-oxaloacetate transaminase (GOT)
2.7.3.2	Creatine kinase*	ATP:creatine N-phosphotransferase	CK	CPK
2.3.2.2	γ-Glutamyl transferase*	(5-L-Glutamyl)-peptide: amino-acid 5-glutamyltransferase	GGT	—
Hydrolases				
3.1.3.1	Alkaline phosphatase*	Phosphate-monoester phosphohydrolase (alkaline optimum)	ALP	—
3.2.1.1	Amylase (α-amylase)	4-α-D-Glucan glucanohydrolase	AMY	—
3.1.1.3	Lipase (triacylglycerol lipase)	Triacylglycerol acylhydrolase	LPS	—
Lyases				
4.1.2.13	Aldolase (fructose-bisphosphate aldolase)	D-Fructose-1,6-bisphosphate D-glyceraldehyde-3-phosphate-lyase (glycerone-phosphate-forming)	ALD	—
Isomerases				
5.3.1.1	Triose-phosphate isomerase*	D-Glyceraldehyde-3-phosphate aldose-ketose-isomerase	TPI	—
Ligases				
6.3.2.3	Glutathione synthase*	γ-L-Glutamyl-L-cysteine:glycine ligase (ADP forming)	GSH-S	—

Data from ExplorEnz. The enzyme database. <http://www.enzyme-database.org/class.php> Accessed 13.05.15.
ADP, Adenosine diphosphate; ATP, adenosine triphosphate; NAD+, ionized form of nicotinamide adenine dinucleotide.
*Accepted name and other name are the same.
[†]Standard abbreviations are not part of the International Union of Biochemistry and Molecular Biology (IUBMB) recommendations, but their use is common.

1. Oxidoreductases catalyze an oxidation-reduction reaction.
2. Transferases catalyze the transfer of functional groups.
3. Hydrolases catalyze hydrolysis reactions.
4. Lyases catalyze removal of chemical groups to form double bonds.
5. Isomerases catalyze the interconversion of isomers.
6. Ligases catalyze bond formation coupled with adenosine triphosphate (ATP) hydrolysis.

The second and third digits of the EC number indicate the subclass and sub-subclass to which the enzyme is assigned. They provide information about the type of group or compound involved in the reaction (i.e., subclass) and additional specifications about the type of reaction involved (i.e., sub-subclass). The fourth digit is a serial number that identifies the individual enzyme within a sub-subclass.

A comprehensive list of EC numbers for the various enzyme classes is available online (http://www.enzyme-database.org/class.php). Table 8-1 lists clinically relevant enzymes by class and EC number.

Kinetics

Reaction Rates of Chemical Reactions

The rate of a chemical reaction is described by enzyme kinetics and specific reaction conditions. The rate changes over the course of the enzymatic reaction. The rate of product formation is affected by the concentration of enzyme in the reaction (Fig. 8-1). As long as the substrate concentration exceeds the enzyme concentration, the reaction velocity is proportional to the concentration of enzyme present in the reaction.

Other features that affect the reaction rate are pH, temperature, cofactors, and inhibitors. Each is explained in more detail later in this chapter. Figure 8-1 demonstrates the relationship of the rate of product formation and change in absorbance over time. Enzyme kinetics should always be assessed during the linear phase of a reaction. Enzymatic activity typically is assessed at fixed time points, and preferably at multiple time points or by continuous monitoring (i.e., kinetic assay).

Thermodynamics

A substrate is converted into a product in a chemical reaction. To do this, the reaction must overcome an energy barrier called the transition state. The transition state has a much higher level of free energy than the substrate or product. Enzymes accelerate reactions by lowering the activation energy (i.e., the change in Gibbs free energy [ΔG]) that is needed to overcome the transition state on the way to product formation (Fig. 8-2).

To better understand Gibbs free energy, the reaction can be split into two steps. First, the substrate and the transition state reach equilibrium. (Substrate molecules with the required amount of activation energy reach the transition state.) Second, only molecules in the transition state can form products at a specific product formation rate (*v*). Enzymes lower the activation energy that is necessary for an enzyme–substrate complex to reach the transition state and proceed to product formation. This equilibrium is a new reaction pathway with markedly decreased activation energy. Enzymes make it much more likely for molecules to possess an amount of energy that is sufficient to reach the transition state.

Enzymatically catalyzed reactions follow this equation:

$$E+S \underset{K_3}{\overset{K_1}{\rightleftharpoons}} [ES] \underset{K_4}{\overset{K_2}{\rightleftharpoons}} E+P$$

An enzymatic catalyst (E) acts on the substrate (S) with a reaction rate of K_1 and forms an intermediate enzyme–substrate complex (ES), which then forms the reaction product (P) at rate K_2, with the catalyst E reconstituted. In many cases, the direction of the reaction is reversible, as indicated by the arrows and the rates for the reverse reactions, K_3 and K_4. The equilibrium can be shifted toward the substrate or toward the product. The reaction rate constant depends on the temperature and quantifies the velocity of the reaction.

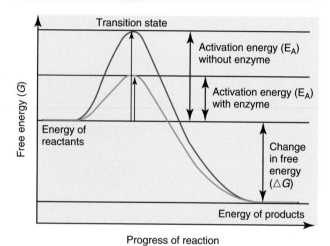

• **Figure 8-2** Enzymes accelerate reactions by lowering the activation energy.

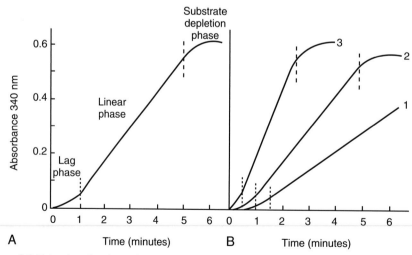

• **Figure 8-1** Rate of product formation. **A,** General scheme of enzyme reaction starting out with lag phase (time needed for enzyme activation), then linear phase (reaction rate is proportional to enzyme activity), and plateau phase (substrate depletion and end of reaction). **B,** Reaction rates with three different amounts of enzyme. Curve 1 has low-enzyme activity, 2 has medium-enzyme activity, and 3 has high-enzyme activity. Increased enzyme activity results in decreased lag phase, decreased linear phase, and a plateau phase of substrate depletion that is reached faster.

Michaelis-Menten Model for Enzyme-Catalyzed Reactions

Leonor Michaelis and Maud Menten proposed the Michaelis-Menten kinetics model to account for enzymatic reaction rates based on the concentrations of an enzyme and its substrate. In the Michaelis-Menten model (Fig. 8-3), v is the initial velocity of an enzyme-catalyzed reaction (i.e., the velocity when the product concentration is near zero), [S] is the substrate concentration, and V_{max} and K_m are two constants that characterize a specific enzyme. V_{max}, the maximum velocity, is the reaction rate when the enzyme is completely saturated with substrate; K_m, the Michaelis constant, is the substrate concentration at which the reaction rate is half of the maximum rate ($v = V_{max}/2$). K_m indicates the affinity of an enzyme for the substrate. A small K_m value indicates high affinity and a high reaction velocity. The maximum rate of product formation is defined by V_{max} in the Michaelis-Menten equation:

$$\nu = V_{max}[S]/K_m + [S]$$

The curve generated from the equation (see Fig. 8-3) describes a reaction rate that steadily increases until all substrate binding sites on the enzyme are saturated and the velocity plateaus.

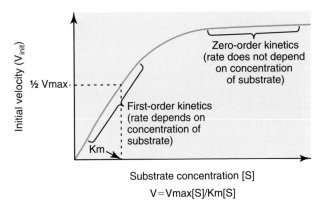

• **Figure 8-3** Michaelis-Menten kinetics. V_{max}, the maximum velocity, is the initial velocity (v) when the enzyme is completely saturated with substrate (S). K_m is the Michaelis constant, which is the substrate concentration at the half-maximum reaction rate.

Lineweaver-Burk Plots

Lineweaver and Burk developed a graphic model to describe enzyme kinetics terms such as K_m and V_{max} in the early 1930s. The Lineweaver-Burk equation is the reciprocal rearrangement of the Michaelis-Menten equation, which yields a linear plot of velocity versus substrate concentration:

$$1/\nu = (K_m/V_{max}[S]) + (1/V_{max})$$

Lineweaver-Burk plots illustrate the effects of different types of inhibitors on K_m and V_{max}. Enzymatic assays in a clinical analyzer most often use competitive inhibition for the determinations. Plots are shown for competitive, noncompetitive, and uncompetitive inhibition in Figure 8-4.

Competitive, Noncompetitive, and Uncompetitive Inhibition

The number of substrate binding sites (i.e., active sites) on enzymes is limited. In competitive inhibition, binding of an inhibitor to the active site of an enzyme prevents the substrate from binding to the enzyme, which inhibits enzymatic function. Competitive inhibitions are reversible, and the effect can be decreased by increasing the substrate concentration. The affinity of the enzyme for the substrate increases (K_m), but the rate of substrate formation remains the same (V_{max}) (Table 8-2).

In noncompetitive inhibition, the inhibitor binds at a regulatory site (i.e., allosteric site) on the enzyme molecule rather than competing with the substrate for the active site (Fig. 8-5). The regulatory site of an enzyme determines the

TABLE 8-2 Kinetic Effects of Inhibition

Type of Inhibition	Change in K_m	Change in V_{max}
Competitive	Increased	No change
Noncompetitive	No change	Decreased
Uncompetitive	Decreased	Decreased

K_m, Michaelis constant; V_{max}, maximum velocity of a reaction.

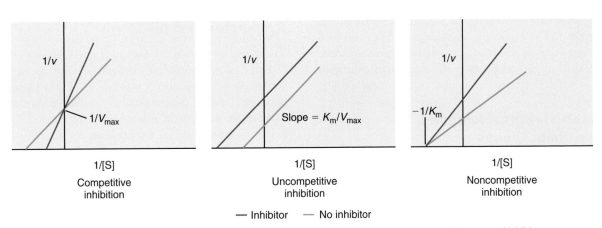

• **Figure 8-4** Lineweaver-Burk plots for competitive, uncompetitive, and noncompetitive types of inhibition. K_m, Michaelis constant; S, substrate; V, velocity.

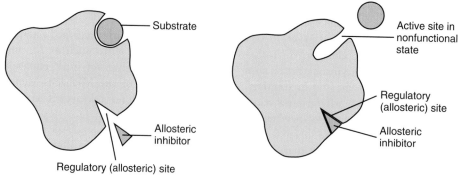

• Figure 8-5 In noncompetitive inhibition, the inhibitor binds at an allosteric site on the enzyme molecule instead of competing with the substrate for the active site.

conformation and activity of the enzyme. This type of inhibition cannot be reversed by an increase in substrate concentration. The K_m remains unaffected because there is no competition for the substrate binding site, whereas the rate of product formation is reduced, resulting in a decreased V_{max}.

Uncompetitive inhibition occurs when the inhibitor binds to the enzyme–substrate complex, preventing the formation of product. Because this type of inhibition is not reversible by adding substrate, K_m and V_{max} are negatively affected.

Drugs as Enzyme Inhibitors

Enzymes can be inhibited by competitive, noncompetitive, and uncompetitive inhibition. Some diseases can be treated by inhibition of enzymes with drugs. A familiar example is the inhibition of angiotensin-converting enzyme (ACE) in the treatment of hypertension. ACE converts angiotensin I to angiotensin II and induces vasoconstriction, promoting hypertension. Captopril is a drug that inhibits ACE through competitive inhibition. Another example is the use of ethanol in the treatment of methanol poisoning. Ethanol competitively inhibits the enzyme alcohol dehydrogenase, preventing methanol metabolism.

The effects of competitive inhibition occur quickly, whereas the onset of noncompetitive enzyme inhibition is prolonged. An example of noncompetitive and irreversible inhibition is the action of salicylate, the active compound in aspirin, on cyclooxygenase isoenzymes to reduce inflammation. Another source of enzyme inhibition is the removal of enzyme activators such as magnesium and calcium by a chelating agent such as citrate or ethylenediaminetetraacetic acid (EDTA). Blood collection in the appropriate collection tube is essential for the determination of enzymatic activity.

Enzyme Activators, Coenzymes, and Prosthetic Groups

Nonprotein substances that are essential for enzyme activity and must bind to the enzyme before the reaction takes place are known as cofactors. Inorganic enzyme activators include magnesium, chloride, manganese, potassium, zinc, iron, and calcium ions. Activators modify enzyme configuration for optimal substrate binding.

Other cofactors for many enzymes are known as coenzymes. Coenzymes are organic substances loosely bound to proteins that are required for enzyme function. Coenzymes participate in the reaction but are not substrates for the enzyme. They carry electrons, specific atoms, or functional groups that participate in the enzymatic reaction. A common coenzyme is nicotine adenine dinucleotide (NAD), which is involved in many dehydrogenation reactions.

Prosthetic groups are tightly bound nonprotein molecules of organic (i.e., sugar, vitamin, or lipid) or inorganic (i.e., metal ion) origin. In contrast to coenzymes, prosthetic groups are tightly bound to proteins and can be linked to the enzyme through a covalent bond. Prosthetic groups play an important role in catalyzing some types of reactions, including oxidation-reduction (redox), oxygenation, and methylation reactions.

The measurement of enzyme activity requires adequate concentrations of the appropriate cofactors. They are usually present in excess to ensure an optimal and complete enzymatic reaction.

Enzyme Reaction Conditions

Various analytical factors affect enzymatic activity. The reaction rate is mainly determined by the pH, the temperature, the concentrations of enzyme and substrate, and the presence of any activators or inhibitors.

Temperature and pH

To catalyze a reaction at maximum speed, the temperature and pH must be carefully controlled. The optimal temperature for most enzymes is below 40° C. At higher temperatures, protein denaturation is possible. Although most enzymes are deactivated at lower temperatures, –5° C seems to be the optimal storage temperature. An increase of about 10° C often results in doubling of the enzymatic activity. Even changes of just a few degrees can lead to major differences in the result.

The pH has similar effects on optimal enzyme activity. Isoforms of the same enzyme possess different optimal pH values. The range can be as low as pH 1.5 for pepsin and up to pH 8.0 for the pancreatic isoform of lipase.

Enzyme Concentration

When the effect of enzyme concentration on the reaction rate is being studied, the substrate must be present in excess. The change in product formation must solely depend on the amount of enzyme in the reaction mixture. The product concentration depends on the enzyme concentration.

Zero-order kinetics ($[S] \gg K_m$) describes a reaction under conditions of substrate excess (see Fig. 8-3). The reaction velocity is independent of the substrate concentration. In zero-order kinetics, all of the enzyme's active sites are saturated with substrate. The activity of the particular enzyme drives product formation at a maximal reaction rate. To determine whether an enzymatic reaction is determined by zero-order kinetics, several product measurements (e.g., absorbance at a specific wavelength) should be obtained.

Substrate Concentration

At a constant enzyme concentration with a steadily increasing substrate concentration, the enzyme velocity will reach its maximum when all substrate binding sites on the enzyme are occupied. First-order kinetics ($[S] \ll K_m$) defines a reaction that depends on the amount of substrate present in the sample (see Fig. 8-3). The rate of product formation is linear and proportional to the substrate concentration. In first-order kinetics, not all enzyme active sites are saturated with substrate, and the substrate concentration is the rate-limiting step.

Isoenzymes

Isoenzymes (or isozymes) are enzymes that catalyze the same reaction but have different structural and biochemical properties. Isoenzymes are genetically distinct variations of an enzyme that have different primary structures. All isoforms of an enzyme have the same EC number.

Commonly Measured Isoenzymes

Before the widespread use of troponin, a commonly measured isoenzyme in the clinical laboratory was the dimer CK-MB, which is a creatine kinase isoform predominantly found in the heart. This isoform consists of two subunits (i.e., M and B) and was used as an early marker for myocardial infarction. Tissue necrosis in response to a heart attack produces a measurable increase in cardiac-specific enzymes such as CK-MB.

Lactate dehydrogenase (LD) is another isoenzyme that used to be frequently measured in the clinical laboratory. This tetramer consists of two different subunits that form five isoenzymes, usually classified as LD1 through LD5. Each isoform is relatively tissue specific and present in different concentrations. In the event of myocardial infarction, the level of the heart-specific isoform LD1 rises above that of the LD2 isoform and creates a flipped pattern on a thin-layer agarose gel electrophoresis system.

Methods Used to Differentiate Isoenzymes in the Clinical Laboratory

The methods used to separate and quantitate the isoforms of a particular enzyme rely on the different structures and post-translational modifications that characterize each isoenzyme. Isoenzymes for most clinically relevant enzymes can be identified with the use of gel electrophoresis assays. The separation of isoenzymes is based on their different physical properties, such as the charge that affects electrophoretic mobility in the gel.

Immunoassays are widely used to target a specific isoform; an antibody specifically recognizes an epitope of a particular subunit. An example is the differentiation of salivary-type and pancreatic-type amylase.

Applying heat to a sample for a defined amount of time can inactivate heat-labile isoforms of an enzyme. The bone-specific isoform of alkaline phosphatase is well known for its heat sensitivity. Less often used methods for isoenzyme analysis include immunoinhibition, chemical inhibition, and substrate specificity.

Specific Enzymes

Enzymes are most commonly measured in serum, plasma, and other body fluids to detect tissue-specific injury, and they are used as markers of tissue damage. Enzymes are commonly measured to detect altered enzyme production by a specific tissue and can also be measured within a tissue to identify abnormalities that may cause disease.

Enzymes occur at very low concentrations in plasma, and this poses a challenge when one is attempting to separate them from other proteins and quantify them. Enzyme concentration is measured by determining catalytic activity. Clinical laboratory assays measure the reaction rate of a particular enzyme, which provides information that is correlated with the enzyme concentration in the sample of interest. Two common methods are used to measure the catalytic activity of enzymes:

1. End-point or one-point method: The reaction is started and allowed to continue for a fixed period of time and then stopped, after which the amount of product generated is measured.
2. Kinetic or multipoint fixed time method: Reaction progression is monitored continuously as a function of time.

Measurements of enzyme catalytic activity must occur during the linear phase (see Fig. 8-1). In this phase, the activity over time remains proportional to absorbance changes. Activity measurements usually begin after the lag phase.

The Enzyme Commission established and standardized the units used to quantitate enzyme activity. The international unit (IU) is the amount of enzyme needed to convert 1 µmol of substrate to product in 1 minute. Enzyme concentration is commonly expressed in units of IU/L (international units per liter).

In the following sections, clinically relevant enzymes are discussed in the context of their physiology, clinical significance, and laboratory assays used to measure them in serum, plasma, and other body fluids.

Aminotransferases

Physiology

The aminotransferases, also known as transaminases, catalyze the transfer of amino groups from amino acids to form 2-oxo-acids. The two clinically relevant aminotransferases are aspartate aminotransferase (AST, EC 2.6.1.1) and alanine aminotransferase (ALT, EC 2.6.1.2).

AST and ALT catalyze the transfer of an amino group from L-aspartate or L-alanine, respectively, to 2-oxoglutarate. The reaction products are L-glutamate and oxaloacetate (AST) or pyruvate (ALT). Pyridoxal phosphate is the coenzyme. The following equations illustrate the transfer reactions:

AST and ALT are found in all major organ tissues. AST is primarily distributed in the heart, liver, skeletal muscle, and kidney. ALT is primarily found in the liver and kidney and is less concentrated in the heart and skeletal muscle. Inside the cell, AST is found in the cytoplasm and mitochondria, whereas ALT is exclusively found in the cytoplasm. In the cytoplasm, AST is two to three times more abundant than ALT.

Clinical Significance

The clinical applications of aminotransferases are exclusively related to the evaluation of liver disease. ALT activity usually is higher than AST activity in most forms of liver disease except alcoholic hepatitis, hepatic cirrhosis, and hepatocellular carcinoma.

Liver disorders associated with destruction of hepatic tissue (i.e., necrosis), including viral hepatitis, display elevated AST and ALT activity before clinical signs and symptoms appear. AST and ALT elevations are usually on the order of 10 to 40 times normal and can reach up to 100 times the value of the upper limit of the reference interval. Nonalcoholic fatty liver disease is a common cause of aminotransferase activity, along with viral and alcoholic hepatitis.

Elevated ALT activity has increased specificity for the liver (compared with AST). Elevations in ALT activity are rare in nonliver disorders. Elevated ALT activity persists longer than that of AST because of the longer half-life of ALT in serum.

Laboratory Procedures and Limitations

Assay methods for measuring aminotransferase activity involve coupling the aminotransferase reaction to a specific dehydrogenase reaction and measuring the change in the concentration of NADH (the reduced form of NAD) by spectrophotometry.

The oxaloacetate formed in the AST-catalyzed reaction is reduced to malate by malate dehydrogenase (MD). Similarly, the pyruvate formed in the ALT-catalyzed reaction is reduced to lactate by lactate dehydrogenase (LD). As both dehydrogenase reactions proceed, NADH is oxidized, and its disappearance is measured by a decrease in absorbance at 340 nm, which is directly proportional to the activity of AST or ALT, as illustrated in the following equations:

$$\text{Aspartate} + \alpha\text{-ketoglutarate} \xrightarrow{\text{AST}} \text{Oxaloacetate} + \text{Glutamate}$$

$$\text{Oxaloacetate} + \text{NADH} + \text{H}^+ \xrightarrow{\text{MD}} \text{Malate} + \text{NAD}^+$$

$$\text{Alanine} + \alpha\text{-ketoglutarate} \xrightarrow{\text{ALT}} \text{Pyruvate} + \text{Glutamate}$$

$$\text{Pyruvate} + \text{NADH} + \text{H}^+ \xrightarrow{\text{LD}} \text{Lactate} + \text{NAD}^+$$

Hemolysis is a significant cause of error because both AST and ALT are present in high concentrations in the cytoplasm. Determination of AST and ALT activity in hemolyzed specimens should be avoided.

Alkaline Phosphatase

Physiology

Alkaline phosphatase (ALP, EC 3.1.3.1) catalyzes the hydrolysis of numerous substrates at alkaline pH. ALP releases inorganic phosphate from the substrate and requires divalent cations (e.g., Zn^{2+}, Mg^{2+}) as cofactors.

ALP activity exists in most organs, particularly on membranes and cell surfaces of the small intestine, kidneys, liver, bone (i.e., osteoblasts), and placenta. ALP occurs in several isoforms, some of which share a common primary structure. The liver isoenzyme is the most abundant in adult serum, followed by the bone isoenzyme and a small amount of ALP of intestinal origin.

Clinical Significance

Increases in ALP activity are clinically significant in the investigation of obstructive hepatobiliary disease and osteoblast-mediated bone disease. ALP activity elevations of 3 to 10 times the upper limit of the reference interval are commonly observed in biliary tract obstruction. However, a single increase in the ALP level is not considered diagnostic, and the evaluation of hepatobiliary disorders must include other markers of hepatic function.

ALP activity elevations related to bone disease are common in osteoblast-related disorders, including Paget disease, osteomalacia, and rickets. A transient physiologic increase in the serum ALP concentration is observed in infants and children and is attributed to normal bone growth.

ALP activity elevations can be detected in the serum of pregnant women starting at 16 weeks' gestation, with increases of two to three times the upper limit of the reference interval observed in the third trimester. These increases reflect the placental origin of the ALP isoenzyme.

Laboratory Procedures and Limitations

Various methods are available for ALP activity determination. The most widely employed method uses 4-nitrophenyl phosphate (4-NPP) as the substrate. ALP catalyzes the hydrolysis of 4-NPP to 4-nitrophenol (4-NP), releasing phosphate. The colorless 4-NP is converted to the yellow 4-nitrophenoxide ion under alkaline conditions. The rate of formation of 4-NP is measured by spectrophotometry at 405 nm, as illustrated in the following equation:

4-Nitrophenol phosphate (colorless) → 4-Nitrophenoxide (yellow)

Hemolysis is a significant cause of error because ALP is more concentrated in red blood cells than in serum. Determination of ALP activity in hemolyzed specimens should be avoided. Chelating anticoagulants (e.g., citrate, oxalate, EDTA) should also be avoided because they complex the cofactors Zn^{2+} and Mg^{2+}, which are essential for ALP activity.

Special Considerations

ALP isoenzymes can be separated and quantitated by a variety of methods. Isoenzyme assays are necessary in certain clinical scenarios:
- Unclear source of elevated ALP levels
- Detection of bone or liver involvement
- Monitoring of therapy for metabolic bone disorders
Table 8-3 lists the methods used to separate and quantitate ALP isoenzymes and their characteristics and clinical use.

TABLE 8-3 Methods for Separation of Alkaline Phosphatase Isoenzymes

Method	Characteristics
Electrophoresis	The method is similar to serum protein electrophoresis. Liver alkaline phosphatase (ALP) migrates fastest; intestinal ALP migrates slowest. Bone ALP migrates at a speed between liver and intestinal ALP. Placental ALP migrates as a distinct band over a diffuse bone ALP band. Widely used with modifications to improve electrophoretic separation
Heat inactivation	Total ALP is measured before and after incubation of a sample at 56° C for 10 minutes. Liver ALP is more stable than bone ALP at 56° C. If <20% of total ALP remains after heating serum, the total activity results from the bone fraction. If >20% of total ALP remains after heating serum, the total activity results from the liver fraction. Placental ALP is the most heat stable. Tumor-related ALP isoforms are heat stable. Imprecise assay due to many variables. Widely used largely to differentiate bone from other heat-stable forms. Not specific for placental or tumor-related isoforms
Chemical inhibition	Uses phenylalanine as an inhibitor. Cannot differentiate bone and liver fractions
Immunoassays	Available for placental and intestinal isoenzymes. Not widely used

γ-Glutamyl Transferase
Physiology

γ-Glutamyl transferase (GGT, EC 2.3.2.2) catalyzes the transfer of a γ-glutamyl residue from a peptide or another compound to an acceptor.

γ-Glutamyl-p-nitroaniline + Glycylglycine $\xrightarrow{\text{GGT}}$

Donor (substrate)   Acceptor

p-Nitroaniline + γ-Glutamylglycylglycine

GGT activity exists in kidney, liver, pancreas, and intestine. The enzyme is largely found on the cell surface and in the cytoplasm. Although the exact function of GGT is unknown, it is thought to be involved in some aspects of glutathione metabolism and in membrane-related transport of amino acids and peptides. The GGT activity in serum primarily has a hepatic origin.

Clinical Significance

Increased GGT levels are not specific and are seen in most individuals with liver disease. The highest increases are seen in hepatobiliary disorders. Patients with primary and metastatic hepatocellular carcinoma display unusually high GGT activity. Other patients with elevated GGT activity are those with alcoholic hepatitis and chronic alcohol drinkers.

Determination of GGT activity can be useful in the context of elevated ALP activity. GGT activity is normal during pregnancy and in patients with bone disorders, conditions that exhibit elevated ALP activity.

Laboratory Procedures and Limitations

The most widely available method uses L-γ-glutamyl-3-carboxy-4-nitroanilide as substrate. Glycylglycine is the acceptor, and the production of 5-amino-2-nitrobenzoate at 37° C is measured by spectrophotometry at 410 nm.

$$\text{L-}\gamma\text{-Glutamyl-3-carboxy-4-nitroanilide + Glycylglycine} \xrightarrow{\text{GGT}}$$

$$\text{5-Amino-2-nitrobenzoate} + \gamma\text{-Glutamylglycylglycine}$$

GGT is a stable enzyme. Determination of enzyme activity is not affected by hemolysis.

Creatine Kinase

Physiology

Creatine kinase (CK, EC 2.7.3.2) catalyzes the reversible phosphorylation of creatine to creatine phosphate by ATP.

$$\text{Creatine + ATP} \xrightarrow{\text{CK}} \text{Creatine phosphate + ADP}$$

The forward reaction occurs in mitochondria, in which CK catalyzes the conversion of ATP to adenosine diphosphate (ADP) and stores energy as creatine phosphate. In the cytoplasm, CK phosphorylates ADP (i.e., reverse reaction) to produce the high-energy ATP that is necessary for muscles to contract. CK activity exists in most tissues. The highest activity is found in skeletal muscle and heart muscle, and less activity is found in brain tissue, intestines, and bladder.

The CK molecule is composed of two subunits: M and B. Different subunit combinations generate three major isoenzymes: CK-BB (CK1), CK-MB (CK2), and CK-MM (CK3). CK-BB is found primarily in brain and intestines, and it is found in extremely low concentrations in serum. CK-MB is found in small amounts in skeletal muscle and is abundant in heart muscle. It represents 2% to 3% of the total CK activity in serum. CK-MM is the most abundant isoenzyme; its activity is distributed primarily in skeletal and heart muscles. Between 97% and 98% of the total CK activity in serum is attributed to CK-MM.

Clinical Significance

Because of its high concentration in skeletal muscle, total CK activity in nondiseased individuals varies depending on age, gender, race, percentage of muscle mass, and physical condition.

Increases in total CK activity are common in pathological conditions involving skeletal and cardiac tissue, including muscular dystrophy, acute rhabdomyolysis, and acute myocardial infarction (AMI). CK elevations are commonly seen when direct muscle injury occurs, such as after intense physical activity, a severe fall, or surgery. The pathophysiology of CK and the CK-MB isoform in the context of AMI are discussed in Chapter 18. Separation and quantitation of CK isoenzymes provide information about specific disorders that exhibit elevated total CK activity.

Laboratory Procedures and Limitations

The most commonly used assay method for CK activity in serum or plasma is a coupled reaction that starts with the reverse conversion of creatine phosphate to creatine by CK and the synthesis of ATP. The generated ATP is used to phosphorylate glucose to glucose-6-phosphate by hexokinase (HK). During the final step, glucose-6-phosphate dehydrogenase (G6PD) oxidizes nicotine adenine dinucleotide phosphate NADP+ to its reduced form, NADPH, the production of which is measured by spectrophotometry.

$$\text{Creatine phosphate + ADP} \xrightarrow{\text{CK, pH 6.7}} \text{Creatine + ATP}$$

$$\text{ATP + Glucose} \xrightarrow{\text{HK}} \text{Glucose-6-phosphate + ADP}$$

$$\text{Glucose-6-phosphate + NADP}^+ \xrightarrow{\text{G6PD}}$$

$$\text{6-Phosphogluconate + NADPH + H}^+$$

Serum CK activity is unstable. Samples must be appropriately processed and stored immediately after collection. Moderate or severe hemolysis affects CK activity results and should be avoided.

Special Considerations

CK isoenzymes can be separated and quantitated by various methods, among which electrophoresis and immunoassay are the most widely used.

Electrophoretic separation of CK isoenzymes is the method of reference. CK-BB migrates the fastest, and CK-MM the slowest, with CK-MB migrating at an intermediate speed. After separation, isoenzyme bands are detected using an overlay reaction and quantitated by fluorescence densitometry using ultraviolet (UV) light. The occasional appearance of an unusual diffuse band that migrates between CK-MM and CK-MB has been attributed to the presence of immunoglobulin-complexed CK-BB, which is called *macro-CK*. Macro-CK is not associated with a particular pathology, and its incidence is uncommon.

CK-MB mass determinations are accomplished with the use of immunoassays. The immunoassays have been designed with antibodies against the M subunits, the B subunits, and the MB dimer, providing high specificity for the isoenzyme. The assays measure the concentration of CK-MB rather than its enzymatic activity and allow sensitive detection of CK-MB increases resulting from myocardial damage. They are widely used in clinical laboratories.

Lactate Dehydrogenase

Physiology

Lactate dehydrogenase (LD, EC 1.1.1.27) catalyzes the reversible oxidation of lactate to pyruvate, with NAD^+ acting as the hydrogen acceptor.

The reverse pyruvate reduction to lactate is strongly favored by the reaction equilibrium. The forward and reverse reactions have distinct reaction conditions and are optimized for temperature, pH, substrate, and buffer concentrations.

LD activity exists in all cells and is found in the cytoplasm at much higher concentrations than in serum. Significant enzyme activity is found in heart, liver, red blood cells, kidney, and skeletal muscle.

The LD molecule is a tetrapeptide with two types of subunits: type M (muscle) and type H (heart). Different subunit combinations generate five major isoenzymes: LD1 (H4), LD2 (H3M), LD3 (H2M2), LD4 (HM3), and LD5 (M4). LD2 is the most abundant isoenzyme in serum, followed by LD1, LD3, LD4, and LD5. The LD1 and LD2 isoforms are distributed in myocardial tissue and red blood cells, with higher relative concentrations of LD1 than LD2 in these cells.

Clinical Significance

Because of its presence in a variety of tissues, increases in LD activity are seen in numerous disorders. Moderate to slight elevations in LD activity levels are common in AMI, pulmonary embolism, leukemia, hemolytic anemia, liver disease, and renal disease. Significantly elevated LD activity is found in pernicious anemia, megaloblastic anemia, and some cancers.

Separation and quantitation of LD has been used to differentiate disorders that exhibit elevated total LD activity. However, this practice is becoming obsolete.

Laboratory Procedures and Limitations

The reactions that mediate the conversion of lactate to pyruvate (i.e., forward reaction) or pyruvate to lactate (i.e., reverse reaction) in the previous equation are widely used

in the clinical laboratory to measure LD activity. Although the reverse reaction progresses faster and results in shorter reaction times, its use is limited by the potential for substrate depletion with loss of linearity. As a result, use of the forward reaction is significantly favored. It is important to understand that the reaction used in the clinical laboratory for reference intervals for LD activity will differ according to the direction of the enzymatic reaction.

Special Considerations

LD isoenzymes can be separated and quantitated. Electrophoretic separation is the most widely used method for this purpose. LD1 migrates the fastest, and LD5 migrates the slowest, with the other three isoenzymes following LD1 sequentially.

After separation, isoenzyme bands are detected using an overlay reaction and quantitated by fluorescence densitometry using UV light. The LD2 band is predominant in the sera of nondiseased individuals, with LD1 second most prevalent. However, in pathologies that affect the heart and red blood cells (e.g., AMI, intravascular hemolysis), the LD1 band is the predominant one. This phenomenon is commonly known as an *LD-flipped pattern,* and it was used in the past as a sensitive marker of AMI when the more specific markers of cardiac damage were not available. The occasional appearance of an atypical diffuse band between LD3 and LD4 has been attributed to immunoglobulin-complexed LD, which is called *macro-LD.* Like macro-CK, macro-LD is not associated with a particular pathology, and its incidence is uncommon.

Amylase

Physiology

α-Amylase (AMY, EC 3.2.1.1) catalyzes the hydrolysis of 1,4-α-glycosidic bonds in straight and branched polysaccharides, releasing various types of sugars.

Amylase activity is found in a variety of tissues, with the highest concentrations found in the acinar cells of the pancreas and in the salivary glands. Amylase is the only enzyme that is filtered through the glomerulus and occurs in urine—a result of its small size. The salivary isoform of amylase (s-AMY) initiates starch digestion in the mouth and esophagus and becomes inactivated by the acidic pH in the stomach. The pancreatic isoenzyme of amylase (p-AMY) continues the hydrolysis of polysaccharides after the stomach contents reach the small intestine, where p-AMY is secreted from the pancreas.

Clinical Significance

Amylase activity in the sera of nondiseased individuals is low. The greatest increases are seen primarily in cases of acute pancreatitis and salivary gland inflammation.

During the progression of acute pancreatitis, transient increases in amylase activity are observed 5 to 8 hours after the onset of symptoms, with a peak seen 12 hours and a return to normal after 3 to 4 days. Because elevated amylase activity is observed in other disorders with similar symptoms, it is considered a nonspecific test when used alone. Additional tests, including urinary amylase and lipase activity determinations, increase its diagnostic specificity. The magnitude of the enzyme activity increase can indicate pancreatic involvement. Elevations of four to six times the upper limit of the reference interval are not unusual in patients with acute pancreatitis. Other pathologies with elevated amylase activity levels include renal insufficiency, biliary tract disorders, ectopic pregnancy, and diabetic ketoacidosis.

Laboratory Procedures and Limitations

Methods commonly used to determine amylase activity utilize small oligosaccharides as substrates. Several variations of coupled-enzyme assays are commercially available. Substrates include maltopentose, maltotetraose, and 4-nitrophenyl glycosides. In the following example of a coupled-enzyme, continuous reaction–monitoring assay, absorbance changes for NAD^+ are measured by spectrophotometry at 340 nm.

$$\text{Maltopentose} \xrightarrow{\text{AMY}} \text{Maltotriose} + \text{Maltose}$$

$$\text{Maltotriose} + \text{Maltose} \xrightarrow{\alpha\text{-glucosidase}} \text{5-Glucose}$$

$$\text{ATP} + \text{Glucose} \xrightarrow{\text{HK}} \text{Glucose-6-phosphate} + \text{ADP}$$

$$\text{Glucose-6-phosphate} + NADP^+ \xrightarrow{\text{G6PD}} \text{6-Phosphogluconate} + \text{NADPH} + H^+$$

Differentiation of s-AMY and p-AMY is usually achieved by measuring total amylase activity in the presence and absence of wheat germ lectin, which inhibits s-AMY activity. The concentrations of the two isoenzymes are mathematically estimated. More specific immunoassays are commercially available for this purpose.

Most Ca^{2+}-chelating anticoagulants (e.g., EDTA, citrate, oxalate) inhibit amylase activity; only heparin use is acceptable. Amylase activity should be determined in serum or heparinized plasma. Otherwise, activity of amylase in serum and urine is stable at most routine storage conditions.

Lipase
Physiology

Lipase (LPS, EC 3.1.1.3) catalyzes the hydrolysis of triglycerides to produce glycerol and fatty acids. The enzymatic activity of human lipase is specific for the ester bonds at positions 1 and 3; it generates a 2-acylglycerol and releases fatty acids.

$$\text{Triglyceride} + 2\,H_2O \underset{\text{Colipase, bile salts}}{\overset{\text{LPS}}{\rightleftharpoons}} \text{2-Monoglyceride} + \text{2 Fatty acids}$$

Lipase exists almost exclusively in the pancreas, which has concentrations up to 5000 times higher than in other tissues. The complete catalytic activity of lipase is achieved in the presence of bile salts and the coenzyme colipase.

Clinical Significance

Lipase activity in the sera of nondiseased individuals is low. Any increase of lipase activity indicates primarily pancreatic involvement. Lipase activity determinations are used to diagnose acute pancreatitis. During an acute pancreatitis episode, lipase activity increases are observed 5 to 8 hours after the onset of symptoms, with a peak at 24 hours and a return to normal after 8 to 14 days. Lipase and amylase activity measurements behave similarly at disease onset, but lipase activity remains elevated for longer periods than amylase activity.

Increased serum lipase levels are seen in other acute disorders with intraabdominal involvement, although less frequently than the nonspecific serum amylase elevations. Serum elevations of lipase activity are more specific than increases in amylase activity for the diagnosis of acute pancreatitis.

Laboratory Procedures and Limitations

Methods commonly used to determine lipase activity consist of estimating the liberation of fatty acids (i.e., titrimetric methods) and measuring light scattering by turbidimetry. Newer synthetic substrates are used in commercially available methods. One coupled-enzyme, continuous reaction–monitoring assay uses the following reactions:

$$\text{1,2-Diacylglycerol} + H_2O \xrightarrow{\text{LPS, Colipase}} \text{2-Monoacylglycerol} + \text{Fatty acid}$$

$$\text{2-Monoacylglycerol} + H_2O \xrightarrow{\text{Monoglyceride lipase}} \text{Glycerol} + \text{Fatty acid}$$

$$\text{ATP} + \text{Glycerol} \xrightarrow{\text{Glycerol kinase}} \text{L-}\alpha\text{-glycerophosphate} + \text{ADP}$$

$$\text{L-}\alpha\text{-glycerophosphate} + O_2 \xrightarrow[\text{kinase}]{\text{L-}\alpha\text{-glycerophosphate}} \text{Dihydroxyacetone phosphate} + H_2O_2$$

$$H_2O_2 + \text{4-Aminoantipyrine} \xrightarrow{\text{Peroxidase}} \text{Colored dye} + 2\,H_2O$$

Lipase activity is stable in serum at most routine storage conditions.

Summary

Enzymes are vital for all living organisms. They catalyze many important physiologic reactions by decreasing the activation energy necessary for a substrate to convert to a product. The velocity of the reaction is defined by substrate and enzyme concentrations, temperature, pH, and the presence of cofactors. Enzyme activity should always be measured under zero-order kinetics (i.e., substrate excess) to ensure that all substrate binding sites are covered with substrate.

In laboratory medicine, enzymes are most commonly measured in serum, plasma, and other body fluids to detect tissue damage and altered enzyme production. Clinical laboratory assays measure the reaction rate of a particular enzyme, which correlates with the amount of enzyme in the sample of interest. Determination of clinically relevant enzymes in serum and plasma is widely embedded in routine clinical practice to diagnose a variety of liver, bone, pancreas, and musculoskeletal disorders.

Review Questions

1. The activity of enzymes is expressed as IU/L (international units per liter) and is measured under which of the following conditions?
   a. Zero-order kinetics and enzyme excess
   b. First-order kinetics and enzyme excess
   c. Zero-order kinetics and substrate excess
   d. First-order kinetics and substrate excess

2. How do enzymes catalyze many physiologic processes?
   a. By increasing the activation energy
   b. By lowering the activation energy
   c. By eliminating the activation energy
   d. By adding energy to the reaction

3. Which of the following does *not* apply to competitive inhibition?
   a. Reversible reaction
   b. Inhibitor binding of the active site of an enzyme
   c. Commonly used in the clinical laboratory
   d. Decreased V_{max}

4. Enzyme activity is often measured in IU/L (international units per liter). Which statement defines the activity of 1 IU/L of enzyme?
   a. Conversion of 1 mmol substrate per second
   b. Conversion of 1 μmol substrate per second
   c. Conversion of 1 mmol substrate per minute
   d. Conversion of 1 μmol substrate per minute

5. Noncompetitive inhibitors of enzymes
   a. Physically bind enzyme at a place other than the active site
   b. Physically bind to the active site of an enzyme
   c. Are displaced by increasing substrate to reverse inhibition
   d. Physically bind to the enzyme–substrate complex

6. A patient is admitted to the emergency department with severe abdominal pain, and pancreatitis is part of the differential diagnosis. Which enzymes should be measured to rule in or rule out pancreatitis?
   a. Acid phosphatase and alkaline phosphatase
   b. CK and LD
   c. Amylase and lipase
   d. AST and ALT

7. Which method of reference is used to separate and quantitate most clinically relevant isoenzymes?
   a. Liquid chromatography
   b. Electrophoresis
   c. Immunofluorescence microscopy
   d. Immunoinhibition

8. Which transaminase has activity most specific to liver tissue?
   a. ALP
   b. GGT
   c. ALT
   d. AST

9. Which of the following factors affects the activity of total creatine kinase in serum?
   a. Brain activity
   b. Physical activity
   c. Digestive activity
   d. Emotional activity

10. Which of the following preanalytical factors commonly affects enzyme activity measurements in the clinical laboratory?
    a. Centrifugation conditions
    b. Patient fasting conditions
    c. Sample hemolysis
    d. Sample icterus

Critical Thinking Questions

1. Compare and contrast classes of enzyme inhibitors and their kinetic effects on the inhibition mechanism.

2. Compare and contrast enzymes that are used in clinical practice to assess liver-related disorders.

CASE STUDY

A 21-year-old female college student is admitted to the Student Health Center complaining of general discomfort and fatigue that started a few days earlier. She states that she woke up feeling nauseous and has not had any food in the past 12 hours. She also complains of pain in the right upper quadrant. Her vital signs indicate she has a fever, and on further questioning, she reveals that she returned from a charity mission trip to rural South America 3 weeks ago.

Physical examination reveals a slight yellow tint of the sclera. Results for several laboratory tests are obtained:

AST, 1211 IU/L (reference interval, 0 to 37 IU/L); ALT, 1542 (reference interval, 0 to 40 IU/L); ALP, 295 (reference interval, 35 to 115 IU/L); GGT, 15 IU/L (reference interval, 5 to 55 IU/L); and total bilirubin 2.5 mg/dL (reference interval, 0 to 1.1 mg/dL).

What diagnosis should be considered for this patient based on the initial laboratory results? What diagnosis can be ruled out based on the initial laboratory results? Which additional laboratory tests should be performed to confirm the suspected diagnosis?

Bibliography

Bais R, Edwards JB. Creatine kinase. *Crit Rev Clin Lab Sci*. 1982; 16(4):291–335.

Bais R, Panteghini M. Principles of clinical enzymology. In: Burtis CA, Ashwood ER, Bruns DE, eds. *Tietz Textbook of Clinical Chemistry and Molecular Diagnostics*. 4th ed. Philadelphia: WB Saunders; 2006.

Baron DN, Moss DW, Walker PG, Wilkinson JH. Abbreviations for names of enzymes of diagnostic importance. *J Clin Pathol*. 1971;24(7):656–657.

Baron DN, Moss DW, Walker PG, Wilkinson JH. Revised list of abbreviations for names of enzymes of diagnostic importance. *J Clin Pathol*. 1975;28(7):592–593.

Berg JM, Tymoczko JL, Stryer L. Enzymes: basic concepts and kinetics. In: Berg JM, Tymoczko JL, Stryer L, eds. *Biochemistry*. 5th ed. New York: WH Freeman; 2002.

Caffo AL. Laboratory calculations. In: Clarke W, ed. *Contemporary Practice in Clinical Chemistry*. 2nd ed. Washington, DC: AACC Press; 2011.

Enzyme Nomenclature Committee. *1978 Recommendations of the Nomenclature Committee of the International Union of Biochemistry on the Nomenclature and Classification of Enzymes*. New York: Academic Press; 1979.

Hohnadel DC. Clinical enzymology. In: Kaplan LA, Pesce AJ, eds. *Clinical Chemistry: Theory, Analysis and Correlation*. 5th ed. St. Louis: Mosby; 2009.

Johnson-Davis KL. Enzymes. In: Bishop ML, Fody EP, Schoeff LE, eds. *Clinical Chemistry: Principles, Techniques and Correlations*. 7th ed. Philadelphia: Wolters Kluwer; 2013.

Lewars EG. *Computational Chemistry*. New York: Springer; 2011. 9–43.

McDonald AG, Tipton KF. Enzyme classification and nomenclature. *FEBS J*. 2014;281:583–592.

Odufalu FD, Chacha P, Mudda G, Iskandar A. *Reaction Rate: The Dynamic Chemistry E-Textbook*. Davis, CA: UC Davis ChemWiki. <http://chemwiki.ucdavis.edu/Physical_Chemistry/Kinetics/Reaction_Rates/Reaction_Rate> Accessed 17.05.15.

Panteghini M, Bais R, van Solinge WW. Enzymes. In: Burtis CA, Ashwood ER, Bruns DE, eds. *Tietz Textbook of Clinical Chemistry and Molecular Diagnostics*. 4th ed. Philadelphia: WB Saunders; 2006.

Royal Society of Chemistry. *Chemistry for Biologists: Enzymes*. London: Royal Society of Chemistry; 2005. <http://www.rsc.org/Education/Teachers/Resources/cfb/enzymes.htm> Accessed 17.05.15.

Sanhai WR, Christenson RH. Isoenzymes and isoforms. In: Kaplan LA, Pesce AJ, eds. *Clinical Chemistry: Theory, Analysis and Correlation*. 5th ed. St. Louis: Mosby; 2009.

9

Clinical Chemistry and Disease

DONNA LARSON

CHAPTER OUTLINE

Introduction

Definition of Disease
  Influence of Culture on Definition of Disease
  Evolution of Disease

Pathology
  The Role of Cells in Disease

Disease Mechanisms

Biochemistry of Disease
  Tests and Diagnoses
  Laboratory Analytes and Assays

Summary

OBJECTIVES

At the completion of this chapter, the reader will be able to:

1. Define disease.
2. Describe how culture influences the definition of disease.
3. Define pathology.
4. Compare and contrast healthy, normal, abnormal, and sick.
5. Describe reference range.
6. Compare and contrast disease mechanisms: inflammation, immunity, cell death, necrosis, cellular adaptations, neoplasia, and cancer.
7. Describe the role laboratory tests play in confirming or ruling out a diagnosis.
8. Compare and contrast false positive and false negative.
9. Describe the sections of a clinical laboratory and examples of tests performed in each.

KEY TERMS

Abnormal	Disease mechanism	Neoplasia
Analyte	False negative	Normal
Assay	False positive	Nucleus
Cancer	Health	Organ
Cell death	Hyperplasia	Pathology
Cell membrane	Immunity	Plasma membrane
Cellular adaptation	Inflammation	Reference range
Cytoplasm	Metaplasia	Tissue
Disease	Necrosis	

❖ Case in Point

Laurie came to see her doctor because she had a stuffy nose, a sinus headache, and a scratchy throat. She was miserable. Breathing through her nose was difficult, and her frontal sinus was aching. Her physician explained that she probably had a cold and that this was caused by a virus. Laurie could use over-the-counter cold medications to relieve her symptoms, and she needed to get plenty of rest and drink lots of fluids until her symptoms subsided. If Laurie's physician had drawn blood to test for a basic metabolic panel, what do you think her chemistry results would have been—normal or abnormal? Why do you think that? If her blood chemistry results were normal, would that mean that she is not sick? Why or why not?

Points to Remember

- The terms *health* and *disease* qualitatively describe the condition of an individual.
- *Normal* and *abnormal* are objective interpretations of data used to determine whether an individual has a disease.
- Reference ranges are constructed by drawing blood from many individuals, performing a test, then calculating a mean and reference interval around the mean (±2 standard deviations).
- Cells contain nuclei, cytoplasm, plasma membranes, and many more organelles.
- Processes or conditions that cause disease include inflammation, immunity, cell death, necrosis, and cellular adaptation.
- Cellular injury causes alterations of body function and chemistry.
- Two types of errors that occur in laboratory measurements are false-positive and false-negative results.
- Ordering of laboratory tests is based on a patient's medical history, physical examination, and objective test results.
- Routine chemistry laboratories perform tests such as glucose, blood urea nitrogen (BUN), creatinine, electrolytes, enzymes, calcium, phosphate, magnesium, liver function tests, and lipid panels.
- Clinical chemistry laboratories also contain sections such as therapeutic drug monitoring, arterial blood gases, special chemistry, and body fluids.

Introduction

Clinical chemistry is a clinical laboratory science discipline that tests specific body substances to determine whether an abnormal condition exists in a living body. Clinical chemistry tests are performed on specimens from all kinds of living creatures, not just human beings. This chapter focuses on tests performed on humans and discusses an overall conceptual definition of disease, the study of disease and its change throughout history, the role of cells in disease, disease mechanisms, the biochemistry of diseases, correlation of laboratory tests to clinical observations, and the laboratory analytes and assays used to detect diseases. It is important to understand the definition and mechanisms of disease to understand the role of clinical chemistry in disease management.

Definition of Disease

Disease is defined as "any deviation from or interruption of the normal structure or function of a part, organ, or system of the body as manifested by characteristic symptoms and signs." The word is derived from an Old French word meaning "lack of ease." Taken literally, the word *disease* indicates that an individual is experiencing something that is putting them not at ease or making them not comfortable.

Influence of Culture on Definition of Disease

The definition of the word *disease* is interpreted through a cultural lens. Disease as it is conceptualized by most people in the United States is not the same as in many other cultures. In the United States, individuals believe that diseases are caused by natural phenomena that can be explained through science. In other cultures, the cause of disease may be viewed differently: Native Americans believe diseases are caused by an imbalance between the affected individual and nature, the Chinese belief is that diseases are caused by an imbalance in the energy that flows through a person, and many Vietnamese people believe that diseases are caused by an imbalance between the hot and cold poles that govern body functions. Cultural perceptions affect how diseases are diagnosed and treated.

Evolution of Disease

The diagnosis and treatment of diseases has evolved through the years and continues to change today. Technology also plays a major role in changing the objective data available to diagnose and treat diseases.

Hippocrates, often considered the father of Western medicine, believed that the body was composed of four "humors": yellow bile, black bile, phlegm, and blood. A shortage of any of these humors would cause disease in the affected individual. This belief lasted through the 19th century, when medical research began in Europe. Medical researchers linked disease to bacteria, viruses, and other natural phenomena.

Spontaneous generation—the belief that microbes could spontaneously appear in an otherwise sterile liquid—was disproven by Louis Pasteur in the 19th century. He identified microbes in the air that were indistinguishable from those that caused disease. This established disease as a condition produced by something external to the human body that could be viewed under the microscope and grown in the laboratory.

In the early 20th century, as scientists like Karl Landsteiner and Frank Macfarlane Burnet learned more about antibodies, they learned that disease can be produced by something internal to the human body as well as by external phenomena. Our modern explanation of disease continues to evolve as research discovers more and more about the human body.

Pathology

Pathology is the study of changes in the body's structure and function that are produced by disease. Pathologists discovered that "healthy" may not be the same as "normal," and "diseased" may not be the same as "abnormal." Health and disease qualitatively describe the condition of an individual. Normal and abnormal refer to the objective interpretations of data used to determine whether an individual has a disease. Most of the time, sick individuals have abnormal laboratory results, but this is not always true. There may be times when individuals have normal results on a standard metabolic panel but other laboratory tests indicate illness. For example, most people with a cold (i.e., stuffy nose, itchy eyes, and scratchy throat) appear to be "sick" but have "normal" results on their standard metabolic panel. Additional tests may show an infection or an allergic response, which could explain the symptoms.

Many years ago, laboratories printed ranges for "normal" results on laboratory slips. The test result was considered "normal" if it was within the range of values printed on the slip. This terminology has now evolved into the concept of a reference range. A reference range is determined by drawing many specimens on seemingly normal individuals, then using statistics to calculate the mean and range (±2 standard deviations from the mean) of those results.

Reference ranges allow health care providers to determine the extent of an abnormality. If an individual has a myocardial infarction, the higher the enzyme test values, the more severe the damage sustained by the person's heart. Reference ranges differ from laboratory to laboratory because each laboratory draws from a different population. References ranges are a good monitoring system for health care providers.

The Role of Cells in Disease

Cells are the building blocks of the human body. Cells group together to form tissues, tissues group together to form organs, and organs group together to form the body. Simply, cells are composed of a nucleus, cell membrane, and cytoplasm (Fig. 9-1).

The cell's nucleus contains the chromosomes, which contain the DNA or genetic material for the organism. DNA enables cells to produce many different proteins and to maintain cell structure and viability. The genes also allow the organism to maintain its integrity and its likeness to other organisms with the same genes (Fig. 9-2).

The cell membrane, or plasma membrane, keeps the cytoplasm, nucleus, and other parts of the cell isolated from the rest of the organism. The plasma membrane is selectively permeable, allowing specific chemicals to enter and exit the cell under particular conditions. (Fig. 9-3). The plasma membrane contains small channels that allow negative ions such as chloride to flow into the cytoplasm when a like negative ion, such as bicarbonate (HCO_3^-), flows out of the cytoplasm into the surroundings. This is a normal biochemical pathway that is regulated by the cell. However, a cell's regulation of this process can be thrown off by infection with a microorganism, a tumor, an injury, or cancerous cells. This is when laboratory tests can detect an abnormality and alert the health care provider to a possible abnormal condition, even a disease state.

The balance of biochemicals in the body is very tightly regulated. When a process is affected by an external condition, laboratory tests, especially those performed in the clinical chemistry laboratory, can provide objective data that

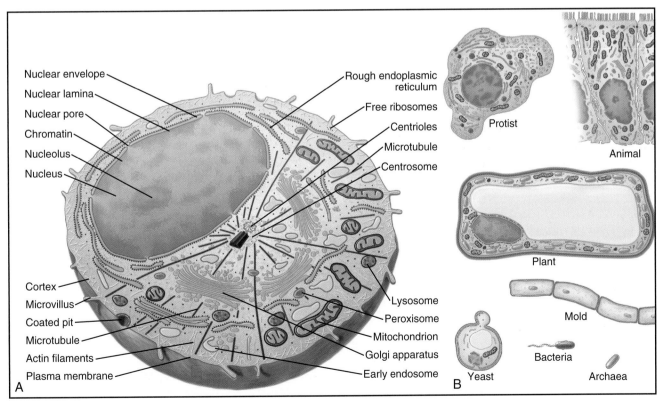

• **Figure 9-1** Basic cellular architecture. **A,** A section of a eukaryotic cell shows the internal components. **B,** Comparison of cells from the major branches of the phylogenetic tree. (From Pollard TD, Earnshaw WC, Lippincott-Schwartz J. *Cell Biology.* 2nd ed. Philadelphia: Saunders; 2007.)

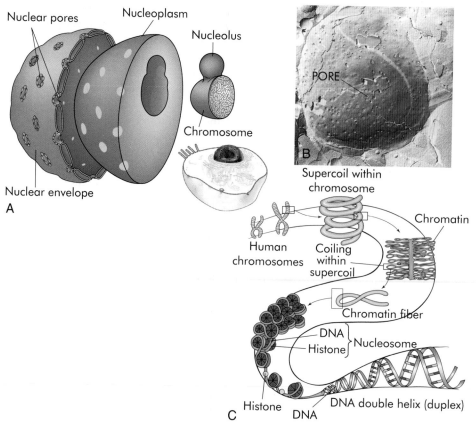

- **Figure 9-2** The Nucleus. The nucleus is composed of a double membrane, called a nuclear envelope, that encloses the fluid-filled interior, called nucleoplasm. The chromosomes are suspended in the nucleoplasm (illustrated here much larger than actual size to show the tightly packed DNA strands). Swelling at one or more points of the chromosome, shown in **A,** occurs at a nucleolus where genes are being copied into RNA. The nuclear envelope is studded with pores. **B,** The pores are visible as dimples in a freeze-etching of a nuclear envelope. **C,** Histone folding of DNA to make up a chromosome. (A and C, From McCance KL, Huether SE. *Pathophysiology: The Biologic Basis for Disease in Adults and Children.* 7th ed. St. Louis: Mosby; 2015; Fig. 1-2. B, From Raven PH, Johnson GB. *Biology.* 3rd ed. St Louis: Mosby Year Book; 1992.)

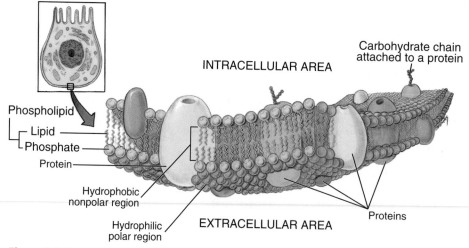

- **Figure 9-3** Structure of the cell membrane. Note the bilayer of phospholipids with the proteins scattered throughout. (From Applegate E. *The Anatomy and Physiology Learning System,* 4th ed. St. Louis: Saunders; 2011.)

health care providers use to aid in diagnosis of a condition or a disease. Because many conditions manifest with the same or similar symptoms, health care providers can also rule out conditions based on the results of clinical chemistry tests.

Disease Mechanisms

There are many processes or mechanisms which, if altered in some way, can cause disease. Disease mechanisms include inflammation, immunity, cell death, necrosis, cellular adaptations such as hyperplasia and metaplasia, neoplasia, and cancer. Inflammation releases neutrophils and macrophages as well as chemicals to repair an injury or destroy a foreign invader. Immunity usually involves immune cells that produce antibodies against a foreigner invader, but these cells can also produce antibodies against the body's own tissues. Cell death involves a process by which cells die in an orderly, programmed fashion. Cells age and die naturally, after a specific life span. The death of cells before their natural time alters body functions and can cause problems. Macrophages, neutrophils, and the spleen handle dead cells and recycle the chemicals within them for use in new cells. Necrosis involves cellular death and the release of chemicals from the cell after death. In this condition, cells die faster than they can be removed, and the cellular chemicals damage the living tissue surrounding the necrotic cells. Hyperplasia is an increase in number of a certain type of cells. Hyperplasia occurs after an injury or stress from an injury. Metaplasia occurs when a cell changes from one type of cell to another due to an injury. When the injury stops, the cell returns to its normal type. Neoplasia is uncontrolled growth of cells resulting in a tumor (benign or malignant); a malignant neoplasm is called cancer.

Much research funding goes into exploring the disease mechanisms for chronic and acute diseases. The understanding of disease mechanisms is always evolving, improving or even changing earlier concepts. An example is diabetes mellitus. In type 1 diabetes mellitus, the beta cells found in the islets of Langerhans of the pancreas do not produce insulin. At first, the mechanism was attributed to environmental influences. In the 1990s, researchers discovered that it involved an autoimmune process in which the body produces antibodies against its own cells. There are still many idiopathic diseases for which medical science has not yet discovered the mechanism.

Biochemistry of Disease

Cellular injury causes alteration of body function and chemistry. For each disease mechanism, body chemistry changes according to the effect on the living tissues surrounding the injury. Cellular death releases intracellular chemicals into the bloodstream, where the levels of these chemicals can be measured. With knowledge of the concentrations of these chemicals, along with a medical history and physical examination findings, the clinician can compose an accurate diagnosis of a disease. These test results can also rule out a disease. This is why clinical chemistry is such an important part of a diagnostic process. Although the reliability of diagnostic tests continues to improve, no clinical chemistry test will be 100% sensitive (i.e., detect all cases) and 100% specific (i.e., detect only the target disease) at the same time.

Tests and Diagnoses

Physicians order clinical chemistry tests to help diagnose disease in individuals. However, these tests do not always produce an accurate result. Two different types of errors occur in laboratory testing: false positives and false negatives. As the name implies, a false-positive test result occurs when an individual does not have a condition even though the laboratory test result indicates that the condition is present. A false-negative result occurs when an individual does have a condition but the test indicates that he or she does not have it. In contrast, true-positive test results occur when a test is positive for a condition and the individual actually does have the condition. With true-negative test results, the test is negative for a condition and, indeed, the individual does not have it. Every laboratory test is evaluated by the manufacturer to determine the percentage of false-negative and false-positive results produced when using the test. This fact also enters into the physician's decision-making process when he or she is attempting to make a diagnosis (Table 9-1).

How does a health care provider determine which laboratory tests to order for an individual? This is a complicated process that relies on a medical history, physical examination findings, and objective test results. In general, health care providers perform the most sensitive test first, then follow up with more specific tests, as necessary. By performing a highly *sensitive* test, providers will not miss many people who have the disease. If the result of the sensitive test is positive, the provider will order an additional, highly *specific* test to identify those individuals who actually have the disease and those who actually do not (i.e., whose result on the first test was a false positive). Usually no single test is 100% sensitive and specific in diagnosing disease. This is why the objective test results must be combined with the results of the medical history and physical examination—several pieces of the puzzle must come together to reveal the whole picture. Many diseases and conditions share similar symptoms, making it extremely hard to come to a correct diagnosis without obtaining all the pieces.

TABLE 9-1	**True and False Test Results**	
Type of Individual	**Positive Test**	**Negative Test**
Individual with disease	True positive	False negative
Individual without disease	False positive	True negative

Laboratory Analytes and Assays

The clinical chemistry test menu expands every year with the addition of more tests and assays to detect specific diseases. Medical researchers discover a substance that is present in a group of individuals with the same symptoms or disease, usually by comparison with a negative "control" group without the symptoms or disease (i.e., seemingly normal individuals). If a test can be developed that allows detection of a substance or substances that are present at a lower (or higher) level in normal individuals than in those with the disease, that test may be useful in helping clinicians make a diagnosis.

Researchers and medical device companies seek methods for determining which substances allow differentiation of normal individuals from those with the disease. Once an accurate and precise method for analyzing the substance is available, the new clinical chemistry test is introduced to the laboratory. In reality, the process of translating research into practice takes approximately 10 years to complete. The federal government is working with researchers to shorten this period.

Clinical chemistry laboratories are divided into sections or areas, depending on the types of instruments used, analytes examined, and tests performed. The composition of the sections varies from laboratory to laboratory. Laboratories commonly have sections devoted to

- Routine chemistry
- Therapeutic drug monitoring or toxicology
- Blood gas analysis
- RIA/EIA
- Special chemistry
- Body fluids

The routine chemistry section is usually the most automated section of the clinical chemistry laboratory. The instruments used in this section are high-throughput analyzers and are considered the workhorses of the laboratory. The types of tests performed here include basic metabolic profiles (e.g., glucose, blood urea nitrogen [BUN], creatinine, electrolytes, enzymes, calcium, phosphorus, magnesium, total cholesterol, triglycerides, total protein), liver function tests, renal function tests, and lipid panels.

The therapeutic drug monitoring section can be a stand-alone section or can be combined with toxicology, blood gases, or other small-volume specialty sections. Some drugs used to treat patients can harm the liver or kidneys with side effects. Patients taking these drugs must have the concentration of the drug in their body monitored to ensure that it stays within a therapeutic range and does not rise up to a toxic level or dip below therapeutic levels and prevent successful therapy. Because of the specialized nature of testing for toxic substances, smaller laboratories may combine the therapeutic drug monitoring section and the toxicology section of a laboratory for improved throughput or efficiency. Both sections use specialized instruments to test for therapeutic drugs, drugs of abuse, and other toxic substances. Testing for sweat chlorides is sometimes grouped in this section.

The blood gas section of a laboratory can be physically located in the clinical chemistry laboratory, or it can be located in a specialized department of the hospital such as the respiratory therapy department. In smaller hospitals, the respiratory therapist draws the arterial blood gas specimen and then transports it, on ice, to the laboratory. In other situations, clinical laboratory professionals are the ones who draw the specimen. Larger facilities may locate the blood gas laboratory in the intensive care unit, with respiratory therapists drawing the specimen and running the tests there instead of transporting the specimen to a separate laboratory.

The RIA/EIA section of a clinical chemistry laboratory is categorized by the method used to evaluate a particular analyte. RIA/EIA tests are performed on automated analyzers that use radioimmunoassay (RIA), enzyme immunoassay (EIA), or enzyme-linked immunoassay (ELISA) techniques to measure hormones, tumor markers, and other similar substances.

The special chemistry section of the clinical chemistry laboratory is where all the other tests that do not use similar methods or analyzers are performed. Such a section typically performs tests for sweat chlorides, aldolase, acid phosphatase, electrophoresis, DNA testing, immunoglobulins, microalbumin, human immunodeficiency virus (HIV), hepatitis, mass spectrometry, and other low-volume specialty tests. This section may also perform clinical procedures such as adrenocorticotropic hormone (ACTH) or growth hormone stimulation tests.

Body fluids are also tested in a clinical chemistry laboratory. Body fluids that are sent to the clinical chemistry laboratory for testing may include cerebrospinal fluid (CSF), peritoneal fluid, synovial fluid, and urine. A large proportion of these specimens require glucose or protein testing or both. Body fluids typically require special specimen handling and may not be suitable for testing on a high-throughput analyzer. These fluids are often more viscous than serum or plasma and may cause a clog in the specimen probe. Most clinicians request fluids to be run immediately (stat) or as soon as possible (ASAP), so running specimens on a separate analyzer can save time and money.

Summary

The clinical chemistry section of a clinical laboratory performs biochemical tests to assist clinicians with diagnosing or ruling out diseases. *Disease* is usually defined as a condition that can be detected by medical history, physical examination, and objective data, although culture can also play a role in how individuals define, diagnose, and treat disease. As medical researchers study diseases, specific causes, symptoms, and treatments evolve. Reference ranges can help clinicians determine whether an individual has a particular disease.

Injuries to cells can result in spillage of cellular contents into the bloodstream and can lead to benign and neoplastic growth, inflammation, infection, and autoimmune responses. Each disease mechanism produces biochemical analytes that are measured and correlated with a disease. Many tests exist to confirm and rule out diseases. Some common tests include those that measure glucose, BUN, creatinine, electrolytes, calcium, phosphorus, or hormones; liver function tests; renal function tests; lipid panels; and tests for immunoglobulins, proteins, and drugs (therapeutic medications and drugs of abuse). However, there are literally thousands more biochemical tests that are available for clinicians to choose from. Unfortunately, no biochemical test is 100% sensitive and 100% specific. As a result, diagnostic tests can produce false-positive and false-negative results. The test result must be combined with the medical history and physical examination findings to produce the most comprehensive picture of a patient's condition. One drawback to this system of diagnosis is that if a clinician is not looking for the patient's disease, he or she will not find it.

Review Questions

1. A condition that is considered a deviation from or an interruption of the normal structure or function of a part, organ, or system of the body, with characteristic symptoms and signs is called a
   a. Condition
   b. Syndrome
   c. Disease
   d. Pathology

2. What affects how diseases are diagnosed and treated?
   a. Cultural perceptions
   b. Laboratory test results
   c. Medical history
   d. Clinical signs

3. Which terms are used to describe the condition of an individual?
   a. Normal and abnormal
   b. Health and disease
   c. Health and normal
   d. Disease and abnormal

4. Blood from many patients is drawn, a specific test is run on the samples, and then the mean and range (±2 standard deviations) is calculated. The result of this process is called the
   a. Confidence interval
   b. Objective data
   c. Reference range
   d. False negative

5. Which of the following differs from laboratory to laboratory according to the population served?
   a. Confidence interval
   b. Objective data
   c. False negative
   d. Reference range

6. All of the following are components of a cell EXCEPT
   a. Nucleus
   b. Cell membrane
   c. Cytoplasm
   d. Biochemicals

7. All of the following processes or conditions can produce disease EXCEPT
   a. Homeostasis
   b. Inflammation
   c. Immunity
   d. Necrosis

8. All of the following are considered cellular adaptations EXCEPT
   a. Hyperplasia
   b. Metaplasia
   c. Necrosis
   d. Neoplasia

9. A malignant neoplasm is
   a. Cancer
   b. Metaplasia
   c. Hyperplasia
   d. Dysplasia

10. Which type of test has occurred when an individual does not have a condition even though the laboratory test indicates that the condition is present?
    a. False negative
    b. True positive
    c. True negative
    d. False positive

Critical Thinking Questions

1. Does healthy mean normal, and does diseased mean abnormal? Why or why not?
2. How are clinical chemistry test results used to confirm or rule out a presumptive diagnosis? Why is this important?
3. What are false-positive and false-negative test results, and why is it important for a clinical to understand these concepts?

CASE STUDY

A 32-year-old woman presents with exhaustion, swollen lymph nodes, and a sore throat. Her physician orders a test for mononucleosis. The test comes back positive. The physician performs a confirmatory test (more specific test), and it is negative. How could this happen?

Bibliography

Bodansky M, Bodansky O. *Biochemistry of Disease*. New York: Macmillan; 1940.

Burtis CA, Bruns DE. *Tietz Fundamentals of Clinical Chemistry and Molecular Diagnostics*. 7th ed. St. Louis: Saunders; 2015.

De Paolo C. Pasteur and Lister: A chronicle of scientific influence. *The Victorian Web*. Updated. July 2012. <http://www.victorianweb.org/science/health/depaolo.html> Accessed 15.05.15.

Dorland's Illustrated Medical Dictionary. 32nd ed. Philadelphia: Saunders; 2012.

Guyton AC, Hall JE. *Human Physiology and Mechanisms of Disease*. 6th ed. Philadelphia: Saunders; 1997.

Hart GD. Descriptions of blood and blood disorders before the advent of laboratory studies. *Br J Haematol*. 2001;115(4):719–728.

Lupton D. *Medicine As Culture: Illness, Disease and the Body*. 3rd ed. London: SAGE; 2012.

Mandal A. What is pathology? *Medical News*. Updated September 2014. <http://www.news-medical.net/health/Pathology-What-is-Pathology.aspx> Accessed 15.05.15.

Peck R, Devore JL. *Statistics: The Exploration and Analysis of Data*. 7th ed. Independence, KY: Cengage Learning; 2012: 464–465.

10

Cell Injury and Its Relationship to Disease

DONNA LARSON

CHAPTER OUTLINE

Introduction

Overview of Cellular Injury

Causes of Cellular Injury

    Hypoxia

    Trauma, Heat, and Cold

    Radiation

    Toxic Substances

    Microbes

    Immune Reaction

    Nutrition

    Genes

    Aging

    Cancer

Changes in Body Chemistry

    Loss of Energy: ATP and Oxygen Depletion

    Mitochondrial Damage

    Loss of Calcium Homeostasis

    Defects in Membrane Permeability

    Generation of Free Radicals

Laboratory Tests

Summary

OBJECTIVES

At the completion of this chapter, the reader will be able to:

1. Identify three ways a cell can adapt to external stimuli such as changes in cell size and cell numbers.
2. Describe ten types of external stress that can injure cells and the specific effects on cells.
3. Identify five biochemical mechanisms that cause cellular injury.
4. Explain how specific chemicals in the blood can be used to diagnose disease.
5. Identify the specific substances that can be measured to diagnose an acute myocardial infarction.

KEY TERMS

Acute myocardial infarction
Apoptosis
Atrophy
Creatine kinase
Creatine kinase isoenzymes
Endotoxins
Free radicals

Homeostasis
Hyperplasia
Hypertrophy
Hypoxia
Ischemia
Lactate dehydrogenase
Lysosomal enzymes

Malignant cells
Metaplasia
Myoglobin
Necrosis
Oncogenic viruses
Troponin I
Troponin T

❖ Case in Point

Robert has wine and other alcoholic drinks on a regular basis and has done so for many years. Because alcohol is processed through the liver, he is at risk for liver damage. Using the mechanisms described in this chapter, explain how damage can occur to Robert's liver and which laboratory test results could indicate that damage has already occurred.

Points to Remember

- Stress causes injuries to the body that lead to disease.
- Cellular adaptations to stress include hyperplasia, metaplasia, and dysplasia.
- Stimuli that can lead to injury include hypoxia, physical actions, radiation, toxic substances, microbes, immune reactions, nutrition, genes, aging, and cancer.
- Five distinct biochemical mechanisms cause injuries to cells.
- When cells die, they release cytoplasmic chemicals into the bloodstream.
- Specific cells release specific chemicals into the bloodstream, and measurement of these chemicals can aid in diagnosing diseases.
- During a myocardial infarction, the creatine kinase MB isoenzyme, troponin I, troponin T, and lactate dehydrogenase are released into the bloodstream.

Introduction

Clinical chemistry is the study of chemicals in the blood and other bodily fluids. Many chemicals are normally produced by organs in the body, but some chemicals in the blood are the result of direct injury or chronic stress that leads to injury. Such injuries affect clinical chemistry test results, which therefore can be used to detect disease and monitor therapy. The chapter begins by discussing cellular adaptations to stress, followed by a discussion of reversible and irreversible injury to cells. The types of stress that cause injuries are discussed along with mechanisms that produce the injury. Finally, some examples of injuries and results for clinical chemistry tests are discussed.

Overview of Cellular Injury

The body's cells automatically function within specific parameters to maintain homeostasis, which is a steady state of equilibrium. Cells are injured by physiologic stress and other pathologic stimuli. When a cell experiences stress, it adapts. Methods of cellular adaptation include atrophy (i.e., decrease in cell size), hypertrophy (i.e., increase in cell size), hyperplasia (i.e., increase in cell number), and metaplasia (i.e., change in cell type) (Figs. 10-1 and 10-2). Cellular adaptations often can be reversed if the source of stress is removed, but severe or prolonged stress can irreversibly injure or kill cells.

Smoking cigarettes and drinking alcohol are examples of activities that stress cells and promote cellular adaptations, although we do not detect any stress on our cells when we engage in these behaviors. Smoking cigarettes leads to lung damage and heart disease, and drinking alcohol leads to liver damage after prolonged exposure.

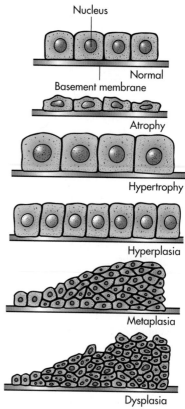

• **Figure 10-1** Cellular adaptations to injury and stress. (From Lewis SM, Heitkemper MM, Dirksen SR. *Medical-Surgical Nursing: Assessment and Management of Clinical Problems.* 7th ed. St Louis: Mosby; 2015.)

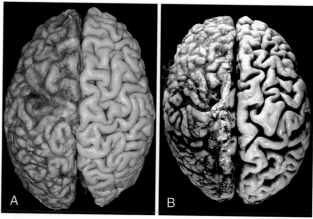

• **Figure 10-2** Atrophy. **A,** Normal brain of a young adult. **B,** Atrophy of the brain in an 82-year-old man with atherosclerotic disease. Atrophy of the brain is a result of aging and reduced blood supply. Notice that loss of brain substance narrows the gyri and widens the sulci. The meninges have been stripped from the right half of each specimen to reveal the surface of the brain. (From Kumar V, Abbas A, Aster JC. *Robbins and Cotran Pathologic Basis of Disease.* 9th ed. Philadelphia: Saunders; 2015.)

Both of these stressors can produce altered clinical chemistry test results.

Injury can cause disease either directly or indirectly, through attempts to repair the damage. Injuries can occur at the molecular, cellular, tissue, or organ level. Molecular injury occurs in the genes of an organism, causing a genetic mutation. The effects of the injury are translated to cells, tissues, and organs. Local injuries can have far-reaching effects in the body. Some injuries go undetected by clinical chemistry tests, but some produce large deviations from reference ranges. This chapter discusses various types of injuries, changes to clinical chemistry test results, and specific tests that can be altered as a result of an injury.

Causes of Cellular Injury

Cells can be injured by many stimuli, including hypoxia, physical actions, radiation, toxic substances, microbes, immune reactions, nutrition, genes, aging, and cancer (Table 10-1). Cellular injury occurs on a continuum, producing many local and systemic effects (Table 10-2).

The body is in a dynamic state in which cells normally grow, adapt, and die. When old cells die, they are removed from the circulation or sloughed off, and new cells take their place. In **apoptosis,** or programmed cell death, the nucleus fragments, and the cell remains mostly intact. This phenomenon is not always associated with injury. Some malignancies alter cells to the extent that the normal, anticipated apoptosis does not occur, and damaged cells continue to proliferate. Mild injuries usually lead to reversible cellular changes (Fig. 10-3), but the cellular changes in severe injuries are irreversible, and the injured cells die.

Necrosis is the result of a pathological process. The cell membrane is severely damaged, allowing the **lysosomal enzymes**

TABLE 10-1	Types of Cellular Injury
Type of Injury	**Examples**
Genetic	Gene defects, chromosomal anomalies
Nutritional	Deficiency or excess of dietary substances (e.g., iron, vitamins)
Immune	Damage caused by the immune system (e.g., autoimmunity)
Endocrine	Deficient or excessive hormone activity
Physical	Mechanical trauma, thermal damage, UV or ionizing irradiation
Chemical	Toxicity due to many agents (e.g., metals, solvents, drugs)
Infectious	Infection by viruses, bacteria, parasites, fungi, and other organisms
Ischemic (hypoxic)	Deficient blood supply or direct oxygen deficit

From McCance K, Huether S. *Pathophysiology: The Biologic Basis for Disease in Adults and Children.* 7th ed. St Louis: Mosby; 2014.

TABLE 10-2	Systemic Manifestations of Cellular Injury
Manifestation	**Cause**
Fever	Release of endogenous pyrogens (e.g., interleukin-1, tumor necrosis factor-α, prostaglandins) from bacteria or macrophages; acute inflammatory response
Increased heart rate	Increase in oxidative metabolic processes resulting from fever
Increase in number of leukocytes (i.e., leukocytosis)	Increase in total number of white blood cells because of infection; normal concentration is 5000 to 9000 cells/mm^3 (increase is directly related to severity of infection)
Pain	Various mechanisms, including release of bradykinins, obstruction, and pressure
Cellular enzymes in extracellular fluid	Release of enzymes from tissue cells*
Lactate dehydrogenase (LDH), LDH isoenzymes	Release from red blood cells, liver, kidney, skeletal muscle
Creatine kinase (CK), CK isoenzymes	Release from skeletal muscle, brain, heart
Aspartate aminotransferase (AST)	Release from heart, liver, skeletal muscle, kidney, pancreas
Alanine aminotransferase (ALT)	Release from liver, kidney, heart
Alkaline phosphatase (ALP)	Release from liver, bone
Amylase	Release from pancreas
Aldolase	Release from skeletal muscle, heart

From McCance K, Huether S. *Pathophysiology: The Biologic Basis for Disease in Adults and Children.* 7th ed. St. Louis: Mosby; 2014.
*The rapidity of enzyme transfer is a function of the weight of the enzyme and the concentration gradient across the cell membrane. The specific metabolic and excretory rates of the enzymes determine how long enzyme levels remain elevated.

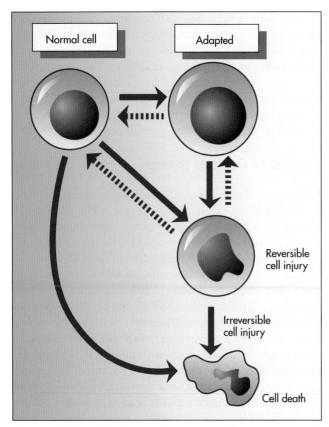

• **Figure 10-3** Cellular injury and responses. After injury, previously normal myocardial cells may adapt through hypertrophy. Reversibly injured cells may heal, but irreversible damage leads to cell death. (From McCance K, Huether S. *Pathophysiology: The Biologic Basis for Disease in Adults and Children.* 7th ed. St. Louis: Mosby; 2014.)

to enter the cytoplasm and digest the cell. The contents spill out into surrounding tissue, causing more damage.

Hypoxia

Hypoxia means *oxygen deficiency.* Oxygen deficiency in cells occurs when too little oxygen is carried in the blood (e.g., anemia, carbon monoxide poisoning, hemoglobinopathy) or too little blood is circulating around the cells (i.e., ischemia). An acid-base imbalance occurs when cells are deprived of oxygen. This imbalance can be reversed, and the cell can return to normal if oxygen is restored to the cell. If oxygen is not restored, the cell dies.

Trauma, Heat, and Cold

Cells can be injured by physical force, which includes trauma, heat, and cold. Trauma disrupts cells, tissues, and organs, simultaneously resulting in hemorrhage and ischemia. Exposure to mild heat causes leakage of adenosine triphosphate (ATP), and intense heat exposure liquefies the cell membrane. Prolonged exposure to cold temperatures can freeze the water in cells, causing frostbite. The ice crystals that form in the cytoplasm rupture the cell membrane, leading to necrosis.

Radiation

The type of radiation that damages cells in the body is called *ionizing radiation* (e.g., gamma rays). This type of radiation is strong enough to dissociate water into H^+ and OH^- ions. The hydroxyl ions attach to DNA and prevent replication. Rapidly dividing cells in the body (i.e., blood cells and intestinal epithelium cells) are most affected by reduced replication. The red and white blood cell counts drop dramatically after radiation exposure, and the lining of the intestines sloughs off. All of these injuries leave the body vulnerable to infection.

Toxic Substances

Damage to cells can occur through direct chemical injury or generation of toxic metabolites after exposure to natural or synthetic chemicals. Strong acids and bases can directly disrupt cells and cause major damage to tissues and organs. Ingestion of strong acids or bases may change the blood pH, resulting in death. Chronic exposure to heavy metals (e.g., lead, mercury) can injure organs such as the liver. Toxic substances also include legal and illegal drugs, chemical warfare agents, alcohol, and carbon monoxide.

Microbes

Pathogenic bacteria, viruses, parasites, and fungi routinely invade the human body. The body can identify and remove small numbers of these organisms, but an infective dose of a microorganism that enters the body can produce disease. Some bacterial species produce toxins that damage the body's cells. The cell walls of gram-negative organisms contain substances that become toxins when the bacteria die. These endotoxins cause vascular collapse or blood clotting within blood vessels. Viruses can directly invade a cell and produce disease, and they can elicit an immune response that kills the virus but also kills the cell containing the virus.

Immune Reaction

Immune reactions are generated by the body to kill invaders. Although the reactions usually kill the invader, the surrounding tissue can also be damaged. For example, when the body sends neutrophils to neutralize foreign materials by releasing digestive enzymes, the enzymes also digest nearby tissue. When the body mounts an immune response, it can also attack joints and produce rheumatoid arthritis.

Nutrition

The correct amounts of nutrients help keep a cell in homeostasis. Too many or too few nutrients can cause disease. Too many nutrients of one type can cause obesity. Too little protein or calories can cause protein-calorie deficiency, a major worldwide illness that often leads to death. Vitamin

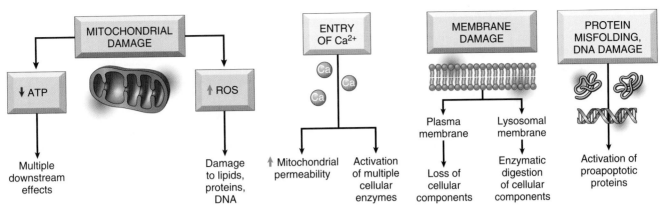

• Figure 10-4 Principal biochemical mechanisms and sites of damage in cell injury. *ATP,* Adenosine triphosphate; *ROS,* reactive oxygen species. (From Kumar V, Abbas A, Aster JC. *Robbins & Cotran Pathologic Basis of Disease.* 9th ed. Philadelphia: Saunders; 2015.)

or mineral deficiencies injure cells by interfering with or blocking important metabolic processes.

Genes

There are two main types of genetic defects: addition or deletion of a nucleotide base, which leads to an abnormal sequence of nucleotide bases, and addition or deletion of an entire chromosome or part of a chromosome. Genetic mutations can lead to altered or missing products (i.e., proteins, chemicals, and structures), affecting physiologic function. Sickle cell disease is an example. In the gene for hemoglobin, a thymine replaces an adenine, resulting in substitution of a valine for glutamic acid in the protein. Valine replacement causes the hemoglobin structure to collapse on itself, prompting cells to assume a sickle-like shape that compromises their oxygen-carrying capacity.

The deletion or omission of an entire chromosome usually occurs during fertilization and therefore is not heritable. Turner syndrome is an example of this type of condition. Extra chromosomes cause conditions such as trisomy X and Down syndrome (trisomy 21).

Aging

Aging affects all cells and ultimately leads to their death. Cells normally have a finite life span and die at the end of it. This "programmed" cell death (i.e., apoptosis) is coupled to the generation of new cells to replace the cells that die. Necrosis, in contrast, is cell death caused by severe or prolonged cellular injury.

Cancer

Cancer arises from genetically damaged cells that continue to proliferate instead of undergoing apoptosis. Uncontrollable cell division creates a tumor as more and more cells are produced. These malignant cells can affect any cell line and may produce the same chemicals as the normal cells. For example, an insulinoma, which is a type of pancreatic tumor, produces an excess of the hormone insulin.

Changes in Body Chemistry

Cellular injury can be produced by five biochemical mechanisms: loss of energy (i.e., ATP and oxygen depletion), mitochondrial damage, loss of calcium homeostasis, defects in membrane permeability, and generation of free radicals (Fig. 10-4).

Loss of Energy: ATP and Oxygen Depletion

Cells use oxygen to carry out aerobic respiration, which produces energy for the cell. Although the cell can also use anaerobic respiration to produce energy, this process produces only one eighth of the energy that aerobic respiration does. Moreover, the end products of anaerobic respiration are toxic and may kill a cell that is forced to use anaerobic respiration for an extended period. After the cell dies, lysosomes and other substances in the cytoplasm are released into the bloodstream.

Mitochondrial Damage

Mitochondrial damage can lead to cell death by several mechanisms. Injury to the mitochondrial membranes causes ions in the cytoplasm to enter and accumulate, disrupting oxidative phosphorylation and energy production. If the permeability of the outer mitochondrial membrane increases, proteins are released from the intermembrane space into the cytoplasm, where they activate other molecules that lead to cell death.

Loss of Calcium Homeostasis

Free calcium levels in a cell's cytoplasm are 10 times lower than extracellular calcium levels. Much of the calcium in a cell is found in the mitochondria and endoplasmic reticulum, but injury can release calcium into the cytoplasm. Increased calcium levels activate ATPases, phospholipases, proteases, and endonucleases. These enzymes can increase ATP levels and damage the membrane, cytoskeleton, and chromatin (Fig. 10-5).

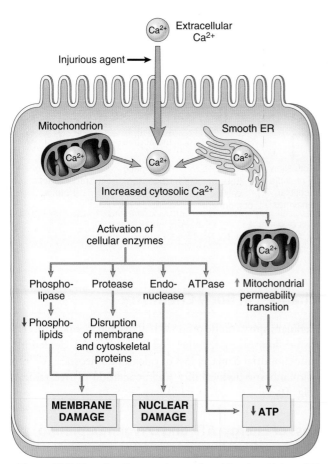

• **Figure 10-5** The role of increased cytosolic calcium in cell injury. *ATP,* Adenosine triphosphate; *ATPase,* adenosine triphosphatase; *ER,* endoplasmic reticulum. (From Kumar V, Abbas A, Aster JC. *Robbins & Cotran Pathologic Basis of Disease.* 9th ed. Philadelphia: Saunders; 2015.)

Defects in Membrane Permeability

Most injuries impede the plasma membrane's ability to maintain a balance of ions between the intracellular and extracellular compartments. Loss of cellular compartments and lysosome disruption leading to the digestion of cellular contents ultimately cause cell death.

Generation of Free Radicals

Free radicals are chemically unstable molecules that readily react with other molecules, resulting in chemical damage. Free radicals initiate autocatalytic reactions: Molecules that react with free radicals are converted to free radicals. Damage caused by free radicals includes membrane injury, DNA strand breaks, faulty protein folding, and protein degradation (Fig. 10-6).

Laboratory Tests

When ischemia causes hypoxia, the muscle tissue or organ cells can die. When muscle tissue dies, substances such as myoglobin, creatine kinase (CK), lactate dehydrogenase, and electrolytes (e.g., potassium, calcium, magnesium) are released into the surrounding tissues and blood. Levels of these chemicals can be measured to diagnose cellular damage.

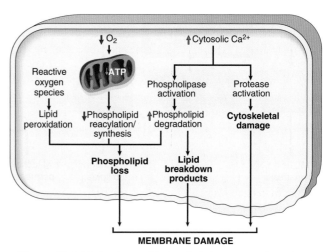

• **Figure 10-6** Mechanisms of ischemia-induced cell injury. Cellular damage often occurs through the formation of reactive oxygen radicals. *ATP,* Adenosine triphosphate. (From Kumar V, Abbas A, Aster JC. *Robbins & Cotran Pathologic Basis of Disease.* 9th ed. Philadelphia: Saunders; 2015.)

Although lactate dehydrogenase is released by dying tissue, it is nonspecific and is not frequently used as an indicator of cellular damage except in hemolytic anemias.

Tissue cells contain various types of chemicals, some of which are tissue specific. For example, in an acute myocardial infarction, part of a coronary artery is blocked and the heart tissue served by this artery becomes hypoxic due to ischemia. If the blockage does not resolve in a short period, the affected heart tissue begins to die and releases substances such as myoglobin, CK, CK-MB fraction, troponin I, troponin T, and lactate dehydrogenase into the blood.

Myoglobin is a protein found in all muscles. An elevated myoglobin value in a blood sample indicates muscle damage somewhere in the body. Unfortunately, this protein is not specific because it does not indicate which muscle is damaged.

The enzyme CK is found in all muscles and in the brain, and the total value for CK is not a specific indicator. However, the levels of creatine kinase isoenzymes (i.e., CK-MM, CK-MB, and CK-BB) can be more specific. For example, normal skeletal muscle contains mostly CK-MM, but the presence of some CK-MB and a large amount of CK-MM can indicate muscle damage. Heart muscle contains mostly CK-MB and some CK-MM, so heart muscle damage can be indicated by the presence of a large amount of CK-MB. Brain damage can be indicated by a large amount of CK-BB.

A good way to pinpoint injury is to order a test for a substance that is found in a particular tissue or organ. For example, a test for the CK-MB isoenzyme can provide information about damage to heart tissue caused by a myocardial infarction. However, two cardiac-specific molecules, troponin T (cTnT) and troponin I (cTnI), also are liberated by heart muscle damage. Current practice relies on cTnT and cTnI instead of CK-MB to diagnose myocardial infarction because they are more specific for cardiac muscle injury.

If there is no tissue damage caused by hypoxia (as in ischemia), other laboratory tests can be used to determine low levels of oxygen in the blood. The most common of these tests is an arterial blood gas determination. An arterial puncture is performed to obtain a well-oxygenated blood sample for testing. (Venous blood is deoxygenated blood that returns to the lung to pick up oxygen and is then circulated through the arteries.) Low blood oxygen levels can be caused by decreased numbers of red blood cells, variant types of hemoglobin, or a poorly functioning respiratory system.

Toxic chemicals can be detected by laboratory testing. For example, in cases of mercury poisoning, the mercury molecule binds directly to the cell membrane and compromises its functions. Analyses of blood, urine, or other tissues can be performed to detect heavy metals such as mercury. In some cases, otherwise harmless chemicals may damage cells indirectly through their metabolites, which can be measured in the clinical laboratory. For example, blood tests for exposure to carbon monoxide (a poisonous gas) would include determination of carboxyhemoglobin, an abnormal form of hemoglobin caused by the attachment of a carbon monoxide molecule.

Microorganisms can injure and kill cells. Cytolytic and cytopathic viruses attach to the cell membrane, enter the cell, and then use the cell's organelles to create new viruses. This process interferes with the cell's normal metabolism and causes death when the cell bursts to release the new viruses. Viral attachment to a cell elicits an immune response to the virus that may also injure and kill the cell. Rapid viral replication results in cell lysis and release of the new viral particles. **Oncogenic viruses** disrupt normal expression of the host cell's genes in favor of expressing the viral genes; this may stimulate the host cell to reproduce uncontrollably and create a malignant tumor. Other microorganisms, such as *Rickettsia* bacteria and malarial parasites, also cause cellular injury and lysis,

Summary

Physiologic stress on the body's cells can result in cellular adaptation, injury, or death. Injury can occur at the molecular, cellular, tissue, and organ levels. Ten types of stimuli cause cellular injury: hypoxia, physical actions, radiation, toxic substances, microbes, immune reactions, nutrition, genes, aging, and cancer. Several chemical mechanisms lead to cellular death. When a cell dies, chemicals in the cytoplasm are released into the bloodstream. For example, an acute myocardial infarction releases CK-MB, lactate dehydrogenase, troponin I, and troponin T into the bloodstream, and tests for these substances can aid in diagnosis.

Review Questions

1. When a cell experiences stress, it adapts in all of the following ways EXCEPT
   a. Meterotrophy
   b. Atrophy
   c. Hypertrophy
   d. Hyperplasia
2. Cellular injuries can cause disease
   a. Directly and through metabolites
   b. Indirectly and through chemical abnormalities
   c. Immunologically and chemically
   d. Directly and indirectly
3. Molecular injuries cause
   a. Apoptosis
   b. Cancer
   c. A mutation
   d. Necrosis
4. Mild injuries lead to
   a. Irreversible cellular change
   b. Reversible cellular change
   c. Severe cellular damage
   d. Hypoxia
5. In necrosis, the cell membrane is damaged, allowing which of the following to enter the cytoplasm and digest the cell?
   a. Lysosomal enzymes
   b. IgM antibodies
   c. Free radicals
   d. Acidic molecules
6. If a cell uses anaerobic respiration for an extended period, what is the end result?
   a. Cellular death
   b. Hypoxia
   c. Free radicals
   d. Lysosomal enzymes
7. All of the following are biochemical mechanisms that can cause cell injury EXCEPT
   a. Mitochondrial damage
   b. Generation of free radicals
   c. Genetic mutations
   d. Loss of calcium homeostasis
8. Free radicals cause damage to cells by which of the following mechanisms?
   a. Normal ion accumulation
   b. Accumulation of too many nutrients
   c. Faulty protein folding and degradation
   d. Antibody neutralization
9. Which of the following chemicals are released from cells when they die?
   a. Free radicals
   b. Antibodies
   c. Fluids
   d. Enzymes
10. What types of virus cause a cell to produce a malignant tumor?
    a. Benign
    b. Oncogenic
    c. Trisomy X
    d. Mediator

Critical Thinking Questions

1. Many people climb Mt. Everest every year. The sheer height of the mountain and the thin air at higher elevations adversely affect climbers. What type of stress and corresponding injuries would you expect to find in these climbers? Name at least three stresses and their corresponding injuries.

2. In 2011, the Sendai region of Japan experienced a 9.0 earthquake and a massive tsunami. The Fukishima Daiichi nuclear plant suffered several fires that crippled the plant, forcing the evacuation of all but 50 employees. Fearing a core reactor meltdown, these 50 men stayed behind to work on the reactor, even though it meant exposing themselves to ionizing radiation far above the permissible exposure limits. What kind of stress did these workers endure? How does ionizing radiation above the permissible exposure limit stress and possibly injure cells in the body?

3. According to the Centers for Disease Control and Prevention, approximately 600,000 people die of heart disease every year in the United States. Of the approximately 715,000 people who experience a heart attack (acute myocardial infarction, or AMI) each year, 385,000 die. Health care, medications, and lost productivity associated with coronary heart disease cost about $108.9 billion annually. How does an AMI interrupt normal body function, and how is an AMI detected in the clinical chemistry laboratory?

CASE STUDY

As a standard procedure, Hannah, a newborn, is screened for genetic conditions before she leaves the hospital. Two of the tests, which are performed in all states, are for phenylketonuria and hypothyroidism. Describe how these diseases can injure cells and harm a newborn.

Bibliography

Campisi J. Aging, cellular senescence, and cancer. *Annu Rev Physiol.* 2013;75:685.

Delanghe JR, De Buyzere ML, Speeckaert MM, Langlois MR. Genetic aspects of scurvy and the European famine of 1845-1848. *Nutrients.* 2013;5:3582–3588.

Favaloro B, Allocati N, Graziano V, Di Ilio C, De Laurenzi V. Role of apoptosis in disease. *Aging (Albany NY).* 2012;4:330.

Kumar V, Abbas A, Fausto N. *Robbins and Cotran Pathologic Basis of Disease.* 7th ed. Philadelphia: Saunders; 2005.

Langley–Evans SC. Nutrition in early life and the programming of adult disease: a review. *J Hum Nutr Diet.* 2015;28(suppl 1):1–14.

Moon K, Guallar E, Navas-Acien A. Arsenic exposure and cardiovascular disease: an updated systematic review. *Curr Atheroscler Rep.* 2012;14:542–555.

Osborn O, Olefsky JM. The cellular and signaling networks linking the immune system and metabolism in disease. *Nat Med.* 2012;18:363–374.

Parsons K. *Human Thermal Environments: The Effects of Hot, Moderate, and Cold Environments on Human Health, Comfort, and Performance.* Boca Raton, FL: CRC Press; 2014.

Pauwels EK, Bourguignon M. Cancer induction caused by radiation due to computed tomography: a critical note. *Acta Radiol.* 2011;52:767–773.

Prüss-Ustün A, Vickers C, Haefliger P, Bertollini R. Knowns and unknowns on burden of disease due to chemicals: a systematic review. *Environ Health.* 2011;10:9.

Semenza GL. Oxygen sensing, hypoxia-inducible factors, and disease pathophysiology. *Annu Rev Pathol.* 2014;9:47–71.

Wilson BA, Salyers AA, Whitt DD, Winkler ME. *Bacterial Pathogenesis: A Molecular Approach.* 3rd ed. Washington, DC: ASM Press; 2011.

11

Inflammation

DONNA LARSON

CHAPTER OUTLINE

Introduction

Defense Mechanisms

The Inflammation Process

    The Complement System

    The Clotting System

    The Kinin System

    Chemical Mediators of Inflammation

    Cellular Mediators of Inflammation

Acute Inflammation

Chronic Inflammation

    Tissue Destruction, Tissue Repair, and Regeneration

Laboratory Procedures and Limitations

    C-Reactive Protein

    Complement Proteins

    Fibrinogen

    α_1-Antitrypsin

    Immunoglobulins

    Cytokines

    Blood Cells and Constituents

Summary

OBJECTIVES

At the completion of this chapter, the reader will be able to:

1. Describe the defense mechanisms used by the body maintain health.
2. Describe the inflammatory process.
3. Differentiate the roles of the complement, clotting, and kinin systems in the inflammatory process.
4. List the signs of inflammation and describe how each is produced.
5. Compare and contrast acute and chronic inflammation.
6. Summarize the hallmarks of chronic inflammation.
7. Compare tissue repair in tissues with a high regenerative capacity with repair in tissues with a low capacity.
8. Assess the clinical usefulness of the C-reactive protein (CRP), complement, fibrinogen, α_1-antitrypsin, cytokines, erythrocyte sedimentation rate (ESR), and white blood cell (WBC) counts in the diagnosis of inflammation.
9. List the laboratory methods used to measure CRP, complement, fibrinogen, α_1-antitrypsin, cytokines, ESR, and WBC differential.

KEY TERMS

Acute inflammation
Acute phase proteins
Alternative pathway
Angiogenesis
Bradykinins
Chronic inflammation
Classical pathway
Complement
C-reactive protein

Cytokines
Edema
Endothelial cells
Fibrinogen
Granuloma
Histamine
Inflammation
Lectin pathway
Leukotrienes

Macrophage
Mediator
Prostaglandin
Protease
Reactive oxygen species
Serapins
Vascular permeability
Vasodilation

◆ Case in Point

Mr. C., a 45-year-old Hispanic man, complains to his physician about a sore on his chin. While he was clearing away yard debris at home, a dirty branch poked him in his chin and broke the skin. Within 36 hours, his lower jaw became red, swollen, and painful with a pus-like discharge. Discuss why this wound would be described as an inflammation.

Points to Remember

- Natural barriers help the body protect itself.
- Inflammation is the response of the body to injury.
- Inflammation involves chemicals and cells and is considered a nonspecific response.
- The goal of inflammation is to prevent further injury and infection and begin healing.
- The complement, clotting, and kinin systems are responsible for an effective inflammatory response.
- The complement cascade destroys pathogens directly or in conjunction with the clotting and kinin systems.
- The classical complement system is activated by antibody–antigen complexes, the lectin pathway by specific bacterial carbohydrates, and the alternative pathway by gram-negative and fungal cell wall polysaccharides.
- The clotting system is responsible for forming a lattice around the injured tissue to stop the bleeding, prevent the spread of infection, trap organisms at the injury site, and provide a structure for repair and resolution.
- Bradykinin is the biologically active molecule in the kinin system that dilates blood vessels and acts with E-series prostaglandins to induce pain, contract smooth muscles, increase vascular permeability, and increase leukocyte migration to the injury site.
- Many chemical mediators are released during inflammation, and the actions of these mediators include increased blood flow, blood vessel dilation at the injury site, increased blood vessel permeability, and leakage of fluid and cells into the extracellular spaces.
- Cells involved in inflammation include neutrophils, monocytes, eosinophils, basophils, lymphocytes, and platelets. They work to confine the damage, kill the organisms, and remove debris.
- Cells secrete chemokines and cytokines to regulate inflammation.
- Mast cells play a central role in inflammation through degranulation and synthesis.
- The liver produces many acute phase proteins during the inflammatory response, including fibrinogen, α_1-antitrypsin, complement components, and C-reactive protein.
- Acute inflammation lasts less than 2 weeks, and chronic inflammation lasts longer than 2 weeks.
- Chronic inflammation is controlled by cells as the body switches from a nonspecific to a more specific response.
- The main cells involved in chronic inflammation are monocytes, macrophages, B and T lymphocytes, and plasma cells.
- The end product of inflammation is repair and resolution.
- The signs of acute inflammation are heat, redness, pain, and swelling.
- The hallmarks of chronic inflammation include migration of cells, infiltration of inflammatory cells, tissue destruction, and repair processes.

Introduction

This chapter examines inflammation, the process by which the human body responds to tissue injury. The three systems that are integral to inflammation—the complement, clotting, and kinin systems—are each summarized individually, and their interactions are highlighted. Acute and chronic inflammation processes are compared, and the characteristics and products of each process are examined. The laboratory procedures for determining acute phase proteins, cytokines, erythrocyte sedimentation rate (ESR), and white blood cell (WBC) counts are described.

Defense Mechanisms

Human defense mechanisms include natural barriers (physical, mechanical, and biochemical) and inflammation. Physical and mechanical barriers include the skin and the mucous membranes of the respiratory, gastrointestinal, and genitourinary tracts. The sloughing of skin cells and the washing mechanism of mucous membranes help keep these areas free of pathogens. In addition, the ciliated epithelial cells of the upper respiratory tract release pathogenic organisms into the environment through coughing or sneezing.

Biochemical barriers in the body include tears, sweat, saliva, mucus, and earwax. These substances can trap and kill pathogenic organisms. In addition, sebaceous glands in the skin secrete antimicrobial (antibacterial, antifungal) agents as well as lactic acid. Sweat, tears, and saliva contain lysozyme, an enzyme that disrupts the cell wall of gram-positive bacteria.

The human body also harbors many bacteria in a commensal relationship (i.e., one that provides benefit to one organism without harming the other). The bacteria live on the body while preventing colonization by pathogenic bacteria. The bacteria in the gut are another good example because they help digest fatty acids; help the body to absorb calcium, iron, and magnesium; and produce vitamin K and biotin. If the body's defenses are compromised and the tissue is injured, inflammation ensues (Fig. 11-1).

The Inflammation Process

Inflammation is the body's response to injury. It is a protective response that is designed to rid the body of the offending agent and repair injury resulting from it. The most

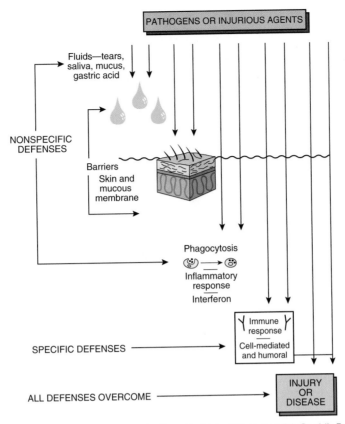

• Figure 11-1 Defense mechanisms in the body. (From VanMeter KC, Hubert RJ. *Gould's Pathophysiology for the Health Professions,* 5th ed. St. Louis: Elsevier, 2015.)

common causes of injury are infection, mechanical damage, oxygen deprivation (ischemia), nutrient deprivation, genetic or immune defects, chemical agents, temperature extremes, and ionizing radiation.

Inflammation involves cells and chemicals and is considered a nonspecific response mechanism. *Nonspecific* means that the response is the same regardless of what is causing the injury. When injury occurs, inflammation immediately affects the arterioles, capillaries, and venules. The process continues through the following steps:

1. The vessels constrict and then dilate to increase the flow of blood.
2. Blood flow coupled with increased permeability of the vessel leads to leakage of fluid from the vessel, causing edema.
3. The fluid leakage makes the blood more viscous, causing warmth and redness.
4. The leukocytes that migrate to the site adhere to the vessel walls.
5. At this point, powerful chemical mediators (e.g., prostaglandins, histamine, leukotrienes, bradykinins) are released; they cause endothelial cells in capillaries and venules to retract, allowing leukocytes and fluid to enter the interstitial spaces.

Once the cells and fluid are in the interstitial spaces, the goal of inflammation is to prevent further injury and infection and to begin healing (Fig. 11-2). That is accomplished through the following processes:

1. Dilution of bacterial toxins with increased fluid in tissues

2. Activation of the complement and clotting cascades to destroy and contain bacteria
3. Attraction of cells (leukocytes, monocytes, macrophages) to ingest bacteria and debris
4. Control of the response so that it does not spread to healthy tissues
5. Interaction with the cellular portion of the immune system to produce a specific immune response
6. Removal of debris and dead bacteria through the lymph system to begin healing

The complement, clotting, and kinin systems are responsible for an effective inflammatory response. To ensure that the proteins involved in these systems do not constantly injure healthy tissue, proteins in the blood circulate in an inactive form. Products of tissue damage activate a few specific proteins in each system. Activation of the first component of each of these systems causes the next component in the system to become activated, producing a sequential effect called a *cascade* (i.e., the complement, clotting, and kinin cascades).

The Complement System

The complement cascade (Fig. 11-3) is an important system because it can destroy pathogens directly or in conjunction with the clotting and kinin systems. This system is the body's defense against bacterial infection. There are three different methods for activating this system, known as the classical,

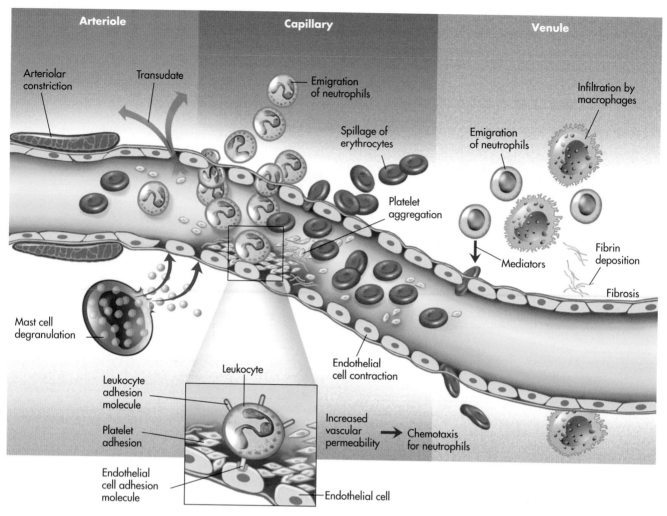

• **Figure 11-2** Sequence of events in the inflammatory response. (From McCance KL, Huether SE. *Pathophysiology: The Biologic Basis for Disease in Adults and Children.* 7th ed. St. Louis: Mosby; 2015.)

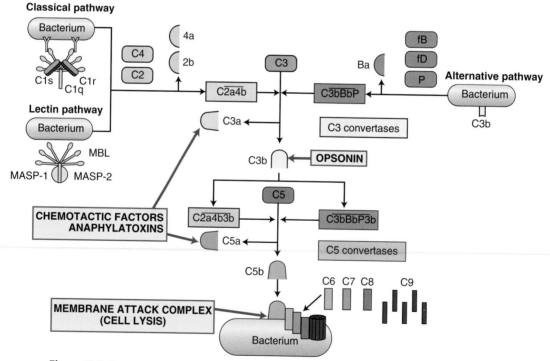

• **Figure 11-3** Complement cascade activation. (From McCance KL, Huether SE. *Pathophysiology: The Biologic Basis for Disease in Adults and Children.* 7th ed. St. Louis: Mosby; 2015.)

lectin, and alternative pathways. The classical pathway is activated by antibody–antigen complexes, the lectin pathway is activated by specific bacterial carbohydrates, and the alternative pathway is activated by gram-negative bacterial and fungal cell wall polysaccharides.

Complement C1 is the first component in the classical pathway. The C1 molecule has a total of six antibody binding sites. Efficient activation of the cascade requires binding of at least two sites to antibody–antigen complexes. Structurally, C1 is composed of one molecule of C1q and two molecules of C1r and C1s. Activation of C1 transforms the molecule into an active enzyme with substrates of C4 and C2. The combined C1, C4, and C2 macromolecule (called C3 convertase) uses C3 as a substrate to produce C3a and C3b. All these molecules together are called the C5 convertase. C5 convertase activates C5, resulting in the production of C5a and C5b. C5 is the molecule responsible for activating the membrane attack complex (MAC), which leads to lysis of the bacterial cell.

The alternative pathway is activated when gram-negative cell wall lipopolysaccharide or yeast cell carbohydrates (zymosan) naturally bind C3b. The lectin pathway is activated when mannose-binding lectin interacts with C4 and C2 to create C3 convertase.

Overall, there are three different ways to activate the complement system, and four outcomes are possible: mast cell degranulation, leukocyte chemotaxis, opsonization, and cell lysis.

The Clotting System

The clotting system is responsible for forming a lattice structure around the injured tissue. This lattice structure is used as a foundation for clot formation. The clotting system can be activated by collagen, proteinases, kallikrein, plasmin, and bacterial products. There are two different pathways for activating the clotting system: the extrinsic (tissue factor) pathway and the intrinsic (contact activation) pathway. The extrinsic pathway is activated by tissue thromboplastin (tissue factor), and the intrinsic pathway is activated by Hageman factor (factor XII) released from a damaged vessel wall. Both pathways lead to a common pathway in which activation of factor X results in formation of a fibrin clot (Fig. 11-4). In summary, the clotting system can be activated in several ways and results in the formation of fibrin at the injury site. The functions of the clotting system that are important in the inflammatory response include preventing the spread of infection, trapping organisms at the site of the injury, stopping bleeding through clot formation, and providing a structure for repair and resolution.

The Kinin System

The kinin system is the final system involved in inflammation. Bradykinin is the primary molecule in this system (Fig. 11-5). Bradykinin dilates blood vessels, acts with prostaglandins (E series) to induce pain, contracts

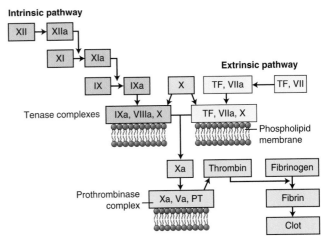

• **Figure 11-4** Clotting cascade. (From McCance KL, Huether SE. *Pathophysiology: The Biologic Basis for Disease in Adults and Children.* 7th ed. St. Louis: Mosby; 2015.)

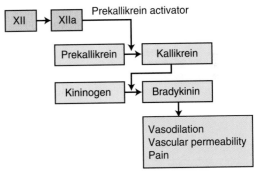

• **Figure 11-5** Kinin cascade. (From McCance KL, Huether SE. *Pathophysiology: The Biologic Basis for Disease in Adults and Children.* 7th ed. St. Louis: Mosby; 2015.)

smooth muscles, increases vascular permeability, and increases leukocyte migration to the injury site. This system is activated by the conversion of prekallikrein to kallikrein by prekallikrein activator (also called factor XIIa in the clotting system). Kallikrein then converts kininogen to bradykinin.

The three systems are interconnected so that the activation of one system produces potent, active substances that can also activate the other systems. Molecules from one system that can affect other systems include the following:

Thrombin	→	Converts C5 to C5a + C5b
Thrombin	→	Converts C3 to C3a + C3b
Plasmin	→	Converts C3 to C3a + C3b
Plasmin	→	Converts C1 to activated C1
Plasmin	→	Converts Hagman factor (XII) to XIIa
Elevated C1	→	Converts Hagman factor (XII) to XIIa
Kallikrein	→	Converts C1 to activated C1
Kallikrein	→	Converts plasminogen to plasmin

The body must control the inflammatory process because inflammation produces such potent, disruptive chemicals that it can potentially harm the body. The body must also

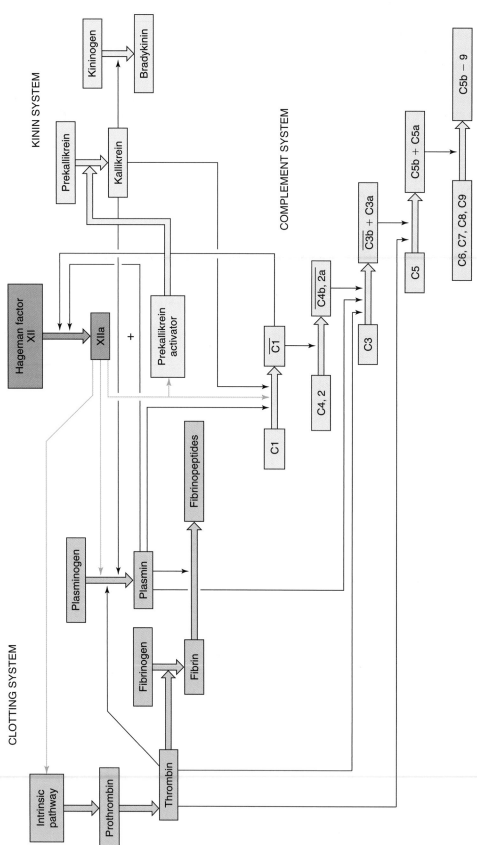

• **Figure 11-6** Interactions between the complement, clotting, and kinin systems. *Thick arrows* denote activation of factors within a system. *Thin arrows* indicate where a particular factor activates a different system. (From McCance KL, Huether SE. *Pathophysiology: The Biologic Basis for Disease in Adults and Children.* 7th ed. St. Louis: Mosby; 2015.)

ensure that the production of these chemicals is confined to the area of an injury and does not spread throughout the body. Ways in which the body keeps inflammation under control include production of activator molecules in an inactive state and circulation of enzymes such as carboxylases that inactivate C3 and C5, kininases, and enzymes that degrade histamine, activated complement components, kallikrein, and plasmin. C1 esterase is a regulator molecule that can inhibit the complement, clotting, and kinin systems (Fig. 11-6).

Chemical Mediators of Inflammation

Many chemical mediators are involved in the inflammatory process (Table 11-1). Chemical mediators can be produced by a variety of body cells in response to injury and by leukocytes that take part in the inflammatory process. Chemical mediators can be released immediately (body cells) or later during the inflammatory process (leukocytes). The primary chemical mediators of acute inflammation are complement, prostaglandins, bradykinins, histamine, leukotrienes, and cytokines such as interleukin-1 (IL-1), IL-6, interferon-γ (IFN-γ), and tumor necrosis factor-α (TNF-α). The actions of these mediators are described in Table 11-1 and include increased blood flow, dilation of blood vessels at the site of the injury, increased blood vessel permeability, and leakage of fluid and cells from blood vessels into the extracellular spaces. The fluids that enter the extracellular spaces contain proteins such as immunoglobulins and cytokines. Cells such as neutrophils, lymphocytes, eosinophils, and monocytes move from the blood vessel to the extracellular space, where they promote chronic inflammation.

Cellular Mediators of Inflammation

In addition to chemical mediators, inflammation involves cellular mediators—some of which (mast cells) are found in the surrounding tissues (Table 11-2). Other cells involved in inflammation secrete and respond to the chemical mediators of inflammation. These cells include basophils, eosinophils,

TABLE 11-1 Chemical Mediators of Inflammation

Mediator Name	Acute or Chronic	Mediator Action
Complement	Acute	Enhanced migration of WBCs, phagocytosis
Prostaglandins	Acute and chronic	Vasodilator
Histamine	Acute	Vasodilation and vascular permeability
Leukotrienes	Acute and chronic	Vasodilation and vascular permeability
Cytokines (IL-1, IL-6, IL-18, TNF-α)	Acute and chronic	Vasodilation and vascular permeability, migration of WBCs
Bradykinins	Chronic	Vasodilation
Adhesion molecules* (ICAM, VCAM, selectins)	Acute and chronic	Help in migration of WBCs

ICAM, Intercellular cell adhesion molecule; IL, interleukin; TNF-α, tumor necrosis factor-α; VCAM, vascular cell adhesion molecule; WBCs, white blood cells.
*Found on leukocytes and blood vessels.

TABLE 11-2 Cellular Mediators of Inflammation

Mediator Name	Acute or Chronic	Mediator Action	Comment
Neutrophils	Acute	Migration, infiltration, phagocytosis	Neutrophils found in peripheral blood and tissues
T lymphocytes	Acute and chronic	Destroys infected cells	T lymphocytes found in peripheral blood and tissues
B lymphocytes and plasma cells	Acute and chronic	Produce antibodies	B lymphocytes found in peripheral blood and tissues, plasma cells found in tissue
Eosinophils	Acute and chronic	Chemicals enhance migration of WBCs	Found in tissues
Monocytes	Chronic	Immature cells	Found in peripheral blood, move to tissues to mature
Macrophages	Chronic	Phagocytosis, tissue destruction/repair, reactive oxygen species	Tissue cells develop from monocytes

WBCs, White blood cells.

lymphocytes, neutrophils, monocytes (precursors to tissue macrophages), and platelets. The cells are activated by products of the three systems of inflammation, and they work with those systems to confine the damage, kill the microorganisms, and remove debris.

These same cells also produce chemicals that enhance or reduce inflammation. Cells secrete chemokines and cytokines to regulate inflammation at a local level and affect the function of target cells. A few cytokines act systemically, such as those that produce fever. Important cytokines belong to the interleukin and interferon groups. Two major proinflammatory cytokines are IL-1 and IL-6. IL-1 acts systemically to produce fever, whereas IL-6 produces fever, signals the liver to produce acute phase reactants, and signals the bone marrow to produce and mature blood cells. IL-10 is antiinflammatory and inhibits cytokine production. Interleukin molecules

protect against pathogens. Interferons are produced to protect against viral infections and regulate inflammation. Chemokines are produced to begin leukocyte chemotaxis. The specific role of each cell is discussed below:

- Mast cells play a central role in inflammation. Mast cells are located in connective tissue and contain many different types of granules. These cells have two major mechanisms of response: degranulation (immediate response) and synthesis (long-term response) (Fig. 11-7). Degranulation enhances the inflammatory response by releasing tryptase, cytokines, histamine, neutrophil chemotactic factor, and eosinophil chemotactic factor. Synthesis releases leukotrienes, prostaglandins (E series), cytokines, and growth factors.
- Platelets circulate in the blood until an injury occurs, after which platelets aggregate at the site of the injury and form (along with the clotting system) the structure for healing.

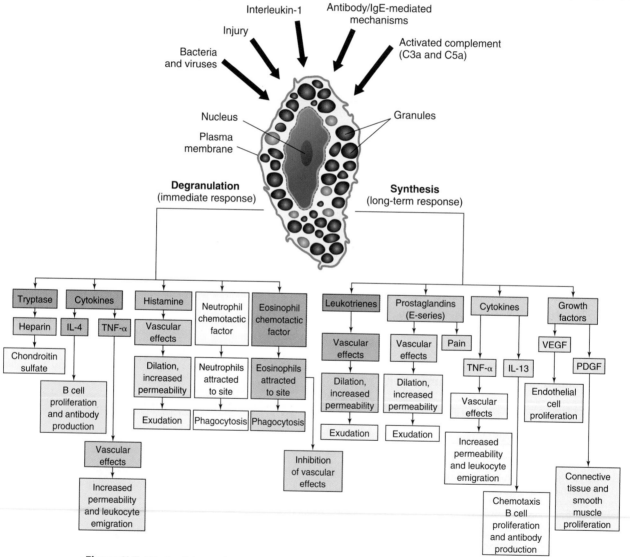

• **Figure 11-7** Effects of degranulation *(left)* and synthesis *(right)* by mast cells. The depiction of a tissue mast cell shows darkly stained granules in the cytoplasm. *IgE,* Immunoglobulin E, *IL,* interleukin; *PDGF,* platelet-derived growth factor; *TNF-α,* tumor necrosis factor-α; *VEGF,* vascular endothelial growth factor. (From McCance KL, Huether SE. *Pathophysiology: The Biologic Basis for Disease in Adults and Children.* 7th ed. St. Louis: Mosby; 2015.)

- Neutrophils phagocytize organisms and debris in the area of the injury.
- Eosinophils play two roles in inflammation: primary defense against parasites and regulation of vascular mediators released from mast cells.
- Basophils are associated with allergies and asthma, but their exact role is not clear.
- Lymphocytes release chemical mediators and control the immune response; some (B cells) mature into plasma cells and produce antibodies.
- Monocytes develop into macrophages once they reach the site of inflammation. Macrophages can also be initiators of the inflammatory response.

Plasma proteins produced by the liver during the inflammatory response are called acute phase proteins. Acute phase proteins include fibrinogen, prothrombin, factor VII, plasminogen, α_1-antitrypsin, α_1-antichymotrypsin, inter-α-antitrypsin, haptoglobin, ceruloplasmin, ferritin, hemopexin, transferrin, complement proteins (C1s, C2, C3, C4, C5, C9), factor B, C1 inhibitor, properdin, α_1-acid glycoprotein, fibronectin, serum amyloid A, C-reactive protein (CRP), albumin, prealbumin, α_1-liprotein, and β-lipoprotein. The laboratory procedures for measuring fibrinogen, α_1-antitrypsin, complement proteins, and CRP are discussed later in this chapter (Fig. 11-8).

Acute Inflammation

The inflammation processes discussed at the beginning of this chapter produce all characteristics of inflammation (local and systemic) and determine the duration of inflammation (acute or chronic). Local inflammation occurs in all cellular and tissue injuries and initiates healing. Acute inflammation is usually a localized and short-lived response after injury to the body, but it can also be systemic (Fig. 11-9).

Characteristics of local inflammation include swelling, pain, heat, and redness. Vasodilation and increased blood flow at the injury site result in heat and redness. Leakage of fluid and cells into the interstitial spaces results in

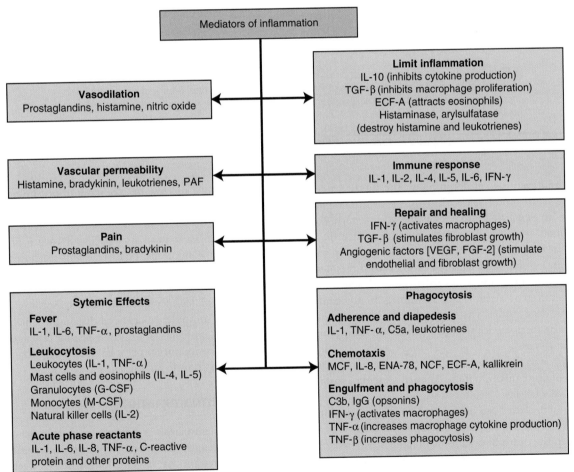

• Figure 11-8 Principal mediators of inflammation. *C3b,* Large fragment produced from complement component C3; *C5a,* small fragment produced from complement component C5; *ECF-A,* eosinophil chemotactic factor of anaphylaxis; *ENA,* epithelial-dermoid neutrophil attractant; *FGF,* fibroblast growth factor; *G-CSF,* granulocyte colony-stimulating factor; *IFN,* interferon; *IgG,* immunoglobulin G (predominant class of antibody in the blood); *IL,* interleukin; *MCF,* monocyte chemotactic factor; *M-CSF,* monocyte colony-stimulating factor; *NCF,* neutrophil chemotactic factor; *PAF,* platelet-activating factor; *TGF,* T-cell growth factor; *TNF,* tumor necrosis factor; *VEGF,* vascular endothelial growth factor. (From McCance KL, Huether SE. *Pathophysiology: The Biologic Basis for Disease in Adults and Children.* 7th ed. St. Louis: Mosby; 2015.)

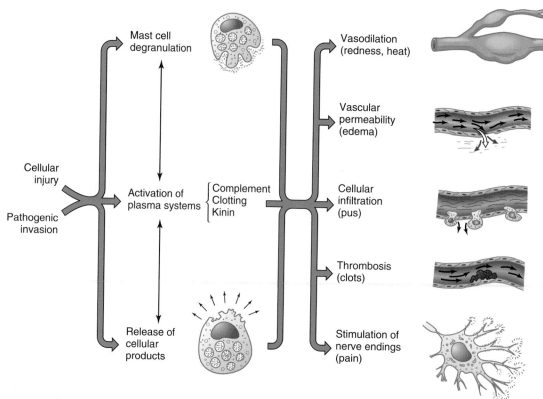

• Figure 11-9 Acute inflammatory response. Inflammation is usually initiated by cellular injury, which results in mast cell degranulation, the activation of three plasma systems, and the release of subcellular components from the damaged cells. These systems are interdependent, so that induction of one (e.g., mast cell degranulation) can result in activation of the other two. The result is the development of microscopic changes in the inflamed site and characteristic clinical manifestations. (Modified from McCance KL, Huether SE. *Pathophysiology: The Biologic Basis for Disease in Adults and Children.* 7th ed. St. Louis: Mosby; 2015.)

swelling, and swelling results in pain. The fluid and cells that move from blood vessels into the interstitial spaces constitute an *exudate.* Exudates can be very watery, containing small amounts of plasma proteins and cells, or they can be very thick and full of leukocytes, as in pus. The exudate can be filled with red blood cells if it is hemorrhagic. Local inflammation can produce different end results in different tissues. For example, in myocardial infarctions, dead cardiac tissue is replaced with scar tissue, whereas a brain tissue injury forms an abscess containing dead brain tissue.

In addition to these local effects, there are systemic manifestations of acute inflammation. An early systemic response is associated with fever, leukocytosis, and large amounts of plasma protein. Fever can be initiated by specific cytokines released from neutrophils and macrophages. This response may lead to the death of organisms that are highly sensitive to body temperature increases. It may also make an individual more susceptible to endotoxins generated by gram-negative bacteria.

Leukocytosis results from inflammation products such as C3a, which stimulates the bone marrow to produce and release increased numbers of leukocytes and monocyte precursors. The number of leukocytes in the blood increases, and this increase may be associated with a so-called shift to the left, in which the bone marrow releases more immature neutrophils to participate in the inflammatory response (see Fig. 11-14).

In the early stages of inflammation, IL-1 increases the amount of plasma proteins (specifically acute phase reactants) in the blood. Acute phase reactants reach their highest levels within 10 to 40 hours after the inflammatory process begins. The increased plasma protein levels, coupled with the fever and leukocytosis, produce symptoms including drowsiness (somnolence), general discomfort (malaise), loss of appetite (anorexia), and muscle aching (myalgia). When an acute inflammatory process lasts for longer than 2 weeks, it becomes a chronic inflammation.

Chronic Inflammation

Chronic inflammation is differentiated from acute inflammation by length of occurrence: Chronic inflammation is any inflammation that lasts for longer than 2 weeks. Sometimes chronic inflammation appears after acute inflammation is unsuccessful at removing the microorganisms or foreign objects, and incomplete wound healing may result. Chronic inflammatory processes can be histologically and mechanically different from those of acute inflammation. Chronic inflammation events are controlled by cells as the body switches from a nonspecific defense mechanism to a

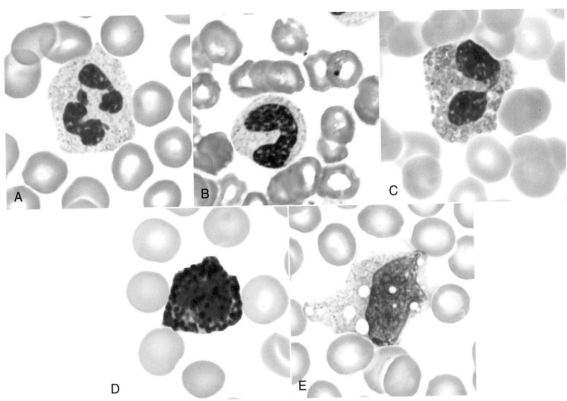

• **Figure 11-10** Cells involved in inflammation. **A,** Segmented neutrophil. **B,** Band neutrophil. **C,** Eosinophil, **D,** Basophil. **E,** Monocyte. (From Carr JH, Rodak BF. *Clinical Hematology Atlas,* 4th ed. St. Louis: Saunders; 2013.)

more specific defense mechanism involving the differentiation of B lymphocytes into plasma cells that produce antibodies against the foreign invaders.

Chronic inflammation may occur without much previous acute inflammation. This is common in mycobacterial infections, in which the bacteria's unique cell wall protects it from degradation, or in leprosy, syphilis, or brucellosis, in which the bacteria survive in the macrophage. Other microorganisms produce toxins that may persist after the bacteria is removed and continue the inflammatory process.

Chronic inflammation produces a dense infiltration of an area with lymphocytes and macrophages. Sometimes the body walls off an area with an excessive migration of macrophages to protect the rest of the body. The accumulation of macrophages around a walled-off infection is called a **granuloma.** Granulomas can eventually become calcified and are easily detectable on radiographic imaging.

Characteristic processes of chronic inflammation include initial migration of cells out of the blood vessels toward the site of injury, infiltration of the injured site by inflammatory cells, and destruction of tissues by these inflammatory cells. The main cells involved in chronic inflammation are monocyte/macrophages, B and T lymphocytes, and plasma cells (Fig. 11-10).

Monocytes are in their immature form while circulating in the blood. Once they leave the blood vessel and migrate to the site of injury, they mature and differentiate into fully functioning macrophages. The mature macrophages engulf

microorganisms and release additional amounts of TNF-α, IL-1, and various prostaglandins that promote the chronic inflammatory process. The death of a phagocyte is accompanied by cell lysis and the release of lysosomal enzymes into the tissue. These enzymes break down the proteins in the tissue, causing much tissue damage. In addition, these enzymes can increase vascular permeability, attract more monocytes, and activate the complement and kinin cascades. Natural inhibitors, such as α_1-antitrypsin, can minimize the amount of tissue damage caused by the lysosomal enzymes. α_1-Antitrypsin is elevated in inflammatory disorders.

B and T lymphocytes migrate to the injury in chronic inflammation (Fig. 11-11). T cells kill viruses and fungi. B cells, part of the specific inflammatory response of the body, differentiate into antibody-producing plasma cells. These antibodies bind to remaining microorganisms (viruses or bacteria) at the injury site. This binding increases the phagocytosis of the microorganisms by macrophages and neutrophils and their removal from the tissues.

Tissue Destruction, Tissue Repair, and Regeneration

Macrophages and lymphocytes are part of the nonspecific inflammatory response because they release substances that will damage any foreign object as well as healthy tissue. Macrophages and lymphocytes release **proteases** and **reactive oxygen species** (ROS) at the site of inflammation to

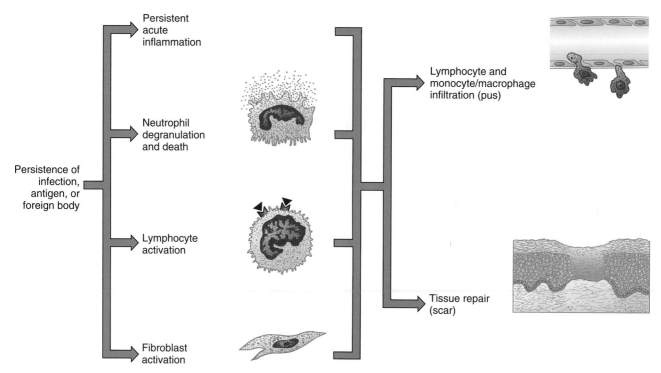

• **Figure 11-11** The chronic inflammatory response. Inflammation usually becomes chronic because of the persistence of an infection, an antibody, or a foreign body in the wound. Chronic inflammation is characterized by the persistence of many of the processes of acute inflammation. In addition, the presence of large amounts of neutrophil degranulation and death, the activation of lymphocytes, and the concurrent activation of fibroblasts result in release of mediators that induce the infiltration of more lymphocytes and monocytes/macrophages and the beginning of wound healing and tissue repair. (Modified from McCance KL, Huether SE. *Pathophysiology: The Biologic Basis for Disease in Adults and Children.* 7th ed. St. Louis: Mosby; 2015.)

help destroy the infectious agents responsible for the original injury. At the same time, the proteases and ROS cannot distinguish healthy tissue from injured tissue, resulting in damage to the body's own tissues. In fact, tissue damage is a consistent result of chronic inflammation. Chronic inflammation is not a healthy state for the body.

While the macrophages and other cells are destroying tissue, chronic inflammatory processes are beginning to repair tissue and form new blood vessels to serve that tissue (**angiogenesis**). Some tissues of the body have a high regenerative capacity (i.e., can replace or repair themselves) to easily overcome the cell and tissue destruction associated with chronic inflammation. Epithelial and gastrointestinal tract cells are easily repaired. Cells with a low regenerative capacity include neurons and skeletal and cardiac muscle cells. These cells are vulnerable to damage from chronic inflammation, and the injured cells are usually replaced with fibrous connective tissue instead of the original tissue. This can inhibit the normal functioning of the repaired areas.

Resolution and Repair

Healing of tissue that was destroyed in acute or chronic inflammatory responses can take as long as 2 years. The best-case scenario for healing is tissue *regeneration*—that is, complete return to normal structure and function. The return of tissues to an approximation of the original structure and function is called *resolution*.

With extensive damage, tissues are not able to regenerate. This is the case with an abscess or granuloma or when much fibrin is present in the inflamed area. In these situations, the body's best option is to *repair* the tissue or to *replace* the original damaged tissue with scar tissue. Scar tissue is composed of collagen, which cannot reproduce the function of the original tissue.

Healing consists of filling in, sealing, and shrinking the wound through reconstructive and maturation phases. The reconstructive phase begins 3 to 4 days after the injury and progresses for up to 2 weeks. The maturation phase begins weeks after the initial injury and continues for up to 2 years.

Laboratory Procedures and Limitations

C-Reactive Protein

A serum CRP measurement is the most often ordered laboratory test to detect inflammation. CRP is synthesized in the liver and is composed of five polypeptide chains linked together to form a disk-shaped cylinder. It binds with the polysaccharide cell walls of many bacteria, fungi, and parasites.

Function

CRP participates in the nonspecific inflammatory response in infection by activating the classical complement pathway. This activation usually results in phagocytosis of the invaders.

Clinical Correlation

CRP levels are increased during the inflammatory response as well as in other conditions. A 2000-fold rise over normal levels is seen in myocardial infarction, stress, trauma, infection, surgery, or spread of neoplasms. Serum CRP levels can rapidly increase 1000-fold or more in the presence of acute inflammation. The level of this protein rises within 6 to 12 hours after the beginning of the inflammatory response and peaks at 48 hours. Levels of serum CRP also rapidly decrease after the acute inflammation is resolved. The CRP level tends to correlate with the amount of tissue damage sustained. CRP tests are sometimes performed for individuals with rheumatoid arthritis or systemic lupus erythematosus (SLE) to determine the inflammatory activity of the disease.

Slightly elevated CRP levels are used to detect increased risk for cardiovascular disease because atherosclerosis is characterized by low-grade chronic inflammation. Detection of CRP elevations in this instance requires a high-sensitivity CRP (hs-CRP) assay. Increased risk for cardiovascular disease occurs when hs-CRP levels are greater than 2.0 mg/L.

Laboratory Procedures and Limitations

CRP can be detected by qualitative and quantitative methods. The qualitative methods involve mixing a drop of serum and a drop of a latex-coated antibody reagent, rotating the mixture for a period of time, and observing the mixture for a precipitate. CRP can be quantitated with the use of an enzyme-linked immunoassay (ELISA), immunoturbidimetry, or immunoprecipitation. The hs-CRP is measured by sensitive immunochemical methods such as particle-enhanced immunoturbidimetry, nephelometry, immunofluorescence, and immunochemiluminescence.

Complement Proteins

Function and Clinical Correlation

The complement system (see Fig. 11-3) is one of the body's nonspecific immune defense systems. As described earlier, the complement system is divided into classical, alternative, and lectin pathways. The classical pathway is usually activated by antibody–antigen complexes, the alternative pathway by several components including properdin, and the lectin pathway by molecules such as CRP, lipopolysaccharide (bacterial walls), and mucopolysaccharide.

Complement C3

C3 is the complement component that is present in largest concentration in the blood. It is synthesized by liver cells. During activation, it is cleaved to C3b and C3a. C3a acts as an anaphylatoxin and a chemotoxin when released into the circulation. C3b acts as an opsonin, resulting in phagocytosis of bacteria, viruses, and other foreign particles. Increased levels of C3 are seen in inflammation and in cases of biliary obstruction. Decreased levels of C3 are seen in autoimmune disease, neonatal respiratory distress syndrome, bacteremias, tissue injury, and chronic hepatitis.

Complement C4

C4 has the second highest concentration of any complement component in the blood. It is the activating enzyme for C3 in the classical pathway. C4 is increased in inflammation, trauma, and tissue injury. It is decreased in disseminated intravascular coagulation (DIC), acute glomerular nephritis, chronic hepatitis, and SLE.

Laboratory Procedures and Limitations

Tests for complement proteins include CH50 (total complement proteins), C3, and C4. These proteins are quantitated with the use of nephelometry and ELISA methods. Hemolytic assays are also available for assessing the function of individual complement components. Because some complement components are labile, serum specimens should be frozen at −70° C if the test cannot be run within a couple of hours.

Fibrinogen
Function

Fibrinogen is cleaved by thrombin to produce fibrin, the major structural component of a clot. Fibrinogen consists of six polypeptide chains arranged in an elongated fashion. Thrombin cleaves small peptides from two of the polypeptide chains, forming fibrin. Fibrin binds with platelets and red blood cells to build the clot.

Clinical Significance

Low plasma concentrations of fibrinogen are directly related to depletion as circulating molecules are used up by the body. Low concentrations are present in severe bleeding or DIC. Liver disease can lead to fibrinogen disorders. The large size of the fibrinogen molecule contributes to the viscosity of plasma. Chronic elevated fibrinogen levels are associated with increased risk for cardiovascular disease as well as increased risk for thrombosis.

Laboratory Procedures and Limitations

Functional clotting assays are the preferred method for measuring fibrinogen. Reference ranges are 150 to 350 mg/L. Fibrin fragments, such as those generated in DIC, are measured with the use of fibrin degradation products or D-dimer assays.

α₁-Antitrypsin

α_1-Antitrypsin is an acute phase protein that is synthesized in the liver and has a normal half-life of 6 to 7 days. It belongs to a group of proteins called **serapins,** which block the enzymatic activity of serine proteases. α_1-Antitrypsin also plays a role in blocking an enzyme, leukocyte elastase, that is released when leukocytes engage in phagocytosis. Elevated concentrations of leukocyte elastase can produce emphysema in the lungs.

Clinical Significance

Increased concentrations of α_1-antitrypsin are found in inflammatory reactions. Its synthesis is stimulated by cytokines. Decreased levels of α_1-antitrypsin are more clinically significant than increased levels. Decreased levels can be caused by a genetic deficiency, increased utilization, or urinary or gastrointestinal loss. Individuals with a genetic deficiency that results in no measureable α_1-antitrypsin develop pulmonary emphysema as early as 20 to 30 years of age. In addition, deficiencies of this protein are associated with neonatal cholestasis (hepatitis), cirrhosis, Wegener granulomatosis, and liver carcinoma. A couple of disorders, neonatal respiratory distress syndrome and severe preterminal disease of the pancreas, display low levels of α_1-antrypsin. Finally, this protein can be lost through the kidneys or the gastrointestinal tract. It is a small protein, so it can easily be lost after proximal tubule damage or in protein-losing enteropathies.

Laboratory Procedures and Limitations

Common methods for quantitating α_1-antitrypsin are immunoturbidimetry and immunonephelometry. α_1-Antitrypsin also appears as the major constituent in the α_1-globulin band on serum electrophoresis. Falsely decreased test results may occur if the serum is allowed to sit on the clot too long or if there is bacterial contamination.

Immunoglobulins

The characteristics, function, clinical significance, and laboratory procedures and limitations for immunoglobulins are discussed in detail in Chapter 15.

Cytokines

Cytokines are commonly measured with the use of bioassays, immunoassays, and flow cytometry. Bioassays are used to measure bioactivity in a particular cell line, chemotactic activity, proliferation, and cytotoxicity. Advantages of bioassays include good sensitivity and the ability to measure the bioactive molecule; disadvantages include lack of specificity, long turnaround time, and poor precision.

Immunoassays are the method of choice for quantitating cytokine levels. ELISA is the most commonly used immunoassay. Cytokine antibody arrays allow the simultaneous detection of 100 or more molecules on one microtiter plate. ELISAs feature excellent sensitivity, high specificity, shorter turnaround time, and automated assays.

Flow cytometry can also be used to detect the presence of intracellular cytokines. This method's turnaround time is less than 2 hours, but the method cannot identify and quantitate the cytokines present in the cell.

Blood Cells and Constituents

The most common hematology tests used to diagnose inflammation are the ESR, leukocyte counts, and the WBC differential. The ESR (Fig. 11-12) is a nonspecific test that is often used to indicate the presence of inflammation. Fibrinogen is a large protein that is increased during the inflammatory response. The ESR measures the distance red blood cells fall in a long test tube over a period of 1 hour. The farther the red blood cells fall, the greater the inflammatory

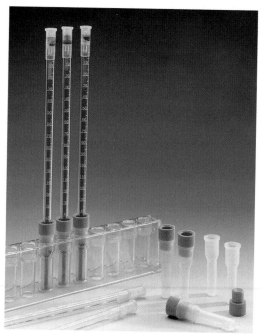

• **Figure 11-12** Erythrocyte sedimentation rate test. (From Keohane EM, Smith LJ, Walenga JM. *Rodak's Hematology: Clinical Principles and Applications.* 5th ed. St. Louis: Saunders; 2016. Courtesy Polymedco, Cortlandt Manor, NY.)

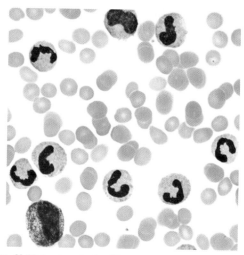

• **Figure 11-13** Leukocytosis. (From Carr JH, Rodak BF. *Clinical Hematology Atlas.* 4th ed. St. Louis: Saunders; 2013.)

response present in the body. The increase in plasma proteins leads to an enhanced erythrocyte rouleaux formation (due to decreased zeta potential for each cell), thereby increasing the sedimentation rate of the red blood cells. Although increased erythrocyte sedimentation is a nonspecific reaction, it is considered a good indicator of an acute inflammatory response. However, the ESR should not be used as the only laboratory parameter to detect inflammation.

The WBC count is very useful in predicting infection or inflammation. Acute inflammation can cause the WBC count to increase significantly. An increased WBC count is called leukocytosis (Fig. 11-13). Values as high as 10 times the reference range may be seen in certain inflammatory states.

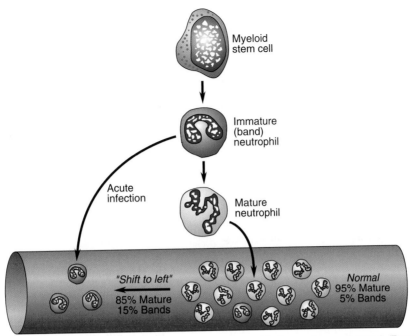

• Figure 11-14 Shift to the left (more bands or immature neutrophils than mature neutrophils). (From Copstead LC. *Pathophysiology,* 5th ed. St. Louis: Saunders, 2013.)

Neutrophils are associated with inflammation, so the level of these cells is quite high in inflammation. When the neutrophil count rapidly increases, as in infection or inflammation, the bone marrow begins releasing all mature and almost-mature neutrophils to assist the body. A WBC differential, in which each type of WBC is identified and counted, can assist in diagnosing inflammation. The presence of immature neutrophils on a WBC differential is called a shift to the left; it may be present in many types of inflammation (Fig. 11-14).

Summary

Inflammation is a very complex process that involves chemicals as well as cells. The body has natural defenses to prevent microorganisms or foreign objects from invading the body. When the natural defenses fail, the inflammatory process begins. Three systems are activated in inflammation: complement, clotting, and kinin systems. Each is a separate system, but they are interconnected and work synergistically to rid the body of the invading microorganism or foreign object. Inflammation can be acute (immediate and lasting up to 2 weeks) or chronic (lasting for longer than 2 weeks). Hallmarks of acute inflammation include redness, heat, swelling, and pain. Acute inflammation can also include systemic consequences such as fever, myalgia, and general malaise. Chronic inflammation is governed by cells and the chemicals produced by them.

Chemical mediators that play a part in inflammation include acute phase proteins (e.g., CRP, fibrinogen, α_1-antitrypsin, complement proteins), clotting proteins (especially fibrinogen), kinin system proteins, leukotrienes, enzymes, cytokines, prostaglandins, and chemokines. Cells involved in inflammation include leukocytes, basophils, eosinophils, monocytes, macrophages, platelets, mast cells, and lymphocytes.

Laboratory tests used to assess inflammation include CRP, fibrinogen, α_1-antitrypsin, complement proteins, clotting factors, immunoglobulins, and cytokines. CRP can be performed qualitatively and quantitatively; it can also be automated. Fibrinogen can be performed with the use of a fibrinometer or an optical coagulation instrument. α_1-Antitrypsin can be quantitated by immunoassay or through serum protein electrophoresis. Complement proteins are assessed automatically, usually by an ELISA test method. Clotting factors are measured on automated coagulation instruments. Immunoglobulins can be quantitated with the use of immunoassay techniques or serum protein electrophoresis techniques. Cytokines are also quantitated by immunoassay techniques.

Review Questions

1. Leakage of fluid to the tissue space most likely leads to which of these cardinal signs of inflammation?
   a. Pain
   b. Redness
   c. Swelling
   d. Heat

2. All of the following are steps in the acute inflammation process EXCEPT
   a. Blood becomes more viscous
   b. Chemical mediators released
   c. Body produces antibodies to invader
   d. Vessels lead fluid causing edema

3. An increase in vascular permeability results in all of the following EXCEPT
   a. Edema
   b. Migration of leukocytes
   c. Destruction of tissue
   d. Leakage of fluids

4. Which property of monocyte/macrophages is most likely to be associated with tissue damage?
   a. Monocytes are immature in blood and mature into macrophages in tissues.
   b. Macrophages release proteases and reactive oxygen species.
   c. Macrophages release TNF-α, interleukin-1, and interleukin-6.
   d. Macrophages are efficient at phagocytizing viruses and bacteria.

5. The erythrocyte sedimentation rate is useful in detecting inflammation in all of the following situations EXCEPT
   a. Traumatic injury
   b. Wound infection
   c. Anemia (low red blood cell count)
   d. Chronic inflammation due to rheumatoid arthritis

6. All of the following activate the complement cascade EXCEPT
   a. Hagman factor
   b. Classical
   c. Lectin
   d. Alternative

7. The primary molecule in the kinin system is
   a. C1 convertase
   b. Hagman factor
   c. Kallikrein
   d. Bradykinin

8. Basophils are known for secreting which of the following substances?
   a. C1 convertase
   b. Histamine
   c. Kallikrein
   d. Hagman factor

9. Which of the following are the phagocytic cells that help engulf microorganisms and foreign objects?
   a. Macrophages
   b. Lymphocytes
   c. Eosinophils
   d. Mast cells

10. Which of the following tests is used most often to detect inflammation?
    a. Cytokines
    b. Complement proteins
    c. CRP
    d. Fibrinogen

Critical Thinking Questions

1. How does the complement cascade participate in the inflammatory process?

2. What are the cells involved in inflammation, and what chemicals does each cell secrete or synthesize in inflammation?

3. What methods are used to measure CRP and cytokines?

CASE STUDY

Ms. B., a 56-year-old woman who is a recent immigrant from Vietnam, has a low-grade fever, weight loss of more than 15 lb in the last month, a persistent cough, and blood-tinged sputum. Sputum testing and chest radiography confirm a diagnosis of tuberculosis. Tuberculosis is a very difficult disease to treat and resolve because of the resistance of the infection to the body's immune response. Chronic inflammation is usually the course of the disease for many months or even years. Describe the hallmarks of chronic inflammation and how macrophages play a role in granuloma formation as seen with tuberculosis.

Bibliography

Abbas AK, Lichtman AH, Pillai S. Cellular and Molecular Immunology With STUDENT CONSULT Online Access. St. Louis: Elsevier Health Sciences; 2011.

Aoki T, Narumiya S. Prostaglandins and chronic inflammation. *Trends Pharmacol Sci*. 2012;33(6):304–311.

Bain BJ. The peripheral blood smear. In: Goldman L, Schafer AI, eds. *Cecil Medicine*. 24th ed. Philadelphia: Saunders Elsevier; 2011: Chapter 160.

Burtis CA, Ashwood ER, Burns DE. *Tietz Textbook of Clinical Chemistry and Molecular Diagnostics*. 5th ed. St. Louis: Elsevier Health Sciences; 2012.

Filep J, Gjorstrup P. El Kebir D. Resolvin E1 modulates Mac-1 signaling and promotes neutrophil apoptosis and the resolution of acute inflammation (P5064). *J Immunol*. 2013;190(Meeting Abstracts 1): 180–115.

Hauser G, Tkalcic M, Pletikosic S, Grabar N, Stimac D. Erythrocyte sedimentation rate: possible role in determining the existence of the low grade inflammation in irritable bowel syndrome patients. *Med Hypotheses*. 2012;78(6):818–820.

Kennelly PJ, Murray RF, Rodwell VW, Botham KM. *Harper's Illustrated Biochemistry*. 28th ed. New York: McGraw-Hill Medical; 2009.

Kumar V, Abbas AK, Fausto N, Aster JC *Robbins Cotran and Pathologic Basis of Disease, Professional Edition: Expert Consult-Online*. St. Louis: Elsevier Health Sciences; 2014.

McPherson RA, Pincus MR. *Henry's Clinical Diagnosis and Management by Laboratory Methods*. 22nd ed. Philadelphia: Saunders Elsevier; 2011.

Sozzani S, Prete AD. Chemokines as relay signals in human dendritic cell migration: serum amyloid A kicks off chemotaxis. *Eur J Immunol*. 2015;45(1):40–43.

St-Onge MP, Zhang S, Darnell B, Allison DB. Baseline serum C-reactive protein is associated with lipid responses to low-fat and high-polyunsaturated fat diets. *J Nutr*. 2009;139(4):680–683.

Tripodi A. The laboratory and the new oral anticoagulants. *Clin Chem*. 2013;59(2):353–362.

Windgassen EB, Funtowicz L, Lunsford TN, Harris LA, Mulvagh SL. C-reactive protein and high-sensitivity C-reactive protein: an update for clinicians. *Postgrad Med*. 2011;123(1):114–119.

Zacho J, Tybjaerg-Hansen A, Jensen JS, et al. Genetically elevated C-reactive protein and ischemic vascular disease. *N Engl J Med*. 2008;359(18):1897–1908.

Zweifach BW, Grant L, McCluskey RT, eds. *The Inflammatory Process*. San Diego, CA: Academic Press; 2014.

12

Body Fluids and Electrolytes

DONNA LARSON

CHAPTER OUTLINE

Introduction

Fluid Balance and Body Fluid Compartments

Electrolytes
- Anion Gap
- Sodium
- Potassium
- Chloride
- Bicarbonate
- Lithium

Colligative Properties
- Osmotic Pressure
- Osmolality

Fluid Imbalances
- Lymphatic System
- Edema

Summary

OBJECTIVES

At the completion of this chapter, the reader will be able to:

1. Describe the two body water compartments.
2. List the common cations and anions in the body.
3. Evaluate the anion gap.
4. Compare and contrast sodium (Na^+) and potassium (K^+) ions in terms of location, regulation, functions, and effects of high and low concentrations.
5. Compare and contrast chloride (Cl^-) and bicarbonate (HCO_3^-) ions in terms of location, regulation, functions, and effects of high and low concentrations.
6. Describe the clinical significance of lithium.
7. Describe colligative properties of solutions.
8. Describe osmolality, its calculation, and use.
9. Describe mechanisms that produce edema.
10. Compare and contrast exudates and transudates and their clinical significance.

KEY TERMS

Aldosterone
Anasarca
Anion gap
Anions
Ascites
Atrial natriuretic peptide
Bicarbonate
Cations
Cell permeability
Colligative properties
Colloidal osmotic pressure
Dehydration
Edema
Electrolytes

Extracellular fluid
Extravascular compartment
Exudate
Exudation
Hydrostatic edema
Hydrostatic pressure
Hyperchloremia
Hyperkalemia
Hypernatremia
Hypochloremia
Hypokalemia
Hyponatremia
Interstitial fluid
Intravascular compartment

Intracellular fluid
Iontophoresis
Lithium
Lymphatic system
Lymphedema
Osmotic edema
Osmolality
Osmotic pressure
Pericardial effusion
Pitting edema
Pleural effusion
Pulmonary edema
Sodium pump
Transudates

❖ Case in Point

A 75-year-old man arrived in the emergency department in a confused mental state. He was a type 2 diabetic who had fallen in his kitchen 2 days earlier and was unable to get up. The man had had nothing to eat or drink for 2 days. The physician diagnosed him with hyperosmolar hyperglycemic nonketotic syndrome. Which chemistry laboratory results were likely abnormal?

Points to Remember

- Water balance in the body is maintained by pressure gradients and electrolytes.
- The two main compartments in the body that contain water are the intravascular and extravascular compartments.
- The extravascular compartment contains intracellular and extracellular water.
- Electrolytes are charged particles (e.g., Na^+, K^+, Cl^-, HCO_3^-, Ca^{2+}, Mg^{2+}, PO_4^{3-}, Li^{2+}) that sustain life by transmitting electrochemical impulses in nerves and muscles (e.g., heart), playing a role in osmotic pressure, distributing water in the body, and controlling cell permeability.
- The sodium (Na^+) ion is the major cation in plasma and interstitial fluid.
- The potassium (K^+) ion is the major cation in intracellular fluid.
- Chloride (Cl^-) and bicarbonate (HCO_3^-) ions are found in high levels in the plasma and interstitial fluid.
- Osmotic pressure is the pressure created by ions of a greater concentration passing through a semipermeable membrane to an area of lower concentration of that ion.
- The anion gap represents the difference between unmeasured anions and unmeasured cations after major electrolytes have been accounted for.
- Lithium is not normally found in humans, but it is used to treat bipolar disorders.
- Colligative properties—those that depend on the ratio of the number of particles of solute and solvent in solution rather than the identity of the solute—include osmotic pressure, freezing point, boiling point, and vapor pressure.
- Osmolality is the concentration of a solution expressed as the total number of solute particles per kilogram of solvent; for example, serum osmolality = $(2 \times [Na^+])$ + $(BUN/2.8)$ + $(glucose/18)$.
- Edema is the accumulation of excess fluid in tissues or body cavities.
- A transudate is a fluid with a low protein and high water content.
- An exudate is a fluid with a high protein and low water content.
- Important types of edema include lymphedema, pulmonary edema, ascites, pleural effusion, and anasarca.

Introduction

The bodies of animals and other life forms contain mostly water. The human body is approximately 60% water, and this means that 60 of every 100 molecules in the body are water molecules. Approximately 83% of blood is water. The body's cells, tissues, and organs have physical barriers to keep water inside, and its distribution throughout the body is maintained by pressure gradients and electrolyte concentrations. Fluid compartments, composition of body fluids, electrolytes, fluid movement, regulation of fluids and electrolytes, colligative properties, hormone imbalances, and the effect of pathophysiologic conditions on clinical chemistry tests are discussed in the following sections.

Fluid Balance and Body Fluid Compartments

Body water exists in two major compartments, the *intravascular compartment* (i.e., inside the lymph and blood vessels) and the *extravascular compartment* (i.e., outside the lymph and blood vessels). The two compartments are separated by a thin layer of cells called the *capillary epithelium*. Blood flowing through the veins and arteries is similar to water flowing through a hose when the valve is opened; however, the movement of water through tissues or organs of the extravascular compartment is more complicated. The extravascular compartment contains intracellular and extracellular water and water found in the interstitial space. The intracellular and extracellular compartments are separated by plasma membranes (Fig. 12-1).

Sufficient intravascular water is needed to ensure that blood is pumped throughout the body to deliver nutrients and retrieve metabolic wastes. Because the circulation is a closed system, it can handle only a finite amount of water. Excess water diffuses through the capillary epithelium and enters the extravascular compartment. Too little intravascular water (due to excessive water loss or decreased water intake) results in *dehydration;* this makes the blood more viscous and more difficult to pump throughout the body.

Although there can be small variations in the amount of intravascular body water, the volume of extracellular body water remains constant. The rate of water lost from the body

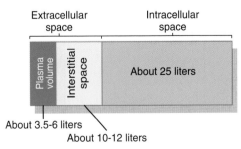

• **Figure 12-1** Normal distribution of total body water in adults. (From Ignatavicius DD, Workman ML. *Medical-Surgical Nursing: Patient-Centered Collaborative Care.* 8th ed. St. Louis: Elsevier; 2016.)

must equal the rate of water intake to maintain the *water balance*. An average adult ingests approximately 2.5 L of water through food and drink every day, and another 200 to 300 mL is generated by metabolic processes. Because the body is efficient and strives to maintain the water balance, the same amount is released daily by the body through urine, feces, sweat, and aerosols during respiration. The body regulates the water balance through the thirst mechanism, electrolyte gradients, antidiuretic hormones, and excretion or resorption by the kidneys. Understanding the basic concepts of water homeostasis is necessary to convert the results of chemical laboratory tests (i.e., data) into information that is meaningful and important in diagnosing disease, monitoring treatment, and maintaining health.

Electrolytes

Emergency room dramas on television portray doctors yelling orders such as "Lytes, stat!" Electrolytes ("lytes") are charged atoms or molecules (i.e., ions) found in body fluids that sustain life through regulation of water distribution, osmotic pressure, nerve transmission to muscles (e.g., heart), cell permeability (i.e., passage of solvents and solutes into and out of cells), oxidation-reduction reactions, and maintenance of blood pH in the narrow range of 7.35 to 7.45. Electrolytes include sodium (Na^+), potassium (K^+), chloride (Cl^-), and bicarbonate (HCO_3^-) ions. Other cations (i.e., positively charged ions) and anions (i.e., negatively charged ions) that influence body processes include phosphorus, magnesium (see Chapter 27), and lithium.

Electrolyte imbalances are life-threatening situations. Recovery from a traumatic event or illness depends on the body's ability to regulate body water and electrolytes. Vomiting, excessive urination, sweating, diarrhea, bleeding, and exudation (i.e., oozing of fluids) from burns or other skin injuries can cause fluid imbalances.

Each type of body fluid contains specific amounts of cations and anions, and fluids can be identified by their ion compositions. For example, sodium is the major cation in plasma and interstitial fluid (that part of the extracellular fluid found between the body's cells). A fluid with a high sodium level is most likely plasma or interstitial fluid. Similarly, potassium is the major cation in intracellular fluid, and high concentrations of chloride and bicarbonate are found in plasma and interstitial fluid. Body fluids also contain protein; high concentrations are found in intracellular fluid, and lower concentrations are found in plasma and interstitial fluid (Fig. 12-2).

Osmosis is the movement of solvent molecules from a higher-concentration solution through a semipermeable membrane to a lower-concentration solution to achieve a balanced solution. In the human body, the cell membrane serves as a semipermeable membrane for osmosis. One of the most important solvents that passes through a cell membrane is water. The physical force exerted from this process is osmotic pressure (Fig. 12-3). Osmotic pressure is created by the many ions inside and outside of the cell. Because intracellular ions are difficult to measure, it is more practical to measure the ion concentration in serum or plasma instead. The extracellular electrolytes measured in serum or plasma indicate the functional integrity of the cell membrane.

Although serum and plasma are the most common body fluids tested, valuable information can be obtained by measuring ion concentrations in urine, spinal fluid, and sweat. The kidneys are responsible for resorbing water and electrolytes. They also excrete excess ions and decrease water excretion when the body is dehydrated. If water intake is reduced and the body cannot compensate, dehydration results and has an extreme effect on ionic concentrations. Fever, diarrhea, inadequate fluid intake, and other clinical problems can cause dehydration. Dehydration affects the extracellular fluid volume, causing blood pressure to fall, which can lead to vascular collapse or shock.

Water from the extracellular compartment transfers into cells by osmosis when the concentration of intracellular ions is greater than the concentration of extracellular ions.

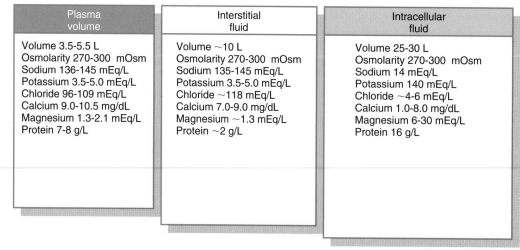

Plasma volume	Interstitial fluid	Intracellular fluid
Volume 3.5-5.5 L	Volume ~10 L	Volume 25-30 L
Osmolarity 270-300 mOsm	Osmolarity 270-300 mOsm	Osmolarity 270-300 mOsm
Sodium 136-145 mEq/L	Sodium 135-145 mEq/L	Sodium 14 mEq/L
Potassium 3.5-5.0 mEq/L	Potassium 3.5-5.0 mEq/L	Potassium 140 mEq/L
Chloride 96-109 mEq/L	Chloride ~118 mEq/L	Chloride ~4-6 mEq/L
Calcium 9.0-10.5 mg/dL	Calcium 7.0-9.0 mg/dL	Calcium 1.0-8.0 mg/dL
Magnesium 1.3-2.1 mEq/L	Magnesium ~1.3 mEq/L	Magnesium 6-30 mEq/L
Protein 7-8 g/L	Protein ~2 g/L	Protein 16 g/L

• **Figure 12-2** Electrolyte concentrations in body fluids. (From Ignatavicius DD, Workman ML. *Medical-Surgical Nursing: Patient-Centered Collaborative Care*. 8th ed. St. Louis: Elsevier; 2016.)

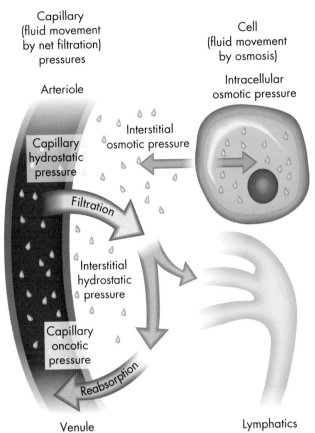

Figure 12-3 Capillary hydrostatic pressure is the primary force for fluid movement out of the arteriolar end of the capillary and into the interstitial space. At the venous end, capillary oncotic pressure (from plasma proteins) attracts water into the vascular space. Interstitial hydrostatic pressure promotes the movement of fluid and proteins into the lymphatic vessels. Osmotic pressure accounts for fluid movement between the interstitial space and the intracellular space. Normally, intracellular and extracellular fluid osmotic pressures are equal (280 to 294 mOsm), and water is equally distributed between the interstitial and intracellular compartments. (From Huether SE, McCance KL. *Understanding Pathophysiology.* 5th ed. St. Louis: Mosby; 2013.)

Conversely, if water loss creates a hypertonic extracellular fluid, intracellular water leaves the cell and enters the extracellular fluid (Fig. 12-4).

The electrolyte concentration does not provide information about the fluid volume or electrolyte gains or losses. If sodium and potassium are lost from the body along with a proportional loss of water, the electrolyte concentration will appear to be constant. The concentration of these ions depends on the amount of solute and the volume of solvent; if each is lost in proportional amounts, the health care provider must combine the laboratory results with the clinical profile to determine the extent of the electrolyte deficit (Table 12-1). The laboratory technician must review results in context.

Anion Gap

Electrolyte determinations are ordered as a panel because the results for sodium, potassium, chloride, and bicarbonate are interrelated. Automated chemistry analyzers are used to quickly and inexpensively derive this information and clinically useful supplemental data such as the **anion gap.** The anion gap can be calculated from the concentrations of various electrolytes and other data by several equations. A commonly used one is the following:

$$\text{Anion gap} = [Na^+ + K^+] - [Cl^- + HCO_3^-]$$

For example, for a patient with sodium concentration of 145mEq/L, potassium concentration of 4.0 mEq/L, chloride concentration of 110 mEq/L, and bicarbonate concentration of 25 mEq/L, the anion gap is calculated by plugging these values into the equation:

$$\text{Anion gap} = (145 + 4) - (110 + 25) = 14$$

Anion gap is an inaccurate term. To keep body fluids balanced, the total positive charges must equal the total negative charges of electrolytes. Because anions must always equal cations and only a few ions are directly measured, the anion gap represents the difference between the unmeasured anions and the unmeasured cations.

What constitutes a normal anion gap is a topic of much disagreement in medicine. Differences in normal values for anion gap are also rooted in the inherent variability in human populations. Because reference ranges are determined for the specific population of individuals served by a clinical laboratory, the "normal" value is based on the reference range for that laboratory. Most patients are in a balanced state and have an anion gap value within the reference range. This normal balance can be altered by increased production or retention of organic acids, as in ketoacidosis or lactic acidosis (Table 12-2).

When anion gap values are found to be outside of reference ranges, the clinical laboratory work must be rechecked. If the anion gap is calculated manually, it should be recalculated. Samples may need to be rerun to verify results. If possible, a different instrument or method should be used when retesting the sample. An abnormal anion gap may not appear to be significant, but when it is combined with other clinical data, such as the clinical history, other laboratory tests, and physical examination findings, the results may be significant. Increased anion gaps that are very high are usually associated with renal failure. Moderately increased anion gaps can be associated with diabetic ketoacidosis.

Although calculation of the anion gap can help a health care provider determine a specific type of electrolyte disorder, it can also be used as a quality control tool for electrolyte testing. For example, a trend of increased or decreased anion gaps in a run of patient specimens may indicate a consistent testing error in one or more analytes. One should always review calculations and procedures and rerun the sample before reporting a significant anion gap value. An abnormal anion gap can indicate either a testing error or a severe health problem in a patient. It is the technician's responsibility to ensure that the testing procedure is sound before reporting the result.

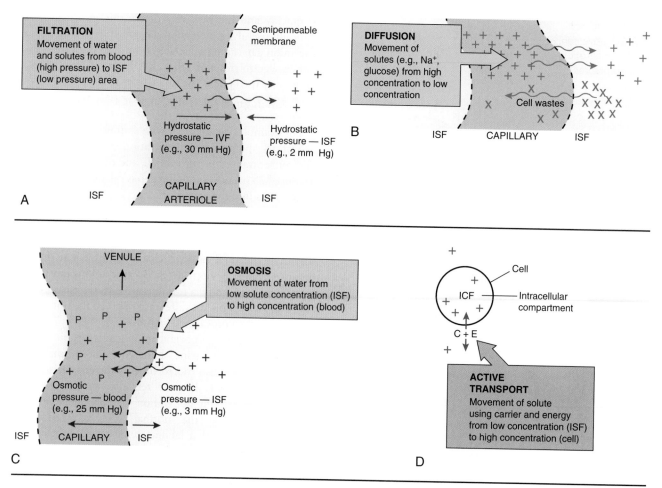

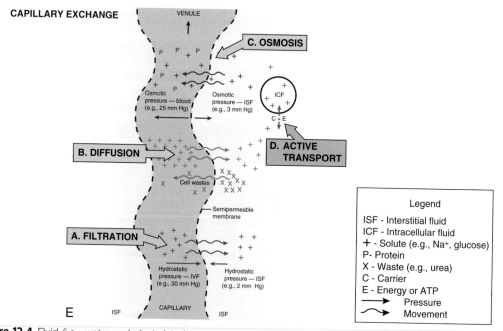

• **Figure 12-4** Fluid (i.e., water and electrolytes) movement among body compartments. **A,** Filtration. **B,** Diffusion. **C,** Osmosis. **D,** Active transport. **E,** Overview of all processes. *IVF,* Intravascular fluid. (From VanMeter KC, Hubert RJ. *Gould's Pathophysiology for the Health Professions.* 5th ed. St. Louis: Elsevier; 2015.)

TABLE 12-1   Electrolyte Levels in Common Conditions

Diagnosis	Sodium (Na⁺) Level	Potassium (K⁺) Level	Chloride (Cl⁻) Level
Dehydration	>145 mEq/L	Normal	>105 mEq/L
Excessive intravenous therapy with sodium chloride (NaCl)	>145 mEq/L	Normal	>105 mEq/L
Fluid retention	<135 mEq/L	Normal	>105 mEq/L
Vomiting	<135 mEq/L	<3.5 mEq/L	<95 mEq/L
Diarrhea	<135 mEq/L	<3.5 mEq/L	Normal
Burns	<135 mEq/L	>5.5 mEq/L	Normal
Excessive use of diuretics	<135 mEq/L	Normal	Normal
Addison's disease	<135 mEq/L	>5.5 mEq/L	<95 mEq/L
Renal disease	<135 mEq/L	Normal	Normal
Excessive antidiuretic hormone (ADH) release	<135 mEq/L	Normal	Normal
Excessive water consumption	<135 mEq/L	Normal	Normal
Renal failure	Normal	>5.5 mEq/L	Normal
Cushing's disease	Normal	<3.5 mEq/L	Normal
Starvation	Normal	<3.5 mEq/L	Normal
Hyperaldosteronism	Normal	<3.5 mEq/L	Normal
Diuretic therapy	Normal	<3.5 mEq/L	Normal
Metabolic acidosis	Normal	Normal	>105 mEq/L
Metabolic alkalosis	Normal	Normal	<95 mEq/L
Hyperparathyroidism	Normal	Normal	>105 mEq/L

Na⁺: 136-145 meq/L
K⁺: 3.5-5.1 meq/L
Cl⁻: 98-107 meq/L
tCO₂ (also called HCO₃): 23-29 meq/L

TABLE 12-2   Anion Gap Results for Various Conditions

Condition	Anion Gap Results
Ketoacidosis (e.g., diabetic, alcoholism, starvation)	Increased
Lactic acidosis	Increased
Aspirin poisoning	Increased
Methanol poisoning	Increased
Ethanol poisoning	Increased
Ethylene glycol poisoning	Increased
Renal failure	Increased
Hypoalbuminemia	Decreased
Lithium toxicity	Increased

Sodium

Sodium is the major cation in extracellular fluid, and it constitutes approximately 90% of all cations in plasma. Sodium enters the body in many forms. The most common sodium-containing food additive is table salt, or sodium chloride (NaCl), which is 40% sodium. Other food additives containing sodium include monosodium glutamate (MSG), sodium bicarbonate, sodium benzoate, and sodium nitrite or nitrate. Even though the amount of sodium ingested by a person varies with the amounts and types of food, the amount of sodium in the body remains constant. Excess sodium is excreted in the urine or lost through perspiration.

After salt is ingested, it is absorbed by the body, causing a temporary increase in extracellular fluid volume. This occurs because the absorbed sodium atoms and the water molecules carrying them equilibrate between the plasma and the interstitial fluid. In addition, the cell temporarily exchanges a small amount of sodium for potassium: Because the sodium concentration of fluid outside the cell is 10 times that inside the cell, sodium ions are pumped out of the cell across the semipermeable cell membrane, and potassium ions are pumped in.

The kidneys ultimately regulate sodium levels in the body by resorbing sodium in an amount required to maintain balance and excreting the excess molecules. Hormones also play a part in maintaining the body's sodium balance.

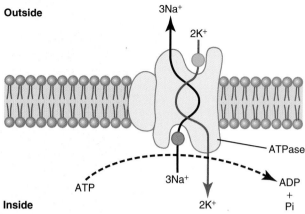

Outside

3Na⁺

2K⁺

ATPase

ATP

3Na⁺

ADP + Pi

Inside

2K⁺

• **Figure 12-5** Sodium-potassium adenosine triphosphatase (Na⁺/K⁺-ATPase), also known as the sodium-potassium pump, actively transports sodium ions out and potassium ions into the cell against their concentration gradients. This process uses the chemical energy stored in the bonds of intracellular adenosine triphosphate *(ATP),* which is released when the molecule is hydrolyzed to adenosine diphosphate *(ADP)* and an inorganic phosphate *(Pi).* (From Hall J. *Guyton and Hall Textbook of Medical Physiology.* 12th ed. Philadelphia: Saunders; 2011.)

Aldosterone, a hormone that is secreted by the adrenal cortex, influences the kidneys to resorb sodium and accelerates the exchange of sodium and potassium ions across the cell membranes. This exchange helps the body retain sodium and excrete potassium. The heart releases a hormone called atrial natriuretic peptide, which causes the excretion of sodium.

Clinical Significance

Functions of sodium include transmitting nerve impulses, maintaining the osmotic pressure of extracellular fluid and retaining water, facilitating muscle contractions, maintaining acid-base balance, and maintaining blood viscosity. Sodium is actively transported by a sodium pump, which is located in the plasma membranes of all animal cells, including those of the intestines and kidneys. This "pump" is actually an enzyme, sodium-potassium adenosine triphosphatase (Na⁺/K⁺-ATPase), which is active in the presence of sodium and potassium (Fig. 12-5). Excess sodium is excreted in urine, and a high sodium blood level produces more urine.

Common diseases often involve a decreased sodium level (i.e., hyponatremia) rather than an increased sodium level (i.e., hypernatremia) (Table 12-3). Hyponatremia can be caused by not eating properly (i.e., low sodium intake), diarrhea, prolonged vomiting, or sweating due to fever. Other conditions that contribute to the loss of sodium from the body include diabetic ketoacidosis (in which large amounts of sodium are excreted in the urine as salts of ketoacids), renal disease (decreased resorption of sodium in the renal tubules), and decreased aldosterone levels.

Hypernatremia is not as common as hyponatremia. Conditions that contribute to an increased sodium level include severe dehydration, Cushing syndrome (i.e., increased adrenal steroid levels resulting in excessive resorption of sodium in the renal tubules), the recovery state after insulin treatment of comatose diabetic patients (i.e., sodium in cells is replaced by potassium), inappropriate

TABLE 12-3	Symptoms of Common Conditions Caused by Electrolyte Imbalance
Condition	**Symptoms**
Hypernatremia	Thirst, central nervous system dehydration leads to confusion and lethargy progressing to coma, increased neuromuscular irritability (e.g., increased twitching, convulsions)
Hyponatremia	Neurologic dysfunction due to brain swelling, muscular twitching, irritability, convulsions, decreased blood volume, circulatory shock
Hyperkalemia	Nausea, vomiting, diarrhea, bradycardia, cardiac arrhythmias, cardiac depression, cardiac arrest, skeletal muscle weakness, flaccid paralysis
Hypokalemia	Cardiac arrhythmias, flattened T wave, muscular weakness, metabolic alkalosis, mental confusion, nausea, vomiting
Hyperchloridemia	No direct clinical symptoms
Hypochloridemia	No direct clinical symptoms

saline solution therapy, and ingestion of high-sodium foods with little water intake.

Laboratory Procedures and Limitations

Ion-selective electrodes (ISEs) are used to measure sodium in clinical specimens. Sodium electrodes have a glass membrane that allows sodium ions to flow into the tip of the electrode, where they interact with the measuring and reference electrode wires. Measurement of the ion concentration corresponds to the activity of the ion in the water fraction of the specimen because, as ions flow through the glass membrane, a potential-measuring circuit between the reference and measuring electrode senses the change in electromotive force that is proportional to the sodium concentration.

The type of ISE depends on the sample used for analysis. A *direct* ISE analyzes whole blood. The specimen is not usually prepared in any way before analysis. The result is independent of solids in the sample. Direct ISEs are found in blood gas analyzers and in point-of-care instruments inside and outside the clinical laboratory. This method accurately analyzes samples from lipemic patients and avoids falsely decreased results.

An *indirect* ISE analyzes a total plasma or serum sample that is diluted with a large volume of diluent. Red blood cells must be separated from the plasma or serum before the sample can be analyzed. The analyte concentration is calculated by multiplying the readout value by the dilution factor. This is the method used in large chemistry analyzers. The reference range for sodium is 136-145 meq/L.

Two common sources of error for sodium ISEs are electrodes coated with protein and competing ions. Most instrument manufacturers realize that a protein coating causes inaccurate sodium readings. Manufacturers require specific cleaning regimens for ISEs to remove the protein coating and enable more accurate readings. Another source of error is specimens with a high lipid or protein content, because these molecules displace fluid that may contain sodium ions.

Serum, heparinized plasma, whole blood, sweat, urine, feces, and gastrointestinal fluids are suitable specimens for sodium testing. Sodium heparin should not be employed as the anticoagulant in an evacuated tube used to measure electrolytes. Lithium heparin is a good alternative. To determine the rate of electrolyte loss, specimens of urine, feces, and gastrointestinal fluids are measured at specific time intervals. Hemolyzed specimens do not usually affect the sodium level unless the specimen is severely hemolyzed, which can cause a dilutional effect error. Urine, plasma, and serum specimens that are not tested immediately must be refrigerated to maintain the specimen's integrity.

Potassium

Potassium is found in high concentrations in intracellular fluid and in lower concentrations in extracellular fluid. Potassium is the most abundant cation in the body, and it is contained in many foods such as fruits and vegetables and food additives such as potassium chloride. Daily potassium intake is approximately equal to daily potassium excretion. Although potassium is rapidly absorbed in the intestinal lumen, it has little effect on the blood concentration. After the body absorbs as much potassium as it needs, excess potassium is excreted by the kidney. This electrolyte is also under the control of adrenocortical hormones.

Clinical Significance

Potassium helps to control muscle activity in the body. Elevated potassium levels inhibit muscle irritability (the ability of a muscle to contract in response to stretching). When an elevated potassium level paralyzes the heart muscle, it stops beating. Low potassium levels also affect muscle contractions. A low potassium level increases the irritability of the heart muscle, leading to irregular heartbeats (i.e., palpitations). High and low potassium levels can be observed on an electrocardiogram (see Table 12-3). The reference range for potassium is 3.5-5.1 meq/L.

Hyperkalemia is an elevated blood potassium level that results when potassium leaves cells faster than it can be excreted by the kidneys. Hyperkalemia can occur during anoxia, shock or circulatory failure, dehydration, Addison disease, severe in vivo red blood cell lysis, and metabolic or renal tubular acidosis. Renal dialysis removes many toxic metabolic byproducts, including accumulated potassium. Regulation of blood potassium levels in patients with renal failure undergoing dialysis is difficult because excess potassium is usually excreted daily through the kidneys.

Hypokalemia is a decreased level of potassium that can result from low potassium intake over time or increased loss due to vomiting, diarrhea, gastrointestinal problems, or diuretic use. Increased aldosterone production increases potassium secretion by the kidneys. Hypokalemia is often found

in individuals with chronic starvation and after surgery. In chronic starvation, muscle cells are broken down for energy, and the potassium in the cells is excreted. Many postoperative patients have received a large amount of potassium-poor fluid, which dilutes the blood, thereby reducing blood potassium levels. Low potassium levels can damage renal tubules.

Laboratory Procedures and Limitations

Like sodium, potassium is measured by ISEs. The construction of the potassium ISE is similar to that of the sodium ISE, except that the potassium ISE is coated with a liquid ion-exchange membrane containing valinomycin. The potassium ion reacts with the valinomycin to create a change in the electrode potential.

Because the highest level of potassium is found intracellularly, testing of hemolyzed specimens falsely elevates the potassium level. If whole blood is being tested, a small portion of the sample should be spun down to check for hemolysis.

Chloride

Chloride has the highest concentration of any anion in extracellular fluid, and it helps maintain electrical neutrality. Electrical neutrality is required, so the concentration of anions and that of cations in body fluids must be equal. As with most other electrolytes, the concentration of chloride varies in different conditions. The concentration of chloride varies inversely with that of bicarbonate to ensure electrical neutrality. When chloride concentrations are high, as in metabolic acidosis, the bicarbonate levels are low. When bicarbonate levels are high, as in metabolic alkalosis, the chloride levels are low.

The *chloride shift* allows oxygen and carbon dioxide to be exchanged in red blood cells (Fig. 12-6). When blood contains oxygen, chloride shifts from the red blood cells to the plasma,

Diffusion of CO_2 into blood and conversion to HCO_3^-

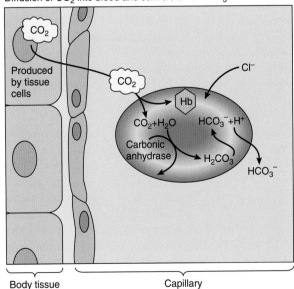

• **Figure 12-6** Carbon dioxide (CO_2) uptake from body tissues by erythrocytes and plasma. Note the chloride shift—Cl^- flows in when bicarbonate (HCO_3^-) flows out. (From Gartner LP, Hiatt JL. *Color Textbook of Histology.* 3rd ed. Philadelphia: Saunders; 2007.)

and bicarbonate leaves the plasma to enter the red blood cell. When the blood contains carbon dioxide, bicarbonate exits the red blood cells, and chloride shifts into the cells.

Chloride is found in extracellular fluids such as serum, plasma, cerebrospinal fluid, tissue fluid, and urine. Chloride does not enter cells, except red blood cells. Two thirds of chloride is found in the plasma, and the remaining one third is found in the red blood cells.

Humans usually ingest approximately 2.5 g of chloride per day as a salt (e.g., sodium chloride, calcium chloride, potassium chloride). The body readily absorbs chloride in the intestines, and excess chloride is excreted in urine or sweat.

The primary functions of chloride are determining osmotic pressure, maintaining the body's acid-base balance, and exchanging oxygen and carbon dioxide in the red blood cell. Osmotic pressure controls the distribution of water among cells, plasma, and interstitial fluids. Acid-base balance is discussed in Chapter 13.

Clinical Significance

The results of chloride testing on an electrolyte panel provide the least amount of clinical information. This value allows the anion gap to be calculated. The anion gap is important in tracking disorders such as severe renal disease and salicylate, ethylene glycol, or methanol poisoning. It is also useful as a quality assurance metric for electrolyte testing. The reference range for chloride is 98-107 meq/L.

Hypochloremia is a decreased level of chloride in plasma. Hypochloremia occurs in many metabolic acidosis syndromes. In diabetic ketoacidosis, ketoacids replace the chloride ions in the blood. In renal disease, damaged kidneys cannot resorb chloride-containing salts properly. In conditions with vomiting or intestinal blockages, chloride does not travel far enough down the intestines to be absorbed. In Addison disease, decreased hormone production leads to low levels of chloride (see Table 12-3).

Hyperchloremia is an increased level of chloride in plasma. Several mechanisms can lead to hyperchloremia, including dehydration, renal tubular acidosis, prolonged diarrhea, and diabetes insipidus. Respiratory alkalosis, which may be caused by hyperventilation brought on by drugs, hysteria, fever, or anxiety, can produce hyperchloremia.

Laboratory Procedures and Limitations

Serum, plasma, urine, and sweat specimens are commonly tested for chloride even though two thirds of chloride is found in plasma. When obtaining specimens for chloride testing, one must be careful to avoid contamination by exogenous chloride. For example, tap water contains high levels of chlorine as a purifying agent, and one must ensure that pipettes and other glassware are free from residual chloride. Another source of error is a common tube anticoagulant, sodium fluoride. Fluoride and chloride are classified as halogens, and both react similarly in laboratory assays. Other precautions that help to preserve the integrity of the specimen are separating plasma or serum from cells as soon as possible and limiting exposure to room air to prevent the

chloride shift. Because chloride is an extracellular anion, moderate hemolysis does not affect the test results.

Chloride ions can be measured with the use of an ISE or a colorimetric method. The ISE used for chloride measurement has an Ag/AgCl electrode and an $AgCl/Ag_2S$ solid membrane. The electrode can be used to measure other halogens such as fluoride, bromide, and iodide. Bromine-containing medications can produce falsely elevated chloride test results.

Automated analyzers may use a colorimetric method instead of an ISE to measure the chloride ion concentration. Chloride ions react with undissociated mercuric thiocyanate to form undissociated mercuric chloride and free thiocyanate ions. Free thiocyanate, when mixed with ferric nitrate, produces a red solution. The degree of red color is directly proportional to the concentration of chloride ions in the sample.

Occasionally, a health care provider requests that a chloride determination be performed on cerebrospinal fluid (CSF). Normally, the chloride concentration in CSF is higher than in serum because CSF has a lower protein concentration, so there are fewer protein anions and more chloride anions in the fluid. Bacterial meningitis raises the protein level in CSF, lowering the concentration of chloride anions in the fluid.

Urine specimens are not routinely tested for chloride concentration. Because the chloride concentration of urine varies with the amount of chloride ingested, urine chloride tests are run only on accurately timed specimens. The timed specimen must have its pH adjusted to 3 with dilute nitric acid.

Sweat contains chloride in amounts that are less than those found in serum. Individuals with cystic fibrosis have high concentrations of chloride in their sweat due to a defective gene and corresponding defective protein, the cystic fibrosis transmembrane conductance regulator. Sweat chloride tests, performed on an iontophoresis machine, are used to screen individuals for this disease. Sweating is usually induced in a very small area on the skin by the drug pilocarpine. The sweat sample (approximately 50 mg) is analyzed by coulometric and amperometric methods. This test is accepted by the Cystic Fibrosis Foundation. The reference range for chloride in sweat is 5-35 meq/L.

Bicarbonate

Bicarbonate is another major anion in extracellular fluids. This anion can is also referred to as *total carbon dioxide* or *carbon dioxide*. Bicarbonate may be found in more than one form in solution, including dissolved carbon dioxide, carbon dioxide bound to amine groups in proteins, bicarbonate ions (HCO_3^-), and carbonic acid (H_2CO_3). Because bicarbonate makes up 90% of the carbon dioxide dissolved in blood, measuring total carbon dioxide provides a good approximation of the total bicarbonate concentration.

Inhalation brings air into the lungs, where oxygen enters the blood and carbon dioxide and water vapor are exhaled into the atmosphere. Metabolic processes can dissociate carbonic acid into hydrogen and bicarbonate ions. Even though bicarbonate is filtered by the kidneys, all of it is resorbed.

Clinical Significance

Bicarbonate and carbon dioxide blood concentrations change dramatically with acid-base imbalances (see Chapter 13). The concentration of these two species alone does not indicate the nature of the imbalance. An analysis of other test results and the patient's clinical picture add meaning to abnormal bicarbonate values. Increased bicarbonate values are found in metabolic alkalosis, compensated respiratory acidosis, and a large potassium deficiency accompanied by alkalosis. Decreased bicarbonate values are found in metabolic acidosis and compensated respiratory alkalosis. The reference range for tCO_2 or bicarbonate is 23-29 meq/L.

Laboratory Procedures and Limitations

Bicarbonate testing should be performed only on serum or heparinized plasma, because other anticoagulants may alter the balance between the red blood cell and plasma carbon dioxide. Venous blood is used as a specimen most often, but capillary blood may also be used. Because room air contains less carbon dioxide than plasma, specimens should be tested as soon as possible after the tube cap is removed. If the tube is left exposed to the air, the carbon dioxide in the specimen can escape, and results for the specimen will be falsely decreased. Bicarbonate is measured by ISEs and by enzymatic and colorimetric methods.

The bicarbonate ISE consists of a glass electrode surrounded by a weak bicarbonate solution enclosed in a silicon membrane. The membrane allows carbon dioxide gas to pass through but keeps out water and ions. When the carbon dioxide enters the weak bicarbonate solution in the electrode, it lowers the pH of the solution. The rate of pH change is directly proportional to the amount of carbon dioxide in the specimen. The pH change rate is compared with a reference electrode, and the concentration in the sample is calculated.

Automated enzymatic methods convert all carbon dioxide in the specimen to bicarbonate by adding a base. Phosphoenolpyruvate carboxylase is then added to the specimen to convert bicarbonate to oxaloacetic acid. Oxaloacetic acid is converted to malate, and the concentration of carbon dioxide is determined by measuring the change in absorbance at 340 nm.

Automated colorimetric methods require the addition of an acid to liberate the carbon dioxide in the specimen. The liberated carbon dioxide passes through a membrane into a solution of cresol red at a pH of 9.2. The carbon dioxide reduces the pH of the dye, decreasing its color intensity. The amount of carbon dioxide in the specimen is directly proportional to the decrease in color intensity.

Lithium

Although lithium is chemically similar to sodium and potassium, the concentration found in animals is small. Lithium tests are routinely ordered by physicians who prescribe lithium carbonate to their patients. Physicians prescribe lithium carbonate to treat manic phases of an affective disorder (in which manic patients respond excessively) and bipolar disorder (in which patients experience mood swings from mania to extreme depression.

Clinical Significance

Lithium enhances the reuptake of neurotransmitters, producing a calming effect on the manic stage and preventing possible attacks. When the neurotransmitters are resorbed, there is less in the nerve junction to transmit the nerve impulses. Physicians monitor lithium levels in patients to ensure that they do not reach or exceed 2 mmol/L, which is a toxic concentration. Lithium levels are measured weekly when treatment begins and then at longer intervals. Symptoms of lithium toxicity include apathy, sluggishness, drowsiness, speech difficulties, and twitching. Patients with severe toxicity (>2.5 mmol/L) exhibit muscle rigidity, hyperactive deep tendon reflexes, and epileptic seizures. Levels greater than 5 mmol/L can cause death.

Laboratory Procedures and Limitations

Lithium can be measured with the use of an ISE, a colorimetric method, or an enzymatic method. The colorimetric and enzymatic methods are popular in clinical laboratories because they can be incorporated into an automated general chemistry analyzer. The colorimetric method uses a porphyrin dye that reacts with lithium in an alkaline solution. This reaction produces a binary compound and a change in absorbance at 510 nm. In the enzymatic reaction, lithium reacts with a lithium-sensitive enzyme, which then reacts with a substrate to form hypoxanthine. The hypoxanthine reacts in a coupled enzyme reaction to generate hydrogen peroxide. Hydrogen peroxide is quantified by using the Trinder reaction, and the lithium concentration is inversely proportional to the amount of hydrogen peroxide generated.

Colligative Properties

Physical properties that depend on the ratio of the number of solute particles to the number of solvent molecules in the solution are called colligative properties. Colligative properties are not based on the identity of the solute or solvent. An important colligative property of blood is osmotic pressure. Freezing point, boiling point, and vapor pressure are colligative properties of solutions.

Osmotic Pressure

Human blood is a solution of cells, chemicals, and water. The solvent in this solution is water, and the chemicals are the solutes. During osmosis, in which two solutions are separated by a semipermeable membrane, water passively moves from an area of lower solute concentration to an area of higher solute concentration in an attempt to equalize the concentrations of water on both sides of the membrane. Lysis of red blood cells in hypotonic solutions is caused by the extracellular-to-intracellular osmosis of water.

Osmotic pressure is the amount of pressure that must be applied to a solution of lower water concentration to prevent osmosis. Solutions that have a high concentration of dissolved substances also have a high osmotic pressure and attract water across a semipermeable membrane from a solution with a low concentration of dissolved substances. Likewise, solutions that have a low concentration of dissolved substances also have a low osmotic pressure and tend to lose water across a semipermeable membrane to a solution with a high concentration of dissolved substances. Because osmotic pressure is difficult to measure, the concentration of dissolved substances, or osmolality, is used to assess the water balance.

Osmolality

Osmolality is the concentration of solutes (in millimoles per kilogram of solvent). When the osmolality of the blood increases, the hypothalamus stimulates antidiuretic hormone (ADH) secretion and causes thirst. ADH increases water resorption through the collecting ducts of the kidney, and thirst causes an individual to drink more water. Both mechanisms result in more water in the blood, decreasing the osmolality of the blood. Serum osmolality is derived from sodium, blood urea nitrogen (BUN), and glucose levels and can be calculated by the following formula:

$$\text{Serum osmolality} = (2 \times [Na^+]) + (BUN/2.8) + (glucose/18)$$

Other formulas are used to calculate osmolality, but this is the most common one. Serum and urine osmolality can also be measured by instruments called *osmometers*.

The reference range for osmolality is 275 to 295 mOsm/kg of plasma water. A random urine osmolality value is between 300 and 900 mOsm/Kg, and a 24-hour urine osmolality value is between 500 and 800 mOsm/Kg. Serum osmolality panel values that indicate disease are those less than 240 mOsm/kg or greater than 321 mOsm/kg. A value of 384 mOsm/kg produces stupor, a value greater than 400 mOsm/kg can cause grand mal seizures, and a value greater than 420 mOsm/kg is fatal.

Clinical Significance

Osmolality plays a key role in homeostasis, and values can be affected by poisons, medications, and diseases. Concentration of toxins such as ethylene glycol, propylene glycol, ethanol, methanol, and salicylates can be approximated by measuring osmolality. For medications such as mannitol, osmolality measurements can be used to prevent toxic renal effects during administration. For burn patients and coma patients, osmolality measurements can be used to optimize hydration. Osmolality is also used to monitor the effectiveness of renal dialysis treatments. Urine osmolality measurement allows a physician to pinpoint the cause of a sodium imbalance (Table 12-4).

The classic hyperosmolar condition is diabetes insipidus, which is caused by an ADH deficiency. Because the kidneys cannot resorb water, the urine becomes very dilute, and the blood contains little water, making it hyperosmotic.

The classic hypo-osmotic condition is the syndrome of inappropriate antidiuretic hormone secretion (SIADH). Excessive secretion of ADH causes resorption of body water, leading to hyponatremia. Excess water resorption dilutes the blood, making it hypo-osmotic.

Laboratory Procedures and Limitations

Osmolality is measured with the use of an osmometer. Osmometers determine the concentration of all molecules and ions in a solution by measuring a solution's colligative properties: colloidal osmotic pressure, boiling point elevation, freezing point depression, and vapor-pressure depression.

The freezing point depression is the easiest and cheapest way to measure osmolality. The freezing point of blood is approximately $-0.53°$ C with an osmolality of 285 mOsm/kg. An aliquot of sample is introduced into a cuvette, which is then placed into a cold block on an osmometer. The thermistor (thermal resistor) is placed into the sample before the process begins. The sample is supercooled rapidly to a temperature below its normal freezing point. Strong stirring causes ice crystals to form in the solution, and heat is released in the process. The heat raises the temperature in the solution to its normal freezing point. The normal freezing point is measured and is inversely related to osmolality. The instrument should be thoroughly rinsed and wiped afterward to reduce carryover. Saline standards are used to calibrate osmometers.

TABLE 12-4	Causes of Increased and Decreased Osmolality	
Increased Osmolality		**Decreased Osmolality**
Serum		
Dehydration (fever, sweating, burns)		Excess hydration
Diabetes mellitus		Hyponatremia
Diabetes insipidus		Syndrome of inappropriate antidiuretic hormone secretion (SIADH)
Uremia		
Hypernatremia		
Ethanol, methanol, or ethylene glycol ingestion		
Urine		
Dehydration		Diabetes insipidus
SIADH		Acute renal insufficiency
Adrenal insufficiency		Glomerulonephritis
Hypernatremia		
High-protein diet		

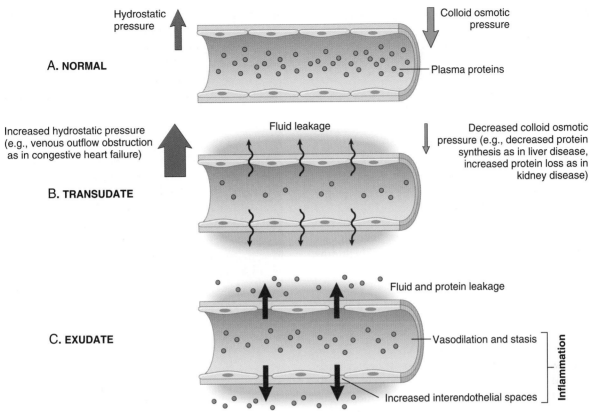

Hydrostatic pressure

Colloid osmotic pressure

A. NORMAL

Plasma proteins

Increased hydrostatic pressure (e.g., venous outflow obstruction as in congestive heart failure)

Fluid leakage

Decreased colloid osmotic pressure (e.g., decreased protein synthesis as in liver disease, increased protein loss as in kidney disease)

B. TRANSUDATE

C. EXUDATE

Fluid and protein leakage

Vasodilation and stasis

Increased interendothelial spaces

Inflammation

• **Figure 12-7** Formation of transudates and exudates. **A,** Normal hydrostatic pressure *(blue arrows)* is about 32 mm Hg at the arterial end of the capillary bed and 12 mm Hg at the venous end. The mean colloid osmotic pressure *(green arrows)* of tissues is approximately 25 mm Hg, which is equal to the mean capillary pressure, and the net flow of fluid across the vascular bed is almost zero. **B,** A transudate is formed when fluid leaks out of vessels because of increased hydrostatic pressure or decreased osmotic pressure. **C,** An exudate is formed in the setting of inflammation because vascular permeability increases as a result of increased interendothelial spaces. (From Kumar V, Abbas A, Fausto N, Aster J. *Robbins & Cotran Pathologic Basis of Disease.* 8th ed. Philadelphia: Saunders; 2010.)

Fluid Imbalances

Lymphatic System

Most of the fluid flowing through the body is found in the vascular system (arteries and veins). The lymphatic system handles a smaller amount of fluid but still plays an important role in fluid balance.

Blood capillaries are composed of thin-walled cells called *endothelial cells.* The endothelial cells are separated by a small space that allows small amounts of fluid to pass. The lymphatic system capillaries collect the leakage from the blood capillaries and empty into larger vessels (collecting ducts). The lymph fluid bathes the lymph nodes and eventually empties into the subclavian veins. The lymphatic system is similar to the venous system because the movement of muscles in the body helps to move the lymph fluids, and the lymph vessels contain valves to prevent backwash.

Some conditions, such as edema, are the result of fluid leakage. Other conditions can cause fluids to enter body cavities, and determining the characteristics of the fluid may aid in diagnosis.

Edema

Edema is an accumulation of excess fluid in interstitial tissues or body cavities. As blood flows through the blood vessels, a certain amount of pressure (flow pressure) is exerted on the inner walls of the vessels. The cells in the surrounding tissues contain intracellular fluid, which exerts a pressure (i.e., hydrostatic pressure) on the outer walls of the blood vessels. In addition, the large proteins and other colloid molecules within the cell exert colloidal osmotic pressure on the outer walls of the blood vessels. In normal fluid balance, all of these forces are in equilibrium. When the forces are not balanced, edema results.

Edema fluid may be a transudate or an exudate. Transudates are fluids that contain low amounts of protein, few cells, and high water content. They are produced in liver and kidney diseases and by cancerous processes. These fluids usually result from low colloidal osmotic pressure or increased hydrostatic pressure, which allows water to leak into the surrounding tissues or body cavities. An exudate is a high-protein fluid with a high number of cells; it is produced by an inflammatory reaction or lymph system blockage (i.e., lymphedema) (Fig. 12-7).

TABLE 12-5	Chemical Characteristics of Transudates and Exudates	
Transudate	**Exudate**	
Low numbers of cells	Moderate to high numbers of cells	
Watery component of plasma (i.e., clear sample)	Large molecules (i.e., cloudy sample)	
Low total protein level	High total protein level	
Low specific gravity (<1.012)	High specific gravity (>1.102)	
Low albumin level	High albumin level	

The four mechanisms that produce edema are increased hydrostatic pressure in vessels (including sodium and water retention), increased vascular permeability, decreased plasma osmotic pressure, and decreased lymphatic effectiveness. The first two mechanisms produce a transudate, and the latter two produce an exudate (Table 12-5).

Edema is caused by disease and is named according to where it occurs in the body. Anasarca is severe generalized edema. Hydrothorax, or accumulation of fluid in the thorax, is also called a pleural effusion. Hemopericardium is a condition in which blood and fluid accumulate in the pericardium; it is commonly called a pericardial effusion. Hydroperitoneum, an abnormal accumulation of fluid in the abdominal cavity, is also called ascites. Accumulation of fluid in the alveoli is called pulmonary edema.

Low-Protein Edema

Pitting edema is a low-protein edema that is usually found in the extremities. When pressure is applied with a finger, water is squeezed out of the swollen tissue, and an indentation (pit) remains until the water returns (Fig. 12-8).

Hydrostatic Edema

Hydrostatic edema occurs when increased hydrostatic pressure in the veins forces water out of the vessels and into the tissue. Varicose veins or congestive heart failure can cause hydrostatic edema in the ankles and feet. Varicose veins result from malfunctioning venous valves that cause blood to pool in the lower extremities. Pooling increases hydrostatic pressure, forcing fluid into the lower-pressure surrounding tissue.

In cases of congestive heart failure, the heart does not efficiently pump blood throughout the body. Inefficient pumping slows the circulation of the blood and increases hydrostatic pressure in the lower extremities, leading to hydrostatic pressure. If the heart failure is left sided, the blood pools in the lungs, and the hydrostatic

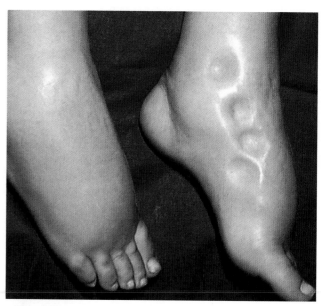

• **Figure 12-8** Edema is an accumulation of excess fluid in tissues. Pitting edema results when pressure is applied and forces fluid out of swollen tissue. The indentation remains until fluid reperfuses the tissue. (From Bloom A, Ireland J. *Color Atlas of Diabetes.* 2nd ed. London: Mosby; 1992.)

pressure causes fluid to leak into the alveoli, resulting in pulmonary edema.

Osmotic Edema

Osmotic edema is another type of low-protein edema, which results from low osmotic pressure. A common cause of low osmotic pressure is a low protein level in blood. A low blood protein level is commonly seen in liver disease (in which proteins are not produced) and in renal glomerular disease (in which large amounts of protein are lost in urine).

The most common cause of osmotic edema is a low plasma sodium concentration. A low sodium level lowers the osmotic pressure, and water leaks into the tissues. The low sodium level also triggers the kidneys to retain sodium, causing water retention and allowing more water into the tissues. This process can be triggered by consumption of salty foods or drinks.

High-Protein Edema

The most common cause of high-protein edema is inflammation. During an inflammatory process, cells and acute phase proteins migrate to the site and leak through the capillaries to form a high-protein edema. High-protein edema can also result from lymphatic obstruction (i.e., lymphedema). Lymph fluid has a high content of protein and cells. Lymphedema does not pit like low-protein edema. The skin has the appearance of an orange peel. Lymphedema usually occurs in the extremities and can be caused by a metastatic tumor.

Summary

Water is the key to life. Water is distributed in compartments, which allows the body to balance water content more effectively. The two major compartments are the intravascular and extravascular compartments. The extracellular compartment is further divided into intracellular and extracellular compartments.

Body water contains electrolytes (e.g., Na$^+$, K$^+$, Cl$^-$, HCO$_3^-$, Ca^{2+}, Mg^{2+}, PO$_4^{3-}$, Li^{2+}), proteins (e.g., colloids), and other molecules. Electrolytes regulate muscle contractions, control water excretion and retention, transmit nerve impulses, maintain osmotic pressure, maintain acid-base balance, serve as intracellular messengers, and are components of high-energy compounds.

The anion gap can be calculated from the normal electrolyte panel of sodium, potassium, chloride, and bicarbonate.

The anion gap can be used to show production or retention of organic acids. Iontophoresis is a special type of electrolyte analysis that is used to determine the chloride content of sweat, which helps in diagnosing cystic fibrosis. Osmolality is the concentration of solutes per kilogram of solvent. The concentration of some substances can be quickly approximated using this measurement.

Body fluid imbalance produces edema when excess fluid leaks into the interstitial or cavity spaces. The fluid can have a high or low protein content. High-protein fluids are called exudates, and low-protein fluids are called transudates. Lymphedema is an example of an exudate. Hydrostatic and osmotic forms of edema lead to accumulation of a low-protein transudate.

Review Questions

1. Name two body compartments.
   a. Intracellular and extracellular
   b. Intravascular and extravascular
   c. Intracellular and extravascular
   d. Intravascular and extracellular
2. The intracellular and extracellular compartments are separated by
   a. An arterial wall
   b. An endothelial membrane
   c. A plasma membrane
   d. An alveolar membrane
3. Electrolytes include all the following EXCEPT
   a. Phosphate
   b. Sodium
   c. Potassium
   d. Chloride
4. Sodium is a major cation in
   a. Interstitial fluid
   b. Intracellular fluid
   c. Exudates
   d. Extravascular fluid
5. Calculate the anion gap given the following electrolyte values: Na$^+$ of 135 mEq/L, K$^+$ of 5 mEq/L, Cl$^-$ of 110 mEq/L, and tCO$_2$ of 28 mEq/L.
   a. 4
   b. 6
   c. 8
   d. 2

6. Which of the following electrolytes accounts for 90% of plasma cations?
   a. Potassium
   b. Sodium
   c. Chloride
   d. Magnesium
7. Which technology is used to measure electrolytes?
   a. Colorimetry
   b. Enzyme reactions
   c. Ion-selective electrodes
   d. Spectrophotometry
8. Potassium is a major cation in
   a. Extracellular fluid
   b. Interstitial fluid
   c. Intracellular fluid
   d. Exudates
9. Which of the following electrolytes is the most common cause of osmotic edema?
   a. Na$^+$
   b. K$^+$
   c. Cl$^-$
   d. HCO$_3^-$
10. The classic hyperosmolar condition is
   a. Diabetes insipidus
   b. Diabetes mellitus
   c. Dehydration
   d. Addison disease

Critical Thinking Questions

1. What happens to the body in dehydration?
2. Evaluate the clinical significance of sodium, potassium, chloride, bicarbonate, and lithium.
3. Define anion gap. Calculate the anion gap for the following set of data, and state whether the anion gap is within normal limits:

Na$^+$ = 145 mmol/L
K$^+$ = 4.2 mmol/L
Cl$^-$ = 100Meq/L
HCO$_3^-$ = 28 mEq/L.

CASE STUDY

An elderly woman was admitted to the emergency department with cardiac issues. Her electrocardiogram result was very abnormal, and she was admitted to the intensive care unit. She told the physician on duty that she had diarrhea for 2 months. The admission laboratory work showed a potassium level of 1.1 mEq/L. What is a likely reason for the woman's cardiac abnormalities? Why was her potassium level so low?

Bibliography

Astle SM. Restoring electrolyte balance. *RN.* 2005;68:34–39.

Burtis CA, Bruns DE. *Tietz Textbook of Clinical Chemistry and Molecular Diagnostics.* 7th ed. Philadelphia: Elsevier; 2014.

Jahnen-Dechent W, Ketteler M. Magnesium basics. *Clin Kidney J.* 2012;5(suppl 1):i3–i14.

Kumar V, Abbas A, Fausto N, Aster J. *Robbins and Cotran: Pathologic Basis of Disease.* 9th ed. Philadelphia: Saunders; 2015.

Thier SO. Potassium physiology. *Am J Med.* 1986;80:3–7.

Verbalis JG. Disorders of body water homeostasis. *Best Pract Res Clin Endorcinol Metab.* 2003;17:471–503.

13

Blood Gases and Acid-Base Balance

DONNA LARSON

CHAPTER OUTLINE

OBJECTIVES

At the completion of this chapter, the reader will be able to:

1. Describe the purpose of measuring blood gases and pH.
2. Describe how gases are exchanged in the body.
3. Interpret the interrelation between pCO_2, pH, and HCO_3^-.
4. Describe the process of collecting a specimen for blood gas testing.
5. Discuss the four electrodes found in a blood gas analyzer.
6. Describe transcutaneous blood gas monitoring and why it works.
7. Name the acid byproducts of metabolism.
8. Compare and contrast the four buffer systems in the body.
9. Describe how the pH changes in arterial blood after the specimen is drawn.
10. Explain how metabolic disturbances in acid-base balance occur.
11. Explain how respiratory disturbances in acid-base balance occur.
12. Describe the respiratory and renal compensation mechanisms.
13. Describe the compensatory mechanisms in respiratory acidosis, respiratory alkalosis, metabolic acidosis, and metabolic alkalosis.
14. Discuss laboratory findings in compensated respiratory acidosis and alkalosis and in metabolic acidosis and alkalosis.
15. Evaluate the clinical significance of respiratory acidosis, respiratory alkalosis, metabolic acidosis, and metabolic alkalosis.

KEY TERMS

Amperometric
Bicarbonate buffer system
Blood gas analysis
Buffer
Carboxyhemoglobin
Central chemoreceptors
Cyanosis
Dalton's law
Elevated anion gap acidosis
External respiration
Henderson-Hasselbalch equation
Henry's law
Hypercapnia

Hyperventilation
Hypocapnia
Hypoventilation
Hypoxemia
Hypoxia
Internal respiration
Lactic acidosis
Metabolic acidosis
Metabolic alkalosis
Normal anion gap acidosis
Oxygen saturation
Partial pressure
pCO_2

Peripheral chemoreceptors
Phosphate buffer system
pO_2
Potentiometric
Pressure gradient
Protein buffer system
Pulmonary diffusion
Respiration
Respiratory acidosis
Respiratory alkalosis
Transcutaneous

❖ Case in Point

A 48-year-old man was admitted to the hospital complaining of abdominal pain. He appeared apprehensive. Other complaints were abdominal bloating and back pain. He was also short of breath. Blood gas results showed the following: pH, 7.58; pCO₂, 22 mm Hg; pO₂, 77 mm Hg. What is the interpretation of these blood gas results? What is hyperventilation? Are the terms *hypoxia* and *ventilation* synonymous? What is the most common treatment for the disorder caused by hyperventilation due to anxiety or hysteria?

Points to Remember

- External respiration is the exchange of oxygen and carbon dioxide that occurs in the lungs.
- Internal respiration is the exchange of oxygen and carbon dioxide that occurs at the tissues.
- The gradients in partial pressure of oxygen and carbon dioxide control the movement of gases between the alveoli and the cells.
- The three factors that control oxygen transport are partial pressure of oxygen (pO_2), diffusion of oxygen into the blood, and the affinity of hemoglobin for oxygen.
- Oxygen saturation ($sO_2\%$) = $[HbO_2]/[Hb] \times 100$
- Henderson-Hasselbalch equation: pH = $6.103 + \log[HCO_3^-]/0.306 \times pCO_2$
- pH is a function of two independent variables: pCO_2 and $[HCO_3^-]$
- Metabolic acidosis: pH is decreased, pCO_2 is normal, HCO_3^- is decreased
- Metabolic alkalosis: pH is increased, pCO_2 is normal, HCO_3^- is increased
- Respiratory acidosis: pH is decreased, pCO_2 is increased, HCO_3^- is normal
- Respiratory alkalosis: pH is increased, pCO_2 is decreased, HCO_3^- is normal
- Compensation for the primary condition will bring the pH close to normal, but the pH will not return to normal until the condition is resolved. Laboratory results showing a near-normal pH and an abnormal pCO_2 or HCO_3^- should be considered compensated.

Introduction

Neonates and patients with cardiopulmonary problems require laboratory tests that can accurately measure oxygen and carbon dioxide in their blood and expired air. With accurate laboratory tests, physicians can optimally mix gases in mechanical ventilators to meet a patient's needs. Most hospitals employ specialized respiratory or cardiopulmonary specialists to draw and run blood gas analyses in a specialized laboratory. There are still a few hospitals that draw and run blood gas samples in the clinical laboratory. Blood gas analysis is integrated with acid-base balance. This chapter discusses the physiology, clinical significance, and laboratory analysis of blood gases and acid-base balance.

Blood Gases

Blood gas analysis (also known as *blood gases*) is performed to determine parameters such as the pH, oxygen content, and carbon dioxide content in arterial or venous blood. The pH of blood is discussed more fully later in the chapter. The amount of oxygen or carbon dioxide in the blood is critical and can mean life or death to trauma patients and other emergency patients. The discussion of blood gases begins with a review of abbreviations and terms.

Physiology

Terms such as *partial pressure, saturation, arterial, venous,* and *capillary* are used when discussing blood gases. **Partial pressure** refers to the amount of pressure contributed by each gas to the total pressure exerted by the mixture. Saturation refers to the percentage of hemoglobin molecules whose binding sites are all filled (saturated) with oxygen molecules (Table 13-1). Arterial blood is the most common specimen for blood gas analysis because blood pumped through arteries is oxygen rich.

Arteries carry oxygen-rich blood to the tissues, where the oxygen is release and metabolic byproducts are picked up. Venous blood contains a lower amount of oxygen and a higher amount of metabolic byproducts than arterial blood. The venous blood returns to the heart via the vena cava, then to the lungs via the pulmonary vein to pick up oxygen, then back to the heart through the pulmonary artery and out to the body through arteries. The process by which oxygen is delivered to the tissues and metabolic byproducts (e.g., carbon dioxide) are removed from the tissues is called **respiration**. The actual exchange of oxygen and carbon dioxide that takes place in the lungs is called **external respiration**. This process occurs each time we take a breath.

External respiration is a complex process. During inhalation, air enters the nose (where it is warmed); it continues moving through the throat into the bronchi, then into the bronchioles, and finally into the alveoli. Alveoli are balloon-like structures that expand and contract during inhalation and exhalation. The alveoli also have very thin walls and are located close to pulmonary arteries and veins.

TABLE 13-1	Blood Gas Notations
Notation	**Definition**
pCO_2	Partial pressure of carbon dioxide in the blood*
pO_2	Partial pressure of oxygen in the blood*
sO_2	Percentage of hemoglobin saturated with oxygen molecules
HCO_3^-	Bicarbonate ion
pH	Measure of the acidity or alkalinity of blood

*The partial pressure of a gas is the amount of pressure contributed by each gas to the total pressure exerted by the mixture.

The gases—oxygen and carbon dioxide—are exchanged through the thin walls of the capillaries (Fig. 13-1). The oxygen is carried in the blood to the tissues, and the carbon dioxide is exhaled. This process is called internal respiration.

Dynamics of gases in the blood are governed by gas laws. The first law that governs gases in the blood is Dalton's law, which states that each gas in a mixture will exert the same pressure as if it were alone in solution. The total pressure of a mixture of gases is the sum of all the partial pressures exerted by all the gases in the mixture. As we consider blood gases, the two gases in the mixture are oxygen and carbon dioxide, and the containers are the lungs and capillaries. The second law, Henry's law, relates the partial pressure of the gas to the concentration of the gas. Henry's law states that, at a constant temperature, the amount of gas dissolved in a solution is directly proportional to the partial pressure of the gas and the solubility of the gas.

Let's look at these two gas laws during breathing:

1. A person breathes in air in which the partial pressure of oxygen (pO_2) is 158 mm Hg and the partial pressure of carbon dioxide (pCO_2) is 0.3 mm Hg.

2. As the air enters, the person's nose and nasopharynx humidify the air, decreasing the pO_2 to 150 mm Hg.

3. As the air continues to advance through the respiratory tract, into the lungs and finally into the alveoli, its pO_2 is reduced to approximately 104 mm Hg, and its pCO_2 increases to 40 mm Hg.

4. The oxygen molecules in the alveoli diffuse into the arteriole, increasing the pO_2 to between 80 and 100 mm Hg; the pCO_2 level remains at 40 mm Hg. This process is called *external respiration.*

5. The newly oxygenated blood (oxyhemgoglobin) returns to the heart, then is pumped throughout the body.

6. When the blood arrives at the tissues, oxygen is released from the hemoglobin (pO_2 is reduced to 45 mm Hg) and migrates into the tissues; the carbon dioxide in the tissues moves into the blood and attaches to hemoglobin (carboxyhemoglobin), increasing the pCO_2 to 50 mm Hg. This process is called *internal respiration.*

7. The blood returns to the lung, where the carbon dioxide is released into the lungs and then into the air. The process begins again (Fig. 13-2).

The pressure gradient between pO_2 and pCO_2 in alveolar blood compared with inhaled air causes oxygen to move into the body and carbon dioxide to move out of the body. The movement of air in and out of the lungs is controlled by the body's respiratory control center. Central chemoreceptors located in the ventral medulla of the brainstem and peripheral chemoreceptors located in the carotid artery and aorta can involuntarily affect breathing rate and depth, as well as other factors. Chemoreceptors located throughout the body are sensitive to the partial pressures of oxygen and carbon dioxide, alerting the brain to increase or decrease the rate of breathing as needed.

Clinical Significance

Oxygen

Life for a human depends on breathing in oxygen and breathing out carbon dioxide. There are diseases that can alter the partial pressures of oxygen and carbon dioxide in the blood, so measuring these gases in the blood is important. Blood gas measurements are used to assess and manage a patient's respiratory and metabolic conditions.

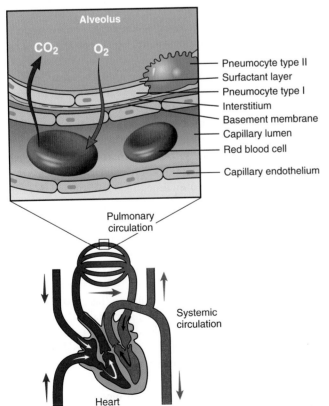

• **Figure 13-1** Respiration. Oxygen enters the blood and is bonded to red blood cells. This releases CO_2, which is then released into the alveolar air destined for expiration. (From Damjanov I. *Pathology for the Health Professions.* 4th ed. St. Louis: Saunders; 2012.)

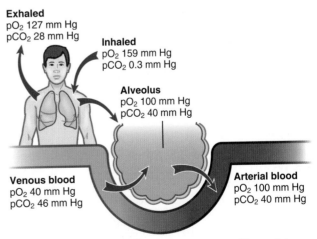

• **Figure 13-2** Gas exchange in normal respiration. The partial pressures of respiratory gases are shown in air inhaled and exhaled from the lungs, at the level of the alveoli, and in pulmonary venous and arterial blood vessels. (Modified from Lewis SL, Dirksen SR, Heitkemper MM, Bucher L. *Medical-Surgical Nursing: Assessment and Management of Clinical Problems.* 9th ed. St. Louis: Mosby; 2014.)

Oxygen is transported by the hemoglobin that is present in red blood cells. There are three factors that can affect oxygen transport: pO_2, diffusion of oxygen across the alveolar membrane, and the affinity of hemoglobin for oxygen. Normally, 95% of the hemoglobin in arterial blood is bound to oxygen (i.e., saturated). Increased pO_2 (>100-120 mm) or 100% binding can result from the administration of oxygen-enriched air or after exercise in healthy individuals. The percentage of hemoglobin bound to oxygen, called the oxygen saturation (sO_2%), can be calculated from $[HbO_2]$, the concentration of saturated hemoglobin in g/dL, and $[Hb]$, the total concentration of hemoglobin (saturated and unsaturated) in g/dL:

$$sO_2\% = \frac{[HbO_2]}{[Hb]} \times 100$$

If an individual's oxygen saturation is less than 95%, either the patient is not receiving enough oxygen or the patient does not have enough functional hemoglobin available to transport the oxygen. The amount of functional hemoglobin available in the blood can be altered by decreased red blood cell numbers or by the presence of nonfunctional hemoglobin (carboxyhemoglobin, methemoglobin, sulfhemoglobin, or cyanmethemoglobin).

Hypoxia refers to decreased pO_2 and decreased sO_2 resulting from lack of oxygen, whereas cyanosis results from decreased sO_2 caused by a high concentration of nonfunctional hemoglobin. Decreased oxygen levels (hypoxia) are considered a medical emergency. There are several conditions that produce hypoxia:

- High altitudes
- Low areas of oxygen (gas-filled room)
- Hypoventilation due to suffocation, water in the lungs (drowning), trauma, or drug overdose with barbiturates or opioids
- Mixing of venous and arterial blood due to congenital heart disease, pneumonia, pulmonary edema, or shock
- Poor blood oxygenation due to pneumonia, respiratory distress syndrome (ARDS), or cancer

Hypoxemia refers to decreased arterial oxygen. Causes include decreased pulmonary diffusion, decreased alveolar spaces due to resection or compression, and poor ventilation/perfusion due to obstructed airways (asthma, bronchitis, emphysema, foreign body, or secretions).

Carbon Dioxide

Carbon dioxide is transported in blood as bicarbonate (HCO_3^-), carbaminohemoglobin, and dissolved carbon dioxide. Carbon dioxide, pH, and pCO_2 are interrelated according to the Henderson-Hasselbalch equation:

$$pH = 6.103 + \frac{\log[HCO_3^-]}{0.306 \times pCO_2}$$

If you know the bicarbonate and pCO_2 concentrations, you can calculate the pH.

Hypercapnia is an increased pCO_2 in arterial blood; it occurs when there is decreased alveolar oxygen caused by breathing carbon dioxide–enriched air. Another mechanism that decreases alveolar ventilation is the use of particular types of drugs that lead to a depressed rate and depth of breathing and increased levels of carbon dioxide in the blood.

Hypocapnia is a decreased pCO_2 in arterial blood; it is caused by increased breathing rates (e.g., hyperventilation). Hypocapnia can also be produced when an individual is on a mechanical ventilator. Hyperventilation has many potential causes, including stress, pain, and emotions.

Laboratory Procedures and Limitations
Specimen Collection

Although collection of all laboratory specimens with care is important, extreme care must be taken when collecting specimens for blood gas analysis. Blood gases can be run on venous or arterial specimens, although venous blood is used only for pH and pCO_2 determinations. Both arterial and venous specimens should be collected without a tourniquet, because stasis causes a lower pO_2 and pH (due to the accumulation of acid metabolites). Arterial blood used for blood gas analysis must be handled with great care to ensure accurate results. Drawing of arterial specimens is extremely difficult and requires special training of personnel (physicians and technicians). In large facilities, respiratory therapists are usually responsible for this procedure; in smaller facilities, laboratory technicians may be required to perform the arterial punctures.

Blood gas samples are collected anaerobically, preferably with liquid heparin as an anticoagulant. Prepackaged kits are typically used for blood gas sampling. They contain a syringe (1 to 5 mL), anticoagulant (already in the syringe), a needle (23 gauge or higher), and a small rubber block to embed the needle after collection. Although this technique may not be used in all hospitals, some method will be used to keep air from entering the syringe (Box 13-1 and Fig. 13-3). After the arterial blood is collected, it is extremely important not to expose the sample to air for any longer than absolutely necessary. Because room air has a higher pO_2 than arterial blood, air exposure will falsely increase the pO_2 in the sample. The only time this is not true is when the blood is drawn from a person who is receiving oxygen therapy; the pO_2 in arterial blood from these individuals will be higher than the oxygen concentration in air. Exposure of an arterial blood specimen to ambient air will also lower the pCO_2 because the concentration of carbon dioxide in the sample is higher than in the air. When a sample loses carbon dioxide, the sample pH will rise (i.e., become more alkaline). Skilled individuals drawing arterial specimens will minimize bubbles, but if bubbles are present, they should be expelled immediately after collection. Medical laboratory technicians should always make a note if a blood gas specimen contains a bubble.

Another critical factor for arterial blood gas samples is temperature. After an arterial specimen is collected, it is placed on ice immediately and transported to the laboratory as soon as possible. In ideal conditions, a blood gas specimen is stable for up to 1 hour; however, the sooner the

• BOX 13-1 Collecting an Arterial Blood Gas Specimen

1. Selection of the site for an arterial puncture is important because there must be collateral blood flow and the artery must be easily accessible. Physicians will collect arterial blood gas specimens from femoral arteries, whereas technicians usually use the radial or brachial sites. The most common site for collecting a blood gas specimen is the radial site because this artery is easily accessible at the wrist. This site is good because there is collateral blood circulation to the hand from the ulnar artery.

2. Before the specimen is collected, the Allen test is performed on the hand above the artery selected for puncture. To perform the Allen test, the technician asks the individual to raise the hand and make a fist. After 30 seconds, pressure is applied to the ulnar and radial arteries to block blood flow to the hand. The technician then asks the individual to open the hand, and the palm is examined for blanching. Next, the technician releases pressure on the ulnar artery; color should return to the individual's palm in about 7 seconds.

3. The arm should be positioned with the palm facing up and the wrist resting on a rolled towel. The wrist should be extended about 30 degrees to stretch and fix the soft tissues over the firm ligaments and bone.

4. The technician opens the kit and ensures that minimal heparin is present in the syringe. Excess heparin can be removed by pulling back on the plunger and then pushing it forward until it stops.

5. The technician performs the puncture using aseptic technique. The site is cleansed with alcohol, and sterile gloves are donned before the puncture is performed.

6. The technician places a finger directly over the artery and then, with the bevel up and at a 45 degree angle, inserts the needle into the skin about 5 to 10 mm below the finger (see Fig. 13-3).

7. The needle and syringe are slowly advanced until blood appears in the syringe.

8. The syringe is held still, and the arterial pressure is allowed to push the blood into the syringe.

9. Once the appropriate amount of sample is collected, the needle is pulled out and pressure is applied with sterile gauze for 5 to 10 minutes.

10. While continuing to apply pressure to the puncture site, the technician makes sure that there are no bubbles in the syringe and inserts the needle into the rubber block provided in the kit. Some kits provide a small rubber cap that is applied to maintain an airtight seal on the syringe.

11. Once the bleeding from the puncture has stopped, the technician applies a pressure bandage to the site, appropriately labels the tube, and places the specimen in a cup of ice for immediate transport to the laboratory.

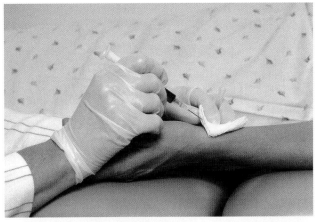

• **Figure 13-3** Arterial puncture. (See Box 13-1 for details.) (From Pagana KD, Pagana TJ. *Mosby's Manual of Diagnostic and Laboratory Tests.* 5th ed. St. Louis: Mosby; 2014.)

These electrodes are encased by a liquid or metal heating block to maintain the electrodes at 37° C. Blood gas analyzers are controlled by microprocessors to carry out periodic calibrations and washings.

The pO_2 electrode contains an oxygen-permeable Teflon or polyethylene membrane. The oxygen electrode is **amperometric** and contains a platinum cathode and a silver–silver chloride anode. The platinum electrode conducts a negative charge that reduces the oxygen in the sample. The change in the ionic current of the sample is measured, and then the pO_2 of the sample is calculated. (See Chapter 3 for more information.)

The pCO_2 electrode uses a glass membrane that is surrounded by a bicarbonate solution which is separated from the sample by a silicone membrane. The carbon dioxide gas diffuses through the silicone membrane, forming carbonic acid and lowering the pH of the solution. The change in the pH of the solution is proportional to the amount of carbon dioxide in the sample, and this pH change is detected by the electrode. The carbon dioxide electrode is **potentiometric.** (See Chapter 3 for more information.)

Once the pO_2 and pCO_2 are known, the HCO_3^- and total CO_2 content can be calculated. Most instruments are programmed to perform these calculations. These values can be displayed, printed, or downloaded to the laboratory information system.

Blood Gas Analyzer General Operating Principles

Once the specimen is well mixed, it is introduced at the sample probe and a command is initiated to aspirate the sample. A pump aspirates the sample into the probe and sends it to a measuring chamber, where the sample contacts the ISEs. The pump pauses to allow the sample to reach body temperature. Once at body temperature, the analytes are measured; then a pump sends the sample to the waste container. Blood gas results from the sample are displayed, printed, or sent to a laboratory information system.

There are noninvasive blood gas monitoring methods that are performed by nurses at the patient's bedside.

specimen is processed, the more accurate the results. Physicians expect the turnaround time for a blood gas sample to be 15 minutes or less.

Measuring Blood Gases

Blood gas analyzers perform the measurement of blood gases. These instruments can measure several parameters simultaneously. Blood gas analyzers are made by a variety of companies using several ion-selective electrodes (ISEs).

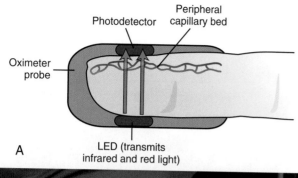

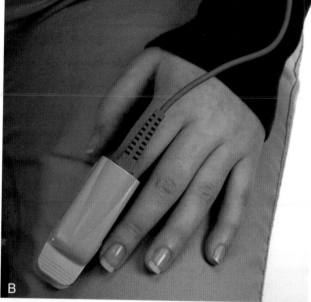

• **Figure 13-4** Pulse oximetry. **A,** The probe of the pulse oximeter is attached to a peripheral capillary bed in the fingertip. The light-emitting diode (LED) transmits light through the capillary bed to a light detector (photodetector) located on the other side of the probe to measure the oxygen saturation of hemoglobin. **B,** Applying the probe to the tip of a finger. (From Bonewit-West K. *Clinical Procedures for Medical Assistants.* 9th ed. St. Louis: Saunders; 2015.)

A common method for measuring blood gases in adults is pulse oximetry. Usually, a sensor is placed on an individual's fingertip and the pO_2 is displayed on a monitor (Fig. 13-4). For neonates, there are transcutaneous monitoring devices. The electrode is placed flat against the baby's skin, usually on the abdomen or chest, and the pO_2 displays on a monitor. These are useful techniques, but abnormal findings or acid-base imbalances can be confirmed only by arterial blood gas analyses.

Acid-Base Theory

Even though the human diet consists of foods that are mostly neutral (in pH terms), organic acids are produced as a byproduct of metabolism, and inhaled carbon dioxide is dissolved in blood to form carbonic acid. The human body is dynamic: It is in a constant state of change that includes maintaining the body's acid-base balance. Acid-base balance is basically a physiologic balance in which the rates of input and output of hydrogen ions are equal for a specific time interval. Acid-base balance involves balancing carbon dioxide and noncarbonic acids and bases in the blood. The acid-base balance is critical for optimal performance of the body. Many chemical reactions rely on enzymes, and enzymes rely on a specific pH to produce the best results. This section looks at the complex mechanisms our bodies use to maintain acid-base balance and the conditions that result from imbalances.

$$pH = \log \frac{1}{[H^+]} \text{ or } pH = -\log[H^+]$$

Buffers

Acids are compounds that donate a hydrogen ion (H^+), and bases are compounds that donate hydroxide ions (OH^-). pH is the negative log of the hydrogen ion concentration: $-\log[H^+]$. Substances with lower pH numbers (e.g., 6.8, 7.2) are acidic, and those with higher pH numbers (e.g., 7.6, 7.8) are alkaline. The human body maintains blood pH in the narrow range of 7.35 to 7.45. This is accomplished through the use of buffer systems as well as the kidneys and the lungs. A buffer is defined as a solution consisting of a weak acid and its conjugate base; when a strong base or strong acid is added to this solution, the pH changes very little. There are four major buffer systems in the human body: bicarbonate, phosphate, protein, and hemoglobin.

Bicarbonate

The bicarbonate buffer system is the most important buffer system in the body because bicarbonate is present in large amounts and can be controlled by both the lungs and the kidneys (Fig. 13-5). When carbon dioxide dissolves in water, it forms carbonic acid, which dissociates into hydrogen and bicarbonate:

$$CO_2 + H_2O \rightarrow H_2CO_3 \rightarrow H^+ + HCO_3^-$$

The effectiveness of the bicarbonate buffer system lies in the fact that there is a lot of bicarbonate available in the body. In addition, the renal tubules can be signaled to increase or decrease bicarbonate absorption, and the lungs can release or retain carbon dioxide.

Phosphate

The phosphate buffer system, which relies on HPO_4^{-2} and $H_2PO_4^-$ ions in the cell, minimizes pH changes inside the cell and in the blood. Although the concentration of this buffer system's components is tiny compared with the concentration of the bicarbonate buffer system's components, the phosphate buffer system ensures acid-base balance inside the cell.

Protein

The protein buffer system comprises the largest concentration of nonbicarbonate substances in the blood (Fig. 13-6). Proteins have many positive and negative charges spread out over the large protein molecule. These charges can help buffer the blood by interacting with hydrogen or hydroxide ions.

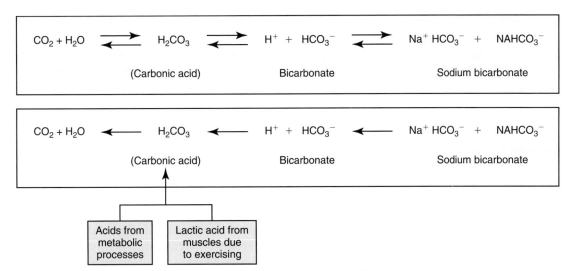

• **Figure 13-5** Bicarbonate buffer system. The *upper panel* shows the dynamic balance of the system. When acids are produced from metabolism (e.g., pyruvic acid, acetic acid, lactic acid from muscles), this buffer system responds. As shown in the *lower panel,* bicarbonate is mobilized from reserves to neutralize the acids, forming more carbonic acid, which dissociates into carbon dioxide and water and is released through the lungs.

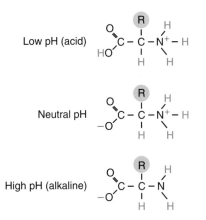

• **Figure 13-6** Protein buffer system. If pH rises from neutral *(top),* the amino acid acts as a base and absorbs the H⁺. If pH drops *(bottom),* the amino acid acts as an acid and releases H⁺.

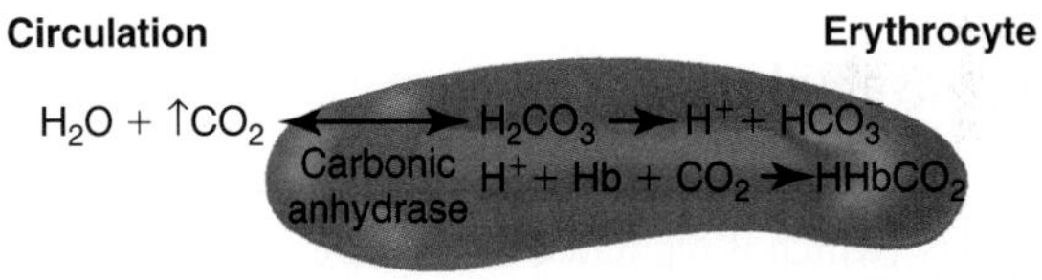

Hemoglobin

The final buffer system in the blood involves the effect of hemoglobin to prevent large pH deviations. Hemoglobin is the major nonbicarbonate component in the red blood cells. Because hemoglobin is a protein, its many positive and negative charges can prevent large changes in pH (Fig. 13-7). In addition to buffer systems, the body can moderate large changes in pH through respiratory or breathing mechanisms as well as renal mechanisms (discussed later).

Laboratory Procedures and Limitations

Blood pH is usually measured along with blood gases in a blood gas analyzer. An ISE with a glass membrane that is filled with potassium chloride is used to measure pH. The H⁺ in the sample causes a change in potential difference between the measuring and reference electrodes. This potential is measured by a voltmeter and converted to pH.

• **Figure 13-7** Hemoglobin buffer system. Carbonic anhydrase takes water and carbon dioxide from the plasma and forms carbonic acid in the red blood cell. It also helps break the carbonic acid in the red blood cell into hydrogen and bicarbonate ions. The hemoglobin in the red blood cells combines with carbon dioxide and hydrogen ions to form carboxyhemoglobin. (Modified from Huether SE, McCance KL. *Understanding Pathophysiology.* 5th ed. St. Louis: Mosby; 2013.)

Blood gas analyzers use two different standard buffers to calibrate the ISEs for measuring pH. These electrodes are similar to the stand-alone pH meters found in a laboratory, with the main difference being that the ISEs used to measure blood pH must be very sensitive and are calibrated to a narrow range.

Arterial blood is the specimen of choice for blood pH measurements, but venous blood may be used occasionally. The specimen is collected by the same method as for collection of an arterial blood gas specimen. Test results can be affected by protein buildup or by bacterial growth, so it is important to keep the sample probe and electrodes on the analyzer very clean.

Measurement of pH is a temperature-sensitive procedure, so it is important that the analyzer be maintained at 37° ± 0.05° C on the heat block. For every 30 minutes that a sample is held at room temperature, the pH will decrease by 0.015 pH units, so it is critical to keep the specimen iced until it is run through the analyzer.

Breathing Mechanisms

As discussed earlier in this chapter, the breathing mechanism brings oxygen from the air into the lungs, where it is picked up by red blood cells and delivered to tissues throughout the body for use in metabolism. The breathing mechanism also allows carbon dioxide, which is a byproduct of metabolism, to be removed from the body through exhalation. If a person breaths very slowly, carbon dioxide will build up in the lungs, causing more carbon dioxide to be dissolved in the blood; this increased carbonic acid in the blood lowers the pH. Conversely, if a person breathes very fast, much carbon dioxide is released from the lungs; this increases the bicarbonate in the blood and raises the pH.

Renal Mechanisms

Many nonvolatile acids produced through metabolism are excreted in urine. The kidneys directly excrete H^+ into the urine and form bicarbonate. The kidneys expel H^+ ions complexed with other molecules: with OH^- to form water, with Na and PO_4^- to form NaH_2PO_4, and as NH_2Cl (ammonium chloride). To excrete additional H^+, kidneys use the sodium-hydrogen pump. In the renal tubules, this system pushes H^+ into the tubular fluid (soon to become urine) in exchange for Na^+ ions.

Acid-Base Balance

The pH of blood is a function of two independent variables: the pCO_2 (which is regulated by the lungs or the respiratory mechanism) and the concentration of HCO_3^- (which is regulated by the kidneys or the renal mechanism). As mentioned earlier, the normal blood pH is 7.35 to 7.45, and the body maintains this physiologic balance such that the

rates of input and output are equal during a timed interval. A person is in *acidosis* if the blood pH is lower than 7.35. If the blood pH is higher than 7.45, the person is in *alkalosis*. These two conditions are further differentiated by cause. Respiratory acidosis describes an acidosis that is caused by a respiratory condition. If the condition is caused by a metabolic problem, it is called metabolic acidosis. Likewise, respiratory alkalosis is caused by respiratory conditions, and metabolic alkalosis is caused by metabolic conditions.

Acid-Base Disorders

When examining acid-base disorders, it is helpful to know the origin of the disorder. Metabolic acid-base disorders primarily involve the bicarbonate concentration, whereas respiratory acid-base disorders primarily involve the dissolved carbon dioxide concentration. The four acid-base disorders covered in this section are metabolic acidosis, metabolic alkalosis, respiratory acidosis, and respiratory alkalosis (Fig. 13-8).

Metabolic Acidosis

Metabolic acidosis represents a bicarbonate deficit. This deficit can be caused by many mechanisms that lead to an elevated anion gap acidosis (e.g., methanol ingestion; renal failure uremia; diabetic ketoacidosis; ingestion of isoniazid, iron, or isopropyl alcohol; lactic acidosis; ingestion of ethylene glycol or ethyl alcohol; salicylate intoxication) or to a normal anion gap acidosis (e.g., diarrhea, renal tubular acidosis, liver failure, sulfur toxicity, ammonium chloride excretion) (Box 13-2).

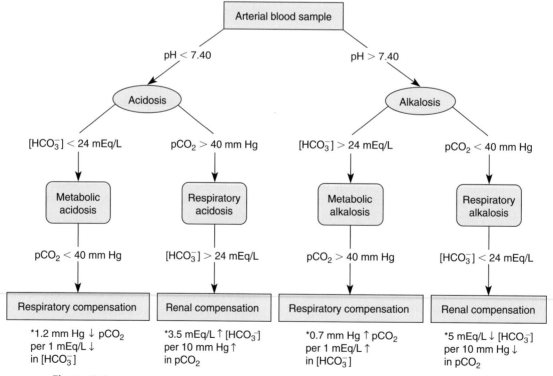

• **Figure 13-8** Approach for the analysis of simple acid-base disorders. *If the compensatory response is not appropriate, a mixed acid-base disorder should be suspected. HCO_3^-, Bicarbonate; pCO_2, partial pressure of carbon dioxide. (From Koeppen BM. *Renal Physiology.* 5th ed. Philadelphia: Mosby; 2013.)

The elevated anion gap acidosis conditions involve the consumption of bicarbonate through buffering of excess hydrogen ions. For example, methanol is metabolized by the liver into formaldehyde and formic acid; accumulation of this acid causes metabolic acidosis. Renal failure uremia is caused by the reduction of H^+ in the renal tubules. This results in a fall in the blood pH leading to metabolic acidosis. Diabetic ketoacidosis results in metabolic acidosis because the body cannot use glucose for energy and must use fats instead. Fat metabolism produces acetoacetic acid, β-hydroxybutyric acid, and acetone; these organic acids result in a metabolic acidosis. Isoniazid toxicity, iron toxicity, and isopropyl alcohol ingestion result in accumulation of lactic acid, causing metabolic acidosis. Lactic acidosis can also be caused by intense exercise, kidney failure, or sepsis. Lactic acid is the end product of anaerobic metabolism and is affected by the rate of metabolism. Ethylene glycol is metabolized into glycolic and oxalic acids; accumulation of these toxic acids may also lead to lactic acid production, making the metabolic acidosis worse. Last, salicylate toxicity (a salicylate level >30 mg/dL) leads to the production of organic acids in the body, producing the metabolic acidosis.

Normal anion gap mechanisms for metabolic acidosis involve the loss of bicarbonate-rich fluid from the body through the kidneys or the gastrointestinal tract. Diarrhea contains much water, potassium, and bicarbonate that is not reabsorbed by the body. Metabolic acidosis results from the loss of these ions. Renal tubular acidosis allows bicarbonate to be lost to the urine instead of being reabsorbed by the kidneys. With the lost buffering power of bicarbonate, the blood's hydrogen ion level increases, causing a metabolic acidosis.

Compensatory Mechanisms

The respiratory mechanism that compensates for metabolic acidosis is stimulated by a low pH. Breathing becomes quick and shallow (hyperventilation) to blow off carbon dioxide

• BOX 13-2 Causes of Metabolic Acidosis

Increased Noncarbonic Acids (Elevated Anion Gap)

Increased H^+ load
Ketoacidosis (e.g., diabetes mellitus, starvation)
Lactic acidosis (e.g., shock)
Ingestions (e.g., ammonium chloride, ethylene glycol, methanol, salicylates, paraldehyde)
Decreased H^+ excretion
Uremia
Distal renal tubule acidosis

Bicarbonate Loss (Normal Anion Gap)

Diarrhea
Ureterosigmoidoscopy
Renal failure
Proximal renal tubule acidosis
Sulfur toxicity

Adapted from McCance KL, Huether SE. *Pathophysiology: The Biologic Basis for Disease in Adults and Children.* 7th ed. St. Louis: Mosby; 2015.

and reduce the pCO_2. The reduced pCO_2 increases the pH, moving it toward the lower limit of normal. In addition, the kidneys try to correct the metabolic acidosis by excreting acid, increasing ammonia formation, and increasing absorption of bicarbonate (Fig. 13-9).

Laboratory Findings

Laboratory findings in metabolic acidosis include an acid pH (<7.35), a low bicarbonate level, decreased pCO_2, and an increased or normal anion gap. In diabetic ketoacidosis, patients have decreased sodium and potassium levels because the kidneys secrete these ions along with organic acids to reestablish the acid-base balance.

Metabolic Alkalosis

Metabolic alkalosis is a primary bicarbonate excess. Three common mechanisms that produce this condition are an increase in bases, decreased excretion of bases, and loss of acidic fluids (Box 13-3). Bases can be increased by massive blood transfusions (i.e., the citrate anticoagulant used in blood collection is a base), by infusion of intravenous solution high in bicarbonate, or by ingestion of large quantities of antacids. In all cases, the amount of bases added to the body causes an alkalotic state.

Secondly, metabolic alkalosis can be caused by decreased excretion of bases resulting in increased bicarbonate levels in the blood. A common example is the prolonged use of diuretics, especially furosemide (Lasix) and bumetanide (Bumex). These diuretics block electrolyte reabsorption and set off a series of reactions that tells the kidney to excrete H^+, which reduces the amount of bicarbonate excreted. Ingestion of a large amount of black licorice also causes alkalosis: Black licorice contains an acid that inhibits an enzyme and causes the kidney to excrete H^+, thus increasing the amount of base in the blood. Hyperaldosteronism and Cushing disease signal the kidney to excrete other electrolytes (e.g., potassium), allowing H^+ to be excreted also. Again, this H^+ excretion increases the base concentration in the blood, resulting in the metabolic alkalosis.

Finally, the loss of acidic fluids can cause the base concentration in the blood to increase. Prolonged vomiting results in loss of acidic fluids to the environment. An upper duodenal obstruction prevents acidic fluids from reaching the intestines where the H^+ in the fluid can be absorbed. In cystic fibrosis, an individual's ability to produce H^+ is reduced, leading to smaller amounts of acid in the individual's body.

Compensatory Mechanisms

To combat the pH increase in the blood, the body attempts to use the respiratory system to decrease blood pH. This is accomplished by retaining carbon dioxide: Slower and deeper breaths bring more carbon dioxide into the lungs and provide additional time for it to diffuse into the blood. The addition of carbon dioxide to the blood results in the formation of carbonic acid, which reduces the pH of the blood. The kidneys also try to combat alkalosis by excreting more bicarbonate and forming less ammonia, thus decreasing the amount of bases that enter the blood (Fig. 13-10).

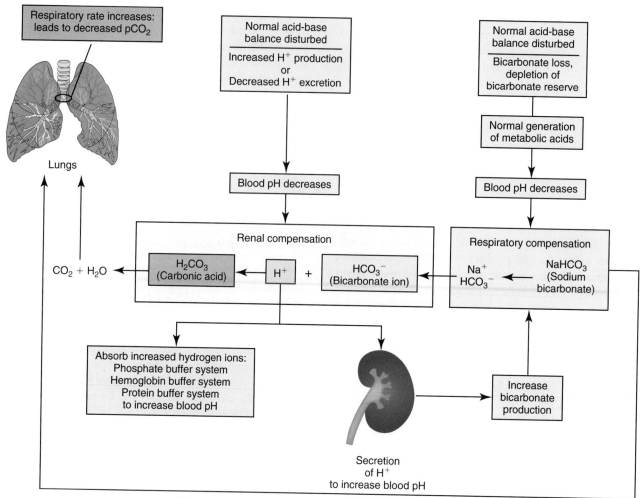

• **Figure 13-9** Metabolic acidosis and compensatory mechanisms.

• BOX 13-3 **Causes of Metabolic Alkalosis**

Excessive licorice ingestion
Cushing syndrome
Hyperaldosteronism
Cystic fibrosis
Prolonged vomiting
Pyloric or upper duodenal obstruction

Laboratory Findings

The blood pH in metabolic alkalosis is higher than 7.45. If it surpasses 7.55, the person may go into tetany, even with a normal calcium level. Because it is a primary bicarbonate excess condition, it follows that the bicarbonate level is also increased. This condition originates in the kidneys, so the pCO_2 is normal.

Respiratory Acidosis

Respiratory acidosis is a condition in which the amount of carbon dioxide eliminated from the lungs is decreased. The causes associated with decreased carbon dioxide elimination

can be either acute or chronic, and they can depress the respiratory center or physically affect the respiratory organs (Box 13-4 and Fig. 13-11). Acute conditions that depress the respiratory center include ingestion of drugs (e.g., narcotics, barbiturates), central nervous system trauma (e.g., cerebrovascular accident), and infection (e.g., meningitis) or inflammation (e.g., encephalitis). An example of a chronic condition that depresses the respiratory center is a comatose state. Acute conditions that affect the respiratory organs include asthma attacks, ARDS, pulmonary edema, pleural effusion, and pneumothorax. The most common chronic condition affecting the respiratory organs is chronic obstructive pulmonary disease. Other diseases that affect respiratory organs and produce respiratory acidosis include sleep apnea and extreme obesity.

Compensatory Mechanisms

Respiratory acidosis is immediately compensated for by the hemoglobin and protein buffers systems in the blood. The kidneys compensate for respiratory acidosis by a method similar to that for metabolic acidosis: excrete more acids, absorb more bicarbonate, and form more ammonia. Renal compensation is slow; it is apparent at 6 to 12 hours but optimal in 2 to 3 days.

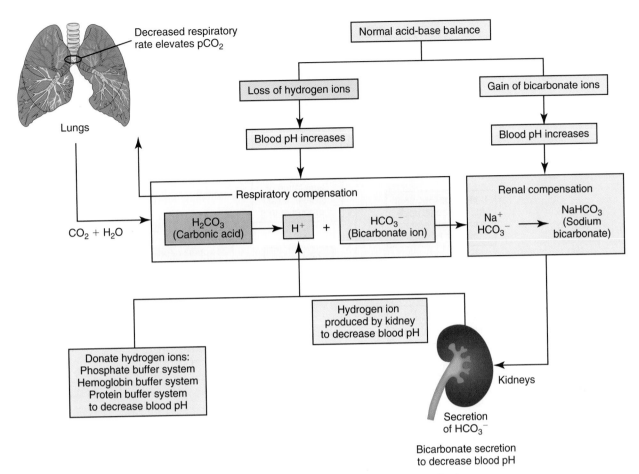

• **Figure 13-10** Metabolic alkalosis and compensatory mechanisms.

Drugs (narcotics and barbiturates)
Comatose states
Chronic obstructive pulmonary states (COPD)
Central hypoventilation
Severe asthma
Adult respiratory distress syndrome (ARDS)
Sleep apnea
Pleural effusion or pneumothorax

Compensation for respiratory acidosis by the respiratory organs depends on their ability to function. For example, if respiratory acidosis is caused by a pneumothorax, limited compensation can be provided by the lungs because one of the lungs is collapsed. If the organs are functional, the respiratory center will change the breathing pattern to increase the rate and depth of breaths. This helps the body eliminate more carbon dioxide to return the blood pH to normal.

Laboratory Findings

In respiratory acidosis, the pH is lower than 7.35, the pCO_2 is increased, and the bicarbonate concentration is normal. In acute respiratory acidosis, the pH drops by approximately 0.10 pH unit for every 15 mm Hg increase in pCO_2. In chronic respiratory acidosis, the pH drops only about 0.05 pH unit for every 15 mm Hg increase in pCO_2.

Respiratory Alkalosis

Respiratory alkalosis results from a primary deficit in pCO_2. This is usually caused by an increased rate or depth of breathing or both (Box 13-5). This means that the basic mechanism is excessive elimination of acid via the respiratory route or hyperventilation faster than the cells can produce carbon dioxide (Fig. 13-12). This condition is caused by anxiety, excessive crying, gram-negative septicemia, meningitis or encephalitis, cerebral vascular accidents, hypoxia, drugs (salicylates, catecholamines, or theophylline), hyperthyroidism, pneumonia, pulmonary emboli, or congestive heart failure. Anxiety and excessive crying cause rapid breathing so that carbon dioxide is blown off, reducing the amount of CO_2 in the blood. Gram-negative septicemia produces acute circulatory failure, which leads to hypoxia and hyperventilation and then to respiratory alkalosis. This mechanism is similar to that of congestive heart failure, which also produces circulatory failure. Meningitis, encephalitis, and cerebral vascular accidents can stimulate the central respiratory receptors and cause hyperventilation. Drugs also stimulate the central respiratory receptors to cause hyperventilation. Hyperthyroidism can lead to anxiety, which can produce hyperventilation, the

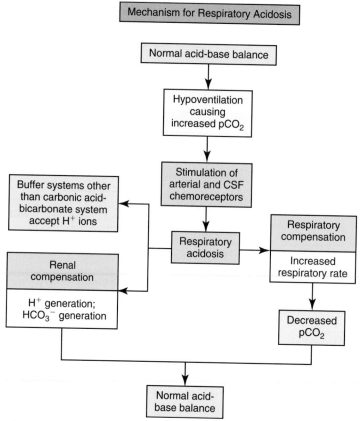

• **Figure 13-11** Respiratory acidosis and compensatory mechanisms. *CSF,* Cerebrospinal fluid.

• **BOX 13-5** **Causes of Respiratory Alkalosis**

Anxiety
Gram-negative septicemia
Meningitis or encephalitis
Cerebrovascular accidents
Hypoxia
Drugs—salicylates, catecholamines
Hyperthyroidism
Pneumonia
Pulmonary embolism
Congestive heart failure

---

hallmark of respiratory alkalosis. Finally, pneumonia or pulmonary emboli can produce a hypoxic state that stimulates central respiratory control centers to increase breathing and may lead to hyperventilation.

Compensatory Mechanisms

The compensatory mechanisms for respiratory alkalosis occur in two stages. First, the hemoglobin and protein buffer systems release H^+ to help combat the rise in pH. Then, in a longer time frame, the kidneys excrete more bicarbonate to help normalize the blood pH.

Laboratory Findings

In respiratory alkalosis, the pH is higher than 7.45, the pCO_2 is decreased, and the bicarbonate level is normal. Individuals who live at high altitudes have low pCO_2 values and are thought to chronically hyperventilate when compared to individuals who live at sea level.

Interpreting Blood Gas Analyses

Interpretation of blood gas results is necessary to determine a patient's acid-base status (Fig. 13-13). Use of a systematic analysis method can help take some of the mystique out of the interpretation:

1. Look at the pH of the blood gas results. Is it normal (7.35 to 7.45)?
2. Is it less than 7.35 (acidosis) or greater than 7.45 (alkalosis)?
3. Is the origin metabolic or respiratory? Look at the relationship between the direction of change (higher or lower) in the pCO_2 and in the pH. The pH and the pCO_2 changes are in the opposite directions for respiratory disorders and in the same direction for metabolic disorders.
4. Is the condition compensated? The primary disorder is the abnormal value that corresponds to the abnormal pH: in alkalosis, it will be a low pCO_2 or a high HCO_3^-; in acidosis, it will be a high pCO_2 or a low HCO_3^-. Once the primary disorder has been identified, the other abnormal parameter is recognized as the compensation, if the direction of the change is the same as for the primary abnormality. Reference/normal values: pH: 7.35-7.45; pO_2: 83-108 mm Hg; pCO_2: 35-48 mm Hg; bicarbonate: 23-30 meq/L.

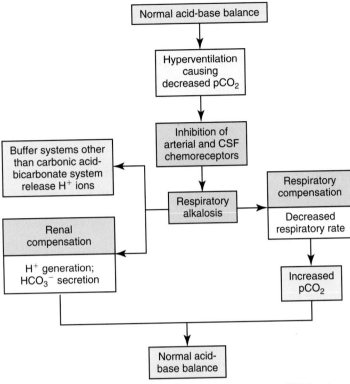

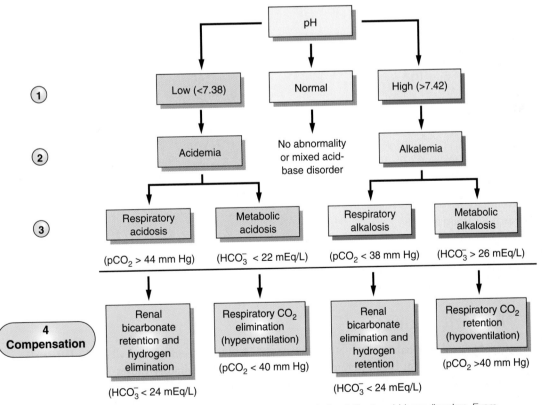

• **Figure 13-12** Respiratory alkalosis and compensatory mechanisms. *CSF,* Cerebrospinal fluid.

• **Figure 13-13** Flow chart for interpreting arterial blood gas results in relation to acid-base disorders. Examine the pH first. Then examine the changes in bicarbonate concentration (HCO_3^-) and partial pressure of carbon dioxide (pCO_2). HCO_3^- is elevated when there is a primary metabolic alkalosis or with renal compensation for primary respiratory acidosis. HCO_3^- is decreased when there is a primary metabolic acidosis or with renal compensation for primary respiratory alkalosis. pCO_2 is elevated when there is primary respiratory acidosis or with respiratory compensation for primary metabolic alkalosis. pCO_2 is decreased when there is primary respiratory alkalosis or with respiratory compensation for metabolic acidosis. (From McCance KL, Huether SE. *Pathophysiology: The Biologic Basis for Disease in Adults and Children.* 7th ed. St. Louis: Mosby; 2015.)

Summary

Acid-base disturbances represent serious medical conditions. Acid-base disturbances are classified as acidosis (pH <7.35) or alkalosis (pH >7.45), with the main cause stemming from the respiratory or metabolic (kidney) components. The main parameters for determining acid-base balance are pH, pCO_2, and HCO_3^-. There are several buffer systems in the blood that help minimize large changes in pH; these are the bicarbonate, protein, hemoglobin, and phosphate systems. There are four acid-base disturbances: metabolic acidosis, metabolic alkalosis, respiratory acidosis, and respiratory alkalosis. It is important to interpret blood gas analyses correctly so that the patient will receive appropriate treatment.

Review Questions

1. A patient's blood gas results are pH, 7.5; pCO_2, 15 mm Hg; HCO_3^-, 40 mmol/L. These results indicate
   a. Respiratory alkalosis
   b. Metabolic acidosis
   c. Metabolic alkalosis
   d. Respiratory acidosis

2. Which set of results is consistent with uncompensated metabolic acidosis?
   a. pH, 7.55; pCO_2, 60 mm Hg; HCO_3^-, 40 mmol/L
   b. pH, 7.25; pCO_2, 60 mm Hg; HCO_3^-, 40 mmol/L
   c. pH, 7.20; pCO_2, 28 mm Hg; HCO_3^-, 15 mmol/L
   d. pH, 7.50; pCO_2, 29 mm Hg; HCO_3^-, 15 mmol/L

3. Which of the following is the primary mechanism of compensation for metabolic acidosis?
   a. Hyperventilation
   b. Aldosterone release
   c. Release of epinephrine
   d. Bicarbonate excretion

4. Determine the anion gap given the following serum electrolyte data: Na, 132 mEq/L; K, 4.5 mEq/L; Cl, 90 mEq/L; CO_2, 22 mmol/L?
   a. 64 mEq/L
   b. 20 mEq/L
   c. 30 mEq/L
   d. 24.5 mEq/L

5. Which of the following is the primary mechanism causing respiratory alkalosis?
   a. Renal failure
   b. Hyperventilation
   c. Too much bicarbonate
   d. Congestive heart failure

6. Respiratory control centers are located in the
   a. Hypothalamus, carotid artery, and aorta
   b. Lungs, carotid artery, and vena cava
   c. Brainstem, lungs, and heart
   d. Brainstem, carotid artery, and aorta

7. A child sleeps with his head under the covers. If blood gases were drawn on this child, what would the results show?
   a. pH decreased, oxygen saturation decreased, pO_2 decreased, and pCO_2 increased
   b. pH increased, oxygen saturation decreased, pO_2 increased, and pCO_2 increased
   c. pH decreased, oxygen saturation decreased, pO_2 decreased, and pCO_2 increased
   d. pH decreased, oxygen saturation increased, pO_2 decreased, and pCO_2 decreased

8. The renal mechanism for maintaining acid-base balance in the body involves which of the following?
   a. The amount of blood flushed through the kidneys
   b. The amount of sodium and chloride retained and excreted by the kidney
   c. The amount of hydrogen ions secreted by the kidney
   d. The amount of urine excreted by the kidney

9. Which of the following are normal blood gas values for people living at high altitude?
   a. pH, 7.40; pCO_2, 20 mm Hg; HCO_3^-, 30 mEq/L
   b. pH, 7.67; pCO_2, 20 mm Hg; HCO_3^-, 15 mEq/L
   c. pH, 7.01; pCO_2, 25 mm Hg; HCO_3^-, (–5) mEq/L
   d. pH, 7.25; pCO_2, 25 mm Hg; HCO_3^-, (–5) mEq/L

10. If a blood gas specimen is left exposed to the air for an extended period, which of the following changes will occur?
    a. pO_2 increases, pH and pCO_2 decrease
    b. pO_2 decreases, pH and pCO_2 increase
    c. pO_2 and pH increase, pCO_2 decreases
    d. pO_2 and pH decrease, pCO_2 increases

Critical Thinking Questions

1. What is meant by "acid-base balance"?
2. What are the normal values for blood pH, pO_2, pCO_2, and bicarbonate in adults?
3. Define acidosis and alkalosis. Relate these to metabolic and respiratory causes. What are some explanations for each?

CASE STUDY

A 52-year-old woman was admitted to the hospital in a semicomatose condition. Her husband reports that she had the flu for 4 days before admission and had been vomiting. In spite of the vomiting, she had continued to drink large quantities of water. She was a known diabetic. Her pulse was weak and rapid, and her blood pressure was normal. Her laboratory values were as follows:

Glucose	454 mg/dL
CO_2	11 mg/dL
Na	130 mEq/L
K	7.6 mEq/L
Cl	93 mEq/L
pH	7.27
pCO_2	24 mm Hg
HCO_3^-	24 mmol/L
pO_2	91 mm Hg

When a patient is vomiting, how does continuing to drink large quantities of water affect the serum electrolyte values? What effect does a high amount of blood sugar have on urinary output? Evaluate the laboratory reports. Describe the results of the low pCO_2 in this case. What condition is this patient in?

Bibliography

Burtis CA, Bruns DE. *Tietz Textbook of Clinical Chemistry and Molecular Diagnostics*. 7th ed. Philadelphia: Saunders; 2015.

McCance K, Huether S. *Pathophysiology: The Biologic Basis for Disease in Adults and Children*. 7th ed. St. Louis: Mosby; 2014.

14

Blood Diseases

SHERYL BERMAN

CHAPTER OUTLINE

Introduction

Hematopoiesis

White Blood Cells

Normal Physiology

Leukemias

Hodgkin and Non-Hodgkin Lymphomas

Red Blood Cells

Hemoglobin

Clinical Correlations

Clinical Chemistry Tests

Summary

OBJECTIVES

At the completion of this chapter, the reader will be able to:

1. Define "hematopoiesis."
2. List the different types of white blood cells.
3. List the characteristics of acute lymphocytic leukemia, acute myelogenous leukemia, chronic lymphocytic leukemia, chronic myelogenous leukemia, hairy cell leukemia, myelodysplastic syndrome, Hodgkin lymphoma, and non-Hodgkin lymphoma.
4. List the chemistry test results that are elevated in leukemia and lymphoma cases.
5. Describe how lymphomas are staged.
6. Describe the structure of hemoglobin.
7. Explain iron homeostasis.
8. Describe ferritin and its function.
9. Describe transferrin and its function.
10. Diagram a porphyrin, and explain how porphyrins form heme.
11. Describe heme synthesis.
12. Discuss the chemistry tests used to determine iron deficiency.
13. Describe hemosiderosis and hemochromatosis.
14. Describe porphyria disorders.
15. Describe three types of modified hemoglobin structures that interfere with normal hemoglobin function.
16. Describe the hemoglobin E, C, S, and SC variants.
17. Describe α-thalassemia, β-thalassemia major, β-thalassemia intermedia, and β-thalassemia minor.
18. Define anemia.
19. Describe aplastic anemia, anemia of chronic renal and endocrine diseases, pernicious anemia, folate and vitamin B_{12} deficiency anemia, iron deficiency anemia, immune hemolytic anemia, hereditary spherocytosis and elliptocytosis, glucose-6-phosphate dehydrogenase deficiency, and paroxysmal nocturnal hemoglobinuria.
20. Describe the tests for iron, total iron-binding capacity, ferritin, and hemosiderin.
21. Calculate the transferrin saturation.
22. Describe normal results for a hemoglobin electrophoresis.
23. Describe abnormal results for a hemoglobin electrophoresis.
24. Describe the hemoglobin electrophoresis procedure.
25. Describe the high-performance liquid chromatography method for separating hemoglobins.
26. Describe how electron spray spectroscopy is used to separate hemoglobins.
27. Describe how DNA analysis is used for patient education in high-risk populations.
28. Describe a test for hemoglobin H.
29. Describe the methods used in sickle cell screening tests.
30. Describe analytic methods for diagnosing and monitoring porphyrias.

KEY TERMS

Acute lymphocytic leukemia
Acute myelogenous leukemia
Anemia of chronic renal and endocrine diseases
Aplastic anemia
Apotransferrin

Carboxyhemoglobin
Chronic lymphocytic leukemia
Chronic myelogenous leukemia
Ferritin
Ferrous protoporphyrin IX
Fetal hemoglobin

Folate and vitamin B_{12} deficiency anemia
Glucose-6-phosphate dehydrogenase deficiency
Hairy cell leukemia
Hemoglobin C

❖ Case in Point

Ms. A, a 21-year-old college student, had been a vegetarian since she was 16 years old. Lately, she had been feeling weak and dizzy and has reported tingling in her feet. Her roommate convinced her to go to the college health center. Her complete blood count showed a 9.4 g/dL hemoglobin level and 28% hematocrit. What type of anemia is the most likely considering her history? What tests would her doctor likely order?

Points to Remember

- Hematopoiesis is the production of new blood cells, including creation, maturation, and differentiation.
- Leukemias are malignant diseases in which the bone marrow and other blood-forming organs produce increased numbers of immature, abnormal white blood cells that are released into peripheral blood instead of mature, normal white blood cells.
- Acute lymphocytic leukemia (ALL) occurs most commonly among children and adolescents.
- Acute myelogenous leukemia (AML) is a malignant disease in which the bone marrow makes abnormal myeloid cell precursors that stop maturing in the early stages of development.
- Chronic lymphocytic leukemia (CLL) is a disease characterized by a large number of small, nonfunctional lymphocytes.
- Chronic myelogenous leukemia (CML) is a malignant disease in which the bone marrow produces increased numbers of mature myelocytes (i.e., neutrophils, basophils, and eosinophils). The cells of CML patients have the Philadelphia chromosome translocation.
- Hairy cell leukemia (HCL) is a chronic lymphoid leukemia in which cells look as if they have hairlike projections.
- Lymphomas are abnormal growths of lymphoid tissue in lymph nodes and vessels. They are classified as Hodgkin and non-Hodgkin lymphomas.
- Staging of lymphomas is important to determine the type of therapy needed and the patient's prognosis.

- Hemoglobin is composed of four globin molecules that each contain one molecule of heme.
- Iron is found in the body as storage iron, tissue iron, myoglobin, and a circulating pool.
- The iron-storage protein ferritin consists of an apoferritin shell and a core of ferric oxyhydroxide.
- Hemosiderin is an iron-containing metabolic byproduct of ferritin degradation by lysozymes.
- Tissue iron consists of iron-dependent peroxidases and cytochromes.
- Myoglobin is a single-chain molecule that resembles hemoglobin and serves as an enzyme.
- Porphyrin consists of four pyrrole rings that bind one iron molecule to form heme.
- The hemoglobin molecule consists of four subunits: two α-proteins and two β-proteins; each subunit contains a heme group.
- Hemoglobin transports oxygen to cells and carbon dioxide away from cells.
- Heme is synthesized in the liver as well as in the bone marrow.
- The heme-containing hemoglobin molecule is synthesized in immature red blood cells in the bone marrow.
- Fetal hemoglobin is composed four subunits, two α-proteins and two γ-proteins, each of which contain a heme group. The γ-subunit is commonly called the fetal hemoglobin subunit.
- Anemia is a deficiency of red blood cells or hemoglobin (<12 g/dL for women and <13 g/dL for men).
- Symptoms of anemia include weakness, tachycardia, pale mucous membranes, and dizziness or lightheadedness.
- Iron deficiency anemia is a condition in which the body lacks enough iron to produce healthy red blood cells. As a result, red blood cells are very small and their oxygen-carrying capacity is decreased.
- Iron deficiency anemia is a microcytic anemia that is diagnosed using tests for serum iron, total iron-binding capacity (TIBC), and ferritin.
- Hereditary hemochromatosis is a genetic disease that causes the body to absorb and store too much iron,

leading to increased transferrin saturation, increased serum iron levels, and possible iron deposits in the liver.

- Carboxyhemoglobin is a hemoglobin molecule which is bound to carbon monoxide Carbon monoxide binds strongly to hemoglobin and cannot be displaced by oxygen, rendering the hemoglobin molecule nonfunctional for oxygen transport.
- Sulfhemoglobin is a form of hemoglobin that contains an irreversibly bound sulfur molecule that prevents normal oxygen binding.
- Methemoglobin is the result of hemoglobin reacting with oxidizing agents to produce heme with Fe^{3+} instead of Fe^{2+}. Because the iron is in the oxidized state, this hemoglobin cannot bind oxygen.
- Hemoglobinopathies result from genetic mutations in hemoglobin proteins. Examples include hemoglobin E, homozygous hemoglobin S (i.e., sickle cell disease), heterozygous hemoglobin S (i.e., sickle cell trait), and hemoglobin SC (i.e., variant of homozygous SS disease).
- Thalassemias are hereditary hemolytic diseases caused by abnormal hemoglobin formation in which a globin protein is missing from the hemoglobin molecule:
  - α-Thalassemia (i.e., Barts hemoglobin) lacks α-globin genes
  - Hemoglobin H has four β-chains
  - β-Thalassemia major (i.e., Cooley anemia) contains hemoglobin F and no hemoglobin A
  - β-Thalassemia intermedia contains decreased α- and β-chains and increased hemoglobin F
  - β-Thalassemia minor is an asymptomatic condition
- Aplastic anemia is a deficiency of all types of blood cells caused by failure of bone marrow development. Red marrow is replaced by fat and non–cell-producing tissue.
- Pernicious anemia is a macrocytic anemia caused by reduced vitamin B_{12} absorption due to lack of intrinsic factor.
- Folate and vitamin B_{12} deficiencies produce a macrocytic anemia. Assays for folate and vitamin B_{12} help to diagnose this condition.
- Immune hemolytic anemia occurs when antibodies form against red blood cells and destroy them before the end of their life span. It is associated with membrane defects, hemoglobinopathies, and immune disorders.
- Glucose-6-phosphate dehydrogenase (G6PD) deficiency can produce a hemolytic anemia, which is diagnosed with a G6PD screening test.
- In paroxysmal nocturnal hemoglobinuria, a genetic defect allows early destruction of red blood cells by complement. This hemoglobin accumulates overnight, leading to dark-colored morning urine.
- Transferrin saturation, is the ratio of serum iron to total iron-binding capacity (TIBC) multiplied by 100 (100 × serum iron/TIBC).
- To test the iron level, the serum pH is reduced, the iron molecules are reduced, and then a chromogen is used to produce a colored complex. The concentration of iron is directly proportional to the serum iron concentration.

- Ferritin is measured by enzyme-linked immunoassay (ELISA), immunoluminescence, and immunoturbidimetric methods.
- Transferrin is measured by immunoturbimetric and immunonephelometric methods.
- Hemoglobin electrophoresis is performed on cellulose acetate with a pH between 8.2 and 8.6.
- High-performance liquid chromatography (HPLC) and electron spray mass spectroscopy can be used to separate hemoglobins and diagnose hemoglobinopathies.
- Sickling tests involve reducing a sample with sodium hyposulfite. If hemoglobin S is present, the resulting solution is cloudy. If there is no hemoglobin S, the solution remains clear.

Introduction

The two major divisions of white blood cell diseases are lymphoma and leukemia. The classification and diagnosis of Hodgkin and non-Hodgkin lymphomas and the major leukemias are discussed in this chapter. Anemia is the primary red blood cell abnormality, and the chemistry tests, methods, and reference ranges used to diagnose and monitor these conditions are described. Other topics include porphyrin physiology, the role of iron in the body, and hemoglobinopathies.

Hematopoiesis

Hematopoiesis is the production of new blood cells, including creation, maturation, and differentiation. There are several types of blood cells, and each is the product of a specific type of parent cell. The multipotent stem cell begins the process of producing blood cells as it differentiates into a myeloid stem cell and a lymphocyte stem cell. The myeloid stem cell further differentiates into megakaryocytes, red blood cells, mast cells, and myeloblasts; myeloblasts transform into basophils, eosinophils, neutrophils, and monocytes. The maturation process from stem cells to mature cells is complex and involves many different types of growth factors. Diseases of white blood cells affect body chemistry.

White Blood Cells

Normal Physiology

Several types of white blood cells are found in peripheral blood: neutrophils (segmented and band), lymphocytes, eosinophils, basophils, and monocytes (Fig. 14-1). Neutrophils engulf and destroy foreign antigens in the blood. Lymphocytes engulf and kill antigens or foreign or defective cells directly or produce antibodies against antigens. Basophils and eosinophils have special granules that release their contents in allergic reactions and against parasites. Monocytes are phagocytic cells that engulf debris and foreign antigens. Two broad classifications of abnormal conditions involving myeloid and lymphoid cells are leukemia and lymphoma.

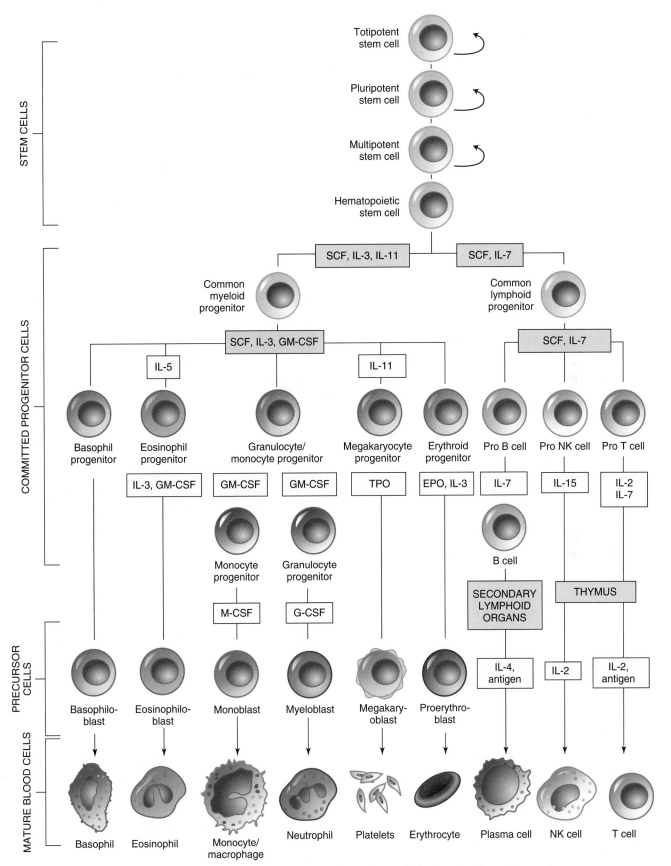

• **Figure 14-1** Differentiation of hematopoietic cells. *Curved arrows* indicate proliferation and expansion of prehematopoietic stem cell populations. *EPO,* Erythropoietin; *G-CSF,* granulocyte colony-stimulating factor; *GM-CSF,* granulocyte-macrophage colony-stimulating factor; *IL,* interleukin; *M-CSF,* macrophage colony-stimulating factor; *NK,* natural killer; *SCF,* stem cell factor; *TPO,* thrombopoietin. (From McCance KL, Huether SE. *Pathophysiology: The Biologic Basis for Disease in Adults and Children.* 7th ed. St. Louis: Mosby; 2015.)

Leukemias

Leukemias are malignant diseases in which abnormal, non-functional white blood cells are released into peripheral blood instead of mature, normal cells. Individuals with acute leukemias have blasts (i.e., primitive, undifferentiated blood cells) in peripheral blood, whereas those with chronic leukemias have immature white blood cells. The total white blood cell count in different leukemias varies from less than $4.5 \times 10^9/L$ to $100 \times 10^9/L$. Because blasts and immature cells do not function like mature cells to phagocytize microorganisms and foreign antigens, affected individuals are prone to infections.

Acute Lymphocytic Leukemia

Acute lymphocytic leukemia (ALL), also called acute lymphoblastic leukemia, is the most common type of leukemia among children and adolescents, but it can also affect adults. In ALL, early lymphoid precursors (i.e., lymphoblasts) proliferate and rapidly replace normal cells in the bone marrow and peripheral blood (Fig. 14-2). ALL patients usually have neutropenia, anemia, and decreased platelet counts. Lactate dehydrogenase (LDH) and uric acid levels are increased. Many patients have disseminated intravascular coagulation (DIC), an elevated prothrombin time, a decreased fibrinogen level, and a positive test result for fibrin split products (or D-dimer) produced by clot degeneration. Other useful diagnostic studies include a chest radiograph, a computed tomography (CT) scan, and an electrocardiogram.

Acute Myelogenous Leukemia

Acute myelogenous leukemia (AML), also called acute myeloid leukemia, is a malignant disease in which the bone marrow makes abnormal myeloid cell precursors that stop maturing in the early stages of development instead of maturing into myelocytes, red blood cells, and platelets. Patients with AML usually have more than 20% blasts in the bone marrow.

AML can be associated with other hematologic disorders, familial syndromes, and exposures to environmental toxins, although many patients have no identifiable risk factors. AML is caused by chromosomal translocations or other genetic factors.

AML patients usually have anemia, thrombocytopenia, and neutropenia because the production of normal blood cells quickly decreases. The abnormal cells do not undergo programmed cell death (i.e., apoptosis), so they accumulate in the bone marrow, blood, spleen, and liver. A complete blood count (CBC) and a differential count of white blood cells are the initial screening tests for this disease (Fig. 14-3). A bone marrow biopsy is necessary for diagnosis. AML patients may have DIC, a prolonged prothrombin time, an increased fibrinogen level, and a positive test result for fibrin split products (or D-dimer). A chemistry metabolic panel reveals elevated LDH and uric acid levels.

Chronic Lymphocytic Leukemia

Chronic lymphocytic leukemia (CLL) is characterized by proliferation of a large number of small, nonfunctional

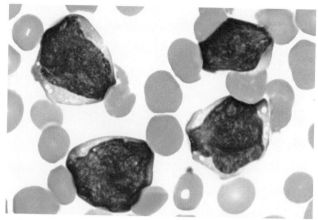

• **Figure 14-2** In acute lymphocytic leukemia, large lymphoblasts with prominent nucleoli and membrane irregularities are seen in peripheral blood (×1000). (From Carr JH, Rodak BF: *Clinical Hematology Atlas.* 4th ed, St. Louis: Saunders; 2013.)

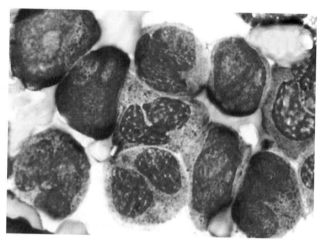

• **Figure 14-3** In acute myelogenous leukemia, blasts constitute 20% or more of the nucleated cells of the bone marrow, and there is maturation beyond the promyelocyte stage in more than 10% of the nonerythroid cells. (From Keohane EM, Smith LJ, Walenga JM. *Rodak's Hematology.* 5th ed. St. Louis: Saunders; 2016.)

lymphocytes. CLL is the most common form of leukemia in adults in Western countries. CLL progresses slowly, and many individuals remain asymptomatic for several years.

Chromosomal mutations on chromosome 17 and other genetic abnormalities exist in some patients with CLL. Flow cytometry and a bone marrow biopsy may be used to establish the diagnosis of CLL. There are no specific clinical chemistry tests for diagnosing or confirming CLL.

Chronic Myelogenous Leukemia

Chronic myelogenous leukemia (CML), also known as chronic myeloid leukemia, is a malignant disease in which the bone marrow produces increased numbers of granulocytes (Fig. 14-4). CML accounts for 20% of all adult leukemias. The result of a CBC with differential usually alerts providers to a leukemia, and a biopsy that finds the Philadelphia (Ph1) chromosome translocation in bone marrow cells is diagnostic for CML. Elevated uric acid levels result from the high turnover

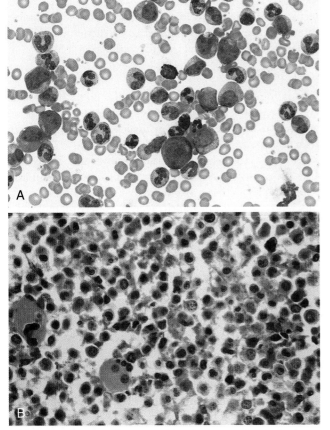

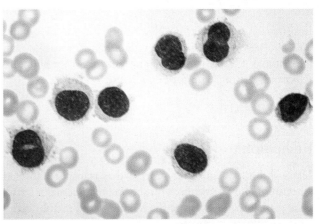

• **Figure 14-5** Hairy cell leukemia. In stained smears, these cells have round or folded nuclei and modest amounts of pale blue, agranular cytoplasm. (From Kumar V, Abbas AK, Aster JC. *Robbins and Cotran Pathologic Basis for Disease.* 9th ed. Philadelphia: Saunders; 2015.)

• **Figure 14-4** Chronic myelogenous leukemia (CML). **A,** Peripheral blood film shows the chronic phase of CML, with a bimodal population of segmented neutrophils and myelocytes (×500). **B,** Bone marrow biopsy specimen shows the chronic phase of CML, with hypercellularity of granulocytes and megakaryocytes (hematoxylin and eosin stain, ×400). (From Keohane EM, Smith LJ, Walenga JM. *Rodak's Hematology.* 5th ed. St. Louis: Saunders;; 2016.)

of bone marrow cells. CML patients also have elevated levels of vitamin B_{12} binding proteins (e.g., transcobalamin I).

Hairy Cell Leukemia

Hairy cell leukemia (HCL) is a chronic lymphoid leukemia in which the abnormal B lymphocytes have hairlike cytoplasmic projections on their surface (Fig. 14-5). Abnormal B cell growth may result from exposure to environmental toxins in some cases.

The diagnosis of HCL is based on examination of blood and bone marrow biopsy specimens to identify cells with the morphologic features of hairy cells. However, bone marrow aspirates may result in a "dry tap" with no marrow obtained. Cytochemical stains are used to confirm the diagnosis. Chemistry tests are not helpful in diagnosing this condition.

Myelodysplastic Syndromes

Myelodysplastic syndromes are a group of malignant hematopoietic stem cell disorders characterized by ineffective blood cell production resulting in a hypercellular or hypocellular marrow and decreased numbers of all blood cells. Erythrocytic, granulocytic, and megakaryocytic cell

lines can be involved. Myelodysplastic syndromes are considered premalignant in some patients and can progress to AML. The diagnosis is made with a CBC with differential, cytochemistry, and bone marrow studies. Clinical chemistry tests are not used in diagnosing this syndrome.

Hodgkin and Non-Hodgkin Lymphomas

Pathophysiology

Lymphoma is an abnormal growth of lymphatic tissue (i.e., cancer) in the lymph nodes and lymphatic vessels. The three primary types of lymphocytes are B cells, T cells, and natural killer cells. B lymphocytes produce antibodies and defend against infections. T lymphocytes kill infected cells and help to regulate other parts of the immune system. Natural killer cells also destroy abnormal cells such as cancer cells. Lymphomas originate from abnormal or transformed B or T cells. Malignant transformation is a multistep, gradual process involving a DNA abnormality. The cancer cells are said to be "transformed."

The two major types of lymphoma are Hodgkin and non-Hodgkin lymphomas. Hodgkin lymphoma originates from abnormal B cells, whereas non-Hodgkin lymphoma originates from abnormal B or T cells. The cause is unknown, but viral infection and DNA mutation are suspected.

Non-Hodgkin lymphoma is eight times more common than Hodgkin lymphoma. There are five classifications of Hodgkin lymphoma and more than 30 classifications of non-Hodgkin lymphoma, based on the type of tumor and the extent of the disease.

Clinical Correlation and Clinical Chemistry Tests

Early-stage lymphomas may have normal hematology and clinical chemistry test results. The diseases are usually differentiated on a lymph node or bone marrow biopsy. Hodgkin lymphoma is marked by the presence of tumor cells called Reed-Sternberg cells. Clinical laboratory studies include a CBC, liver function tests, kidney function tests, and bone marrow biopsies. Other tests used for diagnosis of lymphomas include CT scans, PET scans, chest radiographs, and magnetic resonance imaging (MRI) scans.

Staging

Information gathered from blood tests, imaging tests, and biopsies help with staging of Hodgkin and Non-Hodgkin lymphomas (Table 14-1). Staging allows the provider to select therapies and monitor disease progression.

Red Blood Cells

Hemoglobin

Hemoglobin is a globular protein that transports oxygen and carbon dioxide throughout the body. It is a major structural protein component of the red blood cell membrane.

Hemoglobin structure is complex. The molecule is made up of four globin chains (i.e., two α-proteins and two β-proteins), each of which cradles a molecule of heme in its tertiary structure (Fig. 14-6). Proteins have four levels of structure. The primary structure is determined by the carbon, hydrogen, and oxygen molecules that comprise the molecule;

TABLE 14-1	Stages of Lymphoma
Stage	**Definition**
I	Disease is found in a single lymph node or in a single organ.
II	Two or more lymph nodes are involved, but they are on the same side of the diaphragm.
III	Two or more lymph nodes are involved that are on opposite sides of the diaphragm.
IV	Disease is spread throughout the body, especially in the spleen, bone marrow, skeleton, and central nervous system.

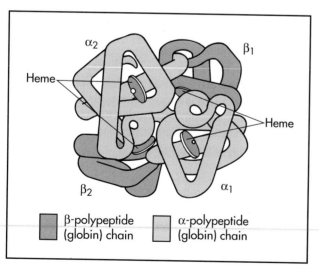

• **Figure 14-6** Structure of hemoglobin. The molecule is a spherical tetramer weighing approximately 64,500 daltons. It contains a pair of α-polypeptide and a pair of β-polypeptide chains and several heme groups. (From McCance KL, Huether SE. *Pathophysiology: The Biologic Basis for Disease in Adults and Children.* 7th ed. St. Louis: Mosby; 2015.)

secondary structure consists of α-helixes and β-pleated sheets; tertiary structure is the folding of the molecule, including intramolecular bonds; and quaternary structure depends on proteins that link together to form complex molecules.

Iron

Iron is found and used throughout the body. It is a vital component of hemoglobin and is also found in myoglobin, attached to enzymes, stored in tissues, and available in an iron circulating pool.

Ferritin and hemosiderin are iron-storage molecules. Ferritin consists of an apoferritin shell surrounding an iron core complex of ferric oxyhydroxide. Hemosiderin granules represent partly degraded, aggregated ferritin molecules whose shells have been digested by lysozymes. Hemosiderin is the end of the intracellular storage iron pathway.

Food consumed in a normal diet contains enough iron to meet average metabolic needs. Iron absorption from digested food in the intestines is regulated through a negative feedback loop. If iron levels in the liver are low, the body increases iron absorption, but if the iron levels are high, the body decreases absorption. Iron absorption is facilitated by regulatory proteins such as β-microglobulin, transferrin, and ceruloplasmin.

Absorbed iron must be transported by a carrier molecule to the liver for heme synthesis. Apotransferrin binds iron (Fe^{3+}) to form transferrin, which transports the iron to the liver and throughout the body. Apoferritin binds ferrous (Fe^{2+}) iron and stores it in the more stable Fe^{3+} form as part of the ferritin molecule.

Tissue iron is found in cellular enzymes and coenzymes, including peroxidases and cytochromes. Myoglobin is a single-chain, iron- and oxygen-binding protein found in muscle. Iron in the blood constitutes the circulating pool. Iron homeostasis is governed by many chemical reactions that are not well understood.

Porphyrins

Heme, the molecule that allows reversible binding of oxygen, consists of porphyrin and an iron atom. Porphyrins are composed of four pyrrole rings that bind to an iron molecule to form heme (Fig. 14-7). The important porphyrins in humans are uroporphyrin, protoporphyrin, and coproporphyrin. Each of these molecules plays a part in heme synthesis. In some disease states, excess porphyrins are excreted from the body. Uroporphyrin is excreted in urine, protoporphyrin in feces, and coproporphyrin in both.

A porphyrin molecule comprises a pyrrole ring and an Fe^{3+} atom. If the iron is reduced (Fe^{2+}), the molecule is called a porphyrinogen. This form is used to make heme. Because porphyrinogens are unstable, porphyrins are measured in the laboratory instead of porphyrinogens.

After the heme prosthetic group is incorporated into a single hemoglobin unit and the two α and two β subunits are assembled, the hemoglobin molecule becomes functional. Oxygen is inhaled into the lungs and passes through the pulmonary epithelium into the bloodstream. Oxygen binding occurs when one oxygen molecule (O_2)

encounters a red blood cell and binds to one heme group in a hemoglobin molecule. The next oxygen molecule binds to another heme group, and the process continues until all four heme groups are bound to oxygen molecules. After one oxygen molecule attaches to hemoglobin, the structure of the hemoglobin molecule is modified, enabling it to attract more oxygen molecules until it is saturated. Conditions in the blood (e.g., pH) can affect the ability of hemoglobin to transport and release oxygen. Similar to the way the iron in hemoglobin attracts and transports oxygen, the amino acids in the protein chains of globins bind carbon dioxide so that it can be picked up in the tissues and released when the red blood cell returns to the lungs (Fig. 14-8).

Heme Synthesis

Heme is the prosthetic group of hemoglobin, myoglobin, and the cytochromes. Most heme is synthesized in developing red blood cells in bone marrow, but about 15% of production takes place in the liver for the formation of heme-containing enzymes. Heme, which is also called ferrous protoporphyrin IX, contains four pyrrole rings surrounding an iron molecule. Four of the six electron pairs in the iron molecule attach to the pyrrole ring nitrogen atoms, one electron pair binds to the globin, and one pair binds to the oxygen molecule. Heme production is regulated by a negative feedback loop.

The heme created by the developing red blood cells in the bone marrow is used to synthesize hemoglobin. One hemoglobin molecule contains four globin molecules, each of which contains one heme group (Fig. 14-9).

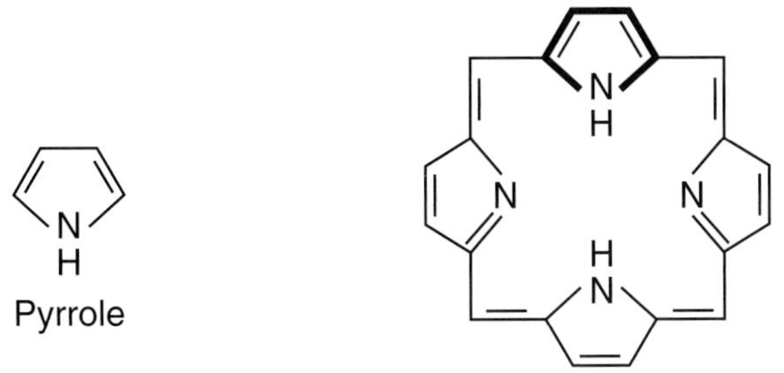

Normal adult hemoglobin is composed of two α- and two β-globin chains. The protein chains fold and compact into a tertiary structure that resembles a globe. The largest portion of the hemoglobin molecule is made of globin chains. Chromosome 16 controls production of the α-globins, and chromosome 11 controls production of the β-globins. DNA mutations produce aberrant proteins, which cause hemoglobinopathies (discussed later). The globin proteins are produced from RNA templates in the endoplasmic reticulum and then linked to a heme to make hemoglobin.

The fetus produces hemoglobin and red blood cells. Fetal hemoglobin is composed of four subunits: two α-proteins and two γ-proteins, each of which contains a heme group. The γ-globin is commonly called the fetal hemoglobin subunit. After the baby is born, the fetal hemoglobin is slowly replaced until, by about 1 year of age, it has all been replaced with hemoglobin A.

Clinical Correlations

Knowing the chemical physiology of iron, porphyrins, and hemoglobin can help a health care provider choose tests to rule out or confirm a diagnosis. The following sections discuss the applicable laboratory tests and results in iron deficiency and overload, acute and nonacute porphyrias, hemoglobinopathies, and anemias.

Iron Deficiency

Because iron plays an integral part in oxygen transport and peroxidase and cytochrome function, decreased iron in the body can cause many problems. Without enough iron, the body cannot produce enough red blood cells to maintain adequate oxygenation, cytochromes do not function properly, red blood cells are small, and individuals become anemic. Measurement of the serum iron level helps a clinician determine whether an individual has adequate iron in the blood.

It is also important to measure storage iron. The workup for iron deficiency includes tests for serum iron level, ferritin level, and total iron-binding capacity. The ferritin level provides a rough idea of the amount of storage iron in the body. The total iron-binding capacity (TIBC) measures the total amount of iron that can be bound by transferrin. The results for serum iron and ferritin may be low, and the TIBC may be high. The cause of a low iron value must be determined before treatment can begin.

• **Figure 14-7** Chemical structures of pyrrole and the porphyrin ring. One of the pyrrole units within the porphyrin ring appears in boldface. (From Kaplan LA, Pesce AJ. *Clinical Chemistry: Theory, Analysis, Correlation.* 5th ed. St. Louis: Mosby; 2010.)

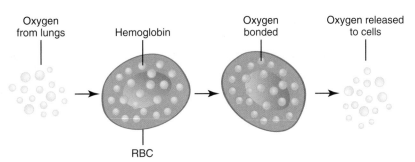

• **Figure 14-8** Oxygen exchange in red blood cells (RBC).

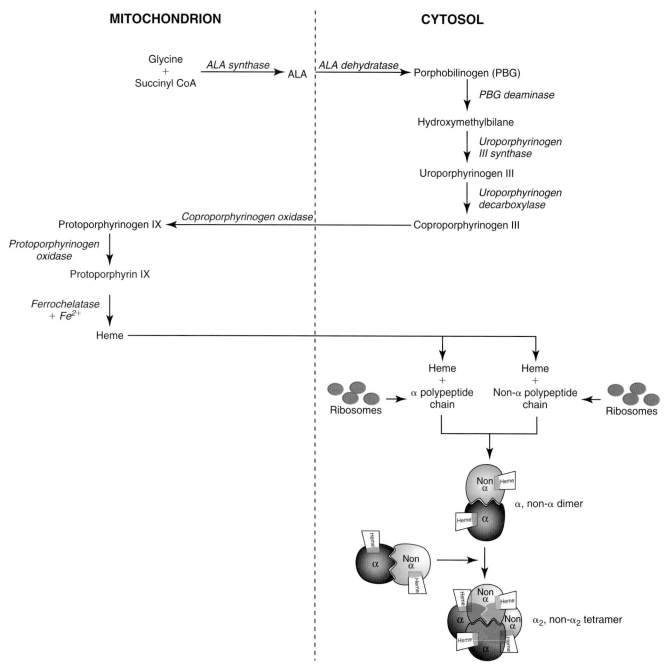

• **Figure 14-9** Hemoglobin assembly begins with glycine and succinyl coenzyme A (CoA), which assemble in mitochondria catalyzed by aminolevulinate synthase to form aminolevulinic acid (ALA). In the cytoplasm, ALA undergoes several transformations from porphobilinogen (PBG) to coproporphyrinogen III, which when catalyzed by coproporphyrinogen oxidase becomes protoporphyrinogen IX. In mitochondria, protoporphyrinogen IX is converted to protoporphyrin IX by protoporphyrinogen oxidase. Ferrous (Fe^{2+}) ion is added, catalyzed by ferrochelatase to form heme. In the cytoplasm, heme assembles with an α-chain and non-α-chain, forming a dimer. Ultimately, two dimers join to form the hemoglobin tetramer. (From Keohane EM, Smith LJ, Walenga JM. *Rodak's Hematology.* 5th ed. St. Louis: Saunders; 2016.)

Iron Overload

In hemosiderosis and hemochromatosis, the body has too much iron. Hemosiderosis is iron overload that results from tissue injury. Hemochromatosis is a complex of diseases, the most common of which is hereditary hemochromatosis.

Hereditary hemochromatosis is a genetic disorder characterized by inappropriately high iron absorption resulting in progressive iron overload. Common symptoms include bronzing of the skin, cirrhosis, and diabetes. Other symptoms include cardiac myopathy, arrhythmias, endocrine deficiencies, and arthropathies. This disease is linked to a human leukocyte antigen (HLA) on chromosome 6. It is most prevalent among people of Northern European descent, but it also occurs in other populations.

Hereditary hemochromatosis is caused by two base-pair alterations in the *HFE* gene on chromosome 6. The affected base pairs are C282Y and H63D. Ten percent of individuals are heterozygous for *HFE* C282Y and 4.4 in 1000 are

TABLE 14-2 Porphyrias

Disease	Defect	Comments
Acute intermittent porphyria	Lack of control of the aminolevulinic acid (ALA) synthase enzyme	
Hereditary coproporphyria	One half of the coproporphyrinogen oxidase level of a normal individual	Affects the liver, autosomal dominant inheritance
Variegate porphyria	Decreased activity of protoporphyrinogen oxidase	Autosomal dominant inheritance of trait
Congenital erythropoietic porphyria (Gunther disease)	Decreased activity of uroporphyrinogen III synthase	Prolonged exposure to sunlight can cause a blistering rash, red urine, and blindness
Erythropoietic porphyria	Protoporphyrin accumulates in the liver	Causes liver disease and moderately elevated liver function test results
Porphyria cutanea tarda	Defective uroporphyrinogen III decarboxylase enzyme	Important extrahepatic manifestation of hepatitis C infection

homozygous for *HFE* C282Y. Laboratory findings include an elevated transferrin saturation value, an increased ferritin level, and possibly excess iron deposits in the liver. Many diabetics have this disease and are not aware of it.

Porphyrias

Porphyrias are a group of clinical syndromes caused by defects in enzymes that catalyze various stages of heme production. *Acute* porphyrias cause periodic neurovisceral attacks with abdominal pain, neurologic deficits, psychiatric symptoms, and red urine. These syndromes include acute intermittent porphyria, hereditary coproporphyria, and variegate porphyria.

Chronic porphyrias are dermatologic diseases that may involve the liver and nervous system but produce no acute attacks. Skin exposed to the sun becomes fragile and blistered, leading to infection, scarring, and changes in skin pigmentation. Chronic porphyrias include congenital erythropoietic porphyria, erythropoietic porphyria, and porphyria cutanea tarda (Table 14-2).

Modified Hemoglobin Structures

Substances such as carbon monoxide, sulfur, and oxidizing agents can modify the structure of hemoglobin. The ferrous iron atom in the heme molecule easily binds and releases an oxygen molecule. Carbon monoxide is a polar molecule that can also bind with heme; once bound, it is difficult to remove (Fig. 14-10). Carbon monoxide poisoning occurs when sustained exposure to carbon monoxide saturates the hemoglobin in the red blood cells, which cannot then bind enough oxygen to keep the brain functioning. Carbon monoxide bound to a hemoglobin molecule modifies the structure to form carboxyhemoglobin.

Sulfhemoglobin is a modified hemoglobin molecule in which sulfur atoms have attached to the hemoglobin, preventing oxygen from attaching to the iron and thus rendering the hemoglobin molecule nonfunctional (Fig. 14-11).

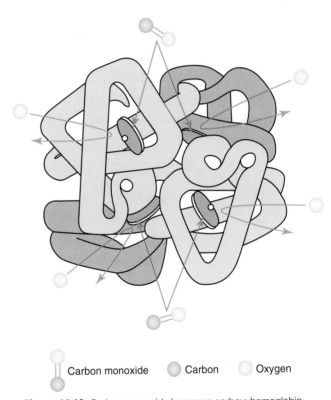

Carbon monoxide Carbon Oxygen

• **Figure 14-10** Carbon monoxide becomes carboxyhemoglobin.

Methemoglobin is the result when hemoglobin reacts with oxidizing agents such as nitrates, quinines, and aniline dyes to produce heme containing Fe^{3+} instead of Fe^{2+}. Oxygen cannot bind to the iron in its oxidized state, so the methemoglobin is nonfunctional. (Fig. 14-12).

Hemoglobinopathies

Construction of a hemoglobin molecule is a multistep process, and errors can occur at any step in the process. The most common clinical conditions result from mutations involving the globins of the hemoglobin molecule. The two main types are thalassemias and hemoglobinopathies. Thalassemias are identified by the globin chain that is not produced, and hemoglobinopathies are identified by the mutation causing the abnormality.

More than 900 hemoglobinopathies have been identified, but only nine have clinical significance. The hemoglobin variants resulting from a mutation are named using letters (e.g., S, D, E), and the diseases are classified according to the type of mutation that causes them.

Abnormal Hemoglobins

Hemoglobin E is a β-globin chain variant in which a lysine residue replaces glutamic acid at position 26. The substitution may produce a mild anemia.

In hemoglobin C, a lysine residue is substituted for glutamic acid at position 6 of the β-globin chain. This mutated form reduces the normal plasticity of red blood cells, causing an asymptomatic condition that can be associated with α-thalassemia and β-thalassemia.

Homozygous hemoglobin S is formed when there is a substitution of valine for glutamic acid at position 6 in the α-helix of the β-globin. Sickle cell disease (i.e., sickle cell anemia), which can be severe, occurs when a person inherits two copies of the gene that encodes hemoglobin S. Hemoglobin S crystallizes when the oxygen tension of blood is reduced. Red blood cells become crescent shaped, and the pointed hemoglobin S crystals that extend from the crescent ends tear blood vessels and organs.

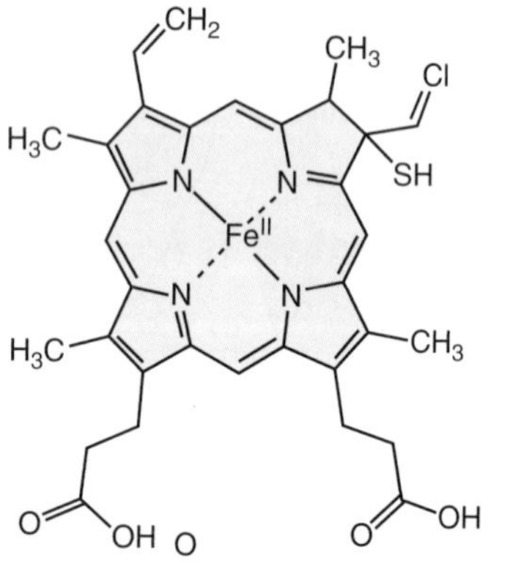

• **Figure 14-11** Structure of sulfhemoglobin.

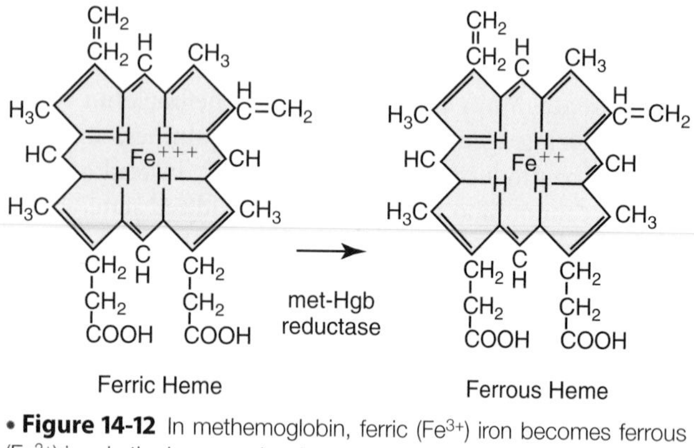

• **Figure 14-12** In methemoglobin, ferric (Fe^{3+}) iron becomes ferrous (Fe^{2+}) iron in the heme molecule.

A person who inherits only a single copy of the hemoglobin S gene (i.e., heterozygous hemoglobin S) is said to have sickle cell trait. The severity of this disease correlates with the amount of hemoglobin S in red blood cells. However, the mutation in the hemoglobin S gene also protects heterozygotes to some extent from malaria caused by *Plasmodium falciparum*.

Persons with hemoglobin SC have inherited one gene for hemoglobin S and one for hemoglobin C. Both β-globin chains have substitutions at position 6: The chain of hemoglobin S has a valine substitution, and the chain of hemoglobin C has a lysine substitution. Persons with hemoglobin SC have fewer sickle cells and fewer acute vaso-occlusive events than those who are homozygous for hemoglobin S, but other effects (e.g., retinopathy, ischemic necrosis of bone) are more severe.

Thalassemias

α-Thalassemia and β-thalassemia are named after the globin chain that is missing from the hemoglobin molecule. These and several other types of thalassemia are clinically significant.

The most severe form of α-thalassemia results from the inheritance of genes for hemoglobin Barts. This type of hemoglobin consists of four γ-chains. Deletion of all four α-globin genes makes hemoglobin Barts incapable of effective oxygen delivery to tissues. Most fetuses with hemoglobin Barts die in utero or a few hours after birth. The condition is common in Southeast Asia.

All α-thalassemias have decreased α-globin production, resulting in an excess of β-chains in adults and excess γ-chains in newborns. The hemoglobin H molecule has four β-globin chains, a condition that produces a chronic anemia of variable severity.

α-Thalassemia major involves two α-chain deletions, but most individuals with this condition are normal. α-Thalassemia trait consists of a single α-chain deletion.

The genetic mutations causing the β-thalassemias produce reduced numbers of β-globins. These thalassemias mild and are prevalent in persons living near the Mediterranean Sea. Scientists think that this condition, like sickle cell trait, reduces the effects of *Plasmodium falciparum* infection.

The mutations in β-Thalassemia major, also called Cooley's anemia, prevent the formation of β-globin chains. The condition is usually noticed in children younger than 1 year of age. Patients have mostly hemoglobin F, have no hemoglobin A, and may have a small amount of hemoglobin A_2. Symptoms include failure to thrive and severe anemia. Diabetes mellitus and hypoparathyroidism are associated conditions, and pericarditis and myocardial hemosiderosis are major causes of death.

β-Thalassemia intermedia is less severe than β-thalassemia major. Patients have some β-chain formation, decreased production of hemoglobin A, and increased production of hemoglobin F.

In β-Thalassemia minor, only one of the two β-globin alleles contains a mutation, and β-chain production is not intolerably compromised. Patients may be relatively asymptomatic.

Anemias

Anemias are conditions marked by a deficiency of red blood cells or hemoglobin in the blood. The World Health Organization defines anemia as a hemoglobin level of less than 13 g/dL in men and less than 12 g/dL in women. The deficiency decreases the ability of blood to carry oxygen to the tissues, resulting in tissue hypoxia. Anemia can be mild, moderate, severe, or life-threatening. Symptoms of anemia, regardless of the cause, include weakness, dizziness, pale mucous membranes, lightheadedness (especially on exertion), and tachycardia (i.e., rapid heart rate).

Many methods are used to categorize anemias, but no one method provides a complete classification system. Anemias can be classified by the size and shape of the red blood cell (i.e., microcytic, normocytic, and macrocytic), the amount of hemoglobin (i.e., hypochromic, normochromic, and hyperchromic), or other factors.

Aplastic Anemia

Aplastic anemia occurs when all cell lines fail to produce mature cells and the red, cell-producing bone marrow is replaced by fat and other tissues that do not produce blood cells. Aplastic anemia can be caused by human immunodeficiency virus (HIV), mycobacteria, cytomegalovirus (CMV), or Epstein-Barr virus (EBV) infection; exposure to solvents or radiation; and chromosomal abnormalities. Fanconi anemia is an inherited bone marrow failure syndrome that includes other chromosomal abnormalities in addition to those for aplastic anemia. The laboratory workup includes a direct antiglobulin test, kidney function tests, and transaminase, bilirubin, and LDH assays.

Anemia of Chronic Renal and Endocrine Diseases

Anemia of chronic renal and endocrine diseases occurs in long-standing systemic disorders such as rheumatoid arthritis, diabetes mellitus, severe trauma, and heart disease. The long-term effects of these diseases include decreased levels of iron in the blood, decreased erythropoietin production, and a decreased red blood cell life span (70 to 80 days instead of 120 days). Individuals with hypotestosteronism or hypothyroidism may also have a mild anemia. These anemias are classified as normocytic, normochromic anemias.

Pernicious Anemia

Pernicious anemia is an autoimmune disease that causes gastric atrophy. It is a macrocytic anemia caused by reduced vitamin B_{12} absorption due to the lack of intrinsic factor. Individuals with pernicious anemia have a markedly increased LDH level and elevated iron saturation and indirect bilirubin values. Pernicious anemia is a hemolytic disorder associated with increased turnover of bilirubin. Potassium, cholesterol, and alkaline phosphatase levels are decreased.

Folate and Vitamin B_{12} Deficiency Anemia

Folate and vitamin B_{12} are coenzymes involved in the production of red blood cells. Because vitamin B_{12} deficiencies result in neurologic lesions and symptoms, a timely and accurate diagnosis is critical. Chemistry assays for serum folate and vitamin B_{12} levels are evaluated to determine the cause of folate and vitamin B12 deficiency anemia. The reference range for vitamin B_{12} is 180 to 914 ng/L, and the reference range for folate is 2 to 20 ng/mL for adults.

Iron Deficiency Anemia

Iron deficiency anemia occurs when there is insufficient iron in the body to support healthy red cell production. The anemia gradually worsens as iron stores are depleted. This is a microcytic anemia (mean corpuscular volume [MCV] < 83 fL) resulting from low blood iron content. Although the anemia may first be suspected from the CBC and differential results, additional tests are needed to make the diagnosis and rule out other conditions that produce a microcytic anemia such as lead poisoning. Table 14-3 shows the chemistry results for iron deficiency anemia and other microcytic anemias.

Immune Hemolytic Anemia

Immune hemolytic anemia is the result of premature destruction of red blood cells by antibodies. This condition can be mild or severe and can be associated with membrane defects, hemoglobinopathies, or mechanical injury. The destruction of the red blood cells can occur in extravascular or intravascular spaces. Extravascular conditions in which the red blood cells are destroyed in the spleen and other tissues include autoimmune hemolytic anemia and hereditary

---

TABLE 14-3   Chemistry Results for Iron Deficiency Anemia and Other Microcytic Anemias

Condition	Iron level	TIBC	Ferritin	Lead	Transferrin Saturation
Iron deficiency anemia	Decreased	Increased	Decreased	Normal	Decreased
Lead toxicity	Normal	Normal	Normal	Increased	Normal
Bleeding (GI or menstrual)	Normal to decreased	Decreased	Decreased	Normal	Normal to decreased
Thalassemia trait	Normal to increased	Normal	Normal to increased	Normal	Normal to increased
Sideroblastic anemia	Normal to increased	Normal	Normal to increased	Normal	Normal to increased

GI, Gastrointestinal; *TIBC*, total iron-binding capacity.

spherocytosis. Hereditary spherocytosis or elliptocytosis, pyruvate kinase deficiency, G6PD deficiency, and paroxysmal nocturnal hemoglobinuria may produce hemolytic anemia. The destruction of red blood cells releases LDH and hemoglobin. The hemoglobin is broken down, increasing levels of indirect bilirubin and **urobilinogen**, a byproduct of bilirubin metabolism.

Hereditary Spherocytosis or Elliptocytosis

Hereditary spherocytosis is an inherited autosomal dominant disease. Many microspherocytes can be seen on the peripheral blood smear. Microspherocytes are caused by a red blood cell membrane defect. Abnormal laboratory assay findings include increased levels of bilirubin, LDH, and unconjugated bilirubin; decreased haptoglobin levels; and an abnormal osmotic fragility test result.

Glucose-6-Phosphate Dehydrogenase Deficiency

Glucose-6-phosphate dehydrogenase (G6PD) **deficiency** is inherited X-linked disorder. It is one of the most common disease-producing enzyme deficiencies. G6PD helps red blood cells to function properly. G6PD deficiency leads to early red blood cell destruction and anemia. It also decreases the haptoglobin level and increases the indirect bilirubin concentration. The disease is diagnosed with a G6PD screening test.

Paroxysmal Nocturnal Hemoglobinuria

Paroxysmal nocturnal hemoglobinuria is a hereditary disease in which red blood cells are lysed by complement, releasing hemoglobin. Accumulation of hemoglobin during the night leads to dark-colored urine in the morning in a minority of individuals. The red blood cells of these individuals have a defective cell membrane that is exceptionally sensitive to the hemolytic action of complement. Ham's acid hemolysis test is used to diagnose this condition.

Clinical Chemistry Tests

Iron and Total Iron-Binding Capacity Tests

Iron and TIBC tests for serum iron levels are based on a colorimetric reaction. Serum pH is reduced, releasing iron from the transferrin molecule. The iron is then reduced (Fe^{3+} to Fe^{2+}) and complexed with a chromogen. The concentration of iron is directly proportional to the color generated. Reference ranges for iron are 65 to 170 µg/dL for men and 50 to 170 µg/dL for women.

The TIBC test determines the amount of available binding sites on the transferrin molecule. Enough iron is added to the sample to saturate the transferrin binding sites. The excess iron is removed, and an iron level is determined for the specimen. The **transferrin saturation** value is calculated using the following equation:

$$\text{Transferrin saturation} = 100 \times \text{serum [Fe]} / \text{TIBC}$$

The TIBC reference range is 255 to 450 µg/dL (Table 14-4).

TABLE 14-4	Effects of Various Conditions on Iron, TIBC, and Transferrin Saturation Values
Condition	**Effect on Iron, TIBC, and Transferrin Saturation**
Diurnal variation	Normal values in morning, low values in mid-afternoon, very low values near midnight
Menses	During menses, low values; before menses, increased values
Pregnancy	May be high due to hormones or may be low due to iron deficiency
Ingestion of iron	High values for iron
Oral contraceptives	High values for iron, may also elevate TIBC
Hepatitis	Very high values
Acute inflammation including abscesses and myocardial infarcts	Low or normal iron, normal or low transferrin saturation
Chronic inflammation	Low or normal iron, normal or low transferrin saturation

TIBC, Total iron-binding capacity.
Modified from Burtis CA, Bruns DE. *Tietz Fundamentals of Clinical Chemistry and Molecular Diagnostics.* 7th ed. St. Louis: Saunders; 2015.

Ferritin

Ferritin levels are measured using immunoluminescence, enzyme-linked immunoassay (ELISA), and immunoturbimetric methods. In the immunoluminescence method, ferritin in the sample reacts with a biotinylated antibody, forming an antigen–antibody complex. This test is performed in a well that is coated with streptavidin, capturing the antigen–antibody complex. The wells are then washed to remove unbound material. A labeled horseradish peroxidase antibody conjugate is added to the well and binds to the ferritin antibody–antigen complex. Unbound material is removed by washing. Substrates containing luminol are added to the wells, causing oxidation of the luminol and light production. The amount of light produced is directly proportional to the ferritin concentration of the sample.

Ferritin is measured with a solid-phase ELISA. Plastic wells are coated with antiferritin antibodies. Antigen–antibody complexes form when ferritin is added to the plastic wells. Antiferritin enzyme labeled with horseradish peroxidase is then added to each well. The ferritin is sandwiched between the solid phase and enzyme-labeled antibodies. An enzyme substrate (i.e., chromogen) is added to the wells, resulting in a blue color. Acid is added to stop the reaction, and it converts the color to yellow. The concentration of ferritin is directly proportional to the intensity of the yellow color.

In the immunoturbidimetric method, latex-bound ferritin antibodies react with the antigen to form an antigen–antibody complex. The turbidity of the solution is measured at 700 nm and is directly proportional to the ferritin concentration. The ferritin reference range is 23 to 336 ng/mL for men and 11 to 306 ng/mL for women.

Hemosiderin

Hemolysis produces hemosiderin in the urine sediment. A urine sample is stained (e.g., with Prussian blue) for hemosiderin and then evaluated under the microscope. Blue staining of the hemosiderin granules indicates that iron is present in the urine sample.

Transferrin

Transferrin is measured with immunoturbidimetric and immunonephelometric methods. The immune complexes in the solution scatter light, and the instrument measures the reduction of incident light caused by reflection, absorption, or scatter. The decrease in transmitted light is proportional to the amount of transferrin in the sample. Transferrin also migrates in the β_1-region on a routine serum electrophoresis. The transferrin reference range is 170 to 370 mg/dL.

Electrophoresis

Electrophoresis is used to separate proteins with various molecular weights in a sample. **Hemoglobin electrophoresis** is used to separate different types of hemoglobin. Hemolysates are prepared from whole blood samples, and small amounts are transferred onto cellulose acetate electrophoresis media. The hemoglobins in the sample are separated by the electrical current using an alkaline buffer (pH 8.2 to 8.6). The media are then stained with Ponceau S stain to visualize the bands. A scanning densitometer is used to determine the relative percentage of each band.

Normal Hemoglobin Electrophoresis

The normal hemoglobin profile of adults is a mixture of the following:

- Hemoglobin A: 95% to 98%
- Hemoglobin A_2: 2% to 3%
- Hemoglobin F: 0.8% to 2%
- Hemoglobin S: 0%
- Hemoglobin C: 0%

Abnormal Hemoglobin Electrophoresis

Many conditions can produce abnormal hemoglobin electrophoresis results. If hemoglobin S is present but the percentage of hemoglobin A is higher than that of hemoglobin S, the diagnosis is sickle cell trait. If hemoglobin S and hemoglobin F are detected but there is no hemoglobin A, the finding indicates sickle cell anemia. If the percentage of hemoglobin A is higher than that of hemoglobin C, the result indicates hemoglobin C trait. If hemoglobin C and hemoglobin F are detected, but there is no hemoglobin A, the diagnosis is hemoglobin C disease. The presence of hemoglobin S and hemoglobin C in the sample indicates hemoglobin SC disease. The finding of hemoglobin H in the sample is diagnostic of hemoglobin H disease. Detection of hemoglobin A_2

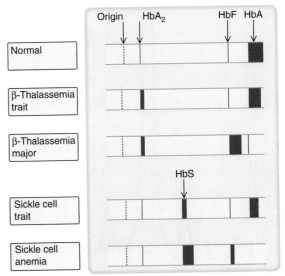

• **Figure 14-13** Hemoglobin electrophoresis. (From Kumar P, Clark ML. *Kumar & Clark's Clinical Medicine.* 8th ed. London: Elsevier. 2012.)

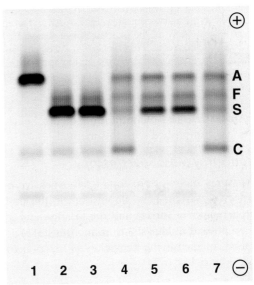

• **Figure 14-14** Electrophoretic separation of hemoglobins (Hb) at alkaline pH. *1,* Normal adult; *2 and 3,* a 17-year-old patient with sickle cell anemia (HbSS); *5 and 6,* patient with sickle cell anemia who was recently transfused (notice the presence of Hb A from the transfused red blood cells); *4 and 7,* Hb A/F/S/C standard for the Hydragel 7 Hemoglobin/Hydrasys System (Sebia Electrophoresis, Norcross, GA). (Modified from Elghetany MT, Banki K. Erythrocytic disorders. In: McPherson RA, Pincus MR. *Henry's Clinical Diagnosis and Management by Laboratory Methods.* 22nd ed. Philadelphia: Elsevier; 2011:578.)

indicates β-thalassemia minor. Increased levels of hemoglobin F indicate hereditary persistence of fetal hemoglobin or that the sample is from an infant (Figs. 14-13 and 14-14).

High-Pressure Liquid Chromatography

High-pressure liquid chromatography (HPLC) is used to identify hemoglobin A_2, hemoglobin F, and other variants. This is accomplished by using a column packed with cation exchange resin. Retention times for many hemoglobin variants are available in the literature (Fig. 14-15).

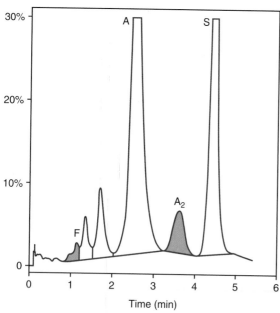

• **Figure 14-15** Ion-exchange high-performance liquid chromatography (HPLC) separation of hemoglobin (Hb) types in a sample from a patient with sickle cell trait demonstrates Hb F, A, A₂, and an abnormal type in the HbS window for the Bio-Rad Variant Classic Hb Testing System (BioRad Laboratories, Philadelphia, PA). (Modified from Elghetany MT, Banki K: Erythrocytic disorders. In: McPherson RA, Pincus MR, eds. *Henry's Clinical Diagnosis and Management by Laboratory Methods.* 22nd ed. Philadelphia: Elsevier; 2011:578.)

Better resolution and quantification of the hemoglobin variants is accomplished with this method.

Electron Spray Mass Spectroscopy

Electron spray mass spectroscopy is an expensive method for identifying various hemoglobins, but it quickly identifies the hemoglobin variant and the location and identity of the amino acid residue substitution. This test is not routinely used for identifying hemoglobinopathies because of its expense (Fig. 14-16).

DNA Analysis

DNA analysis is used to identify individuals in a population with a high incidence of hemoglobinopathies or thalassemias who may benefit from genetic counseling. DNA analysis is used to characterize thalassemias, to identify life-threatening hemoglobin synthesis disorders in the fetus (i.e., chorionic villous samples), and to distinguish among genetic conditions that may have the same symptoms and laboratory results.

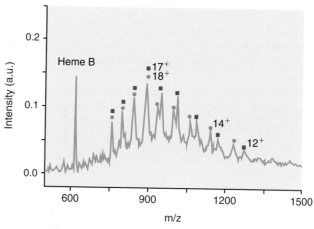

• **Figure 14-16** Electron spray mass spectroscopy.

Hemoglobin H Identification

Hemoglobin H is found in individuals with α-thalassemia. Hemoglobin H inclusions can be detected in a peripheral blood smear if the blood is mixed with new methylene blue or brilliant cresyl blue at 37° C. This is a qualitative, subjective test

Sickling Tests

Sickling screening tests are used to detect hemoglobin S in a sample. Sodium hydrosulfite is added to a sample along with saponin. If the sample becomes turbid, hemoglobin S is present. This method is quick and inexpensive.

Methods for Diagnosing and Monitoring Porphyrias

Samples collected for analysis of porphyrias must be protected from light because the analytes can be destroyed by light, and falsely decreased values result. Urine test methods for porphobilinogen are based on the reaction of Ehrlich reagent with porphobilinogen to produce a magenta-colored product, which is measured at 553 nm. The reference range for random urine specimens is 2 mg/L, and that for 24-hour urine specimens is less than 2.5 mg.

Porphyrins can be analyzed in urine and feces. These analyses are complex, and because they require much time to complete, many laboratories do not perform them. Screening tests are usually performed to justify the more complex analyses. Genetic testing can also be performed.

Summary

Diseases of white and red blood cells include leukemias, lymphomas, anemias, and hemoglobinopathies. Although the LDH and uric acid levels may be increased in leukemias, most leukemias are diagnosed through CBC and bone marrow results. Lymphomas are similar, but they are usually diagnosed with lymph node biopsies. Anemias and hemoglobinopathies are diagnosed with the use of clinical chemistry tests (e.g., total iron, TIBC, ferritin, transferrin); hemoglobin electrophoresis; assays of intrinsic factor, vitamin B₁₂, folate, and G6PD levels; and sickle cell screening tests. Hereditary hemochromatosis is an inherited iron overload condition in which excess iron is stored in the body, especially in the liver. Porphyrias are caused by enzyme deficiencies that affect hemoglobin synthesis, and they are diagnosed on the basis of clinical chemistry test results.

Review Questions

1. Which leukemia is diagnosed by finding the Philadelphia chromosome translocation in bone marrow cells?
   a. CLL
   b. CML
   c. AML
   d. ALL

2. Porphyrins are the building blocks of hemoglobin and are composed of
   a. 4 pyrrole rings bound to an iron molecule
   b. 4 β-globin chains
   c. 4 α-globin chains
   d. 2 pyrrole rings and 2 β-globin chains

3. TIBC measures
   a. The total amount of iron in the blood
   b. The total amount of iron storage in the body
   c. The amount of oxygen that can be carried in the blood
   d. The total amount of iron that can be bound by transferrin

4. Which of the following groups of diseases are caused by defects in enzymes that catalyze the various stages of heme production?
   a. Porphyrias
   b. Leukemias
   c. Lymphomas
   d. Anemias

5. In which hemoglobinopathy is lysine substituted for glutamic acid?
   a. Hemoglobin E
   b. Hemoglobin F
   c. Hemoglobin C
   d. Hemoglobin S

6. A 55-year-old woman has fatigue and pale mucous membranes. Her CBC results are a WBC count, 7.2; hemoglobin, 8.2; hematocrit, 24.1; MCV, 105 fL; and platelet count, 250,000. Her intrinsic factor assay result is 0 mg/dL. What condition does this patient have?
   a. Folate deficiency
   b. Vitamin B_{12} deficiency
   c. Pernicious anemia
   d. Cooley anemia

7. Which of the following conditions is an X-linked disorder and one of the most common disease-producing enzyme deficiencies?
   a. Acute intermittent porphyria
   b. Aplastic anemia
   c. Paroxysmal nocturnal hemoglobinuria
   d. G6PD deficiency

8. Transferrin saturation is calculated using which of the following formulas?
   a. Transferrin saturation = TIBC/100 × serum iron
   b. Transferrin saturation = 100 × serum iron/TIBC
   c. Transferrin saturation = 100 × TIBC/serum iron
   d. Transferrin saturation = serum iron/100 × TIBC

9. The most common method for hemoglobin electrophoresis includes which of the following?
   a. Agarose media at a pH of 7.5 to 7.7
   b. Cellulose acetate media at a pH of 8.2 to 8.4
   c. Agarose media at a pH of 8.2 to 8.4
   d. Cellulose acetate media at a pH of 7.5 to 7.7

10. Complete the following table:

Condition	Effect on Iron, TIBC, and Transferrin Saturation
Diurnal variation	
Menses	
Pregnancy	
Ingestion of iron	
Oral contraceptives	High values for iron, may elevate TIBC
Hepatitis	
Acute inflammation, including abscesses and myocardial infarctions	
Chronic inflammation	

Critical Thinking Questions

1. Compare and contrast iron deficiency anemias with anemias of chronic disease (i.e., anemia of inflammatory states). Discuss the pathophysiology and how laboratory tests can be used to distinguish between the two types.

2. Compare and contrast common hemoglobinopathies, such as sickle cell anemia and the thalassemias, in terms of their pathophysiology and the laboratory tests used to detect each disorder.

CASE STUDY

Little boy J., a 3-year-old boy of African descent, was brought in by his parents and admitted to his local emergency department. The boy was in severe pain due to anoxia. He had been diagnosed recently with sickle cell anemia. Explain how this disease is transmitted. Discuss how it affects hemoglobin and the red blood cells in an affected person. Why are affected persons in pain? Discuss the laboratory tests for identifying the sickle cell anemia. What is sickle cell trait? Is it diagnosed in the laboratory in the same way as sickle cell disease?

Bibliography

Cappellini MD, Fiorelli G. Glucose-6-phosphate dehydrogenase deficiency. *Lancet*. 2008;371:64–74.

Elghetany MT, Banki K. Erythrocytic disorders. In: McPherson RA, Pincus MR, eds. *Henry's Clinical Diagnosis and Management by Laboratory Methods*. 22nd ed. Philadelphia: Elsevier Saunders; 2011.

Giardina PJ, Forget BG. Thalassemia syndromes. In: Hoffman R, Benz EJ, Shattil SS, et al., eds. *Hematology: Basic Principles and Practice*. 5th ed. Philadelphia: Elsevier Churchill Livingstone; 2008.

Golden AK. *Decision Support System*. Rochester, MN: Mayo Clinic; 2014.

Hendrik N, Dörken B, Lenz G. Pathogenesis of non-Hodgkin's lymphoma. *J Clin Oncol*. 2011;29:1803–1811.

Howlader N, Noone AM, Krapcho M, et al. eds. *SEER Cancer Statistics Review*. 1975-2011. Bethesda, MD: National Cancer Institute. <http://seer.cancer.gov/csr/1975-2011> Accessed 07.06.15.

Hvas AM, Nexo E. Diagnosis and treatment of vitamin B12 deficiency—an update. *Haematologica*. 2006;91:1506–1512.

Kurzrock R. Myelodysplastic syndrome overview. *Semin Hematol*. 2002;39(suppl 2):18–25.

Leukemia and Lymphoma Society. *Leukemia*. <http://www.leukemia-lymphoma.org/all_page?item_id=7026&viewmode=print> Accessed 07.06.15.

Little JA, Benz Jr EJ, Gardner LB. Anemia of chronic diseases. In: Hoffman R, Benz Jr EJ, Silberstein LE, et al., eds. *Hematology: Basic Principles and Practice*. 6th ed. Philadelphia: Elsevier Saunders; 2012.

Longo DL. Anemia and polycythemia. In: *Harrison's Principles of Internal Medicine*. Vol 1, 15th ed. New York: McGraw-Hill; 2001:348–354.

National Cancer Institute. *What you need to know about leukemia*. <http://www.cancer.gov/cancertopics/wyntk/leukemia/allpages> Accessed 07.06.15.

National Comprehensive Cancer Network. *Hodgkin lymphoma*. <http://www.nccn.org/professionals/physician_gls/f_guidelines. asp> Accessed 07.06.15.

National Institutes of Health, National Heart, Lung, and Blood Institute. What is anemia? <http://www.nhlbi.nih.gov/health/health-topics/topics/anemia> Accessed 07.06.15.

National Institutes of Health, National Heart, Lung, and Blood Institute. What is aplastic anemia? <http://www.nhlbi.nih.gov/health/health-topics/topics/aplastic/> Accessed 07.06.15.

National Institutes of Health, National Heart, Lung, and Blood Institute. What is Fanconi anemia? <http://www.nhlbi.nih.gov/health/health-topics/topics/fanconi> Accessed 07.06.15.

National Institutes of Health, National Heart, Lung, and Blood Institute. What is pernicious anemia? <http://www.nhlbi.nih.gov/health/health-topics/topics/prnanmia>Accessed 07.06.15.

Price EA, Schrier SS. Extrinsic nonimmune hemolytic anemias. In: Hoffman R, Benz Jr EJ, Silberstein LE, et al., eds. *Hematology: Basic Principles and Practice*. 6th ed. Philadelphia: Elsevier Saunders; 2012.

Seattle Cancer Care Alliance. *Non-Hodgkin's lymphoma*. <http://www.seattlecca.org/diseases/non-hodgkins-lymphoma-overview.cfm?gclid=CKCbmqyM_K8CFUkaQgodgSBWVQ> Accessed 07.06.15.

Shankland KR, Armitage JO, Hancock BW. Non-Hodgkin lymphoma. *Lancet*. 2012;380:848–857.

Steensma DP, Tefferi A. The myelodysplastic syndrome(s): a perspective and review highlighting current controversies. *Leuk Res*. 2003;27:95–120.

Surveillance Epidemiology and End Results. *SEER stat fact sheets: leukemia (ALL)*. <http://seer.cancer.gov/statfacts/html/alyl.html> Accessed 07.06.15.

15

Proteins

DONNA LARSON

CHAPTER OUTLINE

OBJECTIVES

At the completion of this chapter, the reader will be able to:

1. Define protein.
2. Identify the 20 common amino acids.
3. Describe a peptide bond.
4. Compare and contrast the four levels of structure of a protein.
5. Describe conjugated protein.
6. Discuss methods for determining total protein.
7. Discuss the clinical significance of albumin and test methods for determining albumin.
8. Compare and contrast prealbumin, α_1-fetoprotein, α_2-macroglobulin, ceruloplasmin, haptoglobin, transferrin, and myoglobin.
9. Identify the bands in normal serum protein electrophoresis scans and in scans from patients with monoclonal gammopathy, polyclonal gammopathy, nephrotic syndrome, agammaglobulinemia, and multiple myeloma.
10. Review the five classes of immunoglobulins and the characteristics of each class.
11. Compare and contrast immunoglobulin deficiency, polyclonal hyperimmunoglobulinemia, multiple myeloma, Waldenström macroglobulinemia, and cryoglobulin.
12. Describe Bence Jones protein and its clinical significance.
13. Discuss the importance of measuring urine and cerebrospinal fluid (CSF) proteins.
14. Describe two common dye-binding methods used to measure urine and CSF proteins.
15. Describe test methods for 24-hour urine protein determinations.
16. Describe proteins found in CSF and oligoclonal bands.

KEY TERMS

Albumin
α_1-Fetoprotein (AFP)
α_2-Macroglobulin
Amino acid
Apolipoprotein
Ceruloplasmin
Conjugated protein
Glycoprotein
Haptoglobin
IgA

IgD
IgE
IgG
IgM
Immunoglobulin
Isoelectric point
Lipoprotein
Metalloprotein
Microalbumin
Mucoprotein

Myoglobin
Nucleoprotein
Peptide bond
Phosphoprotein
Primary structure
Prosthetic group
Quaternary structure
Secondary structure
Tertiary structure
Transferrin

❖ Case in Point

A 65-year-old man presented to a physician's office with fatigue and bone pain in his hips. The physician ordered laboratory work, with the following results:

Hemoglobin: 10.2 g/dL
Creatinine: 0.9 mg/dL
Albumin: 3.0 g/dL
Total protein: 9.5 g/dL

Which of these laboratory results are considered abnormal? What is the probable diagnosis? What would be a predominant cell in the patient's bone marrow?

Points to Remember

- Proteins are long chains of amino acids linked by peptide bonds.
- There are 20 common amino acids that make up most proteins in the body.
- Proteins have four levels of structure: primary, secondary, tertiary, and quaternary. Structure is linked to function.
- Dye-binding test methods are used to determine total protein.
- Albumin is the most abundant of all plasma proteins. Decreased serum albumin levels can be caused by inflammation, hepatic disease, urinary loss, or gastrointestinal loss, whereas increased albumin levels are linked only to dehydration. Albumin is quantitated with the use of bromocresol green or bromocresol purple dye.
- α_1-Fetoprotein (AFP) is the major protein synthesized by the fetal liver. Screening for AFP is an important indicator for neural tube or open abdominal wall defects in fetuses.
- α_2-Macroglobulin is synthesized in the liver and modulates immunologic and inflammatory reactions. Serum protein electrophoresis is a common method for determining α_2-macroglobulin levels.
- Ceruloplasmin, the major copper-carrying protein in the body, functions as either an oxidant or an antioxidant in chemical reactions. Immunoassays are the test of choice for ceruloplasmin.
- Haptoglobin is a protein that binds to hemoglobin and is synthesized in the liver. This protein can be quantitated by immunochemical assays.
- Transferrin is a small protein that carries two iron molecules in the body. Decreased transferrin is an important clinical state. This protein is measured by immunochemical turbidimetric methods.
- Immunoglobulins are proteins produced by B cells that fall into the following categories: IgG, IgM, IgA, IgD, and IgE. Common hyperimmunoglobulinemias include multiple myeloma, Waldenström macroglobulinemia, and cryoglobulinemia.
- Myoglobin is a small protein that stores oxygen inside the cell. Myoglobin is found in muscle tissue, and its function is to keep iron molecules from oxidizing, thus enabling hemoglobin to bind with oxygen. Muscle-wasting diseases increase myoglobin concentrations in the blood. Immunoassays are used to quantitate this protein.
- Quantitative and qualitative measurements of microalbumin in the urine of diabetics provide a good indicator for renal damage.
- Methods to measure urine protein include sulfosalicylic acid, trichloroacetic acid, Coomassie blue, and pyrogallol red.
- Increased protein concentrations in cerebrospinal fluid (CSF) is an emergency clinical state because it indicates a brain tumor, intracerebral hemorrhage, meningitis, encephalitis, poliomyelitis, or traumatic injury. CSF protein is quantitated with the use of Coomassie blue and pyrogallol red dyes.

Introduction

Proteins are large, multiunit molecules composed of amino acids linked together by peptide bonds. Protein molecules may have primary, secondary, tertiary, and quaternary structures. Proteins are versatile molecules with many functions, including energy production, water distribution, buffering, transport of other molecules, and production of glycoproteins, antibodies, cellular proteins, structural proteins, and enzymes. Protein molecules can be metabolized and used for energy by the body. Proteins are important for water distribution because they affect the colloidal osmotic pressure. The positive and negative charges on the amino acids in a protein can absorb H^+ and OH^- ions, acting as a buffer. Proteins are also responsible for transporting calcium (albumin), iron (ferritin), and other molecules.

Conjugated proteins are large protein molecules that are attached to other molecules such as carbohydrates (glycoproteins) or lipids (lipoproteins). Immunoglobulins (antibodies) are proteins produced by B lymphocytes in response to anything recognized as a "foreign invader" in the blood. Cellular proteins can be found in the endoplasmic reticulum and the Golgi apparatus. Structural proteins make up a cell's cytoskeleton. Enzymes are catalysts that reduce the activation energy for many critical biological reactions occurring in the body.

Laboratory measurement of total and specific proteins is discussed in this chapter. Proteins are electrophoretically separated to expose specific disease conditions based on distinct patterns and their clinical correlations.

Biochemistry of Proteins

Proteins are macromolecules that can weigh as little as 6,000 or as much as 1,000,000 atomic mass units (daltons, or Da). They are polymers composed of a variety of building blocks called **amino acids.** Although proteins have many different shapes and functions, the essence of all proteins is peptide bonds between amino acids. There are approximately 20 common amino acids that combine to form proteins in the human body.

Amino Acids

The empirical formula for an amino acid is $RCH(NH_2)COOH$. The basic structure is illustrated in Figure 15-1. Each amino acid is composed of a carboxyl group (—COOH), an amino group (—NH$_2$), and an R group, which is responsible for the special features of the molecule. Depending on the nature of the R side chain, amino acids may be divided into five groups: nonpolar aliphatic, aromatic, positively charged, polar uncharged, and negatively charged. There are 20 common amino acids: alanine, arginine, asparagine, aspartic acid (aspartate), cysteine, glutamic acid, glutamine, glycine, histidine, isoleucine, leucine, lysine, methionine, phenylalanine, proline, serine, threonine, tryptophan, tyrosine, and valine.

Protein synthesis involves the creation of a long chain of amino acids linked to each other by peptide bonds. A peptide bond occurs when there is covalent bonding of the α-amino group of one amino acid to the α-carboxyl group of a second amino acid, as illustrated in Figure 15-2. The sequence of the amino acids dictates the specific protein. Because the long chains take up much space when arranged linearly, proteins are folded and linked to form more compact molecules.

Structure

Proteins have four distinct structures—primary, secondary, tertiary, and quaternary. Each structural level in a protein possesses distinct characteristics (Fig. 15-3). The primary structure of a protein is the identity and sequence of amino acids in the long polypeptide chain. The secondary structure of a protein consists of one-dimensional assemblies called α-helices and β-pleated sheets. These structures are created by hydrogen and disulfide covalent bonds. The tertiary structure of a protein is the folding of the protein molecule upon itself into a compact, three-dimensional structure. The quaternary structure (spatial arrangement) of a protein occurs when polypeptide subunits aggregate together.

Physical and Chemical Composition

Proteins are classified according to their physical and chemical composition. Proteins are first divided into two major groups—simple and conjugated. **Simple proteins** are those that contain only amino acids biochemicals. There are two subgroups of simple proteins—globular and fibrous. Globins are symmetric and soluble in saline. This group includes albumin, globulins, histones (basic proteins associated with nucleic acids), and protamines (strong basic proteins associated with nucleic acids). Fibrous proteins are asymmetric, water insoluble, and resistant to proteolytic enzymes. This group includes collagens (connective tissue constituents), elastins (found in tendons and arteries), and keratins (found in hair and nails).

Conjugated proteins are proteins that are combined with non–amino acid groups. These proteins have two components—the apoprotein (protein molecule) and the prosthetic group (nonprotein molecule). Types of conjugated proteins include nucleoproteins, mucoproteins, glycoproteins, lipoproteins, metalloproteins, and phosphoproteins. Nucleoproteins contain nucleic acids (DNA and RNA) as the prosthetic group. Mucoproteins contain large amounts of carbohydrates linked to the protein molecule. Glycoproteins also contain carbohydrate molecules, but the amount is less than 4% of the glycoprotein by weight. Lipoproteins are composed of a mixture of cholesterol, triglycerides, and phospholipids linked to apolipoproteins. Metalloproteins have metals bound to proteins as ions or complex metals (e.g., hemeproteins). Phosphoproteins contain a large number of phosphate groups linked to the protein.

The net charge of a protein is determined by combining the ionic charges on the amino acids, carbohydrates, and prosthetic group. The net charge is characteristic of a particular protein but varies with the pH of the environment because the chemical groups composing the protein ionize at different pH levels. The pH at which the net charge of the protein is zero is called the isoelectric point for that specific protein. If the pH of the environment is greater than the isoelectric point, the protein is negatively charged; if it is less than the isoelectric point, the protein is positively charged. Most plasma proteins are negatively charged at normal blood pH (7.35 to 7.45).

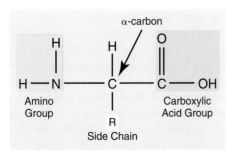

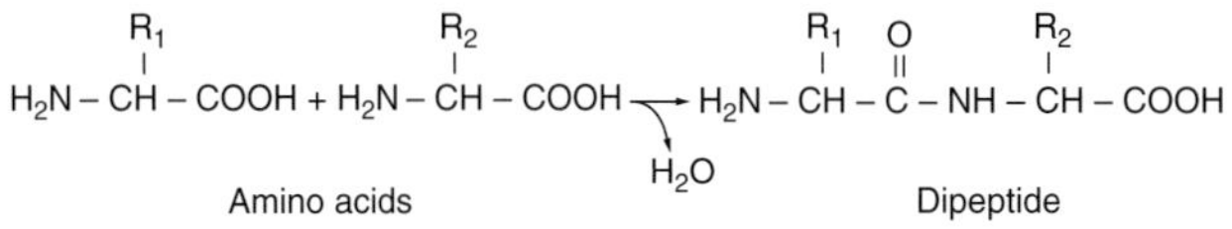

• **Figure 15-2** Peptide bond. Two amino acids are combining to form a dipeptide molecule. During the combination of the amino acids, a water molecule is produced. (From Baynes JW, Dominiczak MH. *Medical Biochemistry.* 4th ed. Edinburgh: Saunders/Elsevier Limited; 2015.)

• **Figure 15-1** Structure of an amino acid.

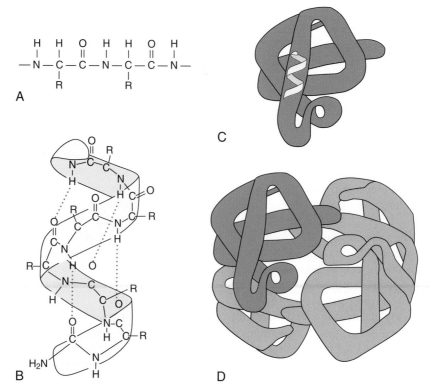

• **Figure 15-3** Structure levels of proteins. **A,** Primary structure. **B,** Secondary structure. **C,** Tertiary structure. **D,** Quaternary structure. (From Baynes JW, Dominiczak MH. *Medical Biochemistry.* 4th ed. Edinburgh: Saunders/Elsevier Limited, 2015.)

Properties

The easiest way to differentiate proteins is according to their properties. Some of the properties used for separation, identification, and assay of proteins include molecular size, differential solubility, electrical charge, adsorption onto inert materials, and specific binding to antibodies. The molecular size of a protein can be used to separate it from smaller molecules. Dialysis, ultrafiltration, gel filtration chromatography, and density-gradient chromatography can separate proteins based on molecular size. Differential solubility can be used precipitate proteins from a solution by changing the pH, ionic strength, temperature, or dielectric constant of the solvent. Changing these parameters affects the solubility of the protein. Another method for differentiating proteins uses electrical charge to change the speed and species of proteins that migrate in serum electrophoresis and isoelectric focusing. Ion-exchange chromatography uses electrostatic interactions to attract proteins to solid media. Adsorption onto inert materials uses hydrophobic, ionic, and hydrogen bonding to attract and separate proteins. Finally, the specificity of protein binding to antibodies, coenzymes, or hormone receptors can be used to quantitate proteins (i.e., immunoassays). Laboratory procedures for individual proteins are discussed in the following sections.

Function

Proteins function in many different ways in the body, most importantly as transporters, receptors, and catalysts.

Proteins can transport small molecules to specific areas. The transporter proteins tend to be globulins, because their structure lends itself for easy linking to molecules. Transporter proteins transport thyroxine (thyroid-binding globulin), cortisol (transcortin), fatty acids (albumin), unconjugated bilirubin (albumin), and calcium (albumin); lipoproteins transport lipids through the blood. Some proteins (receptors) bind to hormones and then transmit the hormonal signal into the cell. Receptor proteins are usually glycoproteins. Proteins can also act as biological catalysts or enzymes. Globulins and metalloproteins are the protein types most likely to be found as enzymes.

Proteins play a part in the structure of body tissues (collagen) as well as hair and nails. They serve as a nutritional source for calories or amino acids. Proteins are responsible for maintaining the colloid osmotic pressure throughout the body as well as body water balance. (Recall that the colloid osmotic pressure is a form of pressure exerted by proteins in plasma that tends to pull water into the blood vessel—see Chapter 12). Proteins are antigenic molecules, meaning that immunologically competent hosts will produce antibodies against them when they are recognized as antigens. Antibodies are globular proteins that are produced by B lymphocytes to protect the body from foreign invaders. Proteins can also be hormones—regulatory substances that are produced by the body to initiate action in specific cells. Finally, proteins are involved in the coagulation system; for example, fibrinogen is a protein.

Plasma Proteins

Serum proteins can be divided into two groups: albumin (54% of serum proteins) and other proteins. The other proteins in the serum are collectively referred to as *globulins*. The globulin concentration is calculated by subtracting the concentration of albumin from the total protein concentration:

Globulin concentration = Total protein concentration − Albumin concentration

Increases or decreases in individual plasma protein concentrations can be affected by nutritional status, physiologic changes, synthesis rate, extracellular distribution, and clearance rate (Table 15-1). Because total protein levels remain relatively constant regardless of nutritional status, measurements of albumin and, more recently, prealbumin are used to assess for protein nutrition. Inflammation is a physiologic change that increases the levels of acute phase reactants and decreases albumin levels. Most plasma proteins are synthesized in the liver, except for immunoglobulins (which are produced by B lymphocytes) and protein hormones (produced by glands). A decrease in the rate of synthesis will affect the amount of protein in the plasma. Albumin is distributed between the vascular and interstitial compartments, with redistribution of the protein occurring frequently. More than half of the body's albumin is in the extravascular space.

Proteins can be cleared from the body by catabolism and protein-losing states. Proteins are broken down by

TABLE 15-1 Plasma Proteins: Reference Ranges and Conditions in which the Protein Is Increased or Decreased

Protein	Reference Range	Increased	Decreased
Prealbumin	10-20 mg/dL	See Table 15-2	See Table 15-2
Albumin	3.5-5.2 g/dL	See Table 15-3	See Table 15-3
α-Fetoprotein	Varies according to gestational age	Trisomy 21 Trisomy 18	Neural tube defect Multiple fetuses Fetal demise Low birth rate
α_1-Globulins	100-300 mg/dL	Acute inflammation Chronic inflammation Hypoproteinemia	Severe hepatitis α_1-Antitrypsin
α_2-Macroglobulin	150-420 mg/dL	Estrogen Age Nephrotic syndrome	Acute phase response Pancreatitis Prostate cancer
α_2-Globulins	600-1000 mg/dL	Acute inflammation Chronic inflammation Nephrotic syndrome Hypoproteinemia	Severe hepatitis Chronic cirrhosis
β-Globulins	700-1200 mg/dL	Chronic inflammation	Severe hepatitis Chronic cirrhosis Hypoproteinemia
Ceruloplasmin	15-60 mg/dL	Estrogen	Menkes disease Wilson disease
Haptoglobin	100-200 mg/dL	Acute phase reaction Protein-losing conditions	Hemolytic disease Hepatocellular disease Neonates
Transferrin	200-320 mg/dL	See Table 15-4	See Table 15-4
γ-Globulins (total)	700-1600 mg/dL	Chronic inflammation Chronic cirrhosis Hypergammaglobulinemia	Acute inflammation Severe hepatitis Nephrotic syndrome Hypogammaglobulinemia
IgG	800-1800 mg/dL	See Table 15-5	See Table 15-5
IgM	60-250 mg/dL	See Table 15-5	See Table 15-5
IgA	90-450 mg/dL	See Table 15-5	See Table 15-5
IgD	0-384 ng/mL		
IgE	0-160 kIU/L		

Continued

TABLE 15-1 Plasma Proteins: Reference Ranges and Conditions in which the Protein Is Increased or Decreased—cont'd

Protein	Reference Range	Increased	Decreased
Myoglobin	10-95 ng/mL	Rhabdomyolysis Muscle injections Strenuous exercise Kidney failure	Not clinically significant
Serum protein (total)	6.4-8.3 g/dL		
Urine protein (total)	Random: 0-20 mg/dL 4-hour: 0-6 mg/dL 24-hour: 0-0.15 g/day	Kidney failure Nephrotic syndrome Glomerulonephritis	Not clinically significant
CSF protein (total)	15-60 mg/dL	Cerebral atrophy Malignancies Meningeal hemorrhage Degenerative disorders Meningitis Encephalitis Inflammation Multiple myeloma Hypothyroidism Stroke Cerebral infarct Guillain-Barré syndrome	Not clinically significant

CSF, Cerebrospinal fluid; *Ig,* immunoglobulin.

nonspecific proteases into amino acids. Protein-losing states such as the nephrotic syndrome, which allow large amounts of proteins to be excreted in the urine, can significantly reduce the concentration of protein in the blood. The reference range for total protein in serum is 6.4 to 8.3 g/dL (see Table 15-1).

This section discusses the function, clinical correlation, and laboratory procedures and limitations for several common plasma proteins: prealbumin, albumin, α-fetoprotein, α$_2$-macroglobulin, ceruloplasmin, haptoglobin, transferrin, immunoglobulins, and myoglobin. Three others—C-reactive protein, complement proteins, and α$_1$-antitrypsin—are discussed in Chapter 11.

Prealbumin

Prealbumin is a small transporter protein with four identical subunits, each of which contains two binding sites. (Despite its name, it is not a precursor for albumin.) This protein binds and transports 10% of the total concentration of the thyroid hormones triiodothyronine (T$_3$) and thyroxine (T$_4$), with each subunit capable of binding to one molecule of thyroid hormone. Prealbumin is also important in the transport of vitamin A (retinol): Prealbumin binds with retinol-binding protein and then enters the circulation. Retinol-binding protein is much smaller than prealbumin and would be filtered out of the circulation through the glomerulus if it did not bind with prealbumin while in the blood. Prealbumin is synthesized in the liver and in the choroid plexus of the central nervous system. Synthesis is stimulated by glucocorticoid hormones, androgens, and nonsteroidal antiinflammatory drugs (NSAIDs).

Prealbumin crosses the blood–brain barrier into the cerebrospinal fluid (CSF) more readily than other proteins. As a result, prealbumin is a normal constituent in CSF. If CSF is concentrated before electrophoresis, a distinct prealbumin band will be present. This prealbumin peak confirms that the specimen is CSF. Normal CSF will also have a major peak of albumin and a small amount of other proteins on the electrophoresis medium (Fig. 15-4).

Clinical Correlation

Prealbumin is used as an indicator of protein nutrition because it responds more rapidly to changing nutrition than albumin does. Prealbumin may be increased in conditions such as severe renal failure, corticosteroid use, and oral contraceptive use, but the test is not used for diagnosing or monitoring in these conditions. This protein is decreased after surgery and in liver disease, hepatitis, infection, stress, inflammation, dialysis, hyperthyroidism, pregnancy, and hyperglycemia (Table 15-2).

Laboratory Procedures and Limitations

Prealbumin, as the name implies, migrates anodally to albumin on serum protein electrophoresis (SPEP). Because serum levels of prealbumin are so small, immunonephelometry or immunoturbidimetry is the method of choice for quantitation. The reference range is 0.0 to 3.1 mg/dL in CSF and 10 to 20 mg/dL in serum (see Table 15-1).

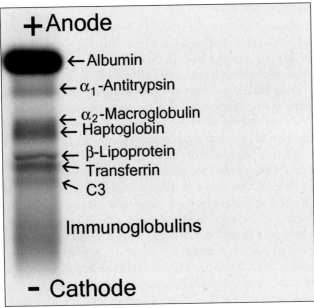

• **Figure 15-4** Normal serum protein electrophoresis result (in agarose) shows the positions of major serum proteins. Individual proteins separate according to their electrical charge between the anode (positive pole) and the cathode (negative pole). (From McPherson RA, Pincus MR. *Henry's Clinical Diagnosis and Management by Laboratory Methods.* 22nd ed. Philadelphia: Saunders; 2012.)

Albumin

Albumin has the highest concentration of any protein in blood. About 50% of protein found in blood is albumin. Because it is a small protein, it is also found in CSF, interstitial fluid, urine, and amniotic fluid. Albumin is synthesized in the liver, and its concentration in the blood is controlled by colloidal osmotic pressure and protein intake. (Recall from Chapter 12 that colloidal osmotic pressure is the pressure exerted on the outer walls of the blood vessels by large proteins and other colloid molecules within the cell.) Sixty percent of the body's albumin is found in the extravascular space.

Function

The primary function of albumin is to maintain the colloidal osmotic pressure in the intravascular and extravascular spaces. Albumin also serves as a transport protein for fatty acids, phospholipids, metallic ions, amino acids, drugs, hormones, and bilirubin.

Clinical Correlation

Albumin levels are elevated in cases of dehydration, marasmus, blood transfusion, exogenous albumin administration, anabolic steroid use, androgen administration, growth hormone administration, and increased insulin levels (Table 15-3). A decreased albumin concentration is very significant and can indicate the presence of a serious disease. The most common disease mechanisms for decreased albumin are overhydration, ascites, edema, hepatic failure, inflammation, nephrotic syndrome, protein-losing states,

trauma, burns, kwashiorkor, cancer, corticosteroid use, zinc deficiency, pregnancy, and collagen diseases.

Inflammation causes low albumin levels because the body shifts priorities and begins producing acute phase proteins in mass while reducing the amounts of other proteins produced. Liver disease affects albumin synthesis because liver cells are destroyed, rendering the cells unable to continue normal albumin production. Serum albumin levels may also be reduced when albumin is lost from the body in large amounts; this is commonly seen with diseases of the urinary

TABLE 15-2 Factors Affecting Prealbumin Levels

Factors Increasing Prealbumin Levels	Factors Decreasing Prealbumin Levels
Severe renal failure	Post-surgery
Corticosteroid use	Liver disease
Oral contraceptives	Hepatitis
	Infection
	Stress
	Inflammation
	Dialysis
	Hyperthyroidism
	Pregnancy
	Hyperglycemia

TABLE 15-3 Factors Affecting Albumin Levels

Factors Increasing Albumin Levels	Factors Decreasing Albumin Levels
Dehydration	Overhydration
Marasmus	Ascites
Blood transfusions	Edema
Exogenous albumin	Hepatic failure
Anabolic steroids	Inflammation
Androgens	Nephrotic syndrome
Growth hormone	Protein losing states
Insulin	Trauma
	Burns
	Kwashiorkor
	Collagen diseases
	Cancer
	Corticosteroid use
	Zinc deficiency
	Pregnancy

tract such as nephrotic syndrome and glomerulonephritis. Finally, hypoalbuminemia can result when large amounts of protein are lost through the gastrointestinal tract, such as in congestive heart failure, connective tissue diseases, amyloidosis, or protein dyscrasias.

Laboratory Procedures and Limitations

Albumin in serum or heparinized plasma is usually measured colorimetrically by a dye-binding method using bromocresol green or bromocresol purple dye. At a pH of 4.2, bromocresol green will turn from yellow-green to blue-green after binding with albumin. This color change is measurable at 623 nm, and this method is linear to 6 g/dL. A high concentration of bilirubin, hemolysis, or lipemia will interfere with this method. This method is sensitive to 1 g/dL of albumin in serum; the reference range is 3.5 to 5.2 g/dL (see Table 15-1).

α-Fetoprotein

α-Fetoprotein (AFP) is a small glycoprotein consisting of one peptide chain. It is the major protein in fetal plasma and is synthesized by the fetal liver. AFP reaches its peak in fetal plasma at the end of the first trimester, whereas the level in maternal plasma peaks at about week 30 of gestation.

Clinical Correlation

Screening of pregnant women for an elevated AFP level at specific gestation times can indicate whether certain birth defects, such as a neural tube defect or an open abdominal wall defect, are present in the fetus. Other conditions that produce elevated AFP levels in maternal serum include multiple fetuses, low birth weight, and fetal demise. Low AFP levels are seen in trisomy 21 (Down syndrome) and trisomy 18 (Edwards syndrome).

Laboratory Procedures and Limitations

The two most common methods for quantitating AFP are the immunofluorescent liquid-phase binding assay and the chemiluminescence immunoassay. For more information on these tests, see Chapter 26.

α₂-Macroglobulin

α₂-Macroglobulin is a serine protease inhibitor and can inhibit many different types of proteinases. This protein, unlike α₁-antitrypsin, is a very large protein molecule that cannot diffuse out of the plasma. It contains four identical polypeptide chains that are linked together to form two dimers. This protein is synthesized in the liver and has a half-life of several days. Functions of α₂-macroglobulin include interfering with proteinases by blocking their access to proteins. It also inhibits enzymes in the kinin, complement, coagulation, and fibrinolytic pathways. α₂-Macroglobulin may be a carrier protein for cytokines and growth factors as well as cations such as zinc. Finally, this protein modulates immunologic and inflammatory reactions.

Clinical Correlation

Estrogen, age, and the nephrotic syndrome correlate with an increased α₂-macroglobulin level. Women normally have higher levels of this protein than do men. The levels of α₂-macroglobulin in infants and children are three times higher than in adults. α₂-Macroglobulin levels are increased in the nephrotic syndrome because the massive amount of proteins lost through the kidneys signals the liver to synthesize more of all proteins to compensate for the loss.

Decreased levels of α₂-macroglobulin are found in acute phase response, pancreatitis, and prostate cancer. Release of interleukin-1 (IL-1) inhibits the synthesis of α₂-macroglobulin. In acute pancreatitis, α₂-macroglobulin levels are markedly decreased through an unknown mechanism. α₂-Macroglobulin levels are decreased in advanced prostate cancer because this protein binds to the excess prostate-specific antigen (PSA) and therefore is reduced in plasma. α₂-Macroglobulin levels do return to normal with successful treatment of prostate cancer (i.e., the PSA levels in the plasma drop).

Laboratory Procedures and Limitations

α₂-Macroglobulin levels are determined through SPEP (Fig. 15-5). It is one of the major proteins comprising the α₂-globulin band. The reference range is 150 to 420 mg/dL (see Table 15-1).

Ceruloplasmin

Ceruloplasmin transports copper ions. Each molecule of ceruloplasmin contains six to eight copper molecules, accounting for 95% of the copper found in the plasma. The protein consists of a single peptide chain linked to carbohydrate side chains. Most ceruloplasmin is synthesized by the liver, but small amounts are synthesized by macrophages and lymphocytes. Its half-life is 4 to 5 days.

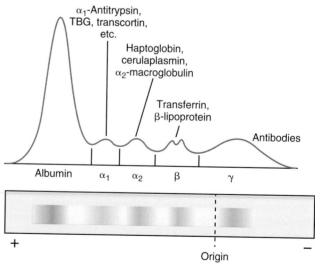

• **Figure 15-5** Serum protein electrophoresis separates the sample into several standard bands, allowing quantitation. Typical proteins found in each band are shown. *TBG,* Thyroxine-binding globulin.

Function

Ceruloplasmin functions as either an oxidant or an antioxidant in chemical reactions. It is important for the incorporation of iron into transferrin because it receives a proton during the oxidation of Fe^{+2} to Fe^{+3}, preventing the formation of toxic iron products. It also functions in membrane lipid oxidation.

Clinical Correlation

Increased levels of ceruloplasmin are seen in women taking estrogen-containing medications and in pregnant women. Low levels of ceruloplasmin are classified as primary (genetic) or secondary deficiencies. In primary deficiencies, the clinical picture is similar to that of hereditary hemochromatosis: increased tissue iron stress and decreased serum iron. Secondary deficiencies may be caused by low serum copper (malnutrition or malabsorption), malfunction of gastrointestinal epithelial cells (preventing release of copper into the circulation), or a defective synthesis process (inability to incorporate copper ions into the molecule).

Menkes disease is an X-linked inherited disorder in which absorbed copper cannot be transported to the blood due to an intracellular enzyme deficiency. (For more information see Chapter 29.) Wilson disease is a genetic disorder that prevents the body from getting rid of excess copper ions. As a result, copper ions are deposited in the liver, eyes, brain, and other body tissues, causing life-threatening organ damage. Patients develop cirrhosis and Kayser-Fleischer rings (dark brown circles around the iris). This disease is fatal if not treated. (For more information, see Chapter 21.)

Laboratory Procedures and Limitations

Ceruloplasmin has a short half-life, so serum must be stored at 4° C (for up to 3 days) or frozen at –70° C for longer storage. Immunoassays are the test of choice for ceruloplasmin, but it can also be functionally assayed. A functional assay determines copper oxidase activity and is more complicated to perform. The reference range is 15 to 60 mg/dL (see Table 15-1).

Haptoglobin

Haptoglobin binds to hemoglobin. It is synthesized in the liver and has a configuration similar to hemoglobin when it is first synthesized. Before entering the bloodstream, the haptoglobin molecule is cleaved into monomers. When hemolysis releases hemoglobin into the extravascular space, it immediately bonds to a haptoglobin molecule. This helps prevent loss of hemoglobin through the kidneys. The half-life of haptoglobin is approximately 5.5 days.

Function and Clinical Correlation

In addition to conserving hemoglobin, haptoglobin kills leukocytes at inflammatory sites; coordinates activity of lymphocytes, monocytes, and granulocytes; acts as a bacteriostatic agent; and controls angiogenesis.

Haptoglobin levels are increased in acute phase reactions and in protein-losing conditions. In acute phase reactions, its synthesis is stimulated by cytokines. The level of haptoglobin increases 4 to 6 days after initiation of the inflammatory process. It seems odd that haptoglobin would be increased in protein-losing conditions, but the massive amount of protein lost in these syndromes stimulates the liver to synthesize more proteins, and all proteins are increased as a result.

Haptoglobin is decreased in hemolytic diseases, in hepatocellular disease, and in neonates. Haptoglobin is used to indicate in vivo extravascular hemolysis because it combines quickly with free hemoglobin. Hepatocellular disease reduces the function of liver and that includes the synthesis of all proteins; haptoglobin and other plasma proteins have reduced levels in this condition. Neonates have absent or very low haptoglobin levels because their livers are immature and cannot synthesize this protein.

Laboratory Procedures and Limitations

Haptoglobin migrates in the α_2 region on SPEP. Immunochemical turbidimetric and nephelometric methods are used to quantitate haptoglobin. Anti-haptoglobin antibodies are mixed with a sample; there they bind with haptoglobin to produce insoluble complexes. The absorbance of the resulting solution is measured and compared with a standard to determine the level of haptoglobin present in the sample. The reference range is 100 to 200 mg/dL (see Table 15-1).

Transferrin

Transferrin is a small protein that contains two iron (Fe^{+3}) binding sites and is used to transport iron in the body. The liver is the major site of synthesis for transferrin, and its concentration depends on the plasma iron level. Its half-life is 8 to 10 days.

Function and Clinical Correlation

Transferrin carries iron to all areas of the body and maintains the iron homeostasis in the body. High transferrin levels are present in iron deficiency, and low levels are present with iron overload. It is also decreased in protein-losing syndromes such as nephrotic syndrome and severe liver disease and in any inflammatory state. There is a genetic condition, called atransferrinemia, in which no transferrin is present in the body. Anemia and hemosiderosis in the liver and heart are the hallmarks of this disease. The hemosiderosis in the heart can lead to heart failure (Table 15-4).

Laboratory Procedures and Limitations

This protein is measured by immunochemical turbidimetric methods. In this technique, anti-transferrin antibodies are mixed with the serum sample in an aqueous solution. The antigen–antibody interaction produces a precipitate that decreases the absorbance of the solution. The concentration of the protein in the sample is determined by comparing the absorbance of the sample solution with that of a standard solution. The reference range is 200 to 320 mg/dL (see Table 15-1).

Immunoglobulins

Function

Immunoglobulins are proteins that function as antibodies. As monomers, they are composed of two light protein chains and two heavy protein chains. They are produced by B lymphocytes and are grouped into five classes: IgG, IgM, IgA, IgD, and IgE (Fig. 15-6). **IgG** makes up 70% to 75% of the immunoglobulins found in the body. Sixty-five percent of IgG is found in the extravascular compartment and 35% in the blood. IgG consists of one immunoglobulin molecule (monomer). **IgM** is the largest and least specific immunoglobulin in the blood. One IgM molecule is composed of five immunoglobulin monomers connected at their bases. It does not cross the placenta, and it is an activator of complement. **IgA** makes up about 15% of the immunoglobulins present in the blood; it exists as a monomer and as a dimer. Some of the IgA in the body is secreted in tears, sweat, saliva, milk, colostrum, and gastrointestinal and respiratory secretions. IgA can activate complement through the alternative pathway.

IgD makes up only about 1% of the immunoglobulins in the blood. It is a monomer, and its function is unknown. **IgE**, another monomer is usually found attached to mast cells; there is very little IgE present in the blood. When an antigen forms a crosslink between two bound IgE molecules, the mast cell is activated to release histamine into the blood. This histamine produces the allergic reactions seen in hay fever, asthma, hives, and eczema. Reference ranges for all immunoglobulin types are as follows: IgG, 800-1800 mg/dL; IgM, 60-250 mg/dL; IgA, 90-450 mg/dL; IgD, 0-384 ng/mL; and IgE, 0-160 kIU/L (see Table 15-1).

Clinical Correlation

At any point in time, the blood contains many different types of antibodies. Several clinical conditions involve immunoglobulins (Table 15-5). There can be an immunoglobulin deficiency, in which one or more classes of immunoglobulins are decreased or absent. There also can be increases in the amounts of all classes of immunoglobulins or of an individual class. Conditions in which all classes are increased at the same time are usually referred to as *polyclonal hyperimmunoglobulinemias*. If the increased concentration involves only one specific type of immunoglobulin, it is a *monoclonal immunoglobulinemia*.

TABLE 15-4	Factors Affecting Transferrin Levels	
Factors Increasing Transferrin Levels	**Factors Decreasing Transferrin Levels**
Iron deficiency	Pernicious anemia
Dehydration	Anemia of chronic disease
Pregnancy	Folate deficient anemia
Oral contraceptives	Overhydration
Estrogen	Chronic infection
Chronic blood loss	Iron overload
Hepatitis	Acute catabolic states
Hypoxia	Uremia
Chronic renal failure	Nephrotic syndrome
	Severe liver disease
	Kwashiorkor
	Zinc deficiency
	Corticosteroids
	Cancer

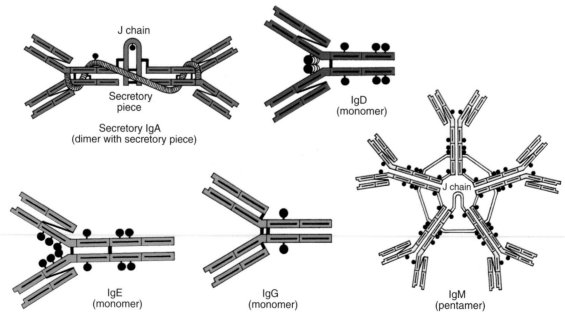

• **Figure 15-6** Secretory immunoglobulins IgA, IgD, IgE, IgG, and IgM. The black circles attached to each molecule represent carbohydrate residues. (From McCance KL, Huether SE. *Pathophysiology: The Biologic Basis for Disease in Adults and Children.* 7th ed. St. Louis: Mosby; 2015.)

Immunoglobulin Deficiency

Most immunoglobulin deficiencies manifest in infancy; those manifesting in adulthood are the result of either another primary disorder (e.g., a monoclonal gammopathy) or immunosuppressive therapy. These disorders can involve particular immunoglobulin classes, subclasses, or light chains. Signs and symptoms include recurrent infections, family history, age at onset, sites of infection, types of microorganisms, blood product reactions, gastrointestinal symptoms, musculoskeletal symptoms, and autoimmune and collagen vascular disease.

The most common types encountered in the laboratory are selective IgG immunodeficiency, selective IgA immunodeficiency, and X-linked agammaglobulinemia. The most common immunodeficiency is selective IgG immunoglobulin deficiency, in which the individual's IgG levels are decreased but levels of the remaining immunoglobulins are within normal limits. In selective IgA immunoglobulin deficiency, the second most common type, IgA is the only immunoglobulin level decreased. In X-linked agammaglobulinemia, all immunoglobulin levels are markedly reduced. (For further details, see Chapter 32.)

Polyclonal Hyperimmunoglobulinemia

If the levels of all immunoglobulins are increased, the body is responding to an infection, although in some situations a particular immunoglobulin is more increased than the others. For example, in autoimmune diseases, all immunoglobulin levels are increased, but the IgG is especially increased. Primary biliary cirrhosis leads to a greatly increased level of IgM. In acute hepatitis, IgG is greatly increased and sometimes IgM can also be markedly increased.

Monoclonal Immunoglobulinemia

A single group or clone of B lymphocytes produces identical immunoglobulins (i.e., monoclonal immunoglobulins). There are conditions in which the size of a particular clone increases and produces a sharp peak on SPEP. These monoclonal immunoglobulins are called *paraproteins*. One paraprotein of particular interest to clinicians is Bence Jones proteins, which are actually protein fragments (light chains). They are considered tumor markers and are found in the urine of individuals with multiple myeloma or Waldenström macroglobulinemia.

Multiple Myeloma. Plasma cell cancer is called multiple myeloma. In multiple myeloma, a single clone of cells produces markedly increased amounts of immunoglobulins. Malignant plasma cell clones grow in the bone marrow, crowding out all the normal cells (Fig. 15-7). They also form

TABLE 15-5	Immunoglobulin Levels in Various Disorders		
	IgG	IgA	IgM
Agammaglobulinemia	↓	↓	↓
Lupus erythematosus	↑	↑	↑
Rheumatoid arthritis	↑	↑	↑
Lymphoid aplasia	↓	↓	↓
Selective IgG-IgA deficiency	↓	↓	N
Selective IgA-IgM deficiency	N	↓	↓
Anti-IgA globulinemia	N	↓	N
Ataxia-telangiectasia	N	↓	N
IgG myeloma	↑	↓	↓
IgA myeloma	↓	↑	↓
Waldenström macroglobulinemia and IgM myeloma	↓ or N	↓ or N	↑
Acute lymphocytic leukemia	↓	↓	↓
Chronic lymphocytic leukemia	↓	↓	↓
Acute myelocytic leukemia	N	N	N
Chronic myelocytic leukemia	N	↓	N
Hodgkin disease	N	N	N
Laennec cirrhosis	↑	↑	N
Biliary cirrhosis	N	N	↑
Acute hepatitis	↑	↑	↑
Hepatocellular carcinoma	N	N	↓
Pulmonary tuberculosis	↑	N	N
Trypanosomiasis	↓	↓	↑↑↑
Gastrointestinal protein loss	↓	↓	↓
Nephrotic syndrome	↓	↓	↓

N, Normal; ↓, decreased; ↑, increased.

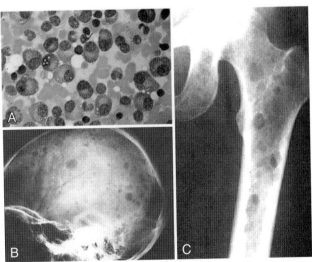

• **Figure 15-7 A,** Malignant plasma cells in multiple myeloma. Most show a dark blue cytoplasm, peripherally located nuclei, and perinuclear clearing. Some cells have vacuoles containing immunoglobulin. **B,** Radiograph of a skull showing multiple "punched out" lytic lesions in multiple myeloma. **C,** Multiple lytic lesions in the femur and pelvis in multiple myeloma. (**A,** From Goldman L, Schafer AI. *Goldman's Cecil Medicine.* 24th ed. Philadelphia: Saunders; 2012:1238, Fig. 193-4. **B,** From Damjanov I, Linder J. *Anderson's Pathology.* 10th ed. St. Louis: Mosby; 1996:1105, Fig. 41-61. **C,** From Doherty M, George E. *Self-Assessment Picture Tests in Medicine: Rheumatology.* London: Mosby-Wolfe; 1995:7, Fig. 4.)

tumors that destroy the bone tissue. Plasma cells secrete immunoglobulins, and the malignant plasma cells secrete monoclonal proteins (called *M proteins*) that resemble immunoglobulins (Fig. 15-8). The most common type of immunoglobulin produced is IgG, followed by IgA and IgD. IgM myelomas are rare; when IgM is markedly increased, Waldenström macroglobulinemia is usually suspected.

Multiple myeloma affects 5.6 of every 100,000 people. The highest incidence occurs at about 70 years of age, with those 40 years and older the predominant population. Multiple myeloma is the result of a chromosomal translocation. The clone cells cause damage by crowding the bone marrow and squeezing out red blood cell precursors to produce anemia; overproducing interleukin-6 (IL-6); causing in-bone destruction; thickening the blood, which results in kidney damage and even renal failure; and depositing light chains in nerve sheaths, causing nerve damage. Eighty percent of the clones produce immunoglobulin light chains (Bence Jones proteins) that can be found in the blood and urine. Bence Jones proteins are reported to damage renal epithelial cells.

Most patients with multiple myeloma have bone pain, pathologic fractures, weakness, anemia, infection, hypercalcemia, spinal cord compression, renal failure, or some combination of these features. In 30% of cases, the condition is discovered through routine blood work or while the patient is seeking care for another, unrelated condition. A large gap (globulin level) between total protein and albumin indicates a possible problem. Other patients seek care because of a fracture that has no known cause; increased bone resorption causes weak bones that fracture under normal conditions. Still other patients seek medical care for bone pain in the back, long bones, skull, or pelvis. Some patients with back pain have spinal cord compression, especially when the back pain is accompanied by weakness or numbness.

Occasionally, patients seek care for bleeding that is caused by thrombocytopenia. With so many plasma cells crowding

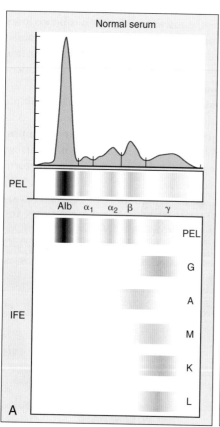
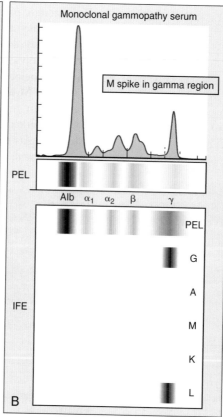
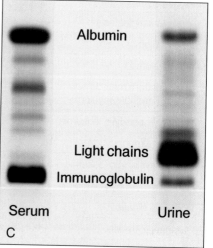

• **Figure 15-8** M protein. Serum protein electrophoresis *(PEL)* is used to screen for M proteins in multiple myeloma. **A,** In normal serum, the proteins separate into several regions between albumin *(Alb)* and a broad band in the gamma (γ) region, where most antibodies (γ-globulins) are found. Immunofixation *(IFE)* can identify the locations of IgG *(G)*, IgA *(A)*, IgM *(M)*, and kappa *(K)* and lambda *(L)* light chains. **B,** Serum from an individual with multiple myeloma contains a sharp M protein *(M spike)*. The M protein is monoclonal and contains only one heavy chain and one light chain. In this instance the IFE identifies the M protein as an IgG containing a lambda light chain. **C,** Serum and urine protein electrophoretic patterns in a client with multiple myeloma. Serum demonstrates an M protein *(Immunoglobulin)* in the γ region, and the urine has a large amount of the smaller-sized light chains with only a small amount of intact immunoglobulin. (**A** and **B,** From Niederhuber JE, Armitage JO, Doroshow JH, Kastan MB, Tepper JE. *Abeloff's Clinical Oncology.* 5th ed. Philadelphia: Saunders; 2014. **C,** From McPherson R, Pincus M. *Henry's Clinical Diagnosis and Management by Laboratory Methods.* 22nd ed. Philadelphia: Saunders; 2012.)

the bone marrow, megakaryocytes can also be squeezed out of the bone marrow, resulting in a very low platelet count, which can lead to bleeding.

Patients who exhibit confusion, sleepiness, bone pain, constipation, nausea, and thirst may have hypercalcemia. Hypercalcemia is produced when the malignant cells stimulate the bone to resorb calcium, leading to bone lesions. The large number of plasma cells that replace normal red and white blood cells may result in leukopenia and altered immunity, which in turn lead to infections. *Streptococcus pneumonia, Haemophilus,* and herpes zoster infections are common in patients with multiple myeloma. When the serum viscosity is greater than 4 times that of normal serum, individuals experience generalized malaise, infection, fever, sluggish mental functions, sensory loss, headaches, and sleepiness. If the protein level is high enough, stroke, myocardial ischemia, or infarction may occur.

Waldenström Macroglobulinemia. Waldenström macroglobulinemia, a chronic lymphoproliferative disease, is one of the malignant monoclonal gammopathies. This disease produces a high level of IgM in the blood, which increases the serum viscosity. As in multiple myeloma, a large number of plasma cells are present in the bone marrow. According to the classification scheme of the World Health Organization, Waldenström macroglobulinemia is a lymphoplasmic lymphoma because it arises from a clone of B lymphocytes. The onset of this disease is insidious and nonspecific; it is often diagnosed through routine blood work. On initial diagnosis, patients exhibit weakness, anorexia, peripheral neuropathy, weight loss, fever, and Raynaud phenomenon.

The hallmark of Waldenström macroglobulinemia is the hyperviscosity syndrome produced by the increased monoclonal IgM in the blood; this leads to vascular complications due to the physical, chemical, and immunologic properties of the protein. This monoclonal IgM paraprotein also causes cryoglobulinemia, coagulation abnormalities, sensorimotor peripheral neuropathy, cold agglutinin disease, anemia, and primary amyloidosis. In addition to the symptoms caused by the IgM paraprotein, the malignant plasma cells infiltrate the bone marrow, spleen, and lymph nodes. In some cases, they also permeate the liver, lungs, gastrointestinal tract, kidneys, skin, eyes, and central nervous system. As in multiple myeloma and other monoclonal gammopathies, the IgM paraprotein appears as a large peak on SPEP. Two conditions differentiate Waldenström symptoms from those of multiple myeloma: (1) Waldenström cells permeate tissues and organs, causing organomegaly, whereas multiple myeloma does not cause this symptom; and (2) Waldenström macroglobulinemia does not produce the bone lesions that are commonly found in multiple myeloma.

Individuals with Waldenström macroglobulinemia experience many complications in addition to the hyperviscosity syndrome, including blurry vision; dizziness; diarrhea and malabsorption; renal disease; amyloidosis of the heart, kidney, liver, lungs, and joints; bleeding; Raynaud phenomenon; cardiac failure; and increased chance of developing additional white blood cell dyscrasias.

Cryoglobulinemia. Cryoglobulinemia occurs when the body produces immunoglobulins that undergo reversible precipitation at low temperatures. Cryoglobulins can cause a systemic inflammation affecting the kidneys and skin. Cryoglobulins can exist with no known underlying disease, or they can be found with an underlying disease such as Waldenström macroglobulinemia.

Laboratory Procedures and Limitations

Immunoglobulin conditions can be identified by SPEP (see Table 15-5). Immunoglobulin levels are quantitated by immunoturbidimetry or immunonephelometry (Fig. 15-9). Further classification is accomplished through immunoelectrophoresis or immunofixation. Other methods used to identify proteins include the Western blot and capillary electrophoresis.

Myoglobin

Myoglobin is a small, single-polypeptide (monomeric) protein that intracellularly stores oxygen. It makes up the skeletal muscle of vertebrates and colors the muscle red. It is related to hemoglobin, which contains four monomer proteins similar to myoglobin.

Function

Myoglobin coordinates the oxygenation of hemoglobin by protecting hemoglobin from other molecules, thus keeping the iron molecules in the hemoglobin in the ferrous (Fe^{2+}) state. Once the iron is oxidized to the ferric (Fe^{3+}) state, hemoglobin loses the ability to bind oxygen. Because myoglobin contains a heme group, it can also bind oxygen. The myoglobin molecule can then release the oxygen to bind with hemoglobin when necessary.

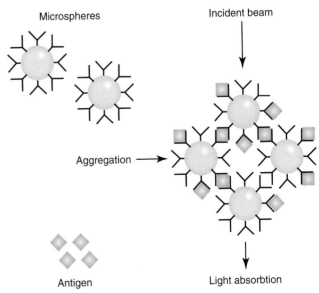

• **Figure 15-9** Immunoturbidimetry.

Clinical Correlation and Laboratory Procedures

Myoglobin is released into the blood when muscle tissue is damaged. It can be found in the urine after muscle trauma. In rhabdomyolysis, a disease that occurs after skeletal muscle is injured, large quantities of toxic intracellular contents (myoglobin) spill into the blood. Myoglobin is toxic to the renal tubular epithelium, and high concentrations can cause acute renal failure.

Semiquantitative methods such as nephelometric, turbidimetric, and fluorescence immunoassays are used to quantitate myoglobin. Two-site immunoassays using monoclonal assays can also be used and are sensitive and specific with reasonable assay times. The reference range is 10 to 95 ng/mL (see Table 15-1).

Proteins in Other Body Fluids

Urine Protein

Normally, very small amounts of protein are excreted in the urine. Tamm-Horsfall protein is a small protein that is normally excreted in urine in small amounts (approximately 40 mg/24 hours). In some diseases, other proteins, such as albumin, may be excreted in large quantities. In addition to measuring albumin in serum, there are instances when a clinician needs information about albumin in the urine. This is especially true for diabetic patients, who are prone to gradual renal damage leading to end-stage kidney disease. If the process can be detected and treated early, the individual may never develop that final stage.

In diabetes, the kidneys start losing tiny amounts of protein at first, and then, as the damage increases, larger amounts are lost. The **microalbumin** test was developed to detect these tiny amounts of protein (albumin), providing an early indication of diabetic and other neuropathies. The most common microalbumin method is a dipstick method, in which reagents are present on absorbent material at the end of a urine dipstick, and a color change appears that is proportional to the concentration of albumin in the urine sample. The strip methodology is based on dye binding and uses sulfonephthalein dye. The presence of albumin changes the dye from a white color to a pale green or aqua-blue color. Microalbumin can also be measured quantitatively with the use of immunochemical methods.

In addition to microalbumin determinations, there are qualitative and quantitative tests for determining the amount of protein in random and timed urine specimens. Qualitative tests include the urine dipstick method, in which protein turns the strip green to green-blue, and the salicylic acid method, in which equal parts of urine and 3% sulfosalicylic acid are added and, if protein is present, the compound precipitates out of solution. In both of these qualitative methods, the concentration of protein is indicated as trace, 1+, 2+, 3+, or 4+ (Fig. 15-10).

Quantitative tests are usually performed on timed urine collections, such as a 24-hour urine. Because the protein level can vary with randomly collected urine specimens, the 24-hour collection ensures a more accurate measurement of the amount

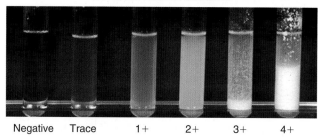

SSA Test: Albumin Standards

Negative   Trace   1+   2+   3+   4+

• **Figure 15-10** Concentrations of protein indicated by the sulfosalicylic acid (SSA) turbidimetric method. (From Brunzel NA. *Fundamentals of Urine and Body Fluid Analysis*. 3rd ed. St. Louis: Saunders; 2013.)

of protein being lost in the urine. Quantitative test methods include trichloroacetic acid–biuret reaction, Coomassie blue, ponceau S, and pyrogallol red–molybdate. Each of these methods involves combining the reagent and the specimen, then determining the change in absorbance at a particular wavelength. The results are calculated from a standard curve. The reference range for a random urine specimen is 0 to 20 mg/dL; for a 4-hour timed specimen, it is 0 to 6 mg/dL, and for a 24-hour specimen, it is 0 to 0.15 g/24 hours (see Table 15-1).

Limitations

For all urine protein determinations, dilute specimens will lead to inaccurate results. Also, ascorbic acid and drugs or other substances that change the color of urine can limit the accuracy of dipstick and quantitative tests. One example is pyrimidine, a drug that is usually given to individuals with urinary tract infections; it changes the color of urine from yellow to bright, fluorescent orange. Interpreting urine dipstick and quantitative test method color changes can be quite challenging with non-yellow urine.

Cerebrospinal Fluid Protein
Function and Clinical Correlation

The CSF bathes the central nervous system, including the brain and spinal column, and then is reabsorbed through the arachnoid. CSF is secreted by the choroid plexuses and the brain ventricles. The volume of the CSF varies with age, with the normal range being 140 ± 30 mL.

Approximately 95% of CSF proteins enter the central nervous system through active transport of plasma proteins across the blood–brain barrier. The remaining proteins are synthesized in the central nervous system. Low-molecular-weight proteins such as albumin are mainly found in CSF. IgG (a small molecule) is found in CSF, whereas IgM (a large molecule) is not. If the blood–brain barrier is altered (e.g., mechanical compression, lesions, tumors, vascular damage, traumatic injury, infection), large amounts of plasma proteins can enter the CSF. The permeability of the blood–brain barrier can be estimated by comparing the protein concentrations in CSF and in plasma. The ratio of CSF albumin to serum albumin is calculated by dividing the former by the latter and multiplying by 100. A normal ratio is less than 0.65%.

The fractions of CSF proteins seen on electrophoresis represent prealbumin, albumin, α_1-globulins, α_2-globulins, β_1-globulins, β_2-globulins, and γ-globulins (Table 15-6).

TABLE 15-6	Fractions of Cerebrospinal Fluid Proteins on Electrophoresis
Fraction	**Interpretation**
Prealbumin	Ventricular origin: low levels in spinal blockage, increased in cerebral atrophy
Albumin	Indicates permeability of blood–brain barrier
α_1	α_1-Antitrypsin α_1-Acid glycoprotein: increased due to tumors and cerebral vascular damage
α_2	α_2-Macroglobulin: elevated in infection and inflammation, with no proteins crossing the blood–brain barrier
β	β_1: increased in meningeal hemorrhage β_2: increased in some degenerative disorders
γ	Quantitation of IgG to determine presence of an immune reaction Qualitative analysis reviews polyclonal and monoclonal gammopathies as well as oligoclonal bands

Prealbumin is produced by the choroid plexus. This fraction is elevated in cerebral atrophy. There is an elevated percentage of prealbumin in CSF of ventricular origin. Prealbumin is decreased or absent in spinal blockage. Albumin is a good indicator of the permeability of the blood–brain barrier. The α_1- and α_2-globulins are elevated in malignant processes. Elevated concentrations of β_1-globulins are found in meningeal hemorrhage. The β_2-globulins have a rounded appearance on the electrophoresis tracing and are elevated in degenerative disorders.

The γ-globulins can be quantified, but this information is not sufficient for a clinical diagnosis. A qualitative analysis of using CSF electrophoresis can provide data to assist in the diagnosis of a polyclonal or monoclonal gammopathy or oligoclonal bands (Fig. 15-11). A polyclonal gammopathy is visible on the electrophoresis tracing as a round and regular contour in the γ-globulin area. In an inflammatory disorder, there is a heterogeneous increase in immunoglobulins (especially IgG). A monoclonal gammopathy is indicated by a classic pointed peak in the γ-globulin region. This peak is identical to the peak seen in the serum electrophoresis

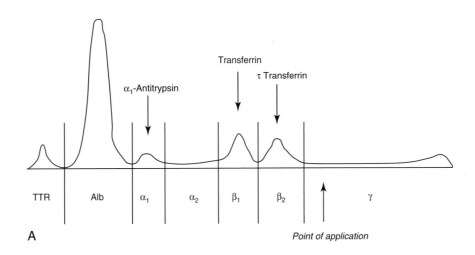

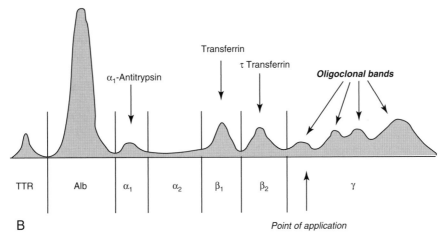

• **Figure 15-11** Cerebrospinal fluid (CSF) protein patterns resulting from high-resolution electrophoresis. **A,** A "normal" CSF protein pattern. The presence in the β_2 region of τ transferrin, a protein unique to CSF, is noteworthy. **B,** An "abnormal" cerebrospinal fluid protein pattern demonstrates the presence of oligoclonal bands in the γ region. These bands will not be present on electrophoresis of the patient's serum. *Alb,* Albumin; *TTR,* prealbumin (transthyretin). (From Brunzel NA. *Fundamentals of Urine and Body Fluid Analysis.* 3rd ed. St. Louis: Saunders; 2013.)

γ-globulin region. The monoclonal protein is synthesized in the central nervous system by the abnormal plasma cells.

Four immunopathologic nervous system disorders can produce two to five bands that appear as oligoclonal bands in the γ region on CSF electrophoresis. These disorders are neurosyphilis, subacute sclerosing panencephalitis, trypanosomiasis, and multiple sclerosis. The first three diseases can be diagnosed through microbiological, parasitologic, or immunochemical testing. In younger individuals, the appearance of oligoclonal bands leads to a diagnosis of multiple sclerosis. In multiple sclerosis, there is an increase in IgG.

Laboratory Procedures and Limitations

CSF proteins are studied to permit classification of the proteins as normal, inflammatory, noninflammatory transudative, inflammatory transudative, or meningitis. The tests needed to classify such conditions include a total CSF protein test, a cellulose acetate or agarose gel electrophoresis, and immunochemical quantitation of IgG and albumin in CSF and serum (see Fig. 15-11). The reference range for total CSF protein is 15 to 60 mg/dL (see Table 15-1). Coomassie blue and pyrogallol red are used to quantitate CSF protein. For more information see Chapter 28.

Summary

Amino acids are building blocks for proteins. Proteins consist of long chains of amino acids (polypeptides) that are linked and folded to form the final protein structure. Proteins have four structural levels—primary, secondary, tertiary, and quaternary. Plasma proteins include prealbumin, albumin, α_1-antitrypsin, AFP, α_2-macroglobulin, ceruloplasmin, C-reactive protein, haptoglobin, transferrin, complement, immunoglobulins, and myoglobin. Abnormal protein levels in other body fluids may be signs of diseases also: An elevated urine protein concentration may indicate kidney disease or nephrotic syndrome, and an elevated protein level in CSF may indicate an infection.

Review Questions

1. Which of the following disease states is characterized by a hyperviscosity syndrome, a monoclonal gammopathy, and Bence Jones proteins present in the patient's urine?
   a. Multiple sclerosis
   b. Glomerulonephritis
   c. Scarlet fever
   d. Multiple myeloma
2. All of the following are common amino acids EXCEPT
   a. Pyrolysine
   b. Alanine
   c. Arginine
   d. Tryptophan
3. The folding of the protein molecule upon itself into a compact three-dimensional shape is known as which kind of structure?
   a. Tertiary
   b. Quaternary
   c. Primary
   d. Secondary
4. Conjugated proteins are proteins that combine with
   a. Collagen
   b. Globulins
   c. Non-amino groups
   d. Fibrous proteins
5. Which of the following techniques uses electrical charge to change the speed and species of proteins that migrate in media?
   a. Ion-exchange electrophoresis
   b. Adsorption bonding
   c. Density-gradient electrophoresis
   d. Isoelectric focusing

6. Which of the following types of proteins are transporter proteins?
   a. Lipoproteins
   b. Hormones
   c. Fibrous
   d. Globulins
7. Where are plasma proteins synthesized?
   a. Liver
   b. Spleen
   c. Bone marrow
   d. Choroid plexus
8. Which of the following proteins is used as an indicator of protein nutrition?
   a. Albumin
   b. Prealbumin
   c. Transferrin
   d. α_2-Macroglobulin
9. Which of the following proteins is found in serum, CSF, interstitial fluid, urine, and amniotic fluid?
   a. Transferrin
   b. α_2-Macroglobulin
   c. Albumin
   d. β-Globulin
10. The level of which protein, measured at particular points during a woman's pregnancy, can indicate whether certain birth defects (neural tube or trisomy 21) are present in the fetus?
    a. α_2-Macroglobulin
    b. Transferrin
    c. α-Fetoprotein
    d. Albumin

Critical Thinking Questions

1. What is the arrangement of serum proteins on agarose gel after serum protein electrophoresis? What electrophoretic pattern would be obtained if the patient had an inflammatory condition? Liver disease?

2. List the five classes of immunoglobulins and briefly discuss each one.

3. What is the difference between monoclonal and polyclonal antibodies?

CASE STUDY

A patient visits the emergency room complaining of being sick for 2 weeks. The patient's symptoms include fever, cough, postnasal drainage, and sinus pressure. Further investigation reveals that the patient has been sick on and off for the past 3 months. The figure illustrates the results of the serum protein electrophoresis that was ordered. The γ portion was markedly decreased. What is the probable diagnosis? What other tests might the provider order to confirm the diagnosis?

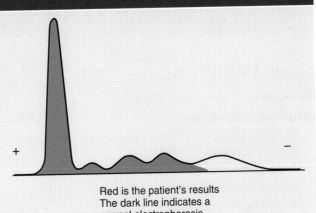

Red is the patient's results
The dark line indicates a
normal electrophoresis

Bibliography

Brunzel NA. *Fundamentals of Urine and Body Fluid Analysis*. 3rd ed. St. Louis: Saunders; 2013.

Burtis CA, Ashwood ER, Bruns DE. *Tietz Textbook of Clinical Chemistry and Molecular Diagnostics*. 5th ed. St. Louis: Elsevier Health Sciences; 2012.

Challand GS, Jones JL. The chemical analysis of urine. In: Williams DL, Marks V, eds. *Scientific Foundations of Biochemistry in Clinical Practice*. 2nd ed. Philadelphia: Elsevier; 1994:317–324.

Centers for Disease Control and Prevention. Collaborative Laboratory Services: Laboratory Procedure Manual—Albumin in Refrigerated Serum, Beckman UniCel DxC800 Synchron. *NHANES*. 2010-2011. <http://www.cdc.gov/nchs/data/nhanes/nhanes_11_12/BIOPRO_G_met_albumin.pdf> Accessed 01.06.15.

Kirschfink M, Mollnes T. Modern complement analysis. *Clin Diagn Lab Imunol*. 2003;10(6):982–989.

Strasinger SK, Di Lorenzo MS. *Urinalysis and Body Fluids*. Philadelphia: FA Davis; 2014.

U.S. National Library of Medicine: Genetics Home Reference: Brain and Nervous System. <http://ghr.nlm.nih.gov/conditionCategory/brain-and-nervous-system> Accessed 01.06.15.

16
Cancer and Tumor Markers

DONNA LARSON

CHAPTER OUTLINE

OBJECTIVES

After completion of this chapter, the reader will be able to:

1. Define the terms *cancer, benign,* and *malignant.*
2. Describe the classifications of tumors.
3. Describe the mechanisms that produce cancer.
4. Describe metastases and the types of cancers that most frequently produce them.
5. Describe the grading and staging systems for cancerous tumors.
6. Describe the first tumor marker discovered and the disease that produced it.
7. Define the term *tumor marker,* and describe the diagnostic tests for tumor markers.
8. Describe what substances are designated as tumor markers.
9. State why tumor markers are not used to screen the general population.
10. Describe analytical methods for detecting tumor markers.
11. Describe the tumor markers associated with the following diseases and how they are used: breast cancer, colon cancer, lung cancer (small cell, non–small cell, and large cell), melanoma, multiple myeloma, ovarian cancer, pancreatic cancer, prostate cancer, and pancreatic cancer.

KEY TERMS

Adenocarcinoma

Adenoma

Adrenocorticotropic hormone

Alkaline phosphatase

α-Fetoprotein

Apoptosis

Bence Jones protein

Benign tumors

β-Human chorionic gonadotropin

BRCA1

BRCA2

CA 15-3

CA 19-9

CA 27.29

CA 72-4

CA 125

CA 242

CA 549

Calcitonin

Carcinoembryonic antigen

Carcinoma

Carcinoma in situ

Degree of differentiation of a tumor

Estrogen receptors

Fibroma

Fibrosarcoma

Grading

HER2

Large cell lung cancer

Lymphoma

Malignant tumors

Melanoma

Metastasize

Neoplasm
Neuron-specific enolase
Non–small cell lung cancer
Oncofetal antigens

Progesterone receptors
Prostate-specific antigen
Proto-oncogenes
Sarcoma

Small cell lung cancer
Staging
Tumor markers
Tumor suppressor genes

 Case in Point

A 65-year-old man went to his provider because he was having trouble urinating. Only a small amount of urine came out when he tried to urinate. He was very uncomfortable because his bladder constantly felt full. The provider examined the man and discovered that his prostate was enlarged. The provider catheterized the man, and much urine was produced. Because this man had an enlarged prostate, the provider ordered a prostate-specific antigen (PSA) test. The test result was 40 µg/L. Is this result normal or abnormal? What should the provider do next? Is the PSA test used to routinely screen men for disease? Why or why not?

Points to Remember

- Tumors can be benign or malignant; a malignancy is called a neoplasm or cancer.
- Normal cells are transformed by genetic alterations into cancer cells.
- The incidence of cancer increases with age.
- Malignant tumors can metastasize and cause death.
- Staging is the clinical evaluation of a primary tumor's size and extent of spread from the primary lesion.
- Tumor markers are substances produced by tumor or by the body in response to a tumor that can be used for differentiating malignant from normal tissue. Tumor markers can be measured in blood, urine, spinal fluid, and tissues to detect cancer or monitor therapy.
- Tumor markers are not used for cancer screening of the general population because levels also can be elevated in noncancerous conditions.
- Tumor markers can be oncofetal antigens, enzymes, hormones, carbohydrates, or DNA.
- Examples of oncofetal antigens are carcinoembryonic antigen (CEA) and α-fetoprotein (AFP).
- Examples of enzyme tumor markers are alkaline phosphatase, neuron-specific enolase (NSE), and prostate-specific antigen (PSA).
- Examples of hormone tumor markers are β-human chorionic gonadotropin and calcitonin.
- Carbohydrate tumor markers include CA 15-3, CA 27.29, CA 549, CA 125, CA 19-9, CA 242, and CA 72-4.
- DNA markers include oncogenes (i.e., mutated genes that prompt proliferation) and tumor suppressor genes.
- The mutated *HER2* gene is detected in about 20% of advanced breast cancers.

- Mutated *BRCA1* and *BRCA2* genes are DNA markers for breast and ovarian cancers.
- Tumor markers include estrogen and progesterone receptors. Breast cancer cells with these receptors depend on the hormones to grow.
- The three main types of lung cancer are small cell carcinoma, non–small cell carcinoma, and large cell carcinoma. Small cell carcinoma is the most aggressive type.

Introduction

Cancer is the second most frequent cause of death for Americans. As individuals age, the probability of developing cancer increases. In addition to age, factors such as gender, lifestyle, ethnicity, infection, environment, and genetics also influence the development of cancer. Cancer comprises more than 100 forms of the disease. The pathophysiology of selected cancers is discussed in this chapter along with detection methods and disease classification.

The lethality of cancer fuels the search for cures and for noninvasive early detection methods. Laboratory tests provide relatively inexpensive, noninvasive methods for diagnosing or ruling out cancer. Researchers have identified tumor markers, elevated levels of which are often found in people with malignancies. Tumor markers are proteins, DNA, hormones, and other substances that are produced by tumor cells and that can be isolated from blood, urine, tissues, and spinal fluid. Many, however, are also elevated in people with other diseases. The characteristics and uses of tumor markers are discussed in the following sections.

Cancer and Tumor Markers

Tumors

A tumor, whether benign or malignant, is an abnormal growth of cells that serves no physiologic purpose. The cells grow uncontrollably because their growth cycle does not receive a stop signal from the genes to cease replication (Fig. 16-1). As a result, cells continue to grow, forming a mass or lump of abnormal cells called a tumor or neoplasm.

Tumors are classified as benign or malignant. Table 16-1 lists the characteristics of benign and malignant tumors. Benign tumors are usually well encapsulated, and the cells retain their normal structure. Malignant tumors are invasive and not encapsulated. They grow rapidly and possess the microscopic hallmarks of nuclear irregularities and abnormal tissue structure (Fig. 16-2). Malignant tumors also metastasize, or spread, to distant parts of the body

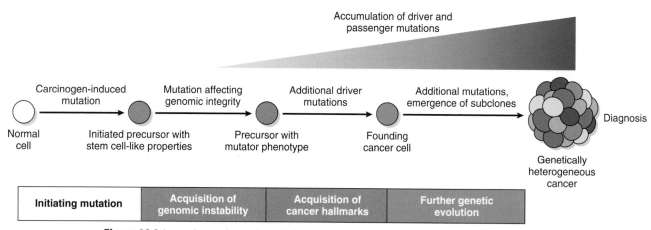

• **Figure 16-1** Loss of normal growth control and development of a cancer through progression of mutations. (From Kumar V, Abbas AK, Aster JC: *Robbins and Cotran Pathologic Basis for Disease.* 9th ed. Philadelphia: Saunders; 2015.)

TABLE 16-1	Benign and Malignant Tumor Characteristics	

Benign Tumor Characteristics	Malignant Tumor Characteristics
Slowly grows larger	Rapidly grows larger
Has a well-defined capsule	Not encapsulated
Composed of well-differentiated cells	Composed of poorly differentiated cells; microscopic hallmarks include nuclear irregularities, and cell type is not the same as surrounding tissues
Does not invade surrounding tissue	Invades local structures and tissues
Microscopically, dividing cells rarely found	Microscopically, many dividing cells seen
Does not metastasize	Spreads throughout the body, often through blood vessels and lymphatics

Adapted from McCance KL, Huether SE. *Pathophysiology: The Biologic Basis for Disease in Adults and Children.* 7th ed. St. Louis: Mosby; 2015.

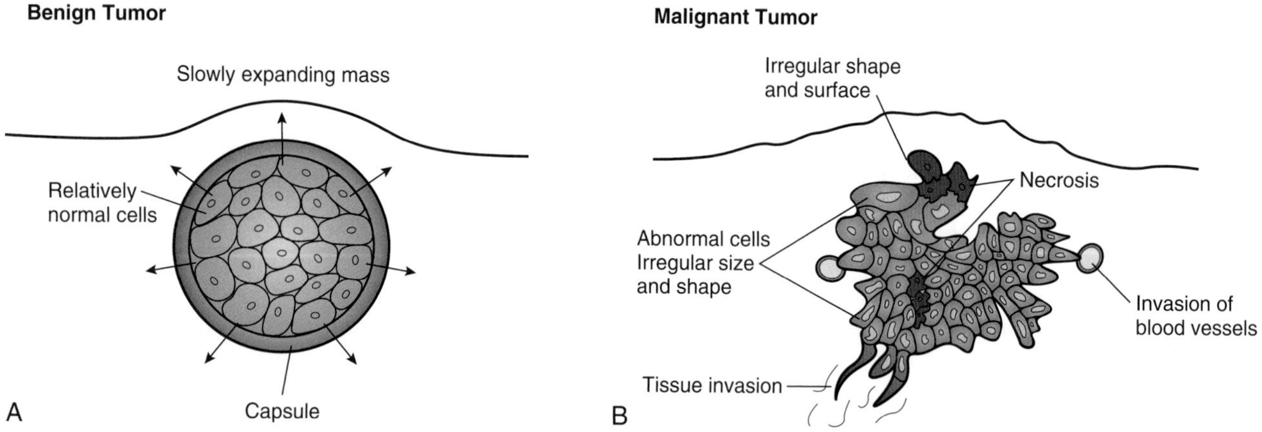

Benign Tumor

Slowly expanding mass

Relatively normal cells

A   Capsule

Malignant Tumor

Irregular shape and surface

Necrosis

Abnormal cells Irregular size and shape

Invasion of blood vessels

Tissue invasion

B

• **Figure 16-2** Characteristics of benign **(A)** and malignant **(B)** tumors. (From VanMeter KC, Hubert RJ. *Gould's Pathophysiology for the Health Professions.* 5th ed. St. Louis: Saunders; 2015.)

and form new malignant tumors. For every type of benign tumor, there is a corresponding malignant tumor.

A tumor may be identified as a **carcinoma in situ,** which is a preinvasive cancer. Carcinomas develop from epithelial cells (including squamous cells), which line the cavities and surfaces of blood vessels and glands. The atypical epithelial cells grow at an increased rate compared with normal cells (Fig. 16-3) but do not spread to neighboring tissues. Carcinomas in situ can be found in the cervix, skin, oral cavity, esophagus, bronchus, stomach, endometrium, breast, and

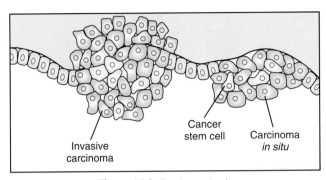

• Figure 16-3 Carcinoma in situ.

TABLE 16-2	Tumor Names	
Tissue of Origin	Benign Name	Malignant Name
Fat	Lipoma	Liposarcoma
Bone	Osteoma	Osteosarcoma
Cartilage	Chondroma	Chondrosarcoma
Blood vessels	Hemangioma	Hemangiosarcoma
Skeletal muscle	Rhabdomyoma	Rhabdomyosarcoma
Hepatocytes	Hepatoma	Hepatocarcinoma

large bowel. In the breast, ductal carcinoma in situ fills the mammary ducts but does not spread further.

Classification of Tumors

Tumors are named after the type of cell from which they arise. For example, a benign tumor originating from a gland is called an **adenoma**, and a malignant tumor originating from a gland is called an **adenocarcinoma**. A benign tumor of fibrous tissue is called a **fibroma**, whereas a malignant tumor originating from fibrous tissue is called a **fibrosarcoma**. **Carcinoma** is added to the name if the tumor originates in the epithelium, and **sarcoma** is added if the tumor originates in connective tissue or other nonepithelial tissue, such as bone, cartilage, fat, muscle, or fibrous tissue. There are exceptions to these naming conventions, such as **lymphoma** (malignant tumor of lymphoid tissue) and **melanoma** (malignant tumor of melanocytes) (Table 16-2).

Pathology of Cancer

In response to genetic damage, a normal cell undergoes a process of transformation to become a cancer cell. The transformation involves disruption of the normal (standard) cellular controls of growth. Cancer cells often require smaller amounts of external growth factors to promote division and development. For example, when normal cells are placed in a tissue culture dish, they stop dividing after the dish is covered with a single layer of cells. Normal cells exhibit *contact inhibition* when they encounter another cell. When

grown in culture, cancer cells show no contact inhibition and continue to divide until they become piled on top of one another (Fig. 16-4). Growth of normal cells is also controlled by anchorage to extracellular matrix proteins. Cancer cells are said to be *anchorage independent* because they continue to divide whether they are anchored or not. Cancer cells can even divide when suspended in a soft agar gel.

Normal cells have a limited life span; they are preprogrammed to undergo a specific number of divisions before they stop dividing. Cancer cells are said to be immortal because they continue to divide for years under appropriate laboratory conditions.

Differentiation is the process by which a less specialized cell acquires additional structures and functions to become a more specialized cell type, such as a muscle, nerve, or bone cell. Cancer cells lack the specialized functions and structures of normal differentiated cells and are said to be anaplastic. Anaplasia is loss of the structural differentiation of mature cells. Anaplastic cells also have larger than normal nuclei and lose their orientation with respect to each other and to normal endothelial cells. Normal cells are uniform in size and structure, whereas cancer cells vary in size and structure and are said to be pleomorphic (Fig. 16-5).

Cancer Metabolism

Cancer cells are continuously dividing and lack normal cell structure and function. It follows that they have different nutritional requirements and metabolic end products than normal cells. The environment for cancer cells is more hypoxic and acidic than a normal cell's environment. Cancer cells are considered parasitic because they pull nutrients from the blood to fuel their cellular processes. Nonmalignant cells break down glucose through mitochondrial oxidative phosphorylation. Cancer cells perform glycolysis but do not use mitochondrial oxidative phosphorylation. Cancer cells can use lactate and its metabolites to produce the chemicals needed for rapid cell growth.

Causes of Cancer

If not repaired, mutations of DNA can transform normal cells into cancer cells. Some genetic mutations are inherited. Acquired genetic mutations can result from viral or bacterial infections, dietary deficits, hormonal imbalances, or exposure to environmental carcinogens (Fig. 16-6). **Proto-oncogenes** are normal genes that become cancer-causing oncogenes when altered by mutations. For example, chronic myelogenous leukemia (CML) is caused by translocation of genetic material between two chromosomes in a bone marrow cell. The resulting abnormality is called the Philadelphia chromosome, and the genetic exchange produces a mutation that leads to CML

Although cancer occurs in people of all ages, it is mostly a disease of aging. The number of individuals diagnosed with cancer increases greatly with advanced age. Massively parallel high-throughput; DNA sequencing; high-density,

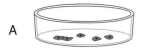
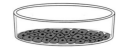
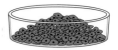

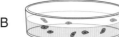

Noncancerous cells are anchorage dependent and proliferate only when attached to a surface.

When these cells form a complete monolayer, they stop dividing due to contact inhibition.

Cancer cells do not exhibit contact inhibition and continue to divide, piling up on each other.

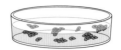

Normal cells suspended in soft agar cannot attach and therefore cannot proliferate.

Cancer cells are anchorage independent and can proliferate suspended in soft agar.

• **Figure 16-4** Cancerous cells show abnormal growth in the laboratory. **A,** Cancer cells, unlike most normal cells, usually continue to grow and pile on top of one another after they have formed a confluent monolayer in culture (loss of contact inhibition). **B,** Cancer cells can grow without being attached to a surface (anchorage independence). (From McCance KL, Huether SE. *Pathophysiology: The Biologic Basis for Disease in Adults and Children.* 7th ed. St. Louis: Mosby; 2015.)

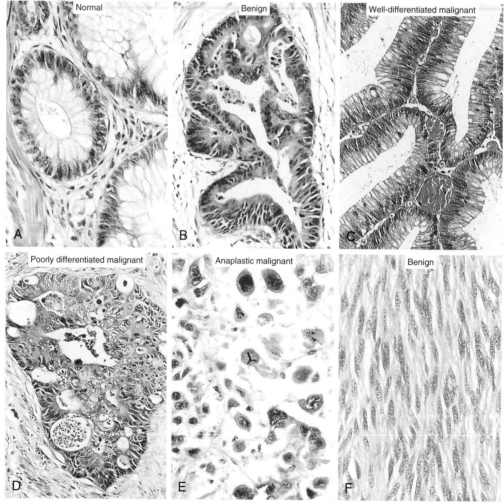

• **Figure 16-5** Loss of cellular and tissue differentiation during the development of cancer. The cells of a benign neoplasm **(B)** resemble those of normal colonic epithelium **(A)** in that they are columnar and have an orderly arrangement. Loss of some degree of differentiation is evident in that the neoplastic cells do not show much mucin vacuolization. Cells of a well-differentiated malignant neoplasm **(C)** of the colon have a haphazard arrangement; although gland lumina are formed, they are architecturally abnormal and irregular. Nuclei vary in shape and size, especially when compared with those in **A.** Cells in a poorly differentiated malignant neoplasm **(D)** have an even more haphazard arrangement, with very poor formation of gland lumina. Nuclei show greater variation in shape and size compared with the well-differentiated malignant neoplasm in **C.** Cells in an anaplastic malignant neoplasm **(E)** bear no relation to the normal epithelium, and there is no recognizable gland formation. Tremendous variation is found in the size of cells and their nuclei, with very intense staining (hyperchromatic nuclei). If the site of origin were not known, it would be impossible to classify this tumor by microscopic appearance alone. Well-differentiated tumors often resemble their cell of origin, as shown in the example of a benign tumor of smooth muscles **(F).** (From Stevens A, Lowe J. *Pathology.* 2nd ed. London: Mosby; 2000.)

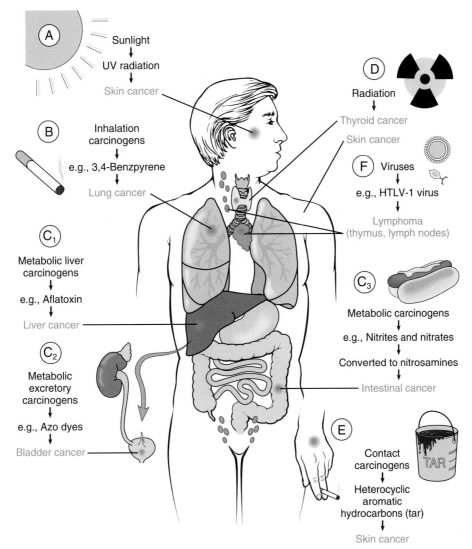

• **Figure 16-6** Causes of cancer. Human carcinogens include UV radiation from sunlight, inhaled carcinogens (3,4-benzpyrene), aflatoxins, azo dyes, gamma radiation, HTLV-1 virus, nitrites, nitrates, and heterocyclic aromatic hydrocarbons (contact causes skin cancer). *HTLV-1,* Human T-cell lymphoma/leukemia virus 1; *UV,* ultraviolet. (From Damjanov I. *Pathology for the Health Professions.* 4th ed. St. Louis: Saunders; 2012.)

single-nucleotide polymorphism; and chromosome copy number analyses are used to discover common genetic alterations in cancer cells.

Genetic alterations can transform normal cells into cancer cells. The transformed cells continue to rely on the mutated genes for growth and sustainability (Fig. 16-7). If the cancer-promoting genes are blocked, cancer cells die.

A gene that prevents mutation and inhibits a damaged cell from proliferating is called a **tumor suppressor gene.** When tumor suppressor genes are inactivated, normal cell functions are disrupted, and uncontrolled cell division occurs.

Epigenetic gene silencing can contribute to cancer. The accessibility of large regions of DNA depends on chromatin structure, which can be altered by chemical modifications of histones and other chromatin components such as cytosine molecules. These modifications can greatly upregulate the expression of oncogenes or downregulate tumor suppressor genes, promoting the immortality of cancer cell lines.

Guardians of the Genome

DNA can be damaged in many ways. Genetic integrity can be maintained by repair mechanisms, which can correct DNA replication errors and damage from radiation, chemicals, and drugs. Molecules (e.g., polymerase) encoded by caretaker genes can identify and repair the damage. However, caretaker genes are subject to inherited mutations that can alter their capacity to repair other defective genes. In that case, mechanisms such as senescence or apoptosis may be able to stop cell division or kill the defective cell.

Chronic Inflammation as a Cause of Cancer

Inflammation and the immune response may create an environment that promotes the transformation of normal cells into cancer cells. Chronic inflammation has been associated

EXAMPLES

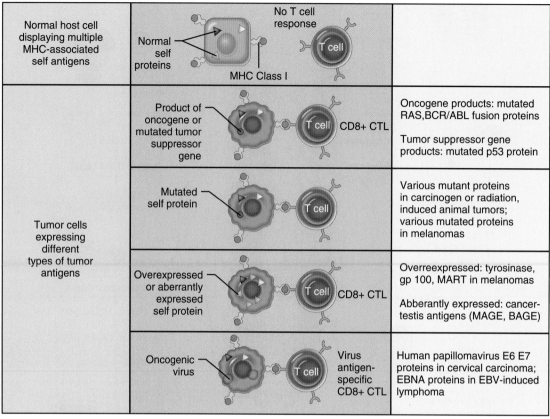

			EXAMPLES
Normal host cell displaying multiple MHC-associated self antigens	Normal self proteins / No T cell response / MHC Class I / T cell		
Tumor cells expressing different types of tumor antigens	Product of oncogene or mutated tumor suppressor gene	T cell CD8+ CTL	Oncogene products: mutated RAS,BCR/ABL fusion proteins Tumor suppressor gene products: mutated p53 protein
	Mutated self protein	T cell	Various mutant proteins in carcinogen or radiation, induced animal tumors; various mutated proteins in melanomas
	Overexpressed or aberrantly expressed self protein	T cell CD8+ CTL	Overreexpressed: tyrosinase, gp 100, MART in melanomas Abberantly expressed: cancer-testis antigens (MAGE, BAGE)
	Oncogenic virus	Virus antigen-specific CD8+ CTL	Human papillomavirus E6 E7 proteins in cervical carcinoma; EBNA proteins in EBV-induced lymphoma

• **Figure 16-7** T cells recognize various types of tumor antigens. Tumor antigens that are recognized by antigen-specific T lymphocytes may be tumor-specific neoantigens (e.g., mutated forms of normal host proteins, viral proteins). T cells can also recognize tumor-associated antigens that are expressed at higher levels on tumors compared with normal cells or are expressed at different stages of development or differentiation. *BAGE,* B melanoma antigen; *CTL,* cytotoxic T lymphocyte; *EBNA,* EBV nuclear antigen; *EBV,* Epstein-Barr virus; *MAGE,* melanoma antigen E; *MART,* melanoma antigen recognized by T cells; *MHC,* major histocompatibility complex. (From Goodman CC, Fuller KS. *Pathology: Implications for the Physical Therapist.* 4th ed. St. Louis: Saunders; 2015.)

with cancer for hundreds of years. Carcinogenesis and chronic inflammation involve many of the same processes. The gastrointestinal tract, pancreas, prostate, thyroid, bladder, skin, and pleurae seem to be more susceptible to developing cancer in the setting of chronic inflammation.

Cancer and inflammation involve neutrophils, leukocytes, and macrophages migrating to the injury site. The cells release cytokines and growth factors that increase cell division and blood vessel growth. In inflammation, the cells also release reactive oxygen species that can cause DNA mutations. Other chemicals increase the production of prostaglandins, which can damage DNA and are associated with colon cancer. Successful tumor cells can manipulate inflammatory cells to produce chemicals that support cellular division, local immune suppression, and blood vessel growth (Fig. 16-8).

Metastasis

Cancer cells spread (i.e., metastasize) from the primary site to other parts of the body and cause disease. The first step of metastasis is invasion of local tissues. The cells break loose from the main tumor and invade the surrounding tissue. Further spread is facilitated when viable tumor cells enter the circulatory or lymphatic systems and travel to a new site, where they attach, begin dividing, and form a new tumor (Fig. 16-9).

Diagnosis and Staging of Cancer

Tumors are a growing part of the body, and they become detectable when the expanding mass exerts pressure on nearby tissue. For example, as a brain tumor grows, it exerts pressure on the normal tissue, producing noticeable symptoms.

All tumors are the result of uncontrolled cell division, and the degree to which tumor cells resemble normal cells is referred to as the degree of differentiation of a tumor. Tissue that is 100% differentiated is normal tissue. Tumor cells are said to be well differentiated if they have some resemblance to normal cells microscopically or are poorly differentiated if they do not (Fig. 16-10). Benign tumors are well differentiated. Well-differentiated malignant tumors grow slowly and metastasize slowly, whereas poorly differentiated malignant tumors grow rapidly and metastasize rapidly.

EXAMPLES

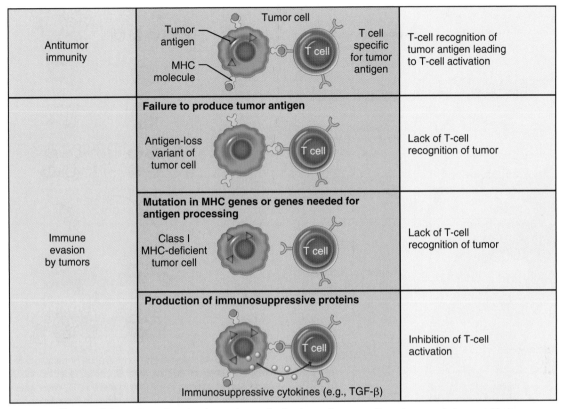

• **Figure 16-8** T cell-mediated antitumor immunity develops after recognition of a cognate tumor antigen and lymphocyte activation. Tumor cells have the capacity to evade immune responses by losing expression of antigens or MHC molecules or by elaboration of immunosuppressive factors. *MHC,* Major histocompatibility complex; *TGF-β,* transforming growth factor-β. (From Goodman CC, Fuller KS. *Pathology: Implications for the Physical Therapist.* 4th ed. St. Louis: Saunders; 2015.)

Tumor Grades and Stages

After a biopsy removes tumor tissue from the body, it is graded and staged to help providers choose the best treatment for patients and establish a prognosis. Cancer grading is performed by a pathologist, who considers the degree of differentiation and other characteristics. Tumors are usually graded on a scale of 1 to 4 or 1 to 3, depending on the type of cancer and the grading system used (Table 16-3). For example, the Gleason system for grading prostate cancer uses a five-level grading system (i.e., GX, G1, G2, G3, G4). In a three-level grading system, grade 1 indicates that tumors are well differentiated with few atypical cells. Grade 1 tumors are considered the least aggressive. Grade 2 indicates that tumors are moderately differentiated, and grade 3 tumors are poorly differentiated or undifferentiated with highly atypical cells. Grade 3 tumors are the most aggressive types and metastasize early in the disease course.

Cancer staging evaluates the size, invasiveness, and spread of tumors. Cancer staging is based on a physical examination, medical history, and diagnostic imaging. A stage I tumor is small and confined to the organ of origin, a stage II tumor is locally invasive, a stage III tumor has spread to lymph nodes, and a stage IV tumor has metastasized to distant sites. The World Health Organization uses the tumor spread–node involvement–metastasis (TNM) system (Table 16-4) to assess stage. The prognosis is worse for a large primary tumor with local lymph node involvement or metastases to other sites.

Some cancers produce hormones that cause a paraneoplastic syndrome. The paraneoplastic syndrome may be the first symptom of an unknown cancer. Table 16-5 lists cancers and the paraneoplastic syndromes they produce.

Treatment

Cancer is usually treated with combinations of chemotherapy, radiotherapy, immunotherapy, and surgery. Patients undergoing treatment may experience pain; fatigue; anorexia; weight loss; taste alteration; altered protein, lipid, and carbohydrate metabolism; anemia; leukopenia; thrombocytopenia; infection; malabsorption; diarrhea; and hair loss.

Tumor Markers

Tumor markers are substances that are produced by a tumor or by the body in response to the tumor, and they can be measured in blood or other samples to detect cancer (Table 16-6). Tumor markers that are elevated in people

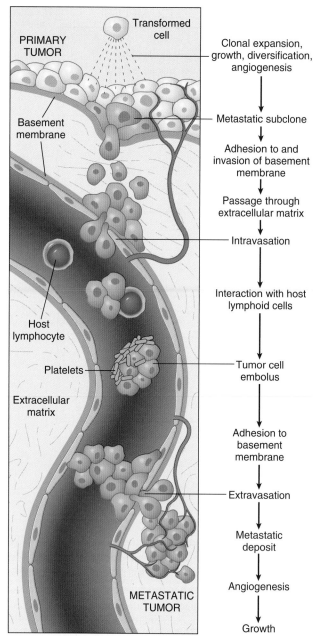

• **Figure 16-9** The metastatic cascade, showing the sequential steps of the spread of a tumor. (From Kumar V, Abbas AK, Aster JC. *Robbins and Cotran Pathologic Basis for Disease.* 9th ed. Philadelphia: Saunders; 2015.)

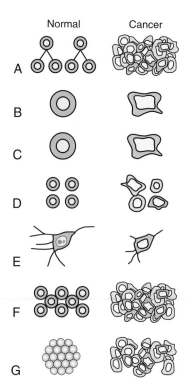

• **Figure 16-10** Microscopic appearance of cancer cells. **A,** Plentiful irregularly shaped, dividing cells. **B,** Large, varied nuclei. **C,** Decreased cytoplasmic volume, in relation to nucleus. **D,** Wide variety of cell size and shape. **E,** Loss of specialization. **F,** Disorganized arrangement. **G,** Lack of definition in tumor boundary.

TABLE 16-3	Grades of Neoplasms
Grade	**Description**
Grade 1	Cells slightly abnormal and well differentiated
Grade 2	Cells more abnormal and moderately differentiated
Grade 3	Cells very abnormal and poorly differentiated
Grade 4	Cells immature and undifferentiated

From Lovaasen KR, Schwerdtfeger J. *ICD-9-CM Coding: Theory and Practice with ICD-10, 2013/2014 edition.* St. Louis: Saunders, 2013.

with malignancies may also be elevated in people without a malignancy or in those with conditions such as chronic inflammation. Levels of tumor markers are usually elevated when the malignancy is well established but not during the early stages of cancer, when early diagnosis and treatment could positively affect the prognosis. This means that measurement of tumor marker levels is not ideal for screening populations but can be used for monitoring therapy or tumor recurrence. Researchers continue to search for tumor markers that are elevated early in the cancer course and only in individuals with cancer.

Blood levels of tumor markers vary during the cancer life cycle of malignant transformation, proliferation, dedifferentiation, and metastasis. Tumor markers can be used for targeted screening, diagnosis, and monitoring of many cancers. For example, prostate-specific antigen (PSA) is used to screen high-risk populations for prostate cancer. Some breast cancer cells test positive for the human epidermal growth factor receptor 2 (HER2), a protein produced by a *HER2* gene mutation. *HER2* amplification is a prognostic factor and can be used to monitor therapy. Tumor marker test results are always combined with medical and surgical information and can be helpful in detecting recurrences.

Discovery

The first tumor marker, the **Bence Jones protein,** was discovered in 1847. This protein is found in the urine of

TABLE 16-4   TNM Staging

TNM Classification*	Description
Primary Tumor (T)	
TX	Primary tumor not assessable
T0	No evidence of primary tumor
Tis	Carcinoma in situ
T1, T2, T3, T4	Increasing size and/or local extent of the primary tumor
Regional Lymph Nodes (N)	
NX	Regional lymph nodes not assessable
N0	No regional lymph node metastasis
N1, N2, N3	Increasing involvement of regional lymph nodes
Distant Metastasis (M)	
MX	Presence of distant metastasis not assessable
M0	No distant metastasis
M1	Distant metastasis

From American Joint Committee on Cancer: *AJCC Cancer Staging Manual,* 7th ed. Chicago: American Joint Committee on Cancer; 2010. *TNM,* Tumor, node, metastasis.
*Tumor stages are derived from combining these parameters. Stage 0 is carcinoma in situ. For stages I, II, and III, higher TNM numbers indicate larger tumor size and more extensive disease or spread beyond the primary site to nearby lymph nodes or adjacent tissues. Stage IV cancer has spread to distant tissues or organs.

TABLE 16-5   Clinical Syndromes Associated With Cancer

Clinical Syndrome	Type of Cancer
Cushing syndrome	Small cell lung carcinoma Pancreatic carcinoma
Syndrome of inappropriate antidiuretic hormone secretion	Small cell lung carcinoma
Hypercalcemia	Small cell lung carcinoma Breast cancer Renal cancer Adult T-cell leukemia/lymphoma Ovarian cancer
Hypoglycemia	Fibrosarcoma Hepatocellular cancer
Carcinoid syndrome	Bronchial adenoma Pancreatic cancer Gastric cancer
Polycythemia	Renal cancer Cerebellar hemangioma Hepatocellular carcinoma
Myasthenia	Bronchogenic cancer Lung cancer Uterine cancer

TABLE 16-6   Common Clinical Tumor Markers

Type of Cancer	Clinical Marker
Breast	CA 125, CEA, HER2
Colon	CEA
Liver	AFP
Lung	CA 124, CEA
Ovary	CA 125, CEA
Pancreas	CA 125, CEA
Prostate	PSA
Stomach	CEA
Testicular	AFP, β-hCG

AFP, α-Fetoprotein; *β-hCG,* β-human chorionic gonadotropin; *CA,* carbohydrate or cancer antigen; *CEA,* carcinoembryonic antigen; *HER2,* human epidermal growth factor receptor 2; *PSA,* prostate-specific antigen.

patients with multiple myeloma. Positive Bence Jones protein test results confirm the diagnosis of multiple myeloma. In 1965, **carcinoembryonic antigen** (CEA) was discovered in patients with colon cancer. The plan was to use CEA as a screening marker, but experience revealed that CEA levels are elevated in other conditions as well.

Monoclonal antibodies are used to detect cancer antigens (CAs) such as CA 125, CA 15-3, and CA 27.29. Advances in molecular genetics have allowed the use of tumor markers at the molecular level. Further developments in genomics, proteomics, and information technology may lead to the use of multiple analytes for cancer diagnosis.

Uses of Tumor Markers

Tumor markers are used for cancer screening (e.g., screening of high-risk prostate cancer patients), for diagnosis (e.g., high-risk patients), and for monitoring the effectiveness of treatment. Because of their low diagnostic sensitivity and specificity, not all tumor markers can be used for screening, diagnosis, or monitoring treatment, and not all cancers have approved tumor markers.

Tumor markers approved by the U.S. Food and Drug Administration (FDA) include CEA, α-fetoprotein (AFP),

PSA, prostatic acid phosphatase (PAP), CA-125, CA 15-3, and CA-27-29. PSA is the only FDA-approved tumor marker that can be used to screen the general population. Clinical correlation of tumor markers and cancers occurs on a case-by-case basis.

The clinical laboratory plays a major role in educating providers on the appropriate use of tumor markers. Clinical guidelines for the appropriate use have been developed by the National Academy of Clinical Biochemistry (NACB),

TABLE 16-7 Clinical Guidelines

Cancer Type	NACB	EGTM	ACS	ASCO
Breast	CA 15-3/CA27.29 for monitoring advanced disease	Steroid receptors in tissue for predicting response to hormone therapy CEA and one *MUC1*-encoded protein in serum for prognosis, follow-up, and monitoring therapy HER2 overexpression in tissue for predicting response to Herceptin (trastuzumab) in patients with advanced disease	None	Routine use of CA 15-3 or CA 27.29 alone not recommended Increasing CA 15-3 or CA 27.29 level may suggest treatment failure Routine use of CEA not recommended Steroid hormone receptors used in selected patients for endocrine therapy HER2 protein overexpression or gene amplification used to select patients for Herceptin (trastuzumab) therapy
Prostate	Percent free PSA when level is between 4 and 10 ng/mL	Total PSA for screening, case finding, or prognosis; used in follow-up and monitoring therapy if additional means of therapy can be offered in case of rising levels Percent free PSA for differential diagnosis when total PSA is between 4 and 10 ng/mL	PSA for screening and detection	Guidelines under development for metastatic disease
Colon	CEA for monitoring therapy	CEA for case finding, prognosis, follow-up, and monitoring therapy	None	CEA for prognosis, detecting recurrence, and monitoring therapy
Lung	None	NSE in differential diagnosis CYFRA 21-1, CEA, and/or NSE for follow-up and monitoring therapy	None	None

ACS, American Cancer Society; *ASCO,* American Society of Clinical Oncology; *CEA,* carcinoembryonic antigen; *CYFRA 21-1,* cytokeratin 19 fragment; *EGTM,* European Group on Tumor Markers; *HER2,* human epidermal growth factor receptor 2; *NACB,* National Academy of Clinical Biochemistry; *NSE,* neuron-specific enolase; *PSA,* prostate-specific antigen.

the European Group on Tumor Markers (EGTM), the American Cancer Society (ACS), and the American Society of Clinical Oncology (ASCO). Table 16-7 summarizes the clinical guidelines from these groups.

Types of Tumor Markers

Tumor markers include many types of molecules such as oncofetal antigens, enzymes, hormones, carbohydrates, and DNA. As the research in this area expands, more types of molecules will be added to the list of tumor markers.

Oncofetal Antigens

Oncofetal antigens are produced by a fetus. During gestation, high levels of these antigens are found in fetal blood. After birth, the antigen levels become very low or disappear. In cancer, these antigens reappear in the blood. α-Fetoprotein (AFP) and CEA are the two major oncofetal antigens used as tumor markers. Both were discovered in the 1960s, and both are glycoproteins.

Serum AFP levels are usually less than 10 µg/L in adults, and a concentration of more than 400 µg/L indicates that

TABLE 16-8 Oncofetal Antigens

Oncofetal Antigen	Cancer	Reference Range
α-Fetoprotein (AFP)	Primary hepatocellular carcinoma Hepatoblastoma Testicular germ cell tumor Choriocarcinoma	10-20 µg/L >1000 µg/L indicates cancer
β-Human chronic gonadotropin (β-hCG)	Germ cell tumors Trophoblastic tumors Hydatidiform mole	<5 mIU/mL

cancer is present. CEA reference values are 3 µg/L for healthy adult nonsmokers and 5 µg/L for smokers. In symptomatic patients, levels greater than 10 µg/L may indicate cancer. AFP and CEA are measured through automated immunoassays (Table 16-8).

Enzymes

Enzymes were determined to be tumor markers soon after the discovery of AFP and CEA. Usually, an increase in enzyme concentration signals an abnormal condition. Most enzymes are not specific or sensitive enough to use for identifying specific cancers. The one exception is **prostate-specific antigen,** an organ-specific tumor marker that is approved by the FDA for screening of general population. PSA is measured using automated immunoassays with enzyme, chemiluminescent, or fluorescent labels (Table 16-9).

Alkaline phosphatase originates in the liver, bone, or placenta. Many individuals with liver or bone cancer or metastases to liver or bone have an elevated alkaline phosphatase level. Alkaline phosphatase is measured using colorimetric assays. Isoenzymes can also be used to determine the origin of the enzyme. More information on test methods can be found in Chapter 27.

Neuron-specific enolase is another enzyme that is used as a tumor marker. NSE is found in small cell lung cancer, neuroblastoma, pheochromocytoma, medullary carcinoma of the thyroid, and melanoma. The level of this enzyme is measured using enzyme-linked immunosorbent assay (ELISA) or automated immunoassay techniques.

Hormones

For more than 50 years, physicians have used hormones as tumor markers (Table 16-10). Hormone levels often are used to monitor the treatment of cancer patients. Common hormones used as tumor markers include adrenocorticotropic hormone, calcitonin, and human chorionic gonadotropin.

Tumors can secrete excess hormones through two mechanisms. First, endocrine tissue in a gland can excrete excess amounts of normally produced hormones. Second, nonendocrine tissue outside of a gland can produce an excess amount of the hormone (i.e., ectopic syndrome).

Elevated hormone levels may indicate the existence of a tumor but provide no clues about its location. For example, **adrenocorticotropic hormone** (ACTH) is normally produced by the pituitary gland, and a tumor in the pituitary gland can produce excess hormone, but ACTH can also be produced by a small cell tumor of the lung (i.e., ectopic syndrome). Elevated ACTH levels are not specific for cancer because they also can be elevated in benign conditions such as chronic obstructive pulmonary disease, hypertension, diabetes mellitus, and stress.

Calcitonin is a hormone that regulates serum calcium concentrations. Calcitonin is useful in detecting familial medullary carcinoma of the thyroid. Levels may be elevated in other cancers and benign conditions, but its usefulness for diagnosis or monitoring treatment of other conditions is uncertain.

β-Human chorionic gonadotropin (β-hCG) is the tumor marker of choice for gonadal (ovary and testicular) choriocarcinomas. It is often used to monitor treatment of testicular tumors.

TABLE 16-9 Enzymes as Tumor Markers

Enzyme	Cancer	Reference Range
Alkaline phosphatase	Liver, bone	44-147 IU/L
Prostate-specific antigen (PSA)	Prostate	Men 40-49 years: 0-2.5 µg/mL 50-59 years: 0-3.5 µg/mL 60-69 years: 0-4.5 µg/mL 70-79 years: 0-6.5 µg/mL
Neuron-specific enolase (NSE)	Small cell lung cancer, neuroblastoma, pheochromocytoma, medullary carcinoma of thyroid, melanoma	<12.5 µg/mL

TABLE 16-10 Hormones as Tumor Markers

Hormone	Cancer Detected	Reference Range
ACTH	Small cell lung	10-60 pg/mL
Calcitonin	Medullary thyroid	<0.1 µg/L
β-hCG	Choriocarcinoma, testicular cancer	<5 mIU/mL

ACTH, Adrenocorticotropic hormone; *β-hCG,* β-human chorionic gonadotropin.

Carbohydrates

Carbohydrate tumor markers include mucins and blood group antigens. Carbohydrate tumor markers are antigens on the tumor cells or secreted by the tumor (Table 16-11). They tend to be more specific than hormones and enzymes. Mucin markers include CA 15-3, CA 27.29, CA 549, and CA 125, and blood group antigens include CA 19-9, CA 242, and CA 72-4.

CA 15-3 is mostly used in patients with metastatic breast cancer for monitoring therapy and disease progression. It is not used to screen for breast cancer because it is also elevated in pancreatic, lung, ovarian, colorectal, and liver cancers. This marker is detected using a murine monoclonal antibody.

CA 27.29 is approved by the FDA for monitoring recurrent breast cancer in patients with stage II or III disease. The tumor marker is detected using solid-phase competitive immunoassay techniques through ELISA or automated assays.

CA 549 is correlated with clinical data to detect recurrence in patients after therapy. An increased CA 549 level after a decreased value indicates the recurrence of metastases and disease progression. This tumor marker is measured with the use of sensitive immunoassays.

CA 125 is correlated with clinical data to detect stage I, II, or III ovarian cancer. The CA 125 level correlates with

TABLE 16-11	Carbohydrate Tumor Markers		
Tumor Marker	**Type of Marker**	**Cancer Detected**	**Reference Range**
CA 15-3	Mucin	Elevated in metastatic cancer of the pancreas, ovary, colorectal, breast, lung, stomach, and uterus	<30 U
CA 27.29	Mucin	Elevated in recurrent breast cancer (stage II or III disease)	<37.7 U/mL
CA 125	Mucin	Elevated in 50% of patients with stage I, 90% of patients with stage II, and >90% of patients with stage III or IV ovarian cancer; useful for detecting recurrent metastasis and monitoring the course of the disease during therapy	<35 U/mL
CA 19-9	Blood group antigen	Elevated in colorectal and pancreatic carcinomas	<37 U/mL

tumor size and stage. Because CA 125 is not elevated in individuals with benign ovarian tumors, CA 125 levels are reliable for differentiating malignant from benign tumors. CA 125 is also used to detect cancer recurrence after treatment, and levels correlate to disease progression and prognosis. This tumor marker is measured with the use of automated immunoassays.

CA 19-9 is correlated with clinical data to diagnose colorectal and pancreatic carcinomas. Elevated levels help distinguish malignant from benign pancreatic disease, and the levels correlate well with pancreatic cancer stage. The level of CA 19-9 at diagnosis indicates a patient's prognosis. This tumor marker is detected with the use of immunoassays.

CA 242 is correlated with clinical data to detect pancreatic and colorectal cancers. CA 19-9 seems to be more effective than CA 242 in diagnosing pancreatic and colorectal cancers. The tumor marker is measured with the use of immunoassays.

CA 72-4 is correlated with clinical data to detect ovarian and gastrointestinal carcinomas. CA 72-4 may be a useful tool in detecting residual tumor in these diseases. An immunoradiometric assay (IRMA) is used to quantitate the tumor marker.

DNA Markers

Cancer is the result of DNA mutations, which are passed on as the abnormal cells multiply. Two types of genes can lead to cancer: oncogenes and tumor suppressor genes. An oncogene is a normally occurring gene that has been damaged by point mutations, insertions, deletions, translocations, or inversions. Oncogenes can transform a normal cell into a tumor cell and drive abnormal cell proliferation. These genes code for proteins that function in cellular division. Tumor suppressor genes are protective and normally limit the growth of tumors. They can repair damaged DNA and initiate apoptosis (i.e., programmed cell death) to eradicate abnormal cells. Inactivation of these genes can lead to cancer.

The HER2 oncogene is identified in about 20% of advanced breast cancers. Overexpressed HER2 proteins are growth factor receptors involved in cell proliferation, differentiation, and survival. HER2 gene amplification correlates well with prognosis for overall survival of patients with HER2-positive breast cancer. Increased HER2 levels also correlate with decreased response to hormone treatment, and HER2 levels are used by providers to guide treatment. Immunohistochemistry is used to measure HER2 protein levels, and fluorescence in situ hybridization (FISH) is used to measure HER2 gene amplification.

The propensity for developing breast cancer can be inherited as an autosomal dominant trait. For example, two mutated genes are associated a higher risk of breast cancer: BRCA1 and BRCA2. Normally, BRCA1 plays critical roles in DNA repair, cell cycle control, and maintenance of genomic stability. The normal BRCA2 gene makes a protein that acts as a tumor suppressor. Individuals who carry a BRCA1 gene mutation have an 85% chance of developing breast cancer and a 45% chance of developing ovarian cancer by age 85.

If an asymptomatic person tests positive for the mutated BRAC1 gene, an ethical dilemma arises: Should the patient have a double mastectomy or ovariectomy? Should insurance companies charge more for individuals who test positive for the defective gene? In February 2013, the actress and activist Angelina Jolie underwent a double mastectomy to decrease her chance of developing breast cancer; she had tested positive for the mutated BRCA1 gene.

Receptors

Receptors have been successfully used as tumor markers. Two of the most widely used tumor markers in this class are estrogen receptors (ERs) and progesterone receptors (PRs). A woman with a breast cancer that is ER and PR positive is a candidate for hormone treatment and has a better prognosis than a woman with an ER- or PR-negative cancer. Those with ER- and PR-negative cancers are treated with other methods such as chemotherapy. Immunocytochemical assays are used to quantitate ERs and PRs.

Clinical Correlations

Breast Cancer

Many patients with early breast cancer have painless masses. Biopsy can confirm the diagnosis. Early detection before

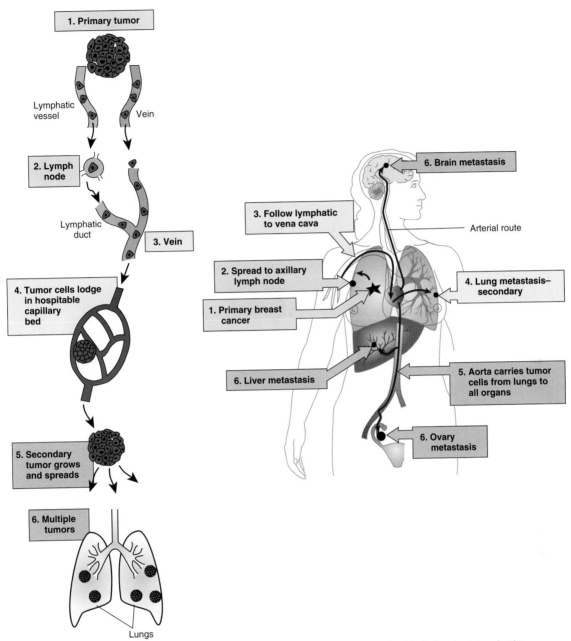

• **Figure 16-11** Metastatic breast cancer. (From VanMeter KC, Hubert RJ. *Gould's Pathophysiology for the Health Professions.* 5th ed. St. Louis: Saunders; 2015.)

breast cancer metastasizes increases survival rates (Fig. 16-11). Tumor markers are not useful for screening, but several are used for selecting therapy, monitoring the results of therapy, and determining the prognosis. Breast examinations and mammograms are used for screening.

Markers used to guide therapy include ERs, PRs, and *HER2.* The density of ERs and PRs indicates whether a tumor is likely to respond to hormone therapy. Receptor-positive patients have a better prognosis. Receptor-negative patients need alternative treatments such as chemotherapy. Amplification of the *HER2* gene indicates that the tumor may be successfully treated with trastuzumab (Herceptin).

CA 15-3 and CA 27.29 are used together to monitor therapy for breast cancer. Increased CA 15-3 and CA 27.29 levels indicate disease progression. For best results, CA 15-3 and CA 27.29 are measured before each course of chemotherapy and every 3 months after beginning hormone therapy.

Colon Cancer

Colon cancer is the most common gastrointestinal cancer and the second most common cause of cancer deaths in the United States. The development of colon cancer is influenced by genetic factors, environmental factors (including diet), and chronic inflammatory conditions (Fig. 16-12). Symptoms of colon cancer include iron deficiency anemia, rectal bleeding, abdominal pain, change in bowel habits, intestinal obstruction, fatigue, weight loss, abdominal tenderness, and ascites.

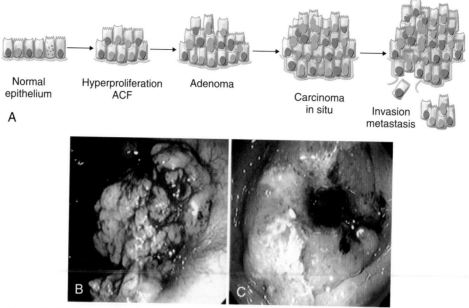

Normal epithelium → Hyperproliferation ACF → Adenoma → Carcinoma in situ → Invasion metastasis

A

• **Figure 16-12** Colon cancer. **A,** The development stages of colon cancer. *ACF,* Aberrant crypt foci. **B,** Large bowel adenocarcinoma; exophytic growth within the lumen. **C,** Large bowel adenocarcinoma; stricturing ("apple core") lesion. (From Goldman L, Schafer AI. *Goldman's Cecil Medicine.* 24th ed. Philadelphia: Saunders; 2012.)

CEA levels are used to monitor colon cancer therapy and disease progression. CEA is not used for screening because levels also can be elevated in benign conditions. Screening is usually accomplished with colonoscopy or sigmoidoscopy. Elevated CEA levels are usually associated with a poor prognosis, but this tumor marker is not used in colorectal staging guidelines.

Hepatocellular Cancer

Hepatocellular carcinoma is a cancer of liver cells (hepatocytes). It usually leads to death in 6 to 20 months. The disease usually occurs concurrently with cirrhosis of the liver (see Fig. 21-19 in Chapter 21). However, 25% of patients who develop hepatocellular carcinoma do not have cirrhosis. Hepatocellular carcinoma remains a common cancer worldwide, but the hepatitis B vaccination program, hepatitis C treatment programs, and alcoholic liver disease reduction are starting to reduce the annual number of cases.

Because this cancer affects the hepatocytes, the function of the liver is compromised, which limits treatment options. The disease takes many years to progress from liver damage to hepatocellular carcinoma. High AFP levels are associated with advanced-stage disease, early recurrence, and a poor prognosis. AFP levels are elevated in 75% of cases. As with most other tumor markers, AFP is not suitable for screening for this disease because levels are also elevated in cases of active hepatitis.

Lung Cancer

Two common types of lung cancer are small cell carcinoma and non–small cell carcinoma (Fig. 16-13). Small cell lung cancer, formerly called oat cell carcinoma, is considered the most aggressive form, and it can cause death within weeks of the diagnosis if not treated. Characteristics include rapid growth, early metastasis, sensitivity to chemotherapy, hypercalcemia, syndrome of inappropriate antidiuretic hormone secretion (SIADH), and ectopic ACTH production. Most patients are symptomatic when diagnosed. Symptoms include shortness of breath, cough, bone pain, weight loss, fatigue, and neurologic dysfunction.

Small cell lung carcinoma is classified as limited-stage or extensive-stage disease. Limited-stage disease, which is treated with chemotherapy and irradiation, has a median survival time of 17 months. Extensive-stage disease is incurable, with a median survival time of 7 months after diagnosis.

Routine laboratory tests can help pinpoint the sites of metastasis. Providers order a complete blood count (CBC) and measurements of electrolytes, blood urea nitrogen (BUN), creatinine, γ-glutamyl transferase (GGT), alanine aminotransferase (ALT), aspartate aminotransferase (AST), bilirubin, albumin, calcium, and alkaline phosphatase as part of the initial workup. Routine chemistry tests also are used to assess organ function before treatment begins. Lactate dehydrogenase (LDH) levels are used for prognosis, and elevated uric acid, BUN, and creatinine levels can indicate rapid tumor lysis syndrome during treatment.

NSE concentrations appear to correlate with the stage of disease and may provide an accurate prognosis. Some research studies indicate that NSE can be used to monitor chemotherapy because it is associated with the disease stage.

Non–small cell lung cancer is the most common type of cancer, with 85% of all lung cancers falling into this classification. Subcategories in this type of cancer include

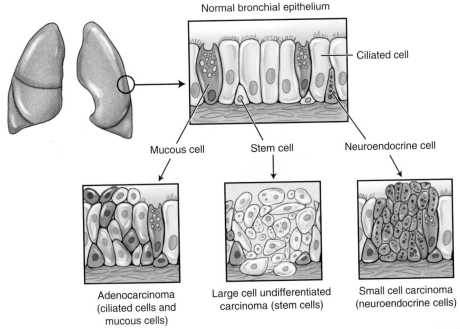

Normal bronchial epithelium

Ciliated cell

Mucous cell   Stem cell   Neuroendocrine cell

Adenocarcinoma
(ciliated cells and
mucous cells)

Large cell undifferentiated
carcinoma (stem cells)

Small cell carcinoma
(neuroendocrine cells)

• **Figure 16-13** Types of lung cancer. (From Shiland BJ. *Medical Terminology and Anatomy for ICD-10 Coding.* 2nd ed. St. Louis: Mosby; 2015.)

adenocarcinoma, squamous cell carcinoma (SCC), and large cell carcinoma (see Fig. 16-13). Unlike small cell carcinoma, the onset of non–small cell carcinoma is insidious, and 55% of patients have widespread disease at diagnosis. Symptoms include cough, chest pain, shortness of breath, coughing up blood, wheezing, hoarseness, recurrent bronchitis and pneumonia, weight loss, loss of appetite, and fatigue.

Clinical chemistry tests may be performed to assess the possibility of metastases, but the chest radiograph is usually the first test performed to detect non–small cell lung cancer. Treatment depends on the stage of disease. Treatment usually involves a combination of surgery, chemotherapy, and radiation therapy.

Large cell lung cancer is rare. It begins in the outer regions of the lungs, and the symptoms associated with it are different from those of small cell and non–small cell cancers. It is strongly linked to smoking. Individuals with large cell lung cancer experience fatigue, mild shortness of breath, and aches in the back, chest, or shoulders. Large cell lung cancer causes fluid to accumulate in the pleural cavity between the outside of the lung and the chest wall, causing chest, back, and shoulder pain.

Chest radiographs are usually the first technique employed to find the tumors. Large cell lung cancer must be staged to ensure proper treatment protocols. Disease onset is insidious, causing it to be diagnosed at a more advanced stage than other lung cancers. Early detection leads to a better prognosis. Advanced-stage disease has a poor prognosis.

Melanoma

Melanoma is the malignant transformation of melanocytes. Melanomas usually occur on the skin but can occur in the gastrointestinal tract, eyes, and brain. Early diagnosis is critical. The 5-year survival rate for individuals diagnosed with stage 0 disease is 97%, whereas it is only 10% for those diagnosed with stage IV disease (Fig. 16-14).

The number of people affected by melanoma increases every year. Because of the importance of early diagnosis, public awareness campaigns use the acronym ABCDE to help people remember the characteristics of malignant moles: asymmetry (A), irregular border (B), color variations (C), diameter greater than 6 mm (D), and elevated surface (E).

A group of proteins (S-100) is used as a diagnostic histologic marker for melanoma and melanoma metastases. S-100 may be useful for diagnosing disease recurrence. This marker is measured by an immunoassay.

Multiple Myeloma

Multiple myeloma is the name given to a spectrum of diseases from monoclonal gammopathy of unknown significance to plasma cell leukemia. It was discovered in 1848 and was described as an overabundance of plasma cells and an increased level of monoclonal paraprotein (M protein).

At clinical presentation, individuals may be asymptomatic or severely symptomatic. Symptoms include bone pain, pathologic fractures, weakness, malaise, bleeding, anemia, infection, hypercalcemia, spinal cord compression, renal failure, and neuropathies.

Routine laboratory tests used to diagnose this disease include a CBC with a differential count; erythrocyte sedimentation rate; a comprehensive metabolic panel; 24-hour urine collection for quantitation of Bence Jones protein, proteins, and creatinine clearance; C-reactive protein; and serum viscosity. Monoclonal gammopathies are diagnosed with serum protein electrophoresis (see Chapter 15).

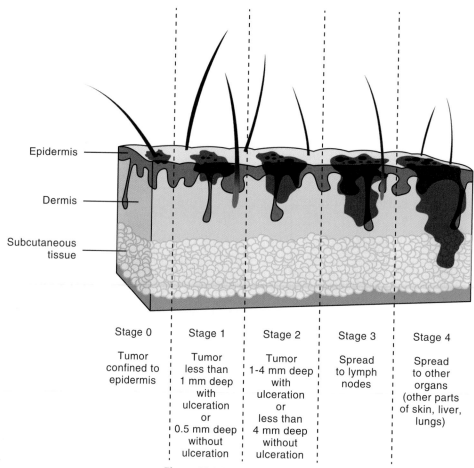

Epidermis

Dermis

Subcutaneous tissue

Stage 0	Stage 1	Stage 2	Stage 3	Stage 4
Tumor confined to epidermis	Tumor less than 1 mm deep with ulceration or 0.5 mm deep without ulceration	Tumor 1-4 mm deep with ulceration or less than 4 mm deep without ulceration	Spread to lymph nodes	Spread to other organs (other parts of skin, liver, lungs)

• **Figure 16-14** Melanoma staging.

Ovarian Cancer

Ovarian cancer is a general term for a group of lesions that includes epithelial ovarian carcinoma (70% of ovarian cancers), germ cell tumors, and sex cord–stromal tumors (Fig. 16-15). Many other cancers metastasize to the ovary, including endometrial, breast, colon, stomach, and cervical cancers.

The most deadly gynecologic cancer in the United States is ovarian cancer, probably because there are minimal, nonspecific, or no symptoms during the early stages of disease. As a result, most individuals have advanced-stage disease at diagnosis. Symptoms include bloating, abdominal distention, abdominal discomfort, pressure on bladder or rectum, constipation, vaginal bleeding, indigestion, acid reflux, shortness of breath, fatigue, and weight loss. Symptoms for individuals with more advanced disease include an ovarian or pelvic mass, ascites, pleural effusion, and bowel obstruction.

The CA 125 level is elevated in ovarian cancer. However, the U.S. Preventive Services Task Force (USPSTF) does not recommend screening of the general population for CA 125 levels because elevated levels also occur in nonovarian carcinomas such as endometrial, pancreatic, lung, breast, colorectal, and other gastrointestinal tumors. CA 125 levels are elevated in 50% of women with stage I ovarian cancer and in 90% of those with stage IV ovarian cancer. This marker is useful for monitoring disease because it correlates directly

with tumor size and stage. A preoperative CA 125 value less than 65 kU/L confers a good prognosis and a 5-year survival rate. CA 125 is useful in detection of recurrent metastases, disease progression, and disease regression. CA 125 is measured with the use of automated immunoassays.

Pancreatic Cancer

Pancreatic cancer is hard to diagnose in its early stages. Because many cases are diagnosed in advanced stages, survival is poor. Pancreatic cancer is ranked as the fourth leading cause of cancer death; it is responsible for 7% of all cancer-related deaths for both men and women.

Between 5% and 10% of pancreatic cancers occur in the tail, 15% to 20% occur in the body, and 75% occur in the head or neck of the pancreas (see Fig. 22-2 in Chapter 22). Symptoms are nonspecific and appear gradually; they include weight loss (often characteristic of this disease), midepigastric pain, nighttime pain, obstructive jaundice, pruritus, depression, diabetes mellitus, thrombophlebitis, and ascites.

Laboratory test results are usually nonspecific and not helpful in diagnosis of this disease. Amylase or lipase results, or both, are elevated in less 50% of patients with pancreatic cancer. CA 19-9 levels are elevated in 75% to 85% of cases, and 40% to 45% of cases have elevated CEA levels.

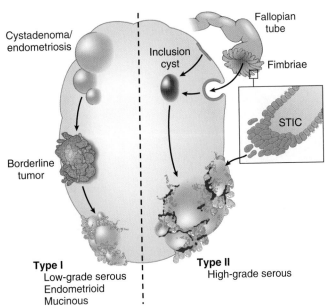

• **Figure 16-15** Pathogenesis of ovarian epithelial tumors. Type I tumors start as benign and may turn into low-grade carcinomas. Type II tumors develop from inclusion cysts or fallopian tube epithelium from unidentified precursors. These often have high-grade features. *STIC,* Serous tubal intraepithelial carcinoma. (From Kumar V, Abbas AK, Aster JC. *Robbins and Cotran Pathologic Basis for Disease.* 9th ed. Philadelphia: Saunders; 2015.)

Prostate Cancer

Prostate cancer is a slow-growing cancer, and most cases are diagnosed in asymptomatic men. It is the most common non-cutaneous cancer among U.S. men, affecting 17% of white men and 20% of African American men. The incidence of prostate cancer diagnosis increases with age. Symptoms include urinary retention, back pain, and hematuria. One of the confounding factors in diagnosing prostate cancer is that these symptoms may also occur in benign prostatic hypertrophy.

Even though PSA is found only in the prostate, there is much controversy about use of this tumor marker as a screening tool for the general population. Men need to discuss the advantages and disadvantages of the various screening methods with providers before deciding to be screened for prostate cancer.

Many studies have been conducted to determine the effectiveness of PSA for detection of prostate cancer in the general population. Initially, 4 ng/mL was thought to be the upper level of normal. Currently, a level of 1 ng/mL equates to an 8% chance of prostate cancer, a level of 4 ng/mL indicates to a 25% chance, and a level greater than 10 ng/mL confers a significantly higher probability of prostate cancer. The USPSTF does not recommend routine screening of PSA in the general population because it has not demonstrated that this results in reduced morbidity and mortality of individuals with prostate cancer. Use of the velocity of the increase in PSA level and the percentage of free PSA in conjunction with other screening methods may improve the accuracy of PSA for detection of prostate cancer (Fig. 16-16).

The velocity of PSA level increase is determined by drawing a specimen at three time points during a period of 18 to 24 month. National Comprehensive Cancer Network Guidelines consider a PSA velocity of 0.35 ng/mL/yr with a total PSA level of less than 2.5 ng/mL to be an indication of cancer. The guidelines also consider a PSA velocity of 0.75 ng/mL/yr with a total PSA level of 4 to 10 ng/mL to be suspicious for cancer. The PSA velocity is a tool for deciding which individuals need a biopsy to confirm or rule out a diagnosis of prostate cancer.

Another tool used by providers to differentiate prostate cancer from benign prostate hypertrophy in individuals with mildly elevated PSA levels is comparing the levels of bound and free PSA. Free PSA is measured with the use of immunoassay techniques. The total PSA and free PSA are measured, and the free PSA is calculated as a percentage of total PSA. The lower the percentage of free PSA, the higher the chances of prostate cancer. This tool is typically used in conjunction with other tools such as digital rectal examination and measurement of the total PSA level. Free PSA levels are particularly useful in men with large glands and in those who have had one negative biopsy. This tool is also used to help the provider decide which individuals need a biopsy to confirm or rule out a diagnosis of prostate cancer.

Testicular Cancer

For men between the ages of 20 and 35 years, testicular cancer is the most common solid malignant tumor. Men in this age group have a 0.033% chance of developing testicular cancer during their lifetimes, and if they do develop the disease, they have a low risk (1 in 5000) of dying from it. The good prognosis is attributable to the fact that the tumor is very sensitive to chemotherapy and can be cured even when there are metastases.

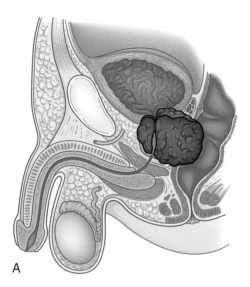

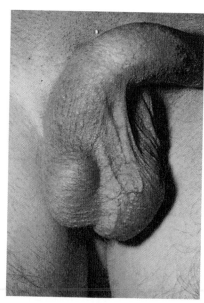

• **Figure 16-17** Testicular tumor. (From McCance KL, Huether SE. *Pathophysiology: The Biologic Basis for Disease in Adults and Children.* 7th ed. St. Louis: Mosby; 2015.)

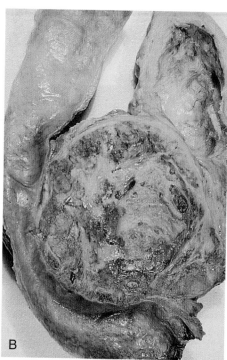

• **Figure 16-16** Carcinoma of the prostate. **A,** Illustration of a prostate tumor. **B,** Carcinoma of the prostate extending into the rectum and urinary bladder. (A, From VanMeter KC, Hubert RJ. *Gould's Pathophysiology for the Health Professions.* 5th ed. St. Louis: Saunders; 2015. B, From Damjanov I, Linder J, eds. *Pathology: A Color Atlas.* St. Louis: Mosby; 2000.)

Patients usually discover a painless swelling or mass in one testicle and may complain of a dull ache or heavy

sensation in the lower abdomen (Fig. 16-17). When the disease metastasizes, the symptoms can include a neck mass, anorexia, nausea, back pain, cough, chest pain, hemoptysis, and shortness of breath.

If a provider suspects testicular cancer, a CBC and measurements of LDH, AFP, and β-hCG are ordered. Between 80% and 85% of individuals with nonseminomatous germ cell tumors have elevated levels of AFP or β-hCG or both. Men with a pure seminoma have elevated levels of β-hCG but not AFP. However, elevated levels of these two tumor markers are not enough to confirm a diagnosis. All suspected cases must be confirmed with a biopsy and histologic examination.

AFP, β-hCG, and LDH levels are instrumental in staging the tumor, monitoring treatment, and determining the prognosis of individuals with testicular cancer. These analytes are also used to determine recurrence of disease after treatment is complete. The reference range for AFP is less than 10 ng/mL. Concentrations of AFP greater than 10,000 ng/mL are found in germ cell tumors. Elevated β-hCG levels are found in seminomas and nonseminomas, and β-hCG levels greater than 10,000 ng/mL are found in germ cell tumors. False-positive elevations may occur after marijuana use. The normal level of β-hCG is 0 ng/mL. LDH levels help determine tumor burden, growth rate, and cellular proliferation.

Summary

Tumors are benign or malignant neoplasms. Malignant tumors can metastasize and cause death. All cancer results from damaged DNA. The growth and spread of neoplasms are controlled by changes in proto-oncogenes and tumor suppressor genes.

Most tumors are graded on a scale of 1 to 4. Grade 1 tumors are the least aggressive, and grade 4 tumors are the

most aggressive. Grading is based on the tumor's microscopic features.

Staging is a clinical evaluation based on the tumor's size, invasiveness, and spread.

Tumor markers are substances that are produced by a tumor or by the body in response to the tumor, and they can be measured in blood or other tissues to detect cancer or monitor therapy. Tumor markers include Bence Jones protein, CEA, AFP, CA 125, CA 15-3, CA 27.29, PSA, NSE, alkaline phosphatase, ACTH, calcitonin, CA 549, CA 242, CA 72-4, estrogen receptors, progesterone receptors, and *BRCA1, BRCA2,* and *HER2* gene mutations. Tumor markers are used to detect colon, hepatocellular, lung (small cell, non–small cell, and large cell), melanoma, multiple myeloma, ovarian, pancreatic, prostate, and testicular cancers.

Review Questions

1. A malignant tumor is
   a. A tumor that metastasizes and causes death
   b. A tumor that does not metastasize or cause death
   c. A tumor that produces substances that can be detected by blood tests
   d. A tumor that is very well differentiated

2. Tumor markers are classified as all of the following EXCEPT
   a. Hormones
   b. Enzymes
   c. Oncofetal antigens
   d. Fats

3. Carbohydrate tumor markers include all of the following EXCEPT
   a. CA 27.29
   b. CA 15-3
   c. CA 52.49
   d. CA 125

4. Which of the following oncogenes is present in breast cancer?
   a. *BRCA1*
   b. *HER2*
   c. *BRCA2*
   d. *TP53*

5. Which of the following tumor markers is elevated in pancreatic cancer?
   a. CA 19-9
   b. CA 15-3
   c. CA 27.29
   d. CA 125

6. Which of the following is the most aggressive type of lung cancer?
   a. Small cell
   b. Non–small cell
   c. Large cell
   d. Well differentiated

7. Grade 1 tumors are
   a. The most aggressive type of tumor
   b. A milder type of tumor
   c. The least aggressive type of tumor
   d. A nonaggressive type of tumor

8. Staging is
   a. A laboratory evaluation of tumor size, invasiveness, and spread
   b. A clinical evaluation of a tumor as well differentiated, moderately differentiated, or poorly differentiated based on microscopic structure
   c. A clinical evaluation of tumor size, invasiveness, and spread
   d. A laboratory evaluation of a tumor as well differentiated, moderately differentiated, or poorly differentiated based on microscopic structure

9. Tumor markers are
   a. Produced by the body in response to a tumor, and they can be measured in blood to detect cancer
   b. Pieces of the tumor wall that slough off into the blood, and they can be measured to detect cancer
   c. A clinical evaluation of a tumor's size, invasiveness, and spread
   d. Produced by a tumor or by the body in response to the tumor, and they can be measured in blood to detect cancer

10. The U.S. Preventative Services Task Force does not recommend PSA screening for the general population because
   a. It is not specific or sensitive enough to ensure that those affected by the disease will receive the correct treatment very soon after diagnosis
   b. It does not reduce the mortality or morbidity of individuals affected by the disease
   c. It is elevated in diseases other than prostate cancer
   d. Prostate cancer cannot metastasize and cause death

Critical Thinking Questions

1. How do cancer cells become immortal?
2. Why are all tumor markers not used to screen the general population for cancer?

3. Discuss the various tumor markers and hormones used to diagnose and treat breast cancer.

CASE STUDY

A 65-year-old woman had loose stools for about 1 year. She noticed that she was a little more fatigued than usual, and she has lost 10 pounds in the past 2 months. What type of cancer might she have? Are there any screening procedures for diagnosing this cancer?

Bibliography

Buggi F, Curcio A, Falcini F, Folli S. Multicentric/multifocal breast cancer: overview, biology, and therapy. In: Schatten H, ed. *Cell and Molecular Biology of Breast Cancer*. New York: Humana Press; 2013:29–42.

Burtis CA, Bruns DE. *Tietz Fundamentals of Clinical Chemistry and Molecular Diagnostics*. 7th ed St. Louis: Saunders; 2015.

Duffy MJ. Carcinoembryonic antigen as a marker for colorectal cancer: is it clinically useful? *Clin Chem*. 2001;47:624–630.

Duffy MJ, Crown J. Companion biomarkers: paving the pathway to personalized treatment for cancer. *Clin Chem*. 2013;59:1447–1456.

Duffy MJ, Lamerz R, Haglund C, et al. Tumor markers in colorectal cancer, gastric cancer and gastrointestinal stromal cancers: European Group on Tumor Markers 2014 guidelines update. *Int J Cancer*. 2014;134:2513–2522.

Hoffman RM, Clanon DL, Littenberg B, Frank JJ, Peirce JC. Using the free-to-total prostate-specific antigen ratio to detect prostate cancer in men with nonspecific elevations of prostate-specific antigen levels. *J Gen Intern Med*. 2000;15:739–748.

Kalemkerian GP, Akerley W, Bogner P, et al. Small cell lung cancer. *J Natl Compr Canc Netw*. 2013;11:78–98.

Kaplan LA, Pesce AJ. *Clinical Chemistry: Theory, Analysis, Correlation*. 5th ed. St. Louis: Mosby; 2010.

Krebs MG, Hou JM, Sloane R, et al. Analysis of circulating tumor cells in patients with non-small cell lung cancer using epithelial marker-dependent and -independent approaches. *J Thorac Oncol*. 2012;7:306–315.

Liu J, Gao J, Du Y, et al. Combination of plasma microRNAs with serum CA19-9 for early detection of pancreatic cancer. *Int J Cancer*. 2012;131:683–691.

Malati T. Tumour markers: an overview. *Ind J Clin Biochem*. 2007;22:17–31.

Rossi G, Mengoli MC, Cavazza A, et al. Large cell carcinoma of the lung: clinically oriented classification integrating immunohistochemistry and molecular biology. *Virchows Archiv*. 2014;464:61–68.

Sevcikova S, Kubiczkova L, Sedlarikova L, Slaby O, Hajek R. Serum miR-29a as a marker of multiple myeloma. *Leuk Lymphoma*. 2013;54:189–191.

Shariat SF, Semjonow A, Lilja H, et al. Tumor markers in prostate cancer I: blood-based markers. *Acta Oncol*. 2011;50(suppl 1):61–75.

Shen J, Todd NW, Zhang H, et al. Plasma microRNAs as potential biomarkers for non-small-cell lung cancer. *Lab Invest*. 2011;91:579–587.

Syring I, Bartels J, Holdenrieder S, et al. Circulating serum miRNA (miR-367-3p, miR-371a-3p, miR-372-3p and miR-373-3p) as biomarkers in patients with testicular germ cell cancer. *J Urol*. 2015;193:331–337.

Zhu CS, Pinsky PF, Cramer DW, et al. A framework for evaluating biomarkers for early detection: validation of biomarker panels for ovarian cancer. *Cancer Prev Res*. 2011;4:375–383.

17

Blood Vessel Diseases

DONNA LARSON

CHAPTER OUTLINE

OBJECTIVES

After completion of this chapter, the reader will be able to:

1. Describe how fatty acids are broken down.
2. Evaluate the role of fatty acids in ketone formation.
3. Describe the structure of triglycerides and their importance.
4. Describe the function of phospholipids, sterols, sphingolipids, and cholesterol.
5. Compare and contrast the structure, function, and importance of chylomicrons, VLDL, LDL, IDL, and HDL.
6. Describe the structure and function of apolipoproteins.
7. Describe lipoprotein (a)—its structure, function, and importance.
8. Describe the absorption of cholesterol.
9. State where cholesterol is synthesized.
10. Describe the transport of cholesterol in the blood.
11. Describe the biological factors that are preanalytical variables in lipid analysis.
12. Discuss the Fredrickson classification system for hyperlipoproteinemias, including types, laboratory values for cholesterol and triglycerides, clinical features, and associated diseases.
13. Discuss the hypolipoproteinemias, including disease symptoms and laboratory values for triglycerides and cholesterol.
14. Compare and contrast the reference values for cholesterol, lipoprotein fractions (HDL, LDL, VLDL), triglycerides, and apolipoproteins and the recommendations from the National Cholesterol Education Program (NECP).
15. Describe the importance of standardized lipid analysis and the guidelines of the NCEP for standardizing this program.
16. Discuss the NRS/CHOL test method.

17. Discuss the enzymatic method for determining triglyceride concentration.
18. Discuss the methods for determining HDL.
19. Discuss the methods for determining VLDL.
20. Discuss the methods for determining LDL (concept and chemical equation).
21. Analyze the relationship between lipoprotein values and clinical vascular disease.

KEY TERMS

Acetoacetic acid
Acetone
Apolipoprotein A-I
Apolipoprotein B-100
Apolipoprotein C-II
Apolipoprotein
Atherogenesis
Atheroma
Atherosclerosis
β-Hydroxybutyric acid
Cardiovascular disease
Cholesterol
Cholesterol Reference Method
   Laboratory Network
Chylomicron
Diastolic

Essential fatty acid
Familial combined hyperlipidemia
Familial hypercholesterolemia
Familial hypertriglyceridemia
Fatty acid
Foam cells
Fredrickson classification of lipid
   disorders
Friedewald formula
High-density lipoprotein
Homocysteine
Hypertension
Ischemia
Lipoprotein
Lipoprotein (a) (Lp(a))
Lipoprotein lipase (LPL)

Low-density lipoprotein
National Cholesterol Education
   Program
Nephrosclerosis
Phospholipid
Plaque
Saturated fatty acid
Sphingolipid
Sterol
Systolic
Tangier disease
Triglyceride
Unsaturated fatty acid
Vasculitis
Very-low-density lipoprotein
Xanthoma

❖ Case in Point

A 50-year-old diabetic comes to the laboratory to have routine bloodwork drawn. His physician orders basic metabolic panel and a lipid profile. After the blood clots, the technician spins down the specimen to find that the serum looks like milk. The test results are as follows:

Na: 140 mEq/L
K: 4.0 mEq/L
Cl: 101 mEq/L
CO_2: 28 mg/dL
Glucose: 455 mg/dL
BUN: 24 mg/dL
Creatinine: 1.1 mg/dL
Phosphate: 3.7 mg/dL
Calcium: 8.8 mg/dL
ALP: 250 IU/L
AST: 35 IU/L
ALT: 29 IU/L
Cholesterol: 500 mg/dL
Triglycerides: 1200 mg/dL
HDL: 35 mg/dL
LDL: 160 mg/dL

What causes the diabetic's serum to look like milk? What lipid test results do you expect to be elevated? How would this specimen fit into Fredrickson's classification scheme?

Points to Remember

- Lipoproteins are linked to cardiovascular disease.
- Lowering lipoproteins can prevent cardiovascular disease and its sequelae.

- Lipids serve as energy sources and as structural components, hormones, and nerve insulators in the body.
- Fatty acids can be saturated (no double bonds between carbons) or unsaturated (double bonds between carbons).
- Essential fatty acids are those that must be ingested because the body cannot make them: α-linoleic acid and linolenic acid.
- Fatty acids used for energy produce three ketone bodies as metabolic byproducts: acetone, acetoacetic acid, and β-hydroxybutyric acid.
- Triglycerides contain a glycerol molecule and three fatty acids (i.e., they are triacylglycerols).
- Glucose is required by cells to synthesize triglycerides.
- Insulin increases the synthesis of triglycerides to be stored in adipose tissue.
- Phospholipids are cell membrane components.
- Sphingolipids are cell membrane components in red blood cells and nerve cells.
- Cholesterol is a sterol with ring compounds, an aliphatic chain, and a hydroxyl group.
- Lipoproteins are molecules that transport lipids in the blood.
- Chylomicrons are used to transport triglycerides from the intestines to muscle and adipose tissue.
- Very-low-density lipoproteins (VLDL) are synthesized in the liver and transported to the muscle and adipose tissue.
- Low-density lipoprotein (LDL) is a cholesterol-rich particle that carries cholesterol to the liver for bile formation.
- High-density lipoprotein (HDL) is synthesized in the liver and intestines and participates in reverse cholesterol transport.
- Apolipoproteins are found on the surface of the lipoproteins.

- Lp(a) is an independent risk factor for cardiovascular disease.
- Lipoprotein lipase breaks down triglycerides.
- When no cholesterol is available, cells and the liver synthesize their own cholesterol.
- Genetic mutations are the cause of many hyperlipoproteins.
- The Fredrickson classification lists six types of hyperlipidemias: types I, IIa, IIb, III, IV, and V.
- Abetalipoproteinemia is a genetic disorder in which apolipoprotein B is produced, resulting in abnormal crenated red blood cells.
- Nongenetic causes for lipoprotein lipase deficiencies include systemic lupus erythematosus, diabetes, and dysgammaglobulinemias.
- Synthesis of lipoprotein lipase depends on the presence of insulin.
- Tangier disease involves production of an abnormal apolipoprotein A-I.
- The National Cholesterol Education Program (NCEP) was established in 1985.
- The NCEP's Expert Panel on Detection, Evaluation, and Treatment of High Blood Cholesterol in Adults established the test result ranges for total cholesterol, HDL, and LDL and their associated treatment protocols.
- The Centers for Disease Control and Prevention created the Cholesterol Reference Method Laboratory Network to standardize measurements for total cholesterol, triglycerides, HDL, and LDL.
- The Friedewald formula is used to calculate LDL using triglyceride, HDL, and total cholesterol test results.
- Atherosclerosis is caused by inflammation and cholesterol deposits in arteries (atheromas).
- Hypertension is abnormally high blood pressure.
- Essential hypertension has no known cause.
- Sequelae associated with hypertension have symptoms, but hypertension does not.
- Vasculitis is an inflammation of arteries and, rarely, veins.

Introduction

Arteries transport oxygenated blood from the heart throughout the body, and veins collect deoxygenated blood from the tissues and organs and return it to the heart. Arteries have thick muscular walls that allow the blood to be pumped from the heart throughout the body. Arteries withstand higher pressures than do veins. Veins are considered a low-pressure system because they fill by gravity and muscle contraction and are less susceptible to disease.

Cardiovascular disease is the leading cause of illness and death in the United States. In 1948, the Framingham research study was initiated to find common factors or characteristics of people with cardiovascular disease. This study was the first to link plasma lipid levels to cardiovascular disease. Lipids are transported through the blood attached to proteins called lipoproteins. Atherosclerosis is caused by the accumulation of lipoproteins and inflammatory cells on the walls of arteries. These accumulations are known as plaques. As the

plaques build up on artery walls, the diameter of the artery decreases, allowing less blood to travel through the artery. As the disease progress, the plaques can become large enough to totally block the artery. The coronary arteries, which supply the heart with blood, are major sites where plaques and blockages form, causing heart attacks. Because of the connection between lipoproteins and cardiovascular disease, accurate measurements of these analytes is important. Lowering plasma lipoprotein levels can prevent cardiovascular disease and its clinical sequelae. This chapter examines lipids, lipoproteins, normal and abnormal lipoprotein metabolism, laboratory procedures for measuring lipoproteins, and the clinical significance of lipoproteins in blood vessel diseases.

Lipids

Lipids are found throughout the body as structural components, hormones, and nerve insulators. As essential as lipids are to our bodies, blood lipids also play a big role in cardiovascular disease, and clinical practice guidelines suggest regular monitoring. The clinical significance of lipids is their link to coronary heart disease, cardiovascular disease, and lipoprotein disorders.

Biochemically, lipids are insoluble in water and soluble in organic solvents. The clinically significant classes of lipids include fatty acids, triglycerides, phospholipids, sterols, sphingolipids, and cholesterol.

Fatty Acids

Fatty acids are carboxylic acids with long chains of carbon groups. The chains can contain single bonds between the carbon groups (saturated fatty acid), or they can have both single and double bonds between the carbon atoms (unsaturated fatty acid). Fatty acids from plant sources are mostly unsaturated, and those from animal sources are mostly saturated (Fig. 17-1). The body uses and produces many fatty acids, but some fatty acids are classified as "essential," meaning that the body cannot synthesize them. Essential fatty acids include α-linoleic acid and linolenic acid.

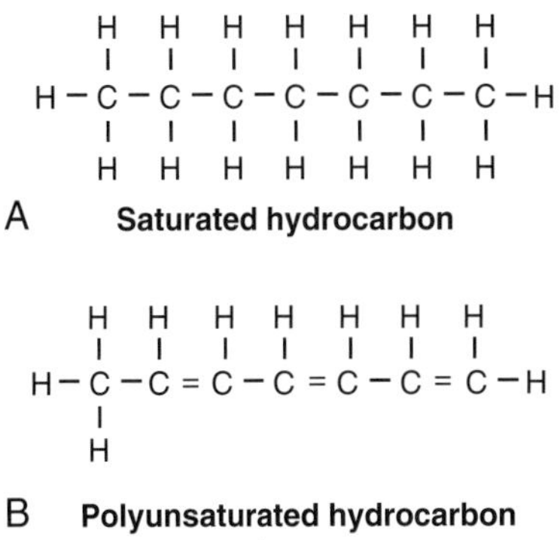

• **Figure 17-1** Saturated and unsaturated fats. **A,** Saturated fat with no double bonds within the carbon chain. **B,** A polyunsaturated fat with several double bonds within the carbon chain. (From VanMeter K, Hubert R. *Microbiology for the Healthcare Professional.* St. Louis: Elsevier; 2010.)

In addition to using fatty acids for structural components, the body also uses long-chain fatty acids as energy sources. A fatty acid produces approximately twice as much energy as a comparable carbohydrate molecule. The body stores fatty acids efficiently, with stored molecules providing excellent insulation.

Excessive starvation or uncontrolled diabetes mellitus may cause the body to use fatty acids from adipose tissue for energy. These fatty acids undergo catabolism in the liver, resulting in the production of three ketone bodies—acetoacetic acid, β-hydroxybutyric acid, and acetone. Ketones are toxic acids, and increased production of these acids leads to ketosis or ketoacidosis or both. *Ketosis* is an increased level of ketones in the blood. *Ketoacidosis* is an extreme case of ketosis in which the body does not regulate ketone production; this causes excessive amounts of ketones to accumulate in the blood, resulting in a lower blood pH.

Triglycerides

Triglycerides are large molecules that contain a glycerol molecule and three fatty acids (Fig. 17-2). The body synthesizes triglycerides to effectively transport fatty acids.

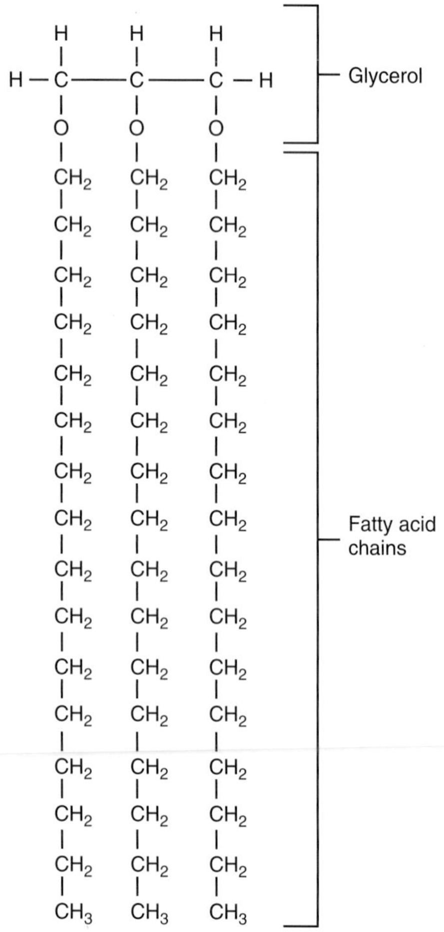

Cells require glucose inside the cell to synthesize triglycerides. If glucose is not present, the triglycerides from fat deposits are broken down to release the fatty acids. Intracellular glucose may not be present in conditions such as starvation, fasting, or uncontrolled diabetes mellitus. Free fatty acids are not soluble in water; once they are released from triglycerides, they attach to albumin for transport.

Excess carbohydrates are stored as triglycerides. Insulin increases the synthesis of triglycerides from carbohydrates. Excess fatty acids in the blood are resynthesized into triglycerides for storage in adipose tissue.

Triglycerides are increased in diabetes mellitus, pancreatitis, alcoholism, glycogen storage diseases, hypothyroidism, nephrosis, pregnancy, gout, and use of oral contraceptives. Triglycerides are decreased in hyperthyroidism.

Phospholipids

Phospholipids are cell membrane components. They are polar compounds with phosphates on one end and lipids on the other; as a result, they position themselves between water (phosphate end) and lipids (lipid end). Phospholipids are a major component of the surfactant that allows the alveoli to distend during breathing. They are important for mitochondrial metabolism, blood coagulation, and lipid transport, in addition to serving as cellular membrane structural units.

Sterols

Sterols consist of several ringed structures connected to a long aliphatic chain and at least one hydroxyl group (Fig. 17-3). Plant sterols resemble cholesterol. However, plant sterols are not well absorbed and can even be used to reduce the absorption of cholesterol.

Sphingolipids

Sphingolipids are cell membrane components in red blood cells and brain and nerve cells. They are involved in the recognition of cells as self and in recognition of blood group antigens.

Cholesterol

Cholesterol is a sterol composed of several ring compounds, an aliphatic chain, and one hydroxyl group (Fig. 17-4). All living organisms contain sterols, and cholesterol is the primary sterol in humans and animals.

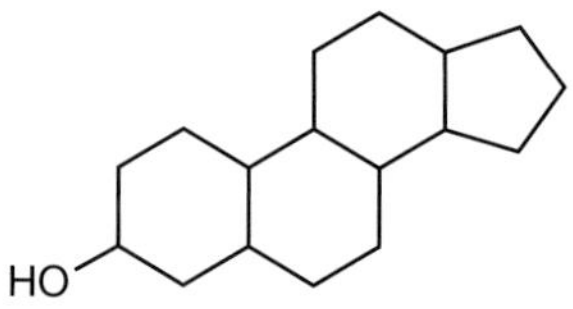

• **Figure 17-2** Glycerol and fatty acid chains.

• **Figure 17-3** Basic chemical structure of sterols.

Cholesterol functions as a structural component in the body as well as a precursor in the synthesis of steroid hormones. Some cholesterol is consumed in the diet, but most of the cholesterol in the body is synthesized by the liver and other body tissues. Cholesterol is required for the production of bile acids, steroids, and cell membranes. The clinical conditions that produce elevated cholesterol levels include hyperlipidemia, atherosclerosis, and liver disease. Measurement of cholesterol and other lipids is routinely ordered to diagnose atherosclerosis.

Lipoproteins

Lipoproteins contain triglycerides, phospholipids, cholesterol, and **apolipoproteins;** they are used by the body to transport insoluble fats through blood (Fig. 17-5). Lipoproteins are classified on the basis of their density as well as the apolipoproteins on their surface. The amount of lipid in a lipoprotein affects its density: the more lipid in a molecule, the lower its density. The five categories of lipoproteins include chylomicrons, very-low-density lipoprotein, intermediate-density lipoprotein (IDL), low-density lipoprotein, and high-density lipoprotein.

The five types of lipoproteins contain differing amounts of cholesterol, triglycerides, phospholipids, protein, and apolipoproteins. **Chylomicrons** are the largest and least dense of all the lipoproteins, and they are synthesized by cells in the small intestine. They transport triglycerides to muscle cells and adipose tissue. Chylomicrons contain 85% triglycerides, 3% cholesterol, 8% phospholipids, and 4% protein. **Very-low-density-lipoproteins** (VLDL) are synthesized in the liver but are a bit smaller and denser than chylomicrons. These lipoproteins carry triglycerides to muscle and adipose tissue. VLDL contain 25% cholesterol, 55% triglycerides, 14% phospholipids, and 6% protein. IDL is formed when VLDL loses its triglyceride molecules. The remaining apoprotein C, free cholesterol, and phospholipids, apoprotein E and B-100, compose the IDL. **Low-density lipoproteins** (LDL) are cholesterol rich and are formed by the removal of triglycerides from VLDLs during catabolism. The major function of LDL particles is to carry cholesterol in the plasma. LDL carries cholesterol to the liver for bile formation, to the tissues for use in the cell membrane, to endocrine organs for steroid hormone production, and to cholesterol storage sites. LDL contains 50% cholesterol, 10% triglycerides, 29% phospholipids, and 11% protein. **High-density lipoproteins** (HDL) are synthesized by the liver and the intestines. They are also formed through the catabolism of chylomicrons and VLDL particles. Their function is to transport cholesterol from the cells to the liver. They are the smallest and densest of the lipoprotein particles. They also have higher concentrations of protein and phospholipid than the other lipoprotein groups. HDL contain 25% cholesterol, 5% triglycerides, 26% phospholipids, and 44% protein (Table 17-1).

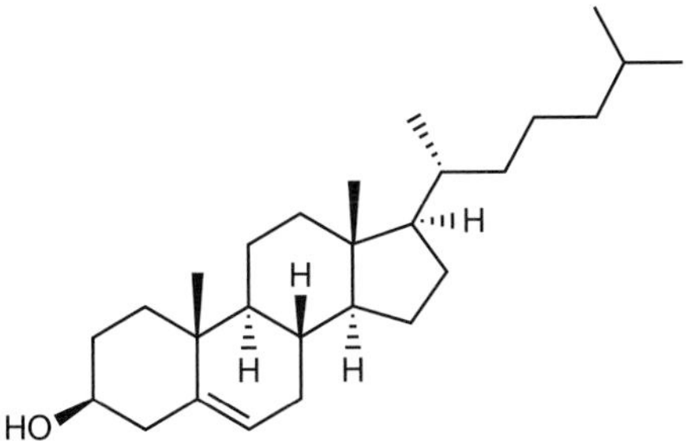

Apolipoproteins

Apolipoproteins are protein portions of lipoprotein molecules. The structure of these molecules is unique because they are soluble in plasma and bind to nonpolar lipids. Certain apolipoproteins are part of specific lipoprotein molecules: **Apo A-I** is found on HDL, apo B-48 on chylomicrons, and **apo B-100** on LDL. Apo C-I, **apo C-II,** apo C-III, and apo E are found on all lipoproteins. The main function of apolipoproteins is to allow lipids (neutral molecules) to be transported through the plasma. Other functions of apolipoproteins include activating or inhibiting enzymes that act on lipoproteins, acting as cofactors to allow lipoproteins to be removed from plasma, and maintaining the structure of a lipoprotein molecule.

Lipoprotein (a) (Lp(a)) is a distinct class of lipoprotein molecules. The Lp(a) structure is similar to that of LDL because both molecules contain an apo B-100 particle. Lp(a) also contains a protein called apolipoprotein(a)

• **Figure 17-4** Structure of cholesterol.

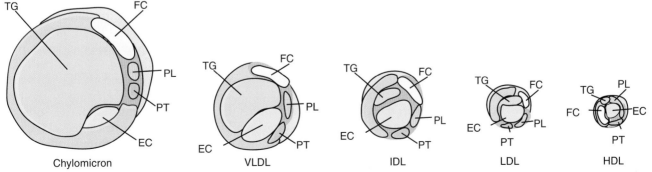

• **Figure 17-5** Lipoproteins *(left to right):* chylomicron, very-low-density lipoprotein *(VLDL),* intermediate-density lipoprotein *(IDL),* low-density lipoprotein *(LDL),* and high-density lipoprotein *(HDL). EC,* Esterified cholesterol; *FC,* free cholesterol; *PL,* phospholipids; *PT,* protein; *TG,* triglyceride.

TABLE 17-1	Lipoproteins			
Name	Composition	Characteristics	Function	
Chylomicrons	85% T 3% C 8% PH 4% P	Largest and least dense of all lipoproteins Synthesized in the intestines	Transport ingested triglycerides to muscle cells and adipose tissue	
Very-low-density lipoprotein (VLDL)	25% T 55% C 14% PH 6% P	Smaller and more dense than chylomicrons Synthesized in the liver	Transport triglycerides synthesized by the liver to muscle cells and adipose tissue	
Low-density lipoprotein (LDL)	50% T 10% C 29% PH 11% P	Smaller and more dense than VLDL particles Synthesized by the liver or in the plasma	Carry cholesterol in the plasma to liver, tissues, endocrine organs, or storage	
High-density lipoprotein (HDL)	25% T 5% C 26% PH 44% P	Smallest and most dense of the lipoprotein molecules Synthesized in intestine and hepatic cells from simple molecules or from breakdown products of chylomicron and VLDL catabolism	Transport cholesterol from the cells to the liver	

C, Cholesterol; *P*, protein; *PH*, phospholipid; *T*, triglyceride.

(apo(a)) that is bound to the apo B-100 particle. Lp(a) is considered an independent risk factor for cardiovascular disease, cerebrovascular disease, atherosclerosis, thrombosis, and stroke. It is most strongly associated with cardiovascular disease and atherosclerosis. An increased Lp(a) predicts early atherosclerosis independent of other cardiac risk factors. In advanced cardiovascular disease, Lp(a) can predict a risk of plaque thrombosis because Lp(a) binds to blood vessel walls and increases the risk of clotting.

Normal Lipoprotein Metabolism

The body uses four main pathways for lipid and lipoprotein metabolism: the exogenous lipoprotein metabolic pathway, the endogenous lipoprotein metabolic pathway, the low-density lipoprotein receptor pathway, and the reverse cholesterol transport pathway. Although each pathway is discussed as a distinct entity, there are overlapping points at which dietary fat intake can influence the synthesis and catabolism of lipids.

Exogenous Lipoprotein Metabolic Pathway

The exogenous lipoprotein metabolic pathway begins after fat is ingested. The intestinal enterocytes assemble chylomicrons from dietary fat and cholesterol. The chylomicrons are encapsulated in secretory vesicles in the Golgi apparatus. The cell uses exocytosis to transport packaged chylomicrons to the extracellular space. The packages are absorbed by the intestinal villi and introduced into the circulation. The packaged chylomicrons acquire additional apo C and apo E from circulating HDL to complete the chylomicron molecules. With the apo C-II attached to

the surface of the chylomicron, lipoprotein lipase (LPL) on the surface of endothelial cells is activated. Triglycerides inside the chylomicron molecule are quickly hydrolyzed into fatty acids. The fatty acids attach to albumin for uptake into muscle or adipose cells. At the same time, circulating HDL molecules absorb phospholipids and apo A from the chylomicron remnants. The apo B-48 and apo E on the chylomicron remnant act as liver cell receptors, allowing the remnant to be taken up by the liver cells. The components of the remnant are broken down into cholesterol, which is made into bile acids, newly synthesized lipoproteins, or cholesterol esters (Fig. 17-6).

Endogenous Lipoprotein Metabolic Pathway

Liver cells can synthesize triglycerides (from fatty acids and carbohydrates) and cholesterol. Insulin promotes triglyceride synthesis by signaling the liver to make triglycerides from carbohydrates and fatty acids. Once these molecules are produced, they are packaged in secretory vesicles and transported (by exocytosis) into the extracellular space. The packages travel to the circulation and begin life as VLDL molecules. VLDL molecules acquire additional apo C from circulating HDL molecules. The apo C-II on the VLDL molecules activates the LPL on the endothelial cells, which hydrolyzes the triglycerides in the VLDL molecule to fatty acids. During the triglyceride hydrolysis, HDL absorbs the apo C on the VLDL molecule. Some remaining VLDL remnants go back to the liver and others form smaller, denser particles called intermediate-density lipoproteins (IDL). Eventually, the IDL is removed from circulation by the liver. The remnant molecules are recycled into newly synthesized lipoproteins (Fig. 17-7).

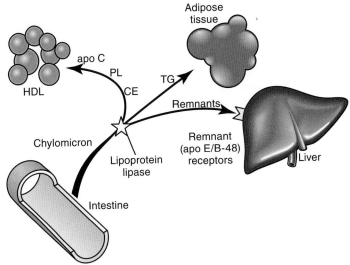

• **Figure 17-6** Metabolism of chylomicrons. Chylomicrons are absorbed by the intestine and enter the blood. In the blood, lipoprotein lipase acts on the chylomicron to produce chylomicron remnants, triglycerides, and cholesterol esters. The remnants go to the liver and combine with apo E/B-48 receptors on the liver. The triglyceride is stored in the adipose tissue and the cholesterol ester is combined with phospholipid and apo C to create HDL molecules. *apo C,* Apolipoprotein C; *apo E,* apolipoprotein E; *B-48,* apolipoprotein B-48; *CE,* cholesterol ester; *HDL,* high-density lipoprotein; *PL,* phospholipid; *TG,* triglyceride.

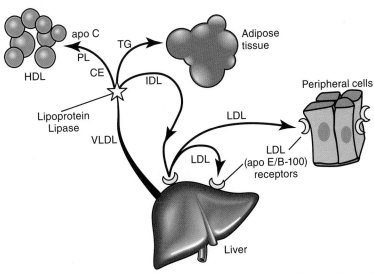

• **Figure 17-7** Metabolism of very-low-density lipoproteins *(VLDL).* VLDL is released into circulation where lipoprotein lipase breaks it into cholesterol ester, phospholipid, triglyceride, and IDL molecules. The cholesterol ester and phospholipid along with apo C are combined together to make HDL. The triglyceride is stored in adipose tissue. The IDL goes to the liver where it is converted to LDL. Some LDL remains in the liver and other LDL goes to the peripheral cells. *apo C,* Apolipoprotein C; *apo E,* apolipoprotein E; *B-48,* apolipoprotein B-48; *CE,* cholesterol ester; *HDL,* high-density lipoprotein; *IDL,* intermediate-density lipoprotein; *LDL,* low-density lipoprotein; *PL,* phospholipid; *TG,* triglyceride.

Low-Density Lipoprotein Receptor Pathway

Cell receptors recognize and bind to the apo B-100 of LDL molecules. After the cell binds to the apo B-100, the LDL molecule is taken into a vesicle that fuses with the LDL to become an endosome. At this point, the LDL receptors separate from the LDL and travel back to the cell surface. The LDL migrates to a lysosome, where the apo B-100 is broken down into peptides, amino acids, and cholesterol. The cholesterol is used by the cell to make cell membranes, steroid hormones (in cells that make them), and bile acids (in liver cells). Cells regulate the amount of free cholesterol by decreasing the amount of endogenous cholesterol produced, increasing the production of cholesterol esters, and inhibiting LDL synthesis when cholesterol levels are high.

Excess cholesterol esters are taken up by macrophages. When macrophages become engorged with cholesterol esters, they are called **foam cells.** Foam cells are the earliest indication of atherogenic lesions.

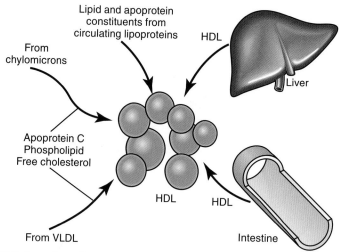

• **Figure 17-8** Formation of high-density lipoproteins (HDL). *VLDL,* Very-low-density lipoprotein.

TABLE 17-2 Fredrickson Classification of Lipid Disorders

Type	Description of Serum	Elevated Particles	Associated Clinical Disorders	Serum TC	Serum TG
I	Creamy top layer	Chylomicrons	Lipoprotein lipase deficiency, apolipoprotein C-II deficiency	N	++
IIa	Clear	LDL	Familial hypercholesterolemia, polygenic hypercholesterolemia, nephrosis, hypothyroidism, familial combined hyperlipidemia	++	N
IIb	Clear	LDL, VLDL	Familial combined hyperlipidemia	++	+
III	Turbid	IDL	Dysbetalipoproteinemia	+	+
IV	Turbid	VLDL	Familial hypertriglyceridemia, familial combined hyperlipidemia, sporadic hypertriglyceridemia, diabetes	N or +	++
V	Creamy top, turbid bottom	Chylomicrons, VLDL	Diabetes	+	++

IDL, Intermediate-density lipoproteins; *LDL,* low-density lipoproteins; *TC,* total cholesterol; *TG,* triglycerides; *VLDL,* very-low-density lipoproteins; *+,* increased; *++,* greatly increased; *N,* normal; *N+,* normal or increased.

Reverse Cholesterol Transport Pathway

HDL is secreted from the liver as crescent-shaped molecules containing mostly phospholipids and apo A-I. HDL molecules gain their spherical shape as they absorb more phospholipids, cholesterol esters, and certain apolipoproteins in the extracellular space. Hepatic cells can take up the cholesterol in the HDL remnants in three ways. First, HDL receptors can attach to HDL cholesterol esters and transfer the cholesterol esters to the liver. Second, HDL remnants can provide the cholesterol esters to lipoproteins containing apo B-100. Third, the apo E present on HDL remnants can be recognized by liver cells. These processes represent a reverse cholesterol pathway that allows cholesterol to be reused by the liver or disposed of (Fig. 17-8).

Abnormal Lipoprotein Metabolism

Abnormal lipoprotein metabolism is the result of genetic or acquired causes. Genetic defects in lipoprotein metabolism usually involve defects in surface apoproteins of the lipoprotein molecules, cell surface receptors of the liver and peripheral cells, or enzymes that regulate synthesis or catabolism. The following sections describe clinically significant conditions involving abnormal lipoprotein metabolism or production. Lipoprotein phenotypes were previously classified by the Fredrickson classification of lipid disorders system, but these conditions are more appropriately classified by metabolic pathways. The Fredrickson classification table is provided for reference (Table 17-2). The laboratory values seen with these conditions are summarized in Table 17-3.

TABLE 17-3	Lipoprotein Laboratory Values in Various Disorders					
Disorder	**Triglycerides**	**VLDL**	**HDL**	**LDL**	**Total Cholesterol**	
Deficiency in lipoprotein lipase	Up to 10,000 mg/dL	N	↓	↑	N	
Apolipoprotein C-II deficiency	500-10,000 mg/dL	↑	↓	↓	150-890 mg/dL	
Familial combined hyperlipidemia						
Type IIa		↑	N	↑	↑	
Type IIb	↑		↓	↑	↑	
Type IV	↑		↓	↑	↑	
Hyperapobetalipoproteinemia	N or ↑	↑	↓	↑ (moderate)	↑	
Familial hypertriglyceridemia	↑	↑	↓	N	N	
Type V hyperlipidemia	↑	↑	N	N	↑	
Dysbetalipoproteinemia (type III)	↑	↑	↓	↓	↑	
Familial hypercholesterolemia	N or ↑	N	↓	↑	↑	
Familial defective apolipoprotein B-100	N	N	N	↑	N or ↑	
Familial hypoalphalipoproteinemia	N	N	↓	N	N	
Defects in the synthesis of apolipoprotein A-I	N	N	↓	N	↓	
Defects in the catabolism of apolipoprotein A-I (Tangier disease)	N	N	↓	N	N	

HDL, High-density lipoprotein; *LDL,* low-density lipoprotein; *VLDL,* very-low-density lipoprotein; ↓, decreased; ↑, increased.

Deficiency in Lipoprotein Lipase Activity

Characteristics of deficient LPL activity include a marked hyperchylomicronemia and hypertriglyceridemia (up to 10,000 mg/dL). The absence of LPL leads to the inability to catabolize dietary fat, and massive amounts of chylomicrons accumulate in the blood. VLDL is usually normal, HDL is decreased, and LDL is increased (see Table 17-3). The condition is usually diagnosed in childhood. Signs and symptoms include severe abdominal pain and acute pancreatitis. When triglyceride levels reach 2000 mg/dL, eruptive xanthomas appear; when they reach 4000 mg/dL, lipemia retinalis appears. The severity of the symptoms is related to the triglyceride level. This condition is a rare (1 in 1,000,000 individuals), autosomal recessive disorder. Individuals with this condition are not predisposed to atherosclerosis.

Apolipoprotein C-II Deficiency

When apolipoprotein C-II is altered or absent, chylomicrons do not break down, and the triglyceride level can increase from 500 to 10,000 mg/dL. The individual's total cholesterol level can vary from 150 to 890 mg/dL, with HDL and LDL values extremely decreased (see Table 17-3). The symptoms of this condition are milder than those seen with deficiency of LPL activity and occur at an older age. Symptoms for this condition do not include eruptive xanthomas or lipemia retinalis. Individuals with this disease are not predisposed to atherosclerosis.

Familial Combined Hyperlipidemia

Characteristics of familial combined hyperlipidemia include increased levels of total and LDL cholesterol (Fredrickson type IIa), increased triglycerides (type IV), or both (type IIb). LDL levels are approximately 190 mg/dL, and triglyceride levels are between 200 and 400 mg/dL. HDL is usually decreased (see Table 17-3). This disease is usually expressed in adolescence, and it is relatively common (1 in 100 individuals). Familial combined hyperlipidemia is associated with coronary heart disease, and atherosclerosis is usually the only symptom.

Hyperapobetalipoproteinemia

Characteristics of hyperapobetalipoproteinemia include increased levels of apo B-100, total cholesterol, triglycerides, and LDL with decreased HDL levels. Elevated lipid levels are caused by the overproduction of VLDL by the liver (see Table 17-3). Atherosclerosis is usually the only symptom, and this condition is associated with coronary heart disease.

Familial Hypertriglyceridemia

Characteristics of familial hypertriglyceridemia include normal LDL, decreased HDL, and increased triglycerides (see Table 17-3). This condition has an autosomal dominant inheritance pattern with delayed expression.

It is a fairly common disease with a frequency of 1 in 500 individuals. The VLDL in this condition is large with an abnormally high triglyceride content. Symptoms include acute pancreatitis if the triglyceride level reaches 4000 mg/dL.

Type V Hyperlipoproteinemia

Characteristics of type V hyperlipoproteinemia include increased chylomicrons and VLDL. This disorder has an autosomal dominant inheritance pattern and is expressed in adulthood. Symptoms include eruptive xanthomas, lipemia retinalis, pancreatitis, and abnormal glucose tolerance with hyperinsulinemia. This condition is not linked to premature atherosclerosis.

Dysbetalipoproteinemia (Type III)

Characteristics of dysbetalipoproteinemia (Fredrickson type III) include increased total cholesterol and triglycerides as well as decreased LDL and HDL (see Table 17-3). This disease is caused by a primary genetic defect in the removal of chylomicrons and VLDL remnants. It is expressed in adulthood. Clinical symptoms include characteristic palmar xanthomas (yellow deposits of cholesterol in the creases of the palms). Eruptive xanthomas also appear on the tendons. Premature atherosclerosis develops in 30% to 50% of the patients affected by this condition, which occurs in 1 in 1000 individuals.

Familial Hypercholesterolemia

Characteristics of familial hypercholesterolemia include increased LDL (two to three times normal), increased total cholesterol (500 to 1200 mg/dL), increased triglycerides, and decreased HDL (see Table 17-3). This condition affects 1 in 500 individuals. It is inherited in an autosomal dominant pattern and is caused by a genetic mutation in the LDL receptor gene. Cholesterol deposits form in the skin, tendons, and arteries. The yellow-orange cutaneous xanthomas are characteristic of this disorder, and they appear before age 30. Homozygotes usually die before 40 years of age from a myocardial infarction.

Familial Defective Apolipoprotein B-100

Characteristics of familial defective apo B-100 include normal or very elevated levels of total cholesterol, increased LDL, normal triglyceride, and normal HDL (see Table 17-3). This condition is caused by a mutation in the apo B-100 gene in individuals of European descent. It occurs in 1 of 500 individuals.

Familial Hypoalphalipoproteinemia

Characteristics of familial hypoalphalipoproteinemia include normal triglyceride, normal LDL, normal VLDL, and decreased HDL levels (see Table 17-3). This condition

is inherited in an autosomal dominant pattern. Affected individuals have a very high incidence of coronary heart disease.

Defects in the Synthesis of Apolipoprotein A-I

Individuals with defects in the synthesis of apo A-I characteristically have normal total cholesterol, normal triglyceride, normal LDL, normal VLDL, and decreased HDL levels; heterozygotes have half the normal HDL value, and homozygotes have only a trace amounts (see Table 17-3). Symptoms include corneal clouding and a risk of developing premature coronary heart disease. Ten percent of the general population have this condition.

Defects in Catabolism of Apolipoprotein A-I (Tangier Disease)

Tangier disease was named for Tangier Island, on which it was first discovered. Characteristics include decreased HDL, decreased total cholesterol (heterozygotes, 170 mg/dL; homozygotes, 70 mg/dL), normal LDL, normal VLDL, and normal triglycerides (see Table 17-3). This condition is inherited in an autosomal dominant pattern. It results in the accumulation of cholesterol esters in body tissue. Symptoms include hyperplastic orange tonsils, splenomegaly, peripheral neuropathy, hepatomegaly, and corneal clouding. Homozygotes show an increased incidence of coronary heart disease.

Lipoproteins and Atherogenesis

Lipoproteins are implicated in the development of atherogenesis. Atherogenesis is associated with elevated LDL levels, elevated VLDL levels and chylomicron remnants, and decreased levels of HDL (Fig. 17-9).

Low-Density Lipoprotein

If LDL cannot be removed from plasma, scavenger cells (macrophages) take in the excess LDL. When these cells gorge themselves on LDL, they become foam cells. Foam cells are found in atherosclerotic plaques.

Very-Low-Density Lipoprotein and Chylomicron Remnants

When humans ingest cholesterol, VLDL and chylomicron remnants in the plasma increase due to increased hepatic synthesis. Even though a person's cholesterol level may never become elevated, the elevated VLDL and chylomicron remnant levels may produce atherosclerotic plaques.

High-Density Lipoprotein

When foam cells are exposed to HDL, they give up their ingested cholesterol and return to their scavenger cell status. This *reverse cholesterol transport* (see earlier discussion) is a function of the HDL. Elevated HDL levels can prevent atherosclerosis.

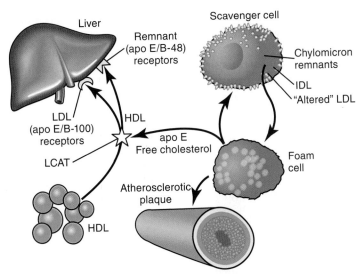

• **Figure 17-9** Lipoproteins and atherosclerosis. One hypothesis linking arthrogenesis with lipoproteins centers on foam cell formation. Foam cells adhere to the walls of blood vessels to form artherosclerotic plaques. Foam cell formation is promoted by chylomicron remnants, IDL, and altered LDL molecules. HDL molecules promote free cholesterol excretion from foam cells, thus preventing the development of atherosclerotic plaque. *apo E,* Apolipoprotein E; *B-48,* apolipoprotein B-48; *B-100,* apolipoprotein B-100; *HDL,* high-density lipoprotein; *IDL,* intermediate-density lipoprotein; *LCAT,* lecithin cholesterol acetyl transferase; *LDL,* low-density lipoprotein.

Laboratory Procedures and Limitations

The Cholesterol Reference Method Laboratory Network

The National Cholesterol Education Program (NCEP) was established by the National Heart, Lung, and Blood Institute in 1985. The purpose of the NCEP is to educate clinicians, patients, and the public about the role played by elevated cholesterol in cardiovascular disease. The NCEP's Expert Panel on Detection, Evaluation, and Treatment of High Blood Cholesterol in Adults released a strategy to identify people at risk for coronary heart disease as well as a strategy for lowering blood cholesterol levels. This panel also created cutoff points for total cholesterol, LDL, and HDL values. Total cholesterol levels of 150 to 180 mg/dL are associated with a low risk of atherosclerotic cardiovascular disease. LDL levels lower than 100 mg/dL are also associated with regression of coronary atherosclerosis. Cholesterol levels of 240 mg/dL or greater are implicated in coronary artery disease (Table 17-4).

The NCEP requires accurate cholesterol measurements so that clinicians can better diagnose coronary heart disease. The Centers for Disease Control and Prevention (CDC) created the Cholesterol Reference Method Laboratory Network to help manufacturers develop a valid method that is traceable to the National Reference System for Cholesterol (NRS/CHOL). The NRS/CHOL is the accuracy base for cholesterol measurements in the United States. The CDC reference method for total cholesterol is a modification of the Abell-Levy-Brodie-Kendall method.

Total Cholesterol

Although total cholesterol can be ordered as a single test, it is more commonly ordered as part of a lipid profile: total

TABLE 17-4	Association of Lipids and Lipoprotein Levels with Atherosclerotic Cardiovascular Disease in Adults 20 Years of Age or Older
Total Cholesterol (mg/dL)	
<200	Optimal
200-239	Borderline high risk
≥240	Very high risk
Low-Density Lipoprotein (mg/dL)	
<100	Optimal
100-129	Near-optimal/above optimal
130-159	Borderline high risk
160-189	High risk
≥190	Very high risk
High-Density Lipoprotein (mg/dL)	
<40 (men) or <50 (women)	Major risk factor for heart disease
≥60	Protection against heart disease
Triglyceride (mg/dL)	
<150	Optimal
150-199	Borderline high risk
200-499	High risk
≥500	Very high risk

Data from National Cholesterol Education Program ATE III Guidelines.

cholesterol, HDL, LDL, VLDL, and triglycerides. Lipid panels usually require a 12-hour fast because the triglyceride level is affected by food intake. Serum is used for lipid panel testing. For best results, specimens should be tested on the day they are collected, but they can be stored at 4° C for 3 to 4 days or at –20° C for several months. The thawed specimen must be thoroughly mixed before testing.

Most clinical laboratories measure total cholesterol using enzymatic methods, which are faster and safer than older methods. Other constituents in the specimen do not cause as much interference with the enzymatic methods. The enzymes serve as catalysts in the following processes:

$$\text{Cholesterol esters} \xrightarrow[\text{(Cholesterol esterase)}]{} \text{Free cholesterol + Fatty acids}$$

$$\text{Free cholesterol} + O_2 \xrightarrow[\text{(Cholesterol oxidase)}]{} \text{Cholest-4-en-3-one} + H_2O_2$$

$$H_2O_2 + \text{Phenol} + \text{4-Aminoantipyrine} \xrightarrow[\text{(Peroxidase)}]{} o\text{-Quinoneimine dye}$$

The colored product (*o*-quinineimine dye) is measured at 480 to 520 nm, and the intensity of the color is directly proportional to the amount of cholesterol in the specimen. Enzymatic methods are usually linear to 500 mg/dL. If a sample result indicates more than 500 mg/dL, the sample should be diluted with saline and retested for a more accurate result.

Triglycerides

Triglyceride tests are performed on clear, unhemolyzed serum specimens. Specimens should be collected after the patient has fasted for at least 12 hours. If testing cannot be performed on the same day, store the specimen at 2° C to 8° C for 1 week or at –20° C for up to 3 months. Specimens should be thawed at room temperature and mixed thoroughly before testing. The enzymatic method for determining triglycerides in serum uses the following steps:

$$\text{Triglycerides} \xrightarrow[\text{(Lipase)}]{} \text{Glycerol + Fatty Acids}$$

$$\text{Glycerol} + \text{ATP} \xrightarrow[\text{(GK)}]{} \text{Glycerol-1-phosphate + ADP}$$

$$\text{Glycerol-1-phosphate} + O_2 \xrightarrow[\text{(GPO)}]{} \text{DAP} + H_2O_2$$

$$H_2O_2 + \text{4-AA} + \text{4-Chlorophenol} \xrightarrow[\text{(POD)}]{} \text{Quinoneimine dye} + \text{HCl} + 2H_2O$$

where ATP is adenosine triphosphate, ADP is adenosine diphosphate, GK is glycerol kinase, DAP is dihydroxyacetone phosphate, GPO is glycerol phosphate oxidase, 4-AA is 4-aminoantipyrine, and POD is peroxidase.

The absorbance of the dye is read at 510 nm and is proportional to the triglyceride concentration. Enzymatic methods are linear to 1000 mg/dL. Specimens with values greater than 1000 mg/dL need to be diluted with saline and retested.

High-Density Lipoprotein

HDL tests are performed on serum specimens. If testing cannot be performed on the same day, the specimen should be stored at 2° C to 8° C for 3 to 4 days or at –20° C for up to 14 days. If specimens are stored for longer than 7 days,

the HDL level will decrease, but this decrease is not clinically significant.

The Beckman Coulter test assay is a two reagent homogenous assay that uses two phases in its direct HDL assay.

Reaction Phase 1

$$\text{LDL, VLDL, Chylomicrons} \xrightarrow[\text{(DSBmT + Peroxidase)}]{\text{(Accelerator + CO)}} \text{Colorless end product}$$

Reaction Phase 2

$$\text{HDL cholesterol} \xrightarrow[\text{(HDL-specific detergent)}]{} \text{HDL disrupted}$$

$$\text{HDL cholesterol} + H_2O + O_2 \xrightarrow[\text{(CE and CO)}]{} \text{Cholest-4-en-3-one} + H_2O_2$$

$$H_2O_2 + \text{DSBmT} + \text{4-AAP} \xrightarrow[\text{(Peroxidase)}]{} \text{Blue color complex}$$

where DSBmT is *N,N*-bis-(4-sulfobutyl)-*m*-toluidine disodium, CE is cholesterol esterase, CO is cholesterol oxidase, and 4-AAP is 4-aminoantipyrine. In the first reaction phase of this assay, free cholesterol from lipoproteins other than HDL is consumed and forms a colorless end product. This end product now contains only HDL cholesterol. The HDL cholesterol is reacted with cholesterol esterase, cholesterol oxidase, and a chromogen to form a blue product. The blue color complex is measured bichromatically at 600/700 nm, and the resulting increase in absorbance is directly proportional to the amount of HDL in the sample. This test methodology was tested in a Cholesterol Reference Method Laboratory Network laboratory to confirm that it meets the guidelines of the NCEP.

Low-Density Lipoprotein

LDL can be measured directly or calculated. The Beckman Coulter method uses a two-reagent homogenous system with two distinct phases. Phase 1 consist of mixing the sample with a detergent to dissolve the cholesterol from non-LDL particles. Cholesterol oxidase (CO), cholesterol esterase (CE), peroxidase, and 4-aminoantipyrine (4-AAP) combine to form a colorless end product. In phase 2, another detergent dissolves the cholesterol in the LDL particles. This cholesterol then reacts with CE, CO, and a chromogen to yield a blue-colored product that is measured bichromatically at 540/660 nm. The LDL concentration in the sample is directly proportional to the resulting increase in absorbance of the blue compound.

Reaction Phase 1

$$\text{HDL, VLDL, LDL, Chylomicrons} \xrightarrow[\text{(CE and CO)}]{} \begin{array}{l}\text{Cholest-4-en-3-one} + \\ \text{Fatty acids} + H_2O_2\end{array}$$

$$H_2O_2 - \text{4-AAP} \xrightarrow[\text{(Peroxidase)}]{} \text{LDL + Colorless end product}$$

Reaction Phase 2

$$\text{LDL} \xrightarrow[\text{(CE and CO)}]{} \text{Cholest-4-en-3-one + Fatty acids} + H_2O_2$$

$$H_2O_2 + \text{DSBmT} + \text{4-AAP} \xrightarrow[\text{(Peroxidase)}]{} \text{Blue color complex}$$

In another approach, the Friedewald formula is used to calculate LDL concentration based on the measured values for total cholesterol, HDL, and triglycerides:

$$LDL = Total\ cholesterol - [HDL + (Triglycerides/5)]$$

An LDL:HDL ratio of less than 3:1 is desirable. As an example, consider a patient whose total cholesterol is 200 mg/dL, HDL is 50 mg/dL, and triglycerides are 200 mg/dL. To calculate the LDL using the Friedewald equation:

$$Triglycerides/5 = 200\ mg/dL \div 5 = 40\ mg/dL$$

$$[HDL + (Triglycerides/5)] = 50\ mg/dL + 40\ mg/dL$$
$$= 90\ mg/dL$$

$$Total\ cholesterol - [HDL + (Triglycerides/5)]$$
$$= 200 - 90 = 110\ mg/dL$$

The patient's LDL is 110 mg/dL. There are some limitations to this formula. If any of the three values used to calculate the LDL are wrong, then the numerical result for LDL will also be wrong. Moreover, this formula cannot be used if the patient's triglyceride level is greater than 400 mg/dL.

Lipoproteins and Clinical Vascular Disease

Lipoprotein levels are determined by genetic and acquired factors. Research conducted over the last 30 years links atherogenesis to serum lipoprotein levels—especially LDL and HDL levels. Experts also agree that lowering lipoprotein levels can lower the risk of coronary atherogenesis. The Expert Panel on Detection, Evaluation, and Treatment of High Blood Cholesterol Levels published recommendations designed to reduce lipoprotein levels to a point sufficient to lower the risk of coronary heart disease. These recommendations included monitoring of serum lipoprotein levels, dietary changes, and drug therapy.

Atherosclerosis

Description

The meaning of atherosclerosis comes from *athero* (thick soup) and *scleros* (hard). This term describes the cholesterol deposits and scarred portion in an arterial plaque or atheroma. Atheromas change with age. Young atheromas are soft and are composed of lipid-containing macrophages and fat deposits. These young atheromas sometimes detach, causing thrombosis and blocked vessels. As an atheroma grows older, scar tissue builds up and calcium is deposited in the lesion. Scar tissue and calcium make the atheroma hard. This is where the term "hardening of the arteries" originated.

Technically, atherosclerosis begins at birth and increases with age. More men than women die before age 50 from atherosclerosis, but after age 50, more women than men die from this disease. Genetics plays a role in this disease, but so do unhealthy lifestyle habits such as high-fat diet, obesity, high-sodium diet, cigarette smoking, and lack of exercise.

Disease Mechanisms

Atherosclerosis begins with endothelial cell damage, which allows an atheroma to form. Endothelial cell damage also allows lipids to be deposited into this area. Macrophages detect the lipids and enter the site to phagocytize the lipids. The macrophages phagocytize the lipids. As this process continues, the macrophages are unable to phagocytize all the LDL, and some LDL ends up accumulated in the damaged vessel. The activity of the macrophages stimulate collagen formation and the macrophage/LDL build up becomes fibrous. This build up can weaken the vessel wall and lead to thrombosis. This process repeats itself as a young, soft atheroma forms. Scarring and chronic inflammation at the site and calcium deposits in the atheroma eventually produce a hard, calcified atheroma.

Risk factors for development of atherosclerosis include age, gender, genetics, high blood cholesterol level, hypertension, smoking, diabetes, high homocysteine levels, and inflammation. As we age, we are more prone to develop atherosclerosis. Women are protected by estrogen until menopause, but after age 60 to 70, women and men have equal chances of developing atherosclerosis. A family history of heart disease or stroke increases the risk of developing this disease. The earlier part of this chapter linked high blood cholesterol levels to atherosclerosis. Hypertension damages endothelial cells and initiates the development of an atheroma. Smoking lowers HDL levels, increases blood pressure, reduces pulmonary function, and damages endothelium in many ways. Diabetics develop vascular disease because they have a deficiency of LPL leading to high levels of cholesterol in the blood, and their high blood glucose levels cause a nonatherosclerotic disease of small blood vessels. Homocysteine is toxic to endothelial cells, and elevated blood levels can produce heart attacks and strokes even in teenagers. The process of inflammation is a key element in the atherogenic process because inflammatory cells (monocytes, macrophages, and others) are drawn to the developing atheroma to unleash the full acute phase response, causing more injury to the area.

Clinical Correlation

Atheromas grow silently over many years or decades; once they become large enough to obstruct blood flow, the individual becomes symptomatic. Coronary atheromas cause ischemia (decreased blood flow) and angina (chest pain) because the heart muscle is not getting enough oxygen to properly function due to clogged arteries. If an atheroma breaks off or grows large enough to totally block a coronary blood vessel, then a myocardial infarction (heart attack) occurs. Heart muscle dies without oxygen. Myocardial infarctions result in heart failure, arrhythmia, and sudden death. If an atheroma occurs in the aorta, it could weaken the artery wall and allow bulges (aneurysms) to occur. These bulges continue to grow until one day they rupture, resulting in a life-threatening situation. Many people die each year from dissecting aortic aneurysms. Atheromas also occur in the brain, causing brain infarctions or strokes. Atheromas in the extremities (e.g., in the toes) can block blood flow, leading to gangrene.

TABLE 17-5	Hypertensive States	
Classification	Systolic Pressure (mm Hg)	Diastolic Pressure (mm Hg)
Optimal	<120	<80
Normal	<130	<85
High-normal or prehypertension	130-139	85-90
Mild hypertension (stage 1)	140-159	90-99
Moderate hypertension (stage 2)	160-179	100-109
Severe hypertension	>180	>110

Data from Seventh Report of the Joint National Committee on Prevention, Detection, Evaluation, and Treatment of High Blood Pressure (JNC 7).

Laboratory Analytes and Assays

Laboratory tests performed to confirm a myocardial infarction include creatine kinase (CK) and its MB isoenzyme (CK-MB), troponin-I, and troponin-T. The laboratory procedures and limitations are covered fully in Chapter 18. Brain infarcts or strokes are usually diagnosed by computed tomography or magnetic resonance imaging but can also be diagnosed through a spinal tap, which is used to sample the cerebrospinal fluid (CSF). If an individual has bled into the CSF, the test will show similar numbers of red blood cells in all four tubes; with a traumatic tap, in contrast, the number of red blood cells in the first tube will greatly exceed the number of red blood cells in the fourth tube.

Hypertension

Normal blood pressure readings are less than 130/35 mm Hg. The top number is the systolic blood pressure—the amount of pressure generated by the heart when it pumps blood into arteries. The bottom number is the diastolic pressure—the amount of pressure in the heart when it is at rest or refilling. Optimal blood pressure is less than 120/80 mm Hg. Systolic values of 130 to 139 mm Hg and diastolic values of 85 to 90 mm Hg are considered high-normal. Stage 1 or mild hypertension is diagnosed with a level of 140 to 159 mm Hg systolic or 90 to 99 mm Hg diastolic; stage 2 or moderate hypertension at 160 to 179 mm Hg systolic or 100 to 109 mm Hg diastolic; and severe hypertension (a medical emergency) at 180/110 mm Hg or greater (Table 17-5).

Description

Hypertension is sustained high blood pressure. Approximately 33% of adults in the United States have high blood pressure, and only 48% of those receiving treatment are able to control their blood pressure. Approximately 95% of diagnosed individuals have *primary hypertension* (not associated with another disease). Primary hypertension is thought to be caused by a combination of genetic and environmental factors. Inherited defects that predispose individuals to primary hypertension include those associated with renal sodium excretion, insulin and insulin sensitivity, activity of the sympathetic nervous system (SNS) and the renin-angiotensin-aldosterone system (RAAS), and cell membrane sodium or calcium transport. Risk factors include family history, advancing age, gender (more common in men younger than 55 years and women older than 70 years), black race, high dietary sodium, glucose intolerance (diabetes mellitus), cigarette smoking, obesity, heavy alcohol consumption, and low dietary intake of calcium, magnesium, and potassium. At a given blood pressure, people with hypertension secrete less sodium in their urine than nonhypertensive individuals. Statistics indicate that people with hypertension have a shorter life expectancy than people without the disease.

Pathophysiology of Hypertension

In healthy individuals, the SNS maintains healthy blood pressure and tissue perfusion by maintaining adequate cardiac output and adequate peripheral resistance. Overactivity of the SNS leads to increased heart rate and increased peripheral resistance due to blood vessel vasoconstriction. This vasoconstriction stimulates renin release, increases tubular sodium reabsorption, and reduces renal flow, thus increasing the blood pressure.

Genetic defects combined with environmental risks cause inflammation and insulin resistance as well as dysfunction of the SNS, RAAS, adducin, and natriuretic hormones (Fig. 17-10). Insulin resistance and the malfunctioning SNS and RAAS cause systemic constriction of blood vessels, leading to increased resistance throughout the arterioles of the body. The malfunction of these systems combines with inflammation to retain salt and water in the kidney, leading to increased blood volume. Increased peripheral resistance and increased blood volume are two of the main causes of sustained hypertension.

Clinical Correlation

Many individuals diagnosed with hypertension already have atherosclerosis, including coronary artery disease. This means that individuals with hypertension are more vulnerable to myocardial infarcts, cerebrovascular accidents, and heart failure. The kidney's blood vessels are also affected by hypertension. With aging, normal blood pressure produces nephrosclerosis (general wear and tear) in renal arterioles. Hypertension accelerates nephrosclerosis, and this condition is called *benign nephrosclerosis*. In severe hypertension, nephrosclerosis causes severe kidney damage leading to *malignant nephrosclerosis*. Recall that hypertension has no symptoms, but the sequelae associated with hypertension have symptoms.

Laboratory Analytes and Assays

Many patients with hypertension will have no abnormal laboratory tests. However, to diagnose hypertension, clinicians will order a battery of laboratory tests to rule out pheochromocytoma, adrenal hyperplasia, and renal disease. These tests include urinalysis (macroscopic and microscopic); a metabolic panel

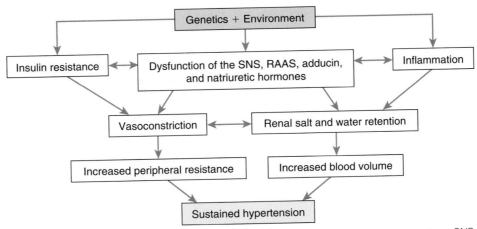

• **Figure 17-10** Pathophysiology of hypertension. *RAAS*, renin-angiotensin-aldosterone system; *SNS,* sympathetic nervous system. (From McCance KL, Huether SE. *Pathophysiology: The Biologic Basis for Disease in Adults and Children.* 7th ed. St. Louis: Mosby; 2015.)

including fasting blood glucose, blood urea nitrogen (BUN), creatinine, sodium, potassium, calcium, thyroid-stimulating hormone (TSH), total cholesterol, HDL, LDL, triglycerides, and hematocrit; 24-hour urine for creatinine and protein; and measurement of catecholamines. The clinician will also obtain an electrocardiogram and a chest radiograph.

Vasculitis

Vasculitis involves inflammation of the arteries and, rarely, the veins. There are several recognized syndromes, each based on the type of blood vessels affected, disease mechanism, and tissues affected. For example, Wegener granulomatosis is a vasculitis that affects the kidneys, lungs, sinuses, and nose. Most vasculitis diseases are caused by an autoimmune process.

Vasculitis can affect any organ in the body. Some sequelae include aneurysm, stroke, gangrene, renal disease, and disseminated intravascular coagulation (DIC). There are no laboratory tests to diagnosis vasculitis, but specific tests can be performed depending on the affected tissue or organ.

Summary

Cardiovascular disease is the leading cause of death in the United States. Lipoproteins are linked to cardiovascular disease, and reducing the levels of lipoproteins can prevent cardiovascular disease and its sequelae. The major classes of lipids in the body are fatty acids, triglycerides, phospholipids, sterols, sphingolipids, and cholesterol. When fatty acids undergo catabolism, three ketone bodies are produced: acetoacetic acid, β-hydroxybutyric acid, and acetone. Triglycerides are composed of three fatty acids and one molecule of glycerol. Excess carbohydrates are stored as triglycerides. Phospholipids are cell membrane components. Sphingolipids are cell membrane components in red blood cells, brain, and nerve cells. Cholesterol is a sterol that is a structural component in cells as well as a precursor of steroid hormones.

There are five categories of lipoproteins: chylomicrons, VLDL, IDL, LDL, and HDL. Apolipoproteins are found on the surface of lipoproteins; they include apolipoproteins A-I, B-48, B-100, C-I, C-II, C-III, and E. Lipoprotein (a), or Lp(a), is an independent risk factor for coronary heart disease. Triglycerides transport fats from the intestines to adipose tissue and muscle tissue. VLDL carries triglycerides produced by the liver to adipose tissue for storage. LDL transports cholesterol to peripheral cells. HDL transports cholesterol from the cells to the liver for conversion into bile acids. The Fredrickson classification of lipid disorders was based on abnormal lipoprotein levels. Hyperlipidemias include deficiency of LPL activity, apo C-II deficiency, familial combined hyperlipidemia (types IIa, IIb, and IV), hyperapobetalipoproteinemia, familial hypetriglyceridemia, type V hyperlipoproteinemia, dysbetalipoproteinemia (type III), familial hypercholesterolemia, familial defective apo B-100, familial hypoalphalipoproteinemia, defects in synthesis of apo A-I, and defects in catabolism of apo A-I (Tangier disease). Lipoproteins play an integral part in atherogenesis.

The National Cholesterol Education Program (NCEP) was founded in 1985 to educate health care professionals and the public about the importance of controlling cholesterol levels and how this can prevent atherosclerosis. The CDC later created the Cholesterol Reference Method Laboratory Network to standardize cholesterol and lipoprotein test methods. Total cholesterol and triglyceride tests use enzymatic methods, whereas HDL and LDL direct measurements use a combination of enzymatic and colorimetric methods. The Friedewald formula can be used to estimate LDL concentrations from the total cholesterol, HDL, and triglyceride test results.

Atherosclerosis is a disease process that damages arteries and causes atheroma formation. Chronic inflammation and calcium deposits cause "hardening of the arteries." Factors that play a role in atherosclerosis development include age, gender, genetics, increased cholesterol, hypertension, smoking, diabetes, and high homocysteine levels. Hypertension is abnormally high blood pressure readings. Normal blood pressure is considered to be 120/80 mm Hg. Severe hypertension is defined as blood pressure greater than 180/110 mm Hg. There is no known cause for most cases of hypertension. Vasculitis, another blood vessel disease, is an inflammation of the arteries and, rarely, the veins.

Review Questions

1. What lipoprotein test methodology is measured bichromatically at 540/660 nm?
   a. HDL
   b. VLDL
   c. LDL
   d. IDL
2. The largest lipoprotein molecule is
   a. LDL
   b. VLDL
   c. Chylomicron
   d. HDL
3. The purpose of which lipoprotein molecule is to transport cholesterol from the liver to the tissues?
   a. VLDL
   b. LDL
   c. Chylomicrons
   d. HDL
4. Elevated levels of which lipoprotein are considered an independent risk factor for coronary heart disease?
   a. HDL
   b. LDL
   c. Lp(a)
   d. VLDL
5. Triglycerides are
   a. Stored in the liver, adipose tissue, and other organs and tissues
   b. Not found in dietary fats
   c. Synthesized in the liver, adipose tissue, and other organs and tissues
   d. Transported by LDL in the blood

6. Risk factors for coronary heart disease include all of the following EXCEPT
   a. Cholesterol >240 mg/dL
   b. Currently smoking cigarettes
   c. Male gender
   d. Taking antihypertensive drugs
7. Seventy percent of which lipid is found in skin, adipose tissue, and muscle cells?
   a. Cholesterol
   b. VLDL
   c. HDL
   d. LDL
8. Which lipid is the major constituent of cell membranes and the outer shells of lipoprotein molecules?
   a. Phospholipids
   b. Cholesterol
   c. VLDL
   d. Lp(a)
9. The function of apolipoproteins is to allow lipoproteins to be
   a. Soluble in the blood
   b. Made into adipose
   c. Soluble in the tissues
   d. Part of the cellular membranes
10. What is the smallest lipoprotein molecule?
    a. Chylomicron
    b. LDL
    c. VLDL
    d. HDL

Critical Thinking Questions

1. What is the formula for estimating LDL? When is this formula not valid?
2. Which general methodology is most often used to determine serum triglyceride levels?
3. Which Fredrickson hyperlipoproteinemia exhibits markedly elevated serum triglyceride levels?

CASE STUDY

A 25-year-old man comes to his physician's office for a routine physical examination. During the examination, the physician notices orange-yellow tonsils and hepatosplenomegaly. The routine blood work ordered by the physician shows a total cholesterol level of 125 mg/dL, triglycerides 300 mg/dL, and HDL 4 mg/dL. What is the most likely diagnosis? What additional tests might the physician order?

Bibliography

Beckman Coulter HDL assay manufacturer information. <https://www.beckmancoulter.com/wsrportal/techdocs?docname=/cis/BAOSR6x95/%25%25/EN_HDL-CHOLESTEROL.pdf> Accessed 14.10.15.

Beckman Coulter LDL assay manufacturer information. <https://www.beckmancoulter.com/wsrportal/techdocs?docname=/cis/baosr6x96/%25%25/en_ldl-cholesterol.pdf> Accessed 14.10.15.

Burtis CA, Bruns DE. *Tietz Fundamentals of Clinical Chemistry and Molecular Diagnostics*. 7th ed. St. Louis: Saunders; 2015.

Chobanian AV, Bakris GL, Black HR, et al. Seventh report of the Joint National Committee on Prevention, Detection, Evaluation, and Treatment of High Blood Pressure. *Hypertension*. 2003;42(6):1206–1252.

Durrington P, Soran H. Hyperlipidemia. In: Lammert E, Zeeb M, eds. *Metabolism of Human Diseases*. Vienna: Springer; 2004:295–302.

Fisher EA, Feig JE, Hewing B, Hazen SL, Smith JD. High-density lipoprotein function, dysfunction, and reverse cholesterol transport. *Arterioscler Thromb Vasc Biol*. 2012;32(12):2813–2820.

Jones RB, Savage CO. Systemic vasculitides: an overview. *Medicine*. 2014;42(3):134–137.

Khera AV, Cuchel M, de la Llera-Moya M, et al. Cholesterol efflux capacity, high-density lipoprotein function, and atherosclerosis. *N Engl J Med*. 2011;364(2):127–135.

Myers GL, Kimberly MM, Waymack PP, et al. A reference method laboratory network for cholesterol: a model for standardization and improvement of clinical laboratory measurements. *Clin Chem*. 2000;46(11):1762–1772.

Pagana KD, Pagana TJ. *Mosby's manual of diagnostic and laboratory tests*. 5th ed. St. Louis: Mosby; 2013. Table 2–38.

Seventh Report of the Joint National Committee on Prevention, Detection, Evaluation, and Treatment of High Blood Pressure (JNC 7). <https://www.nhlbi.nih.gov/files/docs/guidelines/phycard.pdf> Accessed 14.10.15.

Sidney S, Rosamond WD, Howard VJ, Luepker RV. National Forum for Heart Disease and Stroke Prevention. The "heart disease and stroke statistics—2013 update" and the need for a national cardiovascular surveillance system. *Circulation*. 2013;127(1):21–23.

Takahashi H, Yoshika M, Komiyama Y, Nishimura M. The central mechanism underlying hypertension: a review of the roles of sodium ions, epithelial sodium channels, the renin–angiotensin–aldosterone system, oxidative stress and endogenous digitalis in the brain. *Hypertens Res*. 2011;34(11):1147–1160.

U.S. Department of Health and Human Services. Public Health Service; National Institutes of Health; National Heart, Lung, and Blood Institute. National Cholesterol Education Program Report #3. NIH Publication No. 01-3305; May 2001. <https://www.nhlbi.nih.gov/files/docs/guidelines/atglance.pdf> Accessed 14.10.15.

18

Heart Disease

SHERYL BERMAN

CHAPTER OUTLINE

OBJECTIVES

After completion of this chapter, the reader will be able to:

1. Describe the chambers, valves, and major blood vessels associated with the heart.
2. Trace the blood flow of the heart from the right atrium to the aorta.
3. Define myocardial infarction and list the contributing factors.
4. Compare and contrast the blood tests and other tests used for detection of myocardial infarction.
5. Describe the disease processes associated with congestive heart failure.
6. Discuss and evaluate the tests used to diagnose congestive heart failure.
7. Summarize the primary types of congenital heart defects and the tests used to diagnose them.
8. Compare and contrast endocarditis, myocarditis, and pericarditis.
9. Differentiate the laboratory tests that should be used for detection of endocarditis from those used for myocarditis and pericarditis.

KEY TERMS

Atherosclerosis
Atherosclerotic plaque formation
Atrial septal defect
B-type natriuretic peptide
Cardiac catheterization
Cardiac tamponade
Cardiomegaly
Cardiomyopathy
Chronic pericarditis
Congestive heart failure
Constrictive pericarditis

Coronary artery
C-reactive protein
Creatine kinase MB
Diastole
Dyspnea
Electrocardiogram
Endocardial biopsy
Endocarditis
Heart valvular disease
Ischemia
Left-to-right shunting

Myocardial infarction
Myocarditis
Myoglobin
Pericardial effusion
Pericarditis
Procainamide
Systole
Tetralogy of Fallot
Transposition of the great arteries
Troponins I and T
Ventricular septal defect

❖ Case in Point

Mr. H., a 54-year-old African American man, enters the emergency department with left-sided, crushing chest pain; shortness of breath; and dizziness that has lasted 3 hours. His chemistry results are as follows: troponin I >100 ng/mL, creatine kinase (CK) 10,231 IU/L, and CK-MB 598 ng/mL. What is the likely diagnosis? Are there other tests that should be ordered? Describe the mechanism of the condition and why these tests are well suited to its diagnosis.

Points to Remember

- The four chambers of the heart include the right and left atria and the left and right ventricles.
- Blood flows from the right atrium to the right ventricle, pulmonary artery, lungs, pulmonary vein, left atrium, left ventricle, aorta, and systemic circulation.
- Myocardial infarction is the irreversible death of cardiac tissue resulting from a blocked coronary artery.
- Atherosclerosis is a leading cause of myocardial infarction.
- The most specific tests for the diagnosis of myocardial infarction are an electrocardiogram and troponin I and T levels.
- Congestive heart failure is a gradual decrease in the heart's ability to pump blood efficiently.
- Congestive heart failure can be caused by myocardial infarction, hypertension, heart valvular disease, and cardiomyopathy.
- B-type natriuretic peptide is the most specific blood test for detecting heart damage in patients with congestive heart failure.
- Congenital heart diseases are caused by malformations of the heart that are present at birth.
- The most common congenital heart diseases are atrial septal defect, ventricular septal defect, tetralogy of Fallot, and transposition of the great arteries.
- Imaging techniques such as chest radiography, magnetic resonance imaging, and echocardiography are helpful in diagnosing congenital heart defects.
- Endocarditis is inflammation of the innermost layer of the heart.
- The most common cause of endocarditis is bacteria from the bloodstream settling on damaged areas of the heart such as valves.
- Myocarditis is an inflammation of the middle layer or heart muscle.
- Myocarditis is most often caused by viral or bacterial infection.
- Pericarditis is inflammation of the outermost layer of the heart, which is a membranous sac surrounding the heart muscle.
- Pericarditis is caused by underlying conditions such as infection, trauma, and autoimmune diseases.
- A variety of laboratory and imaging tests (e.g., echocardiogram), troponin levels, blood cultures, and other studies are used to diagnose endocarditis, myocarditis, and pericarditis.

Introduction

Diseases that affect the heart include myocardial infarction, congestive heart failure, congenital heart disease, endocarditis, myocarditis, and pericarditis. This chapter explores the laboratory and imaging studies used to diagnose these pathologies.

Heart Structure and Blood Flow

Heart Structure

The heart has four chambers: two atria (right and left) and two ventricles (right and left). The bicuspid (mitral) valve is found between the left atrium and left ventricle, and the tricuspid valve is found between the right atrium and the right ventricle.

All veins carry deoxygenated blood to the heart. All arteries, except the pulmonary artery, carry oxygenated blood away from the heart. The primary large veins that bring blood to the heart are the superior vena cava and inferior vena cava. The superior vena cava carries blood from the upper body, and the inferior vena cava carries blood from the lower body (Fig. 18-1).

Blood Flow through the Heart and Lungs

Deoxygenated blood flows from the body through the superior and inferior venae cavae and into the right atrium. Blood from the superior portion of the body and extremities flows to the heart through the superior vena cava. Deoxygenated blood from the inferior portion of the body and extremities flows to the heart through the inferior vena cava. From the right atrium, blood flows through the tricuspid valve into the right ventricle. From the right ventricle, blood is pumped out of the heart through the pulmonary artery to the lungs. In the lungs, blood becomes oxygenated and flows back to the left atrium of the heart through the pulmonary vein. Blood then travels through the bicuspid (mitral) valve into the left ventricle, from which it is pumped through the aorta to the rest of the body (Fig. 18-2). The arteries that supply oxygenated blood to the heart muscle itself are the coronary arteries.

Myocardial Infarction

Background

Myocardial infarction (MI), also known as a heart attack, is the irreversible death of cardiac muscle tissue, which is most often caused by ischemia (i.e., lack of oxygen) (Fig. 18-3). Ischemia is responsible for the signs and symptoms of MI, including the chest pain, nausea, dizziness, and the shortness of breath, experienced by Mr. H. in the Case in Point.

The most common cause of MI is blockage of one or more blood vessels that supply oxygen directly to the cardiac

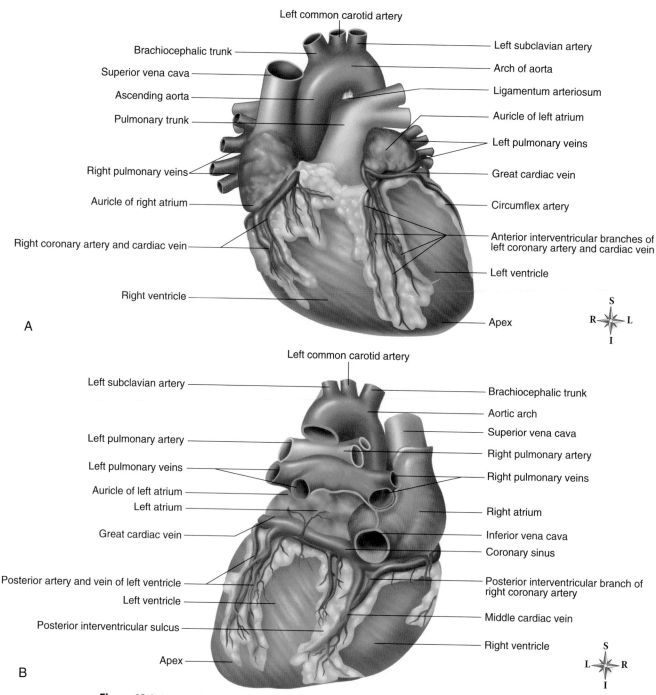

Left common carotid artery

Brachiocephalic trunk

Superior vena cava

Ascending aorta

Pulmonary trunk

Right pulmonary veins

Auricle of right atrium

Right coronary artery and cardiac vein

Right ventricle

Left subclavian artery

Arch of aorta

Ligamentum arteriosum

Auricle of left atrium

Left pulmonary veins

Great cardiac vein

Circumflex artery

Anterior interventricular branches of left coronary artery and cardiac vein

Left ventricle

Apex

A

Left common carotid artery

Left subclavian artery

Left pulmonary artery

Left pulmonary veins

Auricle of left atrium

Left atrium

Great cardiac vein

Posterior artery and vein of left ventricle

Left ventricle

Posterior interventricular sulcus

Apex

Brachiocephalic trunk

Aortic arch

Superior vena cava

Right pulmonary artery

Right pulmonary veins

Right atrium

Inferior vena cava

Coronary sinus

Posterior interventricular branch of right coronary artery

Middle cardiac vein

Right ventricle

B

• **Figure 18-1** Anterior (**A**) and posterior (**B**) view of the heart and the great vessels. (From Patton KT, Thibodeau GA. *Anatomy and Physiology.* 8th ed. St. Louis: Mosby; 2013.)

muscle. These blood vessels are called coronary arteries. Coronary arteries often become blocked due to atherosclerosis, which is an accumulation of lipid plaques and thrombi in the arteries. Atherosclerosis has several genetic and environmental risk factors (Table 18-1).

Diagnosis

Laboratory tests that detect biomarkers in the blood are available for diagnosis of MI. The biomarkers are released from damaged or dying cardiac cells. Each biomarker

appears in the blood in its unique time frame after an MI. Because no laboratory test is 100% specific for MI, the tests should be used in conjunction with an electrocardiogram and the patient's signs and symptoms for the diagnosis. The biomarkers described in Table 18-2 are used to help diagnose an acute MI.

Troponins

Troponins T and I are regulatory proteins in cardiac cells that are integral to muscle contraction. They are released into the blood when myocardial cells are damaged or die.

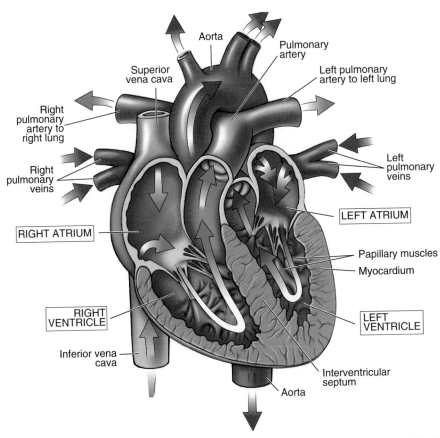

• **Figure 18-2** Chambers of the heart and great vessels. The *arrows* show blood flow through the heart and great vessels. (From Herlihy B. *The Human Body in Health Illness.* 5th ed. St. Louis: Saunders; 2014.)

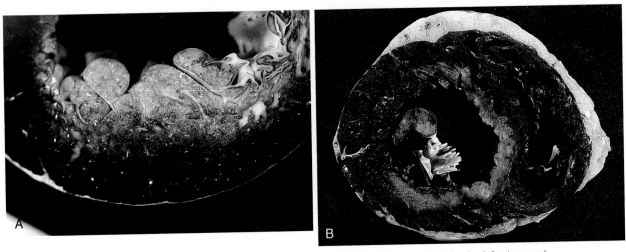

• **Figure 18-3** Myocardial infarction. **A,** Local infarct confined to one region. **B,** Massive infarct caused by occlusion of three coronary arteries. (From Damjanov I, Linder J, eds. *Anderson's Pathology.* 10th ed. St. Louis: Mosby; 1996.)

They are two of the most specific biomarkers for myocardial injury.

Blood troponin levels begin to increase 3 to 12 hours after the onset of an MI and remain elevated for up to 2 weeks. Troponin I levels may remain elevated for up to 10 days, and troponin T levels may be elevated for up to 2 weeks after an MI. Troponin T is not as specific as troponin I for cardiac damage because the troponin T level may also be elevated in skeletal muscle and kidney disorders.

Troponins are usually measured by immunoassay. The normal range for either troponin I or T is 0.01 ng/mL or less. For individuals with cardiac symptoms, troponin levels that are greater than 0.01 ng/mL and rising indicate cardiac injury (Fig. 18-4).

Myoglobin

Myoglobin is found in muscle and can be released into the blood when muscles are damaged. It is a sensitive indicator of cardiac muscle damage but not specific because it is also found in skeletal muscle. The amount of myoglobin in the blood is proportional to the amount of muscle damage.

The absence of myoglobin can be used to rule out MI. Myoglobin levels rise early, usually within 2 to 3 hours after an MI. Myoglobin, like troponins, is measured by immunoassay. Myoglobin reference ranges are 10 to 95 ng/mL for men and 10 to 65 ng/mL for women. Rising levels can indicate cardiac injury (see Fig. 18-4).

Creatine Kinase MB

Creatine kinase (CK) is an enzyme that is found in various tissues. The three subtypes (isoenzymes) are creatine kinase MM, creatine kinase MB, and creatine kinase BB. The MM isoenzyme is found predominantly in skeletal muscle. The MB fraction (CK-MB) is found predominantly in cardiac muscle, and the BB fraction is found predominantly in the brain and lower intestine (i.e., bowel).

CK-MB can be measured to detect an MI. The most common method is immunoassay. CK-MB is less sensitive than troponins, but levels rise in the bloodstream in a similar time frame, usually 3 to 4 hours after an MI. Unlike troponins, CK-MB does not remain elevated and may return to pre-MI levels within 36 hours (see Fig. 18-4). The use of CK-MB is diminishing because of the superior sensitivities and specificities of the previously described tests.

Lactate Dehydrogenase and Alanine Aminotransferase

Levels of lactate dehydrogenase and alanine aminotransferase are rarely used for MI diagnosis because they are nonspecific and rise later than levels of troponins, myoglobin, and CK-MB.

Highly Sensitive C-Reactive Protein

C-reactive protein is an acute phase protein. Levels are elevated in the setting of inflammation. Because atherosclerosis is an inflammatory process, highly sensitive CRP test (hs-CRP) may indicate atherosclerotic plaque formation. The hs-CRP level is used to determine whether someone is at risk for an MI and to diagnose acute coronary events. However, hs-CRP lacks specificity for vascular events.

The hs-CRP level is usually measured with an immunoassay or nephelometry. This measurement may be used alone or in combination with other markers or tests for cardiac

<table>
<tr><td colspan="3">**TABLE 18-1**   **Cardiovascular Risk Factors**</td></tr>
<tr><th>Risk Factors That Cannot Be Changed</th><th>Risk Factors That Can Be Changed</th><th>Protective Factors</th></tr>
<tr><td>Age
Gender
Heredity</td><td>Lipid metabolism–related factors (e.g., diet, hyperlipidemia, obesity)
Diabetes mellitus
Hypertension
Clotting factors
Cigarette smoking
Behavior</td><td>Exercise
Estrogen</td></tr>
</table>

From Damjanov I. *Pathology for the Health Profession.* 4th ed. St. Louis: Saunders; 2013.

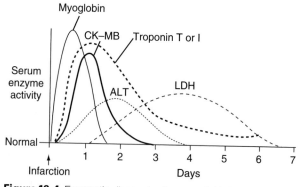

• **Figure 18-4** Enzymatic diagnosis of myocardial infarcts. Troponin T or I are the most important biochemical markers of myocardial infarction. The myoglobin level may rise rapidly after myocardial infarction, but this finding is relatively nonspecific. Creatine kinase (CK-MB) is used less often. Alanine transaminase and lactic dehydrogenase are also used less often and are relatively nonspecific. (From Damjanov I. *Pathology for the Health Profession.* 4th ed. St. Louis: Saunders; 2013.)

TABLE 18-2   **Blood Tests for the Diagnosis of Myocardial Infarction**

Name of Biomarker	Class of Biomarker	First Appears	Disappears	Comments
Troponin I	Protein	3-12 hours	10 days	More specific than troponin T
Troponin T	Protein	3-12 hours	2 weeks	Not as specific as troponin I
Myoglobin	Protein that binds oxygen	2-3 hours	12-24 hours	Found in skeletal and cardiac muscle
Creatine kinase MB	Enzyme	3-4 hours	48-72 hours	Decreasing use due to better sensitivity and specificity of other tests

risk. Low risk for cardiac events is indicated by an hs-CRP value of less than 1.0 mg/L. Average risk is correlated with a value of 1.0 to 3.0 mg/L, and high risk for cardiac events is indicated by values greater than 3.0 mg/L.

Other Diagnostic Tools

Other tools used for the diagnosis of MI include electrocardiography, echocardiography, chest radiography, and angiography. The electrocardiogram (ECG) records the electrical activity (i.e., waves and segments) of the heart. It is considered to be the most important and specific test for the diagnosis of MI. Heart muscle damaged during or after an MI does not conduct electrical impulses in a normal fashion. An ECG abnormality can usually be detected as soon as the MI begins (Fig. 18-5).

An echocardiogram is an ultrasound study in which the reflected sound waves help produce an image of the heart to detect whether it is pumping blood appropriately. The chest radiograph is useful for detecting cardiomegaly (i.e., enlarged heart), which represents compensation for decreased heart function. Radiographs may also detect fluid that is accumulating around the heart, which occurs in heart failure.

Coronary catheterization results, imaged on an angiogram, can show whether the coronary arteries are narrowed or blocked as a result of atherosclerosis or other disease. Contrast dye is injected into the arteries. It helps the physician visualize the coronary arteries to detect a blockage.

Congestive Heart Failure

Background

Congestive heart failure (CHF) is a progressive disease. The ability of the heart to pump blood throughout the body decreases over time. Heart function may decrease because of MI, hypertension, heart valvular disease, or cardiomyopathy.

As the disease progresses, blood flow becomes less efficient, and more stasis occurs in the blood vessels. Stasis increases blood pressure as more fluid moves out of the blood vessels and into the extracellular space. The accumulation of fluid in the lungs and extremities is associated with onset of the signs and symptoms of CHF, such as dyspnea (i.e., shortness of breath) and edema in the extremities (e.g., the hands and feet). CHF can occur at any age but is much more common in the elderly (Fig. 18-6).

Diagnosis

CHF cannot be diagnosed with one test. Instead, physicians use echocardiography, chest radiography, electrocardiography, angiography, and laboratory tests such as B-type natriuretic peptide (BNP), electrolytes, CRP, blood urea nitrogen (BUN), and creatinine.

Echocardiography (i.e., sonogram of the heart) is used in CHF to measure blood volume during systole (i.e., contraction of the ventricles) and during diastole (i.e., refilling of the heart with blood). A decrease in blood volume is expected as the disease progresses. A chest radiograph may show fluid

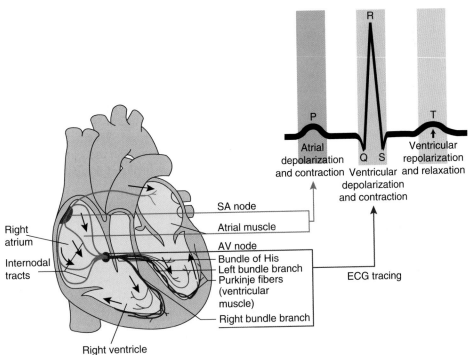

• **Figure 18-5** Conduction system of the heart and its relation to the electrocardiogram (ECG). *AV,* Atrioventricular; *SA,* sinoatrial. (From Gould BE, Dyer R. *Pathophysiology for the Health Professions.* 4th ed. St. Louis: Saunders; 2011.)

around the heart and cardiomegaly (i.e., compensatory increase in heart size due to decreased pumping efficiency).

An ECG measures the electrical conduction systems of the heart. An ECG may help to detect the origin of the events leading to CHF. Events such as MI, arrhythmia, valvular disorders, and ischemic heart disease may interfere with electrical conduction in the heart. Angiography (i.e., an x-ray study of the blood vessels) is used to determine the origins of CHF and can detect blockages in the vasculature (Fig. 18-7).

As CHF progresses, the blood levels of sodium increase and those of potassium decrease. These electrolyte changes result from decreased blood flow through the kidneys. Sodium and potassium levels are usually measured with the use of ion-selective electrodes.

Because kidney failure is common in CHF, BUN and creatinine levels are elevated. Enzymatic reactions are the method of choice to measure both urea and creatinine. These test methods are discussed further in Chapter 24.

B-type natriuretic peptide (BNP) is a substance that is secreted from the ventricles of the heart in response to swelling of the ventricles in CHF. Swelling occurs when heart failure develops and blood pools in the lower chambers of the heart. The level of BNP in the blood increases when heart failure symptoms worsen and decreases when the heart failure condition is stable. The immunoassay for this analyte is sensitive and specific for CHF. The absence of CHF is associated with levels lower than 100 pg/mL, and levels of 100 to more than 900 pg/mL indicate increasing disease severity.

Congenital Heart Defects

Background

A congenital heart defect is a malformation of the heart that is present at birth. The cause of most such defects is unknown, but research has shown that genetic and environmental factors contribute to their development. Congenital heart defects may be minor, life-threatening, or incompatible with life. About 1% of children are born with a congenital heart defect, most commonly atrial septal defect, ventricular septal defect, tetralogy of Fallot, or transposition of the great arteries.

Atrial and Ventricular Septal Defects

Atrial septal defect (ASD) is an abnormal opening in the wall (i.e., septum) that divides the two upper chambers (atria) of the heart. Ventricular septal defect (VSD) is an abnormal opening in the septum that divides the two lower chambers of the heart (i.e., ventricles).

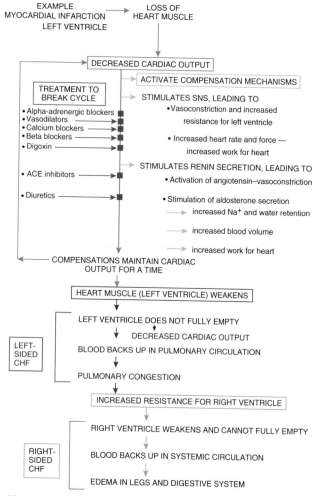

• **Figure 18-6** Course of congestive heart failure. (VanMeter KC, Hubert RJ. *Gould's Pathophysiology for the Health Professions.* 5th ed. St. Louis: Elsevier; 2015.)

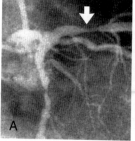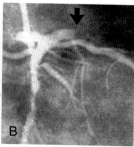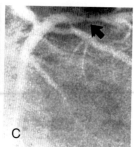

• **Figure 18-7** Angiogram. **A,** Baseline shows narrowing *(white arrow)*. **B,** Transient total occlusion of the left anterior descending branch of the left coronary artery after mental stress *(black arrow)*. **C,** After administration of nitrates and nifedipine, the artery reopened to same diameter as baseline *(black arrow)*. (From Stern S, ed. *Silent Myocardial Ischemia.* St Louis: Mosby; 1998.)

These openings between the chambers of the heart, whether ASD or VSD, allow blood from either side of the heart to cross into the opposite atrium or ventricle. Usually, because the left side of the heart is at a higher pressure than the right side, blood from the left atrium or ventricle flows into the right atrium or ventricle and then back to the lungs. This is called left-to-right shunting. Because the right side of the heart and the blood vessels in the lungs are not built to withstand increased volumes and pressures, left-to-right shunting may result in heart failure, pulmonary arterial hypertension, and heart rhythm problems (Figs. 18-8 and 18-9).

Tetralogy of Fallot

Tetralogy of Fallot (TOF) is a congenital heart defect caused by failure of the right ventricular tract to form properly in the embryo. This results in the four cardiac abnormalities characteristic of TOF:

1. VSD: an abnormal opening between the two lower chambers of the heart
2. Pulmonic stenosis: a narrowed area within the main pulmonary artery that is at, above, or below the pulmonary valve
3. Malpositioned aorta: an aorta that straddles the ventricular septum and overrides the VSD
4. Ventricular hypertrophy: an overly muscular right ventricle

The pH and the partial pressure of carbon dioxide (pCO_2) in TOF patients are usually normal, but the oxygen saturation can vary. Cyanosis results from the shunting. Hypoxemia can result during exercise, bathing, or fever (Fig. 18-10).

Transposition of the Great Arteries

Transposition of the great arteries (TGA) is a congenital heart defect in which the two arteries carrying blood away from the heart are transposed (i.e., reversed). The pulmonary artery, which normally carries deoxygenated blood from the right ventricle to the lungs, is transposed to the left ventricle. The aorta, which normally carries oxygenated blood from the left ventricle to the rest of the body, is transposed to the right ventricle. This congenital heart defect is usually incompatible with life (Fig. 18-11).

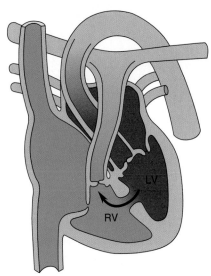

• **Figure 18-9** Blood flow through the ventricular septal defect is usually left to right and produces an acyanotic shunt. *LV,* Left ventricle; *RV,* right ventricle. (From Copstead LC. *Pathophysiology.* 5th ed. St. Louis: Saunders; 2013.)

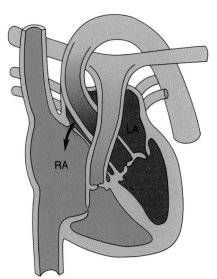

• **Figure 18-8** Blood flow through the atrial septal defect is usually left to right and produces an acyanotic shunt. *LA,* Left atrium; *RA,* right atrium. (From Copstead LC. *Pathophysiology.* 5th ed. St. Louis: Saunders; 2013.)

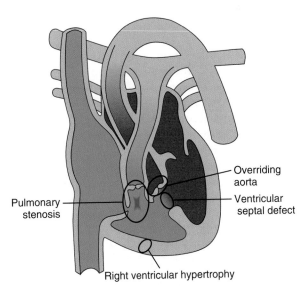

• **Figure 18-10** Tetralogy of Fallot. Dextroposition of the aorta is overriding a ventricular septal defect and is associated with pulmonary stenosis. Because of the congenital stenosis of the pulmonary artery, which prevents the outflow of blood from the right ventricle, there is right-to-left shunting of blood and early cyanosis. (From Copstead LC. *Pathophysiology.* 5th ed. St. Louis: Saunders; 2013.)

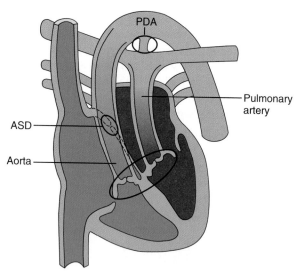

• **Figure 18-11** Transposition of great arteries. Two separate circulations are formed, which is incompatible with life unless mixing of blood occurs through other defects. *ASD*, Atrial septal defect; *PDA*, patent ductus arteriosus. (From Copstead LC. *Pathophysiology.* 5th ed. St. Louis: Saunders; 2013.)

Diagnosis

Several studies are used to diagnose congenital heart defects, including chest radiography, electrocardiography, echocardiography, and blood gas measurements. The chest radiograph provides information about the lungs and about the size and position of the heart. The ECG evaluates the electrical activity of the heart, and the echocardiogram helps to identify heart structures. Blood gas measurements or oximetry indicate a decrease in oxygen saturation to between 65% and 85%.

Endocarditis, Myocarditis, and Pericarditis

Endocarditis

Endocarditis is an infection of the inner layer of the heart (i.e., endocardium). The most common infectious agents involved are *Streptococcus viridians, Staphylococcus aureus,* and *Enterococcus* species. These bacteria originate in a skin wound or from the transient bacteremia in the mouth (due to toothbrushing) and reach the heart through the bloodstream.

Endocarditis rarely affects individuals with a healthy heart. Persons at greatest risk are those with congenital heart defects, heart valve damage, artificial heart valves, or previous cardiac damage. Bacteria and other infectious agents travel to the heart, where they attach to or settle on a damaged area of the heart (Fig. 18-12). Bacteriologic tests such as blood cultures from two separate sites are valuable in diagnosing endocarditis.

Myocarditis

Myocarditis is inflammation of the myocardium, which is the middle layer of the heart wall. This condition results from inflammation caused by chronic infection. Viruses,

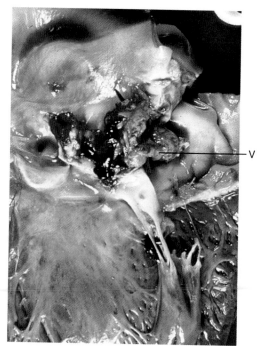

• **Figure 18-12** Bacterial endocarditis. The valves are covered with extensive vegetations (V). (From Damjanov I. *Pathology for the Health Profession.* 4th ed. St. Louis: Saunders; 2013.)

bacteria, parasites, and fungi (Table 18-3) can initiate myocarditis, but it is lymphocytes that do the permanent damage to the heart muscle. Lymphocytes quickly infiltrate the myocardium in response to infection and initiate an inflammatory reaction, which can become chronic and cause much damage.

Myocarditis can be triggered by drugs such as penicillin or the sulfonamides or by recreational drugs such as cocaine. Other diseases in which inflammation may be uncontrolled can also result in myocarditis. Examples include systemic lupus erythematosus, rheumatoid arthritis, and other autoimmune diseases.

If myocarditis becomes severe enough, the heart loses its ability to pump efficiently. Stasis of blood in the heart may occur, and the resulting thromboses can lead to an MI or stroke (Fig. 18-13).

Pericarditis

Pericarditis is swelling and inflammation of the pericardium, a two-layer membrane surrounding the heart. It can be acute (most common) or chronic. Pericarditis may have no known cause (i.e., idiopathic pericarditis), or it may result from many types of pathology. Underlying conditions that can contribute to pericarditis include MI, trauma, viral infection (particularly human immunodeficiency virus [HIV]), fungal infection, metastatic cancer, kidney failure, and sequela of rheumatoid arthritis, systemic lupus erythematosus, and scleroderma. Pericarditis can also occur as a side effect of medications such as procainamide, an antiarrhythmic drug.

TABLE 18-3	**Causes of Infectious Myocarditis**		
Viruses	**Bacteria**	**Fungi**	**Parasites**
Coxsackievirus	*Chlamydia*	*Aspergillus*	*Trypanosoma*
Cytomegalovirus	*Mycoplasma*	*Candida*	*Toxoplasma*
Hepatitis C virus	*Streptococcus*	*Coccidioides*	
Herpesvirus	*Treponema*	*Cryptococcus*	
Human immunodeficiency virus		*Histoplasma*	
Parvovirus			

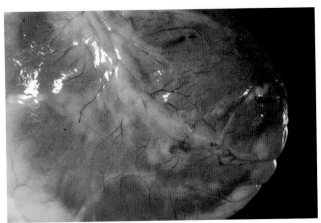

• **Figure 18-13** Myocarditis. (From Klatt EC. *Robbins and Cotran Atlas of Pathology.* 3rd ed. Philadelphia: Saunders; 2015.)

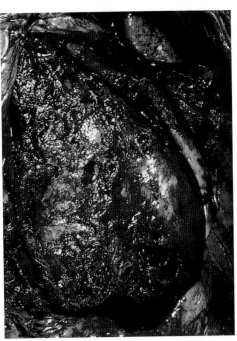

• **Figure 18-14** Pericarditis. The surface of the heart is covered with fibrin and blood, and it appears shaggy. (From Damjanov I. *Pathology for the Health Profession.* 4th ed. St. Louis: Saunders; 2013.)

Potential complications include **cardiac tamponade** (i.e., compression of the heart due to fluid accumulation in the pericardium), **chronic pericarditis,** and **pericardial effusion** (i.e., fluid in the pericardium). Chronic pericarditis can lead to **constrictive pericarditis,** which occurs when the pericardium loses its elasticity because of the accumulation of scar tissue that keeps the heart from working properly. Pericardial effusion and constrictive pericarditis can occur together (Fig. 18-14).

Diagnosis

Blood cultures, complete blood counts, and measurements of troponin, myoglobin, and antibody levels in response to various infectious agents can aid the diagnosis of endocarditis, myocarditis, and pericarditis. Imaging techniques such as echocardiography, electrocardiography, radiography, magnetic resonance imaging (MRI), and angiography can also be helpful. Cardiac biopsy can provide definitive information, but because of its invasive nature, it is not used as often as the other studies.

Blood cultures are used to detect infectious agents in the bloodstream that can be associated with endocarditis, myocarditis, or pericarditis. Blood cultures often are collected from two different sites to detect organisms in the blood. The white blood cell count (part of a complete blood count) can detect inflammation and infection associated with endocarditis, myocarditis, or pericarditis. Troponin and myoglobin levels can identify heart muscle damage, as described earlier.

Antibody titers in response to viruses or bacteria are used to identify a recent or past infection. Increased IgM antibody titers indicate an immune response to a recent or current infection, and IgG levels indicate past exposure to an infectious agent.

Imaging techniques such as echocardiography detect damage and structural abnormalities of the heart. An echocardiogram can also detect fluid surrounding the heart. The electrocardiogram measures the electrical conduction of the heart, which can be impaired by various pathologies and by damage to the heart. Chest radiographs can detect heart enlargement and fluid that may be associated with infection of the heart and lungs. Cardiac MRI can show the size, shape, and gross structure of the heart. MRI can also reveal signs of inflammation of the heart muscle and confirm a diagnosis of myocarditis.

Cardiac catheterization (i.e., angiography) is used to monitor blockages in the heart vasculature and to detect constrictive pericarditis. It can also be used to obtain a tissue sample for endocardial biopsy, which is used to confirm or rule out infection or inflammation.

Summary

This chapter reviewed the normal anatomy, physiology, and blood flow of the heart. Disease processes such as MI, congestive heart failure, congenital heart disease, endocarditis, myocarditis, and pericarditis can damage the heart. Laboratory and imaging studies are used to diagnose these pathologies, monitor therapy, and evaluate prognosis.

Review Questions

1. The bicuspid valve is located
   a. Between the right and left ventricle
   b. Between the right and left atrium
   c. Between the left atrium and left ventricle
   d. Between the right atrium and right ventricle
2. From the right ventricle, where does the deoxygenated blood flow next?
   a. Left atrium
   b. Pulmonary artery
   c. Pulmonary vein
   d. Lungs
3. Which of the following tests is not normally used to diagnose myocardial infarction?
   a. B-type natriuretic peptide
   b. Myoglobin
   c. Troponin I
   d. Creatine kinase MB
4. Which of the following is considered an underlying cause of congestive heart disease?
   a. Tetralogy of Fallot
   b. Myocardial infarction
   c. Transposition of the great arteries
   d. Pericarditis
5. Viral antibody levels are most useful for diagnosing which of the following diseases?
   a. Congenital heart failure
   b. Pericarditis
   c. Myocarditis
   d. Tetralogy of Fallot
6. Which two tests detect swelling of the ventricles that occurs in congestive heart failure?
   a. BNP and electrocardiogram
   b. BNP and echocardiogram

   c. Troponin T and electrocardiogram
   d. Troponin I and echocardiogram
7. Which laboratory test result for myocardial infarction (MI) can be described as rising early, being specific for heart damage, and remaining detectable for up to 10 days after an MI?
   a. Creatine kinase MB
   b. Troponin T
   c. Myoglobin
   d. Troponin I
8. The best study for diagnosis of atrial septal defect is
   a. Electrocardiogram
   b. Echocardiogram
   c. Chest radiograph
   d. Troponins
9. In which of the following diseases does the outermost layer of the heart becomes inflamed and fill with fluid?
   a. Endocarditis
   b. Pericarditis
   c. Myocarditis
   d. Myocardial infarction
10. In which of the following diseases does the pulmonary artery branch from the left ventricle?
    a. Pericarditis
    b. Transposition of the great arteries
    c. Atrial septal defect
    d. Constrictive pericarditis

Critical Thinking Questions

1. Discuss the environmental and genetic risk factors associated with atherosclerosis and coronary disease. Which risk factors can be controlled or modified? Is there a test to determine whether someone is at risk for heart disease? Would this test change an individual's risk factors?

2. Discuss the process for diagnosing myocarditis or pericarditis. Do antibody levels play a role in the diagnosis? Explain why or why not. If yes, which antibody levels?

CASE STUDY

Mrs. M., a 68-year-old woman with a history of rheumatic heart disease diagnosed when she was in her 20s, complains to her physician about increasing shortness of breath on exertion. She also states that the ankle swelling she has experienced for years has become much worse during the past 2 months, making it especially difficult to get her shoes on at the end of the day. In the past week, she has had a decreased appetite, some nausea and vomiting, and tenderness in the right upper quadrant of the abdomen. On physical examination, her jugular veins are noticeably distended. Heart sounds reveals a systolic murmur.

What is the most likely diagnosis? Discuss why rheumatic heart disease is an important part of this patient's history. Which laboratory test should the physician order to detect ventricular damage? What additional tests may help to detect swelling in and around Mrs. M.'s heart?

Bibliography

Amit G, Shiau J, Guyatt G. The ineffectiveness of immunosuppressive therapy in lymphocytic myocarditis: an overview. *Ann Intern Med.* 1998;129:317–322.

Dragoescu EA, Liu L. Pericardial fluid cytology: an analysis of 128 specimens over a 6–year period. *Cancer Cytopathol.* 2013;121:242–251.

Hoffman JI, Kaplan S. The incidence of congenital heart disease. *J Am Coll Cardiol.* 2002;39:1890–1900.

Januzzi JL, Mann DL. Pathophysiology of heart failure. In: Mann DL, Zipes DP, Libby P, Bonow RO, eds. *Braunwald's Heart Disease: A Textbook of Cardiovascular Medicine.* 10th ed. Philadelphia: Saunders Elsevier; 2015.

Kiefer TL, Bashore TM. Infective endocarditis: a comprehensive overview. *Rev Cardiovasc Med.* 2011;13:e105–e120.

Kumar A, Cannon CP. Acute coronary syndromes: diagnosis and management, part I. *Mayo Clin Proc.* 2009;84:917–938.

Kumar A, Cannon CP. Acute coronary syndromes: diagnosis and management, part II. *Mayo Clin Proc.* 2009;84:1021–1036.

Le Winter MM, Hopkins WE. Pericardial diseases. In: Mann DL, Zipes DP, Libby P, Bonow RO, eds. *Braunwald's Heart Disease: A Textbook of Cardiovascular Medicine.* Philadelphia: Saunders Elsevier; 2015.

Liu P, Baughman KL. Myocarditis. In: Bonow RO, Mann DL, Zipes DP, Libby P, eds. *Braunwald's Heart Disease: A Textbook of Cardiovascular Medicine.* 9th ed. Philadelphia: Saunders Elsevier; 2012.

McKenna W. Diseases of the myocardium and endocardium. In: Goldman L, Schafer AI, eds. *Goldman's Cecil Medicine.* 24th ed. Philadelphia: Saunders Elsevier; 2011.

Ridker PM. C-reactive protein, inflammation, and cardiovascular disease: clinical update. *Texas Heart Inst J.* 2005;32:384–386.

Saenger AK, Jaffe AS. The use of biomarkers for the evaluation and treatment of patients with acute coronary syndromes. *Med Clin North Am.* 2007;91:657–681.

Scrica BA, Morrow DA. ST-elevation myocardial infarction: pathology, physiology, and clinical features. In: Mann DL, Zipes DP, Libby P, Bonow RO, eds. *Braunwald's Heart Disease: A Textbook of Cardiovascular Medicine.* 10th ed Philadelphia: Saunders Elsevier; 2015.

Swedberg K, Cleland J, Dargie H, et al. Guidelines for the diagnosis and treatment of chronic heart failure: executive summary (update 2005). The Task Force for the Diagnosis and Treatment of Chronic Heart Failure of the European Society of Cardiology. *Eur Heart J.* 2005;26:1115–1140.

White HD, Chew DP. Acute myocardial infarction. *Lancet.* 2008;372:570–584.

Walter Wilson, Taubert KA, Gewitz M, et al. Prevention of infective endocarditis: guidelines from the American Heart Association: a guideline from the American Heart Association Rheumatic Fever, Endocarditis, and Kawasaki Disease Committee, Council on Cardiovascular Disease in the Young, and the Council on Clinical Cardiology, Council on Cardiovascular Surgery and Anesthesia, and the Quality of Care and Outcomes Research Interdisciplinary Working Group. *Circulation.* 2007;116:1736–1754.

19

Respiratory Diseases

DONNA LARSON

CHAPTER OUTLINE

OBJECTIVES

After completion of this chapter, the reader will be able to:

1. Identify the main structures in the respiratory tract.
2. Illustrate gas exchange in the lungs.
3. Compare and contrast breathing and respiration.
4. State the reference ranges for pH and for the partial pressures of carbon dioxide (pCO_2) and oxygen (pO_2).
5. Describe the pathophysiology and laboratory tests used to diagnose the following conditions:
   a. Respiratory distress syndrome
   b. Acute respiratory distress syndrome
   c. Chronic obstructive pulmonary disease
   d. Cystic fibrosis
   e. Pneumonia
   f. Pulmonary edema
   g. Pulmonary hypertension
   h. Atelectasis
   i. Pulmonary embolism
   j. Idiopathic pulmonary fibrosis
   k. Sarcoidosis
   l. Pleural effusion
6. State pO_2 levels for mild hypoxemia, moderate hypoxemia, severe hypoxemia, loss of consciousness, and anoxia.

KEY TERMS

α_1-Antitrypsin
Asthma
Atelectasis
Chronic bronchitis
Chronic obstructive pulmonary disease
Compression atelectasis
Congestive heart failure

Contraction atelectasis
Elastase
Emphysema
Idiopathic pulmonary fibrosis
Pneumonia
Pulmonary edema
Pulmonary embolism

Pulmonary hypertension
Resorption atelectasis
Right middle lobe syndrome
Sarcoidosis
Spirometry
Status asthmaticus
Thromboemboli

❖ Case in Point

A 70-year-old man goes to see his provider complaining of severe shortness of breath. The man is thin and looks very fatigued. He smoked cigarettes for 40 years but recently quit his habit because he was having trouble breathing. The provider orders a complete blood count (CBC), electrolytes, and an α_1-antitrypsin (ATT) level. The CBC results are normal. The electrolyte results are as follows: Na, 145 mEq/L; K, 4.0 mEq/L; Cl, 107 mEq/L; HCO_3^-, 45 mEq/L. His ATT level is 8 mmol/L. What condition is causing this man's shortness of breath? Interpret his laboratory findings to support the diagnosis.

Points to Remember

- Gas exchange takes place in the alveoli.
- Collagen and elastic fibers are part of alveoli.
- Symptoms of respiratory distress syndrome include hypoxia, tachypnea (rapid breathing), subcostal and intercostal retractions (when the muscles below and between the ribs are sucked in between the ribs during breathing), and diminished breath sounds.
- Arterial blood gas (ABG) analysis in respiratory distress syndrome (in infants) reveals a low partial pressure of oxygen (pO_2), decreased pH, decreased bicarbonate, and increased partial pressure of carbon dioxide (pCO_2).
- Amniotic fluid collected by amniocentesis is the specimen used for determination of fetal lung maturity.
- The major component of the lung surfactant is phosphatidylcholine (lecithin).
- Fetal lungs are considered immature if the result of the fluorescence polarization test result is less than 39 mg/g, intermediate at 40 to 54 mg/g, and mature at greater than 55 mg/g.
- Acute respiratory distress syndrome (ARDS) injures the alveoli, producing massive pulmonary effusions due to acute phase reactants, severe pulmonary edema, and hypoxemia.
- ABG results in ARDS initially show severely decreased pO_2, increased pH, and decreased pCO_2, but when ventilation decreases, the pH becomes decreased and the pCO_2 severely elevated.
- Individuals with cystic fibrosis (CF) produce more mucus than normal and are unable to adequately clear mucus from the lungs. In addition, the mucus they produce is abnormally thick.
- Individuals with CF have chronic bronchial infections with *Pseudomonas aeruginosa*, which readily forms biofilms.
- The standard test for diagnosing CF is the sweat test. A sweat chloride concentration greater than 60 mEq/L is diagnostic of CF.
- Viral pneumonia is a seasonal, mild, and self-limited disease.
- Chronic obstructive pulmonary disease (COPD) includes chronic bronchitis, emphysema, and asthma.

- Chronic bronchitis is present when a person has had a chronic productive cough for 3 months during each of 2 consecutive years.
- Chronic bronchitis is considered obstructive because large amounts of mucus, bronchial inflammation, and infiltration by neutrophils obstruct air flow entering and leaving the lungs.
- Chronic bronchitis leads to hypercapnia and respiratory acidosis ("blue bloaters").
- Emphysema is characterized by destruction of the alveoli and severe dyspnea ("pink puffers").
- α_1-Antitrypsin levels lower than 11 mmol/L lead to destruction of lung tissue and emphysema.
- In asthma, the bronchial tree constricts, obstructing air flow in and out of the lungs.
- Status asthmaticus is a potentially fatal disease that involves a severe asthmatic bronchospasm.
- Pneumonia is an infection in the lungs that causes the lungs to fill with a fluid or pus.
- Pulmonary edema is abnormal fluid collection in the lungs resulting from congestive heart failure.
- Pulmonary hypertension is a progressive disease in which increased pressure in the pulmonary artery leads to right-sided heart failure.
- Atelectasis is a collapsed lung.
- A pulmonary embolus is a thrombus in the pulmonary artery; it can be life-threatening.
- Idiopathic pulmonary fibrosis is a condition in which the lungs become stiff and inelastic.
- Sarcoidosis is a systemic disease characterized by granulomas in the lungs.
- Common symptoms of a pleural effusion include dyspnea, compression atelectasis, and pleural pain.
- An effusion can be a transudate (watery) resulting from conditions that either increase intravascular hydrostatic pressure (e.g., congestive heart failure) or decrease capillary oncotic pressure (e.g., liver or kidney diseases that cause decreased blood protein), or it can be an exudate containing increased white blood cells and plasma proteins.

Introduction

Respiratory diseases affect the lungs, bronchi, and trachea as well as the entire body. The lungs are responsible for exchanging oxygen and metabolic waste products (mainly carbon dioxide) with the environment. This process allows oxygen to be carried throughout the body and carbon dioxide to be released into the environment. Respiratory system diseases affect the oxygen and carbon dioxide exchange process, leading to disruption of functions throughout the body—most notably, the body's acid-base balance. This chapter examines the anatomy of the respiratory system, respiration, the relationships among dissolved gases, and several common respiratory diseases. The detailed discussion of each disease includes the disease mechanism, clinical correlation to chemistry laboratory results, and important laboratory procedures and limitations.

Structure and Function of the Respiratory System

Anatomic Structures

The respiratory system is found in the upper thorax. The upper respiratory system organs are the nose, pharynx, and larynx; the lower respiratory system organs are the trachea, bronchial tubes, and lungs. Air enters the body through the nose, where it is warmed in the spaces and moisturized by the mucous membranes before it travels down the larynx, into the bronchial tubes, and then into the lungs. The gas exchange (oxygen for carbon dioxide) takes place in the smallest component of the lungs, the *alveoli* (Fig. 19-1). Alveoli are composed of epithelial cells surrounded by capillaries. Collagen and elastic fibers are also an integral part of the alveoli; these structures allow for expansion and contraction during inspiration and expiration.

Respiratory Function Review

Inspiration and expiration are governed by intercostal muscles and the diaphragm. The external intercostal muscles contract during inhalation, and the diaphragm moves down to allow the lungs to expand and take in air. A surfactant coats the outer surface of the lungs and allows the pleural membrane to slide over the top of the lungs during inhalation and exhalation.

Respiration

The lungs hold about 6 L of air, but only a fraction of this amount is used during normal breathing. Normal breathing is referred to as *tidal breathing. Tidal volume* is the amount of air that comes into and goes out of the lungs in a single breath. The average respiratory rate is 12 to 20 breaths/min.

Two measurements that help providers differentiate between obstructive and restrictive respiratory disease are the forced vital capacity and forced expiratory volume. The *forced vital capacity (FVC)* measures the amount of air forcefully expelled from maximum inspiration to maximum expiration, whereas the *forced expiratory volume in 1 second (FEV$_1$)* measures the amount of air forcefully expelled from maximum inspiration during the first second of effort. In obstructive lung disease, air flow out of the lungs is slowed while lung volume remains normal; therefore, the ratio FEV$_1$/FVC is reduced. In restrictive lung disease, both air flow and lung volume are decreased, so the FEV$_1$/FVC ratio can be approximately normal or even increased.

Spirometry is used to measure the mechanical function of the lungs through the volumes and capacities (Fig. 19-2). This test measures the function of lung capacity and lung and chest wall physical function to determine whether there is an abnormality.

Blood gas analysis is used to measure the pH of the blood and the amount of oxygen and carbon dioxide present in arterial blood. *Arterial blood gas measurements* (ABGs) indicate how well the lungs exchange oxygen and carbon dioxide with the environment (Table 19-1). (See Chapter 13 for a comprehensive discussion of blood gases.)

Hypoventilation is inadequate alveolar ventilation in relation to demands of the body. The pCO$_2$ levels increase, causing *hypercapnia* (pCO$_2$ > 44 mm Hg). The production of carbon dioxide exceeds the removal of carbon dioxide from the body. This results in respiratory acidosis (see Chapter 13). Alveolar hypoventilation with hypercapnia results in secondary decreased pO$_2$ because the accumulation of carbon dioxide in the alveoli does not allow oxygen to enter the lung.

Hyperventilation is alveolar ventilation that exceeds the demands of the body. The lungs remove carbon dioxide faster than it is produced. This results in decreased pCO$_2$ or *hypocapnia* (pCO$_2$ < 36 mm Hg). Hypocapnia results in respiratory alkalosis (see Chapter 13).

Respiratory Diseases and Pathophysiology

Respiratory diseases include pathologic conditions that affect the organs responsible for gas exchange and oxygenation of the blood. Respiratory diseases can be mild and self-limited (e.g., colds, allergies) or severe and life-threatening (e.g., pulmonary embolism, pneumonia). Respiratory illness causes many deaths all over the world each year. Before antibiotics were in widespread use, pneumonia was one of the most common causes of death in the United States.

Respiratory Distress Syndrome

Respiratory distress syndrome (hyaline membrane disease) is a respiratory disorder in premature infants whose lungs produce insufficient surfactant to keep the alveoli open and functioning. Insufficient surfactant production leads to severe respiratory distress soon after birth. Typically, the fetal lungs are able to produce adequate amounts of surfactant after they reach 32 weeks of gestation. The more premature the neonate, the greater the chance that the infant will experience respiratory distress syndrome after birth.

Symptoms of respiratory distress syndrome include hypoxia, tachypnea (rapid breathing), subcostal and intercostal retractions (i.e., the muscles below and between the ribs are sucked in between the ribs during breathing), and diminished breath sounds.

ABGs reveal a low pO$_2$, decreased pH, decreased bicarbonate, and increased pCO$_2$. Blood cultures are performed to ensure that the infant is not septic. Electrolytes, glucose, and renal and liver function tests are monitored in infants with the disease to ensure that organ failure does not occur.

Fetal lung maturity tests help providers determine whether the fetal lungs are mature. This is important when providers are considering early delivery of the infant due to a medical condition of the mother or fetus. If the fetus's lungs are not mature, providers can administer drugs to stop preterm labor or cancel early delivery of the infant. Sometimes, providers administer corticosteroids to pregnant women to speed up lung maturity in the fetus.

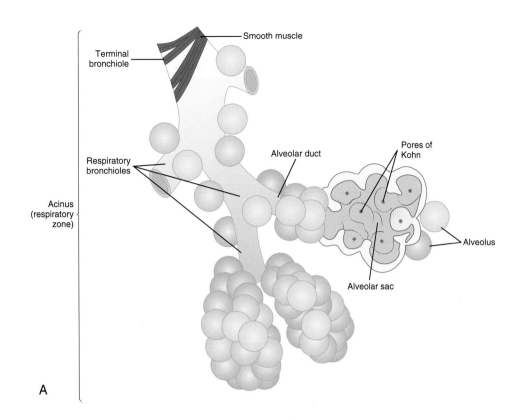

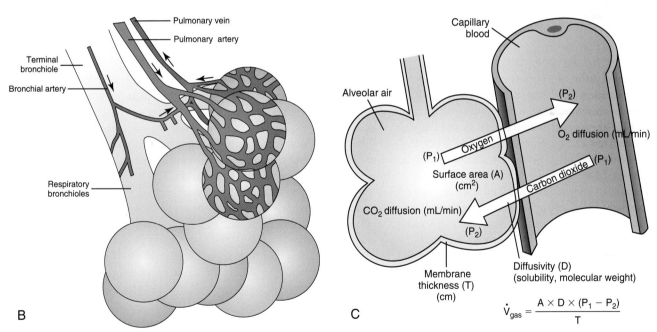

• **Figure 19-1** Structure of the alveoli. **A,** Gas-exchange portion of the lung. Subdivisions of the terminal bronchioles form the acinus. **B,** Pulmonary arteries carry deoxygenated blood *(blue)* to the capillary beds surrounding the alveoli. Oxygenated blood *(red)* flows out of these capillaries to the left atrium and ventricle, where it is pumped into the systemic circulation. **C,** Fick's law of diffusion states that oxygen and carbon dioxide diffuse from high (P_1) to low (P_2) pressures across the alveolar capillary membrane. The flow rate ($\dot{V}_{gas}$) depends on the diffusion constant (D) of the substance as well as the surface area and pressure difference. (From Beachey W. *Respiratory Care Anatomy and Physiology: Foundations for Clinical Practice.* 3rd ed. St. Louis: Mosby; 2013.)

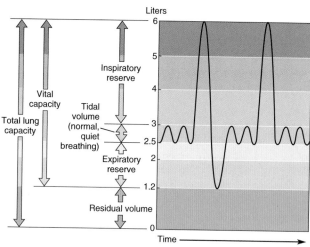

• **Figure 19-2** Pulmonary volumes and capacities. (From Herlihy B. *The Human Body in Health Illness.* 5th ed. St. Louis: Saunders; 2014.)

TABLE 19-1	Arterial Blood Gas Reference Ranges	
Parameter	**Reference Range**
pH	7.35-7.45
pCO_2	35-45 mm Hg
pO_2	75-100 mm Hg

The tests that are commonly used to measure fetal lung maturity or the surfactant concentration are lecithin/sphingomyelin (L/S) ratio, phosphatidylglycerol (PG) concentration, and fluorescence polarization (FP). Rapid tests should be offered on an emergency and routine basis, because the patient's status can change rapidly and the results from this test can help manage labor and delivery.

Amniotic fluid collected by amniocentesis is the specimen used for fetal lung maturity determinations. The fluid is tested as soon as it arrives in the laboratory, or it may be stored at 4° C if testing is delayed for a few hours. The fluid is stable up to 7 days at 4° C; for research purposes, it should be kept at –20° C to –70° C for long-term storage. The condition of the specimen should be noted, and the specimen should be kept on wet ice before and during analysis.

The major component of the lung surfactant is phosphatidylcholine (lecithin). Even though sphingomyelin is not a component of the lung surfactant, it can act as an internal standard for this analysis. The concentration of lecithin increases with gestational age, and as a result, the L/S ratio also increases. This ratio increases dramatically between 34 and 36 weeks of gestation as the fetal lungs mature and much surfactant is produced. Most laboratories use commercially available kits to perform this test. An L/S ratio of 2.5 or greater indicates that the fetal lungs are mature and sufficient surfactant is being produced.

The role of PG in the production of surfactant by the fetal lungs is not well understood. It is measured by a qualitative agglutination test (e.g., agglutination occurs when PG is present). The agglutination level is compared with three control standards—negative, low positive (0.5 to 2 μg/mL), and high positive (2 μg/mL). Mothers with high positive results rarely deliver infants who develop respiratory distress syndrome.

The final method for determining fetal lung maturity is the FP technique. A fluorescent dye is added to the test sample and attaches to both the surfactant and albumin that is present in the sample. In this test method, the albumin acts as an internal standard: When the fluorescent dye attaches to the albumin, there is increased polarization, and when the dye attaches to the surfactant, there is decreased polarization. The overall FP measured in the sample reflects the ratio of surfactant to albumin. Measurements for standards are made, a standard curve is constructed, and sample results are calculated from this curve. Fetal lungs are considered immature if the FP value is lower than 39 mg/g, intermediate if between 40 and 54 mg/g, and mature if greater than 55 mg/g.

Acute Respiratory Distress Syndrome

Acute respiratory distress syndrome (ARDS) injures the alveoli, producing massive pulmonary effusions due to acute phase reactants, severe pulmonary edema, and hypoxemia. This may be caused by direct injury, from aspiration of acidic gastric contents or inhalation of toxic gas, or from indirect injury resulting from acute phase reactants. There are two stages of ARDS—inflammatory and fibroproliferative.

The inflammatory phase occurs within 72 hours of the initial lung injury. The inflammatory process is activated by the lung injury. Neutrophils activated in the inflammatory response release many damaging substances, including proteolytic enzymes, oxygen free radicals, arachidonic acid metabolites, and platelet-activating factor. These chemicals extensively damage the alveolocapillary membranes and greatly increase capillary membrane permeability, which allows fluids, proteins, and cells to leak into the alveoli. Neutrophils release mediators that cause vasoconstriction. The fluid and acute phase proteins inactivate the surfactant, leading to alveolar failure. The fluid also activates the coagulation cascade, leading to fibrin clots within the air spaces. These clots significantly decrease the blood circulation supplying the alveoli. All of these processes lead to hypoxemia, decreased lung compliance, and decreased ventilation and perfusion.

In the fibroproliferative phase, collagen is deposited in the lungs and the alveoli walls thicken. Fibrosis can appear as early as 10 days after the injury and leads to thickening of the arterial walls. Survivors may experience chronic pulmonary hypertension. ARDS can be exacerbated by sepsis, multiorgan failure, or nosocomial pneumonia.

Blood gas results are used to diagnosis and monitor this disorder (Fig. 19-3). Blood gas results initially show severely decreased pO_2, increased pH, and decreased pCO_2, but later change to decreased pH with severely elevated pCO_2 when ventilation decreases. Many individuals with ARDS require mechanical ventilation.

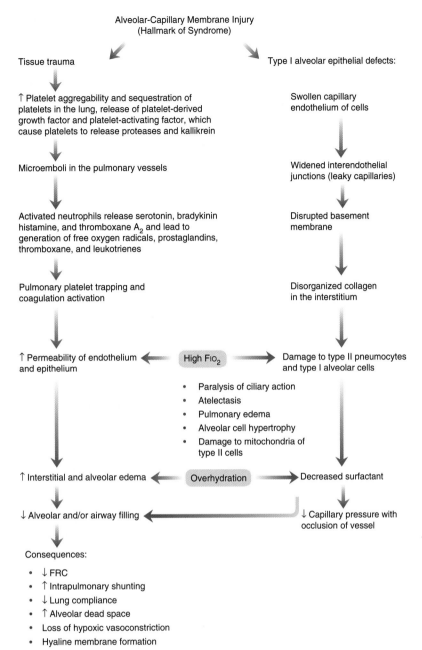

Alveolar-Capillary Membrane Injury
(Hallmark of Syndrome)

Tissue trauma

↑ Platelet aggregability and sequestration of platelets in the lung, release of platelet-derived growth factor and platelet-activating factor, which cause platelets to release proteases and kallikrein

Microemboli in the pulmonary vessels

Activated neutrophils release serotonin, bradykinin histamine, and thromboxane A₂ and lead to generation of free oxygen radicals, prostaglandins, thromboxane, and leukotrienes

Pulmonary platelet trapping and coagulation activation

↑ Permeability of endothelium and epithelium ← High FIO_2 → Damage to type II pneumocytes and type I alveolar cells

- Paralysis of ciliary action
- Atelectasis
- Pulmonary edema
- Alveolar cell hypertrophy
- Damage to mitochondria of type II cells

Type I alveolar epithelial defects:

Swollen capillary endothelium of cells

Widened interendothelial junctions (leaky capillaries)

Disrupted basement membrane

Disorganized collagen in the interstitium

↑ Interstitial and alveolar edema ← Overhydration → Decreased surfactant

↓ Alveolar and/or airway filling ← ↓ Capillary pressure with occlusion of vessel

Consequences:
- ↓ FRC
- ↑ Intrapulmonary shunting
- ↓ Lung compliance
- ↑ Alveolar dead space
- Loss of hypoxic vasoconstriction
- Hyaline membrane formation

• **Figure 19-3** Pathogenesis of acute respiratory distress syndrome. *FiO₂*, Fraction of inspired oxygen; *FRC*, functional residual capacity. (From Copstead-Kirkhorn LC, Banasik JL. *Pathophysiology.* 5th ed. St. Louis: Saunders; 2014.)

Chronic Obstructive Pulmonary Disease

Chronic obstructive pulmonary disease (COPD) is a group of diseases including chronic bronchitis, emphysema, and asthma. All three of these diseases obstruct the flow of air into and out of the lungs and therefore are considered types of COPD.

If a person has a chronic productive cough lasting for as long as 3 months during each of 2 consecutive years, he or she has chronic bronchitis. Chronic bronchitis is characterized by enlargement of mucous cells as well as inflammation and neutrophil infiltrations (Fig. 19-4). Chronic bronchitis is considered to be an obstructive disease because the large amounts of mucus in the bronchi, inflammation of the bronchi and alveoli, and neutrophil infiltration in the airways all lead to obstruction of air flow in and out of the lungs. In chronic bronchitis, the alveoli are normal, so the body compensates for the disease by decreasing ventilation and increasing cardiac output, leading to hypoxemia and polycythemia. If this continues long enough, hypercapnia and respiratory acidosis result. These patients also show signs of right-sided heart failure and are known as "blue bloaters."

In emphysema, the alveoli are destroyed to the point that the air spaces in the lung enlarge (Fig. 19-5). The destruction of the alveoli also leads to loss of elasticity and poor gas exchange. The low blood oxygen results in lowered

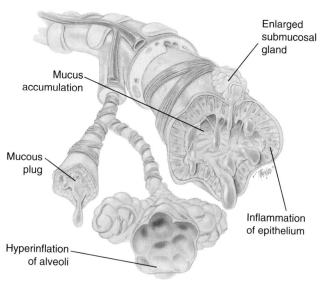

• **Figure 19-4** In chronic bronchitis, there is inflammation and thickening of mucous membrane with accumulation of mucus and pus leading to obstruction characterized by productive cough. (Modified from Des Jardins T, Burton GG. *Clinical Manifestations and Assessment of Respiratory Disease.* 3rd ed. St. Louis: Mosby; 1995.)

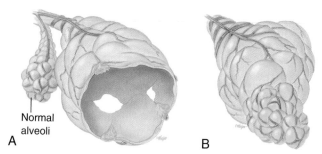

• **Figure 19-5** In emphysema, enlargement and destruction of alveolar walls leads to loss of elasticity and trapping of air. **A,** Panlobular emphysema exhibits abnormal weakening and enlargement of all air spaces distal to the terminal bronchioles; normal alveoli are shown for comparison. **B,** Centrilobular emphysema exhibits abnormal weakening and enlargement of the respiratory bronchioles in the proximal portion of the acinus. (Modified from Des Jardins T, Burton GG. *Clinical Manifestations and Assessment of Respiratory Disease.* 3rd ed. St. Louis: Mosby; 1995.)

cardiac output and hyperventilation, leading to tissue hypoxia throughout the body. These patients suffer from wasting and weight loss and are called "pink puffers." Most cases of emphysema occur in smokers, but individuals with an α_1-antitrypsin (ATT) deficiency are also affected. ATT deficiency is an autosomal codominant condition that leads to development of emphysema. ATT inhibits neutrophils' release of elastase—the enzyme that breaks down the elastic fibers in lung tissue. Levels of ATT below the protective threshold (11 mmol/L) lead to destruction of lung tissue.

In asthma, the bronchial tree constricts especially during exhalation, causing obstruction of air flow. Chronic inflammation is responsible for constriction of the bronchial tree (Fig. 19-6). The inflammation can be caused by allergies, exposure to inhaled irritants such as cigarette

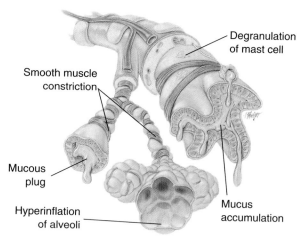

• **Figure 19-6** In bronchial asthma, thick mucus, mucosal edema, and smooth muscle spasm cause obstruction of small airways; breathing becomes labored and expiration is difficult. (Modified from Des Jardins T, Burton GG. *Clinical Manifestations and Assessment of Respiratory Disease.* 3rd ed. St. Louis: Mosby; 1995.)

smoke or polluted air, exercise, viral infections, stress, or drug reactions. Repeated exposure to these irritants can cause airways to become hyperreactive so that bronchospasms occur any time there is exposure to any irritant. The bronchi in chronic asthma are different from normal bronchi. The bronchial lumen is narrow and contains a lot of mucus and fluid from edema, inflammatory cells, and hypertrophied smooth muscle. Status asthmaticus is a potentially fatal condition that involves a severe asthmatic bronchospasm. The individual's bronchi become plugged with thick mucus, which blocks air from entering or leaving the lungs. Gas exchange is minimal, leading to hypoxia and an acidotic state in which the individual becomes cyanotic. This is a medical emergency that requires immediate treatment.

Laboratory Analytes and Assays

Tests used in diagnosing and monitoring of individuals with COPD include ABGs, hematocrit, ATT, electrolytes, sputum evaluation, chest radiography, high-resolution computed tomography (HRCT), and pulmonary function tests (PFTs). Initially, individuals with COPD demonstrate mild to moderate hypoxemia without hypercapnia. As the disease progresses and more lung tissue damage occurs, pCO_2 values increase, but the pH remains normal owing to renal compensation. ABGs are performed on blood gas analyzers that use electrode technology to determine values for pO_2, pCO_2, pH, HCO_3^-, and other parameters (Table 19-2).

Serum chemistry levels may be abnormal, with elevated sodium, possibly decreased potassium, low calcium, and low magnesium. The calcium and magnesium levels may be low due to side effects from drugs used to control the disease.

Sputum evaluations can provide much information for the physician. In stable chronic bronchitis, the sputum is mucoid with macrophages as the dominant cell. In a crisis, the amount of sputum is dramatically increased, neutrophils

TABLE 19-2	Clinical Interpretation of Oxygen Tension (pO$_2$) Levels	
Condition	**Laboratory Values (mm Hg)**	
Mild hypoxemia	60-79	
Moderate hypoxemia	40-59	
Severe hypoxemia	<40	
Loss of consciousness	<30	
Anoxia (brain injury likely)	<20	

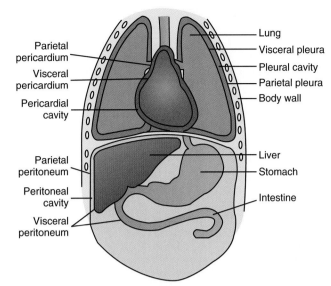

• **Figure 19-7** Relationships of serous membranes, body cavities, and viscera. The heart is enclosed within the pericardial sac. The outer layer of pericardium is called the parietal pericardium. Lining the exterior surface of the heart is the visceral pericardium, which also is called the epicardium. Parietal peritoneum lines the wall of the abdominal cavity. Visceral peritoneum invests stomach, liver, and intestines. The peritoneal cavity is the space between the two layers of peritoneum. (Modified from Kaplan LA, Pesce AJ. *Clinical Chemistry: Theory, Analysis, Correlation.* 5th ed. St. Louis: Mosby; 2010.)

are present, and a mix of bacteria are present, including *Streptococcus pneumonia, Haemophilus influenzae, Moraxella catarrhalis,* and *Pseudomonas aeruginosa.*

Chest radiographs show signs of overinflation in emphysema and increased bronchovascular markings and cardiomegaly in chronic bronchitis. An HRCT scan is more sensitive than a chest radiograph and is often used because it is highly specific for emphysema.

PFTs are used to confirm a suspected diagnosis of COPD. PFTs are also used for assessing the severity of the disease and for following the disease course.

Hematocrit measurements are performed to determine whether the individual is polycythemic. Recall that individuals with chronic bronchitis produce more red blood cells to increase the oxygen in the blood because the airways are obstructed and enough oxygen cannot get into their lungs.

AAT is a protein that is quantitated by several test methods. AAT shows up in the α_1 region on serum protein electrophoresis, and a deficiency can be observed with this method. Quantitative methods for AAT measurement include enzyme-linked immunoassay (ELISA), nephelometry, and immunoturbidimetry. Reference ranges for AAT vary with test methodology but are generally accepted to be between 100 and 300 mg/dL or 20 to 60 µmol/L. The lungs are considered to be protected by an AAT level of 11 µmol/L. Electrolytes, specifically sodium, potassium, calcium, and magnesium, are monitored in individuals diagnosed with COPD because medications used to treat this disease can lead to low levels of electrolytes. Reference ranges for electrolytes in these patients are as follows: sodium, 135 to 145 mEq/L; potassium, 3.5 to 5.1 mEq/L; chloride, 98 to 107 mEq/L; calcium, 8.6 to 10.2 mEq/L; and magnesium, 1.6 to 2.6 mg/dL). PFTs are required for the differential diagnosis of COPD.

Cystic Fibrosis

Cystic fibrosis (CF) is an autosomal recessive genetic disease. It is one of the most common lethal genetic diseases. CF is distinguished by abnormal secretions that block the respiratory, digestive, and reproductive systems (Fig. 19-7). The fundamental abnormality is in transport of the chloride ion (Fig. 19-8). The lungs are the main organs affected, and respiratory failure is the usual cause

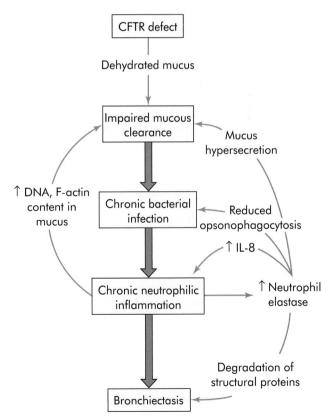

• **Figure 19-8** Pathogenesis of cystic fibrosis lung disease. *CFTR,* Cystic fibrosis transmembrane conductance regulator; *IL-8,* interleukin-8. (From Huether SE, McCance KL. *Understanding Pathophysiology.* 5th ed. St. Louis: Mosby; 2013.)

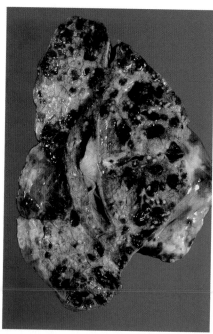

• Figure 19-9 Lung from a patient with cystic fibrosis. The lung shows widespread bronchopneumonia with pus from dilated bronchi and bronchioles. (From Cooke RA, Stewart B. *Colour Atlas of Anatomical Pathology.* 3rd ed. Sydney, Australia: Churchill Livingstone; 2004.)

of death in people diagnosed with CF. Over time, the hypoxic state causes the alveolar arteries to form new branches in an effort to oxygenate more red blood cells (Fig. 19-9).

Individuals with CF produce more mucus than normal and are unable to adequately clear mucus from the lungs. In addition, the mucus they produce is abnormally thick. This thick mucus retains bacteria which form biofilms that can be hard to treat with antibiotics. This mucus contributes to the chronic inflammation present in the lungs of individuals with CF. The fluids in the airways contain large numbers of neutrophils, which release oxidants (i.e., myeloperoxidase and proteases); these oxidants damage lungs, destroy immunoglobulin G, and stimulate mucus-producing cells to produce more mucus.

Individuals with CF have chronic bronchial infections with *P. aeruginosa,* which readily forms biofilms. These biofilms inhibit local immune responses and antibiotics from reaching and destroying the bacteria. Anaerobic bacteria may also play a part in the chronic inflammation seen in CF.

Laboratory Procedures and Limitations

There are several ways to screen for CF. The standard test for diagnosis of CF is the sweat test. A sweat chloride concentration greater than 60 mEq/L is diagnostic of CF. (See Chapter 12 for details.) In addition, CF can be diagnosed by the immunoreactive trypsinogen (IRT) blood test. The test is performed on newborns, and the IRT level is elevated in CF. Genotyping for mutations in the cystic fibrosis transmembrane conductance regulator gene *(CFTR)* is also used to diagnose individuals with CF. Because there are

more than 1900 specific mutations and standard laboratory panels test for only the most common 100 mutations, it is possible for a mutation to be missed. All newborns in the United States are tested for CF.

Pneumonia

Pneumonia is an infection of the lungs that can be caused by viruses, bacteria, or fungi. It is the sixth leading cause of death in the United States. Risks for developing pneumonia include advanced age, immunocompromise, underlying lung disease (especially COPD), alcoholism, impaired swallowing, smoking, intubation, malnutrition, immobilization, cardiac disease, liver disease, or residence in a nursing home. Bacterial pneumonia is usually more severe than viral pneumonia. The acute phase proteins and immune complexes that are released when microbes enter the lungs can damage the mucous and alveolar membranes, causing the bronchioles to fill with exudates and debris (Fig. 19-10). Also, some microbes release toxins that cause additional lung damage. The accumulation of debris and exudates results in hypoxemia and dyspnea. Infection is usually limited to one or two lobes.

Viral pneumonia is a seasonal, mild, and self-limited disease. It can predispose a person to a secondary bacterial pneumonia. The influenza virus is the most common cause of viral pneumonia. Pneumonia is usually diagnosed by sputum culture (bacteria), blood cultures, white blood cell count, chest radiograph, and viral culture or rapid viral detection methods (immunofluorescence, ELISA, or polymerase chain reaction [PCR]). The white blood cell count is elevated and chest radiographs show infiltrates in the lungs. The blood culture, Gram stain, and sputum culture usually reveal the same organism. *Streptococcus pneumonia* is a common isolate.

Pulmonary Edema

Pulmonary edema is an abnormal buildup of fluid in the alveoli; it is usually caused by congestive heart failure (Fig. 19-11). Congestive heart failure is a condition in which the heart struggles to pump blood throughout the body. As a result, blood flow slows down and hydrostatic pressure in the pulmonary capillaries increases; fluid leaks out into the alveoli, interfering with gas exchange in the lungs. Pulmonary edema can also be caused by decreased plasma oncotic pressure, increased negative interstitial pressure, damage to the alveolus/capillary barrier, lymphatic obstruction, mitral stenosis, acute myocardial infarction, cardiomyopathies, medications, high altitude, kidney failure, and other, unknown mechanisms.

Laboratory Tests

Radiographs are used to diagnose pulmonary edema, but laboratory tests can help pinpoint the cause. ABGs can be used to determine the severity of the pulmonary edema: The lower the pO_2, the more severe the case. ABGs are determined on

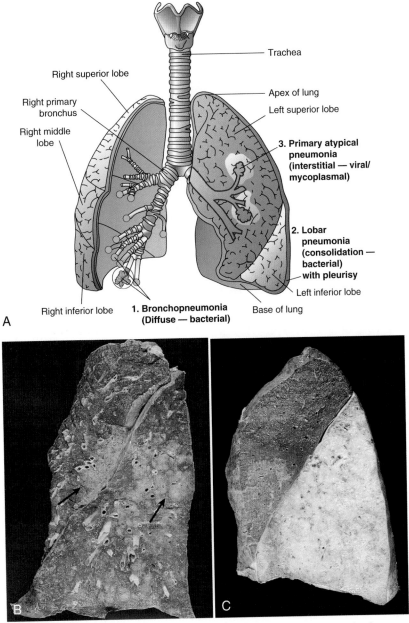

• **Figure 19-10 A,** Types of pneumonia and lobes of the lung. **B,** Bronchopneumonia. Gross section of lung shows patches of consolidation *(arrows).* **C,** Lobar pneumonia. The lower lobe is uniformly consolidated *(light color).* (**A,** From VanMeter KC, Hubert RJ. *Gould's Pathophysiology for the Health Professions.* 5th ed. St. Louis: Elsevier; 2015; **B** and **C,** From Kumar V, Abbas AK, Aster JC. *Robbins and Cotran Pathologic Basis of Disease.* 9th ed. Philadelphia: Saunders; 2015.)

a electrochemical blood gas analyzer. Blood urea nitrogen (BUN) and creatinine determinations are used to assess renal status, because renal failure can lead to pulmonary edema. BUN and creatinine are determined by colorimetric methods, usually on an automated chemistry analyzer. Electrolytes are used to determine whether a chemical imbalance is responsible for a patient's abnormal cardiac function. Most patients with congestive heart failure are taking antidiuretics, and ensuing hypokalemia and hypomagnesemia may alter heart function. Kidney failure can cause hyperkalemia and lead to altered heart function. Complications of pulmonary edema are respiratory fatigue and respiratory failure.

Pulmonary Hypertension

Pulmonary hypertension is a progressive disease that causes elevated pulmonary artery pressure (>25 mm Hg at rest or >30 mm Hg during exercise) which can eventually lead to right ventricular failure. The average pressure in the pulmonary artery is 15 mm Hg. Pulmonary artery pressure is a combination of blood flow and vascular resistance, with vascular resistance as the most common cause of increased pulmonary artery pressure. Primary pulmonary hypertension is rare, whereas secondary pulmonary hypertension can result from COPD, heart disease, collagen vascular diseases, or recurrent pulmonary thromboemboli (Fig. 19-12).

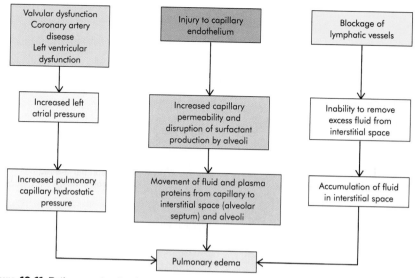

• **Figure 19-11** Pathogenesis of pulmonary edema. (From Huether SE, McCance KL. *Understanding Pathophysiology.* 5th ed. St. Louis: Mosby; 2013.)

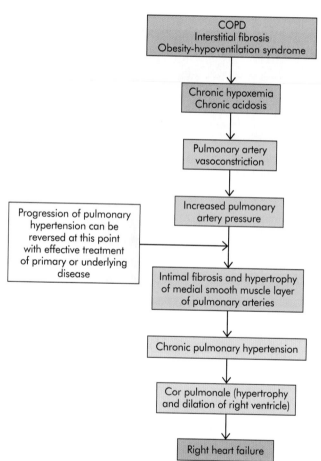

• **Figure 19-12** Pathogenesis of pulmonary hypertension and cor pulmonale. *COPD,* Chronic obstructive pulmonary disease. (From Huether SE, McCance KL. *Understanding Pathophysiology.* 5th ed. St. Louis: Mosby; 2013.)

This disease usually leads to right-sided heart failure, and the only effective therapy is a lung transplant.

Laboratory tests are useful to help assess the cause of pulmonary hypertension, but they are not used to diagnose this condition. ABGs are useful in assessing hypoxemia. Screening tests are helpful to rule out collagen vascular diseases; these tests include erythrocyte sedimentation rate, rheumatoid factor, antinuclear antibody, anti-neutrophil cytoplasmic antibody, and Scl-70 antibody. Liver function tests can detect liver disease associated with portal hypertension.

Atelectasis

Atelectasis is partial collapse of a lung (Fig. 19-13). There are several different types of atelectasis: resorption, compression, and contraction. In resorption atelectasis, a bronchial obstruction blocks air from entering part of a lung, and the gas present in the alveoli is reabsorbed into the blood, thus deflating the alveoli. This is a common condition after surgery: A mucous plug present after general anesthesia may cause an obstruction. Asthma, bronchitis, and tumors may also cause this condition. Compression atelectasis occurs when the lungs are compressed due to upward pressure on the diaphragm from any space-occupying lesion in the thorax. The pressure exerted on the lungs forces air out of a small portion, leading to the collapse. Pleural fluid, blood, or air present in the abdominal cavity may also exert pressure on the diaphragm and cause this condition. Contraction atelectasis decreases lung volume because of the contraction of scars in the lung. These scars can result from necrotizing pneumonia, granulomatous disease, tuberculosis, or other scarring conditions. Contraction atelectasis is not reversible due to the permanent nature of scarring. Resorption and compression atelectasis are both reversible. Infections can occur if atelectasis is a recurrent condition.

Right middle lobe syndrome, another syndrome that involves partial lung collapse, is caused by bronchus obstruction. The right middle lobe is located between the larger upper and lower lobes. The bronchus that transports air into the right middle lobe is long and slender and can easily be obstructed by mucus or inflammatory debris. This syndrome

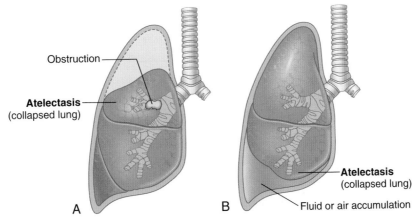

• **Figure 19-13** Two forms of atelectasis. **A,** An obstruction prevents air from reaching distal airways, and alveoli collapse. The most frequent cause is blockage of a bronchus by a mucous or mucopurulent (pus-containing) plug, as might occur postoperatively. **B,** Accumulations of fluid, blood, or air within the pleural cavity can collapse the lung. This may occur with congestive heart failure (in which poor circulation leads to fluid buildup in the pleural cavity), pneumonia, trauma, or a pneumothorax. (From Chabner DE. *The Language of Medicine.* 10th ed. St. Louis: Saunders; 2014.)

is also found in Sjögren syndrome. Individuals with recurrent atelectasis may develop right middle lobe pneumonia or an abscess.

Most often, atelectasis is diagnosed from radiographs. If the atelectasis is large enough, hypoxemia may result and can be detected by ABG analysis. The pO_2 will be low due to decreased oxygenation of the blood from the collapsed portion of the lung.

Pulmonary Embolism

A **pulmonary embolism** is an embolus that has moved from another location in the body to the pulmonary artery (Fig. 19-14). Most thrombi originate in the deep veins of the knee, upper leg, or pelvis. A pulmonary embolism is a complication of venous thrombosis: A portion of the thrombus breaks off to form an embolus that travels to the pulmonary artery. Thromboemboli can be caused by major surgery, trauma, infection, congestive heart failure, pregnancy, birth control pills, prolonged bed rest, metastatic cancer, genetic defect, or the lupus anticoagulant. Many thromboemboli are small and do not cause symptoms. Some cause chest pain and dyspnea when they lodge in the lung, resulting in a small lung infarct. Larger thromboemboli can completely obstruct the pulmonary artery bifurcation, causing immediate death. Routine laboratory test results are nonspecific and are helpful only in that they rule out other possible diagnoses.

Idiopathic Pulmonary Fibrosis

Idiopathic pulmonary fibrosis is a form of chronic, progressive, fibrosing interstitial pneumonia. The cause is unknown. The patient's lungs become stiff and inelastic, limiting both the lung expansion volume and the rates of expansion and contraction. This causes less air to move in

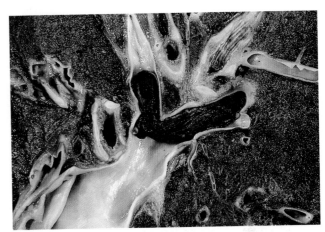

• **Figure 19-14** Pulmonary embolus. The embolus extends into major branches of the pulmonary artery. (From Kumar V, Abbas AK, Aster JC. *Robbins and Cotran Pathologic Basis for Disease.* 9th ed. Philadelphia: Saunders; 2015.)

and out of the lungs, leading to less gas exchange in the alveoli. Laboratory test results are nonspecific for diagnosis of this condition but are often used to rule out other possible diagnoses.

Sarcoidosis

Sarcoidosis is a chronic inflammatory disease that affects many body systems (Fig. 19-15). Disease hallmarks include noncaseating granulomas that occur in the lungs and lymph nodes. Patients can have a continuum of complaints, from asymptomatic to pulmonary and systematic effects. Many patients recover from this disease after treatment with steroids, but some develop lung disease. A very few develop progressive lung disease and die from pulmonary fibrosis or hypertension. Diagnostic imaging procedures are key to diagnosing this disease.

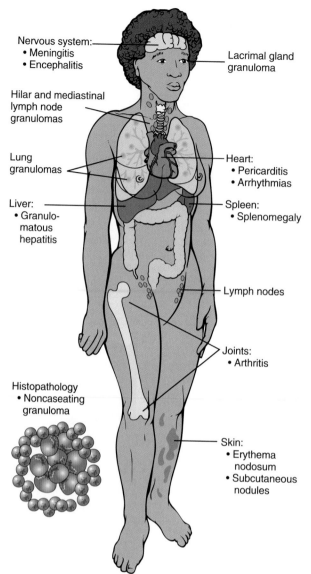

Nervous system:
• Meningitis
• Encephalitis

Lacrimal gland granuloma

Hilar and mediastinal lymph node granulomas

Lung granulomas

Heart:
• Pericarditis
• Arrhythmias

Liver:
• Granulo-matous hepatitis

Spleen:
• Splenomegaly

Lymph nodes

Joints:
• Arthritis

Histopathology
• Noncaseating granuloma

Skin:
• Erythema nodosum
• Subcutaneous nodules

• **Figure 19-15** Sarcoidosis. The most common sites of granulomas are the lungs and the thoracic lymph nodes. Other extrathoracic sites are less commonly involved. The inset shows a granuloma composed predominantly of epithelioid cells, macrophages, and lymphocytes. In contrast to tuberculosis, there is no central necrosis. (From Damjanov I. *Pathology for the Health Professions.* 4th ed. St. Louis: Saunders; 2012.)

Pleural Effusion

A pleural effusion is fluid in the pleural cavity (Table 19-3). Fluid may leak from blood or lymph vessels into the pleural cavity, or an abscess or lesion may drain into the pleural cavity. One type of pleural effusion is a transudate (watery), which may result from conditions that either increase intravascular hydrostatic pressure (e.g., congestive heart failure) or decrease capillary oncotic pressure (e.g., liver or kidney diseases that cause decreased blood protein). A pleural effusion can also be an exudate, containing increased white blood cells and high concentration of plasma proteins. This type of an effusion occurs in inflammatory disorders, infection, or malignancy. Other types of pleural effusions are empyema (pus), hemothorax (blood), and chylothorax (chyle).

Commons symptoms of a pleural effusion include dyspnea, compression atelectasis, and pleural pain. If an effusion happens quickly and involves a large amount of fluid, cardiovascular symptoms are also possible. A provider would hear decreased breath sounds, dullness to percussion, and a pleural friction rub in the affected area.

A chest radiograph confirms the presence of the effusion. The following tests are usually ordered for a pleural fluid workup: CBC with differential, total protein, glucose, lactate dehydrogenase, amylase, pH, cytology, culture and sensitivity (for acid-fast bacteria, aerobes, anaerobes, and fungi), and a Gram stain. In addition to the laboratory tests run on the fluid, blood tests are also ordered: blood cultures, total protein, glucose, lactate dehydrogenase, amylase, and arterial pH.

Table 19-4 shows ABG results for specific diseases.

TABLE 19-3   Types and Causes of Pleural Effusions

Cause	Finding	Pathogenesis
Transudates		
Congestive heart failure	↑ Hydrostatic pressure	Systemic and pulmonary venous hypertension
Hepatic cirrhosis	↑ Hydrostatic pressure	Portal and inferior vena cava hypertension
	↓ Colloid osmotic pressure	Hypoalbuminemia
Nephrotic syndrome	↓ Colloid osmotic pressure	Hypoalbuminemia
Exudates		
Pancreatitis	↑ Capillary permeability	Inflammation caused by chemical injury
Bile peritonitis	↑ Capillary permeability	Inflammation caused by chemical injury
Rheumatoid disease	↑ Capillary permeability	Inflammation of serosa
Systemic lupus erythematosus	↑ Capillary permeability	Inflammation of serosa
Infection (bacterial, tuberculous, fungal, viral)	↑ Capillary permeability	Inflammation caused by microorganisms
Infarction (myocardial, pulmonary)	↑ Capillary permeability	Inflammation caused by extension of the process to the serosal surface
Neoplasms	↑ Capillary permeability	Increased permeability of capillaries that supply tumor implants; pleuritis related to obstructive pneumonitis
	↓ Lymphatic drainage	Lymphatic obstruction secondary to lymph node infiltration

Adapted from Kaplan LA, Pesce AJ. *Clinical Chemistry: Theory, Analysis, Correlation*. 5th ed. St. Louis: Mosby; 2010.
↓, Decreased; ↑, increased.

TABLE 19-4   Summary of ABG Results for Specific Diseases

Condition	ABG Results	Other Significant Laboratory Test Results
Respiratory distress syndrome (in infants)	pH < 7.35, pCO_2 > 55 mm Hg, HCO_3^- < 18 mmol/L	Fetal lung maturity test; chest radiograph reveals a "ground glass" appearance
Acute respiratory distress syndrome (ARDS)	*Initially,* severely decreased pO_2, ↑ pH, ↓ pCO_2 *Progressing* to severely decreased pO_2, ↓ pH, ↑ pCO_2	
Chronic obstructive pulmonary disease (COPD)		↑ RBCs, ↑ hematocrit, ↑ hemoglobin, ↓ chloride
Emphysema	↓ pO_2, ↓ pH, ↓ HCO_3^-, ↑ pCO_2	
Asthma	↓ pO_2, ↑ pH, ↓ HCO_3^-, ↓ pCO_2	
Chronic bronchitis	↓ pO_2, normal but acidic pH (≈7.40), ↑ HCO_3^-, pCO_2 > 45 mm Hg	
Cystic fibrosis	pH 7.4, pCO_2 43-53 mm Hg, pO_2 52-60 mm Hg, HCO_3^- 27-31 mg/dL	Na 135-137 mEq/L, K 3.8-4.6 mEq/L, Cl 94-100 mEq/L, albumin 2.5-3.7 g/L
Pneumonia	↓ pO_2, ↓ to normal pCO_2	*Complete blood count:* ↑ WBCs in bacterial pneumonia, ↓ WBCs in viral pneumonia, anemia present, ↑ platelets, positive blood cultures *Pulse oximetry:* <90-92%
Pulmonary edema	↓ pO_2, ↓ to normal pCO_2	*Heart workup:* most common cause of pulmonary edema is congestive heart failure
Pulmonary hypertension	Normal arterial blood gas results	
Atelectasis	↓ pO_2, ↓ or normal pCO_2	
Pulmonary embolism	↓ pO_2, ↓ pCO_2, respiratory alkalosis	

TABLE 19-4	Summary of ABG Results for Specific Diseases—cont'd	
Condition	**ABG Results**	**Other Significant Laboratory Test Results**
Idiopathic pulmonary fibrosis	↓ pO_2	Antinuclear antibody, rheumatoid factor
Sarcoidosis	Normal	Radiographs can detect air trapping; biopsy needed for diagnosis
Pleural effusion	Normal	Thoracentesis analysis needed for diagnosis

HCO_3^-, Bicarbonate; pCO_2, partial pressure of carbon dioxide; pO_2, partial pressure of oxygen; *RBCs*, red blood cells; *WBC*, white blood cells; ↓, decreased; ↑, increased.

Summary

COPD is a group of diseases that are responsible for many hospital visits every year; it includes chronic bronchitis, emphysema, and asthma. Other respiratory diseases that bring people to the hospital include pneumonia, pulmonary edema, pulmonary hypertension, atelectasis, pulmonary embolism, idiopathic pulmonary fibrosis, and sarcoidosis. Pneumonia is a lung infection that causes the alveoli to fill with fluid, mucus, and pus, thus impairing gas exchange. Pulmonary edema is abnormal fluid buildup in the alveoli due to congestive heart failure. Pulmonary hypertension is increased pressure in the pulmonary artery, which leads to right ventricular failure. Atelectasis is a collapsed lung. A pulmonary embolism is a thrombus in the pulmonary artery. Idiopathic pulmonary fibrosis is a condition that causes a person's lungs to become stiff and inelastic. Sarcoidosis is a chronic inflammatory disease that affects many body systems; the hallmark of the disease is granulomas in the lungs and lymph nodes.

Review Questions

1. Which of the following conditions is the result of an α_1-antitrypsin level lower than 11 mmol/L?
   a. Emphysema
   b. Asthma
   c. Pulmonary edema
   d. Sarcoidosis

2. Which of the following conditions produces large quantities of mucus, neutrophil infiltrates, and inflammation of the bronchi?
   a. Emphysema
   b. Pulmonary hypertension
   c. Chronic bronchitis
   d. Pulmonary edema

3. Which of the following conditions is potentially fatal and is caused by a severe bronchospasm?
   a. Asthma
   b. Status asthmaticus
   c. Emphysema
   d. Pulmonary hypertension

4. Pneumonia is
   a. An abnormal accumulation of fluid in the alveoli that can lead to right-sided heart failure
   b. A collapsed lung
   c. A systemic disease with granulomas in the lungs
   d. An infection that causes the alveoli to fill with pus or fluid

5. Which of the following conditions causes the bronchial tree to constrict, thus obstructing air flow entering and leaving the lungs?
   a. Atelectasis
   b. Pulmonary emboli
   c. Emphysema
   d. Asthma

6. Hypoxemia is considered severe when the pO_2 is
   a. 60-79 mm Hg
   b. <40 mm Hg
   c. 40-59 mm Hg
   d. <20 mm Hg

7. In which of the following diseases do the lungs become stiff and inelastic?
   a. Idiopathic pulmonary fibrosis
   b. Atelectasis
   c. Pulmonary edema
   d. Emphysema

8. People with which of the following conditions are called "blue bloaters"?
   a. Emphysema
   b. Asthma
   c. Chronic bronchitis
   d. Pulmonary hypertension

9. People with which of the following conditions are called "pink puffers"?
   a. Chronic bronchitis
   b. Asthma
   c. Pulmonary hypertension
   d. Emphysema

10. Which of the following conditions is found in Sjögren syndrome?
    a. Constriction atelectasis
    b. Right middle lobe syndrome
    c. Compression atelectasis
    d. Resorption atelectasis

Critical Thinking Questions

1. How is cystic fibrosis produced, and why do individuals with this disease have many lung infections?
2. Why is a pulmonary embolism considered a medical emergency?
3. Explain why the blood gas values for emphysema, chronic bronchitis, cystic fibrosis, and asthma differ from normal values.

CASE STUDY

A 65-year-old woman was diagnosed with cirrhosis of the liver several years ago. Recently, she noticed that her abdomen was distended and she was short of breath, so she went to her provider to find out why. Her provider told her that her stomach was distended due to the presence of fluid. Why do you think she was short of breath? Explain the condition that is causing this symptom.

Bibliography

Davis MD, Walsh BK, Sittig SE, Restrepo RD. AARC clinical practice guideline: blood gas analysis and hemoximetry—2013. *Respir Care*. 2013;58(10):1694–1703.

Drancourt M, Gaydos CA, Summersgill JT, Raoult D. Point-of-care testing for community-acquired pneumonia. *Lancet Infect Dis*. 2013;13(8):647–649.

Inglis SC, Davidson PM, Disler RT. Cochrane overview: comprehensive approaches to chronic obstructive pulmonary disease management. *Am J Respir Crit Care Med*. 2015;191. A1113.

Kacmarek RM, Stoller JK, Heuer AH. *Egan's fundamentals of respiratory care*. St. Louis: Elsevier Health Sciences; 2014.

King TE, Pardo A, Selman M. Idiopathic pulmonary fibrosis. *Lancet*. 2011;378(9807):1949–1961.

McDonough JE, Yuan R, Suzuki M, et al. Small-airway obstruction and emphysema in chronic obstructive pulmonary disease. *N Engl J Med*. 2011;365(17):1567–1575.

Murdoch DR, O'Brien KL, Driscoll AJ, Karron RA, Bhat N. Laboratory methods for determining pneumonia etiology in children. *Clin Infect Dis*. 2012;54(suppl 2):S146–S152.

Pedersen F, Holz O, Lauer G, et al. Multi-analyte profiling of inflammatory mediators in COPD sputum: the effects of processing. *Cytokine*. 2015;71(2):401–404.

Ruppel GL, Enright PL. Pulmonary function testing. *Respir Care*. 2012;57(1):165–175.

Ryerson CJ, Hartman T, Elicker BM, et al. Clinical features and outcomes in combined pulmonary fibrosis and emphysema in idiopathic pulmonary fibrosis. *Chest*. 2013;144(1):234–240.

Sharma O. Defining sarcoidosis. *Sarcoidosis*. 2012;13(3):12.

Takahashi T, Muro S, Sato S, et al. Multiple dimensional analysis of arterial blood gas and pulmonary function in patients with COPD. *Eur Respir J*. 2012;40(suppl 56). P2911.

Wiener RS, Schwartz LM, Woloshin S. Time trends in pulmonary embolism in the United States: evidence of overdiagnosis. *Arch Intern Med*. 2011;171(9):831–837.

20
Gastrointestinal Disease

SHERYL BERMAN

CHAPTER OUTLINE

OBJECTIVES

After completion of this chapter, the reader will be able to:

1. Identify the primary and secondary organs of the gastrointestinal system.
2. Describe the digestive process.
3. Explain the physiology of the gastrointestinal system, including carbohydrate digestion, protein digestion, and lipid digestion.
4. Compare the various tests for identifying *Helicobacter pylori* infection and how *H. pylori* infection is associated with gastric and duodenal ulcers.
5. Explain how the calcium infusion test, the octreotide test, and the secretin test are used in the diagnosis of Zollinger-Ellison syndrome.
6. Compare and contrast acute versus chronic diarrhea as to possible disease correlations.
7. Discuss the tests used to diagnose the etiologies of acute or chronic diarrhea.
8. Discuss the two main divisions of inflammatory bowel disease and how they differ with regard to disease presentation.
9. Evaluate laboratory results with regard to Crohn disease and an ulcerative colitis diagnosis.
10. Discuss all blood and imaging tests used for diagnosis of malabsorption and what values may be expected.
11. Discuss tests to diagnose diverticulitis and diverticulosis.
12. Describe steatorrhea and identify the appropriate diagnostic test.
13. Compare and contrast tropical sprue and celiac sprue with regard to disease mechanism, laboratory tests for diagnosis, and treatment.
14. Discuss the test for fecal fat and the D-xylose absorption test and when they are used.

KEY TERMS

Bile
Celiac disease
Celiac sprue
Cholecystokinin
Chyme
Chymotrypsin
Clostridium difficile
Crohn disease
Diarrhea
Digestive enzymes
Diverticulitis
Diverticulosis

D-xylose absorption
Fecal fat
Gastrin
Gastrinoma
Helicobacter pylori
Inflammatory bowel disease
Irritable bowel syndrome
Malabsorption
Maldigestion
Microvilli
Pancreatic amylase
Pancreatic elastase

Pepsin
Pepsinogen
Peptidase
Polyps
Salivary amylase
Secretin
Steatorrhea
Tropical sprue
Trypsin
Ulcer
Ulcerative colitis
Zollinger-Ellison syndrome

❖ Case in Point

Mr. H. is a 58-year-old man of Syrian descent. He complains to his doctor about abdominal pain, especially in the middle of the night, and loss of appetite. After an additional extensive history, his physician orders an endoscopy of his stomach and duodenum. The endoscopy reveals lesions in the stomach. The endoscope is used to obtain a tissue sample. A urease test is performed with positive results.

1. What is the urease test methodology used in this case?
2. What is the causative agent? What is the pathophysiology behind the production of gastric and duodenal ulcers?

Points to Remember

- The primary purpose of the gastrointestinal tract is to ingest food and turn it into energy for the body.
- The primary classes of molecules that are digested in the body are carbohydrates, proteins, and lipids (fats).
- Ulcers are holes or erosions in the gastrointestinal tract; they are usually found in the duodenum or stomach.
- Most ulcers are associated with infection by pathogenic forms of the bacterial species, *Helicobacter pylori.*
- In Zollinger-Ellison syndrome, one or more gastrinomas are present in the pancreas or duodenum.
- Gastrinomas produce excessive stomach acid and can become malignant.
- Laboratory tests for Zollinger-Ellison syndrome detect increased gastrin levels.
- Acute diarrhea is usually short lived and caused by infectious agents.
- Chronic diarrhea persists and can be caused by infectious agents, malabsorption, inflammatory bowel disease (IBD), chemotherapy, laxative use, celiac disease, or food intolerances.
- The primary tests for acute diarrhea detect the presence of microorganisms, whereas the tests for chronic diarrhea are used to identify the etiology.
- *H. pylori* can be detected by biopsy and culture or by urease breath tests and stool antigen tests.
- IBD refers to either ulcerative colitis or Crohn disease.
- Ulcerative colitis occurs in the large intestine, whereas Crohn disease is characterized by lesions and inflammation anywhere in the gastrointestinal tract.
- The primary tests for diagnosis of IBD are sigmoidoscopy and colonoscopy.
- Blood tests for malabsorption focus on finding decreased levels of iron, zinc, vitamin B_{12}, and vitamin D.
- Tropical sprue, a disease found in the tropics, is caused by a microbial infection that responds positively to antibiotics.
- Celiac disease is an inflammatory reaction to gluten; it is diagnosed by measuring antibody levels and responds positively to a gluten-free diet.
- Diverticulosis indicates weak outpouchings of the large intestine.
- Diverticulitis is an infection of the diverticula.
- Steatorrhea is a condition in which excessive fat in the stool causes it to become greasy and foul smelling.
- The D-xylose test is used to differentiate maldigestion from malabsorption.

Introduction

This chapter introduces gastrointestinal (GI) diseases and the laboratory tests used to diagnosis them. The structure and function of the GI tract and the pathophysiology of significant GI conditions are reviewed. These conditions include ulcers, Zollinger-Ellison syndrome, inflammatory bowel diseases, tropical sprue, celiac disease, and diverticulitis. Malabsorption, steatorrhea, and diarrhea; their disease mechanisms; and the diagnostic assays or techniques used to confirm or rule out these conditions are also discussed.

Gastrointestinal System

The GI system is responsible for turning food into energy. The primary organs of the GI tract are the mouth, esophagus, stomach, small intestine, and large intestine. Accessory GI organs, which aid in digestion, include the liver, gallbladder, and pancreas. The functions of the GI tract include the ingestion of food, digestion of food, absorption of nutrients from food, and waste elimination.

Anatomic Review

The GI tract (Fig. 20-1) is divided into upper and lower portions. The upper GI tract includes the mouth, esophagus, stomach, and part of the small intestine. The lower GI tract includes the remaining portion of the small intestine, the large intestine, the rectum, and the anus. The pancreas, liver, and gallbladder are not technically part of the GI tract although they play important roles in digestion and in the absorption of nutrients.

The mouth is the first organ of the GI system. Ingestion and the beginnings of digestion occur here. In the mouth, chewing breaks the food into pieces and mixes it with saliva. Enzymes in saliva begin to break down the foodstuffs, primarily the carbohydrates. The food travels from the mouth and pharynx through a long tube called the *esophagus* and into the stomach. The esophagus is posterior to the trachea; it passes through an opening in the diaphragm called the *esophageal hiatus.* Peristalsis, or the rhythmic contractions of muscles in the esophagus, helps the food travel through the esophagus to the stomach. Upper and lower sphincters in the esophagus control the movement of food in and out of the esophagus.

The stomach, a hollow organ at the end of the esophagus, receives food from the esophagus. The stomach is divided into four regions: fundus, cardia, body, and pylorus. There are four different types of cells that line the stomach and secrete various substances. The mucosal cells, parietal cells, and chief cells are classified as exocrine cells; they produce gastric secretions or "gastric juice." The mucosal cells secrete

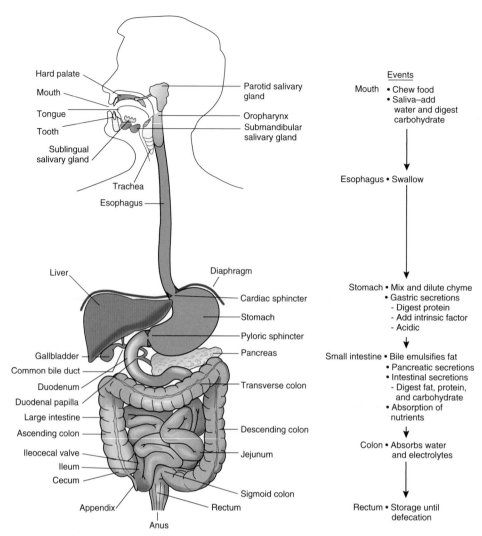

• Figure 20-1 Anatomy of the gastrointestinal tract. (From VanMeter KC, Hubert RJ. *Gould's Pathophysiology for the Health Profession.* 5th ed. St. Louis: Saunders; 2015.)

mucus, the parietal cells secrete hydrochloric acid, and the chief cells secrete pepsinogen and chymosin. The fourth type of cell in the stomach is the endocrine cell, which secretes gastrin.

Food leaving the stomach travels to the small intestine. The small intestine is approximately 22 ft long and is composed of three main sections: duodenum, jejunum, and ileum. Both digestion and absorption take place in the small intestine. The ileum progresses into the large intestine through the ileocecal valve. Like the small intestine, the large intestine has various regions, including the cecum, ascending colon, transverse colon, descending colon, sigmoid colon, rectum, anal opening, and appendix. The cecum is the beginning of the large intestine; it is followed by the ascending, transverse, descending, and sigmoid colon segments and the rectum. The appendix is a small section that protrudes from the cecum at the beginning of the large intestine. The end of the large intestine opens to the environment via the anus. Functions of the large intestine include water absorption, limited digestion of B vitamins, and removal of waste from the body.

The remaining organs of the GI tract, referred to as accessory organs, are the liver, gallbladder, and pancreas. The liver and gallbladder are located in the right upper quadrant of the abdomen. The pancreas is located in the left upper quadrant, just posterior to the stomach and anterior to the spine. The liver, gallbladder, and pancreas are connected to the GI tract via ducts that transfer many substances from these organs to the small intestine to aid digestion.

Normal Physiology

The purpose of the GI tract is the ingestion of food, digestion of the food into small subunits called nutrients, then absorption of these nutrients in the body. There are three primary categories of nutrients that are key to body function: carbohydrates, proteins, and fats. Each nutrient is digested in its own unique way.

Carbohydrate Digestion

Digestion of carbohydrate begins in the mouth, when food mixes with saliva containing salivary amylase. The three

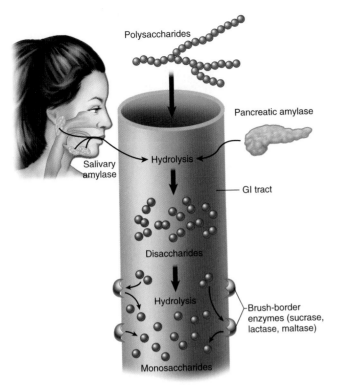

• **Figure 20-2** Carbohydrate digestion. Amylase in saliva and pancreatic juice hydrolyzes polysaccharides into disaccharides. Brush border disaccharidases in the lining of the small intestine then promote hydrolysis of the disaccharides into monosaccharides. (From Patton KT, Thibodeau GA. *Anatomy and Physiology.* 8th ed. St. Louis: Saunders; 2013.)

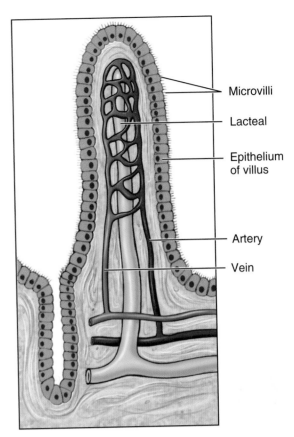

Single villus

• **Figure 20-3** Cross-section of single villus in the small intestines. (From Herilhy B. *The Human Body in Health and Illness.* 5th ed. St. Louis: Saunders; 2014.)

pairs of salivary glands—the parotid glands, submandibular glands, and sublingual glands—secrete mucus and enzymes to begin digestion in the mouth. Salivary amylase breaks starch and glycogen (both polysaccharides) into disaccharides.

Mucus, secreted by the salivary glands and esophagus, helps moisten the food and allows it to move from the mouth and pharynx to the esophagus and stomach. The mixture of food and saliva passes through the cardiac sphincter, which separates the esophagus and stomach, into the first section of the stomach. The stomach mixes and churns the food with gastric juices, further aiding in carbohydrate digestion. This mixture is now called chyme. The chyme travels from the stomach through the pyloric sphincter into the duodenum of the small intestine, where the majority of carbohydrate digestion takes place. As the chyme moves into the duodenum, pancreatic amylase is released through the pancreatic duct into the duodenum. This enzyme breaks down the remaining starch and glycogen into disaccharides (Fig. 20-2).

The interior wall of the small intestine is covered with tiny projections called villi. The villi increase the surface area of the intestines and thus play an important part in the absorption of nutrients (Fig. 20-3). The cells of the villi contain even smaller extensions, called microvilli. In the microvilli are additional digestive enzymes needed to further break down oligosaccharides to monosaccharides.

These enzymes—sucrase, maltase, and lactase—break down the disaccharides sucrose, maltose, and lactose, respectively, into monosaccharides. The monosaccharides are absorbed by the villi and then enter the bloodstream.

The liver plays an important role in carbohydrate digestion. The liver is responsible for converting glycogen to glucose, thereby increasing the blood glucose concentration. It also converts glucose to glycogen, decreasing the blood glucose level. The liver can also convert other organic molecules, such as lipids and proteins, into glucose, if needed by the body for energy.

Protein Digestion

When the food arrives in the stomach, gastrin (a hormone secreted by endocrine cells) stimulates the secretion of gastric juices. The chief cells in the stomach secrete an enzyme precursor called pepsinogen, which is converted to pepsin by the hydrochloric acid in the stomach. Pepsin begins to digest protein as the stomach contents churn and become chyme. The chyme moves into the duodenum, where enzymes break down the proteins into peptides. At this point, cholecystokinin is released from the intestinal walls, stimulating release of trypsinogen, chymotrypsinogen, and procarboxypeptidase from the pancreas. These enzymes further break down proteins into peptides and amino acids. Trypsinogen is converted to trypsin by enterokinase, which is secreted by the mucosal cells of the small intestine. One function of trypsin is to activate and convert procarboxy-peptidase and chymotrypsinogen into carboxypeptidase and chymotrypsin, powerful enzymes that directly break down proteins into oligopeptides. The mucosal cells also secrete an enzyme called peptidase, which is responsible for splitting peptide bonds in oligopeptides to form amino acids.

Protein digestion is completed in the duodenum. The villi of the small intestine absorb the amino acids resulting from protein digestion. Products of protein digestion stimulate the production of secretin. Secretin is produced by the S cells of the duodenum to prevent the pH in the small intestine from remaining below 4.5. It inhibits secretion of hydrochloric acid by parietal cells and stimulates the pancreas to secrete bicarbonate.

The liver also has three roles to play in protein metabolism: deaminating amino acids, forming and excreting urea nitrogen, and synthesizing proteins, including albumin and enzymes.

Lipid Digestion

Lipid digestion is problematic because lipids are not soluble in water. Dietary lipids are composed of triacylglycerol (95%), cholesterol, phospholipids, free fatty acids, and fat-soluble vitamins. Cholecystokinin is secreted in the small intestine, and its function is to slow gastric motility to enhance fat digestion. As the chyme passes into the duodenum, cholecystokinin stimulates the gallbladder to release bile through the common bile duct into the duodenum. Bile is composed of bile salts of cholesterol. Bile salts are formed in the liver from cholesterol and secreted into the gallbladder for storage. This is the only way cholesterol is excreted from the body. The function of bile is to emulsify fats into smaller globules called *micelles*. This process increases the surface area of the fat so that lipid-hydrolyzing enzymes can break down fats more effectively.

Cholecystokinin also stimulates the release of pancreatic lipase and intestinal lipase, both of which hydrolyze the triglycerides into monoacylglycerols and fatty acids. This is an important step in lipid digestion because triglyceride is a large molecule and is unable to diffuse across the cells of the small intestine. Instead, the monoacylglycerols and fatty acids diffuse across the cell membrane, and then triglycerides are reassembled within the intestinal epithelial cells.

Once the fats have been broken down into smaller molecules, they must be transported through the blood (water-based) to different parts of the body. The liver assists in the transportation process by synthesizing albumin, which helps transport fatty acids, and lipoproteins, which help transport most other lipids. Lipoproteins are covered in more detail in Chapter 17.

Abnormal Conditions
Peptic Ulcers

A peptic ulcer is a mucosal break of 3 mm in diameter in the stomach or duodenum. Some untreated ulcers may

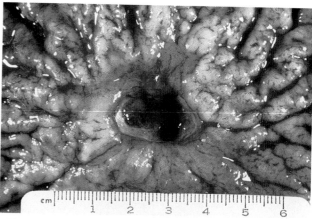

• **Figure 20-4** Chronic peptic ulcer. Gross photograph of a chronic peptic ulcer located in the lesser curvature, straddling the antrum and corpus of the stomach. (From Damjanov I, Linder J, eds. *Anderson's Pathology.* 10th ed. St. Louis: Mosby; 1996.)

continue to erode the mucosal layer and eventually perforate or form a hole through the stomach or duodenum. Duodenal and gastric ulcers can be caused by *Helicobacter pylori*. *H. pylori* stimulates the inflammatory process, thus increasing the chances of intestinal lining erosion (Fig. 20-4).

GI ulcers are diagnosed with the use of gastroscopy, serology tests, breath tests, or stool antigen tests. Gastroscopy uses an endoscope to view the stomach and take tissue samples from an inflamed area. Urease tests, microbiological cultures, and histologic tests are performed on the extracted tissue. The tests for urease are based on the breakdown of urea in the presence of urease:

$$CO(NH_2)_2 + 2H_2O \xrightarrow[\text{(Urease)}]{} H_2O + CO_2 + 2NH_3$$

The urease breath test is a unique test that detects the ability of certain pathogenic types of *H. pylori* to secrete the enzyme urease. In this test, patients drink a urea solution containing radioactively labeled carbon atoms (^{14}C or ^{13}C). If urease-producing *H. pylori* is present, the urea will be broken down by the bacterial urease, and the ^{14}C or ^{13}C will be incorporated into carbon dioxide molecules. The level of radioactivity is measured in the patient's exhaled carbon dioxide. Breath testing has a high sensitivity and high specificity (94% to 98%) for *H. pylori* infection. It can also be used to monitor the effectiveness of treatment because it detects only active or present infections.

Stool tests for *H. pylori* antigen also detect active or very recent infections. Like the breath tests, the stool *H. pylori* antigen tests can be used to monitor the efficacy of antibiotic treatment. The American Gastroenterological Association and the American College of Gastroenterology recommend the urease breath and stool antigen tests as reliable, noninvasive tests for *H. pylori* infection.

Zollinger-Ellison syndrome is a condition characterized by benign, non–β-islet cell, gastrin-secreting tumors (gastrinomas) located in the pancreas or duodenum. These tumors stimulate excessive hydrochloric acid production by the parietal cells in the stomach, leading to the formation of peptic ulcers in the stomach and duodenum. Over time, these gastrinomas may become malignant.

Symptoms of Zollinger-Ellison syndrome include fulminant peptic ulcers, massive gastric hypersecretion, hypergastrinemia, diarrhea, and steatorrhea. Gastrin levels in affected individuals are 2 to 2000 times the normal range. Gastrin levels more than 10 times the upper reference range level accompanied by gastric acid hypersecretion are considered diagnostic of gastrinoma. Fasting gastrin levels provide good prognostic value because the levels correlate well with the size and site of the gatrinoma. Treatment of this condition usually requires surgical intervention.

The diagnostic tests for Zollinger-Ellison syndrome include gastrin levels and imaging techniques. Gastrin is measured in the laboratory with the use of immunoassay techniques. Because gastrin is unstable in serum or plasma, special care should be taken when collecting these specimens. Tubes containing heparin and aprotinin should be used to collect blood specimens, and the tubes should be put on ice after the specimen is mixed and rapidly transported to the laboratory. Plasma separation should take place in a refrigerated centrifuge, and the separated specimen should be frozen immediately. The specimen should be collected, transported, separated, and frozen within 15 minutes of collection. The reference range for gastrin is less than 100 pg/mL.

Diarrhea

Diarrhea is characterized by loose, watery, and frequent stools. Diarrhea is considered chronic when frequent stools are present for more than 4 weeks. Diarrhea may be accompanied by abdominal pain, cramping, nausea, blood, or mucus. Usually, acute diarrhea is short lived and self-limited. However, when diarrhea is severe or persistent (chronic), it can lead to dehydration due to large water loss and dangerously low potassium levels resulting in serious complications or even death. Some patients affected by diarrhea require hospitalization. In infants, significant dehydration can occur within hours.

The causes of acute diarrhea are divided into bacterial, viral, or parasitic causes. Table 20-1 lists some etiologic agents of acute diarrhea. Acute diarrhea can also be caused by the effects of antimicrobial use: Broad-spectrum antimicrobials can destroy the normal gut bacteria and allow opportunistic bacteria to multiply, causing diarrhea. *Clostridium difficile* is an example of such an opportunistic infectious agent.

Chronic diarrhea can persist for weeks, months, or longer. The primary causes of chronic diarrhea are ulcerative colitis and Crohn disease, irritable bowel syndrome, celiac disease, malabsorption, food intolerances, and chemotherapy or radiation. In addition, parasitic infection, colon cancer, polyps, and excessive laxative use can also cause chronic diarrhea.

Laboratory Tests for Diarrhea

Many laboratory tests are available to diagnosis diarrhea, including stool cultures, immunoassays, ova and parasites,

TABLE 20-1	Causes of Acute Diarrhea	
Name of Infectious Agent	**Class of Infectious Agent**
Salmonella	Bacteria
Shigella	Bacteria
Campylobacter	Bacteria
Yersinia	Bacteria
Staphylococcus	Bacteria
Bacillus	Bacteria
Escherichia coli	Bacteria
Clostridium	Bacteria
Calcivirus	Virus
Adenovirus	Virus
Cytomegalovirus	Virus
Human immunodeficiency virus (HIV)	Virus
Noroviruses	Virus
Entamoeba	Parasite
Cryptosporidium	Parasite
Giardia	Parasite

fecal fat, and antibody assays. In a stool culture, stool bacteria in are grown on selective and differential media to identify an infectious agent. For some infectious agents, such as *C. difficile*, rotavirus, and *E. coli* O1:57, enzyme-linked immunoassays (ELISAs) detect the presence of the infectious agent without culturing. The ova and parasites test detects the presence of parasites in stool.

The fecal fat test is a nonspecific test to determine whether there is increased fat in the stool, which would be indicative of malabsorption or maldigestion. A spot fecal fat test is done via microscopy using a Sudan stain. Fecal fat tests can also be performed on 24- or 72-hour stool collections. Individuals follow a high-fat diet for 3 days before the collection, then collect all stool for the next 24 or 72 hours. The stool is delivered to the laboratory, and a small aliquot is used for testing. The reference range is less than 7 g fat in 24 hours.

Tests for celiac disease include a panel of antibody tests: tissue transglutaminase antibodies (TTG), endomysial antibodies (EMA), anti-gliadin antibodies (AGA), and deaminated gliadin peptide antibodies (DGP) are most commonly measured. The anti-EMA is usually an immunofluorescence test, whereas the anti-AGA, anti-DGP, and anti-TTG are usually enzyme immunoassays. The anti-TTG test is usually preferred to the anti-EMA test, and it is the primary test used to detect celiac disease. Sensitivities range from 80% to 100%, and specificities are greater than 95% for all of these antibody tests in the diagnosis of celiac disease (Table 20-2).

TABLE 20-2	Comparison of Serologic Tests for Celiac Disease			
Antibody	Method		Sensitivity (%)	Specificity (%)
Antireticulin antibody (R1-ARA)	Immunofluorescence on rat or mouse kidney		25-30	>90
IgA-antiendomysial antibody	Immunofluorescence on monkey esophagus or human umbilical cord		80-100	>99
IgA-antigliadin antibody	Quantitative ELISA		75-95	95
IgA-antitissue transglutaminase antibody (human antigen)	Quantitative ELISA		>90	>99
IgA-deamidated gliadin peptide antibody	Quantitative ELISA		90	90

From Burtis CA, Ashwood ER, Bruns DE, eds. *Tietz Textbook of Clinical Chemistry*. 5th ed. St. Louis: Elsevier, 2012. *ELISA*, Enzyme-linked immunoassay; *IgA*, immunoglobulin A.

TABLE 20-3	Inflammatory Bowel Disease: A Comparison Between Crohn Disease and Ulcerative Colitis	
Characteristic	Crohn Disease	Ulcerative Colitis
Region affected	Terminal ileum, sometimes colon	Colon, rectum
Distribution of lesions	Transmural, all layers Skip lesions	Mucosa only Continuous, diffuse
Characteristic stool	Loose, semiformed	Frequent, watery, with blood and mucus
Granuloma	Common	No
Fistula, fissure, abscess	Common	No
Stricture, obstruction	Common	Rare
Malabsorption, malnutrition	Yes	Not common

From VanMeter KC, Hubert RJ. *Gould's Pathophysiology for the Health Professions*. 5th ed. St. Louis: Elsevier; 2015.

Inflammatory Bowel Disease

The term **inflammatory bowel disease** (IBD) includes ulcerative colitis and Crohn disease. Ulcerative colitis produces inflammation of the colon, whereas Crohn disease produces inflammation primarily in the small intestines, although it can also affect any place in the GI tract. The characteristics of both diseases are summarized in Table 20-3. Their pathology and appearance are shown in Figures 20-5 and 20-6. Both ulcerative colitis and Crohn disease exhibit bouts of remission and bouts of exacerbation or "flare-ups." The causes of ulcerative colitis and Crohn disease are not known. Both appear to have autoimmune components; the body attacks its own tissue or fails to stop the inflammatory process once it has begun. There appears to be a genetic link or susceptibility to both diseases. Environmental factors such as infectious agents, food antigens, or medications also appear to play a role. Both ulcerative colitis and Crohn disease are associated with abdominal pain, cramping, anorexia, bloody diarrhea, and anemia.

Diagnostic Tests for Inflammatory Bowel Disease

Diagnostic tests for IBD include a complete blood count (CBC) showing anemia or an increased white blood cell count. Fecal examinations will reveal red and white blood cells. White blood cells can signify infection or inflammation, whereas red blood cells are indicative of bleeding. Blood can also be detected by occult blood tests. Imaging and endoscopy are also used to diagnose these conditions.

Malabsorption Syndrome

Malabsorption is defective absorption of nutrients by the GI tract. The absorption defect can be associated with a single nutrient or all nutrients. An example of single-nutrient malabsorption is lactase deficiency. Lactase is an enzyme that breaks down lactose into monosaccharides that can be easily utilized by the body. In lactase deficiency, there is no enzyme to break down lactose, and the result is excretion of lactose. Examples of widespread

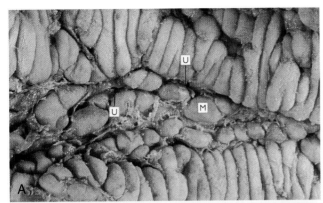

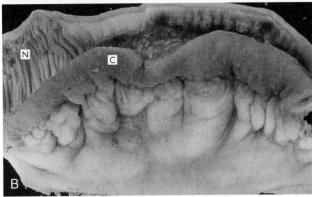

• **Figure 20-5** Crohn disease. **A,** The mucosa in Crohn disease demonstrates a cobblestone pattern as a result of fissured ulcers *(U)* with intervening areas of edematous mucosa *(M)*. **B,** Compared with normal small bowel wall *(N)*, the Crohn segment *(C)* shows wall thickening that has caused a stenosis. (From Kumar V, Fausto N. *Robbins and Cotran Pathologic Basis of Disease.* 7th ed. Philadelphia: Saunders; 2004.)

deficiencies that affect all nutrients include celiac disease and Crohn disease. Most patients with malabsorption conditions experience diarrhea, abdominal discomfort, and weight loss. Treatment depends on the underlying etiology.

Diagnostic laboratory tests for malabsorption may include a CBC, a chemistry screen, prothrombin time, and vitamin or mineral assays. Other tests, such as pancreatic elastase, celiac antibodies, fecal fat, a stool culture, or ova and parasites, are also used to diagnose these conditions.

A CBC is used to detect anemia. Anemia can be present in malabsorption due to lower amounts of iron, vitamin B_{12}, and folate. Malabsorption can also cause a vitamin K deficiency, which can be detected by the prothrombin time. Various vitamins and minerals, such as iron, folate, vitamin B_{12}, magnesium, calcium, vitamin D, and vitamin A are measured to detect malabsorption and are usually decreased. Other useful chemistry tests include albumin, triglycerides, cholesterol, sodium, and potassium.

Serologic tests are needed to detect celiac disease. Tests such as anti-AGA, anti-TTG, anti-DGP, or anti-EMA may help rule out celiac disease as a cause of malabsorption. Pancreatic elastase 1 is an enzyme detected in stool that can help providers understand a patient's exocrine pancreatic status to differentiate between maldigestion and malabsorption.

Stool cultures can rule out bacterial infections, and ova and parasites examinations help rule out parasitic infection. The fecal fat test is a nonspecific test for

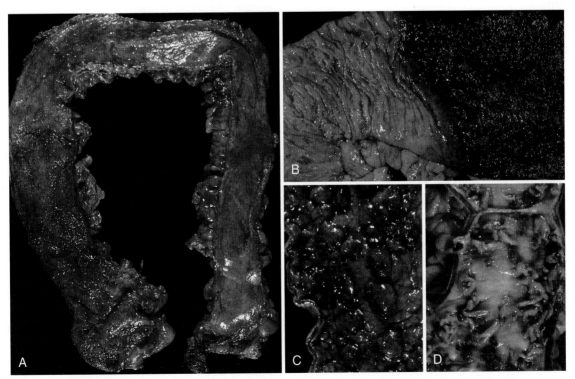

• **Figure 20-6** Gross pathology of acute ulcerative colitis. **A,** Total colectomy shows active pancolitis with red, granular mucosa in the cecum *(left)* and smooth, atrophic mucosa distally *(right)*. **B,** Sharp demarcation between active ulcerative colitis *(right)* and normal mucosa *(left)*. **C,** Inflammatory polyps. **D,** Mucosal bridges. (From Kumar V, Abbas AK, Aster JC. *Robbins and Cotran Pathologic Basis of Disease.* 9th ed. Philadelphia: Saunders; 2015.)

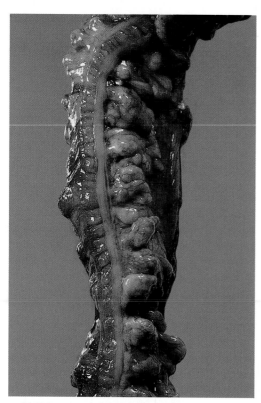

• **Figure 20-7** Diverticulosis of the sigmoid colon. (From Cooke RA, Stewart B. *Colour Atlas of Anatomical Pathology.* 3rd ed. Sydney, Australia: Churchill Livingstone, 2004.)

increased fat in the stool, which is indicative of malabsorption. High fecal fat content supports the diagnosis of malabsorption.

Imaging techniques such as endoscopy, upper and lower GI radiography, and endoscopic retrograde pancreatography may also be used for diagnosis.

Diverticulosis and Diverticulitis

A small pouch in the lining of the large intestine that bulges outward is called a diverticulum (Fig. 20-7), and multiple pouches are called diverticula. This condition is called diverticulosis. About half of all people older than 60 years of age have diverticulosis. When the pouches become inflamed, the condition is called diverticulitis. Diverticulosis and diverticulitis together are called diverticular disease.

Diagnostic Tests for Diverticulosis and Diverticulitis

There are two primary tests for diverticulitis and diverticulosis. An elevated white blood cell count can detect the infection or inflammation of diverticulitis. Diverticulosis is best visualized by a CT scan; sometimes the outward pouching can be seen on a radiograph if inflammation is present as well.

Steatorrhea

Steatorrhea is the presence of excess fat in stools, usually associated with a greasy or oily appearance of the stools. It can be caused by lack of pancreatic enzymes, pancreatitis,

malabsorption, celiac disease, cystic fibrosis, bacterial overgrowth in the bowel, a decrease in bile acids, certain medications, or abnormal mucosal cells. Fecal fat analysis is usually the best test used for diagnosis of steatorrhea.

Tropical Sprue and Celiac Sprue

Tropical sprue is a bacterial condition seen in residents of, or visitors to, tropical areas. An infection or overgrowth of bacteria in the small intestine causes an inflammatory state leading to malabsorption. Celiac sprue or celiac disease is an autoimmune disease in which the body produces antibodies to gluten (a component of wheat, barley, rye, and oats); this results in an inflammatory state leading to malabsorption. Although both diseases are called "sprue," they have different etiologies, require different diagnostic tests for diagnosis, and have different treatment regimens. Tropical sprue is treated with antibiotics, and celiac disease is avoided through a gluten-free diet.

Diagnostic Testing for Tropical Sprue and Celiac Sprue

A history of living in or visiting tropical regions for a prolonged period is key to diagnosing tropical sprue. Signs and symptoms associated with ingestion of gluten-containing foods are the key to the diagnosis of celiac disease. The gold standard for diagnosing both diseases is a biopsy of the small intestine, which is usually performed during endoscopy. Celiac disease shows flattening of the intestinal villi (Fig. 20-8), and tropical sprue shows lesions accompanying villi flattening. However, because of the invasive nature of a biopsy, the diagnosis may be based on patient history, stool culture, and serologic tests.

Gastrointestinal Function Tests

Fecal Fat

Fat is normally reabsorbed back into the body, but fat malabsorption is present in pancreatitis, cystic fibrosis, celiac disease, and intestinal bacterial overgrowth syndrome. Both qualitative and quantitative fecal fat measurements are useful for diagnosis. In the fecal fat screening test, a microscope is used to examine a stool sample mix with Sudan III stain to look for fat globules. Quantitative measurements use a 72-hour stool collection. The stool is well mixed and then analyzed to determine its fat content. The reference range for fecal fat is less than 7 g/day in stool.

D-Xylose Absorption

The D-xylose absorption test is used to determine whether malabsorption in a patient is caused by intestinal malabsorption or nonintestinal causes. D-Xylose is a monosaccharide that is easily absorbed in individuals with normal intestinal integrity and can be found in the blood and urine. In those with intestinal impairment (e.g., celiac disease, intestinal bacterial overgrowth), decreased amounts of D-xylose may be seen in the urine.

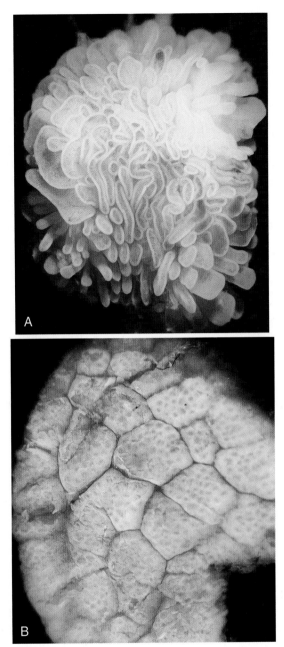

• **Figure 20-8 A,** Normal small intestinal mucosa with villi appearing as fingers and leaves. **B,** Celiac disease produces flat intestinal mucosa with total villus atrophy. (From Cooke RA, Stewart B, *Colour Atlas of Anatomical Pathology.* 3rd ed. Sydney, Australia: Churchill Livingstone, 2004.)

Summary

This chapter began with a GI anatomy and physiology review and a discussion of the primary and accessory organs of the GI tract. The functions of the GI tract include the processes of ingestion, digestion, and absorption of carbohydrates, proteins, and fats. Peptic ulcers may be caused by *H. pylori* infection. Zollinger-Ellison syndrome produces gastrinomas in the pancreas or duodenum that may become malignant. IBD comprises Crohn disease and ulcerative colitis. Infectious agents are often responsible for acute or chronic diarrhea. Blood tests are available for detection of mineral and vitamin deficiencies related to malabsorption. Diverticulitis is an infection of the diverticula. Celiac disease can be prevented in susceptible individuals by a gluten-free diet, whereas tropical sprue is treated with antibiotics. Steatorrhea results from excessive fat in the stool. The D-xylose test is used to differentiate maldigestion from malabsorption.

Review Questions

1. Which of the following organs is the site of bile storage?
   a. Pancreas
   b. Duodenum
   c. Liver
   d. Gallbladder

2. Which of the following cell types secrete hydrochloric acid in the stomach?
   a. Chief cells
   b. Mucosal cells
   c. S cells
   d. Parietal cells

3. Trypsinogen, cholecystokinin, and peptidase are all involved in the digestion of
   a. Fats
   b. Proteins
   c. Lipids
   d. Carbohydrates

4. All of the following tests are associated with the detection of *Helicobacter pylori* EXCEPT
   a. Serologic tests
   b. Urease breath tests
   c. Histologic slides
   d. Fecal fat

5. Which of the following diseases is associated with the formation of gastrin-producing tumors?
   a. *Helicobacter pylori* disease
   b. Zollinger-Ellison syndrome
   c. Pancreatitis
   d. Tropical sprue

6. Bacterial infections, parasite infections, laxative use, colon cancer, and polyps are all possible causes of
   a. Inflammatory bowel disease
   b. Chronic diarrhea
   c. Malabsorption
   d. Acute diarrhea

7. Which of the following is the best test to differentiate ulcerative colitis from Crohn disease?
   a. Sigmoidoscopy
   b. Colonoscopy
   c. Complete blood count
   d. Pancreatic elastase 1

8. Which of the following statements concerning celiac disease is *not* true?
   a. The intestinal villi are flattened.
   b. Antibiotics usually help cure this condition.
   c. Anti-transglutaminase levels and anti-endomysial antibodies are usually diagnostic.
   d. Removal of gluten from the diet usually helps slow or stop this disease.

9. In malabsorption, all of the following blood measurements are likely to be low EXCEPT
   a. Iron level
   b. Prothrombin time
   c. Folate level
   d. Vitamin B_{12} level

10. Which of the following is an infection of the outpouchings of the large intestine?
    a. Diverticulitis
    b. Diverticulosis
    c. Duodenal ulcer
    d. Malabsorption

Critical Thinking Questions

1. Discuss the primary and accessory organs of the GI tract and their functions. Speculate on why the accessory organs are called by that name.

2. Compare and contrast acute and chronic diarrhea with regard to possible causes and the laboratory tests (and results) used for diagnosis.

3. Discuss the difference between malabsorption and maldigestion. Discuss what tests are usually ordered and what tests would be abnormal in both maldigestion and malabsorption.

CASE STUDY

Mr. L., a 21-year-old man of Ukrainian descent, was admitted to the emergency department of a local hospital complaining of recurrent abdominal pain, nausea and vomiting, and rectal bleeding. A colonoscopy demonstrated ulcerations of the ileum and colon consistent with Crohn disease; the ileum was notably stenotic, and only the distal few centimeters could be visualized. A small bowel follow-through study with barium contrast showed that the stenoses and ulcerations extended over the distal 30 cm of the ileum, confirming a diagnosis of Crohn disease. Discuss the laboratory test results that would be abnormal in someone with extensive Crohn disease and why.

Bibliography

Chan FKL, Lau JYW. Peptic ulcer disease. In: Feldman M, Friedman LS, Brandt LJ, eds. *Sleisenger and Fordtran's Gastrointestinal and Liver Disease*. 9th ed. Philadelphia: Saunders Elsevier; 2010: Chapter 53.

Chey WD, Wong BC. American College of Gastroenterology guideline on the management of *Helicobacter pylori* infection. *Am J Gastroenterol*. 2007;102:1808–1825.

Clarke G, Cryan JF, Dinan TG, Quigley EM. Review article: probiotics for the treatment of irritable bowel syndrome—focus on lactic acid bacteria. *Aliment Pharmacol Ther*. 2012;35(4):403–413.

Dickinson B, Surawicz CM. Infectious diarrhea: an overview. *Curr Gastroenterol Rep*. 2014;16(8):1–6.

Erickson RH, Kim YS. Digestion and absorption of dietary protein. *Ann Rev Med*. 1990;41(1):133–139.

Gray GM. Carbohydrate absorption and malabsorption. In: Green M, Greene HL, eds. *The Role of the Gastrointestinal Tract in Nutrient Delivery. Bristol-Myers Nutrition Symposia*. Vol. 3 (Moore JL, series ed.) Orlando, FL: Academic Press; 1984:133–144 .

Hawker P, Sinha R. Overview of medical management of Crohn's disease. In: Rajesh A, Sinha R, eds. *Crohn's Disease: Current Concepts*. Cham, Switzerland: Springer International Publishing; 2015:163–171.

Jeffery IB, O'Toole PW, Öhman L, et al. An irritable bowel syndrome subtype defined by species-specific alterations in faecal microbiota. *Gut*. 2012;61(7):997–1006.

Johnson LR. *Gastrointestinal Physiology*. St. Louis: Elsevier Health Sciences; 2013.

Kergaravat SV, Beltramino L, Garnero N, et al. Magneto immuno-fluorescence assay for diagnosis of celiac disease. *Anal Chim Acta*. 2013;798:89–96.

Lanza FL, Chan FK, Quigley EM. Practice Parameters Committee of the American College of Gastroenterology. Guidelines for prevention of NSAID-related ulcer complications. *Am J Gastroenterol*. 2009;104:728–738.

Lash RH, Genta RM. Gastritis. In: Hawkey CJ, Bosch J, Richter JE, Garcia-Tsao G, Chan FKL, eds. *Textbook of Clinical Gastroenterology and Hepatology*. 2nd ed. Malden, MA: Wiley-Blackwell; 2012:234–247.

Lovell RM, Ford AC. Global prevalence of and risk factors for irritable bowel syndrome: a meta-analysis. *Clin Gastroenterol Hepatol*. 2012;10(7):712–721.

McColl KEL. Helicobacter pylori infection. *N Engl J Med*. 2010; 362:1597–1604.

Mubarak A, Houwen RH, Wolters VM. Celiac disease: an overview from pathophysiology to treatment. *Minerva Pediatr*. 2012;64(3): 271–287.

Munro HN, ed. *Mammalian Protein Metabolism*. Vol. 4. St. Louis: Elsevier; 2012.

National Institute of Diabetes and Digestive and Kidney Diseases. *Celiac disease*. NIH Publication No. 08–4269. Updated January 27, 2012. <http://www.niddk.nih.gov/health-information/health-topics/digestive-diseases/celiac-disease/Pages/facts.aspx> Accessed 08.06.15.

National Institute of Diabetes and Digestive and Kidney Diseases. *Diverticular disease*. NIH Publication No. 13–1163. Updated September 19, 2013. <http://www.niddk.nih.gov/health-information/health-topics/digestive-diseases/diverticular-disease/Pages/facts.aspx> Accessed 08.06.15.

Noto JM, Peek Jr RM. Helicobacter pylori: an overview. In: Houghton J, ed. *Helicobacter Species: Methods and Protocols. Methods in Molecular Biology*. Vol. 921. New York: Humana Press; 2012:7–10.

Schiller RL, Sellin JH. Diarrhea. In: Feldman M, Friedman LS, Brandt LJ, eds. *Sleisenger and Fordtran's Gastrointestinal and Liver Disease*. 9th ed. Philadelphia: Saunders Elsevier; 2010. Chapter 15.

Schubert ML. Gastric physiology. In: Reinus JF, Simon D, eds. *Gastrointestinal Anatomy and Physiology: The Essentials*. Hoboken, NJ: John Wiley & Sons; 2014:58–77.

Semrad CE, Powell DW. Approach to the patient with diarrhea and malabsorption. In: Goldman L, Ausiello D, eds. *Cecil Medicine*. 23rd ed. Philadelphia: Saunders; 2007. Chapter 143.

Soll AH, Vakil NB. Peptic ulcer disease: genetic, environmental, and psychological risk factors and pathogenesis. In: Feldman M, ed. *UpToDate. Alphen aan den Rijn*. The Netherlands: Wolters Kluwer; 2013.

Verburgh P, Reintam-Blaser A, Kirkpatrick AW, De Waele JJ, Malbrain MLNG. Overview of the recent definitions and terminology for acute gastrointestinal injury, intra-abdominal hypertension and the abdominal compartment syndrome. *Réanimation*. 2014;23(2):379–393.

Wilder–Smith CH, Materna A, Wermelinger C, Schuler J. Fructose and lactose intolerance and malabsorption testing: the relationship with symptoms in functional gastrointestinal disorders. *Aliment Pharmacol Ther*. 2013;37(11):1074–1083.

21

Diseases of the Liver

DONNA LARSON

CHAPTER OUTLINE

OBJECTIVES

After completion of this chapter, the reader will be able to:

1. List the anatomy of the liver and the biliary system.
2. Discuss the liver's role in the metabolism of carbohydrates, proteins, and lipids.
3. Explain the liver's role in the excretion of metabolic products such as ammonia and urea.
4. Discuss the major functions of the liver including synthesis of proteins, bile, and coagulation factors; detoxification and metabolism of porphyrins; and storage of various compounds.
5. Compare and contrast the terms direct bilirubin, indirect bilirubin, total bilirubin, conjugated bilirubin, and unconjugated bilirubin.
6. Compare and contrast Gilbert syndrome, Crigler-Najjar syndrome, and Dubin-Johnson syndrome.
7. Define and describe hyperbilirubinemia, jaundice, and kernicterus.
8. Discuss the causes of hepatitis and the difference between acute and chronic hepatitis.
9. List the various types of hepatitis, how they are transmitted, and how each of them is accurately diagnosed using laboratory methods.
10. Analyze the laboratory test results of ferritin, serum iron, and transferrin saturation with regard to hemochromatosis.
11. Identify the causes of Wilson disease and describe the disease mechanisms and tests used to diagnose this condition.
12. Describe the disease mechanisms of liver cirrhosis, which diseases lead to cirrhosis of the liver, and the tests that are used to diagnose cirrhosis.
13. Define and distinguish between cirrhosis and liver failure.
14. Discuss alcohol- and drug-induced liver disease and summarize the tests that best diagnose these conditions.
15. Discuss what liver cancer is, the normal progression of liver disease, and how liver cancer is diagnosed.
16. Identify the consequences of α_1-antitrypsin deficiency and explain how to diagnose this condition.

KEY TERMS

Alanine transaminase (ALT)
Albumin
Alkaline phosphatase (ALP)
α_1-Antitrypsin
α-Fetoprotein
Ascites
Aspartate transaminase (AST)
Bilirubin
Ceruloplasmin

Cirrhosis
Conjugated bilirubin
Copper levels
Coproporphyrin
Cystic duct
Cytochrome P-450
Deamination of amino acids
Ferritin
Fibrosis

γ-Glutamyl transferase (GGT)
Gilbert syndrome
Globulin
Gluconeogenesis
Glucoronyl transferase
Glycogenesis
Glycogenolysis
Haptoglobin
Hemochromatosis

Hemopexin
Hepatic artery
Hepatic duct
Hepatic encephalopathy
Hepatic portal vein
Hepatitis
Hepatomegaly

Hereditary hemochromatosis
Hyperbilirubinemia
Jaundice
Kernicterus
Liver biopsy
Liver enzymes
Liver failure

Porphyria
Porphyrin
Prothrombin time
Transferrin saturation
Transferrin
Unconjugated bilirubin
Wilson disease

❖ Case in Point

A 54-year-old Hispanic man with fatigue, diarrhea, and a fever suspected he had the flu, so he stayed home and rested for a few days. His symptoms continued for more than a week, so he decided to see his provider. He told his physician about his symptoms and that his stools were a lighter color than usual. The provider examined him and thought that his sclerae appeared a bit yellow. His liver function and bilirubin tests showed the following:

Total bilirubin, 5 mg/dL
AST, 350 IU/L
ALT, 450 IU/L

What is the probable condition? What tests would be ordered next? Why?

Points to Remember

- The functions of the liver include the metabolism of many substances; synthesis of bile, proteins, and clotting factors; detoxification; excretion of waste products; and storage of various substances.
- Bile is synthesized in the liver, stored in the gallbladder, and used in digestion of lipids.
- Insulin and glucagon are the two hormones secreted by the pancreas that control hepatic carbohydrate metabolism.
- The two phases of liver detoxification are through cytochrome P-450 and the conjugation pathway.
- Glycogen, iron, lipids, and vitamins are stored in the liver.
- Ammonia, a toxic end product of metabolism, is converted to urea in the liver.
- The accumulation of bilirubin may cause jaundice, which is yellowing of eyes or skin.
- Kernicterus, a syndrome seen in newborn babies, occurs when very high amounts of unconjugated bilirubin cross the blood–brain barrier and can do irreparable damage to brain tissue.
- Gilbert syndrome, Crigler-Najjar syndrome, and Dubin-Johnson syndrome are inherited forms of hyperbilirubinemia.
- Hepatitis, or inflammation of the liver, is caused by chemicals, trauma, drugs, and viruses such as cytomegalovirus, Epstein-Barr virus, and hepatitis A, B, C, D, and E viruses.
- Hepatitis B and C are the most serious types of viral hepatitis because of the incidence of serious complications such as cirrhosis. They are transmitted through the exchange of blood and body fluids.
- The blood tests that are most commonly used to detect liver damage are alanine transaminase (ALT), aspartate transaminase (AST), alkaline phosphatase, γ-glutamyl transferase (GGT), and bilirubin levels.
- Bilirubin is a breakdown product of hemoglobin that is conjugated (attached to glucoronic acid) in the liver.
- In the laboratory, conjugated bilirubin is called direct bilirubin, and unconjugated bilirubin is called indirect bilirubin. Indirect bilirubin plus direct bilirubin equals total bilirubin.
- Cirrhosis is end-stage liver disease accompanied by fibrosis, scarring, and loss of organ function.
- Liver biopsy is the gold standard for diagnosis of cirrhosis, but it is not often done in cases of suspected end-stage liver disease because of the risk of hemorrhage.
- Alcohol is the leading cause of liver disease in the Western world; it often results in fatty liver, hepatitis, and cirrhosis.
- Drug-induced liver disease can be caused by hypersensitivity reactions of the liver to a drug or reactions of the liver to the toxic metabolite of the drug.
- Hemochromatosis is caused by an autosomal recessive genetic defect that causes abnormally high absorption of iron from the gastrointestinal tract and iron deposition in the liver and other organs.
- Wilson disease is an autosomal recessive defect of copper metabolism that causes excessive deposition of copper in the liver and subsequent fibrosis and cirrhosis of the liver.
- Liver cancer is diagnosed via liver biopsy.
- α_1-Antitrypsin deficiency leads to failure to block the effects of neutrophil elastase and may manifest as lung or liver disease.

Introduction

This chapter explores the normal structure and function of the liver and biliary system, disease mechanisms, and the laboratory diagnosis of hepatobiliary disease. Common heptobiliary diseases are Gilbert disease, Crigler-Najjar syndrome, Dubin-Johnson syndrome, acute and chronic

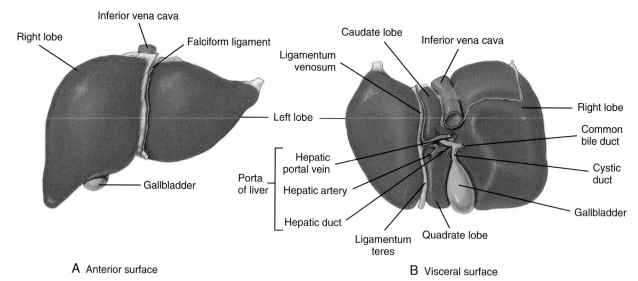

A Anterior surface　　　　　　　　　　　　　　　B Visceral surface

• **Figure 21-1** Anatomy of the liver. (From Applegate EMS: *The Anatomy and Physiology Learning System.* 4th ed. St. Louis: Saunders; 2011.)

hepatitis, end-stage liver disease, cirrhosis, and liver failure. In addition, hereditary diseases of the liver such as Wilson disease, hemochromatosis, and α_1-antitrypsin deficiency are discussed. Finally, an overview of liver cancer and the associated diagnostic tests is presented.

Liver and Biliary Tract

Anatomy

The liver is a triangular organ that is located in the right upper quadrant of the abdominal cavity. It consists of four lobes: left, right, caudate, and quadrate. Two primary sources of blood flow into the liver. Oxygenated blood flows into the liver from the hepatic artery, and nutrient-rich but oxygen-poor blood comes into the liver from the hepatic portal vein. The hepatic duct transports bile out of the liver; it joins with the cystic duct from the gallbladder to empty into the small intestine. The liver is a complex organ that performs many functions that are necessary to the health of the body (Fig. 21-1).

Physiology

Functions of the liver include the metabolism of carbohydrates, lipids, and proteins; production of bile; chemical detoxification; porphyrin catabolism; bilirubin metabolism; and protein synthesis, including albumin, acute phase proteins, and coagulation factors. The liver also is essential in the formation of waste products such as urea and for storage of substances such as glycogen, lipids, and vitamins for use by the body.

Metabolism of Carbohydrates

Carbohydrate metabolism begins with digestion in the mouth, continues into the stomach, and ends in the small intestine, where monosaccharides are absorbed into the

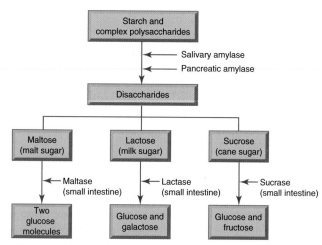

• **Figure 21-2** Carbohydrate digestion. (From Applegate EMS: *The Anatomy and Physiology Learning System.* 4th ed. St. Louis: Saunders; 2011.)

blood (Fig. 21-2). Carbohydrate metabolism and regulation is closely tied to blood glucose levels, which are largely regulated by the liver. The regulation of glucose is influenced by two major hormones, insulin and glucagon, both of which are produced by the pancreas. If the blood glucose concentration is too high, insulin is secreted by the pancreas. Insulin stimulates the transfer of glucose into liver and muscle cells for storage through glyconeogenesis. If blood glucose levels are low, then glucagon is secreted to stimulate the conversion of glycogen to glucose in the liver (glycogenolysis).

In the liver and muscles, most of the glucose is converted into glycogen through glycogenesis, which is an anabolic process. Glycogen is stored in the liver and muscles until the body needs additional glucose. The catabolic process by which glycogen is broken down to glucose, called glycogenolysis, is under the influence of glucagon. Glucagon also stimulates gluconeogenesis, which is the production of glucose from amino acids.

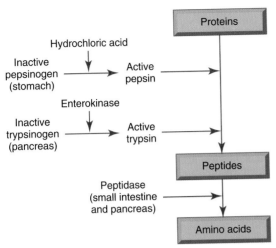

• **Figure 21-3** Protein digestion. (From Applegate EMS: *The Anatomy and Physiology Learning System.* 4th ed. St. Louis: Saunders; 2011.)

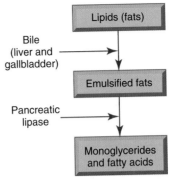

• **Figure 21-4** Lipid digestion. (From Applegate EMS: *The Anatomy and Physiology Learning System.* 4th ed. St. Louis: Saunders; 2011.)

Metabolism of glucose to adenosine triphosphate (ATP) is a primary source of energy in the body. The metabolic process that converts glucose to ATP is called glycolysis. The end products of glycolysis are pyruvic acid and ATP. Pyruvic acid is also converted to acetyl coenzyme A (acetyl CoA), which then enters the citric acid cycle. The citric acid cycle, along with the electron transport chain, produces even more ATP than glycolysis does.

Metabolism of Proteins

Protein regulation and metabolism by the liver takes many forms. The most important functions of the liver in protein metabolism are production of plasma proteins, **deamination of amino acids,** and conversion of amino acids to other compounds useful for the body (Fig. 21-3). Another essential component of protein metabolism in the liver is the formation of waste products such as urea as part of the process of removing toxic metabolites such as ammonia from the body. Almost all plasma proteins are produced by the liver except for immune globulins, which are produced by plasma cells. The liver can produce proteins at a maximum rate of 50 g/day. The loss of plasma proteins causes edema and **ascites** due to the loss of oncotic pressure in the blood vessels.

In addition to production of proteins, the liver also has the ability to produce certain (nonessential) amino acids, and it is the major organ to deaminate amino acids. Deamination is required before the amino acids can be converted into carbohydrates or fats. The deamination process produces metabolic waste products including ammonia, which is toxic to the body; the liver converts ammonia to urea, which is then excreted by the kidney.

Clotting Factors

The liver is the primary site for clotting factor synthesis. The liver also produces proteins involved in the fibrinolytic system, which breaks down blood clots. These clotting factors include both the vitamin K–dependent factors (II, VII, IX, and X) and independent clotting factors. Hemostasis

(clotting and bleeding) abnormalities commonly occur in persons with liver disease. The extent or severity of these abnormalities is related to the severity of liver cell damage.

Metabolism of Lipids

Many types of lipids are stored throughout the body as adipose tissue and serve as a great reserve source of energy to the body. Common lipids include cholesterol, triglycerides, free fatty acids, and phospholipids. Lipids are not soluble in blood, so they are transported throughout the bloodstream as lipoproteins. Most of the lipoproteins, except chylomicrons, are synthesized in the liver. Other roles for the liver in lipid metabolism include the metabolism of fatty acids and triglycerides to produce energy (ATP), the conversion of glycerol into glucose via gluconeogenesis, the conversion of carbohydrates and proteins into fats to be stored as adipose tissue, and the conversion of cholesterol to bile, which is needed for the digestion of fats.

Bile is a yellow-greenish fluid that is produced continuously by the liver. It is concentrated and stored in the gallbladder, then released into the duodenum to aid in fat digestion (Fig. 21-4). Bile is composed of water, bile salts, bilirubin, fatty acids, and cholesterol. Decreased levels of lipids and bile acids are seen as a result of liver disease.

Bilirubin Metabolism

The liver also plays a role in the synthesis and degradation of porphyrins, including heme. Heme, a porphyrin with an iron molecule (Fe^{+2}) at its center, is a major component of hemoglobin, the oxygen carrying analyte in red blood cells (see Fig. 14-6 in Chapter 14).

Heme is formed from δ-aminolevulinic acid (from glycine) and succinyl CoA from the citric acid cycle. **Porphyrias** are caused by defects in heme synthesis. The liver also plays a major role in the degradation of hemoglobin. Hemoglobin is degraded to biliverdin and then to unconjugated bilirubin. The bilirubin is conjugated with glucoronic acid in the liver, which makes it more soluble in water and more easily excreted by the body (Fig. 21-5).

High amounts of unconjugated bilirubin may accumulate in the body and cause cell damage, especially in the central nervous system. The sum of **conjugated bilirubin**

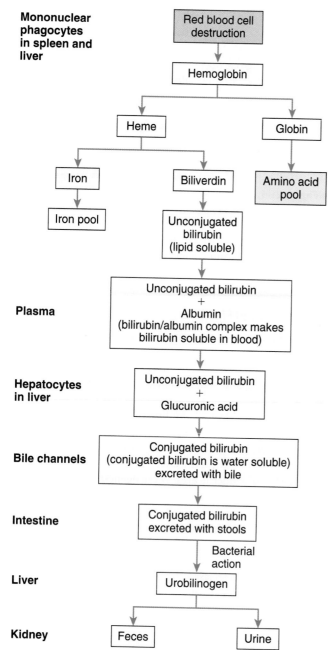

Mononuclear phagocytes in spleen and liver

Plasma

Hepatocytes in liver

Bile channels

Intestine

Liver

Kidney

• **Figure 21-5** Bilirubin metabolism. (From McCance KL, Huether SE. *Pathophysiology: The Biologic Basis for Disease in Adults and Children.* 7th ed. St. Louis: Mosby; 2015.)

(i.e., bilirubin attached to glucoronic acid, also called *direct bilirubin*) and unconjugated bilirubin (also called *indirect bilirubin*) equals total bilirubin.

The Fe^{+2} released from the heme molecule during hemoglobin metabolism is also stored in the liver. The liver synthesizes proteins that help in the transport and storage of iron and heme. These include haptoglobin, transferrin, and hemopexin. Haptoglobin binds free hemoglobin that is released during red blood cell hemolysis. Transferrin transports iron, and hemopexin binds heme after breakdown of the hemoglobin molecule. In addition to storing iron, the liver is also known to store the fat-soluble vitamins D, E, A, and K, as well as glycogen.

Detoxification in the Liver

The liver is the major organ of the body involved in detoxification. Detoxification takes place through two pathways in the liver. Phase I detoxification, also called the cytochrome P-450 pathway, is a pathway of oxidation reduction and hydrolysis that is catalyzed by specific enzymes found in hepatocyte membranes. This pathway is used to convert a toxic chemical to a less toxic form. The process of phase I detoxification creates free radicals which may cause damage to cells if they are not neutralized.

The second pathway, or phase II detoxification, is called the conjugation pathway. In this pathway, the liver adds a chemical group to the toxic chemical, making it less harmful. Often, the toxic chemical becomes more water soluble because of this process and is more easily excreted from the body. Examples of chemical groups that may be added to toxic chemical are glucuronic acid, sulfates, and amino acids.

Liver Diseases

Gilbert Syndrome

Gilbert syndrome is a genetic liver disease caused by reduced activity of the enzyme glucoronyl transferase, which conjugates bilirubin to a water-soluble form. It is the most common cause of hereditary hyperbilirubinemia, with a prevalence of 5% to 10% in the general population. Although there is a higher level of unconjugated bilirubin in the blood of people with this condition, there usually are no serious consequences because 30% of normal enzymatic activity remains. The most common sign of Gilbert disease is jaundice. The disease is usually detected accidently through laboratory evaluation for other pathologies or routine blood work. Values for total bilirubin and unconjugated bilirubin are usually mildly to moderately elevated. Glucoronyl transferase levels are low in this disease.

Crigler-Najjar Syndrome

Crigler-Najjar syndrome type I is a rare autosomal recessive trait in which bilirubin cannot be conjugated into its water-soluble form due to complete absence of the enzyme glucoronyl transferase. This leads to severe unconjugated bilirubinemia and kerniticus. Type I is more serious and potentially life-threatening because the unconjugated (indirect) bilirubin, which is not water soluble, collects in the liver, the spleen, and eventually the central nervous system, causing tissue damage. Liver enzyme results are normal, with low levels of albumin and a total bilirubin level of 20 to 50 mg/dL.

Patients with Crigler-Najjar syndrome type II, an autosomal dominant trait, have decreased levels of glucuronyl transferase that lead to chronic bilirubinemia. Test results for type II include normal liver function tests and a total bilirubin level of 7 to 20 mg/dL. Glucoronyl transferase levels are absent in type I and decreased in type II.

Dubin-Johnson Syndrome

Dubin-Johnson syndrome is an autosomal recessive genetic defect that causes a conjugated bilirubinemia. A result of this defect is that bilirubin is not transported efficiently out of the hepatocytes into the bile. The major sign of this condition, and often the only sign, is jaundice, which usually appears during early adolescence. Some people also experience other signs and symptoms such as upper abdominal pain, anorexia, nausea, or vomiting. Patients with Dubin-Johnson syndrome are known to have characteristic dark pigmentation in their liver and an unusual pattern of urinary porphyrin excretion. Laboratory diagnosis includes liver biopsy, elevated serum bilirubin levels, and urinary coproporphyrin levels that show a unique excretion pattern.

Hyperbilirubinemia, Jaundice, and Kernicterus

Hyperbilirubinemia and jaundice in an adult has two primary causes: excess bilirubin production and liver damage. Excess bilirubin production is caused by increased red blood cell destruction, which releases a large amount of unconjugated bilirubin. Bilirubin travels to the liver to become conjugated, producing an excess in both conjugated (direct) and unconjugated (indirect) bilirubin.

Jaundice is the yellow color seen in the skin and eyes. In newborns, jaundice occurs when bilirubin builds up in an infant's blood, causing hyperbilirubinemia. During pregnancy, the mother's liver conjugates the fetal bilirubin to a water-soluble form and removes it for the baby. However, after birth, the infant's liver must remove the bilirubin. In some infants, the amount of bilirubin produced may overcome the capacity of the newborn liver to remove it. This can be caused by excessive red blood cell hemolysis (as in hemolytic disease of the newborn) or by other liver abnormalities. When too much bilirubin builds up in an infant's blood, jaundice develops, and the skin and sclerae appear yellow. Yellowing of the skin is difficult to detect in darker-skinned infants (and adults) of all nationalities. Because of the difficulty in diagnosing jaundice by skin color, the sclerae are used to detect jaundice.

If severe jaundice goes untreated in an infant, it can cause a condition called kernicterus. Kernicterus is a type of brain damage that results from hyperbilirubinemia in an infant. Bilirubin is toxic to brain cells and easily crosses the blood–brain barrier to damage brain cells.

The second cause for hyperbilirubinemia in adults is liver damage. The damage can prevent the flow of bilirubin through the blood vessels of the liver, causing it to pool and then spill into the circulation. This process increases levels of conjugated (direct) bilirubin in the blood. Sequential laboratory test results reveal a pattern showing increases in unconjugated (indirect) bilirubin and total bilirubin followed by increases in direct bilirubin. Liver disease is associated with increases in direct and total bilirubin during the early disease process; as the disease progresses toward liver failure, the indirect bilirubin level increases as well.

Diagnosis of Hyperbilirubinemia, Jaundice, and Kernicterus

Hyperbilirubinemia is diagnosed through blood tests, jaundice is diagnosed by clinical observation, and kernicterus is diagnosed through clinical symptoms.

In liver disease, conjugated (direct) bilirubin enters the bloodstream in high amounts due to blockage of its normal flow through the liver. Detectable levels of all forms of bilirubin increase as liver damage progresses.

Several methods are used to measure bilirubin. Total bilirubin is measured by enzymatic methods and spectrophotometry. The commonly used Jendrassik and Grof method is based on a colorimetric chemical (diazo) reaction. In the diazo test, 3,5-dicholorphenyldiazonium tetrafluoroborate (DPD) reacts with bilirubin to form azobilirubin:

$$\text{Bilirubin} + \text{DPD} \xrightarrow[\text{Sodium benzoate}]{\text{caffeine}} \text{Azobilirubin}$$

Azobilirubin absorbs light at 570/660 nm, and the absorbance is directly proportional to the bilirubin concentration in the sample. A serum blank is run to eliminate serum interferences.

Another method used to measure total bilirubin is an enzymatic method. Bilirubin is oxidized with bilirubin oxidase to biliverdin and molecular oxygen. At a pH of 8 in the presence of sodium cholate and sodium dodecylsulfate, all four bilirubin fractions are oxidized to biliverdin. Biliverdin is further oxidized to a purple product and then to a colorless product. The total bilirubin concentration is then directly proportional to the decrease in absorbance at 425 or 460 nm.

Only conjugated bilirubin is excreted in urine. Chemical dipsticks use a diazo reagent to detect urine bilirubin at a concentration as low as 0.5 mg/dL. If a bilirubin test on urine cannot be performed immediately, the specimen must be protected from light. Light breaks down the bilirubin, leading to a falsely decreased bilirubin test result.

Hepatitis

Hepatitis is an inflammation of the liver. Hepatitis can be caused by viruses, bacteria, toxic chemicals, drugs, or excess alcohol. There are five distinct hepatitis viruses: A, B, C, D, and E. Cytomegalovirus and Epstein-Barr virus also cause hepatitis. Hepatitis was known in classical Greece, but it was not identified as specific disease until the 19th century. Hepatitis A (HAV) and hepatitis B (HBV) were identified as different diseases during World War II. Hepatitis D (HDV) was recognized in 1977. Although HAV and HBV could be identified in units of blood, transfusion-related cases of hepatitis persisted. These cases were caused by other viruses and were designated *non-A, non-B hepatitis.* In the 1980s, the non-A, non-B hepatitis viruses was identified as hepatitis C (HCV) and hepatitis E (HEV).

Hepatitis can follow an acute or chronic disease course. Acute hepatitis lasts 6 months or less, whereas chronic hepatitis lasts for longer than 6 months. Because hepatitis affects

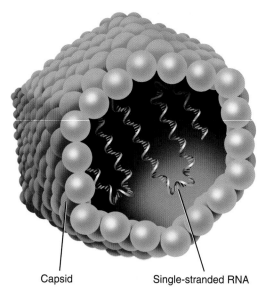

Capsid   Single-stranded RNA

• **Figure 21-6** Hepatitis A virus. (Used with permission of Abbott Laboratories. All rights reserved.)

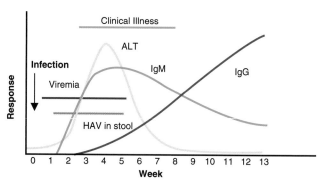

• **Figure 21-7** Time course of hepatitis A virus *(HAV)* infection. *ALT,* Alanine aminotransferase; *IgG,* immunoglobulin G; *IgM,* immunoglobulin M. (Used with permission of Abbott Laboratories. All rights reserved.)

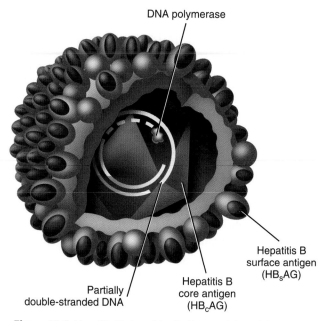

• **Figure 21-8** Hepatitis B virus. (Used with permission of Abbott Laboratories. All rights reserved.)

the liver, which is involved in many metabolic processes, the first symptoms of hepatitis are general. They include fatigue, myalgia, loss of appetite, nausea, diarrhea, constipation, fever, jaundice, chills, weight loss, distaste for food, tea-colored urine, and clay-colored feces. The acute viral hepatitis panel can help a provider distinguish among the different viruses that cause hepatitis. This panel consists of anti-HAV immunoglobulin M (IgM), HB$_s$Ag, anti-HB$_c$ IgM, and anti-HCV (see later discussion). Hepatitis tests are used to screen blood units before transfusion and to evaluate health care personnel (and others) for immunity after HBV vaccination.

Hepatitis A

HAV is a small, single stranded RNA virus (Fig. 21-6). It is transmitted through close person-to-person contact or ingestion of contaminated food or water. Poor personal hygiene or poor sanitation could contribute to the spread of the disease. Children at daycare centers and patients and staff at custodial institutions are at risk for this disease. Once an individual is infected with HAV, the incubation period is 1 to 2 weeks, and symptoms appear suddenly (Fig. 21-7). The risk of spreading HAV infection is greatest during the 2 weeks before symptoms appear. Approximately 70% to 80% of individuals with HAV infection develop jaundice. Good sanitary habits can help prevent infection. The HAV vaccine is available for people who are traveling to endemic areas to help prevent the disease.

Hepatitis B

HBV is a partially double-stranded circular DNA virus. It consists of a central core containing viral DNA and an envelope containing the surface antigen (Fig. 21-8).

Hepatitis B is transmitted by needlesticks with contaminated needles, hemodialysis, transplantation or transfusion of unscreened blood or blood products, acupuncture,

tattooing, body piercing, and sharing of infected razors, as well as by sexual intercourse, perinatally from mother to child, and by contact with infected household objects. In acute hepatitis B, the incubation period is 60 to 90 days with gradual onset of symptoms. Symptoms include anorexia, fatigue, vomiting, abdominal pain, muscle or joint aches, fever, dark urine, skin rashes, and jaundice. Between 30% and 50% of infected individuals develop jaundice. Most adults recover within 6 months and develop antibodies to establish immunity. However, 15% to 25% of those infected with HBV develop chronic liver disease leading to premature death.

Many tests can be performed to appropriately diagnose and monitor HBV infection, including hepatitis B surface antigen (HB$_s$Ag), antibody against the hepatitis B surface antigen (anti-HB$_s$), anti-hepatitis core antigen (anti-HB$_c$), and anti-hepatitis core antigen IgM (anti-HB$_c$ IgM). These tests can be used to monitor seroconversion in two particular instances: Seroconversion from hepatitis B e antigen (HB$_e$Ag) to anti-HB$_e$ indicates progression toward

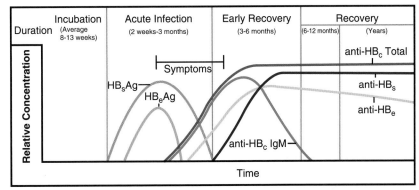

• **Figure 21-9** Acute hepatitis B diagnostic profile, showing the time course for seroconversions. *Ag,* Antigen; *c,* core antigen; *e,* e antigen; *HB,* hepatitis B; *s,* surface antigen; *IgM,* immunoglobulin M. (Used with permission of Abbott Laboratories. All rights reserved.)

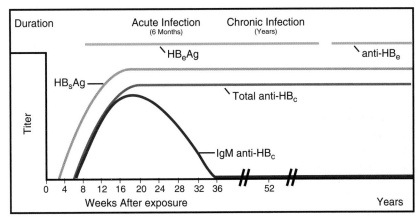

• **Figure 21-10** Progression to chronic hepatitis B virus *(HBV)* infection, showing the typical serologic course. *Ag,* Antigen; *c,* core antigen; *e,* e antigen; *HB,* hepatitis B; *s,* surface antigen; *IgM,* immunoglobulin M. (Used with permission of Abbott Laboratories. All rights reserved.)

resolution of the disease, and seroconversion from HB$_s$Ag to anti-HB$_s$ indicates resolution of the disease (Fig. 21-9).

Chronic hepatitis B occurs when HB$_s$Ag persists in the blood for longer than 6 months. Three markers are used to determine the stage of a chronic infection: HB$_s$Ag, HB$_e$Ag, and anti-HB$_c$ (total). In chronic disease, HB$_s$Ag and anti-HB$_c$ are almost always present. There is a vaccine against HBV and also an HBV immune globulin that can be used as postexposure prophylaxis (Fig. 21-10).

Hepatitis C

HCV is a single, positive-stranded RNA virus with a lipid envelope (Fig. 21-11). It is transmitted by contaminated needlestick, hemodialysis, human bite, transplantation or transfusion of unscreened blood or blood products, acupuncture, tattooing, body piercing, sexual intercourse, perinatally from mother to child, and by contact with infected household products. The clinical course of HCV disease begins with an incubation period of 2 to 26 weeks. The onset is gradual, and 60% to 70% of affected individuals are asymptomatic (Fig. 21-12). Those 30% to 40% with symptoms develop anorexia, malaise, fatigue, abdominal pain,

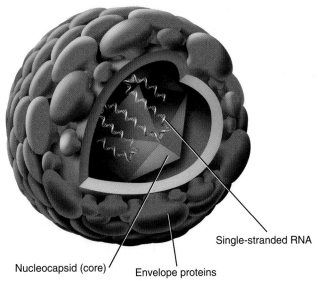

Single-stranded RNA

Nucleocapsid (core) Envelope proteins

• **Figure 21-11** Hepatitis C virus. (Used with permission of Abbott Laboratories. All rights reserved.)

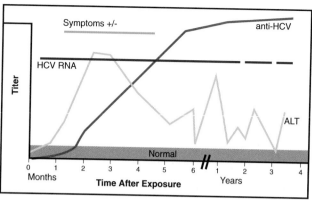

• Figure 21-12 Serologic pattern of acute hepatitis C virus *(HCV)* infection and progression to chronic infection. *ALT,* Alanine aminotransferase. (Used with permission of Abbott Laboratories. All rights reserved.)

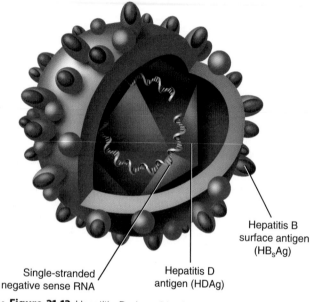

• Figure 21-13 Hepatitis D virus. (Used with permission of Abbott Laboratories. All rights reserved.)

and jaundice. Approximately 60% to 85% of infected individuals develop chronic hepatitis C. Ten to twenty percent of individuals with chronic HCV develop **cirrhosis,** and 1% to 5% develop hepatocellular carcinoma. HCV is the leading reason for liver transplantation in the United States.

Hepatitis C is diagnosed with a positive anti-HCV test. There is no vaccine or immune globulin for this disease. However, pegylated interferon plus ribavirin is the treatment of choice.

Hepatitis D

HDV is a single-stranded RNA virus; its synthesis depends on synthesis of the HB_sAg (Fig. 21-13). HDV cannot infect a person if HBV is not already present. Hepatitis D is transmitted through drug use equipment, transfusion of infected blood or blood products, and sexual intercourse. HDV is a coinfection or a superinfection in individuals already infected by HBV (Figs. 21-14 and 21-15). The incubation period for hepatitis D is 3 to 7 weeks, and the symptoms are the same as for hepatitis B. Approximately 70% to 80% of chronic HBV carriers have an HDV superinfection. Hepatitis D progresses to chronic liver disease with cirrhosis. There is no vaccine for HDV, but because HBV is needed for this virus to replicate and spread, the HBV vaccine will also effectively prevent HDV.

Hepatitis E

HEV is a single-stranded, positive-sense RNA virus and is nonenveloped (Fig. 21-16). Hepatitis E is transmitted enterically through ingestion of contaminated water or food, poor personal hygiene, or person-to-person contact. The clinical course of a HEV infection starts with an incubation period of 15 to 160 days, followed by a sudden onset of symptoms (Fig. 21-17). Symptoms include malaise, anorexia, nausea and vomiting, abdominal pain, and fever. The mortality rate for hepatitis E is 1% to 3 % annually. There is no vaccine or immune globulin.

Table 21-1 compares the characteristics of hepatitis viruses A, B, C, D, and E.

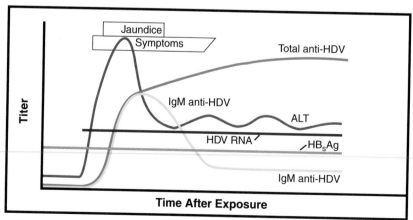

• Figure 21-14 Hepatitis D virus *(HDV)* superinfection of a chronic hepatitis B virus *(HBV)* carrier, showing the typical serologic course. *Ag,* Antigen; *ALT,* alanine aminotransferase; *HB,* hepatitis B; *IgM,* immunoglobulin M; *s,* surface antigen. (Used with permission of Abbott Laboratories. All rights reserved.)

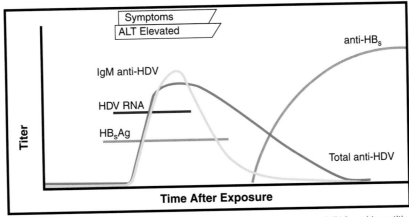

- **Figure 21-15** Typical serologic course with coinfection by hepatitis D virus *(HDV)* and hepatitis B virus *(HBV)*. *Ag,* Antigen; *ALT,* alanine aminotransferase; *HB,* hepatitis B; *IgM,* immunoglobulin M; *s,* surface antigen. (Used with permission of Abbott Laboratories. All rights reserved.)

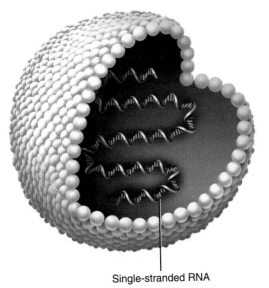

Single-stranded RNA

- **Figure 21-16** Hepatitis E virus. (Used with permission of Abbott Laboratories. All rights reserved.)

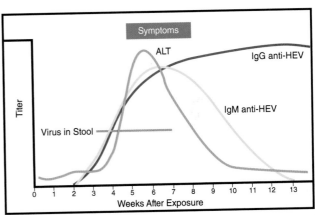

- **Figure 21-17** Hepatitis E virus *(HEV)* infection, showing the typical serologic course. *ALT,* Alanine aminotransferase; *IgG,* immunoglobulin G; *IgM,* immunoglobulin M. (Used with permission of Abbott Laboratories. All rights reserved.)

TABLE 21-1	**Viral Hepatitis Overview**				
Parameter	**Hepatitis A Virus**	**Hepatitis B Virus**	**Hepatitis C Virus**	**Hepatitis D Virus**	**Hepatitis E Virus**
Virus family	*Picornaviridae*	*Hepadnaviridae*	*Flaviviridae*	*Hepadnaviridae*	Not classified
Route of transmission	Fecal-oral route	Percutaneous, permucosal	Percutaneous, permucosal	Percutaneous, permucosal	Fecal-oral (especially contaminated water
Onset	Usually abrupt	Usually insidious	Insidious	Usually abrupt	Usually abrupt
Incubation	15-50 days	Average 60-90 days, range 45-180 days	14-182 days	21-49 days	15-60 days, average 40 days
Chronicity	None	2-10% of everyone ≥5 yr 30-90% of children (0-5 yr)	60-85%	<5% of coinfections ≤80% of superinfections	None reported
Mortality	≤39 yr: ≤0.3% ≥40 yr: 2.1%	0.5-1.0%	10,000-12,000 annually	2-20%	About 1-3%; 15-25% in pregnant women

Laboratory Diagnosis of Viral Hepatitis

Diagnosis of viral hepatitis is best accomplished with various blood tests (Table 21-2), some of which are specific for the diagnosis of liver disease but not specific as to the cause. These analytes include bilirubin and liver enzymes such as alanine transaminase (ALT), aspartate transaminase (AST), alkaline phosphatase (ALP), and γ-glutamyl transferase (GGT). Other blood tests are more specific to the origin of the liver diseases, including antibodies to individual viral antigens (for hepatitis A, B, C, D, and E) and antigens of the viruses themselves (for hepatitis B). With hepatitis B, antibody tests establish a current, chronic, or past infection (Table 21-3). Hepatitis antigen and antibody tests rely on immunoassay or chemiluminescence methodologies.

Recently developed tests include quantitation of the viral genetic material (DNA or RNA) in patients' blood, called the *viral load*. An elevated viral load is associated with a high infectivity potential and a higher potential for advanced liver disease.

Blood Tests

Several enzymes are used in the diagnosis of hepatitis, including ALT, AST, ALP, and GGT (Table 21-4). ALT (formerly known as serum glutamate-pyruvate transaminase [SGPT]) and AST (formerly serum glutamate-oxaloacetate transaminase [SGOT]) are found in various parts of the liver and are released into the bloodstream after liver tissue is damaged. AST is not specific to the liver because it is also found in muscle. More AST than ALT is found in the cytoplasm of the hepatocyte, so the AST level is typically higher than that of ALT in severe hepatocyte injury.

The ALP test actually measures the total activity of a group of isoenzymes that are found in liver, intestine, and placenta. The test is useful in differentiating cholestasis and biliary obstruction from other liver diseases. GGT is considered a liver-specific enzyme. GGT activity is affected by excess alcohol consumption, and enzyme levels are very high in alcohol-induced liver injury.

Liver enzyme test results may alert health care providers that there is an inflammation of the liver, but the diagnosis of hepatitis is made by measurement of specific antigens and antibodies (Table 21-5). Providers use hepatitis B antigen and antibody panels to differentiate an acute from a chronic infection. In acute disease, HB$_s$Ag appears in the blood approximately 1 to 3 months after infection. Anti-HB$_c$ and anti-HB$_s$Ag appear as the disease

TABLE 21-2	Laboratory Diagnosis of Hepatitis A, B, C, D, and E	
Antigen or Antibody Abbreviation	**Antigen or Antibody Name**	**Comments**
HAV IgG	Hepatitis A total antibody	Reflects past infection or immunization
HAV IgM	Hepatitis A IgM	Reflects current infection or infection within the last 6 mo
HB$_s$Ag	Hepatitis B surface antigen	Reflects current infection; a person with a positive HB$_s$Ag result should be considered infectious
Anti-HB$_s$ IgM	Hepatitis B surface antibody	Reflects recent infection (within the last 6 mo)
Anti-HB$_s$ IgG	Hepatitis B surface antibody	Reflects past infection
Anti-HB$_c$ IgM	Hepatitis B Core antibody	Reflects recent infection (within the last 6 mo)
Anti-HB$_c$ IgG	Hepatitis B core antibody (total)	Reflects past infection
HB$_e$Ag	Hepatitis B e antigen	Reflects active viral replication and high level of infectiousness
Anti HB$_e$ IgM	Hepatitis B e antibody	Reflects recent infection (within the last 6 mo)
Anti HB$_e$ IgG	Hepatitis B e antibody	Reflects past infection
Anti-HCV	Hepatitis C antibody (total); this is a screening test only	Reflects past or current infection
Anti-HDV	Hepatitis D antibody (total)	Reflects past or current infection
Anti-HEV IgG	Hepatitis E antibody	Reflects past infection

IgG, Immunoglobulin G; *IgM,* immunoglobulin M.

progresses. As antibody levels in the blood increase, the concentration of antigens decreases. This pattern is associated with acute disease, convalescence, and recovery. Conversely, in patients with chronic HBV disease, the level of HB$_s$Ag stays elevated and never decreases. The only detectable antibody in patients with chronic HBV infection is anti-HB$_c$.

Antibodies to hepatitis viruses are used to detect and diagnose hepatitis A, C, D, and E (see Table 21-2). Anti-HB$_s$Ag, anti-HB$_c$, anti-HB$_c$ IgM, and anti-HB$_c$ are used to diagnose acute and chronic HBV infections. Anti-HAV, anti-HCV, anti-HDV, and anti-HEV are used to diagnose infection with hepatitis viruses other than HBV. IgM antibodies are used to diagnose recent infection (current or within the last several months), and IgG antibodies are used to indicate past (greater than several months) infection. Only hepatitis B has both IgM and IgG tests that help distinguish between current and past infection. The methodologies used for these antibody tests include immunoassays and chemiluminescence.

Hereditary Hemochromatosis

Hereditary hemochromatosis is an autosomal recessive genetic disease that causes an abnormal accumulation of iron in organs, leading to organ injury and toxicity. It is the most common form of iron overload (hemochromatosis). Approximately 75% of patients with hereditary hemochromatosis are asymptomatic, and many are diagnosed when a routine laboratory test (e.g., an iron level) is abnormal or a relative is diagnosed with the disease. Early symptoms of include fatigue, impotence, and arthralgia. However, it takes time before iron deposition in organs causes injury, and usually many years of iron accumulation have occurred before an individual seeks medical attention. At presentation, these individuals have hepatomegaly, skin pigmentation, and arthritis.

Hereditary hemochromatosis is usually diagnosed when there is iron-induced end-organ injury and the individual becomes symptomatic. The clinical manifestations are liver disease (including elevated liver enzymes), skin hyperpigmentation, diabetes mellitus (insulin resistance and impaired insulin secretion), arthropathy, amenorrhea, hypogonadism, cardiomyopathy, osteopenia, osteoporosis, hair loss, and spoon nails. As the disease progresses, cirrhosis and hepatocellular carcinoma

TABLE 21-3 Patterns of Results of Common Laboratory Tests for Hepatitis B

Test	Result	Interpretation of Pattern
HB$_s$Ag Anti-HB$_c$ Anti-HB$_s$	Negative Negative Negative	Susceptible
HB$_s$Ag Anti-HB$_c$ Anti-HB$_s$	Negative Positive Positive	Immune due to natural infection
HB$_s$Ag Anti-HB$_c$ Anti-HB$_s$	Negative Negative Positive	Immune to hepatitis B vaccine
HB$_s$Ag Anti-HB$_c$ Anti-HB$_c$ IgM Anti-HB$_s$	Positive Positive Positive Negative	Acutely infected
HB$_s$Ag Anti-HB$_c$ Anti-HB$_c$ IgM Anti-HB$_s$	Positive Positive Negative Negative	Chronically infected
HB$_s$Ag Anti-HB$_c$ Anti-HB$_s$	Negative Positive Negative	Unclear (four possibilities): Resolved infection (most common) False positive (anti-HB$_c$), thus susceptible "Low-level" chronic infection Resolving acute infection

Ag, Antigen; *HB$_c$,* hepatitis B core antigen; *HB$_s$,* hepatitis B surface antigen; *IgM,* immunoglobulin M.

TABLE 21-4 Laboratory Results for Various Liver and Biliary Tract Diseases

Condition	AST	ALT	ALP	GGT	Total Bilirubin (mg/dL)
Gilbert disease	N	N	N	N	1-5
Crigler-Najjar I	N	N	N	N	20-50
Crigler-Najjar II	N	N	N	N	7-20
Acute hepatitis	500-5000 IU/L	1000-5000 IU/L	N	N	>30
Alcoholic hepatitis	<300 IU/L	N	N	100-500 IU/L	>30
Biliary obstruction	N	N	>200 IU/L	100-500 IU/L	>30
Cirrhosis	N	N	N	N	1-5

ALP, Alkaline phosphatase; *ALT,* alanine aminotransferase; *AST,* aspartate aminotransferase; *GGT,* γ-glutamyl transferase; *N,* normal.

TABLE 21-5 Common Liver Function Tests

Test	Normal Value	Interpretation
Serum Enzymes		
Alkaline phosphatase (ALP)	13-39 U/L	Increases with biliary obstruction and cholestatic hepatitis
γ-Glutamyl transpeptidase (GGT)	Male 12-38 U/L Female 9-31 U/L	Increases with biliary obstruction and cholestatic hepatitis
Aspartate aminotransferase (AST)	5-40 U/L	Increases with hepatocellular injury and injury in other tissues (i.e., skeletal and cardiac muscle)
Alanine aminotransferase (ALT)	5-35 U/L	Increases with hepatocellular injury and necrosis
Lactate dehydrogenase (LDH)	90-220 U/L	Isoenzyme LD_5 is elevated with hypoxic and primary liver injury
5'-Nucleotidase	2-11 U/L	Increases with increase in ALP and in cholestatic disorders
Bilirubin Metabolism		
Serum bilirubin		
Unconjugated (indirect)	<0.8 mg/dL	Increases with hemolysis (lysis of red blood cells)
Conjugated (direct)	0.2-0.4 mg/dL	Increases with hepatocellular injury or obstruction
Total	<1.0 mg/dL	Increases with biliary obstruction
Urine bilirubin	0	Increases with biliary obstruction
Urine urobilinogen	0-4 mg/24 hr	Increases with hemolysis or shunting of portal blood flow
Serum Proteins		
Albumin	3.5-5.5 g/dL	Reduced with hepatocellular injury
Globulin	2.5-3.5 g/dL	Increases with hepatitis
Total	6-7 g/dL	
Albumin/globulin (A/G) ratio	1.5:1 to 2.5:1	Ratio reverses with chronic hepatitis or other chronic liver disease
Transferrin	250-300 µg/dL	Liver damage with decreased values, iron deficiency with increased values
α-Fetoprotein (AFP)	6-20 ng/mL	Elevated values in primary hepatocellular carcinoma
Blood-Clotting Functions		
Prothrombin time (PT)	11.5-14 sec or 90-100% of control	Increases with chronic liver disease (cirrhosis) or vitamin K deficiency
Partial thromboplastin time (PTT)	25-40 sec	Increases with severe liver disease or heparin therapy
Bromsulphthalein (BSP) excretion	<6% retention in 45 min	Increased retention with hepatocellular injury

From McCance KL, Huether SE. *Pathophysiology: The Biologic Basis for Disease in Adults and Children.* 7th ed. St. Louis: Mosby; 2015.

can result. Hepatocellular carcinoma is 200 times more common in patients with hereditary hemochromatosis than in the general public.

Disease Mechanisms

Iron plays a very important role in the body, including formation of the molecule hemoglobin. Normally, about 10% of the iron ingested is absorbed and used. Iron is stored in the liver, pancreas, thyroid gland, heart, adrenal glands, kidneys, skin, spleen, and stomach. Excess iron is stored as hemosiderin. The body normally reduces the amount of iron absorbed by the gastrointestinal tract when sufficient stores of iron are in the tissues. In hereditary hemochromatosis, however, a person may absorb as much as three times the normal percentage of ingested iron, storing the excess mostly in liver tissue but also in the pancreas and other organs. Over years, the accumulated iron can severely damage many organs, leading to organ failure and chronic diseases such as cirrhosis.

Affected individuals typically present clinically between 40 and 60 years of age. Females usually present at an older age than males due to natural blood loss during their reproductive years.

Hereditary hemochromatosis causes diabetes mellitus through two separate mechanisms. Excess iron stores are thought to destroy the beta cells in the pancreas, leading to reduced or no production of insulin. Excess iron in the hepatocytes is also thought to cause insulin resistance. Most hereditary hemochromatosis patients with diabetes mellitus are users of injectable insulin.

Diagnosis of Hereditary Hemochromatosis

Hereditary hemochromatosis typically is not diagnosed early because its symptoms are nonspecific. This condition can be mistaken for chronic fatigue, fibromyalgia, or depression. A transferrin saturation level of 70% or greater is diagnostic of hereditary hemochromatosis. Ferritin is also a good marker, because it increases proportionally to increasing iron stores. Ferritin values greater than 400 µg/L in men and 200 µg/L in women require further investigation. Ferritin is usually used to diagnose this disease, and transferrin saturation is used to monitor treatment. Serum iron and serum ferritin values represent free iron and stored iron, respectively. Transferrin saturation represents the percentage of transport protein molecules whose sites are taken up with iron; it is calculated from the serum iron concentration and the total iron-binding capacity (TIBC).

$$\text{Transferrin saturation} (\%) = 100 \times \text{Serum iron/TIBC}$$

A chemistry panel may be ordered primarily to detect elevations in ALT, AST, ALP, and bilirubin (see Table 21-4). These are usually the first enzymes to increase as the liver is damaged. As more damage occurs in the liver, total protein and albumin levels become decreased. Glucose levels are also useful to detect damage to the pancreas from iron deposition.

Three mutations related to hereditary hemochromatosis have been described in the literature, involving the genes *C282Y, H63D,* and *S65C.* Most individuals with this disease are homozygous for *C282Y* or heterozygous with one *C282Y* or *H63D* mutation.

Secondary hemochromatosis can occur with disorders of erythropoiesis and with disease treatment involving blood transfusions.

Wilson Disease

Wilson disease is an autosomal recessive genetic disease of copper metabolism that leads to copper deposition in body tissues. Over time, the accumulation of copper damages the liver, brain, and eyes. Damage to the heart and kidneys may also occur. Brain damage is progressive over time and manifests both as motor disturbances such as ataxia (unstable gait), tremors, and speech difficulties and as cognitive deficiencies such as personality changes, convulsions, and psychiatric changes. Individuals with Wilson disease are often symptomatic with hepatic disturbances before 10 years of age. However, many of these individuals do not seek medical attention. By the time of presentation later in life, the liver is injured and it is too late to reverse the damage. Wilson disease causes acute active hepatitis, cirrhosis, and fulminant liver failure. Individuals usually seek medical treatment when symptoms appear; as a result, laboratory tests such as AST, ALT, GGT, and bilirubin are typically abnormal and indicate hepatitis, cirrhosis, or liver failure. Patients with unexplained chronic hepatitis should be evaluated for Wilson disease. This disease is fatal if it remains untreated.

Fulminant Wilson disease causes neuropsychiatric illness, musculoskeletal symptoms, and renal symptoms in addition to the liver diseases. Neuropsychiatric symptoms include asymmetric tremor, difficulty speaking, excessive salivation, ataxia, personality changes, clumsiness with the hands, spasticity, grand mal seizures, rigidity, and dystonia. Patients with neuropsychiatric symptoms at presentation often have cirrhosis. Psychiatric symptoms include lack of inhibition, impulsiveness, self-injurious behavior, and emotional swings. Musculoskeletal symptoms include osteopenia, premature degenerative arthritis, and joint disease. Renal symptoms include Fanconi syndrome, which involves defective renal acidification and inadequate excretion of amino acids, glucose, fructose, galactose, pentose, uric acid, phosphate, and calcium. Patients may also have kidney stones and hematuria. Finally, fulminant Wilson disease is characterized by hemolysis and low levels of AST, ALT, and ALP.

Disease Mechanisms

The *ATP7B* gene, found on chromosome 13, is abnormal in Wilson disease. Copper is an important cofactor or coenzyme in the body. Copper links to ceruloplasmin in liver cells and is then excreted by the liver into the blood. Liver cells remove excess copper by secreting it into bile. In Wilson disease, the liver's ability to link copper to ceruloplasmin and to excrete copper in bile is impaired. As a result, copper accumulates in the liver, causing oxidative damage to the liver tissue and resulting in acute active hepatitis, cirrhosis, and, ultimately, liver failure. Copper also settles in the cornea of the eye and in kidney and brain tissue. In the eye, the copper deposits in the cornea cause Kayser-Fleischer rings. Copper oxidizes hemoglobin, resulting in red blood cell hemolysis.

Diagnosis of Wilson disease is not accomplished by one particular laboratory test. Instead, serum ceruloplasmin, urinary copper excretion, presence of Kayser-Fleischer rings, and copper in liver tissue establish the diagnosis. Genetic testing may identify a mutation in the *ATP7B* gene. The results of liver function tests (AST, ALT, GGT, and ALP), bilirubin, total protein, and albumin can be very useful for diagnosis. ALT, AST, and ALP may initially be elevated, but levels fall as the liver becomes more and more fibrotic. The conjugated and total bilirubin levels are elevated, and the albumin is likely to be low due to decreased liver function.

Both blood ceruloplasmin and serum copper levels are low in Wilson disease. These levels are quantitated with the use of enzyme immunoassays. Reference ranges for serum copper are 63.7 to 140.12 µg/dL. Almost all individuals with Wilson disease have a ceruloplasmin level lower than 20 mg/dL. The reference range for ceruloplasmin is 20 to 40 mg/dL. The 24-hour urine copper levels are elevated. The rate of excretion of urinary copper is greater than 100 µg/dL. The reference range of urine copper is less than 40 µg/dL. This test is usually used to confirm the diagnosis.

The gold standard for diagnosis of Wilson disease is the liver biopsy, but, as in hemochromatosis and other advanced liver diseases, the risk of bleeding must be assessed before proceeding.

Cirrhosis and Liver Failure

Cirrhosis is end-stage liver disease characterized by scarring of the liver and decreasing ability of the liver to function (Fig. 21-18). It is classified by histology and appearance as micronodular, macronodular, or mixed. It is often the final phase of chronic liver disease that may be associated with chronic hepatitis B or C, alcohol abuse, hemochromatosis, Wilson disease, α1-antitrypsin (AAT) deficiency, and autoimmune hepatitis. Liver failure occurs when large parts of the liver become damaged and are unlikely to be repaired and the liver is no longer able to function. It may occur rarely as an acute condition but most often occurs after many years of chronic liver disease.

Disease Mechanisms

The liver is a complex organ and has many functions in the body. It synthesizes proteins such as albumin, acute phase proteins, and clotting factors. It also plays a major role in the detoxification of drugs, metabolism of carbohydrates

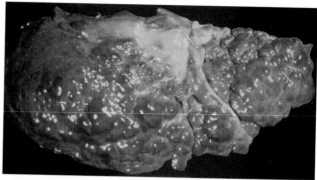

• **Figure 21-18** Cirrhosis resulting from chronic viral hepatitis. Notice the broad scar and the nodular surface. (From Kumar V, Abbas AK, Fausto N, Aster J. *Robbins and Cotran Pathologic Basis of Disease*. 8th ed. Philadelphia: Saunders; 2010.)

and lipids, and storage of many substances (see earlier discussion). The hallmark of cirrhosis is the development of fibrosis or scar tissue that replaces normal liver tissue. This scar tissue not only prevents the normal functioning of the liver but blocks the flow of blood and other substances (e.g., bilirubin) throughout the liver. This results in spillage of bilirubin into the tissues and ascites (the accumulation of fluid in the abdominal cavity). The symptoms of cirrhosis and early liver failure usually include nausea, fatigue, and anorexia. As liver failure progresses, the loss of hepatic function and accumulation of toxic metabolites (especially ammonia) lead to hepatomegaly, petechiae, bleeding, portal hypertension, loss of cognition, disorientation (ammonia-induced hepatic encephalopathy), coma, and death.

Diagnosis of Cirrhosis and Liver Failure

Liver biopsy is used to confirm a diagnosis of cirrhosis. The relevant tests, as discussed earlier, include antigen or antibody tests for hepatitis, serum and urine copper levels and ceruloplasmin levels for Wilson disease, or serum iron and ferritin for hemochromatosis. Imaging tests may also be indicated to detect ascites or to determine the functional status of the liver.

Liver biopsy is considered to be the gold standard for diagnosing cirrhosis. Biopsies involve insertion of a fine needle through the skin between the two lower right ribs into the liver. This test can be risky because there is a danger of excessive hemorrhage (bleeding). If the cirrhosis is advanced and the patient has a low platelet count and low levels of clotting factors, biopsy is not recommended.

Albumin is one of the most important proteins synthesized in the liver. In cirrhosis, decreased albumin synthesis leads to low blood levels. Blood globulin levels can also be low due to decreased synthesis.

The prothrombin time is a clotting test that measures the clotting factors in the extrinsic clotting system. Liver disease leads to low levels of clotting factors because of decreased synthesis in the liver. Prothrombin times in patients with cirrhosis and liver disease are prolonged.

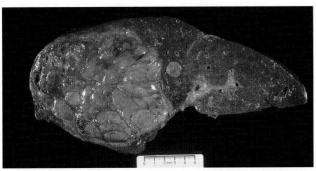

• **Figure 21-19** Hepatocellular carcinoma. A large tumor *(left)* is present in a noncirrhotic liver, with a small metastatic tumor nearby. (From Kumar V, Abbas AK, Fausto N, Aster J. *Robbins and Cotran Pathologic Basis of Disease.* 8th ed. Philadelphia: Saunders; 2010.)

Liver Cancer

Cancer of the liver, or *hepatocellular carcinoma,* is the fifth most common form of cancer in the world. It is also a leading cause of death worldwide. In about one third of cases, individuals have cirrhosis before developing cancer. Major risk factors for liver cancer include chronic infection with HCV, HBV, or both. Hepatocellular carcinoma (Fig. 21-19) occurs more frequently in individuals whose cirrhosis was caused by alcohol abuse, hemochromatosis, AAT, HBV, or HCV. Environmental factors such as tobacco use, arsenic exposure, certain herbicides, and aflatoxins are also implicated in liver cancer.

Liver cancer is diagnosed based on the medical history, physical examination to detect hepatomegaly and jaundice, various imaging techniques, biopsies, and laboratory tests. Laboratory tests help determine the etiology and origin of the tumor and the amount of tissue damage present in the liver. α-Fetoprotein is a tumor marker associated with hepatocellular cancer that can be used for diagnosis and to assess the efficacy of treatment.

α$_1$-Antitrypsin Deficiency

AAT is a serine protease inhibitor that is synthesized in the liver. This enzyme inhibits trypsin as well as other proteolytic enzymes such as neutrophil-derived elastase and proteinase 3. The gene that produces AAT is on chromosome 14. AAT deficiency is an inherited condition. Individuals with this disease develop emphysema at an early age and without a history of smoking. Twenty percent of infants with this disease develop hepatitis, and 25% of those who develop the disease die within 1 year. For infants who survive past 1 year, liver disease is usually nonexistent by age 12. One third to one half of the adults identified with this disease will develop cirrhosis. Because hereditary hemochromatosis was also present in one third of adults with AAT deficiency, the cause of cirrhosis is not clear. As with other liver diseases, cirrhosis can lead to hepatocellular carcinoma. A serum AAT level would be ordered as a screening test, and levels lower than 80 mg/dL suggest the presence of this disease. The reference range for AAT is 100 to 300 mg/dL. Serum AAT is measured by a turbidimetric method. The gold standard for diagnosing AAT deficiency is serum phenotyping by isoelectric focusing.

Summary

The normal functions of the liver and biliary system include metabolism of carbohydrates, lipids, and proteins; synthesis of clotting factors and proteins; storage of numerous compounds; and detoxification and excretion of potentially toxic substances. Disease mechanisms and laboratory diagnosis of hyperbilirubinemia in conditions as such as Gilbert syndrome, Crigler-Najjar syndrome, Dubin-Johnson syndrome, acute and chronic hepatitis, liver cancer, cirrhosis, and liver failure were discussed in this chapter. Hereditary diseases of the liver include Wilson disease, hemochromatosis, and α$_1$-antitrypsin deficiency.

Review Questions

1. Insulin and glucagon are two hormones that play a major role in regulating
   a. Carbohydrate metabolism
   b. Lipid metabolism
   c. Protein metabolism
   d. Porphyrin synthesis
2. Which of the following is *not* a major function of the liver?
   a. Protein synthesis
   b. Production of bile
   c. Production of digestive enzymes
   d. Detoxification
3. All of the following diseases are associated with elevated unconjugated bilirubin EXCEPT
   a. Dubin-Johnson syndrome
   b. Gilbert disease
   c. α$_1$-Antitrypsin deficiency
   d. Crigler-Najjar syndrome
4. Which of the following diseases is a result of chronic scarring of hepatocytes and can be classified as macronodular or micronodular?
   a. Cirrhosis
   b. Jaundice
   c. Hepatitis
   d. Kernicterus
5. A person who is positive for surface antigen, e antigen, and antibodies to surface, core, and e antigen likely has which type of hepatitis?
   a. Hepatitis A
   b. Hepatitis B
   c. Hepatitis C
   d. Hepatitis D

6. High levels of indirect bilirubin, high levels of total bilirubin, and normal levels of direct bilirubin are associated with which of the following conditions?
   a. Gallstones
   b. Red blood cell hemolysis
   c. Hepatitis
   d. Wilson disease

7. An increase in urinary copper but normal or decreased blood copper levels is associated with which of the following conditions?
   a. Hemochromatosis
   b. Wilson disease
   c. Liver failure
   d. Cirrhosis of the liver

8. Which of the following results would likely be associated with primary hemochromatosis?
   a. High serum iron, high ferritin, low transferrin saturation
   b. High serum iron, high serum ferritin, high transferrin saturation
   c. Low serum iron, high ferritin, high transferrin saturation
   d. High serum iron, low serum ferritin, high transferrin saturation

9. Which of the following chemical compounds is converted to urea in the liver and causes encephalopathy with excessive accumulation in brain tissue?
   a. Aspirin
   b. Ammonia
   c. Copper
   d. Iron

10. α-Fetoprotein is used in the diagnosis of which of the following conditions?
    a. Hemochromatosis
    b. Wilson disease
    c. Liver cancer
    d. α$_1$-Antitrypsin deficiency

Critical Thinking Questions

1. Describe the antigens and antibodies that are used for diagnosis in hepatitis B. Differentiate between acute and chronic hepatitis B with regard to presentation, progression of disease, and laboratory results, including antibody results.

2. Describe the many functions associated with the liver. Differentiate between cirrhosis of the liver and liver failure. Speculate on how the functions of the liver may be affected by advanced cirrhosis or liver failure. What changes in ALT, AST, bilirubin, ALP, and GGT levels would be expected in hepatitis compared with liver failure?

CASE STUDY

A 27-year-old male of South American descent is referred to the clinic for evaluation of increased serum aminotransferases (ALT and AST) and bilirubin. Antigen and antibody tests for hepatitis A, B, and C are negative. The patient denies alcohol or drug use of any kind. The patient has noticed a decrease in his ability to concentrate on his graduate school courses over the last year. Liver biopsy suggests an autoimmune hepatitis. The patient denies fevers, chills, nausea, vomiting, gastroesophageal reflux, hematemesis, melena, weight loss, diarrhea, constipation, and change in bowel habits. The family history is noncontributory. Physical examination shows slight hepatomegaly. Serum copper and ceruloplasmin are decreased, but urinary copper is elevated. What is the likely diagnosis?

Bibliography

American Thoracic Society. European Respiratory Society. American Thoracic Society/European Respiratory Society statement: standards for the diagnosis and management of individuals with alpha-1 antitrypsin deficiency. *Am J Respir Crit Care Med.* 2003;168:818–896. <http://www.ers-education.org/lrmedia/2003/pdf/44034.pdf> Accessed 15.06.15.

Bosch FX, Ribes J, Diaz M, Cléries R. Primary liver cancer: worldwide incidence and trends. *Gastroenterology.* 2004;127(5 suppl 1): S5–S16.

Garcia-Tsao G. Cirrhosis and its sequelae. In: Goldman L, Ausiello D, eds. *Cecil Medicine.* 24th ed. Philadelphia: Saunders Elsevier; 2011:Chapter 156.

Grattagliano I, Bonfrate L, Diogo CV, et al. Biochemical mechanisms in drug-induced liver injury: certainties and doubts. *World J Gastroenterol.* 2009;15(39):4865–4876.

Mehta G, Rothstein KD. Health maintenance issues in cirrhosis. *Med Clin North Am.* 2009;93:901–915.

Ostrow JD, ed. *Bile Pigments and Jaundice: Molecular, Metabolic, and Medical Aspects.* Liver: Normal Function and Disease Series; Vol 4. New York: Marcel Dekker; 1986.

Rhoades RA, Bell DR, eds. *Medical Physiology: Principles for Clinical Medicine.* 4th ed. Philadelphia: Lippincott Williams & Wilkins; 2012:Chapter 27.

Rouiller C, ed. *The Liver: Morphology, Biochemistry, Physiology.* New York: Academic Press; 2013.

Sampietro M, Iolascon A. Molecular pathology of Crigler-Najjar type I and II and Gilbert's syndromes. *Haematologica.* 1999;84(2):150–157.

Sherlock S, Dooley J. *Hepatic Cirrhosis. Diseases of the Liver and Biliary System.* 8th ed. Oxford: Blackwell Scientific; 1989:410–424.

Smith Jr LH. Overview of hemochromatosis. *West J Med.* 1990; 153(3):296–308.

Tornheim K, Ruderman NB. Intermediary metabolism of carbohydrate, protein, and fat. In: Ahima RS, ed. *Metabolic Basis of Obesity.* New York: Springer; 2011:25–51.

Zimniak P. Dubin-Johnson and Rotor syndromes: molecular basis and pathogenesis. *Semin Liver Dis.* 1993;13(3):248–260.

22

Pancreatic Diseases and Disorders

DONNA LARSON

CHAPTER OUTLINE

OBJECTIVES

After completion of this chapter, the reader will be able to:

1. Identify the pancreas and describe its function.
2. Compare and contrast acute pancreatitis with chronic pancreatitis.
3. Summarize the disease process in chronic pancreatitis leading to pancreatic failure.
4. Describe the laboratory tests used to diagnose acute pancreatitis.
5. Discuss type 1 diabetes, including symptoms, complications, and pathophysiologic mechanisms.
6. Describe insulin.
7. Describe the metabolic actions of insulin in adipose tissue, muscle, and the liver.
8. Discuss carbohydrate metabolic derangement in type 1 diabetes.
9. Discuss the causes and pathophysiology of hypoglycemia.
10. Describe how ketone bodies are produced.
11. Discuss the clinical significance of ketone bodies.
12. Discuss type 2 diabetes, including symptoms, complications, and pathophysiologic mechanisms.
13. Discuss gestational diabetes, including symptoms, complications, and pathophysiologic mechanisms.
14. List and describe major sequelae and complications of diabetes mellitus.
15. Discuss the factors that determine the blood glucose level.
16. Describe collection and handling of specimens for blood glucose testing, including the additives in the collection tubes and how they affect the specimen.
17. Discuss the hexokinase method for determining glucose, its reference range, and interfering substances.
18. Discuss the glucose oxidase method for determining glucose, its reference range, and interfering substances.
19. Discuss glycohemoglobin, including its definition, use, and appropriate test methods.
20. Discuss the fructosamine test, its reference ranges, and interfering substances.
21. Discuss when the following tests are used, how they are performed, and the necessary patient preparation: fasting blood glucose, 2-hour postprandial blood sugar, 3-hour glucose tolerance test, and 5- or 6-hour glucose tolerance test.
22. Know the normal, mildly abnormal, and severely abnormal glucose tolerance curves.
23. Compare and contrast malabsorption and maldigestion.
24. Explain how pancreatic insufficiency plays a role in maldigestion.
25. Discuss and analyze the tests used to diagnose pancreatic insufficiency.
26. Describe the clinical importance of measuring fecal lipids.
27. Describe the clinical significance of trypsin and chymotrypsin in the stool.
28. Explain the criteria for a diagnosis of chronic diarrhea and identify the common causes for the condition.

KEY TERMS

Acute pancreatitis	Glycohemoglobin	Malabsorption
Amylase	Glyconeogenesis	Maldigestion
Blood glucose levels	Glycosylated hemoglobin	Metabolic syndrome
Cholecystokinin	Hemoglobin A₁c	Pancreatic insufficiency
Chronic diarrhea	Hexokinase method	Secretin-cholecystokinin test
Chronic pancreatitis	Hyperosmolar hyperglycemic	Secretin test
Diabetes mellitus	nonketotic syndrome	Sequelae of diabetes
Diabetic ketoacidosis	Hypoglycemia	Sudan stain IV
Digestive enzymes	Insulin	Trypsin
Fecal fat test	Islets of Langerhans	Trypsinogen
Fecal pancreatic elastase 1 test	Ketone bodies	Type 1 diabetes mellitus
Fructosamine test	Lipase	Type 2 diabetes mellitus
Gestational diabetes mellitus	Lipogenesis	
Glucose oxidase method	Lipolysis	

 ## Case in Point

A 19-year-old college student goes to the emergency department thinking he has the flu. He has a headache, muscle aches, and general fatigue. His laboratory results are the following: glucose level of 800 mg/dL, sodium level of 120 mEq/L, potassium level of 2.9 mEq/L, chloride level of 92 mEq/L, and acetone level of 3+. What is the likely diagnosis? What causes this disease?

Points to Remember

- Acute pancreatitis is inflammation of the pancreas that occurs suddenly and can be a life-threatening illness with severe complications.
- The most important tests for the diagnosis of acute pancreatitis are measurements of serum amylase and lipase levels.
- Serum levels of amylase rise approximately 2 to 12 hours after onset of acute pancreatitis.
- The most common method for determining amylase levels measures activity of the enzyme with specially labeled substrates.
- The amylase reference range is 31 to 107 U/L.
- The serum lipase level rises 4 to 8 hours after the onset of acute pancreatitis. It may rise to 2 to 50 times the normal value, and it decreases in 8 to 14 days.
- Methods for lipase analysis include titrimetric, fluorometric, immunologic, and turbidimetric assays.
- Chronic pancreatitis is inflammation of the pancreas that progresses over time and leads to permanent damage of the pancreas.
- The most common cause of chronic pancreatitis is persistent and heavy alcohol use.
- Pancreatic insufficiency is detected with enzyme tests when 50% of the acinar cells are destroyed, but clinical symptoms do not appear until 90% of acinar cells are destroyed.

- Acute pancreatitis is difficult to diagnose, but the lipase level has good specificity and sensitivity for the diagnosis.
- The secretin test is a functional method used to diagnose pancreatic malfunction.
- Type 1 diabetes mellitus (T1DM) results from beta cell destruction in the islets of Langerhans in the pancreas; destruction leads to absolute insulin deficiency.
- Hyperglycemia occurs in individuals after 80% to 90% of the functional insulin-secreting beta cells in the islets of Langerhans are destroyed.
- Individuals with T1DM experience abrupt onset of classic symptoms, including polyuria (i.e., frequent urination), polydipsia (i.e., excessive thirst and fluid intake), polyphagia (i.e., chronic hunger), fatigue, and weight loss.
- Polyuria occurs in T1DM because the hyperglycemic state acts as an osmotic diuretic; the kidneys filter more glucose than can be reabsorbed by the renal tubules, and the excess glucose is excreted in urine along with large amounts of water.
- Weight loss occurs in T1DM because the body loses fluid through osmotic dieresis and because fat and proteins are used as energy because the body cannot adequately metabolize glucose.
- An individual with insulin deficiency may develop diabetic ketoacidosis. Lipolysis is increased, and more fatty acids are transported to the liver. The liver uses the fatty acids for glyconeogenesis, producing more glucose for the body. Without insulin, the adipocytes (i.e., fat cells) release free fatty acids, which stimulates the liver to produce more ketone bodies i.e., (acetoacetate, hydroxybutyrate, and acetone) than can be used by the body.
- Type 2 diabetes mellitus (T2DM) is a spectrum of disorders ranging from insulin resistance with relative insulin deficiency to a defect of insulin secretion with insulin resistance. Risk factors include increased age, obesity, hypertension, physical inactivity, and family history.
- The metabolic syndrome is a group of disorders (i.e., central obesity, dyslipidemia, prehypertension, and

an elevated fasting blood glucose level) that places an individual at high risk for developing T2DM as well as cardiovascular complications.

- Many individuals with T2DM are obese, and weight loss alone usually lowers blood glucose levels. Control of hyperglycemia may require dietary changes, oral hypoglycemic agents, or insulin administration.
- Symptoms of T2DM are obesity, dyslipidemia, hyperinsulinemia, hypertension, fatigue, itching, recurrent infections, visual changes, numbness, tingling, and weakness.
- Gestational diabetes mellitus is carbohydrate intolerance of various degrees with onset during pregnancy.
- Sequelae of diabetes include renal failure, nontraumatic amputations, blindness, retinopathy, nerve damage, and arthrosclerotic disease.
- Hypoglycemia is a plasma glucose level of 55 mg/dL or less in an adult. Diabetics who inject insulin can expect one to two episodes of symptomatic hypoglycemia per week.
- Hyperosmolar hyperglycemic nonketotic syndrome causes elevated plasma and urine glucose levels, which leads to massive amounts of water loss through the kidneys along with glucose. Water loss causes severe volume depletion accompanied by intracellular dehydration and neurologic changes that may include coma.
- Whole blood glucose test results usually are 10% to 12% lower than results obtained from serum or plasma specimens.
- The hexokinase method uses two enzyme-driven assays (i.e., coupled enzyme assay).
- A common glucose test method is the glucose oxidase method, which is a coupled enzyme assay.
- The glycosylated hemoglobin level indicates the blood glucose level for the preceding 2- to 4-month period.
- The fructosamine test reflects glucose control over a 3- to 6-week period.
- Oral glucose tolerance tests are no longer the gold standard for diagnosing diabetes mellitus, but they are still used by some physicians.
- Cystic fibrosis is a multiorgan disease that affects the lungs and gastrointestinal tract.
- The quantitative 72-hour fecal fat test is used to detect malabsorption disorders.

Introduction

Anatomy and function of the pancreas are reviewed in this chapter, along with the laboratory tests used for diagnosing pancreatic diseases. Although rare, pancreatitis can be very serious or fatal. Most patients with acute or chronic pancreatitis are between 50 and 60 years of age. Diabetes is a serious disease in which the blood glucose level is chronically elevated due to the lack of insulin production by the beta cells in the islets of Langerhans in the pancreas. Maldigestion results from altered production of digestive enzymes by the pancreas.

Overview of the Pancreas

The pancreas is located below the stomach and above the transverse colon. The complex organ is 6 to 9 inches long and contains endocrine and exocrine tissue. Most tissue is exocrine and is composed of acinar (grapelike) cells. Each cell releases pancreatic hormones into a microscopic duct. Several enzymes and bicarbonate, which are essential for digestion, are secreted from the pancreas into the small intestine through the pancreatic duct (Fig. 22-1).

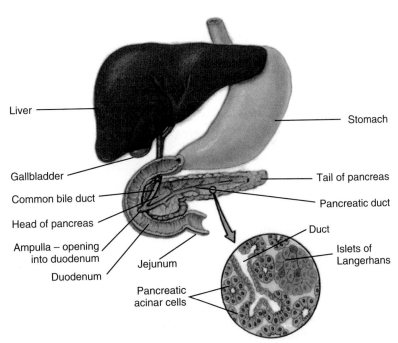

• Figure 22-1 The pancreas in relation to the liver, duodenum, and stomach. (From Applegate EMS: *The Anatomy and Physiology Learning System.* 4th ed. St. Louis: Saunders; 2011.)

The endocrine cells of the pancreas are dotted like islands throughout the organ. Some groups contain alpha cells, and others contain beta cells. Beta cells are found in the islets of Langerhans. The endocrine function of the pancreas regulates glucose metabolism. Pancreatic secretion of insulin and glucagon helps to regulate blood glucose levels and the amount of glucose stored in the liver in the form of glycogen.

Pancreatitis

Pancreatitis is inflammation of the pancreas. Damage occurs when activated digestive enzymes destroy pancreatic tissue. In severe cases, inflammation can result in hemorrhage that damages the pancreas. In acute and chronic forms of pancreatitis, approximately 90% of pancreatitis episodes result from gallstones that block bile ducts or from heavy alcohol ingestion. Fewer episodes are caused by trauma, and in some cases, the cause is unknown.

Acute Pancreatitis

Acute pancreatitis is inflammation of the pancreas that occurs suddenly and can be a life-threatening illness with severe complications. Each year, about 200,000 people in the United States are admitted to the hospital with acute pancreatitis. The most common causes of acute pancreatitis include gallstones that block the common bile duct and heavy alcohol use; other causes are trauma, medications, infections, and tumors (Fig. 22-2, A).

Pain is often severe, and it may become constant and last for several days. It is often described as a "boring pain from front to back." Other symptoms include fever, nausea, and vomiting. In severe cases, hemorrhage (i.e., profuse bleeding) may occur. Hemorrhage may be followed by very low blood pressure and death (see Fig. 22-2, B).

In 80% to 85% of cases, acute pancreatitis resolves on its own or with treatment. However, acute pancreatitis can result in chronic pancreatitis, especially after repeated attacks.

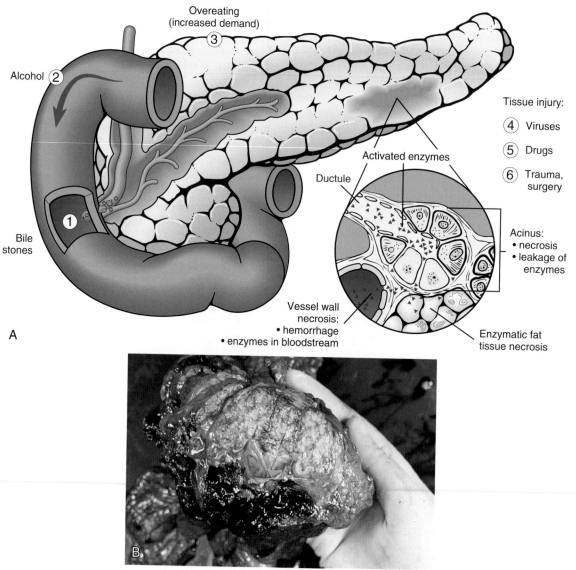

• **Figure 22-2** **A,** Possible causes of acute pancreatitis. **B,** Acute pancreatitis with massive hemorrhage. (From Damjanov I. *Pathology for the Health Professions.* 4th ed. St. Louis: Saunders; 2012.)

Diagnosis

The most important tests for the diagnosis of acute pancreatitis are serum amylase and lipase assays. Another is measurement of trypsinogen activation peptide (TAP) for early diagnosis and determination of severity. Other tests that help predict the severity of the pancreatitis attack include those for phospholipase A_2, procalcitonin, and C-reactive protein.

Amylase

Amylase is an enzyme that converts starch into sugar. It is routinely measured to alert the provider to acute pancreatitis. Levels of amylase in serum rise approximately 2 to 12 hours after the onset of acute pancreatitis. Levels may rise to four to eight times normal, and they return to normal within 3 to 4 days after onset of symptoms. The most common method for measuring amylase is determination of enzyme activity with specially labeled substrates. Although both are used, amylase levels are not as specific as lipase levels for the diagnosis of acute pancreatitis.

Amylase is found in pancreatic secretions and in saliva. It begins the digestion of carbohydrates when food is chewed. Substrates used in amylase assays include maltotetraose, maltopentose, and 4-nitrophenyl-glycosides (Fig. 22-3). The assay takes place at 37° C, and the reference range is 31 to 107 U/L.

Lipase

Lipase is an enzyme that helps to break down fatty acids. The serum lipase level rises approximately 4 to 8 hours after the onset of acute pancreatitis. It may rise to 2 to 50 times the normal value, and it then decreases in 8 to 14 days. Methods for lipase analysis include titrimetric, fluorometric, immunologic, and turbidimetric assays, but by far the most common is direct measurement of lipase activity with modified substrates. The reference range for lipase is <38 U/L.

Chronic Pancreatitis

Chronic pancreatitis is inflammation of the pancreas that progresses over time and leads to permanent damage. Chronic pancreatitis is marked by severe pain and loss of pancreatic function. The most common cause of chronic pancreatitis is persistent and heavy alcohol use.

Chronic pancreatitis, like acute pancreatitis, occurs when digestive enzymes attack the pancreas. In chronic pancreatitis, digestion of the organ causes fibrosis and scarring. The pancreas progressively loses function over time and is slowly destroyed. The loss of function leads to diabetes and pancreatic insufficiency, a form of maldigestion.

Diagnosis

The diagnosis of chronic pancreatitis is challenging because there is no set of tests that can accurately identify the disease. The pancreatic enzymes that are commonly measured to assess pancreatic status are trypsin, amylase, lipase, chymotrypsin, and elastase. Noninvasive tests for assessing pancreatic

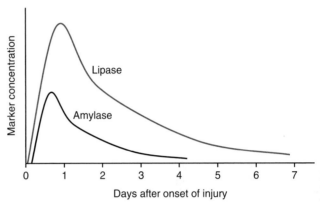

$$5 \text{ ethylidene-4-NP-G}_7 + 5\, H_2O \xrightarrow{\alpha\text{-}amylase}$$
$$2 \text{ ethylidene-G}_5 + 2 \text{ 4-NP-G}_2 +$$
$$2 \text{ ethylidene-G}_4 + 2 \text{ 4-NP-G}_3 +$$
$$\text{ethylidene-G}_3 + \text{4-NP-G}_4$$

$$2 \text{ 4-NP-G}_2 + 2 \text{ 4-NP-G}_3 + 10\, H_2O \xrightarrow{\alpha\text{-}glucosidase} 4 \text{ 4-NP} + 10 \text{ G}$$

• **Figure 22-3** Amylase reactions. *G,* Glycosides; *NP,* nitrophenyl. (From Burtis CA, Bruns DE. *Tietz Fundamentals of Clinical Chemistry and Molecular Diagnostics.* 7th ed. St. Louis: Saunders; 2015.)

• **Figure 22-4** Time-dependent changes in serum amylase and lipase after acute pancreatitis. (From Burtis CA, Bruns DE. *Tietz Fundamentals of Clinical Chemistry and Molecular Diagnostics.* 7th ed. St. Louis: Saunders; 2015.)

function are not very good for detecting early disease because the pancreas has a large functional reserve. Pancreatic insufficiency can be detected using enzyme tests when 50% of the acinar cells are destroyed, but clinical symptoms do not appear until 90% of acinar cells are destroyed (Fig. 22-4).

Lipase

Pancreatitis is difficult to diagnose, but lipase levels have shown good specificity and sensitivity for the disease. Turbidimetric, spectrophotometric, fluorometric, and immunoassay techniques are used to measure lipase. A colorimetric reaction uses 1,2-*o*-dilauryl-rac-glycero-3-glutaric acid-(4 methylresorufin)-ester as a substrate (Fig. 22-5). Lipase hydrolyzes the substrate in an alkaline medium to produce a blue-purple chromogen with peak absorption at 580 nm.

The secretin test is used to diagnose pancreatic malfunction. It is based on the assumption that secretion of pancreatic juice and bicarbonate output are related to the functional mass of pancreatic tissue. The test begins with an overnight fast by the patient, followed by collection of samples from the stomach and duodenum in the morning. After the baseline samples are collected, secretin is administered intravenously, and duodenal fluid is collected at 15-minute intervals for at least 1 hour. The addition of cholecystokinin to the secretin before collecting duodenal fluid gives a more complete assessment of pancreatic function than secretin alone.

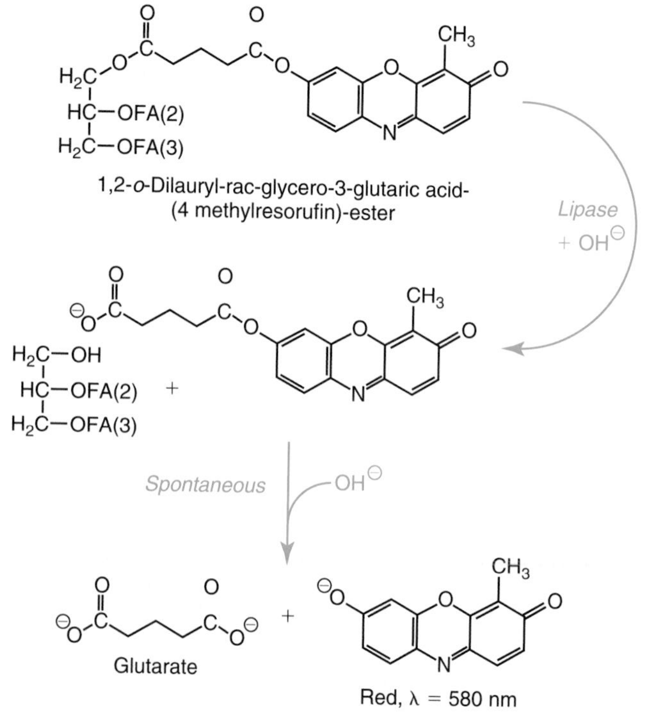

1,2-o-Dilauryl-rac-glycero-3-glutaric acid-
(4 methylresorufin)-ester

Lipase
+ OH⊖

Spontaneous — OH⊖

Glutarate

Red, λ = 580 nm

• **Figure 22-5** Lipase reactions. (From Burtis CA, Bruns DE. *Tietz Fundamentals of Clinical Chemistry and Molecular Diagnostics.* 7th ed. St. Louis: Saunders; 2015.)

Diabetes

Diabetes mellitus is a group of diseases caused by a malfunction of the endocrine pancreas. The diseases are characterized by hyperglycemia resulting from reduced or absent insulin secretion or defects in insulin action, or both.

Types of Diabetes

In 1979, a workgroup of the National Diabetes Data Group reclassified the two major forms of diabetes as type 1 or insulin-dependent diabetes mellitus (IDDM) and type 2 or non–insulin-dependent diabetes mellitus (NIDDM). This terminology replaced the older terminology of juvenile-onset and adult-onset diabetes. In 1997, the American Diabetes Association again revised the classifications to type 1 diabetes mellitus and type 2 diabetes mellitus.

Type 1 Diabetes Mellitus

Type 1 diabetes mellitus (T1DM) is the result of beta cell destruction in the islets of Langerhans in the pancreas that leads to absolute insulin deficiency. T1DM is a T-cell–mediated disease that produces antibodies that destroy beta cells, resulting in low or no insulin production. Most individuals with T1DM have measurable antibodies to the beta cells, but a few do not have autoantibodies, and their disease is considered idiopathic.

T1DM is usually diagnosed before the age of 30 years, but because it can manifest later in life, age is not a criterion. Hyperglycemia occurs only after 80% to 90% of the functional insulin-secreting beta cells in the islets of Langerhans are destroyed. Consequently, T1DM progresses for a long time before acute clinical symptoms are observed. Hyperglycemia can result from lack of insulin or from excess glucagon. Excess glucagon is also responsible for hyperketonemia.

T1DM patients have classic symptoms such as polyuria (i.e., frequent urination), polydipsia (i.e., excessive thirst and fluid intake), polyphagia (i.e., chronic hunger), fatigue, and weight loss. Although the onset of symptoms is abrupt, the disease has a long preclinical course. Polyuria occurs because the hyperglycemic state acts as an osmotic diuretic. The kidneys filter more glucose than can be reabsorbed by the renal tubules, and the excess glucose is excreted in urine along with large amounts of water. Polydipsia occurs because the elevated blood glucose levels attract water from tissue cells into the blood, resulting in intracellular dehydration and a hypothalamic response that increases fluid consumption. Polyphagia results from depleted cellular stores of carbohydrates, fats, and protein, starving the cells and stimulating a response to consume more food. Weight loss occurs because the body loses fluid through osmotic diuresis, and because the body cannot adequately metabolize glucose, fat and proteins are used as energy. Fatigue sets in when poor use of food leads to metabolic changes that leave people lethargic and fatigued. Fatigue can also be caused by severe nocturia and the resulting loss of sleep.

Insulin stimulates lipogenesis (i.e., fat synthesis) and inhibits lipolysis (i.e., fat breakdown). In an individual with insulin deficiency, lipolysis is increased, so more fatty acids are transported to the liver. The liver uses the fatty acids for glyconeogenesis, which produces more glucose for the body. Without insulin, the adipocytes (i.e., fat cells) release free fatty acids, stimulating the liver to produce more ketone bodies (i.e., acetoacetate, hydroxybutyrate, and acetone) than can be used by the body. The ketone bodies accumulate in the blood, decreasing the blood pH and causing metabolic acidosis. This type of metabolic acidosis is called diabetic ketoacidosis (DKA). In DKA, acetone is exhaled, giving the breath an acetone smell or a fruity odor. In severe cases of DKA, brown crystals of acetone can form on the lips (Box 22-1 and Fig. 22-6).

• **BOX 22-1** **Diagnostic Criteria for Diabetes Mellitus**

Only one of the following conditions needs to be satisfied for a diagnosis of diabetes mellitus:
- Hemoglobin A_{1C} (DCCT referenced assay) ≥6.5%
- Fasting blood glucose ≥126 mg/dL (i.e., no calorie intake for at least 8 hours)
- 2-Hour postprandial glucose ≥200 mg/dL during oral glucose tolerance test
- A random glucose sample ≥200 mg/dL for a patient with classic symptoms of hyperglycemia or hyperglycemic crisis

DCCT, Diabetes Control and Complications Trial.

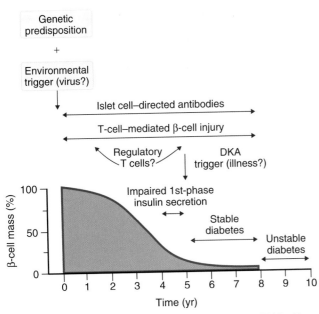

• **Figure 22-6** Development of diabetic ketoacidosis (DKA). (From Goldman L, Schafer AI: *Goldman's Cecil Medicine.* 24th ed. Philadelphia: Saunders; 2012.)

Type 2 Diabetes Mellitus

Type 2 diabetes mellitus (T2DM) is a spectrum of disorders caused by various degrees of insulin resistance in skeletal muscle and defective insulin secretion by the pancreas. Insulin resistance occurs when tissues do not respond normally (i.e., are less sensitive) to insulin, in part because of decreased insulin receptor density. Obesity and higher circulating levels of insulin in the bloodstream promote insulin resistance.

T2DM results from a complex interplay of environmental and genetic factors. Well-recognized risk factors include increased age, obesity, hypertension, physical inactivity, and family history. The metabolic syndrome is a group of disorders (i.e., central obesity, dyslipidemia, prehypertension, and elevated fasting glucose levels) that indicate a high risk of developing T2DM and cardiovascular complications. Individuals with polycystic ovary syndrome (PCOS) demonstrate insulin resistance and have a seven times higher than normal risk of developing T2DM.

Symptoms of T2DM include obesity, dyslipidemia, hyperinsulinemia, hypertension, fatigue, itching, recurrent infections, visual changes, numbness, tingling, and weakness. T2DM can lead to coronary, peripheral artery, and cerebrovascular disease. Diagnostic criteria are similar for T2DM and T1DM (Table 22-1).

Ninety percent of individuals with diabetes mellitus have T2DM. Individuals with T2DM have a more gradual onset of symptoms than those with T1DM, and they usually are not required to inject insulin. Insulin levels in these individuals are variable and can be increased, decreased, or normal. Many people develop T2DM after age 40 years of age, but it can develop in younger individuals. T2DM is becoming more prevalent among adolescents and children as obesity rates increase.

TABLE 22-1	Diagnostic Criteria for Type 1 and Type 2 Diabetes	
Test	**Prediabetes**	**Diabetes**
Fasting blood glucose	100-125 mg/dL	>125 mg/dL
Random blood glucose	175-200 mg/dL	>200 mg/dL
Oral glucose tolerance test	2 hour: 140-200 mg/dL	2 hour: >200 mg/dL
Hemoglobin A$_{1C}$*	6.0-6.5%	>6.5%

*May be falsely elevated in many medical conditions; should not be used to monitor daily glucose levels.

The disease mechanism is impaired insulin action (Fig. 22-7). Many individuals with T2DM are obese, and weight loss alone usually lowers blood glucose levels and improves insulin resistance. Control of hyperglycemia may require a combination of dietary changes, exercise, oral hypoglycemic agents, and insulin administration.

In T2DM, the body compensates for impaired insulin action by producing more insulin, which can happen for years before symptoms appear (Fig. 22-8). Overproduction of insulin leads to beta cell dysfunction, eventually resulting in decreased insulin levels. As the disease progresses, the number of beta cells continues to decrease, in part because glucose and free fatty acids are toxic to beta cells and cause cell death. Cell death triggers an inflammatory response, which causes further beta cell dysfunction. As in T1DM, an individual with T2DM produces more glucose in response to reduced insulin levels and the action of glucagon. In T2DM, there is some functional insulin, which usually prevents the ketoacidosis seen in individuals with T1DM. Tissues in an individual with T2DM do not respond normally to insulin and they are said to have insulin resistance. There are several mechanisms that produce insulin resistance in tissues. Obesity produces insulin resistance in tissues due to decreased insulin receptor density.

Other Types of Diabetes

Some types of diabetes mellitus with hyperglycemia result from genetic defects (e.g., Down syndrome) hormonal defects (e.g., Cushing disease), drugs that alter beta cell function, or infection. The older term for this classification was *secondary diabetes.*

Gestational diabetes mellitus is a form of carbohydrate intolerance with onset during pregnancy. Approximately 6% to 8% of pregnant women develop gestational diabetes mellitus. These women are at high risk for T2DM. Women with gestational diabetes should be evaluated for T2DM with an oral glucose tolerance test. If the test result is negative, they should be reevaluated every 3 years for T2DM (Table 22-2).

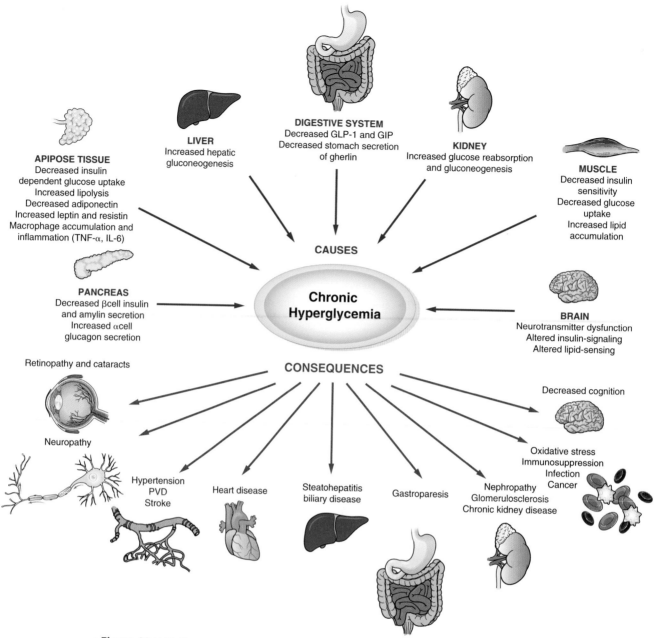

CAUSES

APIPOSE TISSUE
Decreased insulin
dependent glucose uptake
Increased lipolysis
Decreased adiponectin
Increased leptin and resistin
Macrophage accumulation and
inflammation (TNF-α, IL-6)

LIVER
Increased hepatic
gluconeogenesis

DIGESTIVE SYSTEM
Decreased GLP-1 and GIP
Decreased stomach secretion
of gherlin

KIDNEY
Increased glucose reabsorption
and gluconeogenesis

MUSCLE
Decreased insulin
sensitivity
Decreased glucose
uptake
Increased lipid
accumulation

PANCREAS
Decreased βcell insulin
and amylin secretion
Increased αcell
glucagon secretion

**Chronic
Hyperglycemia**

BRAIN
Neurotransmitter dysfunction
Altered insulin-signaling
Altered lipid-sensing

CONSEQUENCES

Retinopathy and cataracts

Neuropathy

Hypertension
PVD
Stroke

Heart disease

Steatohepatitis
biliary disease

Gastroparesis

Nephropathy
Glomerulosclerosis
Chronic kidney disease

Decreased cognition

Oxidative stress
Immunosuppression
Infection
Cancer

• **Figure 22-7** Multiorgan causes and common consequences of chronic hyperglycemia in type 2 diabetes mellitus. *GIP,* Gastric inhibitory polypeptide; *GLP-1,* glucagon-like peptide-1; *IL,* Interleukin; *PVD,* peripheral vascular disease; *TNF,* tumor necrosis factor. (From McCance KL, Huether SE. *Pathophysiology: The Biologic Basis for Disease in Adults and Children.* 7th ed. St. Louis: Mosby; 2015.)

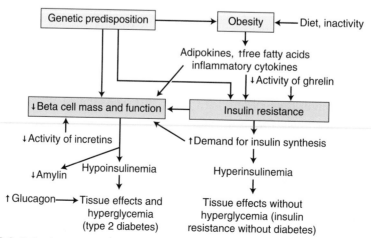

Genetic predisposition → Obesity ← Diet, inactivity

Adipokines, ↑free fatty acids
inflammatory cytokines

↓Activity of ghrelin

↓Beta cell mass and function ⟷ Insulin resistance

↓Activity of incretins

↑Demand for insulin synthesis

↓Amylin   Hypoinsulinemia

Hyperinsulinemia

↑Glucagon → Tissue effects and
hyperglycemia
(type 2 diabetes)

Tissue effects without
hyperglycemia (insulin
resistance without diabetes)

• **Figure 22-8** Pathophysiology of type 2 diabetes mellitus. (From McCance KL, Huether SE. *Pathophysiology: The Biologic Basis for Disease in Adults and Children.* 7th ed. St. Louis: Mosby; 2015.)

TABLE 22-2	Types of Diabetes and Their Characteristics	
Type of Diabetes	**Disease Mechanism**	**Characteristics**
Type 1	Produced by cell-mediated autoimmune destruction of pancreatic beta cells, which leads to absolute insulin deficiency	Little or no insulin secreted Prone to ketoacidosis Insulin dependent Usually develops before age 30 Usually not obese
Type 2	Ranges from predominantly insulin resistant with relative insulin deficiency to a predominantly secretory defect with insulin resistance	Usually not insulin dependent but may be insulin requiring Not prone to ketosis Abdominal obesity common Usually occurs after age 40 Strong genetic predisposition Often associated with hypertension and dyslipidemia
Gestational	Any degree of glucose intolerance with onset or first recognition during pregnancy	Insulin resistance and decreased insulin secretion result in hyperglycemia Obese women Women >25 years old Family history of diabetes Previous gestational diabetes Ethnic groups (e.g., Hispanic, Native American, Asian, African American) at higher risk for gestational diabetes

Sequelae of Diabetes Mellitus

T1DM, T2DM, and gestational diabetes mellitus cause significant morbidity and mortality and an inordinate expenditure of health care dollars. Sequelae of diabetes include renal failure, nontraumatic amputations, blindness, retinopathy, nerve damage, and atherosclerotic disease. Diabetes is the number one cause of renal failure and blindness in the United States. Patients are two to four times more likely to have heart disease (e.g., myocardial infarction) and cerebrovascular disease (e.g., stroke) than people who do not have this disease (Fig. 22-9).

Due to increasing obesity in the American population, the incidence of T2DM has significantly increased every year. In 2007, approximately $174 billion was spent on diabetes, with the total expected to almost double by 2034 (Table 22-3).

Complications of Diabetes Mellitus

Hypoglycemia

Hypoglycemia is a plasma glucose level of 55 mg/dL or lower in an adult (Table 22-4). Diabetics who inject insulin usually have one or two episodes of symptomatic hypoglycemia per week. Severe hypoglycemia occurs in approximately 10% of diabetics every year.

Symptoms of hypoglycemia result from sympathetic nervous system activation (i.e., neurogenic adrenergic symptoms) or reduced blood supply to the brain (i.e., neuroglycopenic symptoms) or both. Neurogenic symptoms include tachycardia, palpitations, diaphoresis, tremors, pallor, and anxiety. Neuroglycopenic symptoms include headache, dizziness, irritability, fatigue, poor judgment, confusion, visual changes, hunger, seizures, and coma. Severe hypoglycemia must be treated quickly, or it can lead

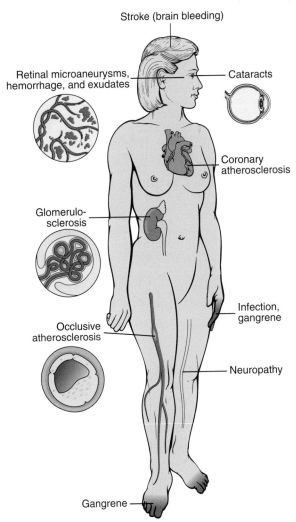

• **Figure 22-9** Complications of diabetes mellitus. (From Damjanov I. *Pathology for the Health Professions.* 4th ed. St. Louis: Saunders; 2012.)

TABLE 22-3   Comparison of Type 1 and Type 2 Diabetes

Characteristic	Type 1	Type 2
Age at onset	Children and young adults	Older but also young adults
Onset	Acute	Insidious
Cause, background	Autoimmune destruction, family history	Familial, lifestyle, and environmental factors, obesity
Body weight	Thin	Obese
Plasma insulin level	Very low	Decreased or normal
Treatment	Insulin replacement	Diet and exercise, oral hypoglycemic agents or insulin replacement
Hypoglycemia or ketoacidosis occurrence	Frequent	Less common

From Gould BE, Dyer R. *Pathophysiology for the Health Professions*. 4th ed. St. Louis, Saunders; 2011.

TABLE 22-4   Complications of Diabetes Mellitus

Characteristics	Hypoglycemia	Diabetic Ketoacidosis	Hyperosmolar Hyperglycemic Nonketotic Coma
Group affected	Individuals taking insulin or sulfonylurea agents	Individuals with type 1 diabetes or with undiagnosed diabetes mellitus	Older adults with type 2 diabetes or with undiagnosed diabetes
Onset	Rapid	Slow	Slowest
Symptoms	Adrenergic reaction: pallor, sweating, tachycardia, palpitations, hunger, restlessness, anxiety, tremors. Neurogenic reaction: fatigue, irritability, headache, loss of concentration, visual disturbances, dizziness, hunger, confusion, transient sensory or motor defects, convulsions, coma, death	Malaise, dry mouth, headache, polyuria, polydipsia, weight loss, nausea, vomiting, itching, abdominal pain, lethargy, shortness of breath, Kussmaul respirations, fruity or acetone odor to breath	Polyuria, polydipsia, hypovolemia, dehydration (e.g., parched lips, poor skin turgor), hypotension, tachycardia, hypoperfusion, weight loss, weakness, nausea, vomiting, abdominal pain, hypothermia, stupor, coma, seizures
Laboratory results	Serum glucose level ≤30 mg/dL in newborns, ≤55-60 mg/dL in adults	Glucose level >250 mg/dL. Decreased bicarbonate level. Increased anion gap. Increased plasma levels of β-hydroxybutyrate, acetoacetone, and acetone	Glucose level >600 mg/dL. Serum osmolality >320 mOsm/L. Increased blood urea nitrogen (BUN) level. Increased creatinine level

From McCance KL, Huether SE. *Pathophysiology: The Biologic Basis for Disease in Adults and Children*. 7th ed. St. Louis: Mosby; 2015.)

to brain death. Several drugs, including insulin, sulfonylureas, repaglinide, and nateglinide, can induce hypoglycemia that results in an altered mental state.

Diabetic Ketoacidosis

DKA is a life-threatening condition of diabetes mellitus that usually results in hospitalization (see Table 22-4). This disorder usually occurs in individuals with T1DM, but it can occur in those with T2DM. DKA results from a very low level of insulin (Fig. 22-10). Counterregulatory hormone levels increase in response to low insulin levels, which decreases glucose uptake, increases the release of fatty acids from stored fats, and triggers gluconeogenesis and ketogenesis. These processes produce a state of metabolic acidosis (Fig. 22-11).

Clinical symptoms of DKA are polyuria, dehydration, Kussmaul respirations (i.e., rapid, deep, and labored breathing), dizziness when standing, central nervous system depression, anorexia, nausea, vomiting, abdominal pain, and thirst. Laboratory test results make the diagnosis: elevated plasma glucose (>250 mg/dL), decreased sodium, decreased phosphorus, decreased magnesium, decreased bicarbonate (<18 mg/dL), serum pH less than 7.30, very decreased potassium, positive plasma ketones, increased anion gap, and positive urine ketones.

DEVELOPMENT OF DIABETIC KETOACIDOSIS

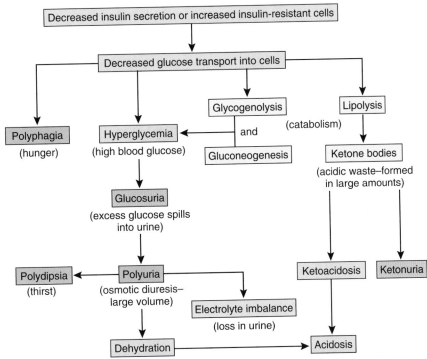

• **Figure 22-10** Development of diabetic ketoacidosis. (From Gould BE, Dyer R. *Pathophysiology for the Health Professions.* 4th ed. St. Louis: Saunders; 2011.)

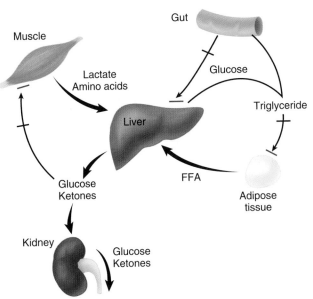

• **Figure 22-11** Effects of severe insulin deficiency on metabolism. Lack of insulin leads to mobilization of substrates for gluconeogenesis and ketogenesis from muscle and adipose tissue, accelerated production of glucose and ketones by the liver, and impaired removal of endogenous and exogenous fuels by insulin-responsive tissues. The results are severe hyperglycemia and hyperketonemia that overwhelm renal removal mechanisms. *FFA,* Free fatty acids. (From Goldman L, Schafer AI. *Goldman's Cecil Medicine.* 24th ed. Philadelphia: Saunders, 2012.)

Treatment for DKA is insulin to reduce the plasma glucose concentration and intravenous fluid administration for rehydration. The electrolyte imbalance is closely monitored until it returns to normal.

Hyperosmolar Hyperglycemic Nonketotic Syndrome

Hyperosmolar hyperglycemic nonketotic syndrome (HHNKS) is considered a medical emergency. HHNKS is caused by infections, medications, and treatment noncompliance, and it is more common in T2DM (see Table 22-4). Insulin deficiency is not as severe in HHNKS as in DKA, but dehydration is worse. HHNKS does not produce large amounts of ketones as DKA does. Insulin levels in HHNKS are high enough to prevent excess fat metabolism but low enough to not use glucose properly. As a result, glucose levels are much higher in HHNKS than in DKA.

In HHNKS, elevated glucose levels in plasma and urine lead to massive amounts of water exiting through the kidneys along with glucose. The result is severe volume depletion accompanied by intracellular dehydration and neurologic changes, up to and including coma. Abnormal laboratory results for HHNKS include increased serum osmolality, decreased electrolyte levels (especially potassium), very high plasma glucose levels (>600 mg/dL), near-normal levels of bicarbonate, near-normal serum pH, and serum osmolarity greater than 320 mOsm/L.

Treatment for HHNKS is similar to that for DKA, but extremely low potassium levels in HHNKS may take days to return to normal. The mortality rate is high for HHNKS patients.

Measurement of Glucose

Glucose can be measured in blood, serum, plasma, urine, and body fluids, including cerebrospinal fluid (CSF).

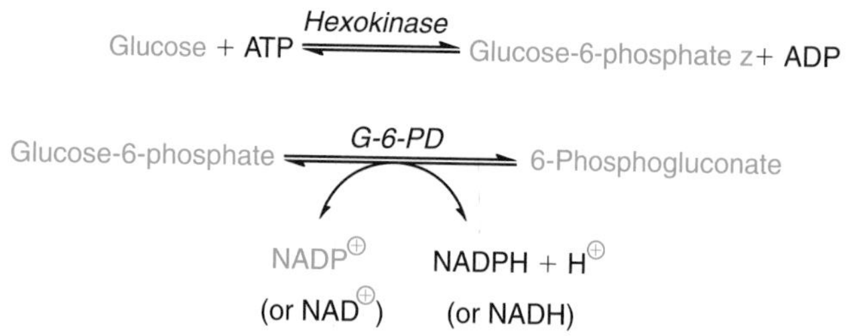

$$\text{Glucose} + \text{ATP} \xrightleftharpoons{\textit{Hexokinase}} \text{Glucose-6-phosphate z+ ADP}$$

$$\text{Glucose-6-phosphate} \xrightarrow{\textit{G-6-PD}} \text{6-Phosphogluconate}$$

$$\text{NADP}^{\oplus} \quad \text{NADPH} + \text{H}^{\oplus}$$
$$(\text{or NAD}^{\oplus}) \quad (\text{or NADH})$$

• **Figure 22-12** Hexokinase methods. *G-6-PD,* Glucose-6-phosphate dehydrogenase. (From Burtis CA, Bruns DE. *Tietz Fundamentals of Clinical Chemistry and Molecular Diagnostics.* 7th ed. St. Louis: Saunders; 2015.)

$$\text{Glucose} + \text{H}_2\text{O} + \text{O}_2 \xrightarrow{\textit{Glucose oxidase}} \text{Gluconic acid} + 2\text{H}_2\text{O}_2$$

$$\textit{o}\text{-Dianisidine} + \text{H}_2\text{O}_2 \xrightarrow{\textit{Peroxidase}} \text{Oxidized } \textit{o}\text{-Dianisidine} + \text{H}_2\text{O}$$

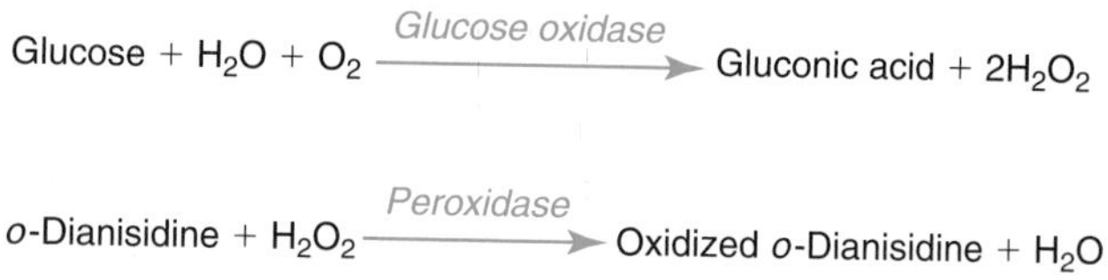

• **Figure 22-13** Glucose oxidase methods. (From Burtis CA, Bruns DE. *Tietz Fundamentals of Clinical Chemistry and Molecular Diagnostics.* 7th ed. St. Louis: Saunders; 2015.)

Normally, whole-blood glucose test results are 10% to 12% lower than results obtained from serum or plasma specimens. Routine laboratory tests use serum or plasma for glucose testing.

When a blood specimen is collected for glucose testing, the serum or plasma should be separated from the cells as soon as possible. The cells in a blood specimen continue to live and metabolize glucose in the tube, and glycolysis lowers the glucose concentration in a sample by 5% to 7% per hour. Because sodium fluoride inhibits glycolysis, the specimen for glucose testing should be placed in a sodium fluoride tube (i.e., gray top). The best way to minimize glycolysis is to remove the plasma from the cells as soon as possible.

Glucose Hexokinase Test Method

Glucose in body fluids is commonly measured by the **hexokinase method** (Fig. 22-12), which uses two enzyme-driven assays (i.e., coupled enzyme assay). The first reaction uses hexokinase to modify glucose to glucose-6-phosphate. The second reaction is the indicator reaction, in which glucose-6-phosphate is acted on by glucose-6-phosphate dehydrogenase to form 6-phophogluconate. In this reaction, NAD⁺ or NADP⁺ is converted to NADH or NADPH + H⁺ and measured at 340 nm. The amount of NADH or NADPH produced is directly proportional to the amount of glucose in the specimen.

This method can be used with serum or plasma samples. Substances that interfere with this test include hemoglobin (>0.5 g/dL), certain drugs, bilirubin, and lipemia (triglycerides >500 mg/dL). This method is usually linear to 500 mg/dL, which means that specimens with glucose concentrations greater than 500 mg/dL must be diluted and reassayed.

Glucose Oxidase Test Method

Another common glucose test method is the **glucose oxidase method,** which is also a coupled enzyme assay. Glucose oxidase catalyzes the reaction of glucose, water, and oxygen to form gluconic acid and hydrogen peroxide. In the second reaction, a chromogen and peroxidase are added to the mixture to produce a colored end product and water. The chemical reaction that produces the chromogen is also referred to as the *indicator reaction* (Fig. 22-13).

TABLE 22-5 Reference Intervals for Fasting Glucose	
Sample Source	**Plasma or Serum Reference Interval (mg/dL)**
Adults	74-100
Children	60-100
Premature neonates	20-60
Term neonates	30-60
Whole blood	65-95
Cerebrospinal fluid	40-70 (60% of plasma value)
Urine (24-hour)	1-15

From Burtis CA, Bruns DE. *Tietz Fundamentals of Clinical Chemistry and Molecular Diagnostics.* 7th ed. St. Louis: Saunders; 2015.

The glucose oxidase method is very specific for glucose. Interfering substances include uric acid, ascorbic acid, bilirubin, hemoglobin, tetracycline, and glutathione, all of which lower test results. This method can be used to measure glucose in CSF. Some instruments eliminate the indicator reaction and use a polarographic oxygen electrode to measure the glucose concentration (Table 22-5). As is true for all chemistry analytes, reference intervals should be determined by each clinical laboratory to better reflect the diversity within the population.

Other methods are used to measure glucose, but glucose hexokinase and glucose oxidase tests are the most commonly used methods.

Glycosylated Hemoglobin

Glycosylated hemoglobin indicates the blood glucose level for the preceding 2- to 4-month period. Glucose nonenzymatically attaches to hemoglobin in a two-step reaction. The result is a stable ketoamine, glycosylated hemoglobin or **hemoglobin A_{1C}** (Fig. 22-14). The gold standard for testing **glycohemoglobin** is high-performance liquid chromatography (HPLC), but glycohemoglobin also can be measured using immunoassay, ion-exchange HPLC, electrophoresis, boronate-affinity HPLC, and enzyme methods. There are also convenient immunoassay-based methods that can be run on a bench-top analyzer. The College of American Pathologists prefers that laboratories use methods that can be traced to a reference standard. Some substances can interfere with these tests.

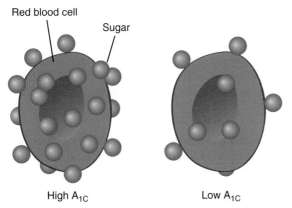

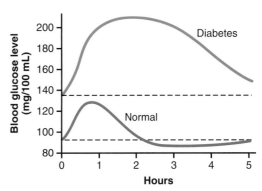

Red blood cell

Sugar

High A$_{1C}$ Low A$_{1C}$

• **Figure 22-14** High hemoglobin A$_{1C}$ and low hemoglobin A$_{1C}$ levels.

• **Figure 22-15** Three-hour glucose tolerance test results plotted for diabetic (*green*) and normal (*red*) curves. (From Hall JE. *Guyton and Hall Textbook of Medical Physiology.* 12th ed. Philadelphia: Saunders; 2011.)

TABLE 22-6	Fructosamine Test Values
Category	**Fructosamine (μmol/L)**
Normal range	<285
Good	<302
Moderate	302-357
Bad	>357

• BOX 22-2	Management Levels for Diabetics

Hemoglobin A$_{1C}$: ≤6.5-7.0%
Fasting glucose: 70-130 mg/dL
Postprandial glucose: ≥140-180 mg/dL

Modified from Burtis CA, Bruns DE. *Tietz Fundamentals of Clinical Chemistry and Molecular Diagnostics.* 7th ed. St. Louis: Saunders; 2015.

Fructosamine Test

The fructosamine test is a laboratory test that reflects glucose control in a 3- to 6-week window (Table 22-6). It is performed on serum samples using an automated instrument; it is convenient and low cost. The test produces reliable results for individuals with normal serum protein levels. If acute illness or liver disease alters serum protein levels, test results can be affected. The fructosamine test is not recommended for specimens with serum albumin levels lower than 3.0 mg/dL. Other interfering substances include hemoglobin and elevated levels of uric acid, triglycerides, and bilirubin. Because heparin interferes with this test, specimens cannot be collected in heparinized tubes.

Oral Glucose Tolerance Tests

Oral glucose tolerance tests are no longer the gold standard for diagnosing diabetes mellitus. Recent American Diabetic Association guidelines allow multiple test results to be used. If a physician orders an oral glucose tolerance test, it is important to know how to perform the test. For the 3 days preceding the test, the individual should eat a diet that contains at least 150 g/day of carbohydrates and then fast for 8 to 14 hours before reporting to the laboratory for the test. The person should refrain from eating food; drinking coffee, tea, or alcohol; and smoking cigarettes before and during the test.

The glucose drink comes in many flavors to aid its consumption. Fasting blood and urine specimens are collected before the individual ingests the glucose drink, which contains 100 g of glucose. A timer is set, and blood and urine specimens are collected every hour for at least 3 hours. If a

physician is looking for confirmation of hypoglycemia, the test will last 5 hours.

From the laboratory test results, a curve is constructed to detail the individual's response to glucose. A normal curve increases rapidly after ingestion, then levels off, and returns to normal within 2 hours. An abnormal curve increases rapidly and stays elevated for a prolonged period (Fig. 22-15). The glucose level often remains elevated (Box 22-2).

Cystic Fibrosis

Cystic fibrosis affects the lungs, liver, pancreas, and gastrointestinal tract. Chapter 19 discusses cystic fibrosis and the lungs. Approximately 65% to 80% of children diagnosed with cystic fibrosis have pancreatic insufficiency. In infants older than 2 weeks, the finding of pancreatic elastase 1 in feces is diagnostic of cystic fibrosis.

Malabsorption and Maldigestion

Maldigestion and malabsorption compromise the body's ability to properly and efficiently absorb nutrients. Maldigestion describes abnormalities that occur in the proximal part of the digestive tract, such as the stomach and exocrine pancreas. It is the inability to break food down into absorbable fragments. Malabsorption describes abnormalities or diseases that affect the distal part of the digestive tract, such as the duodenum or ileum. It involves a failure to absorb properly broken down food.

For diseases of the pancreas that affect the digestive tract, *maldigestion* is the correct term. Maldigestion occurs when the pancreas is damaged by chronic pancreatitis, medications, tumors, or genetic abnormalities. When the pancreas is damaged, the digestive enzymes and bicarbonate that are normally secreted and transported to the small intestine are reduced or lacking. Without them, food is not digested and cannot be absorbed.

Common causes of maldigestion and malabsorption can be found in Box 22-3. Classic symptoms of maldigestion and malabsorption include anorexia, weight loss, fatigue after minor effort, difficulty breathing, edema, weakness, tetany, dehydration, isolated nutritional deficiencies (e.g., iron, folate, vitamin B_{12}, vitamin D, vitamin K), abdominal discomfort, abdominal distention, flatulence, gut rumbling and gurgling sounds, watery diarrhea, and steatorrhea (i.e., fat in stool). The stool passed by individuals with steatorrhea is usually loose, bulky, offensive, greasy, light-colored, and difficult to flush away.

Pancreatic Insufficiency

Early malabsorption conditions may begin with mild gastrointestinal symptoms, and the individual may complain of fatigue and anorexia. At this point, providers rely on laboratory test results to aid in diagnosing the condition. Antibody tests are used for celiac disease, and other useful assays include those for hemoglobin, mean red blood cell volume, folate, ferritin, calcium, albumin, and alkaline phosphatase. Metabolic panels usually are good screening tests. Others that may be useful later in the disease course include fecal fat, fecal pancreatic elastase 1, secretin-cholecystokinin, trypsin, and trypsinogen (i.e., immunoreactive trypsin) tests.

Fecal Fat Test

The fecal fat test is a nonspecific method for detecting increased fat in the stool, which indicates malabsorption or maldigestion. The qualitative test is performed using microscopy and Sudan stain IV. A quantitative 72-hour fecal fat test is also used to detect malabsorption disorders. Individuals follow a high-fat diet for the 4 days before and while they collect specimens. A preweighed collection container is provided to patients. Patients collect all stool specimens for the last 72 hours of the high-fat diet. Fecal fat in the specimen is measured using nuclear magnetic resonance spectroscopy. An elevated level indicates a malabsorption disorder.

• BOX 22-3 Common Disorders Leading to Malabsorption

Zollinger-Ellison syndrome
Chronic pancreatitis
Cystic fibrosis
Pancreatic cancer
Disease or resection of terminal ileum
Small bowel bacterial overgrowth
Celiac disease
Tropical sprue
β-Lipoproteinemia

Fecal Pancreatic Elastase 1 Test

The fecal pancreatic elastase 1 test is performed using an enzyme-linked immunosorbent assay (ELISA). Results of this test are a good indication of exocrine pancreatic function. It is not invasive and is less expensive than the current "gold standard," the secretin-cholecystokinin test.

Secretin-Cholecystokinin Test

The secretin-cholecystokinin test is a combination of the secretin test and the cholecystokinin test. It is used to assess the function of the pancreas and gallbladder. Cholecystokinin (CCK) is a hormone secreted by the small intestine, and it can be given intravenously. Normally, cholecystokinin stimulates the pancreas to secrete the digestive enzymes amylase, trypsin, and lipase. After CCK is administered, the amount of amylase, lipase, and trypsin is measured in the small intestine. If the amount of enzymes secreted into the small intestines is decreased, pancreatic exocrine function is not normal.

Trypsin

Trypsin is an enzyme released by the pancreas during digestion. Smaller than normal amounts can be found in the stool when the pancreas does not produce enough trypsin during digestion.

Trypsinogen

Trypsinogen (i.e., immunoreactive trypsin) is released by the pancreas during digestion. Trypsinogen is converted by substances in the small intestine into trypsin. Blood levels of trypsinogen can be measured to determine whether levels in the blood are increased. Low trypsinogen levels are an indicator of pancreatic sufficiency.

Chronic Diarrhea

Chronic diarrhea is a malabsorption condition. Liquid or loose stools are passed more than three times each day for 4 weeks. Common causes of chronic diarrhea are listed in Box 22-4.

• BOX 22-4 Common Causes of Chronic Diarrhea

Colon cancer
Ulcerative and Crohn colitis
Celiac disease
Tropical sprue
Carbohydrate enzyme deficiency
Lymphoma
Giardiasis
Chronic pancreatitis
Cystic fibrosis
Hyperthyroidism
Diabetes
Addison disease
Drugs
Alcohol

Several mechanisms produce chronic diarrhea. Carbohydrate malabsorption (i.e., unabsorbed solutes in the bowel) produces an osmotic diarrhea as water enters the colon from the tissue. Laxative abuse produces chronic diarrhea through active secretion of water and electrolytes into the bowel (i.e., secretory diarrhea). Irritable bowel disorders such as Crohn disease and ulcerative colitis produce diarrhea as a result of the inflammatory process and loss of fluid in the bowel.

Summary

The pancreas has endocrine and exocrine functions. Acute pancreatitis is inflammation of the pancreas that can be life-threatening. Acute pancreatitis can be caused by gallstones but is more commonly caused by heavy use of alcohol. Chronic pancreatitis occurs when repeated bouts of acute pancreatitis damage the pancreas. Acute and chronic forms of pancreatitis are diagnosed using amylase and lipase test results.

T1DM and T2DM are the major forms of diabetes mellitus. In T1DM, the islets of Langerhans, which contain the beta cells that secrete insulin, are destroyed by autoantibodies. T1DM is usually diagnosed before 30 years of age. Symptoms of T1DM appear suddenly and include polyuria, polydipsia, polyphagia, fatigue, and weight loss. T1DM patients usually have frequent episodes of DKA. DKA is a type of metabolic acidosis that includes increased levels of glucose and increased serum and urine levels of acetone.

T2DM disorders range from insulin resistance with relative insulin deficiency to a secretory defect in insulin with insulin resistance. Ninety percent of diabetics have T2DM. T2DM symptoms develop slowly and include obesity, dyslipidemia, hyperinsulinemia, hypertension, fatigue, itching, recurrent infections, visual changes, numbness, tingling, and weakness. T2DM can lead to coronary artery, peripheral artery, and cerebrovascular disease. Individuals with T2DM can have HHNKS, which is similar to DKA but does not produce elevated ketone levels in blood and urine. Gestational diabetes is carbohydrate intolerance during pregnancy.

Hypoglycemia is a blood glucose level less than 55 mg/dL in adults. It occurs in 10% of diabetics. Glucose is usually measured using glucose hexokinase and glucose oxidase methods. Glycosylated hemoglobin is used to monitor glucose levels over 2 to 5 months, and the fructosamine test monitors glucose levels over 3 to 6 weeks.

Malabsorption and maldigestion conditions are caused by inadequate pancreatic enzymes. Chronic diarrhea is a symptom of malabsorption and maldigestion conditions.

Review Questions

1. The most specific and sensitive blood test for detection of acute pancreatitis is
   a. Serum amylase
   b. Serum lipase
   c. Immunoreactive trypsinogen
   d. Fasting blood glucose
2. A high level of trypsinogen-activated peptide indicates
   a. Progression of acute pancreatitis to chronic pancreatitis
   b. Acute maldigestion
   c. Formation of fibrosis in the pancreas
   d. A severe form of acute pancreatitis
3. Which of the following is the next logical test after a positive result on a newborn screening test of serum immunoreactive trypsinogen?
   a. Sweat test
   b. Fecal fat test
   c. Genetic identification of an abnormal *CFTR* gene
   d. Glucose tolerance test
4. Which of the following is a sensitive, specific, and noninvasive way to detect pancreatic insufficiency?
   a. Fecal fat test
   b. Pancreatic elastase 1 test
   c. Serum trypsin test
   d. Secretin-cholecystokinin test
5. What does the finding of an abnormally high alanine transaminase level and a high lipase level indicate?
   a. The acute pancreatitis is the result of gallstones.
   b. Acute pancreatitis is the diagnosis.
   c. The acute pancreatitis is the result of heavy alcohol use.
   d. The chronic pancreatitis is the result of heavy alcohol use.
6. Quantitative fecal fat tests are performed on a 72-hour stool specimen to diagnose which of the following conditions?
   a. Diarrhea
   b. Chronic pancreatitis
   c. Occult fat
   d. Steatorrhea
7. Chronic pancreatitis is usually caused by
   a. Excessive alcohol consumption
   b. Trauma
   c. Shock
   d. Mumps
8. A 6-year-old boy came to the emergency department complaining of lethargy, nausea, and vomiting for 3 to 4 days. The mother reported that the child was urinating frequently, was thirsty all the time, and was eating a lot. The patient's white blood cell count was 12,500 cells/µL, hemoglobin was 10.2 g/L, acetone value was

large, glucose level was 900 mg/dL, pH was 7.183, Po_2 was 120 mm Hg, Pco_2 was 20 mm Hg, HCO_3^- was 12, and base excess was 14.7. What is the patient's diagnosis?

a. Cystic fibrosis
b. Type 2 diabetes
c. Metabolic syndrome
d. Type 1 diabetes

9. One reason for hyperglycemia in type 1 diabetics is
a. Autoimmune attack of insulin receptors in peripheral tissues
b. Impaired transport and uptake of glucose in peripheral tissues
c. Oversecretion of thyroxin
d. Oversecretion of cortisol

10. A patient's urine tests positive for glucose, with a level of 170 mg/dL. Why does glucose appear in the patient's urine?
a. Renal threshold was exceeded
b. Insulin deficiency
c. Excessive amounts of ketones secreted into the blood
d. Insulin overproduction

Critical Thinking Questions

1. How does insulin decrease blood glucose levels?
2. Discuss the factors that determine the blood glucose level.
3. How is a starch metabolized, starting in the mouth?

CASE STUDY

Mr. K, a 56-year-old man with a long-standing history of alcohol abuse, complains of chronic diarrhea and weight loss to his doctor. He has a history of chronic pain in the epigastric area that has increased in intensity over the years. For the past 9 months, he has experienced bloating with foul-smelling and greasy diarrhea that occurs four to six times each day. He has lost 30 lb over the past 9 months.

Radiographs reveal calcifications in the midportion of the abdomen. Computed tomography of the abdomen showed calcifications located in the pancreas, atrophy of the gland, and mild dilation of the entire pancreatic duct. An endoscopic ultrasound examination showed changes compatible with chronic pancreatitis. What are the Sudan stain and quantitative fecal fat studies likely to show? What is the expected course of illness?

Bibliography

American Diabetes Association. Diagnosis and classification of diabetes mellitus. *Diabet Care.* 2014;37(suppl 1):S81–S90.

Hofmeyr S, Meyer C, Warren BL. Serum lipase should be the laboratory test of choice for suspected acute pancreatitis. *S Afr J Surg.* 2014;52:72–75.

Khan TZ, Wagener JS, Bost T, et al. Early pulmonary inflammation in infants with cystic fibrosis. *Am J Respir Crit Care Med.* 2012;151:1075–1082.

Laterza L, Scaldaferri F, Bruno G, et al. Pancreatic function assessment. *Eur Rev Med Pharmacol Sci.* 2013;17(suppl 2):65–71.

Mayumi T, Inui K, Maetani I, et al. Validity of the urinary trypsinogen-2 test in the diagnosis of acute pancreatitis. *Pancreas.* 2012;41:869–875.

Moore DJ, Forstner GG, Largman C, et al. Serum immunoreactive cationic trypsinogen: a useful indicator of severe exocrine dysfunction in the paediatric patient without cystic fibrosis. *Gut.* 1986;27:1362–1368.

Pagana KD, Pagana TJ. *Mosby's Diagnostic and Laboratory Test Reference.* St. Louis: Elsevier Health Sciences; 2012.

Petersson U, Borgström A. Characterization of immunoreactive trypsinogen activation peptide in urine in acute pancreatitis. *JOP.* 2006;7:274–282.

Picón MJ, Murri M, Muñoz A, Fernández-García JC, Gomez-Huelgas R, Tinahones FJ. Hemoglobin A1c versus oral glucose tolerance test in postpartum diabetes screening. *Diabet Care.* 2012;35:1648–1653.

Pongprasobchai S. Maldigestion from pancreatic exocrine insufficiency. *J Gastroenterol Hepatol.* 2013;28(suppl 4):99–102.

Quinton P, Molyneux L, Ip W, et al. β-Adrenergic sweat secretion as a diagnostic test for cystic fibrosis. *Am J Respir Crit Care Med.* 2012;186:732–739.

Ramsey BW, Davies J, McElvaney NG, et al. A CFTR potentiator in patients with cystic fibrosis and the G551D mutation. *N Engl J Med.* 2011;365:1663–1672.

Saudek CD, Herman WH, Sacks DB, et al. A new look at screening and diagnosing diabetes mellitus. *J Clin Endocrinol Metab.* 2008;93:2447–2453.

Schuetz P, Chiappa V, Briel M, Greenwald JL. Procalcitonin algorithms for antibiotic therapy decisions: a systematic review of randomized controlled trials and recommendations for clinical algorithms. *Arch Intern Med.* 2011;171:1322–1331.

Tenner S, Baillie J, DeWitt J, Vege SS. American College of Gastroenterology guideline: management of acute pancreatitis. *Am J Gastroenterol.* 2013;108:1400–1415.

Vernooij-van Langen AM, Loeber JG, Elvers B, et al. Novel strategies in newborn screening for cystic fibrosis: a prospective controlled study. *Thorax.* 2012;67:289–295.

Wagener JS, Zemanick ET, Sontag MK. Newborn screening for cystic fibrosis. *Curr Opin Pediatr.* 2012;24:329–335.

Wang SS, Lin XZ, Tsai YT, et al. Clinical significance of ultrasonography, computed tomography, and biochemical tests in the rapid diagnosis of gallstone-related pancreatitis: a prospective study. *Pancreas.* 1988;3:153–158.

23

Endocrinology

JIMMY L. BOYD AND DONNA LARSON

CHAPTER OUTLINE

OBJECTIVES

After completion of this chapter, the reader will be able to:

1. Explain the three main classes of hormones.
2. Describe the three general aspects of hormone actions.
3. Describe the two mechanisms of hormonal actions.
4. Compare and contrast the control and command structure for endocrine glands.
5. Describe how a negative feedback loop controls hormone production.
6. Name five each of the peptides, glycoproteins, steroids, amines, and derivatives of arachidonic acid hormones.
7. Describe the mechanism of action for protein hormones.
8. Identify test methods used to measure hormones.
9. Compare and contrast hypopituitarism and hyperpituitarism.
10. Differentiate Graves disease, goiter, Hashimoto thyroiditis, and triiodothyronine (T_3) toxicosis.
11. Compare and contrast Cushing disease, Addison disease, pheochromocytoma, ectopic adrenocorticotropic hormone (ACTH), and congenital adrenal hyperplasia.
12. Describe the measurement techniques for triiodothyronine (T_3), thyroxine (T_4), free T_4, free T_3, and thyroid-stimulating hormone (TSH), and explain how they can be used to differentiate thyroid diseases.
13. List the metabolites of epinephrine and norepinephrine that are measured in the urine.
14. Describe ectopic hormones and explain why their production is problematic.
15. Name the carcinomas that produce ectopic hormones and match the hormone to the carcinoma.
16. Differentiate primary, secondary, tertiary, and ectopic hormone diseases.
17. Describe how the hypothalamic-pituitary-adrenal axis affects physiologic functions.
18. State the purpose of somatostatin.
19. Explain the actions of antidiuretic hormone, oxytocin, ACTH, growth hormone, prolactin, TSH, luteinizing hormone, and follicle-stimulating hormone.
20. Compare and contrast the diseases associated with excess pituitary hormone.
21. State the laboratory tests used to diagnose the syndrome of inappropriate antidiuretic hormone secretion.
22. Describe diabetes insipidus, including the cause, symptoms, and laboratory tests used for the diagnosis.
23. Compare and contrast adrenal cortex disease mechanisms, symptoms, and laboratory tests results.
24. Explain the effect of stress on the adrenal medulla.
25. Describe the laboratory tests used to detect pheochromocytoma and neuroblastoma, and explain why blood tests for epinephrine and norepinephrine are not used.
26. Describe the endocrine hormones secreted by the pancreas and their functions.
27. Describe hypoparathyroidism.
28. Describe the connection between aldosterone, angiotensin, and renin.

KEY TERMS

Acromegaly
Addison disease
Adrenal cortex
Adrenal medulla
Adrenocorticotropic hormone
Aldosterone
Amine hormone
Androstenedione
Angiotensin II/III
Angiotensin-converting enzyme
Angiotensinogen
Anterior pituitary
Antidiuretic hormone
Arachidonic acid–derived hormone
Catecholamine
Circadian rhythm
Congenital hypothyroidism
Cortisol
Cretinism
Cushing syndrome
Dehydroepiandrosterone
Dehydroepiandrosterone sulfate
Diabetes insipidus
Dipsogenic diabetes insipidus
Diurnal variation
Ectopic disease
Eicosanoids
Epinephrine
Euthyroid sick syndrome
Familial hypocalciuric hypercalcemia
Fight or flight response
Follicle-stimulating hormone
Follicular cells
Gastrin
Giantism
Glucagon
Glucocorticoid

Glycoprotein hormone
Graves disease
Growth hormone
Hashimoto thyroiditis
Hirsutism
Hormone
Hyperthyroidism
Hypoparathyroidism
Hypopituitarism
Hypothalamic-pituitary-adrenal axis
Hypothalamus
Hypothyroidism
Insulin
Luteinizing hormone
Melatonin
Metanephrine
Mineralocorticoid
Natriuretic peptide
Negative feedback loop
Nephrogenic diabetes insipidus
Neuroblastoma
Neurogenic diabetes insipidus
Norepinephrine
Normetanephrine
Oxytocin
Panhypopituitarism
Parafollicular cell
Paresthesia
Peptide or polypeptide hormone
Pheochromocytoma
Pineal gland
Pituitary gland
Posterior pituitary
Primary aldosteronism
Primary disease
Primary hyperparathyroidism
Prolactin

Prolactinoma
Pseudohypoparathyroidism
Renin
Secondary aldosteronism
Secondary disease
Secondary hyperparathyroidism
Secondary hyperthyroidism
Secondary hypocortisolism
Secondary hypothyroidism
Serotonin
Somatostatin
Steroid hormone
Subclinical hyperthyroidism
Subclinical hypothyroidism
Syndrome of inappropriate antidiuretic
  hormone secretion
Tertiary hyperthyroidism
Tertiary hypothyroidism
Testosterone
Tetraiodothyronine
Thymopoietin
Thymosin
Thymus gland
Thyroglobulin
Thyroid cancer
Thyroid hormone resistance
Thyroid-stimulating hormone
Thyroid storm
Thyroiditis
Thyrotoxicosis
Toxic multinodular goiter
Transthyretin
Triiodothyronine
Vanillylmandelic acid
Zona fasciculata
Zona glomerulosa
Zona reticularis

❖ Case in Point

A 45-year-old woman consulted a physician after blood pressure screening at a health fair revealed mild to moderate hypertension. The patient had central obesity, thin limbs, and a round, ruddy face. She was not taking any medications. Her blood pressure was 160/100 mm Hg. A fasting blood glucose test performed on a fingerstick sample in the doctor's office showed a level of 120 mg/dL.

The physician ordered serum cortisol samples to be drawn at 8 AM and 4 PM. Laboratory results for cortisol were as follows: 32 μg/dL at 8 AM and 30 μg/dL at 4 PM. What is the patient's probable diagnosis? Why?

Points to Remember

- Endocrine glands release hormones into the blood to assist fetal development of the reproductive and central nervous systems, promote physical growth through childhood into adulthood, coordinate sexual hormones to enable reproduction, support body processes such as metabolism, and direct responses (e.g., fight or flight) to emergency situations.

- Hormones are regulatory substances (usually peptides or steroids) that are secreted into the blood by glands and cause specific responses in target cells.

- The endocrine system works with the nervous system to regulate responses to changing internal and external stimuli.

- The negative feedback loop is a common method for controlling the body's hormone response to a stimulus.

- In the negative feedback loop of the thyroid, the hypothalamus produces thyrotropin-releasing hormone (TRH), which stimulates the anterior pituitary gland to produce thyroid-stimulating hormone (TSH). TSH stimulates the thyroid gland to synthesize and release thyroid hormones into the blood. The increasing blood levels of thyroid hormones stimulate the hypothalamus to stop producing TRH, which curtails the production of TSH by the anterior pituitary gland and thus stops the thyroid from producing thyroid hormones.

- The peptide hormones are mostly synthesized by the anterior pituitary, placenta, pancreas, and parathyroid glands.
- Protein hormones attach to cell membrane receptors and activate a second messenger within the cell that carries out the hormone's function (enzyme activation or protein synthesis).
- The lipid core of steroid hormones is compatible with the structure of the cell membrane and allows the hormone to passively diffuse into the cell. Inside the cell, steroid hormones bind with intracellular receptors, forming a receptor–ligand complex that travels to the nucleus and affects DNA transcription and replication.
- All amine hormones are regulated by a negative feedback mechanism.
- Most hormones are measured with an enzyme-linked immunosorbent assay (ELISA), enzyme-multiplied immunoassay technique (EMIT), fluorescence polarization immunoassay (FPIA), fluorescent immunoassays, or high-pressure liquid chromatography (HPLC).
- The hypothalamic-pituitary-adrenal axis (HPA axis) links the central nervous system to the endocrine system.
- The HPA axis affects physiologic functions through the release of inhibitory, releasing, and tropic hormones.
- The hypothalamus mediates electrolyte balance, fluid balance, body temperature, blood pressure, and body weight to maintain the normal physiologic state of the body.
- Hypothalamic diseases manifest clinically as pituitary diseases.
- The posterior pituitary gland does not synthesize hormones; it instead stores two hormones synthesized by the hypothalamus.
- The anterior pituitary is the active, hormone-synthesizing portion of the pituitary gland.
- In all three forms of diabetes insipidus, the kidney is unable to increase its permeability to water and, as a result, large volumes of dilute urine are excreted.
- Adrenal cortex hormones (i.e., steroid hormones) are synthesized using cholesterol as a base molecule.
- The major glucocorticoid secreted by the adrenal cortex is cortisol, which regulates carbohydrate, protein, and lipid metabolism.
- Aldosterone is regulated by the renin-angiotensin system, potassium level, and natriuretic peptide levels. The major action of aldosterone is to stimulate reabsorption of sodium in the collecting ducts of the kidney and thereby regulate water and salt balance.
- The glucocorticoids, the most important of which is cortisol, affect cell metabolism and nerve function, suppress inflammation, and suppress growth.
- The weak hormones, androstenedione and dehydroepiandrosterone (DHEA), bind to protein and travel through the blood to the gonads, skin, and adipose tissue, where they are converted to sex hormones.
- Hyperaldosteronism is characterized by hypertension, hypokalemia, renal potassium wasting, and neuromuscular changes. It is the most common cause of secondary hypertension.
- In Cushing syndrome, excess secretion of adrenocorticotropic hormone (ACTH) by a pituitary adenoma increases the level of cortisol in the blood, causing symptoms known as Cushing syndrome. Similar symptoms can be produced by excessive intake of glucocorticoids, an ACTH-secreting nonpituitary tumor, or cortisol secretion from an adrenal adenoma or carcinoma.
- The symptoms of Addison disease include hypocortisolism and hypoaldosteronism.
- Stresses such as traumatic injury, hypoxia, and hypoglycemia stimulate the release of epinephrine and norepinephrine into the blood by means of sympathetic nerves.
- When norepinephrine is released in response to a stressful event, specific norepinephrine receptors in the cerebral cortex, limbic system, and spinal cord form a neurotransmitter system that produces alertness, stimulates arousal, and influences the reward system.
- Somatostatin regulates blood glucose, lipids, peptides, vasoactive intestinal peptides, and cholecystokinin.
- Glucagon (reference range, ≤60 pg/mL) regulates blood glucose by stimulating the breakdown of glycogen to glucose (i.e., hepatic glycogenolysis).
- Insulin (reference range, 4 to 20 mU/mL) regulates blood glucose levels by stimulating the conversion of glucose to glycogen (i.e., glycogenesis).
- Serotonin is synthesized from tryptophan and secreted by the gastrointestinal tract. It is a neurotransmitter and contracts smooth muscle. It is transported by platelets and metabolized in the liver into 5-hydroxyindoleacetic acid (5-HIAA).
- Because melatonin has a pivotal role in regulating body temperature, the sleep-wake cycle, female reproductive hormones, and cardiovascular function, its deficiency or excess can produce anxiety, stress, depression, seasonal affective disorder, sleep disorders, immunologic disorders, cardiovascular disease, and cancer.
- Estrogen promotes cellular growth in the uterus, fallopian tubes, vagina, external genitalia, and mammary glands (i.e., breasts) and affects fat distribution in childbearing women.
- The principal function of the thyroid gland is secretion of hormones that regulate metabolic processes, neurologic development, oxygen consumption, heat production, growth, sexual maturity, and protein and carbohydrate metabolism.
- In tissues, free triiodothyronine (free T_3) stimulates heart rate and contractions, accelerates synthesis and degradation of cholesterol and triglycerides, and enhances the adrenergic receptors' response to catecholamines.
- Thyroid hormone production is regulated by the hypothalamic-pituitary-thyroid axis.

- TSH is composed of one α subunit and one β subunit, which are covalently linked. The α subunit is the same as the α subunits in luteinizing hormone (LH), follicle-stimulating hormone (FSH), and human chorionic gonadotropin (hCG). The β subunit specifically stimulates the thyroid gland.
- Triiodothyronine (T_3) diffuses through the cell membrane and binds to thyroid hormone nuclear receptors, which bind to DNA thyroid hormone response elements that inhibit or stimulate gene transcription.
- Primary hyperthyroidism occurs when total T_3, total thyroxine (T_4), free T_3, and free T_4 levels are increased with a simultaneous decrease in TSH levels.
- Secondary or tertiary hyperthyroidism is caused by increased TSH levels or increased TRH levels, or both.
- Graves disease is the most common hyperthyroid disease, accounting for 60% to 80% of cases.
- The symptoms of Graves disease include goiter (i.e., thyroid gland enlargement), infiltrative ophthalmopathy (i.e., exophthalmos or protruding eyes), and dermopathy (i.e., pretibial swelling of the shins).
- Subclinical hyperthyroidism is important to identify because of adverse effects on the cardiovascular system (i.e., increased incidence of atrial fibrillation) and the skeletal system (i.e., osteoporosis and increased fractures).
- In primary hypothyroidism, the TSH level is increased, and the levels of total T_3, total T_4, free T_3, and free T_4 are decreased. Hashimoto thyroiditis is the most common form; it manifests as a chronic autoimmune disorder and often is misdiagnosed.
- In Hashimoto thyroiditis, the autoantibodies cause destruction of the thyroid gland, which can cause the gland to enlarge (i.e., goiter) or to atrophy.
- Third-generation immunoassays using monoclonal and polyclonal antibodies can detect TSH levels as low as 0.05 mU/L.
- Although measurement of TSH is a good screening test for most thyroid diseases, thyroid dysfunction should be confirmed by examining total T_4, free T_4, total T_3, and free T_3 levels.
- A low T_4 level with an increased TSH level usually indicates hypothyroidism, and an increased T_4 level with a decreased TSH level indicates hyperthyroidism.
- Magnesium, calcium, and phosphate levels affect parathyroid hormone levels.
- Primary hyperparathyroidism, a common endocrine disorder, is caused by adenomas, hyperplasia, and carcinomas.

Introduction

The endocrine system is varied and complex. Endocrinology is the study of the glands that produce hormones and the effects of hormones on organs. The hormones produced by the endocrine system coordinate specific responses through cell-to-cell communication and intracellular signaling. These responses assist the body in adapting to internal and external changes.

Endocrinologists study how hormones are synthesized, stored, released, transported, used, and degraded. A hormone secreted into the circulation by a gland at one location has specialized effects on tissues distant from the site of production (Table 23-1). The endocrine system is multifunctional; many hormones can affect a single physiologic function, and one hormone can affect several organs.

Overview of the Endocrine System

Glands located in various places in the body make up the endocrine system (Fig. 23-1). Endocrine glands release hormones into the blood, which carries them to target tissues. Hormones assist fetal development of the reproductive and central nervous systems, direct physical growth through childhood into adulthood, coordinate sexual hormones to enable reproduction, help body processes run efficiently and effectively (i.e., metabolism), and ensure proper responses (e.g., fight or flight) in emergency situations. A **hormone** is a chemical substance (usually a peptide or steroid) formed in endocrine glands that regulates the activity of distant receptive cells and organs. When an endocrine gland receives a chemical signal, it responds by synthesizing and releasing hormones. This action must be controlled to prevent continuous production of hormones. The endocrine system has many ways of regulating hormone synthesis and release:

TABLE 23-1 Pituitary Hormones

Hormone	Action
Antidiuretic hormone (ADH)	Maintains osmolarity of the body
Oxytocin	Causes contraction of mammary glands and milk secretion from the nipple
Adrenocorticotropic hormone (ACTH)	Stimulates the adrenal cortex to secrete glucocorticoids, cortisol, corticosterone, aldosterone, and androstenedione
Growth hormone (GH)	Promotes growth in infants, children, and adolescents
Prolactin (PRL)	Breast milk production during pregnancy and lactation
Thyroid-stimulating hormone (TSH)	Binds with thyroid receptors to signal the thyroid gland to increase secretion of T_4 and T_3
Luteinizing hormone (LH)	Promotes ovulation in women and testosterone production by the testes in men
Follicle-stimulating hormone (FSH)	Initiates spermatogenesis, stimulates testicular growth, and stimulates synthesis and release of testosterone in men; stimulates growth and recruitment of immature ovarian follicles in women

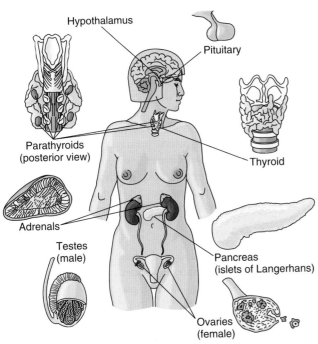

Figure 23-1 Principal endocrine glands. (From Ignatavicius D. *Medical-Surgical Nursing: Patient-Centered Collaborative Care.* 7th ed. St. Louis: Elsevier; 2013.)

- Hormone secretion is dictated by circadian rhythms, diurnal patterns, pulsatile patterns, cyclic patterns, and levels of chemical substances.
- Negative and positive feedback loops control hormone expression.
- Receptive cells have specific receptors that bind to and carry out the action of a hormone.
- Circulating enzymes degrade peptide hormones.
- Hydrophobic (lipid-soluble) hormones such as steroid hormones are secreted by the adrenal cortex directly or after modification in the liver.
- The endocrine system works with the nervous system to regulate responses to internal and external stimuli.

Negative and positive feedback loops are used by the endocrine system to precisely control hormone synthesis and release (Fig. 23-2). The negative feedback loop is a common method for controlling the hormone response to stimuli. A negative feedback loop is associated with thyroid hormone production. The hypothalamus produces thyrotropin-releasing hormone (TRH), which stimulates the anterior pituitary gland to produce thyroid-stimulating hormone (TSH). TSH stimulates the thyroid gland to synthesize and release thyroid hormones into the blood. Increasing levels of thyroid hormones in the blood stimulate the hypothalamus to stop producing TRH, which curtails the production of TSH by the anterior pituitary gland and thus stops the thyroid from

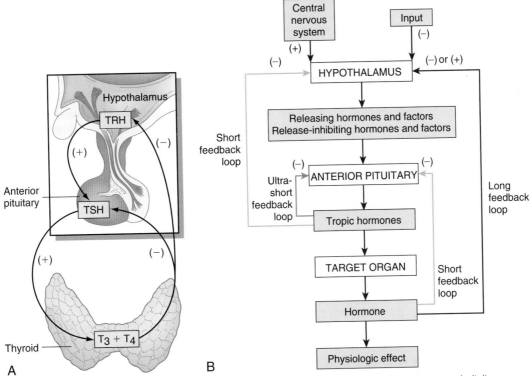

Figure 23-2 Feedback loops. **A,** Endocrine feedback loops involving the hypothalamus and pituitary gland for regulation of the thyroid gland in this example. **B,** General model for control and negative feedback regulation of hypothalamic-pituitary target organ systems. Negative feedback regulation is possible at three levels: target organ (i.e., ultrashort feedback), anterior pituitary (i.e., short feedback), and hypothalamus (i.e., long feedback). *TRH,* Thyrotropin-releasing hormone; *TSH,* thyroid-stimulating hormone; T_3, triiodothyronine; T_4, tetraiodothyronine (thyroxine). (From Huether SE, McCance KL. *Understanding Pathophysiology.* 5th ed. St. Louis: Mosby; 2013.)

TABLE 23-2	Structural Categories of Hormones
Structural Category	**Examples**
Peptides, polypeptides	Growth hormone, insulin, leptin, parathyroid hormone, prolactin, adrenocorticotropic hormone, antidiuretic hormone, calcitonin, endorphins, glucagon, hypothalamic hormones, lipotropins, melanocyte-stimulating hormone, oxytocin, somatostatin, thymosin, thyrotropin-releasing hormone
Glycoproteins	Follicle-stimulating hormone, luteinizing hormone, thyroid-stimulating hormone
Amines	Triiodothyronine (T_3), thyroxine (T_4), epinephrine, norepinephrine
Steroids (derived from cholesterol)	Estrogens, glucocorticoids (e.g., cortisol), mineralocorticoids (e.g., aldosterone), progestins (e.g., progesterone), testosterone
Derivatives of arachidonic acid	Leukotrienes, prostacyclins, prostaglandins, thromboxanes

producing thyroid hormones. This mechanism helps the body maintain normal physiologic levels of hormones.

Types of Hormones

Hormones are classified by structure. They include peptides, glycoproteins, steroids, amines, and derivatives of arachidonic acid (Table 23-2).

Peptide or polypeptide hormones include growth hormone, insulin, leptin, parathyroid hormone (PTH), prolactin, adrenocorticotropic hormone (ACTH), antidiuretic hormone (ADH), calcitonin, endorphins, glucagon, hypothalamic hormones, lipotropins, melanocyte-stimulating hormone, oxytocin, somatostatin, thymosin, and TRH. These hormones circulate freely in the blood and have half-lives of a few minutes.

Glycoprotein hormones include follicle-stimulating hormone (FSH), luteinizing hormone (LH), and thyroid-stimulating hormone (TSH). They have half-lives of a few minutes. These hormones usually do not bind to other proteins in the blood.

Amine hormones include triiodothyronine (T_3), thyroxine (T_4), epinephrine, and norepinephrine. They are derivatives of the amino acid tyrosine. Thyroid hormones have half-lives of a few days, and catecholamines such as epinephrine and norepinephrine have half-lives of a few minutes.

Steroid hormones are derived from cholesterol and include estrogens, glucocorticoids (e.g., cortisol), mineralocorticoids (e.g., aldosterone), progestins (e.g., progesterone), and testosterone. These hormones are synthesized and then quickly secreted from the cell. Very little of them is stored. Because these hormones are made with cholesterol and are hydrophobic, they

must bind with proteins to move through the blood. Some have a low affinity for binding protein and easily reach equilibrium between free and bound states. Some are bound to specific proteins, which affects their half-lives and elimination. These hormones are inactivated through metabolic transformations and are excreted in the urine or bile or both.

Arachidonic acid–derived hormones are made from polyunsaturated fatty acids. These hormones are called eicosanoids, and they include prostaglandins, prostacyclins, leukotrienes, and thromboxanes. Polyunsaturated fatty acids are degraded to arachidonic acid, which is the precursor for these molecules. The hormones are metabolized soon after they are produced, with an expected lifetime of a few seconds.

Protein Hormones

Most hormones produced in the body are protein or polypeptide hormones. Peptide hormones are mostly synthesized by the anterior pituitary, placenta, pancreas, and parathyroid glands. They range in size from nonapeptides (i.e., nine amino acids long) to large protein complexes. They are typically synthesized and then stored in secretory granules until needed.

Peptide hormones have various functions, but they all have the same mechanism of action. They are water soluble and do not need carrier proteins. They are in the blood for a short period (<10 to 30 minutes), and their levels in the blood vary. They attach to cell membrane receptors and activate a second messenger within the cell that effects enzyme activation or protein synthesis.

Steroid Hormones

Steroid hormones are derived from cholesterol. They are not stored but are produced as needed. Steroid hormones must bind to a carrier protein to be transported through the blood. Steroid hormones include cortisol, aldosterone, testosterone, estrogen, and progesterone.

Steroid hormones are lipid soluble and are synthesized by the gonads, placenta, and adrenal glands. The lipid core of the steroid hormones is compatible with the structure of the cell membrane and allows the hormone to passively diffuse into the cell. Inside of the cell, steroid hormones bind to intracellular receptors, forming a receptor–ligand complex that regulates DNA transcription and replication by interacting with nuclear receptors.

Amine Hormones

Amine hormones share a common precursor, the aromatic amino acid tyrosine. They are synthesized by the thyroid gland and the adrenal medulla. The thyroid gland produces thyroid hormones (T_4 and T_3), and the adrenal medulla produces the catecholamines epinephrine and norepinephrine. Catecholamines are neurotransmitters in the central and peripheral nervous systems. Catecholamines are water soluble and do not require carrier proteins, but T_4 is lipid soluble and does require a carrier protein.

Amine hormones exert their action by activating a secondary messenger system in the cell. The thyroid hormones must be free from the carrier protein to function. The free hormone crosses the cell membrane and binds with a specific intracellular receptor and then with nuclear DNA, affecting DNA transcription. Free thyroxine (free T_4) is the active hormone, and its concentration is lower than that of protein-bound T_4. All amine hormones are regulated by a negative feedback mechanism.

Most hormones are measured with an enzyme-linked immunosorbent assay (ELISA), enzyme-multiplied immunoassay technique (EMIT), fluorescence polarization immunoassay (FPIA), fluorescent immunoassays, or high-pressure liquid chromatography (HPLC). Although radioimmunoassay (RIA), immunoradiometric assay (IRMA), and EMIT are rarely used in the clinical setting, reference laboratories still employ these conventional methods. Hormone testing using gas chromatography with mass spectrometry (GC-MS) coupled with tandem mass spectrometry (MS/MS) is gaining popularity in clinical laboratories.

Laboratory test results assist in diagnosing, managing, and treating endocrine disorders. Because of the tiny amounts of hormones present in the blood, hormone assay testing must be able to measure extremely small amounts of these chemicals. Total and free hormone levels pose an intricate puzzle for the provider.

Disease Processes

Diseases and disorders of the endocrine system often result from tumors, inflammatory or degenerative processes, and genetic mutations. Pituitary disorders can be hyperfunctional or hypofunctional processes. Primary disease originates in a specific target organ. In secondary disease, the disease originates in the hypothalamus or pituitary. Tertiary disease can result from a tumor in the hypothalamus or pituitary. The term ectopic disease is used when there is a tumor in the body that is secreting hormones.

Anatomy, Pathophysiology, and Laboratory Testing

Hypothalamic-Pituitary-Adrenal Axis

The hypothalamic-pituitary-adrenal axis (HPA axis) coordinates actions of the neuroendocrine system through secretion of inhibitory, releasing, and tropic hormones and feedback mechanisms. Hypothalamic, pituitary, and adrenal interactions control reactions to stress and regulate digestion, the immune system, mood, sexuality, and energy storage and expenditure.

Hypothalamus

Anatomy and Physiology
The hypothalamus is located at the base of the brain, below the thalamus and above the pituitary, and it is the size of an almond. The major function of the hypothalamus is to maintain homeostasis. The hypothalamus produces TRH, which stimulates the production of TSH and prolactin;

> ### • BOX 23-1 Hormones Produced by the Hypothalamus
>
> - Thyrotropin-releasing hormone
> - Gonadotropin-releasing hormone
> - Somatostatin
> - Growth hormone–releasing hormone
> - Corticotrophin-releasing hormone
> - Dopamine
> - Prolactin-releasing factor

gonadotropin-releasing hormone (GnRH), which stimulates the production of FSH and LH; corticotropin-releasing hormone (CRH), which stimulates the production of ACTH; prolactin-inhibiting factor (i.e., dopamine); and growth hormone–releasing hormone (GHRH), which stimulates the secretion of growth hormone and allows the hypothalamus to control hormones released by the pituitary gland.

The supraoptic and paraventricular nuclei of the hypothalamus produce ADH and oxytocin. The hypothalamus also produces a peptide hormone called somatostatin, which inhibits TSH, GH, gastrointestinal hormones (e.g., gastrin, insulin, glucagon, secretin), and pancreatic hormones. Somatostatin reduces the amount of these hormones secreted by tumors (Box 23-1).

The hypothalamus mediates electrolyte balance, fluid balance, body temperature, blood pressure, and body weight to maintain the normal physiologic state of the body. The gland receives input from the from various body systems and alters functions to maintain homeostatic set points.

Clinical Disorders
Because hypothalamic diseases manifest clinically as pituitary diseases, they are described in later sections.

Pituitary

Anatomy and Physiology
The pituitary gland has two parts with distinct functions: the anterior pituitary (i.e., adenohypophysis) and the posterior pituitary (i.e., neurohypophysis). The pituitary gland attaches to the hypothalamus via a stalklike structure called the infundibulum. The nerves in the infundibulum originate in the hypothalamus and end in the pituitary gland, allowing coordinated functions of the glands (Fig. 23-3).

Posterior Pituitary. The posterior pituitary does not synthesize hormones; instead, it stores two hormones synthesized by the hypothalamus: ADH and oxytocin. It excretes the hormones when directed by the hypothalamus. The hormones are synthesized in the hypothalamus, transported along axons, and then stored in the nerve terminals.

Antidiuretic hormone (ADH), also called vasopressin, maintains the body's osmolarity. When the osmoreceptors in the body detect an increase in plasma osmolarity, the hypothalamus secretes ADH and sends it to the posterior pituitary for release into the circulation. The hormone then travels to the kidneys, where it increases reabsorption of water in the collecting ducts, decreasing the amount of

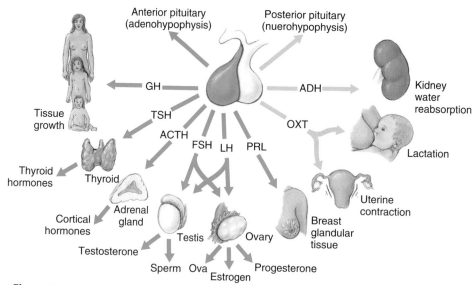

• **Figure 23-3** Effects of pituitary gland hormones. *ACTH*, Adrenocorticotropic hormone; *ADH*, antidiuretic hormone; *FSH*, follicle-stimulating hormone; *GH*, growth hormone; *LH*, luteinizing hormone; *OXT*, oxytocin; *PRL*, prolactin; *TSH*, thyroid-stimulating hormone. (From Applegate EMS. *The Anatomy and Physiology Learning System.* 4th ed. St. Louis: Saunders; 2011.)

water and increasing the amount of sodium in the urine. ADH binds to receptors in blood vessels, causing vasoconstriction and increased blood pressure, and to receptors in the collecting ducts of the kidney cells, causing water retention and increased plasma osmolarity.

Oxytocin is secreted by the hypothalamus, stored in the posterior pituitary, and then released by oxytocin cells in the hypothalamus, which are activated by nipple suckling. The hormone causes mammary glands to contract, leading to milk secretion from the nipple. During childbirth, oxytocin is responsible for stimulating the uterine smooth muscles to contract. In men, oxytocin levels increase during ejaculation, increase smooth muscle contractions, and propel sperm out of the body through the urethra.

Anterior Pituitary. The anterior pituitary is the active, hormone-synthesizing portion of the pituitary gland. The anterior pituitary synthesizes and secretes ACTH, growth hormone, prolactin, TSH, LH, and FSH (Fig. 23-4).

ACTH is under the control of the hypothalamus. Its levels peak before waking and decrease throughout the day. Levels are also influenced by pain, cold exposure, hypoglycemia, trauma, depression, and surgery. ACTH stimulates the adrenal cortex to secrete glucocorticoids, aldosterone, and androstenedione.

Growth hormone (GH) promotes growth in infants, children, and adolescents. To stimulate growth, GH promotes gluconeogenesis and lipolysis, which provide energy for amino acid uptake by cells and subsequent growth.

Thyroid-stimulating hormone (TSH) binds with the thyroid receptors to signal the thyroid gland to increase secretion of T_4 and T_3. Binding also results in increased TSH synthesis and thyroid cell growth.

The presence of luteinizing hormone (LH) and follicle-stimulating hormone (FSH) signals the beginning of ovulation and puberty in girls. In boys, FSH stimulates testicular growth and the synthesis and release of testosterone.

LH is responsible for ovulation and for the production of testosterone by the testes.

Prolactin secretion increases during pregnancy and is responsible for breast milk production. High estrogen levels during pregnancy inhibit the effects of prolactin on lactation. After childbirth, estrogen levels decrease, allowing prolactin to induce lactation. The hormone exhibits sleep-related diurnal variations, with increased levels occurring during the night (see Table 23-1).

Clinical Disorders

The most common pituitary disorders are pituitary tumors. Although most tumors are not a medical emergency, they can alter normal body physiology. Pituitary disorders may result in excess hormone or not enough hormone for normal functioning. The cause of production of an excessive amount of a hormone by the pituitary is abnormal growth of cells (i.e., tumor) in the gland, increased production of tropic hormones by the hypothalamus, or an ectopic tumor elsewhere in the body. Hormonal deficiencies often involve more than one hormone and have many causes.

Excess Pituitary Hormone Disorders

Syndrome of Inappropriate Antidiuretic Hormone Secretion. Syndrome of inappropriate antidiuretic hormone secretion (SIADH) occurs when the pituitary secretes high levels of ADH without being stimulated to do so. SIADH can be caused by secretion of ADH by ectopic tumors, such as small cell carcinoma of the lung, duodenum, stomach, or pancreas; bladder cancer; prostate cancer; endometrial cancer; lymphomas; and sarcomas. SIADH also occurs in cases of tuberculosis, asthma, cystic fibrosis, encephalitis, meningitis, intracranial hemorrhage, and trauma. It may occur in connection with drugs such as antidepressants, antipsychotics, narcotics, general anesthetics, chemotherapeutic agents, nonsteroidal antiinflammatory drugs, and quinolone antibiotics.

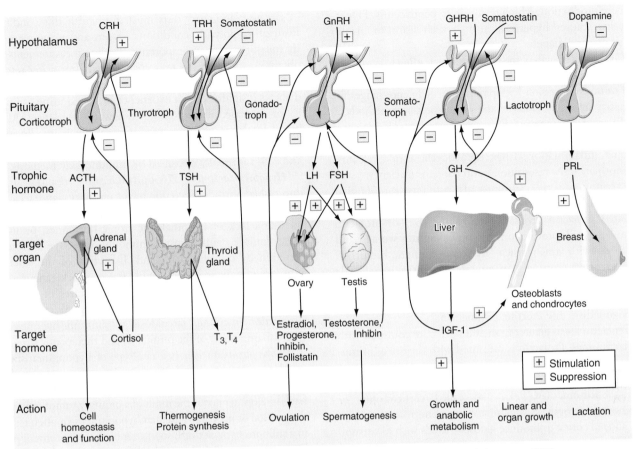

• **Figure 23-4** The hypothalamic-pituitary-target organ axis. *ACTH,* Adrenocorticotropic hormone; *CRH,* corticotropin-releasing hormone; *FSH,* follicle-stimulating hormone; *GHRH,* growth hormone–releasing hormone; *GnRH,* gonadotropin-releasing hormone; *IGF-1,* insulin-like growth factor 1; *LH,* luteinizing hormone; *PRL,* prolactin; T_3, triiodothyronine; T_4, thyroxine; *TRH,* thyrotropin-releasing hormone; *TSH,* thyroid-stimulating hormone. (Modified from Melmed S, Kleinberg D. Anterior pituitary. In: Larsen PR, Kronenberg HM, Melmed S, et al, eds. *Williams Textbook of Endocrinology.* 10th ed. Philadelphia: WB Saunders; 2003:181.)

In SIADH, excessive ADH production leads to water retention. ADH increases the renal collecting ducts' permeability to water, so more water is reabsorbed by the kidneys. Water retention leads to hyponatremia, hypo-osmolarity, and increased urine osmolarity.

Symptoms of SIADH are thirst, impaired taste, anorexia, weight gain, dyspnea on exertion, fatigue, and dulled senses when the sodium level drops from 140 to 130 mEq/L. Although individuals gain weight due to water retention, there is no edema in their legs or arms. When sodium levels decrease from 130 to 120 mEq/L, vomiting and severe abdominal cramps occur. Sodium levels lower than 115 mEq/L cause confusion, lethargy, muscle twitching, and seizures. Sometimes SIADH develops slowly, and when sodium levels drop below 110 to 115 mEq/L, irreversible nerve damage can occur.

Laboratory tests used to diagnose SIADH include measurements of electrolytes and of serum and urine osmolality. The diagnosis is based on a serum osmolality lower than 280 mOsm/kg, a serum sodium level lower than 125 mEq/L, urine osmolality higher than serum osmolality, and normal renal, adrenal, and thyroid function test results. Osmolality is usually measured by the freezing point depression technique, and sodium is measured using ion-specific electrodes (see Chapter 3).

Growth Hormone Excess. Acromegaly is a condition that occurs in adults with excess GH. In children and adolescents, excess GH results in giantism. Excess GH is usually produced by a pituitary adenoma, and 15% of pituitary adenomas produce GH. Acromegaly most often affects women, and if it is not treated, it can result in an early death. Acromegaly is a progressive disease that affects the whole body. It produces cardiac hypertrophy, hypertension, atherosclerosis, and type 2 diabetes. Colon, breast, and lung cancers are more common among people with acromegaly.

Tumors secrete GH irregularly, which interferes with the usual secretory patterns, including baseline levels and sleep-related peaks. Excess GH in children and adolescents causes excessive bone growth, with some individuals reaching 8 or 9 feet in height. In adults, excess GH causes connective tissue growth and bone growth, which results in an enlarged tongue, coarse skin, coarse body hair, nerve damage, swelling and decreased range of motion of the large joints, kyphosis, elongated ribs, and facial, hand, and foot bone enlargement.

GH affects glucose, lipid, and protein metabolism. GH inhibits peripheral glucose uptake and increases hepatic glucose production, which results in hyperglycemia. Hyperglycemia causes hyperinsulinism, which leads to insulin resistance and diabetes.

GH causes growth of the myocardium, leading to cardiomyopathy. As a tumor grows, it can compress the pituitary gland and cause compression hypopituitarism. Reference ranges for GH vary among laboratories and with various test methods.

Hyperprolactinemia. Excessive secretion of prolactin is associated with renal failure, cirrhosis, hypothyroidism, trauma, inflammation, drugs (e.g., tricyclic antidepressants, phenothiazines, reserpine), adrenal insufficiency, and prolactinomas. Prolactinomas are pituitary tumors that secrete prolactin at a constant rate and produce sustained elevated prolactin levels. The constant level of prolactin stimulates milk production in nonpostpartum women and in those with amenorrhea. In some women, hirsutism (i.e., excessive terminal hair growth in a postpubertal male pattern) develops due to decreased estrogen levels and increased testosterone levels. Symptoms in men include hypogonadism and erectile dysfunction.

Prolactin levels greater than 200 ng/dL are common with prolactinomas. Prolactin is measured with the use of immunoassay techniques.

Adrenocorticotropic Hormone Excess. Adrenocorticotropic hormone (ACTH), also called corticotropin or adrenocorticotropin, is a pituitary hormone that stimulates the adrenal cortex to produce glucocorticoids such as cortisol. ACTH is secreted in response to stress. Excessive production of ACTH is a major cause of Cushing syndrome (discussed later).

Luteinizing Hormone and Follicle-Stimulating Hormone Excess. LH and FSH are glycoproteins produced by the anterior pituitary. The hormones are called gonadotropins because they stimulate the ovaries and the testes. Excessive hormone secretion indicates lack of a negative feedback loop due to gonadal failure or a pituitary tumor.

Thyroid-Stimulating Hormone Excess. TSH is secreted by the anterior pituitary gland. As TSH levels increase, more thyroid hormones are produced. When TSH levels are decreased, the production of thyroid hormones decreases (see later discussion).

Pituitary Hormone Deficit Disorders

Antidiuretic Hormone Deficiency. Diabetes insipidus results from a low ADH level. The three forms of this disorder are classified by their causative mechanism: neurogenic diabetes insipidus (low levels of ADH), nephrogenic diabetes insipidus (resistance of renal collecting tubules to ADH), and dipsogenic diabetes insipidus (excessive fluid intake that lowers plasma osmolality to below the ADH secretion threshold).

In all three forms of diabetes insipidus, the kidney is unable to increase its permeability to water. As a result, large volumes of dilute urine are excreted. There is also an increase in plasma osmolality. Urine output can be 8 to 12 L/day. Because urine specific gravity is low (1.005), dehydration ensues. Symptoms of all three forms are similar: polyuria (i.e., frequent urination), nocturia (i.e., urination at night), continuous thirst, and polydipsia (i.e., consuming large amounts of fluids).

Because laboratory tests must distinguish this condition from other polyuric conditions, serum and urine osmolality measurements are important. Baseline measurements are obtained, and then the tests are repeated after water restriction (i.e., fluid intake is severely restricted). Individuals with diabetes insipidus do not experience increased urine osmolality or decreased urine volume with water restriction. ADH blood levels are also measured. Osmolality is usually measured by the freezing point depression method (see Chapter 3), and ADH is usually measured by immunoassay methods.

Hypopituitarism. Hypopituitarism results from diminished hormone secretion by the pituitary gland; it causes dwarfism in children and premature aging in adults. Causes include a lack of hypothalamic tropic hormones, pituitary stalk damage, and, most commonly, defective hormone secretion by the pituitary gland. Infarction of the vascular pituitary can be associated with severe shock, aneurysms, sickle cell disease, or pregnancy. Other causes of pituitary damage include pituitary adenomas, surgical removal or destruction, infections, sarcoidosis, autoimmune hypophysitis (i.e., inflammation of the pituitary), and therapeutic drugs.

Panhypopituitarism is a rare type of hypopituitarism in which the concentrations of all pituitary hormones are low or zero. Panhypopituitarism is an anomaly that occurs during fetal development or as the result of a pituitary tumor or injury. Congenital or neonatal-onset panhypopituitarism often results in a stillborn baby or death soon after birth. Symptoms of panhypopituitarism include cortisol deficiency, thyroid deficiency, and loss of secondary sex characteristics. Specific pituitary hormone deficiencies are discussed in the following sections.

Adrenocorticotropic Hormone Deficiency. ACTH deficiency can be life-threatening because this hormone controls cell metabolism. This disorder usually does not occur alone but is accompanied by general hypopituitarism. Because ACTH controls the production of cortisol, the symptoms of ACTH deficiency are those of cortisol deficiency: nausea, vomiting, anorexia, fatigue, weakness, hypoglycemia, decreased glycogen reserves, decreased gluconeogenesis, and limited maximum aldosterone secretion (see "Adrenal Glands").

Luteinizing Hormone and Follicle-Stimulating Hormone Deficiencies. Women of childbearing age with LH and FSH deficiencies have decreased body hair and decreased libido. They do not have menses, and the vagina, uterus, and breasts atrophy. In men with these deficiencies, the testes atrophy, and beard growth is significantly decreased (see Chapter 25).

Thyroid-Stimulating Hormone Deficiency. TSH deficiency usually occurs together with general hypopituitarism. After the onset of hypopituitarism, symptoms of decreased TSH may take 4 to 8 weeks to appear. Symptoms include an inability to tolerate cold temperatures, mild myxedema (i.e., swelling of skin and underlying tissues giving a waxy consistency), dry skin, lethargy, and decreased metabolism. These symptoms are less severe compared with those of primary hypothyroidism (see later discussion under the heading, "Thyroid").

Growth Hormone Deficiency. GH deficiencies occur in children and adults and may be caused by genetic mutations or tumors. In children, GH deficiency results in growth failure and fasting hypoglycemia. In adults, symptoms include increased body fat, decreased muscle bulk and strength, reduced sweating, dry skin, depression, social withdrawal, osteoporosis, fatigue, loss of motivation, and a diminished sense of well-being. GH levels decrease with age.

Laboratory Evaluation of Hypopituitarism. Hypopituitarism is diagnosed by correlating signs and symptoms with measurements of tropic hormones from the pituitary and the target endocrine gland. The hormones are usually measured with the use of immunoassays.

Adrenal Glands

Anatomy and Physiology

The adrenal glands are composed of the adrenal cortex (i.e., outer portion) and the adrenal medulla (i.e., inner portion). The adrenal cortex is composed of the zona glomerulosa (an outer layer that secretes mineralocorticoids), the zona fasciculata (a middle layer that secretes glucocorticoids), and the zona reticularis (an inner layer that secretes androgens). The adrenal medulla secretes the catecholamines epinephrine and norepinephrine.

Adrenal cortex hormones are synthesized from cholesterol. The hormones alter cellular processes by passing through the cell membrane and binding to intracellular receptors, which then bind to DNA in responsive genes, altering the transcription rates of the genes.

Hormones of the Adrenal Cortex. Hormones produced by the adrenal cortex include mineralocorticoids (e.g., aldosterone), glucocorticoids (e.g., cortisol, cortisone,

corticosterone), and the adrenal androgens, some of which are precursors of estrogens. Aldosterone is the major mineralocorticoid secreted by the adrenal glands. It is responsible for maintaining extracellular fluid volume and regulating sodium reabsorption and potassium excretion by cells of the renal distal convoluted tubules.

The major glucocorticoid secreted by the adrenal cortex is cortisol, which regulates carbohydrate, protein, and lipid metabolism. The half-life of cortisol is approximately 90 minutes, after which the liver deactivates it. Cortisol levels show diurnal variation; levels are highest in the morning on waking and lowest in the late evening. Diurnal variation is affected by the sleep-wake cycle of the individual.

Androgens secreted by the adrenal cortex include dehydroepiandrosterone sulfate (DHEAS), dehydroepiandrosterone (DHEA), and androstenedione (which has androgenic and estrogenic activity). DHEAS has a half-life of 8 to 11 hours compared with 30 to 60 minutes for other secreted androgens. Adrenal androgens are converted to functional sex hormones such as testosterone and estradiol in the gonads and other target tissues.

Synthesis, Regulation, and Physiologic Effects. Synthesis of glucocorticoids and adrenal androgens is stimulated by ACTH. The mineralocorticoids are stimulated through a different mechanism: Renin (an enzyme produced by the kidney) acts on angiotensinogen to produce angiotensin II/III, which stimulates the zona glomerulosa cells to produce more aldosterone. Synthesis of adrenal hormones is shown in Figure 23-5.

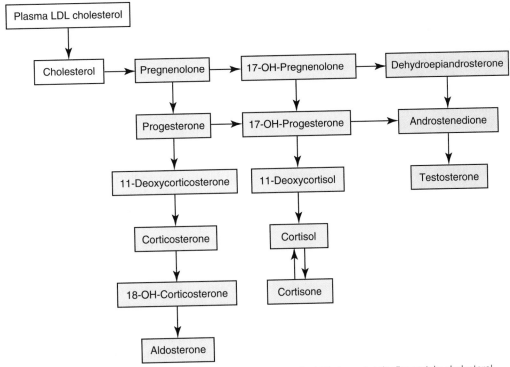

• **Figure 23-5** Principal pathways of adrenal steroidogenesis. *LDL,* Low-density lipoprotein cholesterol. (Modified from Kaplan LA, Pesce AJ. *Clinical Chemistry: Theory, Analysis, Correlation.* 5th ed. St. Louis: Mosby; 2010.)

Cortisol is regulated by the hypothalamus and the anterior pituitary gland. CRH stimulates the anterior pituitary gland to produce ACTH, which acts on the adrenal cortex to produce cortisol (Fig. 23-6).

Aldosterone is regulated by the renin-angiotensin system, potassium level, and natriuretic peptide level (Fig. 23-7). Renin is an enzyme found in the cells of the afferent arteriole in the glomerulus as part of the juxtaglomerular apparatus. Renin is produced when sodium levels or pressure in the afferent arterioles of the glomerulus decreases. Renin converts angiotensinogen to angiotensin I. Angiotensin-converting enzyme (ACE) converts angiotensin I to angiotensin II, a powerful vasoconstrictor that increases blood pressure and stimulates the release of aldosterone. Aldosterone is also released when the blood potassium level rises, and it is inhibited when the blood potassium level falls. Natriuretic peptides inhibit aldosterone release and help to prevent extracellular water accumulation.

Sixty percent of aldosterone and 96% of cortisol are bound to proteins in the blood. These hormones are synthesized from cholesterol, which is not soluble in water, so in order to travel in the blood, they must be bound to a protein that is soluble in water. The free cortisol is biologically active.

Glucorticoids. Glucocorticoids, the most important of which is cortisol, affect metabolism, mediate the function and homeostasis of the central nervous system, suppress inflammation, and suppress growth. The hormones affect carbohydrate metabolism by suppressing the release of insulin, initiating gluconeogenesis in the liver, and decreasing cellular glucose uptake. They also break down proteins and regulate amino acid transport so that the molecules can be used for gluconeogenesis in the liver. Increased protein metabolism leads to increased excretion of nitrogen in the urine and activation of urea cycle enzymes.

The glucocorticoids are immunosuppressive and antiinflammatory (Box 23-2). Because stress increases glucocorticoid production, acute and chronic forms of stress decrease immune system function. Other effects of glucocorticoids are listed in Box 23-3. Glucocorticoids repress the transcription of many genes encoding proinflammatory molecules. They reduce the amount of arachidonic acid released from membrane phospholipids after tissue damage, and they suppress the synthesis of eicosanoids, which reduces inflammation.

Mineralocorticoids. Mineralocorticoids (e.g., aldosterone) control the excretion of electrolytes mostly through the kidneys but also through the colon and sweat glands. Aldosterone regulates reabsorption of sodium in the collecting ducts of the kidney, sweat glands, stomach, and salivary glands. Chloride and water are retained when sodium is retained. When sodium is reabsorbed, potassium and hydrogen ions are excreted. Angiotensin II is a potent vasoconstrictor that further stimulates aldosterone secretion.

Androgens. The adrenal cortex secrets small amounts of androgenic hormones that are regulated by ACTH. The weak hormones, androstenedione and DHEA, bind to proteins and travel through the blood to the gonads, skin, and adipose tissue, where they are converted to sex hormones. DHEA is converted to DHEAS in the liver and adrenal cortex before

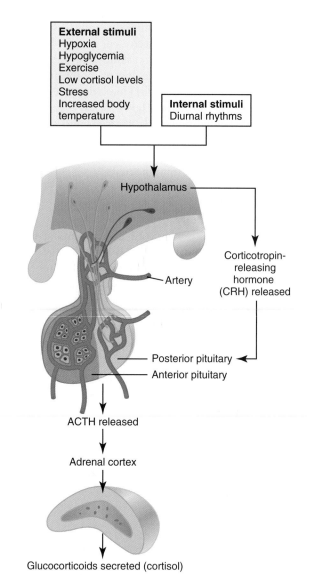

• **Figure 23-6** Regulation of glucocorticoid (cortisol) secretion. *ACTH,* Adrenocorticotropic hormone.

it travels to target organs. In aging and obese individuals, estrogen production from androgens is enhanced.

The active sex hormones are testosterone and estradiol. These lipid-soluble hormones diffuse across cell membranes and bind to intracellular receptors in the cytoplasm and nucleus. Binding alters gene expression, which leads to the development of secondary sex characteristics during puberty (see Chapter 25).

Hormones of the Adrenal Medulla. The adrenal medulla secretes the catecholamines epinephrine (i.e., adrenaline), norepinephrine (i.e., noradrenaline) in conjunction with the sympathetic nervous system. These hormones are stored in the adrenal chromaffin cells or pheochromocytes, which release them into the blood in response to stresses such as traumatic injury, hypoxia, or hypoglycemia. Figure 23-8 details the endocrine response to stress.

Epinephrine and norepinephrine act as neuromodulators in the central nervous system and as hormones in the circulatory system. At their target sites, the catecholamines

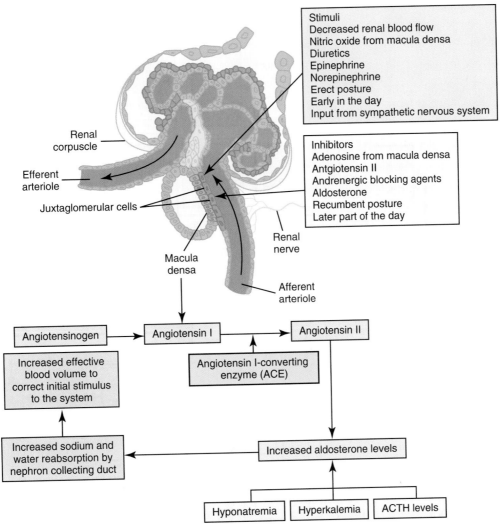

Stimuli
Decreased renal blood flow
Nitric oxide from macula densa
Diuretics
Epinephrine
Norepinephrine
Erect posture
Early in the day
Input from sympathetic nervous system

Inhibitors
Adenosine from macula densa
Antgiotensin II
Andrenergic blocking agents
Aldosterone
Recumbent posture
Later part of the day

Renal corpuscle

Efferent arteriole

Juxtaglomerular cells

Renal nerve

Macula densa

Afferent arteriole

Angiotensinogen → Angiotensin I → Angiotensin II

Angiotensin I-converting enzyme (ACE)

Increased effective blood volume to correct initial stimulus to the system

Increased sodium and water reabsorption by nephron collecting duct ← Increased aldosterone levels

Hyponatremia Hyperkalemia ACTH levels

• **Figure 23-7** Regulation of aldosterone secretion. *ACTH,* Adrenocorticotropic hormone.

• BOX 23-2 **Antiinflammatory Effects of Glucocorticoids**

- Decrease the activity of macrophage receptors
- Decrease proliferation of helper T cells
- Depress cellular immunity more than humoral immunity
- Decrease natural killer cell activity
- Suppress synthesis, secretion, and actions of acute phase reactants (e.g., prostaglandins, thromboxanes, leukotrienes)
- Inhibit inflammatory gene expression
- Stimulate antiinflammatory cytokines
- Stabilize lysosomal membranes

• BOX 23-3 **Effects of Glucocorticoids**

- Inhibit bone formation
- Inhibit antidiuretic hormone secretion
- Stimulate gastric acid secretion
- Sensitize arterioles to vasoconstriction by norepinephrine
- Increase effects of thyroid and growth hormones
- Increase glyconeogenesis
- Increase hepatic glycogen synthesis
- Increase lipolysis
- Increase blood glucose levels
- Increase protein catabolism
- Decrease protein synthesis
- Enhance conversion of norepinephrine to epinephrine in adrenal medulla
- Inhibit thyroid-stimulating hormone release
- Cause depression, psychosis, loss of memory
- Maintain normal blood pressure

---

bind to plasma membrane receptors and activate a secondary messenger system in the cell. The half-life is less than 2 minutes in the circulation. These hormones are responsible for the body's fight or flight response.

Epinephrine plays a major role in the **fight or flight response,** which is a coordinated effort of the nervous and endocrine systems to prevent or resolve a harmful event or threat to survival. In response to perceived danger, epinephrine is released, increasing the heart rate, blood pressure, muscle strength, and glucose metabolism. The fight or flight response prepares the body for strenuous activity.

Norepinephrine is released from sympathetic neurons and affects the heart and peripheral vessels. Increased secretion of norepinephrine from the sympathetic nervous

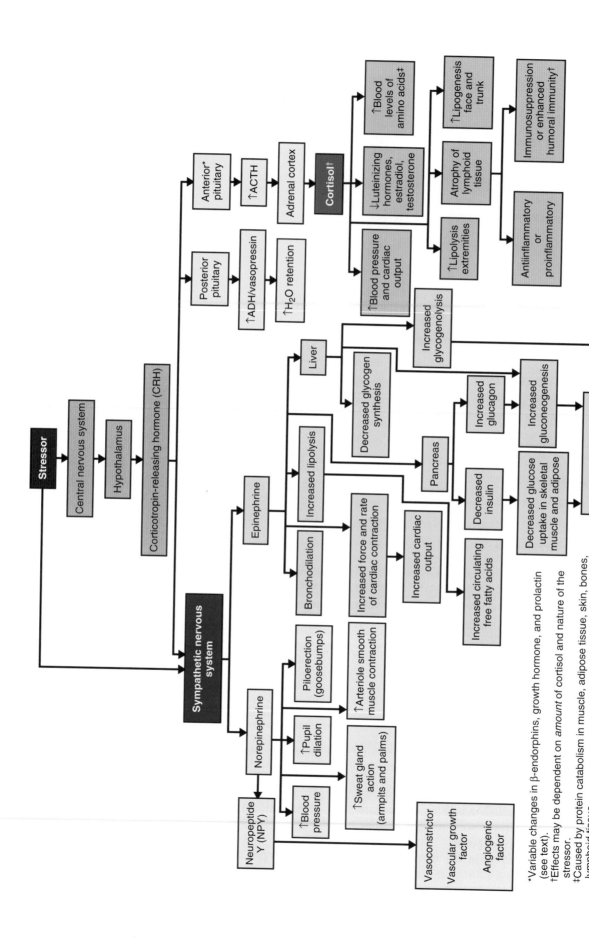

*Variable changes in β-endorphins, growth hormone, and prolactin (see text).

†Effects may be dependent on *amount* of cortisol and nature of the stressor.

‡Caused by protein catabolism in muscle, adipose tissue, skin, bones, lymphoid tissue.

ADH, Antidiuretic hormone; *ACTH*, adrenocorticotropic hormone.

• **Figure 23-8** The stress response. (From McCance KL, Huether SE. *Pathophysiology: The Biologic Basis for Disease in Adults and Children.* 7th ed. St. Louis: Mosby; 2015.)

TABLE 23-3	Effects of Epinephrine, Norepinephrine, and Dopamine	
Hormone	**Effects**	
Epinephrine	Increases heart rate and force of contractions	
	Relaxes gallbladder and ducts	
	Stimulates lipolysis in adipocytes	
	Stimulates kidney to release renin	
	Dilates arterioles	
	Decreases gastrointestinal motility and tone	
	Dilates bronchial muscles	
Norepinephrine	Increases force of heart contractions	
	Venous constriction	
	Sweating	
	Bladder sphincter contraction	
	Spleen contractions	
	Arterioles constriction	
	Dilates pupils	
	Gastrointestinal sphincter contraction	
	Uterine contractions in pregnancy	
	Ejaculation	
	Decreased gastrointestinal motility and tone	
	Inhibits pancreatic islet beta cell secretion of insulin	
	Inhibits lipolysis in adipocytes	
	Inhibits intestinal secretions	
	Stimulates platelet aggregation	

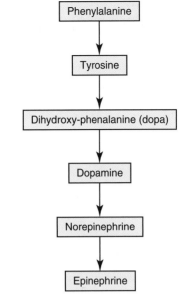

• **Figure 23-9** Synthesis of catecholamines.

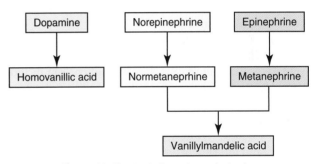

• **Figure 23-10** Metabolism of catecholamines.

system increases the rate of heart contractions. Norepinephrine affects the brain, increasing attention and response pathways. Norepinephrine also increases peripheral blood vessel resistance, which raises blood pressure. When norepinephrine is released in response to a stressful event, interaction with specific norepinephrine receptors in the cerebral cortex, limbic system, and spinal cord (i.e., neurotransmitter system) produces alertness and arousal and influences the reward system (Table 23-3).

Catecholamine synthesis is different from that of the steroid hormones produced by the adrenal glands. The catecholamines are produced from the amino acid phenylalanine (Fig. 23-9). The enzyme that converts norepinephrine to epinephrine is secreted only in the adrenal medulla, and its production is stimulated by cortisol (Fig. 23-10).

To end the activity of epinephrine and norepinephrine, they are taken up by nerve cells, where they are stored and reused when another stressful event arises. Both hormones can be catabolized into end products that are excreted in the urine. Epinephrine is metabolized to metanephrine and then to vanillylmandelic acid (VMA). Norepinephrine is metabolized to normetanephrine and then to VMA.

Because the half-life of both hormones is very short, laboratory assays measure the metabolites in 24-hour urine specimens. Laboratory tests are usually ordered only for patients with catecholamine-secreting tumors. Free urinary catecholamines, metanephrine, normetanephrine, and VMA are measured to rule out a pheochromocytoma, Urinary homovanillic acid (HVA) and VMA are measured to rule

out a neuroblastoma. To exclude a carcinoma, 5-hydroxyindoleacetic acid (5-HIAA) is measured.

The analytical method most widely used for these analytes is HPLC coupled with electrochemical or fluorochemical detectors. Reference intervals for urinary catecholamines are affected by physiologic factors such as sex, sitting, standing, age, hypertension, and hospitalization. Norepinephrine reference ranges are 110 to 410 pg/mL for the supine position, 120 to 680 pg/mL for sitting, and 125 to 700 pg/mL for standing. Epinephrine reference ranges are less than 50 pg/mL for the supine position, less than 60 pg/mL for sitting, and less than 90 pg/mL for standing. Some drugs also increase catecholamine levels (Box 23-4).

Clinical Disorders

Hormonal Disorders of the Adrenal Cortex. Any disease that alters the secretion of adrenal cortex hormones profoundly affects development and homeostasis. Adrenal gland diseases can be caused by secretion of too much or too little hormone to maintain homeostasis (i.e., hyperadrenalism or hypoadrenalism, respectively). For example, overproduction of cortisol by the adrenal glands results in Cushing syndrome, whereas underproduction of

• BOX 23-4 **Drugs That Increase Catecholamine Levels**

Albuterol
Amitriptyline
Amlodipine
Amphetamines
Atenolol
Caffeine
Carbidopa
Cocaine
Diltiazem
Doxazosin
Ephedrine
Hydralazine
Imipramine
Isosorbide
Labetalol
Levodopa

Metoprolol
Minoxidil
Nicotine
Nifedipine
Nortriptyline
Phenelzine
Phenoxybenzamine
Prazosin
Propranolol
Pseudoephedrine
Selegiline
Terazosin
Theophylline
Tranylcypromine
Verapamil

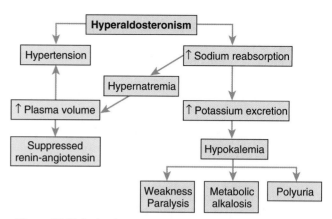

• **Figure 23-11** Pathophysiology of primary hyperaldosteronism. (From Bonow RO, Mann DL, Zipes DP, Libby P, eds. *Braunwald's Heart Disease: A Textbook of Cardiovascular Medicine.* 9th ed. Philadelphia: Saunders; 2012.)

aldosterone leads to Addison disease. If too much androgen or estrogen is produced, the result can be female virilization or male feminization, respectively.

Three conditions result from hyperadrenalism: hyperaldosteronism, Cushing syndrome, and primary adrenal hyperplasia. Conditions caused by hypoadrenalism include hypoaldosteronism (i.e., Addison disease) and autoimmune adrenalitis. Hypoadrenalism can also result from granulomatous diseases (i.e., fungal infections, tuberculosis, histoplasmosis, and cytomegalovirus infection), neoplastic infiltrate, and intraadrenal hemorrhage.

Hyperaldosteronism. There are two types of hyperaldosteronism: primary aldosteronism (i.e., Conn syndrome) and secondary aldosteronism (i.e., secondary hyperaldosteronism). Conn syndrome is uncommon and is usually found in conjunction with an aldosterone-secreting adrenal adenoma (Fig. 23-11).

Hyperaldosteronism is characterized by hypertension, hypokalemia, renal potassium wasting, and neuromuscular changes. It is the most common cause of secondary hypertension that is treatment resistant. Long-term untreated hypertension leads to left ventricular dilation and hypertrophy and vascular disease. The physiologic effects in primary aldosteronism include increased renal absorption of sodium and water, hypovolemia, hypertension, and excretion of potassium. Despite the increased renal reabsorption of water, there is no edema. Metabolic syndrome (i.e., hypertension, obesity, dyslipidemia, insulin resistance, and hyperglycemia) can be associated with primary aldosteronism.

Secondary hyperaldosteronism is caused by increased aldosterone secretion from a source other than the adrenal glands. Most often, the angiotensin II level is elevated through a renin-dependent mechanism that causes increased aldosterone secretion. Increased angiotensin II levels can be caused by dehydration, shock, hypoalbuminemia, renal

artery stenosis, heart failure, or hepatic cirrhosis. Other conditions that cause secondary hyperaldosteronism include renin-secreting tumors and an inherited renal defect in the tubular reabsorption of sodium. Physiologic effects of secondary aldosteronism include hypokalemic alkalosis, altered myocardial conduction, and skeletal muscle changes. Renal tubules become insensitive to ADH, and excessive loss of water causes severe potassium depletion. The reference ranges for aldosterone are 6 to 22 pg/dL for men and 5 to 30 pg/dL for women.

Laboratory tests used to diagnose hyperaldosteronism include serum and urine electrolyte levels, serum and urine aldosterone levels, aldosterone suppression testing, and serum renin levels. Electrolytes are measured using ion-selective electrodes (see Chapter 3), and aldosterone and renin levels are measured using immunoassay techniques.

Cushing Syndrome. Prolonged exposure to increased cortisol leads to a collection of signs and symptoms known clinically as Cushing syndrome (Fig. 23-12). This condition can be produced by a cortisol-secreting adenoma or carcinoma in the cortex of the adrenal gland (sometimes called primary hypercortisolism), an ACTH-secreting pituitary adenoma (Cushing disease) or by an ectopic (nonpituitary) tumor that produces excess plasma ACTH. Cushing syndrome of any cause disrupts the normal feedback control of ACTH secretion, leading to loss of diurnal variation in glucocorticoid levels and failure of ACTH and cortisol to increase in response to stimuli.

The most common symptom of Cushing syndrome is weight gain, especially in the trunk, face, and neck. Patients typically have central obesity and growth of fat pads on the face (i.e., moon face) and on the back of the neck (i.e., buffalo hump). Other symptoms include thinning scalp hair, facial flush, purple striae, easy bruising, skin hyperpigmentation, increased body and facial hair, a protruded abdomen with thin extremities, a decreased immune response, hyperglycemia, hypertension, and

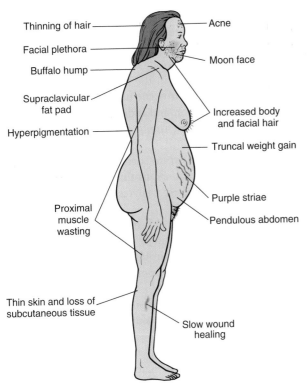

Thinning of hair
Facial plethora
Buffalo hump
Supraclavicular fat pad
Hyperpigmentation
Proximal muscle wasting
Thin skin and loss of subcutaneous tissue

Acne
Moon face
Increased body and facial hair
Truncal weight gain
Purple striae
Pendulous abdomen
Slow wound healing

• **Figure 23-12** Cushing syndrome. (From Monahan FD, Sands JK, Neighbors M, Marek JF, Green-Nigro CJ. *Phipps' Medical-Surgical Nursting.* 8th ed. St. Louis: Mosby; 2007.)

• BOX 23-5 **Symptoms of Cushing Syndrome**

Physical Symptoms

- Weight gain
- Thinning of scalp hair
- Facial flush
- Moon face
- Purple striae
- Pendulous abdomen
- Easy bruising
- Acne
- Increased body and facial hair
- Supraclavicular fat pad (i.e., buffalo hump)
- Skin hyperpigmentation
- Central obesity
- Thin extremities
- Vertebral compression fractures

Physiologic Symptoms

- Decreased immune system function
- Hyperglycemia
- Hypertension
- Muscle wasting
- Osteoporosis

---

muscle wasting (Box 23-5). Breakdown of the protein matrix of the bone by cortisol causes osteoporosis, pathological fractures, vertebral compression fractures, bone and back pain, kyphosis (i.e. curvature of the spine producing a hunchback), and reduced height. Within 5 years after diagnosis, patients have morbidity and mortality rates of 50%. The cause of death is often suicide, infection, or coronary artery disease.

The most common laboratory test to screen for Cushing disease in people with Cushing syndrome is the 24-hour urine free cortisol measurement. A normal level (<100 μg/day) rules out Cushing disease (i.e., pituitary tumor). If the level is abnormal (>120 μg/day), another cause for the Cushing syndrome needs to be sought.

Because serum cortisol levels tend to be abnormal in various pathological conditions, the level of ACTH is measured to help determine the cause. In cases of adrenal tumor, blood levels of ACTH are low (<10 pg/mL), whereas in Cushing disease, they are somewhat elevated (40 to 260 pg/mL). ACTH levels higher than 300 pg/mL indicate ectopic production by an ACTH-secreting tumor elsewhere in the body.

Serum cortisol reference ranges are 5 to 23 μg/dL for morning and 3 to 16 μg/dL for evening. The reference range for ACTH is 10 to 85 pg/mL. Cortisol and ACTH levels are measured with immunoassay techniques.

The standard test for differentiating hypercortisolism caused by an adrenal or ectopic tumor from pituitary Cushing disease is the high-dose dexamethasone suppression test. Dexamethasone is a potent glucocorticoid that exerts negative feedback to suppress pituitary secretion of ACTH but does not affect ACTH-producing cells in ectopic or adrenal tumors. In a normal individual, high-dose dexamethasone produces a 50% suppression of cortisol levels. Levels are also suppressed in most individuals with Cushing disease. However, cortisol is not suppressed in individuals with adrenal or ectopic ACTH production. The result of this test is combined with ACTH measurement to help make the differential diagnosis.

Congenital Adrenal Hyperplasia. Congenital adrenal hyperplasia is an autosomal recessive disorder that disrupts cortisol production due to an enzyme deficiency. Low cortisol production increases ACTH production, which eventually leads to adrenal hyperplasia.

Addison Disease. Primary adrenal insufficiency is called Addison disease. Autoimmune mechanisms produce Addison disease more commonly in women than in men. Other causes include tuberculosis, fungal infections, human immunodeficiency virus infection, neoplastic infiltrates, and bilateral adrenal hemorrhage. Patients with Addison disease have low corticosteroid and mineralocorticoid levels with elevated ACTH levels. Clinical symptoms appear in this disease only after more than 90% of the adrenal tissue is destroyed.

The symptoms of Addison disease include hypocortisolism and hypoaldosteronism. The symptoms usually occur gradually, and individuals with mildly decreased cortisol levels experience weakness and are easily fatigued. The skin is hyperpigmented. As the cortisol level continues to decrease, anorexia, nausea, vomiting, diarrhea,

- Weakness and easy fatigability that gets worse as the day goes on
- Anorexia
- Nausea
- Vomiting
- Diarrhea
- Abdominal pain
- Weight loss
- Hypoglycemia
- Fatigue
- Mental confusion
- Apathy
- Psychosis
- Hyperpigmentation
- Vitiligo (i.e., patches of white, depigmented skin)
- Addisonian crisis (i.e., severe hypotension and vascular collapse)

weight loss, hypoglycemia, mental confusion, apathy, and psychosis develop. This results eventually in addisonian crisis, and hypotension leads to vascular collapse and shock (Box 23-6).

Secondary Hypocortisolism. A few conditions can produce secondary hypocortisolism: prolonged glucocorticoid administration, pituitary infarction, pituitary tumors, and hypophysectomy. Prolonged glucocorticoid use can produce secondary hypocortisolism because the glucocorticoids suppress ACTH secretion. When the adrenal cortex is not stimulated, it atrophies. Pituitary infarction and pituitary tumors destroy pituitary tissue, leaving the pituitary unable to secrete ACTH. In hypophysectomy, the anterior portion of the pituitary is removed, and no tissue is available to produce ACTH.

Hormonal Disorders of the Adrenal Medulla. Catecholamines play a vital role in maintaining health, and excess or deficiency of these hormones affects the entire body. Excess catecholamines can produce stress, a fall in blood pressure or blood volume, thyroid hormone deficiency, congestive heart failure, and arrhythmias. Low levels of catecholamines can produce idiopathic postural hypotension. Two neuroendocrine tumors that produce catecholamines are pheochromocytomas and neuroblastomas.

Pheochromocytoma. Pheochromocytomas are catecholamine-secreting tumors that must be recognized quickly because they can cause cardiovascular complications and death. Pheochromocytomas occur in fewer than 0.2% of individuals with hypertension. Although about 90% of pheochromocytomas are benign, they can have severe health consequences, the most common of which is hypertension. Others include headache, palpitations, diaphoresis, pallor, dyspnea, nausea, anxiety attacks, and generalized weakness. Individuals at high risk for pheochromocytoma are those who have a family history of the disease or have had a previous pheochromocytoma.

Ten percent of pheochromocytomas are malignant. There is no way to differentiate a malignant pheochromocytoma from a benign tumor using catecholamine levels or histopathological features. Instead, malignancy is diagnosed by the finding of metastases in the liver, lungs, lymph nodes, or bones. Metastases can occur up to 20 years after diagnosis of a benign tumor, and individuals with a history of the tumor are at risk for tumor recurrence and should be screened periodically.

Laboratory tests used to detect pheochromocytomas are assays of urinary catecholamines, metanephrines, and VMA. Levels of all of these analytes are greatly increased in this disease.

Neuroblastoma. Neuroblastoma is a malignant, catecholamine-secreting tumor made of postganglionic sympathetic neurons. Neuroblastomas occur mainly in children and are the most common malignancy in those younger than 1 year of age. Most of these tumors are found in the adrenal gland. They usually metastasize to bone marrow, lymph nodes, liver, skin, testis, and intracranial structures.

Hypertension is uncommon with this tumor. Symptoms include a tumor mass and hematologic abnormalities resulting from bone marrow involvement. An excess of catecholamines is produced, but because the ganglion cells in the neuroblastoma do not store as much of the catecholamines as chromaffin cells do, many of the symptoms of pheochromocytomas do not occur.

Laboratory tests used to screen for neuroblastomas are VMA and HVA assays. Because this disease is found mostly in children, 24-hour urine specimens are difficult to collect. Random urine specimens can be used in place of the 24-hour urine specimen.

Pancreas

Hormones and Function

The pancreas functions as an endocrine gland and an exocrine gland. The pancreas secretes endocrine hormones, including glucagon, insulin, gastrin, and somatostatin, and exocrine hormones, including the digestive enzymes trypsin and chymotrypsin, elastase, collagenase, lipase, amylase, and nucleases.

Glucagon (reference range, ≤60 pg/mL) regulates blood glucose by stimulating the breakdown of glycogen to glucose (i.e., hepatic glycogenolysis). Increased glucagon levels are associated with high-protein meals, acute hypoglycemia, and exercise; decreased levels are associated with high-carbohydrate meals. The hormone also stimulates gluconeogenesis and lipolysis.

Insulin (reference range, 4 to 20 mU/mL) regulates blood glucose levels by stimulating the conversion of glucose to glycogen (i.e., glycogenesis). Insulin also promotes carbohydrate transformation into fats (i.e., lipogenesis) and amino acid storage, thereby increasing glycogenesis and decreasing glycogenolysis. Insulin is secreted when blood glucose levels increase. The hormone is inhibited by epinephrine and norepinephrine and by drugs such as thiazides (i.e., diuretics), Dilantin (an antiseizure drug), and diazoxide (a hypoglycemic agent). A full discussion of glucagon and insulin is found in Chapter 22.

Somatostatin is a peptide hormone produced by the delta cells of the pancreas and by the hypothalamus. Somatostatin regulates blood glucose, lipids, peptides, vasoactive intestinal peptides (VIP), and cholecystokinin. Glucagon stimulates somatostatin production and inhibits GH secretion. Somatostatin blocks digestion by reducing gastrointestinal motility and inhibiting the secretion of digestive enzymes (e.g., hydrochloric acid), glucose, triglycerides, insulin, gastrin, and glucagon.

Gastrin (reference range, ≤100 pg/mL) is secreted by the stomach in response to neurogenic brain impulses as food enters the stomach. Zollinger-Ellison syndrome is discussed in Chapter 20.

Serotonin is a neurotransmitter that is synthesized from tryptophan and secreted by the gastrointestinal tract. It contracts smooth muscle. It is transported by platelets and metabolized in the liver to 5-HIAA. Elevated levels are found in celiac disease, tropical sprue, and cystic fibrosis (see Chapters 19 and 22).

The reference range for 5-HIAA is 2 to 8 mg/24 hours. Carcinoid tumors of the appendix and ileum produce levels of 5-HIAA as high as 150 to 625 mg/24 hours. Symptoms of elevated serotonin levels include flushing, hepatomegaly, diarrhea, bronchospasm, and heart disease. Laboratory analyses are performed on preserved 24-hour urine specimens, with patients avoiding foods that contain serotonin, such as bananas, pineapples, and tomatoes, for at least 3 days before the test.

Pineal Gland

Anatomy

The pineal gland consists of a small structure located near the center of the brain. It is about 8.5 mm long, is shaped like a pine cone, and has a reddish gray color. Fluoride, calcium, and phosphorus deposits build up in it with age.

Hormone and Function

The pineal gland secretes melatonin, which helps to maintain the circadian rhythm and regulates LH and FSH levels. The circadian rhythm is a 24-hour biological clock that is influenced by periods of light and dark. Melatonin levels are low during the day because light exposure stops the release of melatonin into the blood, and they are high during dark periods, when the hormone is released. Photoperiods influence sleep patterns. Melatonin is thought to block the secretion of LH and FSH.

The peak melatonin level occurs when the body temperature is at its lowest point. Ovulation raises body temperature and causes melatonin levels to decrease. Body temperature also affects the sleep cycle because it normally rises during the day and decreases at night. The variation between the two temperatures is about 1°, which

is critical for sleep. A falling body temperature promotes sleep, and a rising temperature promotes wakefulness.

Because melatonin is soluble in both water and fat, it is an antioxidant that protects all parts of the cell. Its solubility properties allow it to cross the blood–brain barrier and the placenta barrier. Melatonin scavenges free radicals, protecting DNA, proteins, and lipids from oxidative damage. Melatonin is a more powerful antioxidant than glutathione, mannitol, or vitamin E.

As melatonin levels increase, sympathetic activity decreases. As melatonin levels decrease, sympathetic activity increases, which increases the risk of coronary disease. Increased sympathetic activity releases epinephrine and norepinephrine, which damage blood vessels through increased arthrogenic uptake of low-density lipoprotein (LDL) cholesterol. Melatonin also inhibits platelet aggregation.

Increased or decreased production of melatonin produces anxiety, stress, depression, seasonal affective disorder, sleep disorders, immunologic disorders, and cardiovascular disease and increases the risk of some cancers.

Thymus
Anatomy

The thymus gland is a primary lymphoid organ of the immune system. It is located in the mediastinum (i.e., the area behind the sternum and between the lungs) of the chest wall. It is below the thyroid gland and the fourth costal cartilage of the ribs. The thymus gland reaches its maximum size (about 1 ounce) during puberty and atrophies with age.

Hormones and Function

The thymus produces thymopoietin (TPO) and thymosin (TMO). Thymopoietin plays a role in the differentiation and maturation of lymphoid stem cells into T cells, and thymosin plays a role in late T-cell maturation. During childhood, the thymus provides an environment for development of T cells from progenitor cells. The mature T cells then migrate to the lymph nodes, where they become functional immune cells.

Reproductive System
Ovary and Testis Hormones and Function

Ovaries secrete estrogen, progesterone (a hormone released by the corpus luteum that stimulates the uterus to prepare for pregnancy), and small amounts of androgens (i.e., male sex hormones such as testosterone). The primary estrogen (i.e., female sex hormone) is estradiol, which is bound in the circulation to sex hormone–binding globulin (SHBG). Estrogen is responsible for growth promotion in the uterus, fallopian tubes, vagina and external genitalia, and mammary glands (i.e., breasts) and for fat distribution in childbearing women. Estrogen also functions in the development of puberty, proliferation of the uterine endometrium during the proliferative phase of the menstrual cycle, and thickening of the cervical mucus. It has metabolic effects such as bone growth. Estrogen is regulated by FSH. A full discussion is found in Chapter 25.

Testosterone is a steroid hormone derived from cholesterol. It is produced by the testes. Testosterone is regulated by LH and is bound to SHBG in the blood. The hormone functions in the development and maturation of the male reproductive system. FSH stimulates spermatogenesis and normal development of the seminiferous tubules, whereas LH stimulates production of testosterone in the testicles. A negative feedback mechanism governs the production of FSH and LH by the hypothalamus. A full discussion is found in Chapter 25.

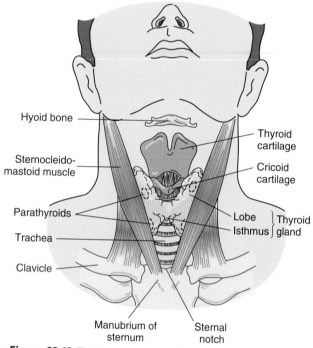

• **Figure 23-13** Thyroid gland and midline neck structures. (From Monahan FD, Sands JK, Neighbors M, Marek JF, Green-Nigro CJ. *Phipps' Medical-Surgical Nursing.* 8th ed. St. Louis: Mosby; 2007.)

Thyroid

Anatomy

The thyroid gland is located at the base of neck. It is shaped like a butterfly, with two main lobes connected by an isthmus (Fig. 23-13). It weighs between 15 and 25 g.

The gland consists of ring-shaped follicles that are composed of follicular cells surrounding colloid, thyroid hormone, thyroglobulin, and other glycoproteins (Fig. 23-14). The follicular cells secrete thyroid hormones. Autonomic nervous system neurons are located on the blood vessels that supply the follicular cells. Substances that stimulate the autonomic nervous system, such as acetylcholine and catecholamines, affect thyroid hormone section. The thyroid gland also contains parafollicular cells (i.e., C cells), which secrete calcitonin. Calcitonin lowers blood calcium levels by inhibiting osteoclasts.

The principal function of the thyroid gland is to secrete hormones that regulate neurologic development, oxygen consumption, heat production, growth, sexual maturity, and metabolism of proteins and carbohydrates. Follicular cells secrete T_3 and T_4. Thyroid hormones are under the regulatory feedback of the pituitary's secretion of TSH. Thyroid hormones use a mechanism similar to that of steroid hormones to affect body processes. They bind to intracellular receptors, then to DNA receptors, and affect the expression of proteins. The hormones help maintain a healthy metabolism and normal growth.

Hormones and Function

Synthesis and Secretion

The thyroid gland produces two major hormones: 3,5,3′5′-tetraiodothyronine or thyroxine (T_4) and triiodothyronine (T_3). T_4 is produced at a higher level than T_3. The follicular cells of the thyroid gland use tyrosine as a base to synthesize both hormones. TSH stimulates the gland, and iodine enters the follicular cells. Iodine attaches to tyrosine,

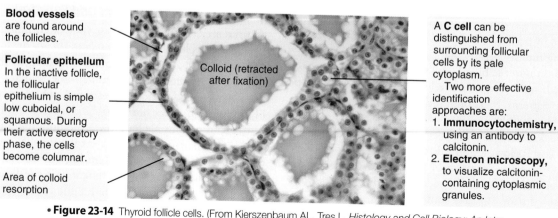

• **Figure 23-14** Thyroid follicle cells. (From Kierszenbaum AL, Tres L. *Histology and Cell Biology: An Introduction to Pathology.* 3rd ed. Philadelphia: Mosby; 2012.)

and tyrosine-iodine molecules couple to produce T_3 and T_4 (Figs. 23-15 and 23-16; Table 23-4).

After thyroid hormones are synthesized, they are attached to **thyroglobulin, transthyretin,** or albumin and stored in the colloid until they are secreted. Approximately 70% of T_4 is bound to thyroxine-binding globulin, 20% is bound to transthyretin, and 10% is bound to albumin. T_3 is bound to thyroid-binding globulin. Small amounts of T_4 and T_3 circulate unbound in the blood, and these free forms of the hormones are metabolically active. In the tissues, free T_3 increases the heart's rate and contractions, stimulates synthesis and degradation of cholesterol and triglycerides, and enhances the response of adrenergic receptors to catecholamines. Free T_3 is almost five times more active than free T_4. To maintain optimal metabolic processes, a minimum of 80 µg of T_4 and less than 10 µg of T_3 is secreted. T_3 can also be formed from T_4 through additional (peripheral) iodination in the liver.

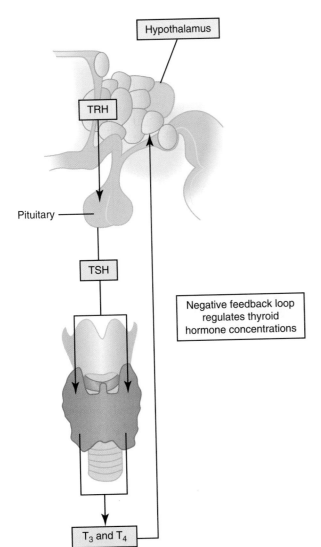

• Figure 23-15 Regulation of thyroid hormone secretion. *TSH,* Thyroid-stimulating hormone; *TRH,* thryrotropin-releasing hormone; *T3,* triiodothyronine; *T4,* thyroxine

Regulation

Thyroid hormone production is regulated by the hypothalamic-pituitary-thyroid axis. The hypothalamus releases TRH, which stimulates the pituitary to produce TSH. TSH stimulates the thyroid gland to secrete T_3 and T_4. Because thyroid hormone secretion is regulated by a negative feedback loop, an increase in T_3 and T_4 inhibits release of TRH from the hypothalamus. Laboratory assays for TRH are not clinically useful.

TSH is composed of one α subunit and one β subunit, which are covalently linked. The α subunit is the same as the α subunits in LH, FSH, and human chorionic gonadotropin (hCG). The β subunit is specific for stimulating the thyroid gland. The most useful laboratory tests for diagnosing and monitoring hyperthyroid and hypothyroid diseases are measurements of TSH and free T_4.

Physiologic Effects

T_3 is more physiologically active than T_4. T_4 can also be deiodinated in the peripheral tissues to produce physiologically active T_3. T_3 diffuses through the cell membrane and binds to the thyroid hormone nuclear receptors, which bind to thyroid hormone response elements and inhibit or stimulate gene transcription. The actions of thyroid hormones are listed in Table 23-5. Thyroid hormones support cell differentiation, growth, and maturation. Severe illness and starvation cause T_3 and T_4 levels to decrease, but TSH levels remain constant. Thyroid hormones are metabolized through deiodination (i.e., removal of iodine from the molecule), or they are conjugated with glucuronide or sulfate and excreted in bile.

Clinical Disorders

Thyroid disease is categorized as **hyperthyroidism** (i.e., overproduction of thyroid hormones) or **hypothyroidism** (i.e., underproduction of thyroid hormones). The disease is further classified as primary (i.e., originating in the thyroid gland) or secondary (i.e., caused by pituitary dysfunction). Because iodine is an integral part of T_3 and T_4, iodine-deficient diets lead to thyroid dysfunction, usually through autoimmune mechanisms.

Hyperthyroidism

Hyperthyroidism, also known as **thyrotoxicosis,** is defined as an increased concentration of the thyroid hormones produced by a hyperfunctioning thyroid gland. Usually, hyperthyroidism is a primary thyroid disease. Causes of hyperthyroidism are found in Table 23-6.

Excess thyroid hormones increase the body's metabolism. Symptoms of hyperthyroidism include weight loss (i.e., increased lipolysis), fatigue, heat intolerance, nervousness, loss of muscle mass (i.e., excessive protein breakdown), and sweating (see Table 23-5). This condition is exacerbated by excessive production of thyroid hormones from nonthyroid sources such as an adenoma and leakage of thyroid hormones from follicles.

In primary hyperthyroidism, levels of total T_3, total T_4, free T_3, and free T_4 are increased, and there is a simultaneous decrease in TSH levels. **Secondary hyperthyroidism**

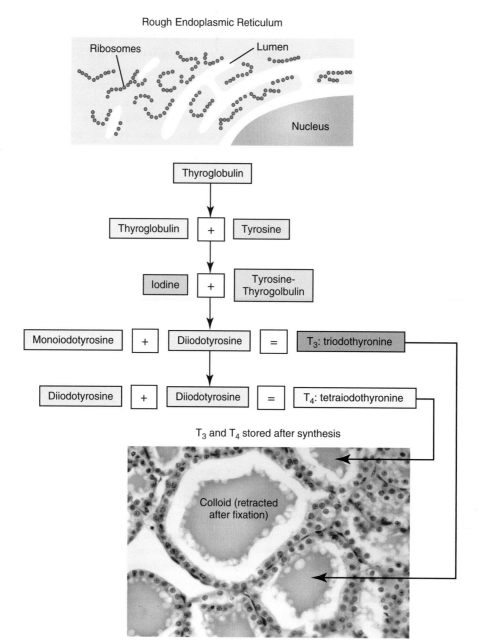

• **Figure 23-16** Synthesis of thyroid hormones. (From Kierszenbaum AL, Tres L. *Histology and Cell Biology: An Introduction to Pathology.* 3rd ed. Philadelphia: Mosby; 2012.)

and **tertiary hyperthyroidism** are caused by increased TSH levels with or without increased TRH. When T_3 and T_4 levels increase substantially, the negative feedback loop causes a decrease in TSH, often to very low (0.02 IU/L) or undetectable levels. Pituitary adenomas cause decreased TSH and increased free T_4 levels. Hyperthyroidism can range from a mild to a moderate condition, and a phenomenon known as a **thyroid storm** can occur when uncontrolled thyrotoxicosis leads to life-threatening complications. Table 23-7 shows the correlations between laboratory hormone levels and thyroid gland disorders.

Graves Disease

Graves disease is the most common hyperthyroid disease, accounting for 60% to 80% of cases. Women between 40

and 60 years of age are the most commonly diagnosed group. More than 80% of individuals diagnosed with this disease have a family member with the disease. Graves disease is an autoimmune disorder in which the body produces antibodies to thyroid TSH receptors, resulting in the overproduction of thyroid hormones. Antibodies to thyroglobulin and thyroperoxidase are found in Graves disease and Hashimoto thyroiditis.

The symptoms of Graves disease include goiter (i.e., enlargement of the thyroid gland), infiltrative ophthalmopathy (i.e., exophthalmos or protruding eyes), and dermopathy (i.e., pretibial swelling of the shins). The autoantibodies produced in Graves disease cross the placenta and can cause a transient Graves disease in the newborn. Laboratory tests results used to diagnose Graves disease are listed in Table 23-7.

TABLE 23-4 **Regulation and Function of Thyroid Hormones**

Hormone	Regulation	Functions
Thyroxine (T_4) and triiodothyronine (T_3)	T_4 and T_3 levels are controlled by TSH	Regulates protein, fat, and carbohydrate catabolism in all cells
	Released in response to metabolic demand	Regulates metabolic rate of all cells
	Influences on amount secreted	Regulates body heat production Insulin antagonist
	Gender	Maintains growth hormone secretion, skeletal maturation
	Pregnancy	Affects central nervous system development
	Increased gonadal and adrenocortical steroids increase levels	Necessary for muscle tone and vigor Maintains cardiac rate, force, and output
	Exposure to extreme cold increases levels	Maintains secretion of gastrointestinal tract Affects respiratory rate and oxygen utilization
	Chemical regulation	Maintains calcium mobilization
	Growth hormone–inhibiting hormone decreases levels	Affects red blood cell production
	Dopamine decreases levels	Stimulates lipid turnover, free fatty acid release, and cholesterol synthesis
	Catecholamines increase levels	
Calcitonin	Elevated serum calcium is major stimulant for calcitonin	Lowers serum calcium by opposing bone-resorbing effects of parathyroid hormone, prostaglandins, and calciferol by inhibiting osteoclastic activity
	Other stimulants	Lowers serum phosphate levels
	Gastrin	
	Calcium-rich foods (regardless of serum calcium levels)	May also decrease calcium and phosphorous absorption in gastrointestinal tract

From Monahan FD, Phipps WJ. *Phipps' Medical-Surgical Nursing: Health And Illness Perspectives*. 8th ed. St. Louis: Mosby; 2007.

TABLE 23-5 **Physiologic Effects of Thyroid Hormones and Syndromes of Thyroid Dysfunction**

System	Thyroid Hormone Effects	Hyperthyroidism	Hypothyroidism
Metabolic	Increased calorigenesis and oxygen consumption	Heat intolerance Flushed skin	Cold intolerance Dry and pale skin
	Increased heat dissipation	Increased perspiration	Coarse skin
	Increased protein catabolism	Increased appetite and food ingestion	Lethargy
	Increased glucose absorption and production (i.e., gluconeogenesis)	Muscle wasting and proximal weakness	Generalized weakness Weight gain
	Increased glucose use	Weight loss Onycholysis (nail disease) Lid lag Proptosis (exophthalmos)	Voice coarsening, slow speech Myxedema
	Lipid metabolism	Decreased serum high-density lipoprotein cholesterol	

Continued

TABLE 23-5	Physiologic Effects of Thyroid Hormones and Syndromes of Thyroid Dysfunction—cont'd		
System	Thyroid Hormone Effects	Hyperthyroidism	Hypothyroidism
Cardiovascular	Increased adrenergic activity and sensitivity	Palpitations Fast heart rate (tachycardia)	Slow heart rate (bradycardia) Low blood pressure
	Increased heart rate	Bouncy, hyperdynamic arterial pulses	Heart failure
	Increased myocardial contractility	Shortness of breath	Heart enlargement Atrial fibrillation
	Increased cardiac output Increased blood volume Decreased peripheral vascular resistance	Widened pulse, increased systolic blood pressure, decreased diastolic blood pressure	
Central nervous system	Increased adrenergic activity and sensitivity	Restlessness, hypermotility Nervousness Fatigue Exaggerated reflexes Tremor	Apathy Mental sluggishness Depressed reflexes Mental retardation
Gastrointestinal tract	Increased motility	Hyperdefecation	Constipation

From Burtis CA, Bruns DE. *Tietz Fundamentals of Clinical Chemistry and Molecular Diagnostics*. 7th ed. St. Louis: Saunders; 2015.

TABLE 23-6	Causes of Hyperthyroidism
Category	Type of Disease
Autoimmune	Graves disease Hashimoto disease Thyrotoxicosis
Thyroiditis (often transient hyperthyroidism)	Painless, sporadic thyroiditis Postpartum thyroiditis Subacute thyroiditis Suppurative thyroiditis Radiation thyroiditis Drug-induced thyroiditis
Nodular disease	Toxic multinodular goiter Toxic adenoma
Thyroid-stimulating hormone (TSH) mediated	TSH-producing pituitary adenoma
Human chorionic gonadotropin (hCG) mediated	Hyperemesis gravidarum Trophoblastic disease
Exogenous thyroid hormone intake	Excessive replacement therapy Intentional suppressive therapy Factitious hyperthyroidism

From Burtis CA, Bruns DE. *Tietz Fundamentals of Clinical Chemistry and Molecular Diagnostics*. 7th ed. St. Louis: Saunders; 2015

Nodular Disease

As individuals age, the chance of developing a thyroid nodule increases. Most nodules are benign, but some individuals develop a toxic multinodular goiter. This is the second leading cause of hyperthyroidism, especially among older individuals. A **toxic multinodular goiter** involves an enlargement of the thyroid gland with low TSH and normal thyroxine levels (i.e., subclinical levels) or with clinical hyperthyroidism. The nodules can be composed of colloid, cysts, adenomas, or carcinomas. Thyroid cancer is a rare cause of hyperthyroidism.

Thyroiditis

Thyroiditis is inflammation of the thyroid gland. There are many types of thyroiditis, and most cause hyperthyroidism (Table 23-6). Postpartum thyroiditis is usually a self-limited disease and occurs 1 to 6 months after delivery. Most women do not receive treatment for this condition. Irradiation of the thyroid gland produces thyroiditis accompanied by a sudden release of thyroid hormones. It is self-limited and usually does not require treatment. Some drugs are also known to cause thyroiditis (Table 23-8).

Subclinical Hyperthyroidism

With the development of more sensitive tests for thyrotropin and TSH, individuals with low TSH concentrations accompanied by normal thyroid hormone concentrations can be identified. They do not have hyperthyroidism symptoms, and they are classified as having **subclinical hyperthyroidism.** The causes of subclinical hyperthyroidism mirror the causes of overt hyperthyroidism (usually nodules and multinodular goiters). It is important to identify subclinical hyperthyroidism because of adverse effects on the cardiovascular system (i.e., increased incidence of atrial fibrillation) and on the skeletal system (i.e., osteoporosis and increased fractures).

Euthyroid Sick Syndrome

Euthyroid sick syndrome is defined as normal functioning of the thyroid gland in the setting of abnormal levels of thyroxine-binding globulin. It is often monitored by TSH levels. The euthyroid sick syndrome is associated with

TABLE 23-7 Results of Thyroid Function Tests in Thyroid Disorders

Disorder	TSH	T$_4$	T$_3$	Free T$_4$
Primary hypothyroidism	↑	↓	N or ↓	↓
Hashimoto thyroiditis, hypothyroidism	↑	N	N or ↓	N or ↓
Graves disease	↓	↑	↑	↑
TSH deficiency	N or ↓	↓	↓	
Thyroid hormone resistance	N or ↑	↑	↑	↑
TSH-dependent hyperthyroidism	↑	↑	↑	↑
Subacute thyroiditis	↑ or ↓	↑ or ↓	↑ or ↓	↑ or ↓
Subclinical hyperthyroidism	↓	N	N	N
Subclinical hypothyroidism	↑	N	N	N
T$_3$ thyrotoxicosis	N	N or ↓	↑	↑
T$_4$ thyrotoxicosis		↑	N or ↓	N or ↓

N, Normal; *T$_3$*, triiodothyronine; *T$_4$*, thyroxine; *TSH*, thyroid-stimulating hormone; ↓, decreased; ↑, increased.
Modified from Burtis CA, Bruns DE. *Tietz Fundamentals of Clinical Chemistry and Molecular Diagnostics.* 7th ed. St. Louis: Saunders; 2015.

TABLE 23-8 Types of Thyroiditis

Autoimmune	Infectious or Postviral	Other
Hashimoto (i.e., chronic lymphocytic thyroiditis) Postpartum thyroiditis Painless sporadic thyroiditis	Subacute thyroiditis Suppurative thyroiditis	Radiation thyroiditis Drug-induced thyroiditis

From Burtis CA, Bruns DE. *Tietz Fundamentals of Clinical Chemistry and Molecular Diagnostics.* 7th ed. St. Louis: Saunders; 2015.

hospitalized patients. There is a characteristic abnormality of the thyroid hormones and a reduction in hormone binding to thyroxine-binding globulin. The syndrome is somewhat nonspecific but can be associated with conditions such as the nephrotic syndrome, decreased protein production, fasting, starvation, liver cirrhosis, diabetic ketoacidosis, and the ingestion of certain drugs.

Hypothyroidism

Hypothyroidism results from decreased levels of thyroid hormones. It usually occurs as primary hypothyroidism. Common causes for hypothyroidism are found in Table 23-9.

Various forms of hypothyroidism exist, and major symptoms include impaired speech and memory, cold intolerance, weight gain, constipation, dry skin, and bradycardia. Hypothyroidism primarily affects older women and manifests initially as an enlarged thyroid gland (i.e., goiter).

Primary hypothyroidism involves thyroid gland dysfunction, whereas secondary hypothyroidism involves pituitary and hypothalamic dysfunction. In primary hypothyroidism, the TSH level is increased, but the total T$_3$, total T$_4$, free T$_3$, and free T$_4$ levels are decreased. Hashimoto thyroiditis, also called chronic lymphocytic thyroiditis or Hashimoto disease, is the most common form. It is a chronic autoimmune disorder that is often misdiagnosed. Secondary hypothyroidism is caused by TSH deficiency (i.e., pituitary disease), and tertiary hypothyroidism is caused by TRH deficiency (i.e., hypothalamus disease).

Hashimoto Thyroiditis

Abnormalities associated with the capacity of the binding proteins to adequately and efficiently bind to the thyroid hormones result in typical development of thyroid antibodies. Thyroid antibodies associated with autoimmune-related thyroid disease are thyroid-stimulating immunoglobulins, thyroid microsomal antibodies, anti-thyroid peroxidase, and anti-thyroglobulin antibodies. In Hashimoto thyroiditis, the autoantibodies cause cell- and antibody-mediated destruction of the thyroid gland, which can cause the gland to enlarge (i.e., goiter) or atrophy.

Congenital Hypothyroidism

Congenital hypothyroidism (i.e., cretinism) causes mental retardation in children, but it is very treatable. Newborns are screened for T$_4$ and TSH to diagnose the condition quickly.

Congenital hypothyroidism is caused by an inborn error of thyroid metabolism or iodine deficiency. Symptoms include decreased activity, large anterior fontanelle, poor feeding and weight gain, small stature or poor growth, jaundice, constipation, hypotonia, and hoarse cry. These infants sleep most of the time. The disease is rare in the United States.

TABLE 23-9	**Thyroid Diseases**	
Condition	**Causes**
Chronic autoimmune thyroiditis	Hashimoto disease
Iatrogenic or treatment-related	After thyroidectomy After radioactive iodine treatment Prior external neck irradiation Use of antithyroid drugs
Transient thyroiditis	Painless sporadic thyroiditis Postpartum thyroiditis Subacute thyroiditis
Congenital hypothyroidism	Thyroid agenesis/dysgenesis Defects in hormone synthesis
Infiltrative thyroid disease	Riedel thyroiditis Hemochromatosis Sarcoidosis Amyloidosis
Iodine deficiency or excess	Error of thyroid metabolism or dietary iodine deficiency
Drugs	Antithyroid drugs Interferon-α Amiodarone Lithium Interleukin-2 Sunitinib

From Burtis CA, Bruns DE. *Tietz Fundamentals of Clinical Chemistry and Molecular Diagnostics.* 7th ed. St. Louis: Saunders; 2015.

Subclinical Hypothyroidism

Subclinical hypothyroidism is a condition with normal thyroid hormones levels and a high TSH level. Individuals may be asymptomatic, or they may have mild symptoms of hypothyroidism. The causes for this condition mirror those for hypothyroidism in general. Individuals with subclinical hypothyroidism have a higher than normal rate of cardiovascular mortality. Sometimes, the condition converts to overt hypothyroidism.

Thyroid Hormone Resistance

Thyroid hormone resistance is an autosomal dominant disorder that is characterized by diminished responsiveness of target tissues to thyroid hormone. A thyroid hormone receptor-β gene mutation is responsible for producing defective T_3 nuclear receptors.

Thyroid Cancer

Thyroid cancer is rare. Tumor types include papillary (differentiated), follicular (differentiated), medullary, and anaplastic (undifferentiated) cancers and primary thyroid lymphoma. The prognosis for undifferentiated cancers is far worse than for differentiated cancers. Thyroid cancers may metastasize from primary melanoma, breast, colon, or renal cancers. Individuals with thyroid cancer usually have a discrete tumor, but the tumor does not usually secrete thyroid hormones.

Thyroglobulin is produced by some carcinomas, but it is not a good malignant tumor marker because benign tumors also produce thyroglobulin. Medullary cancers secrete calcitonin, which can be used as a tumor marker to diagnose and monitor the response to treatment.

Laboratory Tests

Third-generation immunoassays using monoclonal and polyclonal antibodies can detect TSH levels as low as 0.05 mU/L. They have adequate sensitivity to detect most thyroid diseases except in cases of hypothalamic or pituitary damage, medication interference, or thyroid hormone resistance. The reference range is 0.5 to 5.0 mIU/L. Tests can detect thyrotoxicosis in patients with severe hyperthyroidism due to their suppressed TSH values.

Although measurement of TSH is a good screening test for most thyroid diseases, thyroid dysfunction should be confirmed by examining total T_4, free T_4, T_3, and free T_3 levels. T_3 thyrotoxicosis is a disease in which the TSH and T_3 levels are normal but T_4 and free T_4 levels are increased (Table 23-9).

Thyroxine Measurement

T_4 is measured after it is separated from its transport protein. It is used in conjunction with TSH to differentiate thyroid diseases. A low T_4 level together with an increased TSH level usually indicates hypothyroidism, and an increased T_4 level with a decreased TSH level indicates hyperthyroidism. T_4 thyrotoxicosis can occur in individuals who are taking certain drugs (e.g., β-blockers, amiodarone, steroids) and in cases of iodine-induced thyrotoxicosis. Laboratory results for T_4 thyrotoxicosis include an elevated T_4 level with a normal or low T_3 level.

Total T_4 can be measured by electron capture gas chromatography, high-performance liquid chromatography (HPLC), and isotope dilution liquid chromatography–tandem mass spectrometry, which is considered the best method for determining T_4 reference values. Routine laboratory testing for total T_4 levels uses competitive immunoassay methods on automated analyzers. The assays can measure total and free T_4. A variety of photometric, fluorescent, and luminescent substrates are used to quantitate T_4. These techniques are adapted for automated analyzers. The cloned enzyme donor immunoassay (CEDIA) is also used to measure T_4 and is also adapted for automated analyzers.

Serum is the preferred specimen for T_4 testing, although ethylenediaminetetraacetic acid (EDTA) and heparinized plasma can be used. Specimens can be stored at 2° to 8° C for up to 7 days or –20° C for up to 30 days.

Triiodothyronine Analysis

T_3 is measured directly by immunoassay, and the reference range is 60 to 160 µg/dL. Compared with T_4, more T_3 exists in the free form because much less is bound to protein. Most individuals with hyperthyroidism have increased T_4 and T_3, with higher levels of the latter. T_3 levels are usually not useful in determining hypothyroidism because they are normal in 15% to 30% of cases. Individuals with conditions such as myocardial infarction and poorly controlled diabetes mellitus may have decreased T_3 levels (Box 23-7).

Parathyroid Glands

Anatomy

Between two and six (usually four) parathyroid glands the size and shape of a grain of rice are located adjacent to the thyroid gland. Their location is curious because the parathyroid and thyroid glands do not interact. The parathyroid glands affect calcium homeostasis only and do not affect metabolism.

Hormone and Function

The parathyroid glands produce PTH (i.e., parathormone), which interacts with vitamin D to increase blood calcium levels. Calcium binds to receptors on the parathyroid chief cells, generating a signal that increases PTH secretion when calcium levels rise and decreases PTH secretion when calcium levels decline.

Magnesium, calcium, and phosphate levels also affect PTH levels. In cases of normal calcium levels and low magnesium levels, PTH secretion is mildly stimulated. In cases of low calcium and low magnesium levels, PTH secretion decreases. Increased phosphate levels lead to decreased calcium levels and increased PTH secretion. PTH levels exhibit diurnal rhythms while regulating calcium and phosphorus (Fig. 23-17).

PTH regulates calcium through the kidneys (i.e., increased retention) and the bone (i.e., increased release). When blood levels of calcium are low, PTH stimulates osteoclast activity, dissolving bone and increasing blood calcium. When calcium levels are high, PTH activates the kidneys to reduce renal calcium clearance and increase its reabsorption. Simultaneously, PTH decreases the amount

of phosphorus reabsorbed and increases its clearance, producing a lower blood phosphorus level. In long-term stimulation of PTH, bone is broken down and reformed; the result is brittle bones that are easily broken. Intact PTH has a half-life of less than 5 minutes.

Clinical Disorders

Diseases involving the parathyroid glands include primary, secondary, and tertiary hyperparathyroidism and hypoparathyroidism. Hyperparathyroidism occurs when the parathyroid glands excrete excess amounts of PTH with resulting hypercalcemia. Hypoparathyroidism occurs when there are decreased levels of or no circulating PTH. The PTH reference range is 9 to 69 pg/mL. Hypoparathyroidism is diagnosed when the level is lower than 20 pg/mL and hyperparathyroidism is when the level greater than 65 pg/mL.

Hyperparathyroidism

Primary hyperparathyroidism is a common endocrine disorder that is caused by adenomas, hyperplasia, and carcinomas (Table 23-10). In the disease state produced by adenomas, PTH production is increased and does not respond to normal feedback mechanisms. The blood calcium level is elevated, but it does not stop PTH secretion. The cause of this disorder is unknown. In primary hyperparathyroidism caused by hyperplasia, an increase in PTH-producing cells seems to be the cause of the increased PTH level.

Although hypercalcemia and hypophosphatemia occur in individuals with primary hyperparathyroidism, most patients are asymptomatic. Others have symptoms related to hypercalcemia: muscle weakness, fatigue, hypertension, bradycardia, headache, depression, confusion, abdominal pain, nausea, and vomiting. Severe cases can lead to coma and death.

Secondary Hyperparathyroidism

Secondary hyperparathyroidism is caused by a chronic disease that lowers blood calcium levels, leading to increased PTH secretion. Examples include intestinal malabsorption

---

• BOX 23-7 Thyroid Hormone Reference Ranges

- T_3: 60-160 µg/dL
- T_4: 5-12 µg/dL

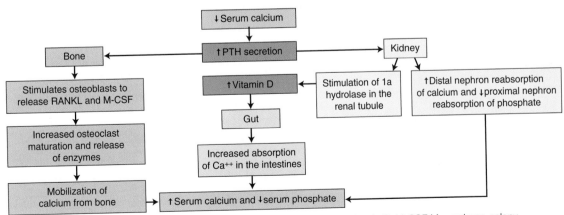

• Figure 23-17 Normal calcium metabolism regulated by PTH and vitamin D. *M-CSF*, Macrophage-colony stimulating factor; *PTH*, parathyroid hormone; *RANKL*, receptor activator of NF-κB ligand. (From McCance KL, Huether SE. *Pathophysiology: The Biologic Basis for Disease in Adults and Children.* 7th ed. St. Louis: Mosby, 2015.)

syndromes (e.g., Crohn disease, irritable bowel syndrome), chronic kidney disease, and vitamin D deficiency. Intestinal malabsorption syndromes lead to poor calcium absorption resulting in low blood calcium levels, and chronic kidney disease leads to lower reabsorption of calcium in the glomerular filtrate or a vitamin D deficiency resulting in low blood calcium levels. Therapeutic drugs such as phenytoin, phenobarbital, and laxatives can also lower blood calcium levels through accelerated vitamin D metabolism or reduced absorption of calcium in the gastrointestinal tract. Chronic secondary hyperparathyroidism can lead to tertiary hyperparathyroidism, as can renal transplantation.

Individuals with chronic renal failure develop secondary hyperparathyroidism before they advance to dialysis. Most patients with secondary hyperparathyroidism also have renal failure. The few who have secondary hyperparathyroidism without renal failure often have a vitamin D deficiency. Secondary hyperparathyroidism can manifest with cardiovascular calcification, a compromised immune system, neurobehavioral changes, osteomalacia, and bone pain.

Useful laboratory tests include measurements of PTH, calcium, phosphorus, and 25-hydroxyvitamin D levels. Individuals with secondary hyperparathyroidism have low to normal calcium levels, elevated PTH levels, phosphorus levels that tend to be in the high-normal range, and low vitamin D levels (<30 ng/mL).

Hypoparathyroidism

Hypoparathyroidism results from injury to the parathyroid or thyroid gland during neck trauma or surgery. Osteomalacia, autoimmune diseases, inborn errors of metabolism, thyroidectomy, and idiopathic atrophy (rare) result in decreased PTH secretion. In addition, hypocalcemia results when either decreased levels of PTH or a deficiency of vitamin D exists. Altered neuromuscular activity occurs with calcium levels lower than 6.0 mg/dL.

Individuals with hypoparathyroidism may have paresthesias (i.e., tingling in the fingertips, toes, or perioral area), hyperirritability, fatigue, anxiety, mood swings, seizures, wheezing and dyspnea, cataracts, muscle cramps (lower back, legs, and feet), diaphoresis, and biliary colic.

TABLE 23-10 Primary Hyperparathyroidism

Symptoms	Changes in Analytes	Mechanisms
Renal colic, nephrolithiasis, recurrent urinary tract infections, renal failure	Hypercalciuria, hyperphosphaturia, proximal renal tubular bicarbonate leak, urine pH >6	Calcium phosphate salts precipitate in alkaline urine, renal pelvis, and collecting ducts; calcium oxalate stones also formed
Abdominal pain, peptic ulcer disease	Hypercalcemia-stimulated hypergastrinemia	Elevated hydrochloric acid secretion
Pancreatitis	Hypercalcemia	Cause is unknown but high calcium levels are implicated
Bone disease, osteitis fibrosis and osteitis cystic osteoporosis	Parathyroid hormone (PTH)-stimulated bone resorption, metabolic acidosis	Osteoporosis more commonly encountered, but other disorders are more specific for hyperparathyroidism
Muscle weakness, myalgia	PTH excess, possible direct effect on striated muscle and on nerves	Characteristic myopathic changes in muscle histology (neuropathy of type I and type II muscle fibers)
Neurologic and psychiatric problems (e.g., impaired memory, confusion, depression, anxiety, psychosis)	Hypercalcemia	Neuropathy; electroencephalographic changes seen
Polyuria, polydipsia	Hypercalcemia	Direct effect on renal tubule to decrease responsiveness to antidiuretic hormone
Constipation	Hypercalcemia	Decreased peristalsis of gastrointestinal tract
Anorexia, nausea, and vomiting	Hypercalcemia	Central stimulation of vomiting center
Hypertension	Renal disease, direct effect of calcium on arterial smooth muscle, pheochromocytoma	Plasma renin activity elevated or normal
Arthralgia and arthritis	Gout, pseudogout, periarticular classification	Hyperuricemia, chronic renal failure with high calcium-phosphate product

Data from McCance KL, Huether SE. *Pathophysiology: The Biologic Basis for Disease in Adults and Children.* 7th ed. St. Louis: Mosby; 2015; Flint PW, Haughey BH, Lund VJ, et al, eds. *Cummings Otolaryngology—Head and Neck Surgery.* 5th ed. St. Louis: Mosby; 2010.

In **pseudohypoparathyroidism,** an inherited disease, the PTH receptors are unable to produce a response when bound with PTH. Peripheral tissue becomes resistant to PTH, leading to normal levels of PTH, low levels of calcium, and increased phosphorus levels.

Laboratory Procedures and Limitations

Screening tests for total calcium, albumin, and ionized calcium levels are performed to determine whether hypercalcemia is present. The tests should be performed at more than one office visit to confirm the result. Elevated PTH and calcium levels are diagnostic of primary hyperparathyroidism. A 24-hour urine test for calcium is performed to rule out a benign condition called **familial hypocalciuric hypercalcemia.** Individuals with primary hyperparathyroidism may also have hyperchloremic acidosis, hypophosphatemia, and an increased urinary calcium excretion rate. Common hormones and their relationship to endocrine disorders are listed in Table 23-11.

TABLE 23-11 Common Hormones

Hormone	Regulation	Action	Diseases	Reference Range
Insulin	Inhibited by hypoglycemia, somatostatins	Facilitates the entry of glucose into cells	Type 1 diabetes mellitus Type 2 diabetes mellitus	2-25 µU/mL
Growth hormone	Hypothalamus	Increases protein synthesis	Excess: acromegaly, pituitary giantism Deficit: dwarfism	<5 ng/mL
Prolactin	Hypothalamus	Initiation and maintenance of lactation	Excess: alterations of fertility	<20 ng/mL
Thyroid-stimulating hormone (TSH)	Hypothalamus, pituitary	Increases and enlarges thyroid follicular cells	Hypothyroidism Hyperthyroidism	<5 µIU/mL
Adrenocorticotropic hormone (ACTH)	Hypothalamus, pituitary	Stimulates adrenal cortex to transform cholesterol to glucocorticoids	Deficit: Addison disease Excess: Cushing disease	25-100 pg/mL
Follicle-stimulating hormone (FSH)	Hypothalamus, anterior pituitary, ovaries	Follicle stimulation	Infertility and irregular menses	Varies in cycle
Luteinizing hormone (LH)	Hypothalamus, anterior pituitary, ovaries	Corpus luteum development	Infertility and irregular menses, menopause, hirsutism	Varies in cycle
Antidiuretic hormone (ADH)	Hypothalamus, posterior pituitary	Elevates blood pressure, reabsorbs water	Syndrome of inappropriate antidiuretic hormone secretion Diabetes insipidus	<2.5 ng/L
Oxytocin	Hypothalamus, posterior pituitary	Muscle contraction for childbirth and sperm ejaculation, milk secretion	None known	1.1 µU/mL
Cortisol	Hypothalamus, pituitary, adrenals	Metabolism of carbohydrates, fats, proteins, and antiinflammatory effects	Addison disease Cushing disease	AM: 5-23 µg/dL PM: 3-16 µg/dL
Aldosterone	Hypothalamus, pituitary, adrenals	Maintains salt and water balance	Primary aldosteronism, hypoaldosteronism	m: 6-22 pg/dL f: 5-30 pg/dL
triiodothyronine (T$_3$)	Hypothalamus, pituitary, thyroid gland	Stimulation of oxygen consumption and metabolic rate of tissues	Hyperthyroidism (thyrotoxicosis), hypothyroidism, Graves disease, Hashimoto disease, myxedema, cretinism	60-160 µg/dL
Thyroxine (T$_4$)	Hypothalamus, pituitary, thyroid gland	Stimulation of oxygen consumption and metabolic rate of tissues	Hyperthyroidism (thyrotoxicosis), hypothyroidism, Graves disease, Hashimoto disease, myxedema, cretinism	5-12 µg/dL
Parathyroid hormone (PTH)	Hypothalamus, pituitary, parathyroid glands	Increases calcium reabsorption, inhibits phosphorus reabsorption, increases production of 1,25-dihydroxy-cholecalciferol	Hyperparathyroidism	9-69 pg/mL

Continued

TABLE 23-11 **Common Hormones—cont'd**

Hormone	Regulation	Action	Diseases	Reference Range
Serotonin	Pineal	Neurotransmitter, stimulates or inhibits smooth muscles and nerves	Increased levels: chronic tension headache, hypertension, schizophrenia, Duchenne muscular dystrophy, preeclampsia	5-HIAA metabolite: 2-8 mg/24 hr
Melatonin	Pineal	Suppression of gonadotropin and GH secretion, induction of sleep	Increased: seasonal affective disorder, decreased estrogen-progesterone ratio, decreased thyroid function, decreased adrenal function, hypotension Decreased: decreased body temperature, insomnia, increased estrogen-progesterone ratio, immune suppression associated with cancer	Varies
Glucagon	Pancreas	Glycogenolysis, gluconeogenesis, ketogenesis, lipolysis	Increased or decreased: diabetes mellitus	≤60 pg/mL
Somatostatin	Hypothalamus	Suppresses many hormones, inhibits insulin and glucagon secretion	Increased: somatostatinoma Decreased: rare	10-22 pg/mL
Gastrin	Stomach	Secretes gastric acid, gastric mucosal growth	Increased: gastrinoma, Zollinger-Ellison syndrome, acid-suppressing drugs	≤100 pg/mL
Secretin	Stomach, pancreas	Secretes pancreatic bicarbonate and digestive enzymes	Increased: Zollinger-Ellison syndrome, peptide, secretin-secreting islet cell tumor Decreased: acholuria, celiac disease	15-150 pg/mL
Cholecystokinin	Pancreas	Stimulates gallbladder contraction, secretes pancreatic enzymes	Diseases resulting from increased or decreased levels are rare	1.03-1.23 pmol/L
Epinephrine	Hypothalamus, pituitary, adrenals	Stimulates sympathetic nervous system, glycogenolysis, lipolysis, ketogenesis, thermogenesis	Increased: pheochromocytoma Decreased: dopamine β-hydroxylase deficiency	Sitting: <60 pg/mL
Norepinephrine	Hypothalamus, pituitary, adrenals	Stimulates sympathetic nervous system, glycogenolysis, lipolysis	Increased: pheochromocytoma Decreased: dopamine β-hydroxylase deficiency	Sitting: 120-680 pg/mL
Dopamine	Adrenals	Neurotransmitter in brain, precursor to epinephrine and norepinephrine	Increased: psychosis, schizophrenia, insomnia Decreased: attention-deficit/hyperactivity disorder (ADHD), depression	1042-2366 pg/mL

Summary

The endocrine system produces most of the hormones in the body and is composed of many organs. It produces protein, steroid, and amine hormones as well as those derived from arachidonic acid (i.e., prostaglandins, prostacyclins, leukotrienes, and thromboxanes). Hormones usually exert their effects by activating secondary messenger systems in cells. The production and release of a hormone is typically governed by a negative feedback loop. Most hormones are measured with the use of ELISA, EMIT, FPIA, fluorescent immunoassay, and HPLC methods.

The hypothalamus produces trophic hormones (i.e., TRH, gonadotropin-releasing hormone, somatostatin, GH-releasing hormone, corticotrophin-releasing hormone, dopamine, and prolactin-releasing hormone), which stimulate organs to produce biologically active hormones. The pituitary produces ACTH, GH, prolactin, TSH, LH, and

FSH. Organs that produce biologically active hormones include the adrenal glands (i.e., glucocorticoids, mineralocorticoids, epinephrine, norepinephrine), thyroid gland (i.e., T_3, T_4), ovaries (i.e., estradiol, progesterone), testes (i.e., testosterone), pineal gland (i.e., melatonin), parathyroid gland (i.e., PTH), stomach (i.e., gastrin), gastrointestinal tract (i.e., serotonin), and pancreas (i.e., insulin, glucagon, and somatostatin).

Excesses or deficiencies of hormones or ectopic production of a hormone can result in many diseases states. Common endocrine disorders include Addison disease, Cushing disease, Graves disease, Hashimoto thyroiditis, SIADH, acromegaly, diabetes insipidus, pheochromocytoma, neuroblastoma, hyperaldosteronism, thyrotoxicosis, cretinism, carcinomas, hyperparathyroidism, dwarfism, giantism, infertility, and Zollinger-Ellison syndrome.

Review Questions

1. Which of the following is *not* a class of hormones?
   a. Steroids
   b. Peptides
   c. Lipoproteins
   d. Amines
2. The hormones epinephrine, norepinephrine, thyroxine, and triiodothyronine belong to a class of hormones known as
   a. Steroids
   b. Peptides
   c. Glycoproteins
   d. Amines
3. Which of the following endocrine glands can perform both endocrine and exocrine functions?
   a. Adrenal
   b. Hypothalamus
   c. Pancreas
   d. Pituitary
4. The hormones that are secreted by the adrenal cortex are derived from which of the following precursors?
   a. Enterochromaffin cells
   b. Cholesterol
   c. Catecholamines
   d. Nucleoproteins
5. Which of the following pairs of hormones are synthesized in the pituitary and regulated by the hypothalamus and the posterior pituitary?
   a. ACTH and ADH
   b. MLT and oxytocin
   c. GH and TSH
   d. ADH and oxytocin

6. Which of the following hormones can be regulated by analysis of the end products catecholamines and vanillylmandelic acid?
   a. Epinephrine and norepinephrine
   b. ADH and oxytocin
   c. T_3 and T_4
   d. ADH and aldosterone
7. Which of the following is *not* a hormone produced by the anterior pituitary?
   a. TSH
   b. FSH
   c. LH
   d. PTH
8. Which of the following is *not* a site of action for calcium regulation associated with parathyroid hormone?
   a. Bones
   b. Kidneys
   c. Adrenal
   d. Small intestines
9. Gigantism, dwarfism, and acromegaly are disorders associated with abnormalities of which of the following hormones?
   a. ACTH
   b. GH
   c. LH
   d. TSH
10. A chemical compound that is secreted into the blood by a gland and causes a specific response in a target cell is called a
    a. Hormone
    b. Neurotransmitter
    c. Satellite cell
    d. Polypeptide

Critical Thinking Questions

1. List the three zones of the adrenal gland. Identify a hormone found in each zone.
2. Describe the effects of parathyroid hormone (PTH) on calcium and phosphorus levels.
3. List the role and specific effects of angiotensin II in the renin-angiotensin-aldosterone system.

CASE STUDY

A 56-year-old, white woman complains to her physician about hot flashes, heat intolerance, bradycardia, hypertension, and hyperactivity. Her height and weight are proportional, and she is within the normal range of body-mass index for her age group. She says that she exercises daily and reports that she does not feel tired and weary from exercise or when retiring for sleep at night. The physician orders blood work from the laboratory, with the following results (reference ranges are given in parentheses):

Bicarbonate: 18 mEq/L (21-32 mEq/L)
Calcium: 11.0 mg/dL (8.5-10.1 mg/dL)
Chloride: 110 mmol/L (98-108 mmol/L)
Estrogen: 200 pg/mL (60-400 pg/mL)
Free T_3: 500 pg/dL (260-480 pg/dL)
Free T_4: 30 pmol/L (10-26 pmol/L)
Glucose: 118 mg/dL (70-110 mg/dL)
Magnesium: 1.1 mg/dL (1.8-2.6 mg/dL)
Phosphorus: 2.0 mg/dL (2.7-4.5 mg/dL)
Potassium: 5.8 mmol/L (3.6-5.2 mmol/L)
Prolactin: 15 ng/mL (0-23 ng/mL)
Sodium: 150 mmol/L (135-148 mmol/L)
Thyroglobulin: normal (3-42 ng/mL)
Thyroid peroxidase antibodies: increased (negative <20 U; positive >26 U)
Thyroid-stimulating hormone: 0.45 mIU/L (0.40-4.2 mIU/L)
Thyroxine-binding globulin: 4.2 mg/dL (1.4-3.0 mg/dL)
Total T_3: 290 ng/dL (80-200 ng/dL)
Total T_4: 240 nmol/L (57-148 nmol/L)
Tyrosine: 0.85 mg/dL (1.41 ± 0.19 mg/dL)

List all tests results that are abnormal. What is the preliminary diagnosis? What are the roles of thyroid-stimulating hormone, triiodothyronine (T_3), thyroxine (T_4), and thyroglobulin? What is the final differential diagnosis? What additional tests can the physician request?

Bibliography

Abrams C. ADH-associated pathologies: diabetes insipidus and syndrome of inappropriate ADH. *MLO Med Lab Obs.* 2000;32: 24–25, 28, 30-33.

Arneson W, Brickell J. *Clinical Chemistry: A Laboratory Perspective.* Philadelphia: FA Davis; 2007.

Backer H, Hollowell J. Use of iodine for water disinfection: Iodine toxicity and maximum recommended dose. *Environ Health Perspect.* 2000;108:679–684.

Beato M, Klug J. Steroid hormone receptors: an update. *Hum Reprod Update.* 2000;6:225–236.

Blick KE, Liles SM. *Principles of Clinical Chemistry.* Albany, NY: Delmar Publishers; 1985.

Chen H, Senda T, Emura S, Kubo K. An update on the structure of the parathyroid gland. *Open Anat J.* 2013;5:1–9.

Christenson RH, Gregory LC, Johnson LJ. *Appleton & Lange's Outline Review of Clinical Chemistry.* New York: Appleton & Lange/McGraw-Hill; 2001.

Cooper MS, Stewart PM. Adrenal insufficiency in critical illness. *J Intensive Care Med.* 2007;22:348–362.

Corwin EJ. *Handbook of Pathophysiology.* 3rd ed. Philadelphia: Lippincott, Williams, & Wilkins; 2008.

Denzer F, Denzer C, Lennerz BS, Bode H, Wabitsch M. A case of phace syndrome and acquired hypopituitarism? *Int J Pediatr Endocrinol.* 2012;20:21–24.

Fleck SK, Wallaschofski H, Rosenstengel C, et al. Prevalence of hypopituitarism after intracranial operations not directly associated with the pituitary gland. *BMC Endocr Disord.* 2013;13: 51–58.

Gardner D, Shoback D. *Greenspan's Basic and Clinical Endocrinology.* 9th ed. Norwalk, CT: Lange Medical Publications; 2011.

Geffner ME. Hypopituitarism in childhood. *Cancer Control.* 2002;9:212–222.

Goldstein S, Simon J, Fagan J. Estrogen deficiency during menopause: its role in the metabolic syndrome. *Suppl OBG Manage.* 2005;(suppl):S1–S12.

Gordon H, Vander-Wyk BC, Bennett RH, et al. Oxytocin enhances brain function in children with autism. *Proceed Natl Acad Sci U S A.* 2013;110:285–291.

Gorman LS, Chiasera JM. Introduction to endocrine focus series. *Clin Lab Sci.* 2013;26:106–125.

Grossman A, Pacak K, Sawka A, et al. Biochemical diagnosis and localization of pheochromocytoma: can we reach a consensus? *Ann N Y Acad Sci.* 2006;1073:332–347.

Herbomez M, Forzy G, Bauters C, et al. An analysis of the biochemical diagnosis of 66 pheochromocytomas. *Eur J Endocrinol.* 2007;156:569–575.

Kaplan A, Jack R, Opheim KE, Toivola B, Lyon AW. *Clinical Chemistry: Interpretation and Techniques.* 4th ed. Philadelphia: Lippincott, Williams, & Wilkins; 1995.

Kaplan L, Pesce A. *Clinical Chemistry: Theory, Analysis, Correlation.* St. Louis: Mosby; 2009.

Koivunen ME, Krogsrud RL. Principles of immunochemical techniques used in clinical laboratories. *Lab Med.* 2006;37:490–497.

Lee MKV, Vasikaran S, Doery JCG, Wijeratne N, Prentice D. Cortisol/ACTH ratio to test for primary hypoadrenalism: a pilot study. *J Postgrad Med.* 2013;89:617–620.

Leung AM, Braverman LE, Pearce EN. History of US iodine fortification & supplementation. *Nutrients.* 2012;4:1740–1746.

Lott JA. The pancreas: a small gland with a big mission. *Advr Med Lab Professional.* 1997:49–52. November.

Lutchman N, Paiker JE. Phaeochromocytomas: an update. *J Endocrinol Metab Diabet South Afr.* 2006;11:68–79.

Molenaar N, Johan Groeneveld AB, Dijstelbloem HM, et al. Assessing adrenal insufficiency of corticosteroid secretion using free versus total cortisol levels in critical illness. *J Intensive Care Med.* 2011;37:1986–1993.

Murray RK, Gramer DK, Mayes PA, Rodwell VW. *Harper's Biochemistry.* 21st ed. Norwalk, CT: Appleton & Lange; 2012.

Ogedegbe H. Thyroid function test: a clinical lab perspective. *MLO Med Lab Obs.* 2007;39:10–19.

Ott DT. Learn to answer troublesome questions about thyroid tests: a primer. *MLO Med Lab Obs.* 1996;28:50–57.

24

Kidney and Urinary Tract Diseases

SHERYL BERMAN

CHAPTER OUTLINE

OBJECTIVES

After completion of this chapter, the reader will be able to:

1. Describe the structure of the kidney.
2. Describe the flow of blood through the nephron.
3. Describe the role of the nephron in filtration and reabsorption.
4. Describe the formation of urine in the kidney.
5. Discuss the renin-angiotensin-aldosterone pathways in the body.
6. Discuss the role of the kidney in homeostasis.
7. Discuss how proteins are conserved in the nephron.
8. Discuss the roles of erythropoietin and how it is affected by kidney function.
9. Describe uremic syndrome and identify the related laboratory tests.
10. Explain the disease mechanisms of acute glomerulonephritis and the laboratory tests used for diagnosis.
11. Identify the causes and characteristics of nephrotic syndrome.
12. Compare and contrast all forms of renal tubular acidosis.
13. Define cystitis and pyelonephritis and the tests used for diagnosing urinary tract infections.
14. Identify the causes and characteristics of polycystic kidney disease.
15. Discuss renal changes in diabetic patients.
16. Describe causes and disease mechanisms of renal failure and the related laboratory tests.
17. Discuss how different forms of renal obstruction occur.
18. Describe all major parts of a urinalysis, and explain what each examination reveals about a patient's health.
19. Discuss urine and serum electrolytes measurements, and explain what they reveal about disease states in the body.
20. Discuss what information the anion gap, osmolality, urine protein, and uric acid measurements provide about kidney function.
21. Compare and contrast the use and limitations of blood urea nitrogen, serum creatinine, and 24-hour creatinine clearance tests.
22. Describe the test methods for blood urea nitrogen, creatinine, 24-hour urine creatinine clearance, 24-hour urine protein, uric acid, urine electrolytes, and osmolality.
23. Compare and contrast hemodialysis and peritoneal dialysis.

KEY TERMS

1,25-Dihydroxyvitamin D$_3$
Acute tubular necrosis
Aldosterone
Angiotensin I
Angiotensin II
Angiotensinogen
Antidiuretic hormone
Azotemia
Blood urea nitrogen
Calcium oxalate crystals
Casts
Creatinine
Creatinine clearance
Cysteine crystals
Cystitis
Cystolithiasis
Diabetes insipidus
Diabetic nephropathy
Erythropoietin

Fat bodies
Glomerular filtration
Glomerular filtration rate
Glomerulonephritis
Hematuria
Hemodialysis
Homeostasis
Ketones
Kidney dialysis
Kidney failure
Kidney transplantation
Leukocyte esterase
Microalbumin
Nephrolithiasis
Nephrotic syndrome
Oliguria
Peritoneal dialysis
Peritubular epithelial cells
Polycystic kidney disease

Proteinuria
Pyelonephritis
Pyonephrosis
Renal calculi
Renal obstruction
Renal threshold
Renal tubular acidosis
Renin
Renin-angiotensin-aldosterone pathway
Tamm-Horsfall protein
Triple phosphate crystals
Ureterolithiasis
Uric acid
Urinalysis
Urine
Urinary tract infection
Urobilinogen
Urosepsis

❖ Case in Point

A 36-year-old diabetic man has foamy urine, fatigue, foot and ankle edema, and neuropathy. After an examination, his provider orders a urine protein test, and the test result is 300 mg/dL. What is the likely diagnosis? What would be the likely diagnosis if the urine protein level was 3 g or greater in 24 hours?

Points to Remember

- The renal system maintains acid-base balance, electrolyte balance, water balance, and hormone production.
- The kidney produces erythropoietin and plays an important role in vitamin D production and protein conservation.
- Glomerulonephritis is inflammation of the glomerulus.
- Urinary tract infections can start with the bladder (i.e., cystitis) and progress to the kidneys (i.e., pyelonephritis).
- Nephrotic syndrome is a condition associated with extreme proteinuria, hypoalbuminemia, and hyperlipidemia.
- Renal tubular acidosis is a condition in which the proximal and distal tubules are unable to regulate bases and acids, respectively.
- Polycystic kidney disease is a condition in which cysts form in and enlarge the kidney, eventually interfering with its function.
- Diabetic nephropathy is a sequela of diabetes mellitus that can lead to renal failure.
- Renal failure can be acute, which is usually reversible, or chronic, which is usually irreversible.

- Renal obstruction is caused by structural abnormalities, disease processes, or calculi (i.e., stones) in the bladder, ureters, or kidneys.
- Urinalysis is a screening tool for renal disease and other metabolic diseases.
- A routine urinalysis consists of physical, chemical, and microscopic examinations.
- Sodium, potassium, protein, and creatinine levels are measured in serum and urine.
- Blood urea nitrogen and creatinine are commonly measured in renal function tests.
- The creatinine clearance test parallels the glomerular filtration rate. It is performed using a 24-hour urine sample and measures 24-hour urine and serum creatinine levels.
- Hemodialysis and peritoneal dialysis remove wastes from the blood when the kidneys are unable to do so.

Introduction

The normal and abnormal structure and function of the urinary tract are described in this chapter. Urine production, fluid homeostasis, acid-base balance, and hormone and vitamin production are discussed in the context of pathological conditions such as glomerulonephritis, nephrotic syndrome, urinary tract infections, polycystic kidney disease, renal tubular acidosis, and renal failure. The techniques and limitations of laboratory procedures are described for the measurement of electrolytes, urinalysis, osmolality, blood urea nitrogen, creatinine, and creatinine clearance. Treatments for renal disease such as hemodialysis and peritoneal dialysis are summarized.

Kidney Anatomy

The urinary or renal system consists of two kidneys, two ureters, one bladder, and one urethra (Fig. 24-1). The kidneys filter blood, concentrate wastes into **urine,** and then excrete the urine. Urine travels from the renal calyx through the ureters to the bladder. Urine is stored in the bladder and excreted through the urethra to the outside.

The functional unit of the kidney is the nephron. The nephron is composed of the glomerulus, Bowman capsule, proximal convoluted tubules, loop of Henle, distal convoluted tubules, and collecting ducts (Fig. 24-2). The kidney has an outer layer called the cortex and an inner layer called the medulla. The glomeruli and the proximal and distal tubules are located in the cortex, and the loop of Henle, collecting ducts, and renal pelvis are located in the medulla.

The glomerulus is a cluster of capillaries supported on a specialized basement membrane. The capillaries and the basement membrane form the filtration membrane through which substances such as water, urea, **creatinine,** and other wastes are filtered from the body and eventually excreted. The basement membrane allows substances to pass through into the filtrate or to be retained in the blood. If the glomerulus is damaged, substances such as proteins and cells may pass through the glomerulus and be excreted in the urine rather than being returned to the bloodstream.

The Bowman capsule surrounds the glomerulus and acts as the beginning of the proximal convoluted tubules. The juxtaglomerular apparatus is an area of the nephron that is vital in maintaining blood pressure through intravascular blood volume and sodium concentration. This area is found where the efferent arteriole, afferent arteriole, early distal tubule, and glomerulus are very close together.

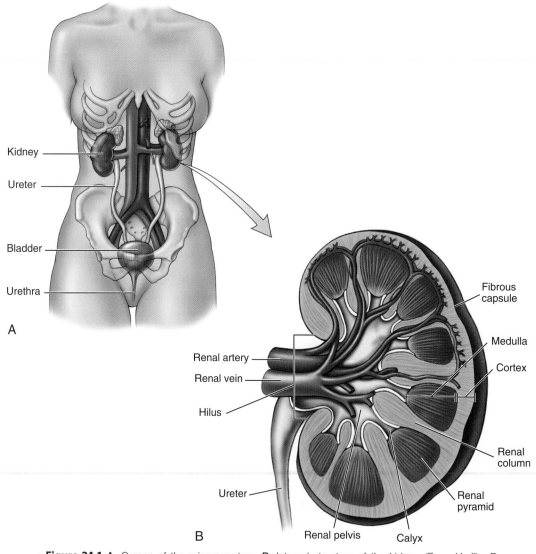

• **Figure 24-1 A,** Organs of the urinary system. **B,** Internal structure of the kidney. (From Herlihy B. *The Human Body in Health and Illness.* 5th ed. St. Louis: Elsevier; 2014.)

The juxtaglomerular apparatus is composed of specialized cells of the afferent arteriole, distal tubule, and the cells between these structures and the glomerulus. The specialized cells contain renin granules and sympathetic nerve fibers.

Renin is a proteolytic enzyme that is released from specialized cells when the pressure in the afferent arteriole and sodium concentration in the tubule decrease. The release of renin converts angiotensin in the blood to angiotensin I. The lungs convert angiotensin I to angiotensin-converting enzyme, which stimulates aldosterone release and increased distal tubular sodium retention. This process is regulated through a negative feedback loop.

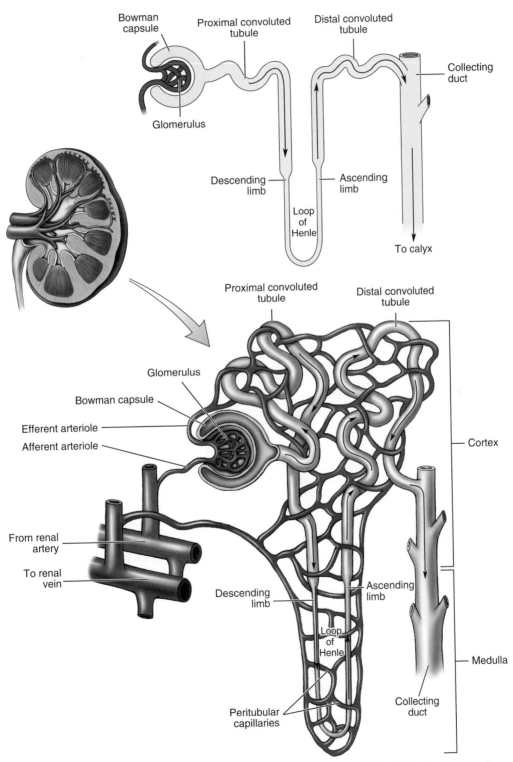

• **Figure 24-2** Tubular and vascular structures of the nephron unit. (From Herlihy B. *The Human Body in Health and Illness.* 5th ed. St. Louis: Elsevier; 2014.)

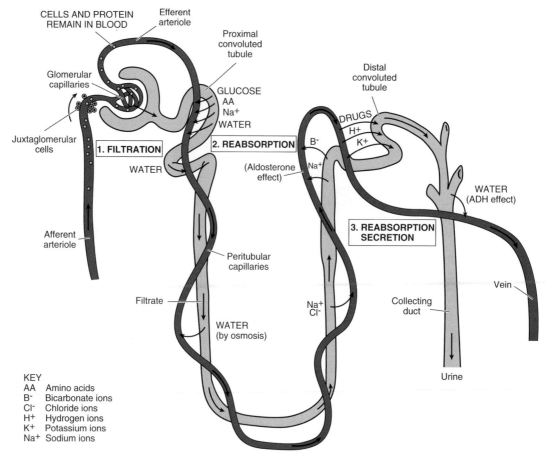

KEY
AA   Amino acids
B⁻   Bicarbonate ions
Cl⁻   Chloride ions
H⁺   Hydrogen ions
K⁺   Potassium ions
Na⁺   Sodium ions

• **Figure 24-3** The formation of urine. (From VanMeter KC, Hubert RJ. *Gould's Pathophysiology for the Health Profession.* 5th ed. St. Louis: Saunders; 2015.)

The proximal convoluted tubules are a major site of reabsorption in the nephron. Reabsorption can be an active process requiring the expenditure of energy, or it can be energy neutral as in passive diffusion (Fig. 24-3). The proximal tubules reabsorb most of the salt, water, glucose, and amino acids in the filtrate. They also reabsorb low-molecular-weight proteins and electrolytes (i.e., potassium, chloride, magnesium, and calcium). The cells of the proximal tubule secrete hydrogen ions and ammonia into tubular fluid. If the level of glucose in the bloodstream is elevated and above the **renal threshold,** the tubules cannot reabsorb the excess glucose, and it may "spill" into the urine, producing elevated urinary glucose levels.

The loop of Henle functions primarily in water absorption. The distal tubules also play a role in limited water and electrolyte reabsorption. The cells of the distal tubules are sensitive to the hormones aldosterone and **antidiuretic hormone** (ADH). Water permeability by the distal tubules is high when ADH is present and low in its absence. ADH also affects the cells of the collecting ducts. When water is reabsorbed in the presence of ADH, the remaining solute concentration of substances such as sodium and chloride rises in the distal tubules. Aldosterone increases reabsorption of sodium by the distal tubules and causes the body to retain water.

The primary function of the renal system is to maintain **homeostasis** in the body. The kidneys maintain homeostasis by removing metabolic waste and organic substances from the plasma and by regulating plasma volume, electrolytes, and hydrogen ion concentration. They also maintain homeostasis by regulating erythropoietin, renin, and vitamin D production.

Normal Physiology

Urine Formation

Urine formation is a complicated process that removes waste products from the blood to keep the body healthy. The three major phases of urine production are glomerular filtration, tubular reabsorption, and tubular secretion (Fig. 24-4, see Fig. 24-3).

Glomerular filtration is passive and nonselective. Hydrostatic pressure forces fluids in blood flowing through the glomerulus out through the membrane. The amount of filtrate that is formed each minute by all of the glomeruli is the **glomerular filtration rate** (GFR). Normal GFR is between 120 and 125 mL/min. The GFR is governed by autoregulation (i.e., feedback loop

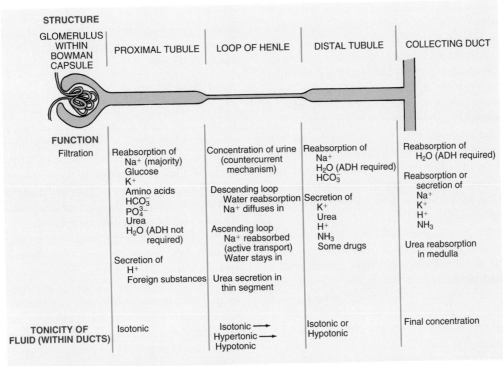

STRUCTURE				
GLOMERULUS WITHIN BOWMAN CAPSULE	PROXIMAL TUBULE	LOOP OF HENLE	DISTAL TUBULE	COLLECTING DUCT
FUNCTION Filtration	Reabsorption of Na$^+$ (majority) Glucose K$^+$ Amino acids HCO$_3^-$ PO$_4^{3-}$ Urea H$_2$O (ADH not required) Secretion of H$^+$ Foreign substances	Concentration of urine (countercurrent mechanism) Descending loop Water reabsorption Na$^+$ diffuses in Ascending loop Na$^+$ reabsorbed (active transport) Water stays in Urea secretion in thin segment	Reabsorption of Na$^+$ H$_2$O (ADH required) HCO$_3^-$ Secretion of K$^+$ Urea H$^+$ NH$_3$ Some drugs	Reabsorption of H$_2$O (ADH required) Reabsorption or secretion of Na$^+$ K$^+$ H$^+$ NH$_3$ Urea reabsorption in medulla
TONICITY OF FLUID (WITHIN DUCTS)	Isotonic	Isotonic ⟶ Hypertonic ⟶ Hypotonic	Isotonic or Hypotonic	Final concentration

• **Figure 24-4** Major functions of nephron segments. *ADH,* Antidiuretic hormone. (Modified from Hockenberry MJ. *Wong's Nursing Care of Infants and Children.* 8th ed. St. Louis: Mosby; 2007.)

that responds to the rate of filtrate flow in the tubules), neural mechanisms (usually stress induced), and the renin-angiotensin mechanism (i.e., increasing sodium reabsorption increases systemic blood pressure and blood volume).

As soon as the filtrate enters the proximal convoluted tubules, organic molecules are almost totally reabsorbed, and water and ions are reabsorbed according to hormonal influence. Sodium reabsorption is accomplished through active transport. Sodium is the most abundant cation in filtrate, and active sodium reabsorption creates an electrical gradient that allows negative ions to be passively reabsorbed. Active sodium reabsorption also creates osmotic gradients in water-permeable sections of the tubules, permitting water reabsorption. Glucose, amino acids, vitamins, and cations are reabsorbed by secondary active transport. Urea, creatinine, and uric acid remain in the filtrate because the first does not have a carrier molecule, the second is not lipid soluble, and the third is too large. The proximal convoluted tubule is where most selective reabsorption occurs.

The descending portion of the loop of Henle reabsorbs water, and the ascending portion reabsorbs electrolytes. Aldosterone, ADH, and atrial natriuretic hormone regulate the water balance and sodium permeability of the distal convoluted tubule and collecting duct.

The final phase of urine formation is tubular secretion. Tubular secretion disposes of unnecessary substances, reabsorbed solutes, and excess potassium and controls blood pH. Tubular secretion occurs in the proximal and distal convoluted tubules and in the collecting ducts. Urine that exits the body through the urethra is clear and pale to deep yellow, slightly aromatic, and usually slightly acidic, and it has a higher specific gravity than water. Excreted urine is 95% water and 5% urea, creatinine, and uric acid.

Regulation of Fluids and Electrolytes

The renin-angiotensin-aldosterone pathway regulates blood pressure, fluid, and electrolytes (Fig. 24-5). Renin is an enzyme that is synthesized and secreted by the juxtaglomerular cells of the kidney. Renin is secreted when there is decreased blood pressure, decreased sodium concentration in the tubules, or decreased nerve impulse transmission to the kidneys. Renin converts angiotensinogen, a precursor protein secreted by the liver, to angiotensin I. Angiotensin I is converted to angiotensin II in the kidney. Angiotensin II is a powerful vasoconstrictor that causes a rise in blood pressure. Angiotensin II also works on the adrenal cortex and stimulates aldosterone secretion. Aldosterone stimulates thirst and increases reabsorption of sodium by the distal tubules, causing the body to retain water. ADH secretion causes further water retention. Angiotensin II stimulates ADH release by the posterior pituitary gland. Increased levels of ADH result in greater reabsorption of water by the collecting ducts and decreased water excretion.

Protein Conservation

Proteins are essential for optimal body functions, and the kidney helps to ensure proteins stay in the blood and do not enter the urine. Protein can enter the urine because of glomerular and tubular damage and as overflow.

The glomerulus filters approximately 12,000 g of protein daily. Most proteins are reabsorbed by the body. Normally, less than 200 mg of protein are detected in urine. Larger proteins are unable to pass through the healthy glomerular membranes, and small-molecular-weight proteins are reabsorbed by the proximal tubules and released into the blood.

Glomerular disease processes may increase the glomerular permeability and result in larger amounts of protein entering the urine. These processes include basement membrane damage from immune complexes (i.e., glomerulonephritis) or increased protein deposits (i.e., diabetic nephropathy). These mechanisms result in high-molecular-weight proteins being released into the urine. As the diseases progress and the permeability increases, large amounts of high-molecular-weight proteins are released into the urine, and kidney function is compromised.

The overflow mechanism also results in proteinuria, but proteins entering the urine are low-molecular-weight proteins. Proteinuria of a low-molecular-weight protein results from an increased blood concentration. For example, the low-molecular-weight Bence Jones protein enters urine when blood protein levels increase dramatically in multiple myeloma. Myoglobin is released into the urine in individuals with rhabdomyolysis.

Proteinuria can result from decreased tubular reabsorption and tubular damage. Glomerular permeability remains normal. Tubular damage can be caused by drugs, heavy metals, or anoxia. Lower-molecular-weight proteins such as α_1-microglobulin appear in urine. Enzymes such as alkaline phosphatase and N-acetyl-β-D-glucosaminidase are often found in the urine of individuals with tubular damage.

Tamm-Horsfall protein is secreted by the kidneys. Although its exact function is unknown, it is thought to help prevent kidney stones. In certain conditions, excessive amounts of Tamm-Horsfall protein may be secreted or may remain in tubules and collecting ducts for prolonged periods. When that occurs, Tamm-Horsfall proteins may solidify and be excreted in the urine as microscopic casts.

Acid-Base Balance

One of the most important functions of the kidneys is maintaining the acid-base balance of blood. Blood acidity increases when levels of acidic compounds rise or levels of alkaline compounds fall. Blood alkalinity increases when levels of alkaline compounds rise or the concentration of acidic compounds falls. Acidity and alkalinity of the blood and urine can change through intake, production, or elimination of acidic or alkaline compounds.

The blood's acid-base balance is strictly controlled because even minor changes from the normal range can severely affect many organs. The normal range for pH is 7.35 to 7.45. The blood's acid-base balance is controlled by buffering systems, the lungs, and the kidneys. The lungs can quickly compensate for acidosis or alkalosis, whereas the kidney and buffering systems compensate more slowly. The kidneys control pH primarily through the secretion and reabsorption of acids such as hydrogen ions and bases such as bicarbonate and ammonia. The kidneys use proximal tubule and distal tubule mechanisms to maintain the acid-base balance.

Tubule Mechanisms

The two main functions of the proximal tubule are bicarbonate reabsorption and ammonia production. Bicarbonate is filtered through the glomerulus, and 85% to 90% is reabsorbed in the proximal tubule, with the remainder reabsorbed in the distal tubule and collecting ducts.

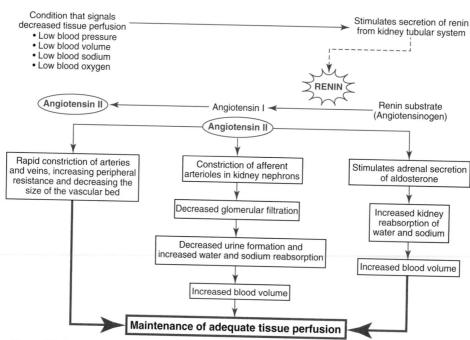

• **Figure 24-5** The renin-angiotensin-aldosterone pathway. (From Ignatavicius D. *Medical-Surgical Nursing: Patient-Centered Collaborative Care.* 7th ed. St. Louis: Elsevier; 2013.)

Bicarbonate cannot be reabsorbed by the proximal tubule cells. Instead, bicarbonate in the filtrate combines with the hydrogen ions (H$^+$) secreted by the proximal tubule cell into the filtrate to form carbon dioxide (CO_2) and water (H_2O). The CO_2 easily diffuses into the proximal tubule cells and combines with hydroxide ions (OH$^-$) to form bicarbonate (HCO_3^-). Sodium ions (Na$^+$) in the filtrate mediate the absorption of H$^+$ and potassium (K$^+$) ions through active transport (i.e., sodium pump). For each molecule of H$^+$ secreted by the proximal tubule cells, one molecule of HCO_3^- and one molecule of Na$^+$ are reabsorbed from the filtrate into the blood. Factors controlling bicarbonate reabsorption include the bicarbonate concentration in the filtrate, filtrate flow rate, arterial PCO_2, and angiotensin II.

The proximal tubules also affect acid-base balance through ammonium ion (NH_4^+) production. Ammonium ions are produced by the proximal tubule to buffer hydrogen ions, and they are then removed from the filtrate in the loop of Henle. The high acid level in the filtrate as it passes through the proximal tubules facilitates the transfer of ammonium ions from the proximal tubule cells into the filtrate, moderating the pH of the filtrate.

The distal tubule mechanism involves reabsorption of H$^+$ and HCO_3^- in the filtrate as it becomes urine and moves on to the collecting ducts. This results in a fluid with properties close to those of excreted urine (Table 24-1).

Hormone Function

The kidney produces three hormones: renin, erythropoietin, and calcitriol. Renin was discussed earlier. **Erythropoietin** (EPO) stimulates the colony-forming units–erythroid (CFUs-E) in bone marrow to increase red blood cell production. Hypoxemia and anemia stimulate the **peritubular epithelial cells** of the renal cortex to synthesize EPO.

EPO binds to EPO receptors on CFUs-E in the bone marrow, which protects the CFUs-E from apoptosis (i.e., programmed cell death). As a result, the CFUs continue their transformation into more functional red blood cells. Recombinant human EPO (rhEPO) is manufactured by pharmaceutical companies and can be used to maintain or increase red blood cell production in people with kidney failure, chemotherapy side effects, and some systemic diseases who can no longer produce EPO.

The third hormone produced by the kidney, calcitriol, regulates calcium absorption. Ultraviolet light captured by the skin converts 7-dehydrocholesterol (i.e., previtamin D_3) to cholecalciferol (vitamin D_3). Vitamin D binding protein carries cholecalciferol to the liver. In the liver, the cholecalciferol is converted to 25-hydroxyvitamin D. The proximal tubule of the kidney secretes 1α-hydroxylase, which converts 25-hydroxyvitamin D to biologically active **1,25-dihydroxyvitamin D$_3$** (i.e., calcitriol). This process is regulated by the parathyroid hormone.

Disease States

Uremic Syndrome

Azotemia occurs when the blood contains increased levels of **blood urea nitrogen** (BUN), creatinine, and other products of protein metabolism. The uremic syndrome encompasses failure of the excretory, regulatory, and endocrine functions of the kidney.

Kidney failure is defined as a GFR of 15 mL/min/m^2 or less or a **creatinine clearance** less than 10 mL/min. Symptoms include azotemia, progressive weakness, easy fatigue, nausea, vomiting, anorexia, weight loss, muscle cramps, pruritus, and change in mental status. Characteristic laboratory results include a BUN greater than 50 mg/dL, creatinine level greater than 3.0 mg/dL, potassium level greater than 6.5 mEq/L, and hemoglobin level less than 10 g/dL.

If uremic syndrome remains untreated, it can progress to stupor, coma, and death. The two possible treatments include dialysis and **kidney transplantation.**

Glomerulonephritis

Glomerulonephritis is inflammation of the glomerulus. It can have a sudden or severe onset (i.e., acute glomerulonephritis) or a gradual or progressive onset (i.e., chronic glomerulonephritis). Antibodies produced against the basement membranes of the glomeruli interfere with their ability to filter out or retain certain substances in the nephron.

Glomerulonephritis can be primary, occurring as an isolated disorder, or secondary, occurring as a known complication of another primary disease. In primary glomerulonephritis, the connection to an accompanying disease may be unclear or unknown. Diseases that are associated with glomerulonephritis include group A β-hemolytic streptococcal infection, bacterial endocarditis, amyloidosis, Goodpasture disease, polyarteritis, lupus erythematosus,

TABLE 24-1	Factors Regulating Renal H$^+$ Excretion
Factor	**Result**
Extracellular volume	Volume depletion leads to increased sodium retention.
Arterial PCO_2	Increased PCO_2 leads to increased H$^+$ secretion and increased HCO_3^- reabsorption.
K$^+$ and Cl$^-$ deficiency	Decreased K$^+$ leads to increased HCO_3^- reabsorption. Decreased Cl$^-$ prevents excretion of excess HCO_3^-.
Aldosterone level	Increased aldosterone leads to Na$^+$ reabsorption and increased urinary excretion of H$^+$ and K$^+$ (i.e., metabolic acidosis)

Cl$^-$, Chloride ion; *H$^+$*, hydrogen ion; *HCO$_3^-$*, bicarbonate ion; *K$^+$*, potassium ion; *Na$^+$*, sodium ion; *PCO$_2$*, partial pressure of carbon dioxide.

hepatitis, measles, mumps, and infectious mononucleosis (Fig. 24-6). Excessive use of nonsteroidal antiinflammatory drugs (NSAIDs) such as aspirin or ibuprofen is associated with glomerulonephritis.

Glomerulonephritis may be temporary and reversible, or it may progress. Progressive glomerulonephritis can lead to chronic kidney failure and end-stage renal disease.

Common signs and symptoms of glomerulonephritis include proteinuria (usually <3 g/day), swelling (i.e., edema) of the extremities, hematuria (i.e., blood in urine), fatigue, abdominal pain, increased BUN level, increased creatinine level, oliguria, many urinary casts (e.g., hyaline casts, granular casts, red blood cell casts), and high blood pressure (i.e., hypertension). The most common findings in glomerulonephritis are blood and protein in the urine. Because blood and protein are normally reabsorbed into the bloodstream, the finding of blood and protein in the urine indicates glomerular damage.

Nephrotic Syndrome

The nephrotic syndrome is caused by several underlying conditions that injure the glomeruli and result in increased glomerular membrane permeability. It is characterized by proteinuria (usually >3 g/day), edema, hypoalbuminemia, lipiduria, and hyperlipidemia. The syndrome usually results in the excretion of fat bodies (i.e., degenerated tubular cells containing abundant lipid) in the urine.

The causes of the nephrotic syndrome are listed in Table 24-2. One characteristic of the syndrome is hyperlipidemia. Hypoproteinemia and low blood oncotic pressure cause reactive protein synthesis in the liver, which includes lipoproteins. This is the body's attempt to replace proteins in the blood. Edema is explained by hypoalbuminemia due to massive protein loss in the urine. Hypoalbuminuria leads to hypoalbuminemia, and as hypoalbuminemia lowers the blood colloid osmotic pressure, more water leaks into surrounding tissues.

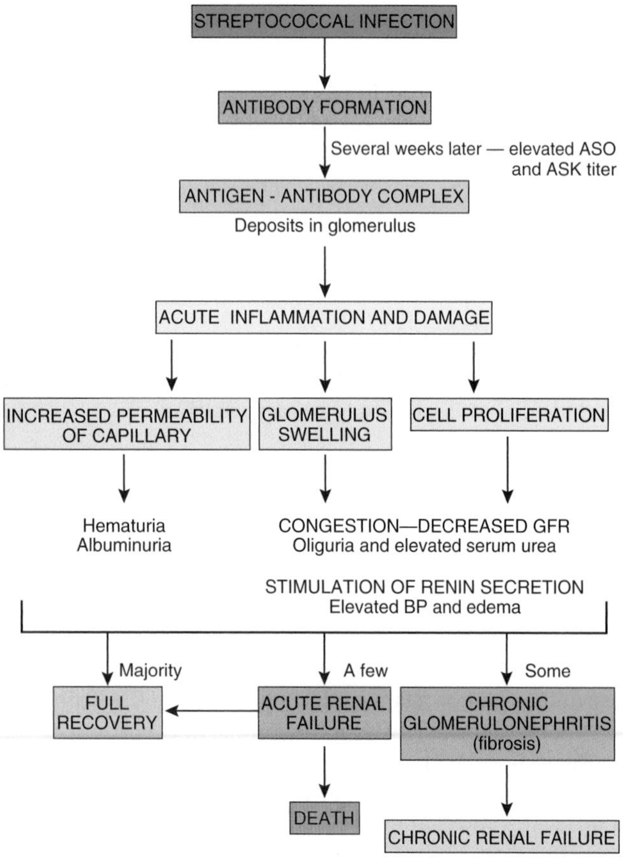

Renal Tubular Acidosis

Renal tubular acidosis (RTA) is a collection of acquired and inherited disorders of the proximal and distal tubules. The mechanism for these disorders is failure to reabsorb bicarbonate or failure to secrete hydrogen ions. Signs and symptoms include increased blood chloride levels, a normal anion gap, metabolic acidosis, and a normal GFR. The three main categories of RTA are classified according to the biochemical (rather than genetic) defect: distal RTA (type 1), proximal RTA (type 2), and combined distal and proximal RTA (type 4).

• **Figure 24-6** Development and course of poststreptococcal glomerulonephritis. *BP,* Blood pressure; *ASK,* antistreptokinase; *ASO,* antistreptolysin O. (From VanMeter KC, Hubert RJ. *Gould's Pathophysiology for the Health Profession.* 5th ed. St. Louis: Saunders; 2015.)

TABLE 24-2 Causes of Nephrotic Syndrome

Disease	Type of Disease	Comments
Minimal change disease	Renal	Common cause of nephrotic syndrome in children
Focal segmented glomerulonephritis	Renal	
Membranous nephropathy	Renal	Usually due to infection or autoimmune disease
Diabetic nephropathy	Renal or autoimmune	Due to diabetes mellitus
Systemic lupus erythematosus	Autoimmune	
Polyarteritis nodosa	Autoimmune	
Amyloidosis	Autoimmune	
Malignancy	Usually carcinoma	
Renal vein thrombosis	Systemic	
Heart failure	Systemic	Right heart failure and constrictive pericarditis

Distal RTA (type 1) is the most common type of RTA, in which the urine cannot be maximally acidified. Despite metabolic acidosis, the urine pH remains greater than 5.5. Causes include genetic abnormalities, autoimmune diseases (e.g., Sjögren disease, systemic lupus erythematosus, thyroiditis), conditions causing nephrocalcinosis (e.g., primary hypoparathyroidism, vitamin D intoxication), drugs or toxins (e.g., amphotericin B, toluene inhalation), and other renal disorders (e.g., obstruction uropathies). Several mechanisms produce distal RTA, such as a weak hydrogen pump that cannot transport hydrogen ions against a high concentration gradient. Leaky membranes cause back diffusion of hydrogen ions, and tubular damage creates insufficient hydrogen ion pumping capacity.

Findings for distal RTA include inappropriately high urine pH (>5.5), low levels of tubular acid secretions, low urine bicarbonate levels despite severe metabolic acidosis, and renal sodium wasting (i.e., secondary hyperaldosteronism increases sodium reabsorption and potassium loss through the urine). The diagnosis is based on a high chloride blood level with metabolic acidosis. It can also cause alkaline urine with kidney stone formation.

Proximal RTA (type 2) results from impaired bicarbonate reabsorption in the proximal tubule. It is caused by vitamin D deficiency, cystinosis, lead nephropathy, amyloidosis, and medullary cystic disease. In individuals with normal blood bicarbonate levels, approximately 15% of bicarbonate is lost in the urine. Individuals with severe acidosis have low blood bicarbonate levels (<17 mmol/L), and this can result in zero bicarbonate levels in urine.

Symptoms of proximal RTA result when the blood bicarbonate levels increase. The proximal tubules cannot absorb the increased bicarbonate in the blood, causing a large amount of bicarbonate to be excreted in the urine. In response, the distal tubule increases hydrogen ion production to neutralize the additional urine bicarbonate, and net urine acid decreases. This results in metabolic acidosis with an inappropriate increased urine pH. In the blood, HCO_3^- is replaced with Cl^-. Increased levels of Na^+ ions from the distal tubule result in hyperaldosteronism with a severely decreased K^+ level.

Type 4 RTA is another renal tubular acidosis that affects the renal interstitium and tubules. Type 4 RTA is caused by a defect in urine cation exchange in the distal tubule, reducing secretion of hydrogen and potassium ions. Clinical findings include a GFR greater than 20 mL/min and hyperkalemia. This disorder is caused by aldosterone deficiency, Addison disease, and bilateral adrenalectomy. Secondary proximal RTA may result from diseases such as multiple myeloma or from kidney transplant rejection (Table 24-3).

Urinary Tract Infection

Cystitis is inflammation of the bladder that is caused by a bacterial infection. Cystitis can also result from other diseases such as bladder cancer. The diagnosis is based on signs and symptoms (i.e., increased frequency of urination and painful urination) and physical, chemical, and microscopic examination of a urine specimen. A urine culture and sensitivity test can identify the etiologic agent and the sensitivity of the bacteria to antimicrobials.

Pyelonephritis is an infection of the kidney that may begin as a lower urinary tract infection such as cystitis or prostatitis and progress to the kidney. Pyelonephritis can also occur without a lower urinary tract infection. The most common causes of pyelonephritis are organisms that originate from the gastrointestinal tract and live on or colonize the surfaces of the urogenital tract. They include *Escherichia coli*, *Enterococcus faecalis*, *Klebsiella pneumonia*, and *Staphylococcus saprophyticus*. Factors that may increase the risk of pyelonephritis include structural abnormalities of the urinary tract or anything that blocks normal urine flow, such as prostatic hyperplasia, kidney stones, or an indwelling urinary catheter. Other risk factors include a family history of recurrent urinary tract infections, changes in sexual behavior, changes in sexual partners, or a compromised immune system.

Symptoms of acute pyelonephritis include fever, malaise, painful urination, vomiting, and abdominal and flank pain. Physical examination reveals tenderness at the costovertebral angle. A urinalysis, white blood cell count and differential, and urine culture are helpful in diagnosing pyelonephritis.

TABLE 24-3	**Types of Renal Tubular Acidosis**		
Findings	Type 1	Type 2	Type 4
Hyperchloremic acidosis	Yes	Yes	Yes
Urine pH	>5.5	<5.5 (usually >5.5 before acidosis is established)	<5.5
Blood K^+ level	Low to normal	Low to normal	High
Renal stones	Yes	No	No
Mechanism	Reduced H^+ excretion in distal tubule	Impaired HCO_3^- reabsorption in proximal tubule	Impaired cation exchange in distal tubule

H^+, Hydrogen ion; HCO_3^-, bicarbonate ion; K^+, potassium ion.

Pyelonephritis can be successfully managed if detected early and treated promptly with appropriate antimicrobials. If left untreated, severe pyelonephritis can result and lead to **pyonephrosis** (i.e., pus around the kidney), **urosepsis** (i.e., systemic infection), kidney failure, and death (Fig. 24-7).

Polycystic Kidney Disease

Polycystic kidney disease (PKD) is a genetic disorder with an autosomal dominant or autosomal recessive pattern of inheritance. In the autosomal dominant form, only one copy of the gene is required for the offspring to have the disease. In the autosomal recessive form, two copies (one from each parent) are required for offspring to have the disease.

The autosomal dominant and autosomal recessive forms of PKD are characterized by cysts in the kidneys. The cysts are often filled with fluid and can be few or numerous. The cysts replace functioning nephrons with nonfunctioning

space. They increase the size of the kidney and decrease kidney function.

Autosomal dominant PKD is an adult-onset disease, and autosomal recessive PKD first appears in childhood. In adult-onset PKD, the accumulation of cysts in the kidney is gradual, whereas in autosomal recessive PKD, the cysts begin growing during early childhood. Patients have hypertension and hematuria, and approximately 50% develop end-stage renal disease by age 35.

PKD is common in the United States and is a leading cause of kidney transplantation (Fig. 24-8). PKD is diagnosed using the family history, genetic testing, and imaging techniques such as ultrasound, magnetic resonance imaging (MRI), and computed tomography (CT). A family history is key in diagnosing genetic diseases. Performing genetic testing for the PKD gene in affected persons or in family members is expensive, but it can yield a diagnosis.

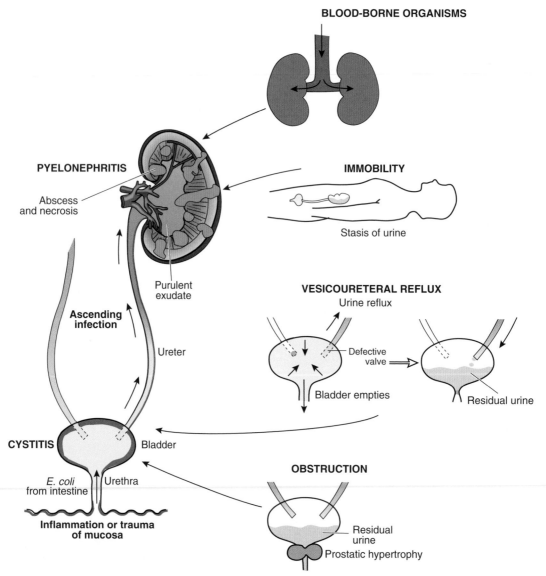

• **Figure 24-7** Causes of infection in the urinary tract. (From VanMeter KC, Hubert RJ. *Gould's Pathophysiology for the Health Profession.* 5th ed. St. Louis: Saunders; 2015.)

Diabetic Nephropathy

Diabetes mellitus is characterized by chronic high blood glucose levels, which over time injure the retina (i.e., retinopathy), kidney (i.e., nephropathy), nerves (i.e., neuropathy), and arteries (i.e., atherosclerosis). One third of diabetics develop end-stage renal disease, making diabetes the most common cause of the disease in the United States. Nephropathy decreases renal function, quickly leading to end-stage renal disease (Fig. 24-9).

Research indicates that early detection of proteinuria leads to early detection of nephropathy. A microalbumin test is often used to detect early proteinuria. An elevated microalbumin level is defined as a higher than normal protein level in urine that is less than detectable by conventional methods. A sustained elevated urinary microalbumin value of 30 to 300 mg/24 hours indicates an increase in the transcapillary escape rate of albumin and indicates microvascular disease. With a microalbumin level of more than 30 mg/dL, a diabetic is 20 times as likely to develop diabetic nephropathy, and this level predicts end-stage renal disease, cardiovascular instability, and an increased all-cause

mortality rate. If proteinuria is diagnosed early, angiotensin-converting enzyme inhibitors can slow the decline in renal function.

Renal Failure

Renal failure occurs as an abrupt or rapid decrease in the kidney's ability to filter the blood. Increased BUN and creatinine levels are characteristics of renal failure, and the BUN to creatinine ratio can exceed 20:1. Renal failure can be acute or chronic.

In acute renal failure, progressive loss of renal function is characterized by oliguria (i.e., decreased urine production), azotemia (i.e., increased nitrogen in the urine), and an electrolyte imbalance. Acute renal failure can be classified as prerenal, renal, or postrenal. Prerenal causes include hypoperfusion due to ischemia, toxins, or trauma to the kidney. Postrenal causes include structural abnormalities or calculi in the bladder or ureters associated with decreased urine flow. Renal causes of acute renal failure include systemic diseases such as systemic lupus erythematosus and diabetes mellitus or progressing kidney disease

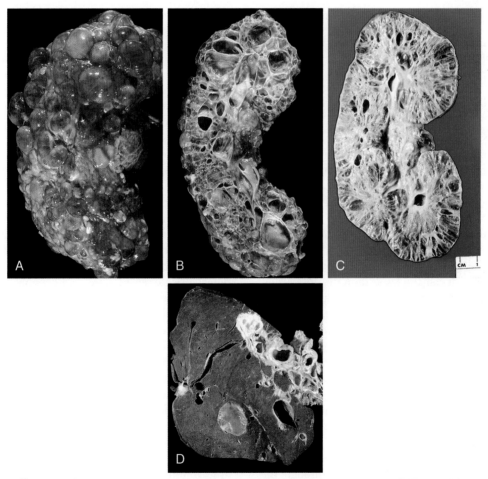

• **Figure 24-8** Polycystic kidney disease (PKD). **A** and **B,** Autosomal dominant adult PKD viewed from the external surface of a bisected kidney. The kidney is markedly enlarged and contains numerous dilated cysts. **C,** Autosomal recessive childhood PKD shows smaller cysts and dilated channels at right angles to the cortical surface. **D,** Liver cysts in adult PKD. (From Kumar V, Abbas A, Fausto N, Aster J. *Robbins & Cotran: Pathologic Basis of Disease.* 9th ed. Philadelphia: Saunders; 2015.)

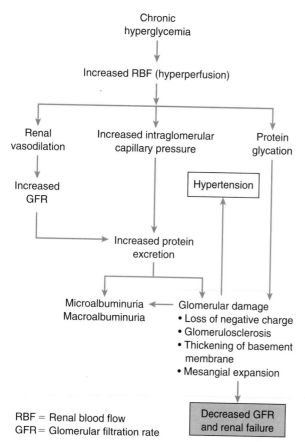

Chronic
hyperglycemia

↓

Increased RBF (hyperperfusion)

↓

Renal
vasodilation — Increased intraglomerular
capillary pressure — Protein
glycation

↓

Increased
GFR — Hypertension

↓

Increased protein
excretion

Microalbuminuria ← Glomerular damage
Macroalbuminuria — • Loss of negative charge
• Glomerulosclerosis
• Thickening of basement
membrane
• Mesangial expansion

↓

Decreased GFR
and renal failure

RBF = Renal blood flow
GFR = Glomerular filtration rate

• **Figure 24-9** Diabetic neuropathy. (From McCance KL, Huether SE. *Pathophysiology: The Biologic Basis for Disease in Adults and Children.* 7th ed. St. Louis: Mosby; 2015.)

such as acute tubular necrosis, glomerulonephritis, and nephrotic syndrome. The underlying cause should be determined, and if possible, it should be removed or repaired. Kidney dialysis may be necessary until the underlying cause is treated and kidney function returns.

Chronic renal failure results from progression of acute kidney failure or the progression of a disease such as diabetes mellitus, prolonged hypertension, PKD, glomerulonephritis, or pyelonephritis. It can also result from the progression of a chronic systemic disease such as systemic lupus erythematosus, amyloidosis, or Goodpasture syndrome. The signs and symptoms of renal failure include nausea, vomiting, muscle cramps, and arrhythmia. Kidney disease can be exacerbated by excessive ingestion of ibuprofen, acetaminophen, and aspirin. Renal failure may result in edema, metabolic acidosis or acidemia, hyperkalemia, hypocalcemia, hyperphosphatemia, and in later stages, anemia and malnutrition. Chronic renal failure is also associated with an increased risk of cardiovascular disease.

Renal failure is diagnosed by a decrease in the GFR, which is the rate at which blood is filtered through the glomeruli of the kidney. A decreased GFR is associated with decreased or absence of urine and with detection of waste products (i.e., creatinine or urea) in the blood. Hematuria and proteinuria are common in renal failure.

Because the creatinine clearance test (discussed later) result is considered a good indicator of the GFR, it is used to detect renal failure. It is important to determine the underlying cause and monitor the systemic effects of renal failure.

Diabetes Insipidus

Diabetes insipidus causes excretion of large volumes (>3 L/24 hours) of dilute urine (<300 mOsm/kg). The disease is caused by decreased production of ADH or a decreased ability to concentrate urine due to ADH resistance in the kidney. Decreased production of ADH can be idiopathic or the result of brain or pituitary tumors, cranial surgery, or head trauma. The decreased ability to concentrate urine due to ADH resistance in the kidney is observed in patients with chronic renal insufficiency, lithium toxicity, hypercalcemia, hypokalemia, glucosuria, or tubulointerstitial disease.

The signs and symptoms of diabetes insipidus include polyuria (3 to 20 L/24 hours), polydipsia, and nocturia. Laboratory tests used to diagnose this disorder include 24-hour urine volume, serum electrolytes, serum glucose, urine specific gravity, simultaneous plasma and urinary osmolality, and plasma ADH levels.

Renal Obstruction

A renal obstruction blocks the flow of urine from the renal pelvis to the ureter. The renal pelvis is the broadened top part of the ureter into which the kidney tubules drain. Renal obstruction can affect one or both kidneys and may be an acute or chronic event.

Renal obstruction can be caused by renal calculi (i.e., kidney stones), prostatic hypertrophy, blood clots, metastatic cancer, structural abnormalities of the ureters, scar tissue in the ureters, or bladder abnormalities. If urine flow is blocked, the backflow creates a pressure that eventually reaches the renal pelvis, tubules, and glomerulus. Urinary infections and the formation of renal calculi may be a complication of urinary stasis. Long-standing (i.e., several weeks) renal obstruction of both kidneys can lead to renal damage, acute renal failure, and possibly death. Early diagnosis of renal obstruction is essential to prevent permanent kidney damage.

Renal calculi or kidney stones are one of the most common causes of urinary obstruction. Kidney stones are crystalline or solid aggregates formed from dietary minerals such as calcium, magnesium, and uric acid. More than 80% of kidney stones occur in men older than age 30. Kidney stones can be found in the kidney itself (i.e., nephrolithiasis), in the bladder (i.e., cystolithiasis), or in the ureter (i.e., ureterolithiasis). Many stones leave the body without causing symptoms. However, when the stone reaches at least 3 mm in diameter, it can cause urinary obstruction and symptoms.

Diagnosis of renal obstruction is accomplished with imaging techniques, urinalysis, tests for BUN and creatinine levels, and a white blood cell count.

Laboratory Procedures

Urinalysis

The three main parts of a **urinalysis** are the physical, chemical, and microscopic examinations of a urine sample. The physical examination detects the color and clarity of the urine, and unusual odors noticed during the physical examination may indicate a particular condition. Color usually ranges from pale yellow to deep amber. The sample may be clear to very cloudy.

The chemistry examination includes specific gravity, pH, protein, glucose, **ketones**, blood, **leukocyte esterase**, nitrites, bilirubin, and **urobilinogen.** It is usually performed using a dipstick test kit (Fig. 24-10).

The microscopic examination looks for cells (i.e., epithelial cells, bacteria, yeast, white blood cells, and red blood cells), casts, and crystals (Fig. 24-11). **Casts** are formed from Tamm-Horsfall proteins in the distal convoluted tubules and collecting ducts of the nephron. Casts can be hyaline, cellular (i.e., red cells, white cells, or epithelial cells), granular, or waxy. Waxy and finely granular casts indicate profound stasis of urine in the kidney tubules or collecting ducts. Included are **calcium**

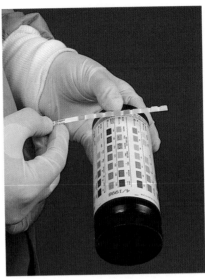

• **Figure 24-10** Chemical examination of urine is usually performed using a dipstick test kit. The colors indicate levels of various chemicals in the urine sample. (From Bonewit-West K. *Clinical Procedures for Medical Assistants.* 9th ed. St. Louis: Saunders; 2015.)

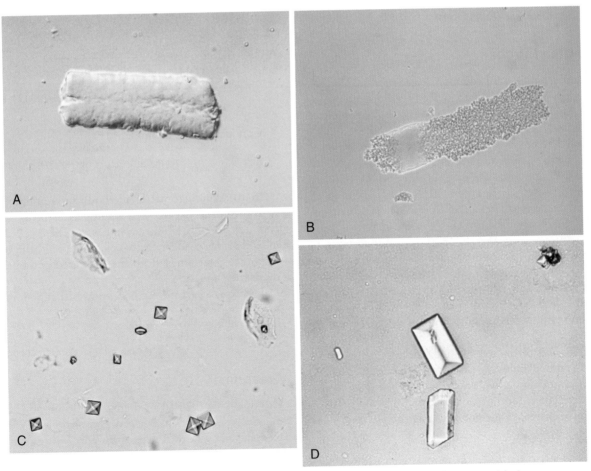

• **Figure 24-11** Microscopic sediment in urine. **A,** Waxy cast. The three-dimensional image uses interference contract (Nomarski) microscopy (×100). **B,** Coarse granular cast (bright-field microscopy, ×100). **C,** Calcium oxalate crystals: octahedral (envelope) form of dihydrate crystals (bright-field microscopy, ×200). **D,** Triple phosphate crystals: typical coffin lid form (bright-field microscopy, ×100). (From Brunzel NA. *Fundamentals of Urine and Body Fluid Analysis.* 3rd ed. St. Louis: Saunders; 2013.)

oxalate crystals, triple phosphate crystals, hippurate crystals, uric acid crystals, cysteine crystals, and tyrosine crystals. Most crystals are considered nonpathogenic, but some, such as cysteine and tyrosine, are considered pathogenic.

A complete urinalysis provides important information with which to diagnosis systemic illnesses such as diabetes mellitus, acute tubular necrosis, and pyelonephritis. A urinalysis is considered a screening test because it is the first step in determining whether the abnormality detected is associated with renal function specifically or an indication of systemic conditions.

Electrolytes

Electrolytes can be measured in serum and urine. A full discussion of serum electrolytes is available in Chapter 13. Sodium, potassium, and chloride are the most commonly measured urine electrolytes. Urine sodium levels reflect the integrity of the tubular reabsorption function. If the urine sodium level is low, the kidney is reabsorbing sodium at a normal rate, and the kidney is stimulated to conserve sodium. If the urine sodium level is high, sodium is not being reabsorbed in the kidneys and is being lost in the urine. This test is ordered to distinguish between the various forms of renal failure (Table 24-4).

Blood Urea Nitrogen

BUN and creatinine are common screening tests for kidney function. BUN is formed in the liver from ammonia. It is the end product of protein catabolism. BUN comprises approximately 45% of nonprotein nitrogen in the blood. It is freely filtered by the glomerulus, and urea excretion is adjusted by the tubules of the kidney.

Excessive amounts of urea in the blood indicate decreased glomerular function. BUN levels are used to differentiate prerenal, renal, and postrenal malfunction. BUN is increased in acute and chronic nephritis, urinary obstruction, metal poisoning, pneumonia, uremia, Addison disease, peritonitis, surgical shock, and cardiac failure. A high-protein diet, stress, and administration of steroids can also produce increased BUN levels. Low BUN levels are found in late pregnancy, starvation, and malnutrition. The reference range for BUN is 6 to 20 mg/dL.

Indirect and direct test methods are used to measure BUN. Common indirect tests include the coupled enzymatic, Berthelot reaction, and conductometric methods, and diacetyl monoxime is used in the direct method.

Coupled enzymatic method (measured at 578 nm):

$$Urea + H_2O \xrightarrow{Urease} 2\ NH_3 + CO_2$$

$$NH_3 + Salicylate \xrightarrow{\substack{Nitroprusside \\ hydrochloride}}$$

$$2,2\text{-Dicarboxy indophenol}$$

TABLE 24-4 · Causes of Increased and Decreased Urine Sodium Levels

Increased Urine Sodium	Decreased Urine Sodium
Excessive dietary salt	Hyperaldosteronism
Diuretic therapy	Hyponatremia
Adrenal insufficiency	Prerenal azotemia
Salt-wasting nephropathy	Glomerulonephritis
Acute tubular necrosis	Hepatorenal syndrome
Analgesic abuse-induced interstitial nephritis	Renal failure
Syndrome of inappropriate antidiuretic hormone secretion	Nephrotic syndrome
Vomiting	Nonsteroidal antiinflammatory drugs
Hypothyroidism	Some corticosteroids
Postobstructive disease	
Hepatic failure	
Congestive heart failure	
Some antibiotics	
Prostaglandins	

Berthelot method (measured at 340 nm):

$$Urea + H_2O \xrightarrow{Urease} 2\ NH_3 + CO_2$$

$$NH_3 + \alpha\text{-Ketoglutarate} + NADH^+ + H^+ \xrightarrow{\substack{Glutarate \\ dehydrogenase}}$$
$$L\text{-Glutamate} + NAD^+ + H_2O$$

Conductometric method:

$$BUN \xrightarrow{Urease} NH_4^+$$

In the conductometric method, ammonium (NH_4^+) is formed after urease (i.e., catalyst) treatment, and the conductivity of the solution increases. The NH_4^+ ions are measured by an ion-selective electrode, and the concentration is determined from the measured potential using the Nernst equation.

Diacetyl monoxime method (measured at 540 nm):

$$BUN + Diacetyl \xrightarrow{Heat\ \&\ H^+}$$
$$Diazine + H_2O\ (yellow\ chromogen)$$

Creatinine

Creatine is synthesized in the liver and transported to the muscles and the brain, where a phosphate group is added to make phosphocreatine, a high-energy compound that donates a phosphate group to the ADP molecule, leaving creatine in the muscle and generating ATP. The energy provided by ATP fuels muscle contraction.

Approximately 1% to 2% of creatine is spontaneously and irreversibly converted to its waste product, creatinine. Creatinine production is constant, related to muscle mass.

It is freely filtered by the glomerulus and not reabsorbed by the tubules. Because diet, age, sex, and exercise do not affect blood creatinine levels, it is a good indicator of renal function. Any condition that obstructs urine elimination or interferes with glomerular filtration results in elevated blood creatinine levels. The reference range for serum creatinine is 0.5 to 1.5 mg/dL, and the reference range for urine creatinine is 800 to 2000 mg/24 hours.

The Jaffe reaction was first described in 1886. In it, creatinine complexes with alkaline picrate to form an orange-red complex:

$$\text{Creatinine} + \text{Picrate} \xrightarrow{\text{Alkaline}} \text{Orange-red complex}$$

This method is not specific for creatinine, and interfering substances include protein, glucose, ascorbic acid, and ketones. To create a creatinine test method that is less susceptible to interfering substances, several multistep enzymatic methods were developed:

Reaction 1:

$$\text{Creatinine} + \text{H}_2\text{O} \xrightarrow{\text{Creatinase}} \text{Creatine}$$

$$\text{Creatine} + \text{ATP} \xrightarrow{\substack{\text{Creatine} \\ \text{kinase}}} \text{Creatine phosphate} + \text{ADP}$$

$$\text{ADP} + \text{Phosphoenolpyruvate} \xrightarrow{\substack{\text{Pyruvate} \\ \text{kinase}}} \text{Pyruvate} + \text{ATP}$$

$$\text{Pyruvate} + \text{NADP} + \text{H}^+ \xrightarrow{\substack{\text{Lactate} \\ \text{dehydrogenase}}} \text{Lactate} + \text{NAD}^+$$

Reaction 2:

$$\text{Creatinine} + \text{H}_2\text{O} \xrightarrow{\text{Creatinase}} \text{Creatine}$$

$$\text{Creatine} + \text{H}_2\text{O} \xrightarrow{\text{Creatinase}} \text{Sarcosine} + \text{Urea}$$

$$\text{Sarcosine} + \text{O}_2 + \text{H}_2\text{O} \xrightarrow{\substack{\text{Sarcosine} \\ \text{oxidase}}} \text{Formaldehyde} + \text{Glycine} + \text{H}_2\text{O}_2$$

$$\text{Indicator (reduced)} + \text{H}_2\text{O} \xrightarrow{\text{Peroxidase}} \text{Indicator (oxidized)} + \text{H}_2\text{O}$$

Reaction 3:

$$\text{Creatine} + \text{H}_2\text{O} \xrightarrow{\substack{\text{Creatinine} \\ \text{deaminase}}} N\text{-Methylhydantoin} + \text{NH}_3$$

$$N\text{-Methylhydantoin} + \text{ATP} + \text{H}_2\text{O} \xrightarrow{\text{L-methylhydantoinase}} \text{Carbamoylsarcosine} + \text{ADP} + \text{Pi}$$

$$\text{Carbamoylsarcosine} + \text{H}_2\text{O} \xrightarrow{\substack{\text{L-carbamoylsarcosine} \\ \text{aminohydrolase}}} \text{Sarcosine} + \text{CO}_2 + \text{NH}_3$$

$$\text{Sarcosine} + \text{O}_2 + \text{H}_2\text{O} \xrightarrow{\substack{\text{Sarcosine} \\ \text{oxidase}}} \text{H}_2\text{O} + \text{Glycine} + \text{HCHO}$$

$$\text{Indicator (reduced)} + \text{H}_2\text{O}_2 \xrightarrow{\text{Peroxidase}} \text{Indicator (oxidized)} + 2\,\text{H}_2\text{O}$$

Reaction 1 suffers from poor sensitivity, poor precision, and relatively expensive reagents. This method is not popular. Reaction 2 is a more popular method that is used in point-of-care instruments. Reaction 3 is used in dry chemistry systems and employs a two-slide system.

Creatinine Clearance

The creatinine clearance rate, or the volume of serum that is cleared of creatinine per unit time, is a useful test for approximating the GFR. The GFR is the best measure of kidney function, but measuring it can be time-consuming and expensive, whereas the creatinine clearance test offers a simple, cost-effective approximation of glomerular filtration.

The creatinine clearance test begins with a 24-hour urine collection and a serum creatinine sample drawn during the 24-hour collection period. The 24-hour collection is the most common, although 12- and 4-hour collections may be used. Urine and serum creatinine values in the specified units are plugged into the creatinine clearance formula:

$$\frac{\text{urine creat. (mg/dL)}}{\text{serum creat. (mg/dL)}} \times \frac{\text{urine volume (mL)}}{\text{min. of collection}}$$
$$\times \frac{1.73\ \text{m}^2\ \text{(avg. person's surface area)}}{\text{patient's surface area (m}^2\text{)}}$$

Reference ranges for creatinine clearance are 74 to 138 mL/min for men and 65 to 123 mL/min for women. Because creatinine levels in urine are much higher than serum values, urine specimens are usually diluted with water 1:20 for testing.

Uric Acid

Uric acid is an end product of purine (i.e., adenosine and guanosine) metabolism. Endogenous purines are broken down in the body to form approximately 400 mg of uric acid, and an additional 300 mg is created from dietary sources. Individuals with gouty arthritis may have very high uric acid blood levels (18,000 to 30,000 mg). One reason for overproduction is the increased synthesis of purine precursors.

Most of the uric acid in the blood is filtered through the glomerulus and then reabsorbed in the proximal and distal tubules. Uricemia is an increased blood level of uric acid;

blood levels are greater than 7.0 mg/dL in men and greater than 6.0 mg/dL in women. Hyperuricemia and hyperuricuria can cause kidney disease, gout, and kidney stones. Causes of hyperuricemia include inherited metabolic disorders, excess dietary purine intake, alcohol, preeclampsia, tissue hypoxia, increased nucleic acid turnover (i.e., leukemia, myeloma, radiotherapy, chemotherapy, and trauma), increased renal absorption, reduced secretion, thiazide diuretics, and lead poisoning. Hypouricemia (<2.0 mg/dL) is much less common but can occur. It is usually caused by conditions such as Fanconi syndrome or exposure to toxic agents.

Uric acid is measured in the laboratory using phosphotungstic acid, uricase, and high-performance liquid chromatography (HPLC) methods. In the phosphotungstic acid method, phosphotungstic acid is reduced by urate in an alkaline media:

$$\text{Phosphotungstic acid} + \text{Uratic acid} \xrightarrow[\substack{\text{Alkaline} \\ \text{medium}}]{} \text{Blue-colored complex}$$

Uricase is an enzymatic method used to quantitate the amount of uric acid in the blood. Uric acid is converted by uricase to allantoin and hydrogen peroxide:

$$\text{Uric acid} + O_2 + H_2O \xrightarrow[\text{Uricase} + O_2]{} \text{Allantoin} + CO_2 + H_2O_2$$

A related method measures the amount of hydrogen peroxide using hydrogen peroxidase and oxygen acceptors to create a chromogen that is measured bichromatically in the visible spectrum. Electrochemical and biosensor systems also use uricase in oxygen electrode. HPLC methods using ion-exchange or reversed-phase columns are used to quantitate uric acid. Reference ranges for uric acid are 3.5 to 7.2 mg/dL for men and 2.6 to 6.0 mg/dL for women.

Urine Protein

Proteinuria can be glomerular or tubular in origin and usually indicates renal disease. In glomerular proteinuria, the protein lost in the urine is usually higher-molecular-weight protein. The loss through the glomerulus most often results from increased permeability of the glomerular membranes. In tubular proteinuria, the proteins lost are low- to medium-molecular-weight proteins that fail to be reabsorbed by the nephron tubules.

Due to the clinical significance of urine protein, a positive protein finding on the urine dipstick should be investigated further. An accurately timed 24-hour urine specimen is preferred for urine protein testing. A random specimen can be accepted if no other specimens are available.

Urine protein is measured using the Lowry, trichloroacetic acid, sulfosalicylic, Coomassie blue, and pyrogallol red methods. The Lowry method combines protein with

TABLE 24-5	Causes of Increased and Decreased Urine Osmolality	
Increased Urine Osmolality	**Decreased Urine Osmolality**
Dehydration	Diabetes insipidus
Syndrome of inappropriate antidiuretic hormone secretion	Excessive fluid intake
Adrenal insufficiency	Acute renal insufficiency
Glycosuria	Glomerulonephritis
Hypernatremia	
High-protein diet	

phosphotungstic and phosphomolybdic acids to form a blue-colored complex:

$$\text{Protein} + \text{copper ions} \xrightarrow[\substack{\text{Alkaline pH and} \\ \text{phenol reagent}}]{} \text{copper-protein complex}$$

Tests with trichloroacetic and sulfosalicylic acids are turbidimetric methods used to measure proteins. The addition of acid to the protein titrates the acidic groups to create insoluble particles. The amount of light transmitted through the solution is used to calculate the amount of protein in the sample.

Coomassie blue and pyrogallol red are dye-binding methods used for quantitating protein in urine. Proteins combined with these dyes produce colored compounds that can be used to quantitate the amount of protein in the sample.

Osmolality

Urine osmolality measures the number of dissolved particles per kilogram of water. Osmolality is an accurate measure of urine concentration and is useful in diagnosing diabetes insipidus and hydration status. Osmolality can be used to diagnose ADH disorders, but serum and urine osmolality values must be measured. The random urine osmolality reference range is 300 to 900 mOsm/kg of water, and the 24-hour urine osmolality reference range is 500 to 800 mOsm/kg of water. Table 24-5 lists the conditions that increase or decrease urine osmolality.

Hemodialysis and Peritoneal Dialysis

Hemodialysis and peritoneal dialysis are used to treat end-stage renal disease. In hemodialysis, a dialysis machine with a semipermeable membrane substitutes as a kidney to remove waste products such as urea, creatinine, salts, and acids (Fig. 24-12). A major limitation of hemodialysis is the inability to do the procedure at home. Regular trips to a hospital or clinic interrupt the process of daily living. There also may be a significant risk of introducing infection through the canula.

In peritoneal dialysis, the blood vessels in the peritoneum and the fluid introduced into the peritoneal cavity help to filter out the waste products. Limitations of peritoneal dialysis include infection and damage to the peritoneal membrane.

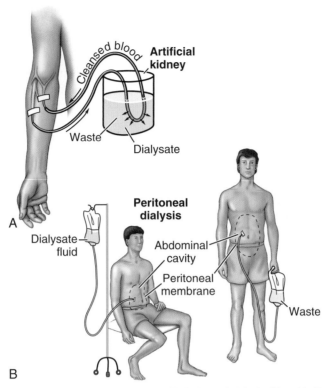

• **Figure 24-12** Types of dialysis. **A,** Artificial kidney. **B,** Peritoneal dialysis. (From Herlihy B. *The Human Body in Health and Illness.* 5th ed. St. Louis: Elsevier; 2014.)

Summary

The renal system is composed of two kidneys, two ureters, a bladder, and a urethra. The functional unit of a kidney is the nephron, which contains the glomerulus, the proximal and distal tubules, and the collecting ducts. The primary job of the nephron is filtration and reabsorption. The kidney is responsible for production of urine, conservation of protein and water, maintaining acid-base and electrolyte balance, and production of red blood cells and vitamin D_3.

Diseases that involve the kidneys include glomerulonephritis, urinary tract infections (i.e., cystitis and pyelonephritis), PKD, nephritic syndrome, tubular acidosis, and renal failure. End-stage renal disease can be treated by hemodialysis or peritoneal dialysis.

Kidney function is measured with laboratory tests for BUN, serum creatinine, and creatinine clearance. The most commonly ordered kidney test is a urinalysis, which can screen for renal abnormalities and systemic diseases such as diabetes. Obstruction of the kidneys may be caused by renal calculi, diseases such as metastatic cancer, or structural abnormalities.

Review Questions

1. Which of the following is *not* normally used to diagnose pyelonephritis?
   a. Kidney biopsy
   b. Urine culture and sensitivity
   c. Urinalysis
   d. Patient's signs and symptoms
2. Which of the following conditions is genetically linked as either autosomal recessive or dominant?
   a. Acute tubular necrosis
   b. Azotemia
   c. Polycystic kidney disease
   d. Acute kidney injury
3. Which of the following is *not* a cause of renal obstruction?
   a. Uremia
   b. Renal calculi
   c. Metastatic cancer
   d. Prostatic hypertrophy
4. Which of the following is a result of hydrogen ion imbalance in uremia?
   a. Metabolic acidosis
   b. Azotemia
   c. Malnutrition
   d. Hypercalcemia
5. Which of the following is associated with nephrotic syndrome?
   a. Proteinuria
   b. Pyuria
   c. Hemorrhage in the body
   d. Bleeding in the urinary tract

6. Which of the following is secreted by the kidney and controls red blood cell formation?
   a. Proteinuria
   b. Erythropoietin
   c. Renin
   d. Vitamin D_3
7. Which of the following laboratory measurements is used to measure glomerular filtration rate?
   a. Creatinine
   b. Creatinine clearance
   c. Uric acid
   d. Blood urea nitrogen
8. Which of the following is a nonserum protein associated with the formation of microscopic casts?
   a. Albumin
   b. Globulin
   c. Microalbumin
   d. Tamm-Horsfall
9. Which of the following hormones helps keep urine concentrated?
   a. Angiotensinogen
   b. Antidiuretic hormone
   c. Phosphate
   d. Erythropoietin
10. Which structure of the nephron is the primary site of filtration?
   a. Proximal tubule
   b. Loop of Henle
   c. Glomerulus
   d. Collecting duct

Critical Thinking Questions

1. Discuss the three parts of a urinalysis. What tests are performed in each part? Name two disease states that can be diagnosed by each part of a urinalysis.
2. Discuss how homeostasis is maintained in the body with regard to the renal system. Name at least three substances that are controlled by the kidney. Discuss in detail how they are controlled.
3. Discuss the similarities and differences between cystitis and pyelonephritis. What are the complications of both diseases?

CASE STUDY

Ms. K, age 23 years, has progressively worsening renal failure due to polycystic kidney disease. Renal failure was diagnosed about 5 years ago, after an episode of hematuria. She has multiple bilateral renal cysts. She also has two cysts in her liver and mild hypertension that is controlled with medication. She has no other health problems. She is likely to require dialysis soon and has been advised to consider renal transplantation. What is polycystic kidney disease? What is the disease mechanism, and how is the disease treated?

Bibliography

Al-Badr W, Martin KJ. Vitamin D and kidney disease. *Clin J Am Soc Nephrol*. 2008;3:1555–1560.

American Diabetes Association. Standards of medical care in diabetes—2013. *Diabetes Care*. 2013;36(suppl 1):S11–S66.

Bellomo R, Kellum JA, Ronco C. Defining acute renal failure: physiological principles. In: *Applied Physiology in Intensive Care Medicine 1*. Berlin: Springer; 2012:115–119.

Chevalier RL. Pathogenesis of renal injury in obstructive uropathy. *Curr Opin Pediatr*. 2006;18:153–160.

Cohen EP, Lemann J. The role of the laboratory in evaluation of kidney function. *Clin Chem*. 1991;37:785–796.

Daugirdas JT, Black PG, Ing TS. *Handbook of Dialysis. 4th*. Philadelphia: Lippincott Williams & Wilkins; 2007.

Dechert T. Fluid, electrolyte, and acid-base disorders. In: *Current Diagnosis and Treatment Surgery*. 14th ed. New York: McGraw-Hill; 2015:104.

Donnelly S. Why is erythropoietin made in the kidney? The kidney functions as a critmeter. *Am J Kidney Dis*. 2001;38:415–425.

El-Hefnawy AS, Shokeir AA. Diagnosis of urinary tract stones: an overview. In: *Urolithiasis*. London: Springer; 2012:243–250.

Florkowski CM, Chew-Harris JS. Methods of estimating GFR—different equations including CKD-EPI. *Clin Biochem Rev*. 2011;32:75.

Guyton AC, Hall JE. *Textbook of Medical Physiology*. Philadelphia: Elsevier Saunders; 2016. 310.

Harris Peter C, Torres VE. Polycystic kidney disease. *Ann Rev Med*. 2009;60:321.

Jarraya F, Lakhdar R, Kammoun K, et al. Microalbuminuria: a useful marker of cardiovascular disease. *Iran J Kidney Dis*. 2013;7:178–186.

Laing CM, Toye AM, Capasso G, Unwin RJ. Renal tubular acidosis: developments in our understanding of the molecular basis. *Int J Biochem Cell Biol*. 2005;37:1151–1161.

Levinsky NG, Davidson DG, Berliner RW. Effects of reduced glomerular filtration on urine concentration in the presence of antidiuretic hormone. *J Clin Invest*. 1959;38:730–740.

Molitoris BA. Acute kidney injury. In: Goldman L, Schafer AI, eds. *Cecil Medicine*. 24th ed. Philadelphia: Saunders Elsevier; 2011.

Schrier RW. Diagnostic value of urinary sodium, chloride, urea, and flow. *J Am Soc Nephrol*. 2011;22:1610–1613.

Sirén AL, Fratelli M, Brines M, et al. Erythropoietin prevents neuronal apoptosis after cerebral ischemia and metabolic stress. *Proc Natl Acad Sci U S A*. 2001;98:4044–4049.

Sterns RH. Disorders of plasma sodium—causes, consequences, and correction. *N Engl J Med*. 2015;372:55–65.

Wada J, Makino H. Inflammation and the pathogenesis of diabetic nephropathy. *Clin Sci*. 2013;124:139–152.

25

Reproductive Diseases and Disorders

DONNA LARSON

CHAPTER OUTLINE

OBJECTIVES

After completion of this chapter, the reader will be able to:

1. Describe the structure and functions of the female and male reproductive systems.
2. Describe the female hormone cycle, hormonal diseases, and laboratory analytes and assays used to aid diagnosis.
3. Describe the male hormone cycle, hormonal diseases, and laboratory analytes and assays used to aid diagnosis.
4. Compare and contrast male and female infertility and laboratory analytes and assays used to aid diagnosis.
5. Identify causes of amenorrhea and laboratory analytes and assays used to aid in diagnosis.
6. Identify causes of hirsutism and laboratory analytes and assays used to aid in diagnosis.
7. List causes and symptoms of Klinefelter syndrome and laboratory analytes and assays used to aid in diagnosis.
8. List pathophysiology and symptoms of Kallmann syndrome and laboratory analytes and assays used to aid in diagnosis.
9. Describe orchitis and laboratory analytes and assays used to aid diagnosis.
10. Describe epididymitis and laboratory analytes and assays used to aid diagnosis.
11. Analyze menopause and laboratory analytes and assays used to aid diagnosis.
12. Describe polycystic ovary syndrome, symptoms, and laboratory assays used to aid diagnosis.
13. Explain the analytical methods used for clinical chemistry testing related to the reproductive system.

KEY TERMS

Anosmia
Congenital idiopathic hypogonadotropic hypogonadism
Corpus luteum
Dehydroepiandrosterone sulfate
Endometrium
Epididymitis
Follicle-stimulating hormone

Gonadotropin-releasing hormone
Hirsutism
Kallmann syndrome
Klinefelter syndrome
Luteinizing hormone
Menopause
Orchitis
Osteoporosis

Ovulation
Perimenopausal period
Polycystic ovary syndrome
Primary amenorrhea
Primary infertility
Secondary amenorrhea
Secondary infertility

❖ Case in Point

A 24-year-old woman and her 26-year-old husband are unable to conceive. The couple has had unprotected intercourse for approximately 18 months, with no resulting pregnancy. The husband's infertility workup is completely normal. Both individuals are avid runners and participate in marathons at least four times each year. The wife's infertility workup came back with a repeat follicle-stimulating hormone (FSH) level of more than 40 IU/L. She had an FSH determination about a month earlier that was also more than 40 IU/L. What condition accounts for the couple's inability to conceive? Are follow-up hormonal tests necessary? Why or why not?

Points to Remember

- Gonadotropin-releasing hormone stimulates release of follicle-stimulating hormone (FSH) and luteinizing hormone (LH) from the pituitary.
- FSH stimulates the ovary to release an ovum.
- LH stimulates the testes to produce testosterone; FSH and testosterone stimulate spermatogenesis.
- Estrogen is the main female hormone for normal reproductive organ function.
- Testosterone is the main male hormone for normal reproductive organ function.
- Semen analysis measures ejaculation volume, pH, sperm count, motility, and sperm morphology.
- Infertility is defined as not conceiving after 1 year of unprotected intercourse.
- Male infertility can be caused by a low sperm count, abnormal sperm motility, hormonal dysfunction, or psychosocial factors.
- Female infertility is evaluated using serum analysis, endocrine hormone levels, and anti-sperm antibody detection.
- Primary testicular failure can be determined from an increased FSH level with a decreased testosterone level.
- Anti-sperm antibodies are detected using an immunobead technique.
- Female infertility is caused by hormonal disease, tubal, cervical, uterine, psychosocial, and iatrogenic factors.
- The most common cause of female infertility is failure to ovulate.
- A FSH level that remains greater than 40 IU/L over several months is considered diagnostic of primary ovarian failure. Ovulation cannot be measured directly using laboratory tests.
- Hirsutism is caused by increased androgen levels in women.
- Klinefelter disease (genotype XXY) is a common genetic disorder that causes hypogonadism and infertility in men.
- Providers may order many laboratory tests to rule out other conditions when trying to diagnose hypogonadotropic hypogonadism syndrome.
- Orchitis and epididymitis are abnormal conditions that do not require chemistry tests for diagnosis.
- Menopause is preceded by a perimenopausal period as the ovary response to gonadotropins decreases.
- Estrogen deficiency in postmenopausal women can lead to osteoporosis.
- Polycystic ovary syndrome is caused by hormonal dysfunction.

Introduction

Many diseases affect the physical and chemical components of the male and female reproductive systems. Hormones causing masculinization are called androgens, and hormones causing feminization are called estrogens. The normal functions of the male and female systems and the abnormal conditions affecting them are described in this chapter. Abnormal conditions include infertility, amenorrhea, hirsutism, Klinefelter syndrome, Kallmann syndrome, orchitis, epididymitis, menopause, and polycystic ovary syndrome (PCOS).

Reproductive System Structure and Function

The female lower urinary tract and reproductive system are separate. The urethra is located between the clitoris and the vaginal opening. The male lower urinary tract and reproductive system use common structures to accomplish reproductive and urinary functions. Some reproductive system diseases can affect the urinary system.

Female System and Normal Function

The female reproductive system is composed of the ovaries, fallopian tubes, uterus, clitoris, labium major, labium minor, and vagina. During the reproductive years, a complex hormonal cycle develops an ovum that passes through the fallopian tubes each month (Fig. 25-1). The hormonal cycle begins in the hypothalamus with the secretion of gonadotropin-releasing hormone. The gonadotropin-releasing hormone stimulates the anterior pituitary gland to release follicle-stimulating hormone (FSH) and luteinizing hormone (LH). FSH causes ovulation, and LH causes the ovary to produce progesterone.

Ovulation occurs when FSH stimulates the ovary to release an ovum into the peritoneal cavity. The follicle that released the ovum becomes a corpus luteum. As the corpus luteum disintegrates, the cells along its margin release estrogen. Estrogen develops and maintains female reproductive organs and causes development of secondary sex characteristics, such as fat deposits in breasts, buttocks, and thighs; axillary and pubic hair; mammary glands; and a broadened pelvis. The LH released by the pituitary gland prepares the lining of the uterus (i.e., endometrium) for implantation of a fertilized ovum. If

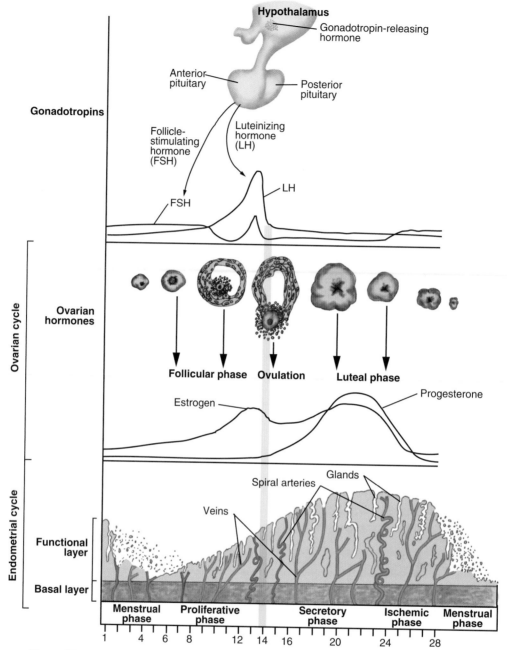

• **Figure 25-1** The female reproductive cycle, showing the changes in secretion of hormones from the anterior pituitary during the course of a cycle and interrelated changes in the ovary and uterine endometrium. (From McKinney ES, James SR, Murray SS, Nelson K, Ashwill J. *Maternal-Child Nursing.* 4th ed. St. Louis: Saunders; 2013.)

there is no implantation, the LH level falls, and the corpus luteum disintegrates. The thick endometrial layer is shed as menses.

Male System and Normal Function

The male reproductive system consists of testes, epididymis, vas deferens, seminal vesicles, prostate, and the penis. The hypothalamus produces gonadotropin-releasing hormone, which causes the pituitary to produce FSH and LH, both

of which act on the testes. LH acts on the Leydig cells to produce testosterone, and FSH and testosterone initiate spermatogenesis. A small amount of testosterone is produced from a precursor molecule, dehydroepiandrosterone (DHEA), which is produced by the adrenal glands. As the blood testosterone level increases, a negative feedback loop stops production of the gonadotropin-releasing hormone in the hypothalamus (Fig. 25-2). Testosterone production also results in facial hair, a deep voice, increased muscle mass, and other masculine features.

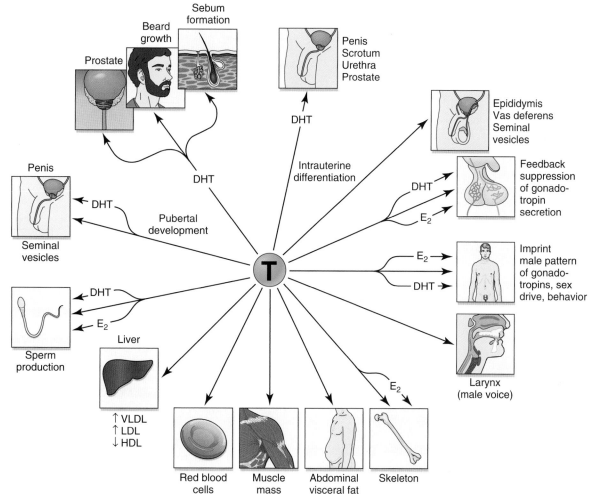

• **Figure 25-2** Testosterone action affects the male body in different ways. In the uterus, testosterone stimulates the creation of a penis, scrotum, urethra, and prostate. During puberty, testosterone also stimulates sebum formation, deep voice, beard growth, prostate, penis, sperm, and seminal vesicle development. Testosterone also promotes increased VLDL and LDL, with decreased HDL levels. Increased red blood cells, bone strengthening, and muscle mass are also a result of testosterone action. Testosterone allows for abdominal visceral fat. Estrogen and testosterone produce a male pattern of gonadotropins leading to sex drive and specific behaviors. Testosterone and estrogen levels are regulated through a negative feedback loop of gonadotropin secretion from the pituitary gland. *DHT,* Dihydrotestosterone; E_2, estradiol; *HDL,* high-density lipoproteins; *LDL,* low-density lipoproteins; *T,* testosterone; *VLDL,* very-low-density lipoproteins. (From Koeppen B, Stanton B. *Berne and Levy Physiology.* Updated 6th ed. Philadelphia: Mosby; 2010.)

Diseases and Disorders

Infertility

Infertility is defined as not conceiving after 1 year of unprotected intercourse. Primary infertility is defined as a couple with no successful pregnancies, and secondary infertility describes a couple with previous conceptions but who are not able to conceive currently. Many infertility issues are caused by dysfunction of the hypothalamic-pituitary-gonadal axis.

Male Infertility

Male infertility may go undetected because when it is mild and combined with normal female fertility, conception may be delayed. Many factors may cause male infertility: endocrine disorders (e.g., hypothalamic dysfunction,

pituitary failure, thyroid disorders, testicular failure), anatomic defects, abnormal spermatogenesis (e.g., low sperm count, abnormal sperm motility), and psychosocial factors (e.g., unexplained impotence, decreased libido) (Box 25-1). Laboratory tests play a vital role in diagnosing male infertility.

Testosterone drives normal sperm development. Any condition that affects testosterone levels can result in male infertility. Congenital idiopathic hypogonadotropic hypogonadism is the most common cause of hypothalamic hypogonadism. Congenital idiopathic hypogonadism occurs when the hypothalamus or pituitary fails to stimulate the gonads to produce sex hormones (Fig. 25-3). Disorders that cause hypogonadism include congenital or acquired panhypopituitarism, hypothalamic syndromes, malnutrition or anorexia, adenomas, trauma, metastases,

Poor Sperm Quality

Substance abuse, especially tobacco
Age
Sexually transmitted infections
Exposure to workplace hazards such as radiation or toxic
  substances
Exposure of scrotum to high temperatures
Nutritional deficiencies
Obesity
Anti-sperm antibodies

Structural or Hormonal Disorders

Undescended testes
Hypospadias
Varicocele
Obstructive lesions of the vas deferens or epididymis
Low testosterone levels
Hypopituitarism
Endocrine disorders
Testicular damage caused by mumps infection
Retrograde ejaculation

Other Factors

Genetic disorders (e.g., Klinefelter syndrome)
Decrease in libido (e.g., heroin, methadone, selective serotonin
  reuptake inhibitors, barbiturates)
Impotence (e.g., alcohol, antihypertensive medications)

From Lowderwmilk DL, Perry SE, Cashion MC, Alden KR. *Maternity and Women's Health Care*. 11th ed. St. Louis: Mosby; 2016.

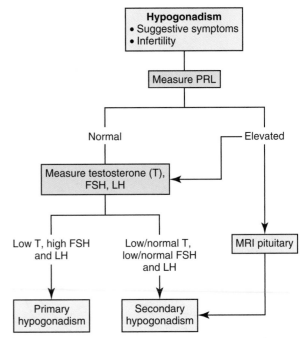

• **Figure 25-3** Clinical approach to the investigation of male hypogonadism. *FSH*, Follicle-stimulating hormone; *LH*, luteinizing hormone; *MRI*, magnetic resonance imaging; *PRL*, prolactin; *T*, testosterone. (Modified from Kaplan LA, Pesce AJ. *Clinical Chemistry: Theory, Analysis, Correlation*. 5th ed. St. Louis: Mosby; 2010.)

and hemochromatosis. Obesity in the infertile male may indicate increased estrogen production.

Laboratory Evaluation

Male infertility is evaluated using semen analysis, endocrine hormone levels, and anti-sperm antibody detection. Semen analysis measures ejaculation volume, pH, sperm count, motility, and sperm morphology. Routine semen analysis is discussed later in this chapter. The clinical chemistry laboratory may also determine fructose, acid phosphatase, zinc, and magnesium levels in semen. A semen analysis can be performed after a vasectomy. A drop of semen is placed on a slide and examined for the presence of sperm.

The laboratory workup for male infertility determines endocrine hormone levels, including total testosterone, free testosterone, LH, and FSH. Testosterone levels affect spermatogenesis. FSH levels can indicate a genetic condition or germ cell failure. Elevated FSH levels with decreased testosterone levels indicate primary testicular failure. Decreased FSH and decreased testosterone levels indicate pituitary or hypothalamic insufficiency (Fig. 25-4).

Anti-sperm antibodies can cause male infertility. Anti-sperm antibodies can also be identified in women and be a cause of infertility. Anti-sperm antibodies are detected using an immunobead technique, which involves attaching rabbit anti-human antibodies to a polyacrylamide bead. The bead is then incubated with semen, allowing the anti-human

antibody to bind to the anti-sperm antibodies on the sperm. Beads that bind to antibody attached to the sperm are detected microscopically.

Female Infertility

Female infertility is caused by ovarian or hormonal disease (e.g., thyroid, liver, PCOS, ovarian failure, hypothalamic or pituitary insufficiency), tubal factors, cervical factors, uterine factors, psychosocial factors (e.g., decreased libido), and iatrogenic factors (Box 25-2). Some conditions that affect the ovary and lead to infertility may be difficult to diagnose.

Failure to ovulate is the most common female infertility problem. In PCOS, complex hormonal dysfunction prevents monthly release of an ovum and menses and causes infertility. Congenital adrenal hyperplasia affects ovulation due to increased androgen levels. Iatrogenic causes include primary ovarian failure, menopause, and pituitary or hypothalamic insufficiency. Tubal, cervical, and uterine abnormalities can be caused by anatomic defects, inflammation, or infection. Anti-sperm antibodies can also contribute female infertility.

Laboratory Evaluation

Evaluation of female infertility begins with a medical history and a physical examination that includes vaginal and cervical Papanicolaou (Pap) tests. Endometriosis, adhesions, and open fallopian tubes are important findings of the physical examination.

In primary ovarian failure (i.e., hypogonadotropic hypogonadism), at least two FSH levels greater than 30 IU/L collected a month apart are diagnostic. Infertility workups also

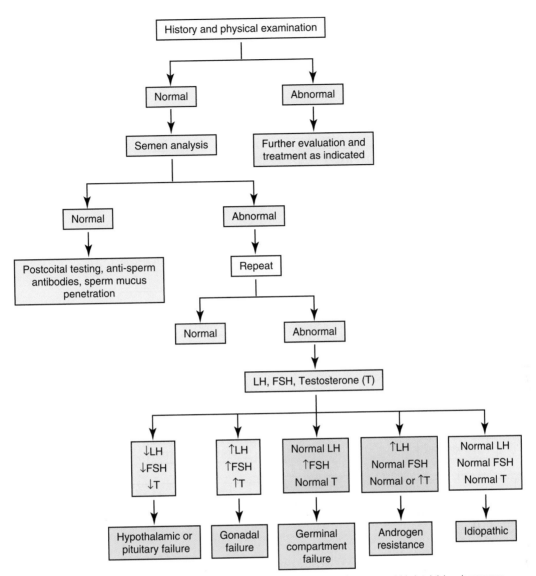

• **Figure 25-4** Diagnosing male infertility. *FSH,* Follicle-stimulating hormone; *LH,* luteinizing hormone; *T,* testosterone. (Modified from Burtis CA, Ashwood ER, Bruns DE, eds. *Tietz Textbook of Clinical Chemistry.* 5th ed. St. Louis: Elsevier; 2012.)

• BOX 25-2 Factors Affecting Female Fertility

Ovarian Factors

Developmental anomalies
Anovulation, primary or secondary
Pituitary or hypothalamic hormone disorder
Adrenal gland disorder
Congenital adrenal hyperplasia
Disruption of hypothalamic-pituitary-ovarian axis
Amenorrhea after discontinuing oral contraceptive pills
Premature ovarian failure
Increased prolactin levels

Uterine, Tubal, and Peritoneal Factors

Developmental anomalies
Tubal motility reduced
Inflammation in the tube
Tubal adhesions
Endometrial and myometrial tumors
Asherman syndrome (i.e., uterine adhesions or scar tissue)
Endometriosis
Chronic cervicitis
Hostile or inadequate cervical mucus

Other Factors

Nutritional deficiencies (e.g., anemia)
Obesity
Substance abuse
Thyroid dysfunction
Genetic disorders (e.g., Turner syndrome)
Anxiety

From Lowderwmilk DL, Perry SE, Cashion MC, Alden KR. *Maternity and Women's Health Care.* 11th ed. St. Louis: Mosby; 2016.)

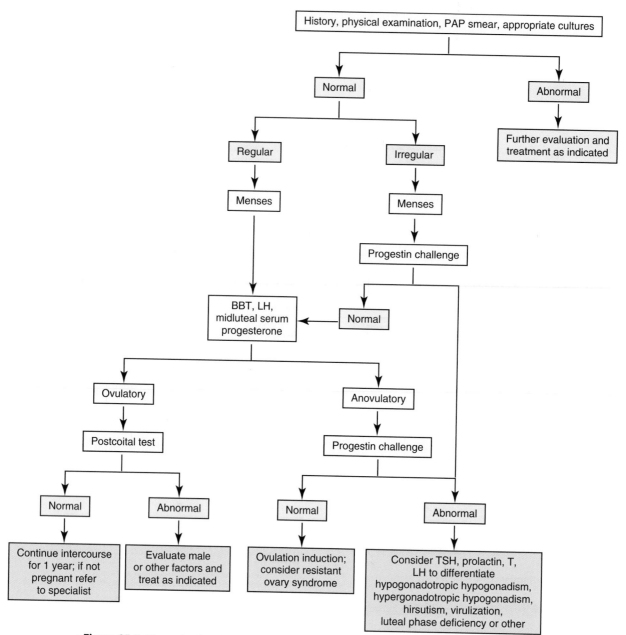

• **Figure 25-5** Diagnosing female infertility. *BBT,* Basal body temperature; *LH,* luteinizing hormone; *PAP smear,* Papanicolaou smear; *T,* testosterone; *TSH,* thyroid-stimulating hormone. (Modified from Burtis CA, Ashwood ER, Bruns DE, eds. *Tietz Textbook of Clinical Chemistry.* 5th ed. St. Louis: Elsevier; 2012.)

include an assessment of ovulation and luteal function. Ovulation cannot be directly measured using laboratory tests, but basal body temperature, LH surge, and a midluteal progesterone level can indicate ovulation. The primary laboratory test used to evaluate ovulation is progesterone because an increased level indicates that a corpus luteum was formed. The increased level does not confirm that an egg was released. A midluteal level greater than 10 ng/mL is seen in normal ovulation.

The LH surge can be used to detect ovulation because the level increases 24 to 36 hours before ovulation. The surge can be detected by home ovulation kits, which are affordably priced and effectively predict ovulation in 70% to 92% of women. The kit uses a double monoclonal enzyme-linked immunoassay technique and a urine dipstick. Urine is drawn

across a test pad and a reference region. A positive result must be as dark or darker than the reference area (Fig. 25-5).

Amenorrhea

Amenorrhea is the failure to start menstrual bleeding by age 16 (i.e., **primary amenorrhea**) or the absence of menses in menstruating women (i.e., secondary amenorrhea). Almost one half of those with primary amenorrhea have genetic conditions such as Turner syndrome or fragile X syndrome. Primary amenorrhea is also caused by hypothalamic dysfunction, which can reduce the amount and frequency of gonadotropin-releasing hormone produced, resulting in low LH levels and abnormal follicular

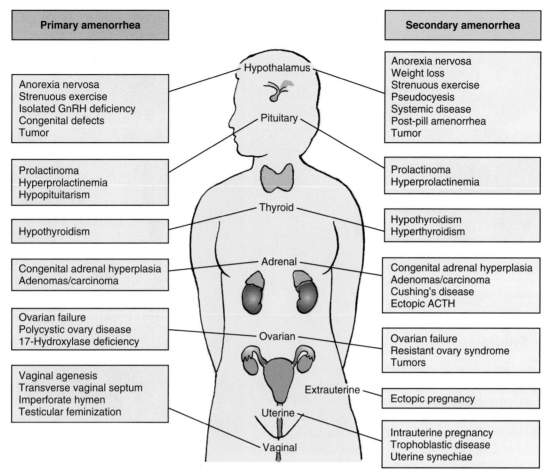

| Primary amenorrhea | | Secondary amenorrhea |

Hypothalamus

Primary amenorrhea:
Anorexia nervosa
Strenuous exercise
Isolated GnRH deficiency
Congenital defects
Tumor

Secondary amenorrhea:
Anorexia nervosa
Weight loss
Strenuous exercise
Pseudocyesis
Systemic disease
Post-pill amenorrhea
Tumor

Pituitary

Prolactinoma
Hyperprolactinemia
Hypopituitarism

Prolactinoma
Hyperprolactinemia

Thyroid

Hypothyroidism

Hypothyroidism
Hyperthyroidism

Adrenal

Congenital adrenal hyperplasia
Adenomas/carcinoma

Congenital adrenal hyperplasia
Adenomas/carcinoma
Cushing's disease
Ectopic ACTH

Ovarian

Ovarian failure
Polycystic ovary disease
17-Hydroxylase deficiency

Ovarian failure
Resistant ovary syndrome
Tumors

Extrauterine

Vaginal agenesis
Transverse vaginal septum
Imperforate hymen
Testicular feminization

Ectopic pregnancy

Uterine

Intrauterine pregnancy
Trophoblastic disease
Uterine synechiae

Vaginal

• **Figure 25-6** Causes of amenorrhea. *ACTH,* Adrenocorticotropic hormone; *GnRH,* gonadotropin-releasing hormone. (Modified from Black JM, Hawks JH. *Medical-Surgical Nursing: Clinical Management for Positive Outcomes.* 8th ed. Philadelphia: Saunders; 2009.)

development. The FSH levels in these individuals are usually within reference ranges.

Secondary amenorrhea can be caused by a chronic medical condition such as hypothyroidism, hyperthyroidism, or sarcoidosis (Fig. 25-6). Eating disorders, depression, exercise, or extended periods of physical or mental stress can also cause amenorrhea. Many female marathon runners experience amenorrhea due to a syndrome known as female athletic triad. Women with athletic triad syndrome exercise vigorously and may have amenorrhea, disordered eating, and osteoporosis. Ovarian tumors, ovarian failure, PCOS, and Cushing syndrome can also cause secondary amenorrhea. Evidence demonstrates that a critical body fat level is necessary for the female reproductive system to function normally.

Because amenorrhea is most often caused by pregnancy, a pregnancy test is usually ordered first. If the pregnancy test result is negative, routine laboratory tests such as a complete blood count, erythrocyte sedimentation rate, liver function tests, blood urea nitrogen and creatinine levels, and urinalysis are ordered to rule out a chronic disease process. Thyroid-stimulating hormone (TSH), prolactin, FSH, and LH tests are usually ordered next to determine whether the woman's hormonal cycle is correctly functioning. If the FSH level is 40 IU/mL or greater and is confirmed by a repeat FSH determination 1 month later, the ovaries are not functioning properly. TSH, prolactin, FSH, and LH are usually measured using immunochemical methods.

Hirsutism

Hirsutism in women consists of excessive terminal hair growth in a postpubertal male pattern (Fig. 25-7). The condition is usually caused by increased androgen levels. Testosterone is converted to dihydrotestosterone, which acts on hair follicles to produce terminal hair (see Chapter 29). Causes of hirsutism include severe insulin resistance, androgen-producing ovarian or adrenal tumors, menopause, PCOS, acromegaly, Cushing syndrome, and drug side effects.

Laboratory tests are used to confirm androgen excess in the blood and to identify the source of excess androgens such as total testosterone, free testosterone, and dehydroepiandrosterone sulfate (DHEAS). Elevated DHEAS levels indicate an adrenal source for the androgens, whereas elevated testosterone levels indicate an adrenal or ovarian source for the androgens. If the testosterone level is less than 2 ng/mL and the DHEAS level is less than 700 μg/dL, cancer is unlikely.

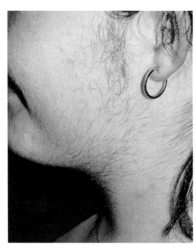

• **Figure 25-7** Facial hirsutism. Terminal hair growth is visible on the chin of this 40-year-old woman with idiopathic hirsutism. (From Lawrence CM, Cox NH. *Physical Signs in Dermatology: Color Atlas and Text.* St. Louis: Mosby; 1993.)

Klinefelter Syndrome

Klinefelter syndrome is a common genetic disorder that causes hypogonadism and infertility in men. Men with this disease have an extra X chromosome, producing an XXY karyotype. The additional X chromosome causes physical and cognitive abnormalities; mental retardation is common. Men with this condition have sparse or absent facial hair, decreased muscle mass, feminine distribution of adipose tissue, enlarged breasts, small testes, azoospermia, oligospermia, hyalinization and fibrosis of seminiferous tubules, decreased libido, osteoporosis, and increased urinary gonadotropin levels (Fig. 25-8). Klinefelter syndrome is thought to be a form of primary testicular failure because the gonadotropin levels are elevated due to a lack of feedback inhibition by the pituitary gland.

The best laboratory test for diagnosing this disease is a cytogenetic analysis to determine the karyotype. Testing hormone levels (e.g., FSH, LH, estradiol, testosterone) can be useful in treating the patient with Klinefelter syndrome.

Kallmann Syndrome

Kallmann syndrome is a rare genetic condition that is characterized by a gonadotropin-releasing hormone deficiency. Other aspects of hypothalamic-pituitary function appear to be normal in individuals with this syndrome. The four subtypes of Kallmann syndrome are caused by different genetic mutations, but all affect the production of hormones that direct sexual development. A hallmark characteristic of this syndrome is hyposmia (i.e. diminished sense of smell) or anosmia (i.e., absent sense of smell). Some individuals also have congenital heart disease and neurologic manifestations. Table 25-1 lists the symptoms for men and women.

As for other hypogonadotropic hypogonadism syndromes, many laboratory tests may be ordered by the provider to help rule out other conditions. Because a common

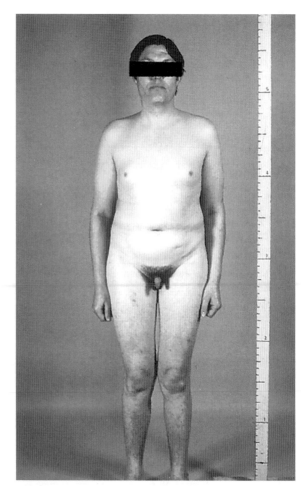

• **Figure 25-8** Klinefelter syndrome in a young man. Limited gynecomastia is present, and the body shape is somewhat feminine. (From Besser GM, Thorner MO. *Clinical Endocrinology.* 2nd ed. London: Mosby-Wolfe; 1994.)

cause for amenorrhea is pregnancy, women with amenorrhea require a human chorionic gonadotropin (hCG) test to rule out pregnancy. Electrolyte determinations are ordered to rule out primary adrenocortical insufficiency. Not everyone with Kallmann syndrome has primary adrenocortical insufficiency, but those who do have hyponatremia and hyperkalemia. Because hemochromatosis can produce a similar biochemical profile, ferritin levels are determined to rule out the disorder. Ferritin levels in Kallmann syndrome are normal.

Testosterone levels (i.e., total and free) in postpubertal boys are usually greater than 100 ng/dL. Estradiol levels in postpubertal girls are decreased. Low-normal or decreased LH and FSH levels are found in postpubertal individuals with Kallmann syndrome. Genetic testing is valuable in diagnosing this syndrome.

Orchitis

Orchitis is an inflammation of the testes usually caused by the mumps virus, but other viruses and bacteria also cause this condition (Fig. 25-9). If caused by the mumps virus,

TABLE 25-1 Male and Female Symptoms and Hormone Levels in Kallmann Syndrome	
Male Symptoms	**Female Symptoms**
Absent or incomplete puberty	Absent or incomplete puberty
Anosmia or severe hyposmia	Anosmia or severe hyposmia
Congenital heart disease	Congenital heart disease
Color blindness, hearing deficit, epilepsy, paraplegia	Color blindness, hearing deficit, epilepsy, paraplegia
Decreased libido and erectile dysfunction	Amenorrhea
Infertility	Dyspareunia (i.e., painful sexual intercourse)
Osteoporosis	Infertility
Primary adrenocortical insufficiency	Osteoporosis
Decreased total and free testosterone levels	Primary adrenocortical insufficiency
Decreased FSH and LH levels	Decreased estradiol levels
	Decreased FSH and LH levels

FSH, Follicle-stimulating hormone; *LH,* luteinizing hormone.

TABLE 25-2 Symptoms of Epididymitis	
Acute Epididymitis	**Chronic Epididymitis**
Scrotal pain and swelling developing over several days	More than 6 weeks of constant or waxing and waning pain
Located on one side	Indurated scrotum but not usually swollen
Dysuria, frequency, or urgency	
Fever and chills	
No nausea or vomiting (differentiates this condition from testicular torsion)	
Urethral discharge	

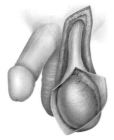

• **Figure 25-9** In orchitis, the testicle is inflamed and swollen. (Ball JW, Dains JE, Flynn JA, Solomon BS, Steward RW. *Seidel's Guide to Physical Examination.* 8th ed. St. Louis: Mosby; 2015.)

orchitis appears 4 to 7 days after the individual develops the mumps. Systemic symptoms associated with orchitis include fatigue, malaise, myalgias, fever, chills, and nausea. The testicles become swollen and painful. Clinical chemistry tests are not helpful in diagnosing this condition, but a urethral culture and Gram stain should be performed.

Epididymitis

Epididymitis is inflammation of the epididymis, which is a tightly coiled portion of the sperm duct that connects each testicle to its vas deferens. This condition is thought to be caused by an infectious agent, but cultures and DNA amplifications are usually negative. Epididymitis is the fifth most common urologic condition in men between the ages of 18 and 50 years. Symptoms are detailed in Table 25-2.

Laboratory tests such as urinalysis, complete blood count, urethral culture, syphilis, and human immunodeficiency virus (HIV) testing are usually ordered to confirm the diagnosis. Clinical chemistry tests are not used for diagnosing epididymitis.

Menopause

Menopause occurs when circulating reproductive hormone levels decrease, menses cease, and reproductive capability ends. Menopause is designated when a previously menstruating woman experiences 12 months without menses. A **perimenopausal period** occurs before menopause due to the decreased response of the ovaries to gonadotropins, leading to physical symptoms such as irregular menses. Other perimenopausal and menopausal symptoms include hot flushes, insomnia, weight gain, bloating, mood changes, depression, and headache. Symptoms can begin 6 to 8 years before the final menstrual period and continue for years afterward. Symptoms decline as the postmenopausal years pass.

As the ovary's response to gonadotropins decreases, FSH levels increase, estradiol levels decrease, and LH and progesterone levels remain unchanged. As estrogen levels continue to decrease, prolactin levels also decrease. Decreased estrogen levels lead to vasomotor instability and hot flushes. After menopause, the ovary responds to the increased LH levels by secreting only testosterone and androstenedione (Fig. 25-10), which can lead to hirsutism in some elderly women. Estrogen deficiency in postmenopausal women leads to increased bone resorption, accelerated bone loss, and **osteoporosis** (i.e., bones become fragile from loss of tissue), and they have a greater risk of cardiac disease. Although estrogen replacement therapy

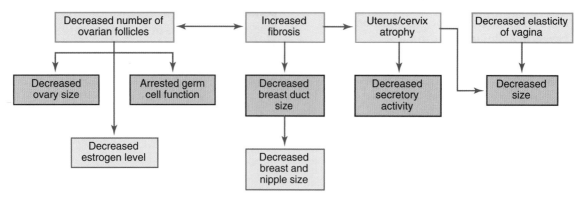

```
┌─────────────────┐     ┌─────────────┐     ┌─────────────┐     ┌─────────────────┐
│Decreased number │◄───►│  Increased  │────►│Uterus/cervix│     │Decreased        │
│of ovarian       │     │  fibrosis   │     │  atrophy    │     │elasticity       │
│follicles        │     │             │     │             │     │of vagina        │
└─────────────────┘     └─────────────┘     └─────────────┘     └─────────────────┘
```

| Decreased ovary size | Arrested germ cell function | | Decreased breast duct size | | Decreased secretory activity | | Decreased size |

Decreased estrogen level

Decreased breast and nipple size

• **Figure 25-10** Changes in the female reproductive system associated with menopause. (From Copstead-Kirkhorn LC, Banasik JL. *Pathophysiology.* 5th ed. St. Louis: Saunders; 2014.)

can slow down but not reverse osteoporosis, it is controversial because it is associated with an increased risk of breast cancer.

Polycystic Ovary Syndrome

Polycystic ovary syndrome (PCOS), also called Stein-Leventhal syndrome, affects a small percentage of women in their reproductive years. Women with PCOS have hormonal abnormalities and ovaries with a thick outer surface because of cysts (Fig. 25-11). It results from factors that lead to a hypothalamic-pituitary dysfunction.

The syndrome is characterized by insulin resistance, excessive androgen hormones, high lipid levels, high insulin levels, obesity, oligomenorrhea, hirsutism, and acne. Women with this syndrome have a high risk of cardiovascular disease and many develop type 2 diabetes. FSH levels are low, and LH levels are high. The elevated LH levels result in increased testosterone and androstenedione levels that are 50% to 150% higher than normal.

Laboratory Procedures and Limitations

Reproductive diseases can be assessed by measuring hormonal imbalances. The history, physical examination, and functional tests are also important in assessing reproductive diseases. Analytical methods include quantitation of testosterone (i.e., total, free, and weakly bound), DHEA, 17-ketosteroids, estrogen, progesterone, LH, and FSH. Semen analysis is also performed.

Total Testosterone

Free, weakly bound, and tightly bound types of testosterone are found in blood. Free testosterone is not attached to a protein, weakly bound testosterone is attached to albumin, and tightly bound testosterone is attached to sex hormone–binding globulin (SHBG). Free testosterone and weakly bound testosterone are considered the biologically active species because both are available to interact with target cells. Total testosterone measurements measure all three types.

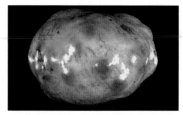

• **Figure 25-11** In polycystic ovary syndrome, the ovary is studded with fluid-filled cysts developed from follicles that have failed to rupture. (From Kumar V, Abbas A, Fausto, Aster J. *Robbins & Cotran Pathologic Basis of Disease.* 8th ed. Philadelphia: Saunders; 2010.)

Immunoassays are the tests of choice for measuring circulating testosterone. The gas chromatography with mass spectrometry (GC-MS) method is used to determine testosterone reference values and measure the bias of immunoassay methods. Serum or heparinized plasma specimens are used for total testosterone measurements. Morning specimens are preferred for testing because testosterone levels in the body reach a peak concentration between 4:00 and 8:00 AM. Reference ranges are 260 to 1000 ng/dL for men and 15 to 70 ng/dL for women.

Free Testosterone

Because free and weakly bound forms of testosterone are the available fractions of testosterone, measuring these compounds may better reflect androgen status. Both types are measured in a free testosterone test, which uses immunoassay methodology. The reference range for free testosterone is 50 to 210 pg/mL for men and 1.0 to 8.5 pg/mL for women.

Dehydroepiandrosterone

Because DHEA is usually produced by the adrenal glands, measurement of DHEA and its sulfated conjugate (DHEAS) is important to gauge the production of adrenal androgens. Women with PCOS have elevated DHEAS levels. Immunoassays measure DHEA and DHEAS using serum or heparinized plasma. Specimens should be collected before 10:30 AM. Reference ranges are shown in Table 25-3.

TABLE 25-3 Comparison of DHEAS and DHEA

DHEAS		DHEA	
Group (yr)	Values (μg/mL)	Group	Values (ng/mL)
Men 18-30	125-619	Men	180-1250
Men 31-50	59-452	Women	130-980
Men 51-60	20-413		
Men 61-83	10-285		
Women 18-30	45-380		
Women 31-50	12-379		
Women, postmenopausal	30-260		

DHEA, Dehydroepiandrosterone; *DHEAS*, dehydroepiandrosterone sulfate.

17-Ketosteroids in Urine

17-Ketosteroids are metabolites of testosterone secreted by the testes and the adrenal glands. Decreased concentrations of 17-ketosteroids in urine are found in primary hypogonadism (i.e., Klinefelter syndrome) and panhypopituitarism. Increased concentrations of 17-ketosteroids in urine are found in people with testicular tumors, adrenal hyperplasia, adrenal cancer, or hirsutism.

17-Ketosteroids are measured in 24-hour urine specimens. The test uses a colorimetric reaction (i.e., Zimmerman). The procedure begins by using an acid to cleave the glucuronic and sulfuric acid conjugates of 17-ketosteroids. Next, these compounds are extracted, washed with alkali, then mixed with a chromophore to develop a colored end product with a maximum absorbance at 520 nm.

Estrogens

The most accurate and reliable method for measuring estrogens is GC-MS. The most commonly used test in clinical laboratories is immunoassay. Serum or plasma (i.e., heparinized or with ethylenediaminetetraacetic acid [EDTA]) can be used for analysis. Reference ranges for women are 20 to 150 pg/mL for the early follicular phase, 40 to 350 pg/mL for the late follicular phase, 150 to 750 pg/mL for the midcycle phase, 30 to 450 pg/mL for the luteal phase, and 20 pg/mL or higher for the postmenopausal period.

Progesterone

Progesterone is the female hormone that prepares the uterus for implantation of the fertilized egg. Progesterone measurements are useful for evaluating ovulation. Progesterone levels rise immediately after ovulation, and the concentration decreases if pregnancy does not occur. If pregnancy occurs, progesterone levels continue to rise because the placenta becomes the major source of this hormone. Serial measurement of progesterone is valuable for detecting luteal defects in women with undefined infertility, monitoring the return of fertility after childbirth, and monitoring oral progesterone treatment.

Immunoassays are used to measure progesterone in serum or plasma (i.e., heparinized or with EDTA). Reference ranges are 13 to 97 ng/dL for men. For women, reference ranges are 15 to 70 ng/dL for the follicular phase and 200 to 2500 ng/dL for the luteal phase.

Luteinizing Hormone and Follicle-Stimulating Hormone

During the follicular phase of the female reproductive cycle, LH production is suppressed. As the follicle matures, LH is produced, resulting in a midcycle surge of LH. LH acts on the cells of the mature follicle and induces production of progesterone. After the corpus luteum is formed, LH production decreases. Measuring LH levels helps to confirm when ovulation should occur because the levels increase dramatically 24 to 36 hours before ovulation.

FSH controls the development and maturation of follicles. FSH peaks slightly a few days before menses begin. The peak stimulates the growth and maturation of follicles in the ovary. Growing follicles result in a fall in the FSH concentration. Progesterone triggers a rise in FSH at midcycle. FSH levels decrease until a small peak occurs near the end of the cycle. This peak stimulates follicular maturation for the next cycle.

Because the α-subunits of LH and FSH are identical, diagnostic test methods must distinguish between the β-subunits. Immunoassays are used to measure both hormones, and some assays are automated. The specimen of choice is serum, and hemolyzed, lipemic, or icteric specimens must not be used. Because these hormones undergo episodic, circadian, and cyclic variations, multiple serial specimens may be required for proper interpretation.

Semen Analysis

Semen analysis begins with a semen specimen that is delivered to the laboratory within 30 minutes of collection. In many instances, physicians collect the specimens, but some physicians allow individuals to collect specimens at the laboratory. The volume of the specimen is measured with a graduated cylinder. Indicator paper is used to determine the pH of the specimen. After observing the motility microscopically, a portion of the specimen is diluted with semen-diluting fluid. The diluting fluid kills the sperm so that they can be counted in a hemocytometer. The morphology of the sperm is observed in the hemocytometer or on a stained slide.

Summary

The male and female reproductive systems are controlled by complex hormonal interactions. In males, these interactions lead to sperm production and the ability to reproduce. In females, they lead to ovulation and monthly menses if conception is absent. Males and females can be genetically infertile or can become infertile during the reproductive years. Many laboratory tests can be performed to pinpoint the source of infertility in both sexes.

Conditions that affect reproduction include amenorrhea, hirsutism, Klinefelter syndrome, Kallmann syndrome, orchitis, epididymitis, menopause, and PCOS. Amenorrhea and hirsutism are caused by dysfunction or lack of hormonal production and interaction with reproductive structures.

Klinefelter and Kallmann syndromes are genetically acquired and are characterized by hormonal imbalances early in life that lead to delayed or absent puberty along with systemic conditions such as type 2 diabetes and cardiovascular disease. Orchitis and epididymitis are inflammatory conditions of the testes that interfere with normal function. Changes in estrogen, gonadotropin, and other hormone production occur with age.

Most reproductive hormones are measured using immunoassays, some of which are automated. Serum or plasma specimens are preferred for many assays. Due to variations in the concentrations of these hormones throughout the reproductive cycle and beyond, serial measurement may be necessary to properly interpret the tests.

Review Questions

1. Which of the following is a cause of infertility in men?
   a. Too much semen
   b. Too many sperm
   c. Abnormal sperm
   d. Too much testosterone
2. Which of the following is the most common cause of female infertility?
   a. Polycystic ovary syndrome (PCOS)
   b. Failure to ovulate
   c. Orchitis
   d. Menopause
3. Which of the following conditions is characterized by testicular swelling and pain on one side?
   a. Epididymitis
   b. Orchitis
   c. Male infertility
   d. Kallmann syndrome
4. Which acute condition is produced by a viral or bacterial infection and often develops 4 to 7 days after an individual comes down with the mumps?
   a. Orchitis
   b. Epididymitis
   c. Klinefelter syndrome
   d. Kallmann syndrome
5. A man with anosmia, congenital heart disease, infertility, and color blindness visits his provider. Laboratory results include total and free testosterone levels of lower than 100 ng/dL, decreased FSH, and decreased LH. Which of the following best describes the patient's symptoms and laboratory results?
   a. Hirsutism
   b. Osteoporosis
   c. Menopause
   d. Kallmann syndrome

6. Which of the following conditions is characterized by a gradual decline in ovarian function and is usually accompanied by hot flushes, absent menses, depression, and weight gain?
   a. Primary infertility
   b. Kallmann syndrome
   c. Polycystic ovary syndrome
   d. Menopause
7. Which of the following conditions is defined as the absence of menses?
   a. Hirsutism
   b. Amenorrhea
   c. Orchitis
   d. Polycystic ovary syndrome
8. When the female body produces too many androgens and terminal hair (especially on the face) that grows in a male pattern, the condition is referred to as
   a. Menopause
   b. Amenorrhea
   c. Hirsutism
   d. Orchitis
9. Which of the following substances indicates an adrenal origin for androgens?
   a. Estrogen
   b. FSH
   c. DHEAS
   d. LH
10. Estrogen deficiency can lead to which of the following conditions?
    a. Osteoporosis
    b. Hirsutism
    c. Polycystic ovary syndrome
    d. Klinefelter syndrome

Critical Thinking Questions

1. Explain why many infertility issues are caused by a dysfunction of the hypothalamic-pituitary-gonadal axis.

2. What is menopause, and why does it only affect women?

CASE STUDY

Most insurance companies pay for women to undergo bone density scans starting at 60 years of ate. Bone density scans are used to detect osteoporosis. What significant event occurs in a women's life that prompts insurance companies to pay for this scan starting at 60 years of age? Why do insurance companies not pay for the bone scan at a younger age? What other conditions may justify doing a bone density scan on a woman younger than 60 years of age?

Bibliography

Bandmann HJ, Breit R, Perwein E, eds. *Klinefelter's Syndrome*. Heidelberg: Springer Science & Business Media; 2012.

Bode D, Seehusen DA, Baird D. Hirsutism in women. *Am Fam Physician*. 2012;85:373–380.

Burtis CA, Bruns DE. *Tietz Fundamentals of Clinical Chemistry and Molecular Diagnostics*. 5th ed Philadelphia: Elsevier Health Sciences; 2014.

Foo JP, Polyzos SA, Anastasilakis AD, Chou S, Mantzoros CS. The effect of leptin replacement on parathyroid hormone, RANKL-osteoprotegerin axis, and Wnt inhibitors in young women with hypothalamic amenorrhea. *J Clin Endocrinol Metab*. 2014;99:E2252–E2258.

Kaplan LA, Pesce AJ. *Clinical Chemistry: Theory, Analysis, Correlation*. 5th ed St. Louis: Mosby; 2009.

Layman LC. Clinical genetic testing for Kallmann syndrome [editorial]. *J Clin Endocrinol Metab*. 2013;98:1860.

Mascarenhas MN, Flaxman SR, Boerma T, et al. Trends in primary and secondary infertility prevalence since 1990: a systematic analysis of demographic and reproductive health surveys. *Lancet*. 2013;381:S90.

Stachenfeld NS. Hormonal changes during menopause and the impact on fluid regulation. *Reprod Sci*. 2014;2:555–561.

Stewart A, Ubee SS, Davies H. Epididymo-orchitis. *BMJ*. 2011;342:d1543.

Wein AJ, Kavoussi LR, Novick AC, Partin AW, eds. *Campbell-Walsh Urology*. 10th ed Philadelphia: Elsevier; 2009.

26

Pregnancy

SHERYL BERMAN

CHAPTER OUTLINE

OBJECTIVES

After completion of this chapter, the reader will be able to:

1. Discuss the process of pregnancy, the parameters, and timing that make human chorionic gonadotropin (hCG) a good marker for normal and ectopic pregnancy confirmation.
2. Discuss the use of amniotic fluid to assess the health of the fetus.
3. Describe the purpose for measuring hCG to determine pregnancy.
4. Describe test methodologies for detecting hCG.
5. Explain the testing process for gestational diabetes.
6. Describe what ectopic pregnancy is, why it usually does not go to term, and why it presents a significant risk for the mother.
7. Contrast the progression of serum hCG levels in a healthy pregnancy with those in an ectopic pregnancy.
8. Identify the symptoms and diagnostic testing for hyperemesis gravidarum.
9. Compare and contrast preeclampsia, eclampsia, and HELLP syndrome and describe the risks posed by each condition for the mother and baby.
10. Explain how maternal Graves disease affects a fetus.
11. Identify the causes, symptoms, and diagnostic testing for fetal complications, including neural tube defects, Down syndrome, respiratory distress syndrome, and hemolytic disease of the newborn.
12. Discuss the dominant, recessive, and sex-linked genetic disorders that are screened for in pregnancy.
13. Discuss the use of the lecithin/sphingomyelin (L/S) ratio in assessing fetal lung maturity.
14. Describe the proper handling of serum or amniotic fluid specimens to protect the integrity of bilirubin in the sample.
15. Discuss the tests used to determine fetal lung maturity and why this testing is important.

KEY TERMS

α-Fetoprotein (AFP)
Amniocentesis
Anencephaly
Chorionic villi sampling
Conception
Down syndrome (trisomy 21)

Eclampsia
Ectopic pregnancy
Edwards syndrome (trisomy 18)
Embryo
Encephalocele
Fetus

HELLP syndrome
Hemolytic disease of the newborn (HDN)
Human chorionic gonadotropin (hCG)
Hyperemesis gravidarum
Lecithin
Lecithin/sphingomyelin ratio

KEY TERMS—cont'd

Meconium
Meningomyelocele
Multiple of the median (MoM)
Neural tube defects

Preeclampsia
Pregnancy
Quantitative hCG
Respiratory distress syndrome

Sphingomyelin
Spina bifida

 Case in Point

A 25-year-old pregnant woman goes to her provider for her first prenatal visit. Her provider orders prenatal laboratory work: glucose, urinalysis, electrolytes, rapid plasma reagin (RPR, test for syphilis), TORCH titer (a test for perinatal infections including toxoplasmosis, rubella, cytomegalovirus, herpes simplex, and human immunodeficiency virus), vaginal culture, and blood type and screen. Her fasting blood glucose level is found to be 140 mg/dL. What test should the provider order next? Why? What disease should be suspected?

Points to Remember

- As the fertilized ovum continues to develop in the uterine wall, cells of its outer membrane (chorion) invade the uterine wall and begin to form chorionic villi.
- The placenta attaches the fetus and the umbilical cord to the uterus, provides the fetus with nutrients, removes wastes, and produces hormones necessary for pregnancy.
- The embryo is surrounded by a cavity filled with amniotic fluid as it continues to develop.
- Maternal immunoglobulin G antibodies readily cross the placenta.
- As the placenta grows larger, it secretes hormones into the mother's circulation: human chorionic gonadotropin (hCG), human placental lactogen, progesterone, estradiol, estriol, and estrone.
- The estrogen hormones (estradiol, estriol, and estrone) produced by the placenta stimulate development of the endometrium, uterine growth, adequate uterine blood supply, and uterine preparation for labor.
- The volume of amniotic fluid is increased in maternal diabetes mellitus, hemolytic disease of the newborn, fetal esophageal atresia, multifetal pregnancy, anencephaly, and spina bifida.
- The fetal lungs are mature when they produce a pulmonary surfactant that allows the lungs to expand and contract during breathing.
- hCG is a reliable marker of pregnancy, and most pregnancy tests use the presence of this marker to confirm pregnancy.
- The common conditions that can affect the mother during pregnancy include gestational diabetes, ectopic pregnancy, hyperemesis gravidarum, preeclampsia, HELLP (hemolysis, elevated liver enzymes, low platelet counts with preeclampsia) syndrome, eclampsia, and Graves disease.
- Blood glucose levels are drawn and tested during the 24th to 28th week of pregnancy to screen for gestational diabetes.
- An ectopic pregnancy occurs when the fertilized egg implants somewhere outside the uterus.
- Ectopic pregnancies can be medical emergencies because the fertilized egg continues to grow and ruptures the fallopian tube; the resulting hemorrhage releases a large volume of blood into the abdominal cavity.
- Preeclampsia is characterized by hypertension (high blood pressure, >140/90 mm Hg on two separate occasions) and proteinuria (protein in the urine) after the 20th week of pregnancy.
- Severe preeclampsia is defined as presence of one of these symptoms in addition to hypertension and proteinuria: blood pressure >160/110 mm Hg, proteinuria (>5 g in 24-hr collection, or >3+ on two random specimens), pulmonary edema, cyanosis, oliguria (<400 mL in 24 hr), persistent headaches, epigastric pain, impaired liver function, thrombocytopenia (platelet count <100,000/ mm^3), and decreased fetal growth or placental abruption (placenta breaking away from uterus).
- A life-threatening manifestation of preeclampsia is eclampsia, in which a mother experiences grand mal seizures or falls into a coma.
- The major characteristics of the HELLP syndrome are thrombocytopenia and disseminated intravascular coagulation (DIC).
- Conditions associated with neural tube defects include meningomyelocele or spina bifida (in which the bottom end of the neural tube fails to fuse), encephalocele (sacs containing brain and membranes that protrude through abnormal openings in the skull), and anencephaly (lack of parts of the brain and skull).
- The biggest contributing factor to neonatal morbidity and death every year is pre-term delivery.
- The premature infants usually have a low birth weight, and their lungs are not mature enough to produce enough pulmonary surfactant, which is necessary for independent breathing.
- Neural tube defects can effectively be screened prenatally through α-fetoprotein (AFP) testing.
- The multiple of the median (MoM) is the tool used to normalize AFP test results during test interpretation.

- Both amniocentesis and chorionic villi sampling carry risks to both the mother and baby; these risks need to be balanced with potential benefits before a decision to pursue such testing is made.
- The quadruple test actually combines the results from several tests (AFP, hCG, unconjugated estriol, and dimeric inhibition) that are correlated with a pregnant woman's age; a single Down syndrome risk estimate is calculated.
- Fetal lung immaturity, or the respiratory distress syndrome (RDS), occurs most often when insufficient lung surfactant is present.
- The fetal lung maturity test evaluates the ratio of lecithin (phosphatidyl choline) to sphingomyelin (a phospholipid) in amniotic fluid.

Introduction

This chapter begins by discussing the fundamentals of pregnancy—conception, embryo development, fetal growth, the role of the placenta, the role of amniotic fluid, and the maturation of the fetus. Some complications of pregnancy and diseases of the developing fetus are then discussed. Laboratory tests used to evaluate maternal health, pregnancy development, and fetal development and health are described.

Pregnancy

A woman's ovaries release one ovum a month. The ovum travels from the ovary, down the fallopian tube, into the uterus. Sperm reach the ovum in the fallopian tube and fertilize it (conception), marking the beginning of pregnancy. The fertilized ovum divides multiple times as it travels down the fallopian tube. By about 5 days after fertilization, it contains 50 to 60 cells and has entered the uterus, where it becomes implanted (Fig. 26-1).

As the embryo continues to develop in the uterine wall, cells of its outer membrane (chorion) invade the uterine wall and begin to form chorionic villi. This forms the basis for the placenta. The placenta attaches the fetus and the umbilical cord to the uterus, provides the fetus with nutrients, removes wastes, and produces hormones necessary for pregnancy. Substances in the mother's circulation must pass through the placenta to the fetal circulation. The placenta blocks large proteins and hydrophobic compounds bound to plasma protein. The fetus is protected by maternal immunoglobulin G antibodies that readily cross the placenta. The embryo is surrounded by a cavity filled with amniotic fluid as it continues to develop. The embryo is termed a fetus at 10 weeks after conception. Week 13 represents the end of the first trimester of pregnancy, week 26 represents the end of the second trimester, and delivery represents the end of the last trimester. As the fetus grows, so does the placenta (Fig. 26-2).

As the placenta grows larger, it secretes hormones into the mother's circulation: human chorionic gonadotropin (hCG), human placental lactogen, progesterone, estradiol, estriol, and estrone. The levels of all of these hormones increase as the placenta continues to grow. hCG is the exception because its concentration peaks at the end of the first trimester. hCG is very important to pregnancy because it stimulates progesterone production by the ovaries, which suspends menstruation to protect the pregnancy. The estrogen hormones (estradiol, estriol, and estrone) produced by the placenta stimulate development of the endometrium, uterine growth, adequate uterine blood supply, and uterine preparation for labor.

Amniotic fluid plays an important role in the development and health of the fetus. Amniotic fluid provides an environment in which the fetus can move, acts as a cushion against possible injuries, and maintains a constant temperature for the fetus. The amniotic fluid volume may vary because the fetus swallows amniotic fluid, urinates into the

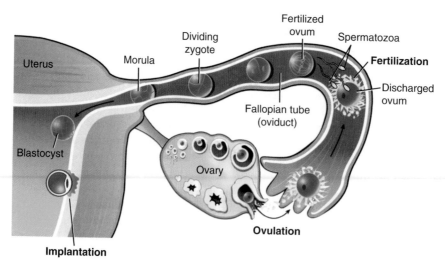

• **Figure 26-1** Fertilization of the ovum and implantation of the blastocyst into the uterine lining. (From Shiland BJ. *Medical Terminology and Anatomy for ICD-10 Coding.* 2nd ed. St. Louis: Mosby; 2015.)

fluid, and excretes fluids through its lungs (fetal breathing). Amniotic fluid is also the major vehicle for transporting nutrients and electrolytes into the fetal circulation. In some conditions, the volume of amniotic fluid is increased; these conditions include maternal diabetes mellitus, hemolytic disease of the newborn, fetal esophageal atresia, multifetal pregnancy, anencephaly, and spina bifida. The concentration of phospholipids in the amniotic fluid reflects the maturity of the fetal lungs. A normal fetus does not defecate into the amniotic fluid. However, if the fetus is stressed during

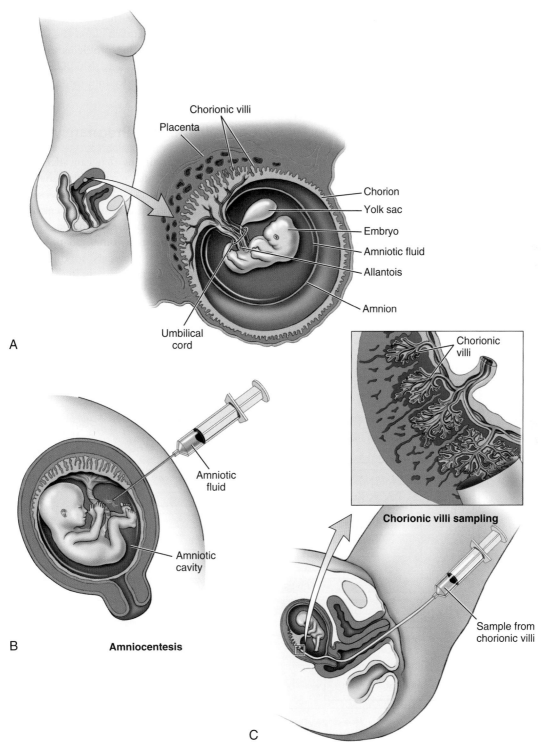

• **Figure 26-2** Extraembryonic membranes and the formation of the placenta. **A,** The embryo is surrounded by the amnion and the amniotic fluid in the amniotic cavity. **B,** Amniocentesis. **C,** Chorionic villi sampling. (From Herlihy B. *The Human Body in Health Illness.* 5th ed. St. Louis: Saunders; 2014.)

pregnancy, it may pass a stool called meconium, which has a large concentration of bile pigments. The bile pigments are green and color the amniotic fluid the same green color. An amniotic fluid that contains meconium indicates that the fetus is under stress.

The organs (lung, liver, and kidneys) of the fetus develop and mature throughout the pregnancy (Fig. 26-3). The fetal lungs are mature when they produce a pulmonary surfactant that allows the lungs to expand and contract during breathing. The pulmonary surfactant is composed of phospholipid (lecithin) and a small amount of sphingomyelin. The fetal liver produces the blood cells during the first two trimesters, but then this function moves to the bone marrow. The liver also produces α-fetoprotein (AFP). The liver becomes the organ that detoxifies the blood and metabolizes bilirubin late in the pregnancy, but sometimes not until after birth. The fetal kidneys excrete urine in the first trimester, but they do not mature fully until after birth.

Laboratory Confirmation of Pregnancy

A pregnancy test detects β-hCG in a woman's blood or urine. As mentioned previously, after 5 days of dividing, the fertilized egg implants and a placenta forms. The placenta produces hCG, and this is what pregnancy tests measure.

Pregnancy tests are generally positive approximately 2 weeks after conception. hCG is a reliable marker of pregnancy (even ectopic pregnancy), and most pregnancy tests use the presence of this marker to confirm pregnancy. A variety of pregnancy tests are available, including very reliable home pregnancy tests, most of which are immunoassay based, although latex agglutination is also a common method of detecting pregnancy. Most laboratories use quantitative β-hCG test methods to determine the exact level of β-hCG in a woman's blood (Fig. 26-4). This is especially crucial for detecting problems early in a pregnancy. hCG peaks at approximately 100,000 IU/L at the end of the first trimester, then declines throughout the remainder of the pregnancy.

Complications of Pregnancy

The common conditions that can affect the mother during pregnancy include gestational diabetes, ectopic pregnancy, hyperemesis gravidarum, preeclampsia, HELLP syndrome (hemolysis, elevated liver enzymes, low platelet counts with preeclampsia), eclampsia, and Graves disease. The bodies of pregnant women adapt to pregnancy, so it is incumbent upon providers to differentiate abnormal changes from the normal changes in the mother's body during pregnancy.

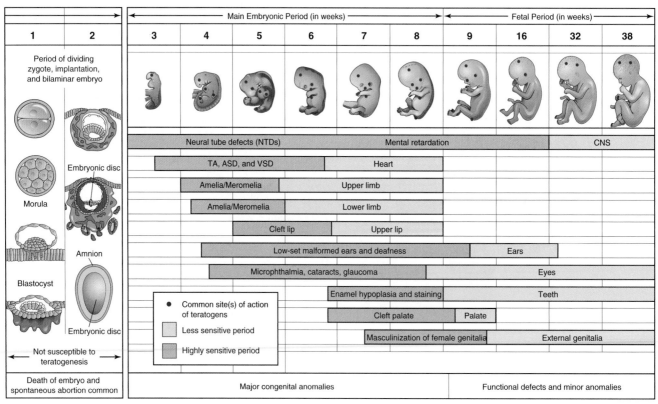

• **Figure 26-3** Critical periods in human development. The dark color denotes highly sensitive periods of development, when birth defects are most common, while the light color indicates stages that are less sensitive. (From Moore KL, Persaud TVN, Torchia MG. *Before We Are Born: Essentials of Embryology and Birth Defects.* 9th ed. Philadelphia: Saunders; 2016.)

Gestational Diabetes

Blood glucose levels are drawn and tested during the 24th to 28th week of pregnancy to screen for gestational diabetes. Many physicians prefer a modified glucose tolerance test as a screen for gestational diabetes instead of a fasting blood glucose level. This modified test can be used to preclude further testing, but it is not sufficient to diagnose gestational diabetes. A glucose tolerance test involves measuring the fasting blood glucose level, after which the patient ingests 75 g of glucose and has blood drawn at 1, 2, and 3 hours after ingestion for glucose level determination. If glucose values exceed set limits for any two of the four samples (fasting, 1 hour, 2 hour, or 3 hour), the test is considered positive for gestational diabetes. (See Chapter 22 for a full discussion of diabetes and glucose testing.) Gestational diabetes occurs in about 18% of pregnancies.

Ectopic Pregnancy

An ectopic pregnancy occurs when the fertilized egg implants somewhere outside the uterus. Usually, the fertilized egg implants in one of the fallopian tubes (Fig. 26-5). The symptoms of ectopic pregnancy include lower abdominal pain, vaginal bleeding, and cessation of menses. Sometimes, the fallopian tubes are damaged because of genetic or sexually transmitted disease, and the fertilized egg is unable to move down the fallopian tube. Ectopic pregnancies can be medical emergencies if the fertilized egg continues to grow and ruptures the fallopian tube; the resulting hemorrhage releases a large volume of blood into the abdominal cavity. The following symptoms suggest a medical emergency: abdominal rigidity, severe tenderness, and evidence of hypovolemic shock (orthostatic blood changes due to hemorrhage).

Diagnostic tests for ectopic pregnancy include a urine pregnancy test and a quantitative hCG measurement. The qualitative test confirms that a pregnancy is present and indicates whether appropriate levels of hCG are being produced to match the estimated gestational age. Serum β-hCG levels can be correlated to gestational age in a normal pregnancy. During the first trimester of pregnancy, β-hCG levels double every 48 to 72 hours until reaching 10,000 to 20,000 mIU/mL. A lower than expected increase can

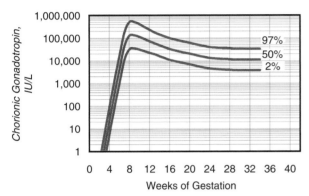

• **Figure 26-4** Concentration of human chorionic gonadotropin (hCG) in maternal serum as a function of gestational age at the 2nd, 50th, and 97th percentiles. The maternal serum values from 14 to 25 weeks are medians calculated from 24,229 pregnancies tested at ARUP Laboratories, Inc., from January to October 1997. (From Burtis CA, Bruns DE. *Tietz Fundamentals of Clinical Chemistry and Molecular Diagnostics.* 7th ed. St. Louis: Saunders; 2015.)

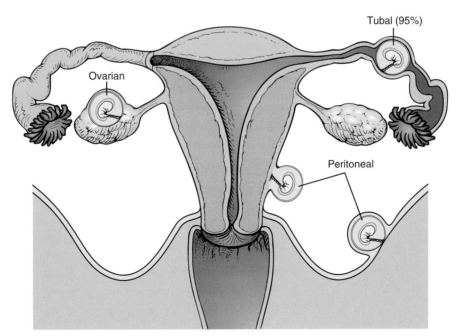

• **Figure 26-5** The fallopian tube is the most common site for ectopic pregnancies, but they can also occur on the ovary or on the peritoneal surface of the abdominal cavity. (From Damjanov I. *Pathology for the Health Professions.* 4th ed. St. Louis: Saunders; 2012.)

indicate an ectopic pregnancy. Serial β-hCG measurements are needed to confirm an ectopic pregnancy and monitor the resolution after surgical removal.

Hyperemesis Gravidarum

Hyperemesis gravidarum is a severe form of nausea and vomiting in pregnancy. The nausea and vomiting is accompanied by ketosis and weight loss. This condition can cause acid-base imbalances, electrolyte imbalances, nutritional deficits, and even death. The symptoms of this disease, in addition to nausea and vomiting, include excessive salivation, fatigue, weakness, dizziness, sleep disturbance, distorted taste, depression, anxiety, irritability, mood changes, and decreased concentration.

To diagnose this condition, a full work-up is required to rule out many more conditions. Commonly ordered laboratory tests include urinalysis, complete blood count, hepatitis panel, basic metabolic panel, liver enzymes and bilirubin, amylase and lipase levels, thyroid-stimulating hormone level, urine culture, and serum ketones. If this condition is not promptly treated, it can lead to death.

Preeclampsia

Preeclampsia is characterized by hypertension (high blood pressure, >140/90 mm Hg on two separate occasions) and proteinuria (protein in the urine) after the 20th week of pregnancy. The exact cause of preeclampsia is unknown, but risk factors for this condition include age greater than 40 years, black race, family history of preeclampsia, chronic renal disease, chronic hypertension, diabetes mellitus, twin gestation, and a high body mass index (>31). Severe preeclampsia is defined as the presence of one of the following symptoms in addition to hypertension and proteinuria: blood pressure 160/110 mm Hg or higher, proteinuria (>5 g in 24 hr collection, or >3+ on two random specimens), pulmonary edema, cyanosis, oliguria (<400 mL in 24 hr), persistent headaches, epigastric pain, impaired liver function, thrombocytopenia (platelet count <100,000/mm^3), and decreased fetal growth or placental abruption (placenta breaking away from uterus).

The only treatment for preeclampsia is delivery. Individuals who have mild preeclampsia can have labor induced after 37 weeks' gestation. Because the fetus must survive after birth, it can be treated with corticosteroids to speed fetal lung maturity. If a woman develops preeclampsia before 34 weeks' gestation, the severity of the disease and its effect on the mother and child must be weighed against the risks of infant prematurity. Providers should consider delivery if the fetal heartbeat is irregular or weak, the mother's membranes have ruptured, the mother's blood pressure is uncontrollable, or there is severe intrauterine growth restriction, oliguria (<500 mL/24 hr), serum creatinine greater than 1.5 mg/dL, pulmonary edema, shortness of breath, chest pain with pulse oximetry of less than 94% on room air, persistent or severe headache, or right upper quadrant tenderness.

Laboratory test results are very helpful in diagnosing and monitoring preeclampsia. Women who are diagnosed with new-onset hypertension should have a complete blood count, alanine aminotransferase (ALT), aspartate aminotransferase (AST), creatinine, and uric acid determinations for their initial work-up. Laboratory values for preeclampsia and HELLP syndrome are shown in Table 26-1.

Eclampsia

A life-threatening manifestation of preeclampsia is eclampsia, in which a mother experiences grand mal seizures or falls into a coma. Eclampsia can lead to intracranial hemorrhage. Eclampsia is rare in the United States and the Western world, but when it does occur, it is most often associated with young mothers (<20 years) or mothers older than 35 years of age. It is also associated to a higher degree with women of lower socioeconomic status due to their lack of prenatal care.

HELLP Syndrome

Another life-threatening manifestation of preeclampsia is the HELLP syndrome. The major characteristics of the HELLP syndrome are thrombocytopenia and disseminated intravascular coagulation (DIC). Although most cases occur between the 27th and 36th weeks of pregnancy, this syndrome can occur after delivery. Women with this disorder have right upper quadrant pain, malaise, nausea, vomiting, headache, and jaundice. Laboratory results include a very high level of lactate dehydrogenase (LD) and ALT and AST levels 2 to 10 times the upper reference values.

TABLE 26-1 **Laboratory Values for Preeclampsia and HELLP Syndrome**

Test	Test Result
Urine protein	>300 mg/24 hr (urine dipstick >1+)
Serum uric acid	>5.6 mg/dL
Serum creatinine	>1.2 mg/dL
Platelet count	<100.000/mm^3
Coagulation tests	Elevated PT or APTT, decreased fibrinogen, increased D-dimer
Indirect bilirubin	>1.2 mg/dL
Lactate dehydrogenase	>600 U/L
Peripheral blood smear	Platelet count <100,000/mm^3

APTT, Activated partial thromboplastin time; *HELLP,* hemolysis, elevated liver enzymes, low platelet counts with preeclampsia; *PT,* prothrombin time.

The only treatment is delivery. After delivery, the mother may require organ transplantation.

Graves Disease

Initially, the fetus is dependent on its mother for a supply of thyroid hormones, which can cross the placenta. If the mother has Graves disease or a low level of thyroid hormones, the fetus can be affected. Adverse outcomes such as preterm delivery, fetal death, and a reduced IQ result from low thyroid hormone levels in the fetus. By the third trimester, the fetus's thyroid gland functions independently from the mother's. If a woman has Graves disease when she becomes pregnant, her anti-thyroid antibodies will cross the placenta and stimulate the fetal thyroid gland, leading to fetal hyperthyroidism.

Fetal Complications

In addition to diseases of the mother, the fetus may develop abnormally or develop abnormal conditions while in the uterus. These conditions include neural tube defects, Down syndrome, and hemolytic disease of the newborn.

Neural Tube Defects

Neural tube defects are life-threatening abnormalities associated with the development of the fetal central nervous system. As the fetus develops, a hollow neural tube with fused ends develops as the precursor of the spinal cord. Failure of the neural tube to fuse produces permanent developmental defects of the brain, spinal cord, or both. Conditions associated with this defect include meningomyelocele or spina bifida (in which the bottom end of the neural tube fails to fuse), encephalocele (a sac containing brain and membranes that protrudes through an abnormal opening in the skull), and anencephaly (lack of parts of the brain and skull). These defects correlate with folic acid deficiency in the mother during pregnancy. Ninety percent of these abnormalities can be detected by screening maternal blood for AFP. AFP is leaked into the amniotic fluid from openings in the fetal neural tubes and then absorbed into the maternal circulation through the amniotic fluid.

Down Syndrome

Down syndrome (trisomy 21) is a common and serious developmental disorder caused by an autosomal chromosome defect. In this disorder, the affected individual has one extra copy of the long arm of chromosome 21. The characteristics of this chromosomal anomaly include moderate to severe mental retardation, hypotonia, congenital heart defects, and a flat facial profile. Because this is a relatively frequent disorder with serious long-term implications, prenatal screening for Down syndrome is common.

Respiratory Distress Syndrome

The biggest contributing factor to neonatal morbidity and death every year is pre-term delivery. If an infant is born before 37 weeks' gestation in the uterus, it will probably suffer from respiratory distress syndrome, also known as hyaline membrane disease. The infants usually have a low birth weight, and their lungs are not mature enough to produce enough pulmonary surfactant, which is required for independent breathing. This is the major life-threatening problem that affects premature babies. These infants require supplementary oxygen and mechanical ventilation to stay alive. The lack of surfactant causes the alveoli to collapse during exhalation. The lungs become still, and the blood that flows around the collapsed alveoli is unoxygenated. Symptoms of this disorder include hyperventilation with or without cyanosis, nasal flaring, exhalation grunting, and intercostal retractions (skin is pulled between the ribs due to difficulty inhaling). Before the infant is born, providers run a fetal lung maturity test to check for lung surfactant in the infant.

Hemolytic Disease of the Newborn

Hemolytic disease of the newborn (HDN) results when a fetus's red blood cells (RBCs) contain an antigen that the mother's RBCs lack (Fig. 26-6). If the mother's RBCs do not have the antigen, then she will develop an antigen against the fetus's RBCs. All pregnant women have a sample drawn for a blood type and antibody screen during their prenatal visit. The purpose of this test is to determine the mother's blood type. The immunogenic antigen system that produces the most cases of HDN per year is the Rh blood antigen system. Usually, mothers are D negative and the fetus is D positive. Most times, the first D-positive child born to a D-negative mother is not severely affected by the maternal antibodies. However, the second child born to a D-negative mother who has been sensitized to the D antigen is severely affected and may not live until birth. To protect the fetus, D-negative women are routinely injected with anti-D during the 28th week of pregnancy. If antibodies are present in the mother's system to ward off the anti-D–positive RBCs, then the mother's body will not produce antibodies of her own against these cells. Rho(D) immune globulin (RhoGAM) prevents anti-D sensitization.

The main concern for the fetus is that the maternal antibodies will destroy its RBCs, resulting in hemolytic anemia and severely elevated bilirubin levels. High bilirubin levels can produce brain damage, so the pregnancy is closely monitored. Bilirubin levels can be estimated from amniotic fluid. The absorbance of amniotic fluid is measured at 450 nm and compared with absorbance readings of the same amniotic fluid at 350 and 550 nm. A baseline is drawn from the absorbance at 350 nm to the absorbance at 550 nm. The deviation of the reading at 450 nm is directly proportional to the amount of bilirubin in the sample.

PATHOPHYSIOLOGY REVIEW

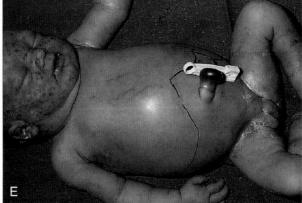

Maternal circulation

Maternal Rh-negative erythrocyte

Fetal Rh-positive erythrocyte enters maternal circulation

A

Fetal Rh-positive erythrocyte

Maternal circulation

Maternal Rh-negative erythrocyte

Rh antibodies

B

C

Agglutination of fetal Rh-positive erythrocytes leads to hemolytic disease of the newborn

Maternal circulation

Maternal Rh antibodies cross the placenta

D

D antigen

Hemolysis

E

• **Figure 26-6　A,** Before or during delivery, Rh-positive erythrocytes from the fetus enter the blood of an Rh-negative woman through a tear in the placenta. **B,** The mother is sensitized to the Rh antigen and produces Rh antibodies. Because this usually happens after delivery, there is no effect on the fetus in the first pregnancy. **C** and **D,** During a subsequent pregnancy with an Rh-positive fetus, Rh-positive erythrocytes cross the placenta, enter the maternal circulation, and stimulate the mother to produce antibodies against the Rh antigen. **E,** The Rh antibodies from the mother cross the placenta, causing agglutination and hemolysis of fetal erythrocytes, and hemolytic disease of the newborn develops. (From McCance KL, Huether SE. *Pathophysiology: The Biologic Basis for Disease in Adults and Children.* 7th ed. St. Louis: Mosby; 2015.)

TABLE 26-2 Laboratory Test Results for Fetal Defects

	α-Fetoprotein	β-Human Chorionic Gonadotropin	Estriol	Inhibin A
Neural tube defects	↑	—	—	—
Trisomy 18	↓	↓	↓	↓
Trisomy 21	↓	↑	↓	↑

Laboratory Diagnosis of Fetal Abnormalities

Clinical laboratories perform prenatal screening tests on maternal blood for many fetal disorders (Table 26-2). Neural tube defects can effectively be screened prenatally through AFP testing. Most AFP assays are enzyme immunoassays performed on maternal serum. The multiple of the median (MoM) is the tool used to normalize values during test interpretation. Because the level of AFP increases throughout the pregnancy, median values for AFP during each week of gestation are established by each laboratory. An individual AFP value is expressed as an MoM by dividing it by the median for that particular gestational week. If the resulting value is higher than a cutoff point, indicating that the test result is much higher than the median, a neural tube defect may be present. If it is lower than the median, Down syndrome may be present.

Chromosomal Abnormalities

Screening for chromosomal abnormalities can be done through blood testing on the mother, amniocentesis, or chorionic villi sampling (see Fig. 26-2, B and C) Amniocentesis is done usually between 15 and 20 weeks of pregnancy. Amniocentesis involves puncturing the amniotic sac with a needle and withdrawing a few milliliters of amniotic fluid into a syringe. Chorionic villi sampling is usually done between weeks 10 and 12, so results can be available to the parents during the first trimester of pregnancy. Chorionic villi sampling involves removing cells from the fingerlike projections (villi) that protrude from the outer membrane surrounding the developing fetus (see Fig. 26-2). Both amniocentesis and chorionic villi sampling carry risks to mother and baby, and these risks need to balance with the potential benefits before a decision to pursue such testing is made. The chromosomal defects most commonly screened for are neural tube defects such as spina bifida and chromosomal abnormalities such as Down syndrome (trisomy 21) and Edwards syndrome (trisomy 18) (see Table 26-2).

In addition to chromosomal tests, there is a quadruple screening test specific for Down syndrome risk assessment. This test combines the results from several tests (AFP, hCG, unconjugated estriol, and dimeric inhibition) that are correlated with a pregnant woman's age, and a single Down syndrome risk estimate is calculated. This is a widely used tool.

Fetal Lung Maturity Testing

The lungs are the last of the organ systems to mature in the fetus. Fetal lung immaturity, or RDS, occurs most often when insufficient lung surfactant is present. There are several methods for measuring lung surfactant to assess fetal pulmonary maturity. They are most often performed on amniotic fluid. These tests include the lecithin/sphingomyelin ratio (L/S ratio), the phosphatidyl glycerol level, and a fluorescent polarization test.

Lecithin/Sphingomyelin Ratio

This test evaluates a ratio of lecithin (phosphatidyl choline) to sphingomyelin (a phospholipid) in amniotic fluid. Lecithin is a major component of airway surfactant, whereas sphingomyelin is a non-lung compound that serves as a good internal standard for this assay. After 32 to 33 weeks' gestation, the concentration of lecithin increases significantly compared with the relatively constant concentration of sphingomyelin. In a normal pregnancy, the ratio of these two substances reaches 2.0 at approximately 35 weeks' gestation. Those infants whose L/S ratio is 2.0 or higher have mature lungs. Laboratories usually use a commercially available test kit with an amniotic fluid sample. Collection of amniotic fluid must be done carefully to avoid contamination of the sample, because contamination with blood, meconium, vaginal secretions, or urine can interfere with testing and produce false results. The specimen must be protected from light because of the bilirubin present in the fluid. It is best to freeze the sample if the test cannot be performed immediately.

Phosphatidyl Glycerol

Phosphatidyl glycerol is thought to be a component of surfactant that appears at 35 to 36 weeks' gestation, shortly after the increase in lecithin concentration. Its presence in the amniotic fluid is thought to indicate an advanced state of fetal pulmonary maturity. Contaminants such as meconium, urine, and vaginal secretions usually do not interfere with the phosphatidyl glycerol test methods, so a vaginal pool specimen (even after the amniotic sac has broken) can still be used as a specimen. Phosphatidyl glycerol assays are usually qualitative rapid agglutination tests. The test is reported as negative, low positive (0.5 to 2 μg/mL), or high positive (≥2 μg/mL).

Fluorescent Polarization Test

A fluorescent polarization test is used to measure the ratio of surfactant to albumin. High values indicate high levels of surfactant and lung maturity. The disadvantage of this technique, as with the L/S ratio, is that blood and meconium interfere with the result. The advantage of this test is that it is simple and more precise than the L/S ratio. A free-flowing vaginal pool or amniotic fluid can be used as a sample. Most laboratories use a commercial assay for this test.

Summary

Pregnancy begins when an ovum is fertilized by a sperm. A woman misses a menses, and this prompts examination of the urine or blood for β-hCG. This hormone is produced by the placenta, and a positive test result signals pregnancy. β-hCG is usually measured by enzyme immunoassay methods. In a normal pregnancy, the ovum implants into the uterus and eventually forms (with the mother) a placenta, umbilical cord, and amniotic sac. The fetus grows and matures before entering the world as a child upon delivery. This is an extremely complex process that occurs in approximately 37 to 39 weeks. During this time, abnormal conditions can appear in the mother or the fetus or both.

Complications of pregnancy include gestational diabetes, ectopic pregnancy, hyperemesis gravidarum, preeclampsia, HELLP syndrome, eclampsia, and Graves disease. Conditions that affect the fetus include neural tube defects, Down syndrome, and HDN. Screening of maternal serum can detect neural tube defects and Down syndrome. For HDN, blood typing of mother and fetus is important.

AFP is measured to detect neural tube defects in a fetus. Assays use enzyme immunoassay methods. The results are reported as MoM to normalize values for interpretation. Low AFP levels indicate Down syndrome. Amniocentesis and chorionic villi sampling are techniques used to collect specimens for chromosome analysis of the fetus. Down syndrome risk assessment is calculated by using AFP, hCG, unconjugated estriol, and dimeric inhibition test results.

Fetal lung immaturity produces RDS because too little lung surfactant is produced by the fetus. Corticosteroids can be given in utero to help the fetus produce adequate lung surfactant. The L/S ratio is a lung maturity test. Measurement of phosphatidyl glycerol also tests for lung maturity in utero.

Review Questions

1. Low levels of AFP, low levels of estriol, and high levels of hCG are often associated with
   a. Trisomy 18
   b. Trisomy 21
   c. Increased rate of miscarriage
   d. Spina bifida
2. High levels of surfactant in amniotic fluid indicate
   a. Increased possibility of miscarriage
   b. Fetal lungs are mature
   c. Meconium contamination of the amniotic fluid
   d. Low levels of lecithin
3. Which of the following is associated only with eclampsia and not with preeclampsia?
   a. Low platelet count
   b. Seizure in the mother
   c. Hypertension
   d. Proteinuria
4. Which of the following structures is formed after the fertilized ovum implants into the uterus?
   a. Chorionic villi
   b. Placenta
   c. Amniotic sac
   d. Fallopian tubes
5. How does a fetus receive essential nutrients and electrolytes?
   a. Through the amniotic fluid
   b. By passive diffusion from maternal blood into fetal blood
   c. By active transport from the meconium
   d. From phospholipids and bilirubin found in amniotic fluid

6. At what point are the fetal lungs considered mature?
   a. When they produce pulmonary surfactant
   b. At 28 weeks' gestation
   c. When lecithin levels are three times as high as sphingomyelin levels
   d. At delivery
7. Which of the following is something that a fetus does *not* do in utero?
   a. Defecate
   b. Urinate
   c. Move
   d. Grow
8. Why are AFP test results interpreted using MoM?
   a. To normalize the test results
   b. There is a logarithmic relationship between the amount of AFP in the blood and Down syndrome
   c. Bilirubin can interfere with AFP, and MoM takes away the bilirubin interference
   d. To minimize the amount of sphingomyelin in the sample
9. Neural tube defects include all the following EXCEPT
   a. Trisomy 18
   b. Meningomyelocele
   c. Encephalocele
   d. Anencephaly
10. What special handling procedures are required for amniotic fluid?
    a. Protect from light
    b. Place in a sterile tube with EDTA anticoagulant
    c. Place in a sterile red top tube and let the specimen clot
    d. Place in a cup of ice and deliver to laboratory immediately

Critical Thinking Questions

1. Why can an ectopic pregnancy be a life-threatening medical emergency?
2. What are the symptoms of preeclampsia, and what is its treatment?

3. What is the difference between preeclampsia and eclampsia, and why is this difference important?

CASE STUDY

Ms. D, a mother approaching her 35th week of pregnancy reports to an urgent care facility with her husband. She complains of diffuse abdominal pain, weakness, and dizziness that started approximately 3 days earlier. Her blood pressure is 145/95 mm Hg. The laboratory technician does a quick urinalysis and detects 1+ protein in the patient's urine. A blood sample is drawn, the physician calls the woman's obstetrician, and the woman and her husband are sent to the hospital. What condition does Ms. D have, and why is this considered a serious situation? What are the possible complications of this condition?

Bibliography

Berg BR, Houseman JL, Garrasi MA, Young CL, Newton DW. Culture-based method with performance comparable to that of PCR-based methods for detection of group B streptococcus in screening samples from pregnant women. *J Clin Microbiol.* 2013;51(4):1253–1255.

Bianchi DW, Platt LD, Goldberg JD, et al. Genome-wide fetal aneuploidy detection by maternal plasma DNA sequencing. *Obstet Gynecol.* 2012;119(5):890–901.

Bodurtha J, Strauss III JF. Genomics and perinatal care. *N Engl J Med.* 2012;366(1):64–73.

Bredaki FE, Poon LC, Birdir C, Escalante D, Nicolaides KH. First-trimester screening for neural tube defects using alpha-fetoprotein. *Fetal Diagn Ther.* 2012;31(2):109–114.

Bustamante-Aragonés A, de Alba MR, Perlado S, et al. Non-invasive prenatal diagnosis of single-gene disorders from maternal blood. *Gene.* 2012;504(1):144–149.

Butler SA, Khanlian SA, Cole LA. Detection of early pregnancy forms of human chorionic gonadotropin by home pregnancy test devices. *Clin Chem.* 2001;47(12):2131–2136.

Centers for Disease Control and Prevention. *Sexually Transmitted Disease Surveillance 2013.* Atlanta: U.S. Department of Health and Human Services; 2014.

Centers for Disease Control and Prevention. Sexually transmitted diseases treatment guidelines, 2010. *MMWR Morb Mortal Wkly Rep.* 2010;59(no. RR-12).

Centers for Disease Control and Prevention. *STDs and pregnancy: CDC fact sheet.* <www.cdc.gov/std/pregnancy/stdfact-pregnancy.htm> Accessed 27.08.15.

Davies S, Byrn F, Cole LA. Human chorionic gonadotropin testing for early pregnancy viability and complications. *Clin Lab Med.* 2003;23(2):257–264.

Ellard S, Kivuva E, Turnpenny P, et al. An exome sequencing strategy to diagnose lethal autosomal recessive disorders. *Eur J Hum Genet.* 2015;23(3):401–404.

Kemp S, Berger J, Aubourg P. X-linked adrenoleukodystrophy: clinical, metabolic, genetic and pathophysiological aspects. *Biochim Biophys Acta.* 2012;1822(9):1465–1474.

Lau TK, Cheung SW, Lo PSS, et al. Non-invasive prenatal testing for fetal chromosomal abnormalities by low-coverage whole-genome sequencing of maternal plasma DNA: review of 1982 consecutive cases in a single center. *Ultrasound Obstet Gynecol.* 2014;43(3):254–264.

Lee SM, Romero R, Park JS, et al. A transcervical amniotic fluid collector: a new medical device for the assessment of amniotic fluid in patients with ruptured membranes. *J Perinat Med.* 2015;43(4):381–389.

Nicolaides KH, Wright D, Poon LC, Syngelaki A, Gil MM. First-trimester contingent screening for trisomy 21 by biomarkers and maternal blood cell-free DNA testing. *Ultrasound Obstet Gynecol.* 2013;42(1):41–50.

Olooto WE, Amballi AA, Mosuro AO, Adeleye AA, Banjo TA. Assessment of total protein, albumin, creatinine and aspartate transaminase level in toxemia of pregnancy. *J Med Sci.* 2013;13(8):791–796.

Pagana KD. *Mosby's Manual of Diagnostic and Laboratory Tests.* St. Louis: Elsevier Health Sciences; 2013.

Paquet C, Yudin MH. Toxoplasmosis in pregnancy: prevention, screening, and treatment. *J Obstet Gynaecol Can.* 2013;35(1):78–81.

Pokhrel T, Sharma S, Bhat SR. TORCH profile: a convenient method for screening infection in pregnancy by ELISA—a review. *Res Rev J Microbiol Virol.* 2014;4(1):16–21.

Ralph SG, Rutherford AJ, Wilson JD. Influence of bacterial vaginosis on conception and miscarriage in the first trimester: cohort study. *BMJ.* 1999;319(7204):220–223.

Rausch ME, Sammel MD, Takacs P, et al. Development of a multiple marker test for ectopic pregnancy. *Obstet Gynecol.* 2011;117(3):573–582.

Reid S, Casikar I, Barnhart K, Condous G. Serum biomarkers for ectopic pregnancy diagnosis. *Expert Opin Med Diagn.* 2012;6(2):153–165.

Tennant C, Friedman AM, Pare E, Bruno C, Wang E. Performance of lecithin-sphingomyelin ratio as a reflex test for documenting fetal lung maturity in late preterm and term fetuses. *J Matern-Fetal Neonatal Med.* 2012;25(8):1460–1462.

Van Mello NM, Mol F, Ankum WM, et al. Ectopic pregnancy: how the diagnostic and therapeutic management has changed. *Fertil Steril.* 2012;98(5):1066–1073.

Wilson H. Advances in prenatal diagnostics. *Biomark Med.* 2014;8(4):453–454.

27

Bone, Joint, and Skeletal Muscle Diseases

DONNA LARSON

CHAPTER OUTLINE

OBJECTIVES

After completion of this chapter, the reader will be able to:

1. Describe the normal anatomy and physiology of bones.
2. Describe the purpose of alkaline phosphatase (ALP) in the body.
3. Compare and contrast the concentration of ALP and the mechanism that causes elevated ALP levels in osteogenesis imperfecta, Paget disease, and rickets or osteomalacia.
4. Compare and contrast clinical chemistry test results for osteogenesis imperfecta, Paget disease, and rickets or osteomalacia.
5. Compare and contrast the location, regulation, functions, and low and high levels of calcium (Ca^{2+}), magnesium (Mg^{2+}), and phosphate (PO_4^{3-}) ions.
6. Describe the laboratory methods for testing calcium, phosphorus, and magnesium levels.
7. Describe the normal anatomy and physiology of joints.

8. Compare and contrast the mechanisms causing osteoarthritis, rheumatoid arthritis, ankylosing spondylitis, and gout.
9. Correlate clinical chemistry test results for osteoarthritis, rheumatoid arthritis, ankylosing spondylitis, and gout.
10. Describe the normal anatomy and physiology of skeletal muscle.
11. Compare and contrast the creatine kinase (CK) concentration and the mechanism releasing CK into the bloodstream in the following diseases: Duchenne muscular dystrophy, Becker muscular dystrophy, rhabdomyolysis, and myasthenia gravis.
12. Correlate clinical chemistry test results for Duchenne muscular dystrophy, Becker muscular dystrophy, rhabdomyolysis, and myasthenia gravis.

KEY TERMS

Ankylosing spondylitis
Anti–cyclic citrullinated peptide
Anti–mutated citrullinated vimentin
Atrophy
Becker muscular dystrophy
Bone resorption
Cardiomyopathy

Cholecalciferol
Duchenne muscular dystrophy
Gout
Hypercalcemia
Hypermagnesemia
Hyperphosphatemia
Hypocalcemia

Hypomagnesemia
Hypophosphatemia
Myasthenia gravis
Osteitis deformans
Osteoarthritis
Osteogenesis imperfecta
Osteoid

❖ Case in Point

A 26-year-old man was working in a welding shop when a large piece of metal fell on his leg and crushed the bottom half. He was taken to the emergency department, and the attending physician ordered laboratory tests. The following results were obtained: creatine kinase level, 1844 IU/L; sodium level, 121 mEq/L; potassium level, 5.0 mEq/L; chloride level, 89 mEq/L; and carbon dioxide level, 32 mg/dL. He also had dark-colored urine. What is the most probable diagnosis for this man?

Points to Remember

- Bones are metabolically active, slightly flexible structures that require mechanical stress to maintain health.
- Osteogenesis imperfecta is a genetic disease with an autosomal dominant inheritance pattern.
- Individuals with osteogenesis imperfecta can have 60 or more fractures in their lifetimes.
- Collagen analysis can be useful for diagnosing osteogenesis imperfecta.
- Paget disease begins with an area of excessive bone resorption. Reparative bone formation occurs in a disorganized manner, resulting in compact, dense bone that is prone to fracture.
- Rickets is a bone disease in which osteoid does not calcify in children and adolescents.
- Osteomalacia is bone disease in which osteoid does not calcify in adults.
- Rickets is caused by a deficiency of vitamin D metabolites or a dietary deficiency of calcium or phosphorus.
- Alkaline phosphatase (ALP) levels are dramatically increased in Paget disease due to increased bone resorption.
- Calcium (Ca^{2+}) is the most prevalent inorganic ion in the body. Most of it is found in the skeleton, along with phosphate (PO_4^{3-}) and magnesium (Mg^{2+}) ions.
- Increased uric acid levels in individuals with severe Paget disease can lead to gouty arthritis.
- Clinical chemistry tests used in the workup for rickets include calcium, phosphorus, ALP, parathyroid hormone, 25-hydroxyvitamin D, and 1,25-dihydroxyvitamin D determinations.
- Osteoarthritis is the most common form of arthritis and results from mechanical wear and tear on joints.
- Rheumatoid arthritis is a chronic autoimmune disease that affects synovial joints.

- Laboratory tests used in diagnosing rheumatoid arthritis include erythrocyte sedimentation rate (ESR), C-reactive protein (CRP), complete blood count (CBC), rheumatoid factor (RF), anti–cyclic citrullinated peptide (anti-CCP), and anti–mutated citrullinated vimentin (anti-MCV) assays.
- Ankylosing spondylitis is one of many spondyloarthropathies and is a chronic, systemic inflammatory condition.
- Ankylosing spondylitis affects the sacroiliac joints and the axial skeletal. Symptoms appear before 40 years of age.
- Gout is an arthritic condition in which monosodium urate monohydrate crystals are deposited in joints.
- Muscle is composed of bundled contractile fibers connected to motor nerves.
- Duchenne muscular dystrophy is a severe type of muscular dystrophy. All types produce progressive muscle weakness, which compromises the ability to walk, breathe, and pump blood.
- Becker muscular dystrophy, a milder form of the disease, was first described in 1955. Duchenne and Becker muscular dystrophies are caused by different mutations in the same gene on the X chromosome. Those with the Becker form display symptoms later than individuals with Duchenne muscular dystrophy.
- Myasthenia gravis is an autoimmune disease caused by the formation of antibodies against acetylcholine nicotinic postsynaptic receptors at the neuromuscular junction of skeletal muscles. This prohibits impulses generated by the brain from reaching muscles, which therefore cease to function.

Introduction

The musculoskeletal system provides structure for the body, protects organs, and enables movement. It mainly consists of bones, joints, and skeletal muscle. Bones are living organs that require mechanical stress to maintain health. Two bones meet and form a joint, which allows movement. Skeletal muscles are arranged with origins and insertions that allow the body to move in a particular way. The brain sends signals to the muscles, causing contraction and relaxation. When all systems work together in harmony, the result is a healthy musculoskeletal system.

Normal Anatomy and Physiology of Bones

Bones are metabolically active, slightly flexible structures that require mechanical stress to maintain health. Bones are

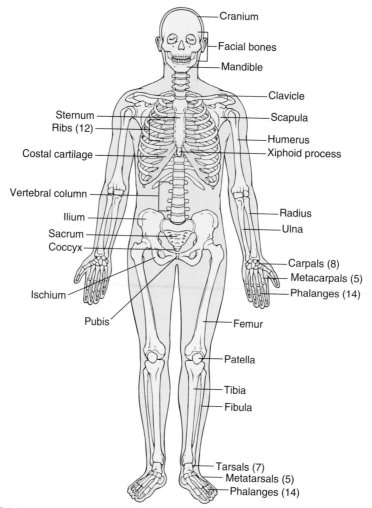

• **Figure 27-1** Anterior view of a normal skeletal system. (From Frazier MS, Drzymkowski JW. *Essentials of Human Diseases and Conditions.* 5th ed. St. Louis: Saunders; 2013.)

affected by hormones and vitamins, especially calcitonin and vitamin D. Bones are affected by a variety of diseases, including bone marrow disorders, osteogenesis imperfecta, Paget disease, and rickets.

The long bones, short bones, and flat bones of the skeletal system are well adapted to their functions. Long bones are found in the legs and arms; short bones are found in the vertebral column, hands, and feet; and flat bones are found in the hips, ribs, and skull (Fig. 27-1).

Each bone is covered by a membrane *(periosteum)* that contains nerves and blood vessels. The bone cavity contains red and yellow bone marrow. *Yellow marrow* is mostly fat and does not produce blood cells. *Red marrow* produces red blood cells, platelets, and most white blood cells. In adults, red marrow can be found in the sternum, ribs, pelvis, and proximal ends of the femur and humerus.

Bone Diseases

Osteogenesis Imperfecta

Osteogenesis imperfecta (sometimes called brittle bone disease) is a genetic disease with an autosomal dominant inheritance pattern that affects collagen throughout the body. It is characterized by blue sclerae (i.e., dark blue with a gray tinge), brittle bones that are easily fractured, defective middle ear bones that lead to deafness, abnormal tooth development, and bone deformity (Fig. 27-2).

Affected individuals usually grow to a normal height but have greatly reduced exercise tolerance and muscle strength. They tend to be pain tolerant, and old fractures often are discovered when radiographs are obtained for other issues. During a lifetime, affected individuals can have 60 or more fractures.

Laboratory test results are usually within reference ranges. Providers can use the routine test results to rule out other bone diseases. A definitive diagnosis is provided by identifying mutations in the *COL1A1* and *COL1A2* genes, which normally produce type I collagen. Collagen analysis can also be useful for diagnosing the disease.

Paget Disease

Paget disease is the second most common bone disorder in the elderly. It was identified by Sir James Paget as osteitis deformans in 1877. The disease begins with an area of excessive bone resorption, which prompts new bone formation.

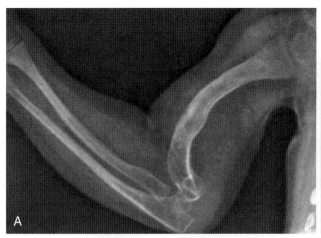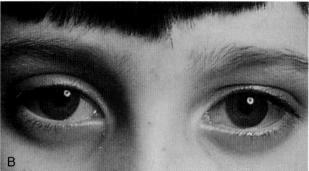

• **Figure 27-2** Osteogenesis imperfecta. **A,** Radiograph of an upper extremity in a person with osteogenesis imperfecta shows severe osteoporosis, slender bones, and multiple healed fractures. **B,** Blue sclerae caused by osteogenesis imperfecta. (**A,** From Bullough PG: *Bullough and Vigorita's Orthopaedic Pathology.* 3rd ed. St. Louis: Mosby 1997;134. **B,** From Swartz MH. *Textbook of Physical Diagnosis: History and Examination.* 7th ed. Philadelphia: Saunders; 2014.)

Because bone tissue is broken down and absorbed much faster than normal, the body speeds up the bone rebuilding process, but the repair process produces abnormal bone that is deposited in a disordered mosaic pattern and is mechanically weaker, less compact, more vascular, and more susceptible to fracture than normal bone.

Paget disease is caused by a combination of genetic and environmental factors. Individuals with the disease are likely to have parents or siblings with it. A latent viral infection (e.g., measles) in bone may trigger Paget disease in people who have inherited certain genes (Fig. 27-3). Most individuals with Paget disease are of European ancestry.

Most affected individuals do not have symptoms, but the disease can cause bone pain, secondary osteoarthritis, bone deformity, excessive warmth, and neurologic complications. Paget disease is most commonly found in the spine, pelvis, femur, sacrum, and skull, but it can affect any bone.

In individuals with Paget disease, blood and urine levels of calcium and phosphorus are normal. Alkaline phosphatase (ALP) levels are dramatically increased (up to 10 times normal) due to increased bone resorption. Chapter 8 discusses ALP test methods and their clinical uses. Due to increased bone resorption, uric acid levels are increased in individuals with severe disease and can lead to gouty arthritis. Chapter 24 discusses uric acid test methods and their clinical uses.

In addition to laboratory tests, diagnosis requires plain radiographs and bone scans. Bone scintigraphy is a more sensitive tool for diagnosing individuals with this disease than whole body radiographs. Approximately 10% of patients with Paget disease also have secondary hyperparathyroidism due to inadequate calcium intake during extensive bone remodeling.

Rickets

Rickets is a bone disease of children and adolescents in which osteoid does not calcify. Defective mineralization and softening of bone causes a similar disease, osteomalacia, in adults. Rickets is most commonly caused by a deficiency of vitamin D metabolites or a dietary deficiency of calcium or phosphorus. Ultraviolet B light reacts with a cholesterol derivative to form vitamin D_3 (i.e., cholecalciferol) in the skin.

Natural sources of vitamin D include wild-caught, cold-ocean fish (e.g., salmon) and ultraviolet light exposure. In the United States, milk is fortified with vitamin D to ensure that children receive adequate vitamin D. Because human milk typically contains low levels of vitamin D, breastfed infants can develop rickets if they do not receive vitamin D supplementation.

Children with rickets may have skeletal deformities and short stature. Female children with rickets can develop pelvic distortion that affects childbirth later in life. Severe rickets may cause respiratory failure. Infants also may have tetany or seizures due to low calcium levels (Fig. 27-4).

Clinical chemistry tests that are useful in the workup for rickets include assays of calcium, phosphorus, ALP, parathyroid hormone (PTH), 25-hydroxyvitamin D, and 1,25-dihydroxyvitamin D. Early in the disease, the level of ionized calcium may be low, but by the time of diagnosis, it is usually within the reference range. As calcium from bone is resorbed during skeletal remodeling, it is replaced by calcium from blood, lowering blood calcium levels. PTH is released in response to the low blood calcium levels, which return to normal. Tests usually find elevated ALP levels and decreased phosphorus levels in patients with rickets (Table 27-1).

Laboratory Procedures for Bone Diseases
Calcium

Calcium is the most prevalent inorganic ion in the body. Ninety-nine percent of the body's calcium is stored in the skeleton, with the remaining 1% located in the soft tissues and extracellular fluid. A tiny amount of calcium can be found intracellularly as an integral part of the cell

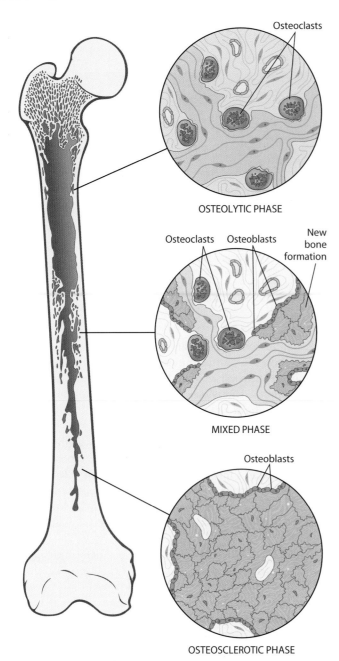

• **Figure 27-3** Diagrammatic representation of the three phases of Paget disease of bone. (From Kumar V, Abbas A, Fausto N, Aster J. *Robbins and Cotran: Pathologic Basis of Disease.* 9th ed. Philadelphia: Saunders; 2015.)

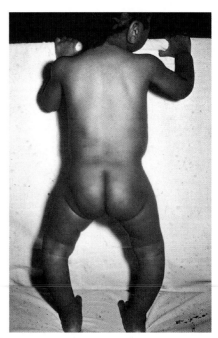

• **Figure 27-4** Rickets. (From Kumar V, Abbas A, Fausto N, Aster J. *Robbins and Cotran: Pathologic Basis of Disease.* 9th ed. Philadelphia: Saunders; 2015.)

membrane, mitochondria, and nucleus. Extracellular calcium is involved in the coagulation cascade, nerve conduction, and muscle contraction.

Calcium in blood can exist in three forms: free or ionized, bound to plasma proteins (primarily albumin), and bound to diffusible anions (phosphate, bicarbonate, lactate, or citrate). About 50% of the calcium in the body is in the free or ionized form, 40% is bound to plasma proteins, and 10% bound to diffusible anions. The calcium cation (Ca^{2+}), binds to negatively charged sites on the albumin molecule. As the pH of the blood increases, more calcium binds to albumin, and there is a smaller amount of free calcium in the blood. As the pH of the blood decreases, less calcium binds to albumin, and there is a larger amount of free calcium in the blood.

Calcium plays an important role in many body processes. For example, extracellular calcium serves as an intracellular messenger by binding and releasing cellular proteins. The proteins change their structure and function upon binding to calcium. Calcium as an intracellular messenger helps regulate muscle contraction, hormone and fluid secretion, mitosis, and ion transfer across cell membranes. Bones are dynamic systems that constantly absorb, reabsorb, and release calcium, and bones serve as a storehouse for calcium. The dynamic balance of calcium in the body is controlled by hormones (Fig. 27-5).

The two major hormones controlling calcium metabolism are PTH and 1,25-dihydroxyvitamin D (i.e., active form of vitamin D) (Fig. 27-6). When plasma calcium concentrations decrease, the parathyroid gland secretes PTH, and calcium from bones is released into the bloodstream. PTH also increases the reabsorption of calcium in the kidneys and intestines. An adult takes in approximately 500 to 1000 mg of calcium daily and excretes the same amount in urine and feces. Dairy products are rich in calcium, as are many leafy green vegetables such as collard greens, turnip greens, and kale.

Clinical Significance

A decreased plasma calcium level is called **hypocalcemia.** Low calcium levels are associated with tetany (i.e., muscle spasms). After pregnancy, women can experience a mild form of tetany during lactation due to the high calcium demands that this condition exerts on the body. Other conditions that cause hypocalcemia include hypoparathyroidism, vitamin D

TABLE 27-1 Laboratory Tests Results for Bone Diseases

Disease	Vitamin D	Alkaline Phosphatase	Calcium	Uric Acid	Phosphorus	Parathyroid Hormone
Osteogenesis imperfecta	Normal	Normal	Normal	Normal	Normal	Normal
Paget disease	Normal	≤10 × normal	Normal	Increased	Normal	Normal
Rickets	Decreased	Increased	Decreased	Normal	Decreased	Normal

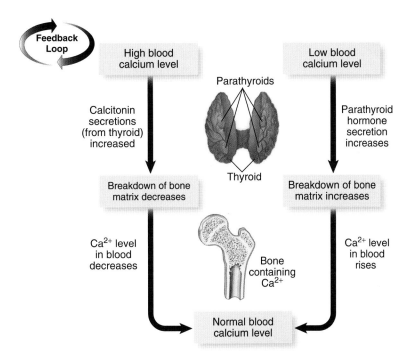

• **Figure 27-5** Parathyroid hormone (PTH) feedback mechanism to maintain calcium homeostasis. (From Patton KT, Thibodeau GA. *Anthony's Textbook of Anatomy and Physiology.* 20th ed. St. Louis: Mosby; 2013.)

deficiency, gastrointestinal malabsorption of calcium or vitamin D, chronic renal failure, and magnesium deficiencies.

An increased plasma calcium level is called **hypercalcemia.** Hypercalcemia is more common in clinical practice than hypocalcemia and can be found in asymptomatic as well as seriously ill patients. Prolonged high calcium levels cause the deposition of insoluble calcium salts in the soft tissues and produce renal calculi. Causes of hypercalcemia include cancer, hyperparathyroidism, vitamin D overdose, excessive use of antacids, Paget disease, and chronic renal disease.

Chronic renal failure can cause hypocalcemia and hypercalcemia. Differentiating hypocalcemia and hypercalcemia caused by chronic renal failure requires serum calcium, phosphate, and ALP test results. PTH levels may also be useful in differentiating the two conditions.

Laboratory Procedures and Limitations

Calcium measurements include total calcium and free (ionized) calcium. Tests for total calcium measure ionized, protein-bound, and complexed calcium in plasma. Ionized calcium measurements provide a better clinical picture by testing for the biologically active calcium molecule. Total calcium, which includes ionized and protein-bound calcium, can be affected by the serum protein level. Most automated instruments perform total calcium assays even though the ionized calcium level provides more clinically useful information. Ionized or free calcium tests must be ordered separately from a routine or total calcium test.

Total Calcium. Total serum calcium is commonly measured with the use of a chelating agent that produces a colored solution that is measured spectrophotometrically. Two common chelating agents are dyes: *o*-cresolphthalein complexone and arsenazo III. The *o*-cresolphthalein complexone method is precise and easy to automate. In the assay for total calcium, the *o*-cresolphthalein complexone solution is maintained at an alkaline pH, which allows the dye to bind to the calcium in the specimen. In addition to the dye, the reagent includes chemicals that

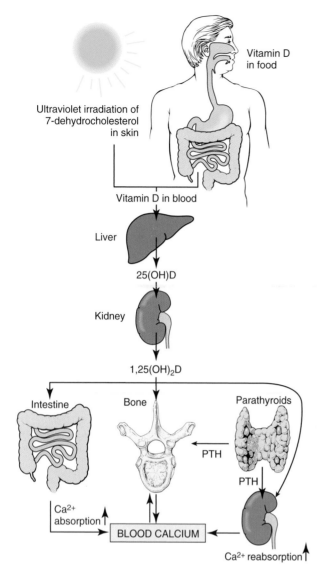

• **Figure 27-6** Vitamin D metabolism and the various pathologic processes that can interfere with it. *PTH,* Parathyroid hormone. (From Damjanov I. *Pathology for the Health Professions.* 4th ed. St. Louis: Saunders; 2012.)

bind magnesium and urea to decrease the amount of interference:

$$Ca^{2+} + o\text{-Cresolphthalein} \xrightarrow{\text{Alkaline pH}} \text{Colored complex}$$

The specimen of choice for calcium testing is serum, but heparinized plasma is acceptable. Tubes containing anticoagulants such as citrate, oxalate, and ethylenediaminetetraacetic acid (EDTA) should not be used for calcium testing because they bind calcium and affect the test results. Serum specimens for calcium testing are stable at 4° C for several days and for several months if stored tightly capped to prevent evaporation and frozen at –20° C. Hemolyzed, icteric, and lipemic samples should not be used for calcium testing because they interfere with the total calcium testing methods.

Ionized Calcium. Ionized calcium provides a better clinical picture than total calcium because ionized calcium is the biologically active portion that acts as an intracellular messenger. One advantage to measuring ionized calcium is that it is not affected by changes in serum albumin concentration. Ionized calcium is measured with the use of a calcium-specific ion-sensitive electrode (ISE). The ISE is a selective membrane that allows calcium ions in a calcium chloride solution to move across the membrane, creating an electrical potential difference. This difference, which can be measured and checked against a reference electrode, is related to the activity of free calcium in the sample.

Ionized calcium analyzers can test samples of serum, plasma, and whole blood. Although the high selectivity of the ISE prevents interference from sodium, potassium, magnesium, lithium, and hydrogen ions, protein deposits on the electrode can enhance the interference of magnesium and lithium.

Because citrates, oxalates, and EDTA bind ionized calcium, they should not be used for sample collection. Heparin may be used for specimens requiring ionized calcium determinations. In addition to anticoagulants, the temperature of the testing environment can affect the electrode and the ability of ionized calcium to bind to proteins. Therefore, most analyzers maintain the sample and testing environment of the ISE at 37° C.

Calcium binding is also affected by the pH of the testing environment. As the pH of the solution increases, the ionization of albumin increases, and more ionized calcium in the specimen binds to albumin, thus lowering the amount of ionized calcium in the specimen. Conversely, if the pH is lowered, less ionized calcium binds with albumin, leading to a falsely elevated ionized calcium level. When uncapped specimens are exposed to air, they become more alkaline due to the loss of carbon dioxide molecules, and this can result in a falsely lower ionized calcium level.

Phosphorus

Approximately 85% of the body's phosphorus is found in insoluble calcium salts in the bones. The remaining 15% exists as phosphate esters in soft tissues. Organic phosphate is found in nucleic acids, phospholipids, phosphoproteins, and high-energy compounds such as adenosine triphosphate (ATP). Nucleic acids are the building blocks of DNA, which provides the blueprint for life. Phospholipids are incorporated into cell membranes, phosphoproteins are enzymes used by hemoglobin to carry oxygen, and ATP is used in all metabolic pathways. All of these compounds are necessary to sustain life.

Because most foods contain phosphorus, supplementation is usually not a concern. Excess absorbed phosphorus is excreted through the kidneys. Because calcium and phosphorus are linked in the bone as calcium phosphate, hormones that affect calcium (i.e., PTH, calcitonin, and vitamin D) also affect phosphate concentrations. For example, if PTH stimulates the kidneys, calcium is reabsorbed, and phosphate is excreted. Because of the inverse relationship between calcium and phosphate concentrations, the phosphate concentration increases whenever the calcium concentration decreases.

Clinical Significance

Hypophosphatemia is a decreased level of phosphate in the blood. The most common mechanism is decreased absorption of phosphate by the kidneys. Hyperparathyroidism, rickets, and some renal diseases can cause decreased absorption of phosphate. Other conditions include prolonged ingestion of antacids, chronic starvation, and malabsorption syndromes, including vomiting and diarrhea. Symptoms of severe hypophosphatemia include neuromuscular disturbances, hemolytic anemia, decreased release of oxygen from hemoglobin, impaired white blood cell and platelet function, and profound muscle weakness. Patients recovering from diabetic ketoacidosis, respiratory alkalosis, acute alcoholism, and serious burns may have severe hypophosphatemia.

Hyperphosphatemia is an increased level of phosphate in the blood. It can be caused by hypocalcemia, bone metastasis, hypoparathyroidism, renal failure, and vitamin D intoxication. Infants and children normally have high phosphate blood levels due to increased levels of growth hormone.

Laboratory Procedures and Limitations

The most common test for phosphorus is the ammonium molybdate method. Phosphorus ions interact with ammonium molybdate in an acidic environment to form a colorless phosphomolybdate complex, which can be measured directly at 340 nm.

$$PO_4 + \text{Ammonium molybdate} \xrightarrow{\text{Acidic pH}}$$
$$\text{Colorless phosphomolybdate complex}$$

A modified method includes reducing the phosphomolybdate complex to a blue phosphomolybdate complex, which can be measured at 600 to 700 nm. The pH of the solution must be tightly controlled because if the solution is less acidic, spontaneous reduction of the phosphomolybdate compound may occur. In either method, the absorbance of the phosphomolybdate complex is directly proportional to the concentration of phosphorus in the specimen. Many automated instruments use the method that measures the complex at 340 nm because of the simplicity, speed, and reagent stability.

The specimen of choice for phosphorus determinations is serum. Anticoagulants such as citrate, oxalate, and EDTA interfere with the testing procedure. For accurate phosphate levels, serum should be separated from the red blood cells as soon as possible after centrifuging. Hemolyzed specimens affect the test results because red blood cells contain high levels of organic phosphate esters. The phosphate concentration of a hemolyzed specimen increases 4 to 5 mg/dL each day the specimen is stored

because the organic phosphate esters are hydrolyzed into inorganic phosphate while in storage.

Icteric or lipemic specimens also interfere with phosphorus testing methods. Because phosphate is a common ingredient in many detergents, glassware used for processing the specimen should be thoroughly rinsed.

Magnesium

Magnesium (Mg^{2+}) has the fourth highest concentration of cations in the body. Most is found in the bones, complexed with calcium and phosphate. The levels of magnesium ions are low in extracellular fluid and almost as high as potassium ions in intracellular fluid. Magnesium exists as 70% ionized and 30% bound to albumin in the extracellular fluid.

The best sources of magnesium are meat and green vegetables. Magnesium is also found in large amounts in avocados, nuts, beans, bananas, and chocolate. Like calcium, magnesium is absorbed in the upper intestines. Calcium requires hormones for absorption, but magnesium does not.

The kidney is responsible for maintaining the magnesium balance. When magnesium levels are low, the kidney resorbs available magnesium, and when the levels are high, the kidney excretes excess magnesium. The detailed mechanism controlling magnesium balance is unknown, but aldosterone appears to play a role because it causes potassium retention and sodium and magnesium excretion.

Many enzymatic reactions in the body require cofactors to carry out a reaction. The cofactor binds to the enzyme but is not considered a substrate. Magnesium acts as a cofactor in more than 350 enzymatic reactions, including phosphorylation, protein synthesis, glycolysis, cell replication, and nucleotide metabolism.

Clinical Significance

Hypomagnesemia is a fairly common condition in which magnesium levels are decreased. Vomiting and diarrhea increase magnesium losses and result in hypomagnesemia. Many patients in intensive care units have hypomagnesemia due to prolonged fluid therapy with fluids that do not contain magnesium supplementation. Other clinically important causes include diuretics, renal diseases, diabetes mellitus, and alcoholism.

Low magnesium levels usually result from a disease or therapy. Symptoms of the primary disease can mask the symptoms of hypomagnesemia. For example, low magnesium levels can cause tetany, but low calcium levels can also cause tetany. Magnesium deficiency is a leading cause of hypocalcemia. Hypomagnesemia can cause tachycardia and fibrillation if left untreated.

Hypermagnesemia is a rare condition in which magnesium levels are increased. Most cases result from excess intake of magnesium salts, which can be used to relieve constipation. Mothers and neonates can exhibit hypermagnesemia after treatment with magnesium for preeclampsia or eclampsia. Other causes of hypermagnesemia include renal diseases, severe dehydration, and aldosterone deficiencies.

The most common symptoms of hypermagnesemia are neuromuscular. Muscles are paralyzed, deep tendon reflexes disappear, and breathing may slow down and even stop. When the heart muscle becomes paralyzed, cardiac arrest results. Because high plasma magnesium levels decrease PTH secretion, hypocalcemia also results.

Laboratory Procedures and Limitations

Heparinized plasma and serum are the specimens of choice. Citrate, oxalates, and EDTA anticoagulants should not be used because they form complexes with the magnesium in the solution and decrease the test results. Serum separator tubes are used for this test, or the serum is removed as soon as possible from the red blood cells, because the cells leak magnesium into the serum and cause falsely elevated test results. Hemolyzed specimens also cause falsely elevated test results.

The calmagite colorimetric method is commonly used to determine magnesium levels. Serum is mixed with calmagite (blue) in an alkaline medium to form a red complex that is measured at 532 nm. As with most colorimetric methods, the color is directly proportional to the amount of magnesium in the sample.

$$Mg^{2+} + Calmagite \xrightarrow{\text{Alkaline medium}} Red\ complex$$

Normal Anatomy and Physiology of Joints

Joints are places where two bones meet (Fig. 27-7). Fibrous joints connect bones by bundles of collagen fibers, and they allow no movement. These joints are found, for example, in the sutures of the skull and the peg and socket joints of teeth.

Cartilaginous joints are found in the spinal column (i.e., intervertebral joints), in the pubic symphysis, and between the first rib and the sternum. The bones are joined together by cartilage, allowing slight movement between them.

Synovial joints allow the greatest amount of movement and are found in the knee, elbow, shoulder, wrist, and hip. Synovial joints contain a space called the synovial cavity between the bones that allows free movement. The cavity is connected by a sheath of fibrous tissue and lined by a fibrous synovial membrane; this membrane contains secretory cells that secrete a thick synovial fluid, which lubricates the joint and decreases friction. The bones are usually bound together by fibrous straps called *ligaments.* The synovial joint has saclike structures call bursae that are filled with fluid and further ensure smooth movement.

Joint Diseases

Osteoarthritis

Joints are susceptible to injury because they tend to be unstable. Osteoarthritis is the most common form of arthritis.

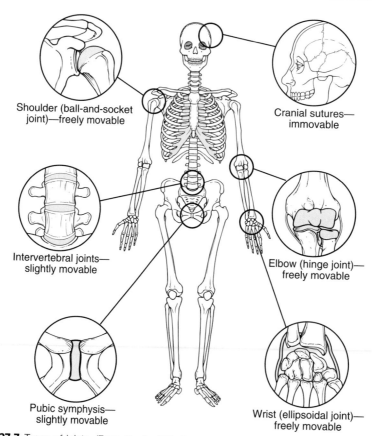

Shoulder (ball-and-socket joint)—freely movable

Cranial sutures—immovable

Intervertebral joints—slightly movable

Elbow (hinge joint)—freely movable

Pubic symphysis—slightly movable

Wrist (ellipsoidal joint)—freely movable

• **Figure 27-7** Types of joints. (From Frazier MS, Drzymkowski JW. *Essential of Human Diseases and Conditions.* 5th ed. St. Louis: Saunders, 2013.)

It results from mechanical wear and tear on the joint that leads to degeneration of cartilage and bone. The prevalence of osteoarthritis increases with each decade of life, presumably because of joint wear. Osteoarthritis affects weight-bearing joints such as the hips, knees, and spine. Obesity can cause osteoarthritis in the hip and knee joints because of the extra stress it exerts on those joints.

Osteoarthritis is diagnosed clinically with the use of radiographs. Laboratory test results are usually within reference ranges and do not help diagnose this condition (Fig. 27-8).

Rheumatoid Arthritis

Rheumatoid arthritis (RA) is a chronic, systemic, autoimmune disease that causes inflammation, deformity, and immobility of synovial joints, especially in the fingers, wrists, feet, and ankles. Rheumatoid arthritis occurs more often in women than in men.

Although the cause is unknown, some researchers think that the Epstein-Barr virus triggers a T-lymphocyte autoimmune reaction against the synovial membrane. The disease process involves the growth of blood vessels and fibrous tissue into the synovium and joint cartilage. A highly vascular, inflamed membrane (i.e., pannus) forms over the cartilage and releases destructive enzymes that dissolve the cartilage in the joint (Fig. 27-9).

Diagnostic laboratory tests for RA include C-reactive protein (CRP), complete blood count (CBC), rheumatoid factor (RF), erythrocyte sedimentation rate (ESR), anti–cyclic citrullinated peptide (anti-CCP), and anti–mutated citrullinated vimentin (anti-MCV) assays. The ESR and CRP levels are elevated in this disease, and the CRP level increases as the disease progresses. Many people with RA also have anemia from the disease process or the medications used to treat it. Disease activity corresponds to the severity of anemia, which can be reversed with therapy.

The most specific tests for RA are the autoantibody tests. The RF test is not specific for RA because it is also elevated in connective tissue diseases, infections, and other autoimmune disorders. RF levels can fluctuate with disease activity, but they tend to remain high even during drug-induced remissions. RF levels predict progression of bone erosions.

Anti-CCP and anti-MCV levels are used to diagnose RA. Elevated anti-CCP levels in conjunction with an elevated RF level are specific for RA. The finding of both antibodies indicates a worse prognosis. RF is detected by latex agglutination or immunoturbidimetric tests. Anti-CCP and anti-MCV are measured by enzyme-linked immunoassay (ELISA) methods.

Ankylosing Spondylitis

Ankylosing spondylitis is one of many spondyloarthropathies. It is a chronic, systemic, inflammatory condition that affects the sacroiliac joints and the axial skeletal. Symptoms appear before 40 years of age and persist for longer than 3 months. Pain is worse in the morning or with inactivity and improves with activity. Symptoms include slow onset of low back pain, kyphosis, fatigue, uveitis, cardiovascular disease, pulmonary disease, renal disease, gastrointestinal disease, neurologic disease, and metabolic bone disease (Fig. 27-10).

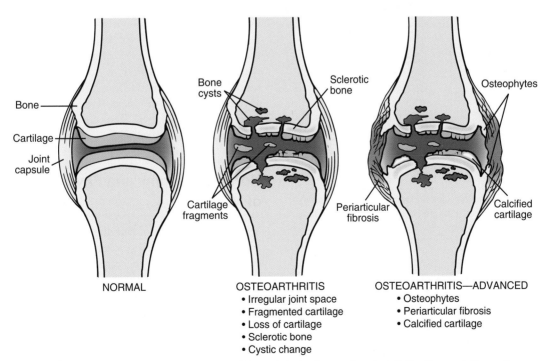

• **Figure 27-8** Schematic representation of the pathologic changes in osteoarthritis. Fragmentation and loss of cartilage denude the subchondral bone, which undergoes sclerosis and cystic change. Osteophytes form on the lateral sides and protrude into the adjacent soft tissues, causing irritation, inflammation, and fibrosis. (From Damjanov I. *Pathology for the Health Professions.* 4th ed. St. Louis: Saunders; 2012.)

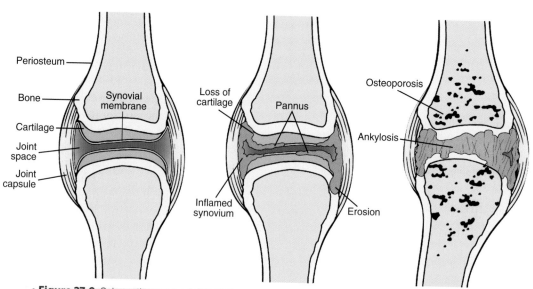

• **Figure 27-9** Schematic representation of the pathologic changes in rheumatoid arthritis. Inflammation (i.e., synovitis) leads to pannus formation, obliteration of the articular space, and ankylosis. The periarticular bone has disuse atrophy in the form of osteoporosis. (From Damjanov I. *Pathology for the Health Professions.* 4th ed. St. Louis: Saunders; 2012.)

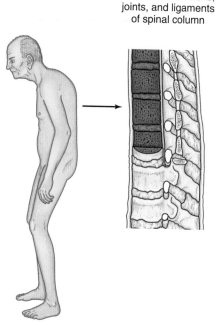

• **Figure 27-10** Characteristic posture and primary pathologic sites of inflammation and damage caused by ankylosing spondylitis. (McCance KL, Huether SE. *Pathophysiology: The Biologic Basis for Disease in Adults and Children.* 7th ed. St. Louis: Mosby; 2015.)

The diagnosis is supported by detection of human leukocyte antigen B27 (HLA-B27); 92% of white patients with ankylosing spondylitis are positive for HLA-B27. However, HLA-B27 is not required, because the diagnosis is based on clinical criteria and radiologic findings.

Gout

Gout is an arthritic condition in which monosodium urate monohydrate crystals are deposited in joints. The crystals are long and thin and have pointed ends. Individuals with gout produce too much uric acid or are unable to clear excess uric acid from the body (Fig. 27-11).

Symptoms include episodes of intense pain, warmth, swelling, redness, and tenderness. Gout most often affects the big toe joint. The knees, fingers, wrists, and ankles can also be affected. Usually, only one joint at a time is affected, but several joints can be affected at the same time. The attacks begin without warning and can last for 8 to 12 hours. If joints affected by gout are not treated, chronic degenerative arthritis can result.

Gout is best diagnosed by aspirating joint fluid from the affected joint and performing a synovial fluid analysis, which uses polarized light to identify monosodium urate monohydrate crystals. Although 90% of gout patients have an elevated serum uric acid level, gout can occur despite a normal uric acid level. Tests for uric acid are detailed in Chapter 24 and Table 27-2.

Normal Anatomy and Physiology of Muscles

Muscle is composed of bundles of contractible fibers connected to motor nerves. Skeletal muscle cells and their motor nerves cannot be regenerated. The motor nerves transmit signals to muscle fibers down an axon and through a synapse. Signals progress down nerve axons as waves of electrical disturbance in the cell membrane. The signal stimulates the release of a neurotransmitter (i.e., acetylcholine), which signals the muscle fiber to contract (Fig. 27-12).

Healthy muscles require an adequate blood supply and healthy nerves. Loss of a nerve supply leads to neurogenic **atrophy,** which occurs most frequently in diabetics. Nerve diseases and nerve trauma can also cause neurogenic atrophy.

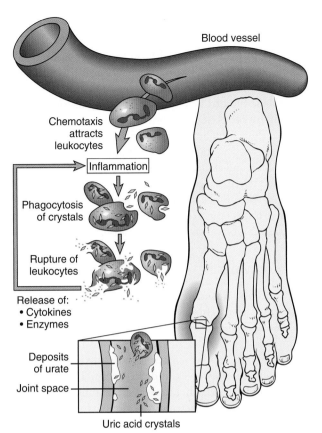

• **Figure 27-11** In gouty arthritis, deposits of uric acid crystals in the connective tissue have a chemotactic effect and cause exudation of leukocytes into the joint. Inflammation most often affects the metatarsophalangeal joint of the big toe. (From Damjanov I. *Pathology for the Health Professions.* 4th ed. St. Louis: Saunders; 2012.)

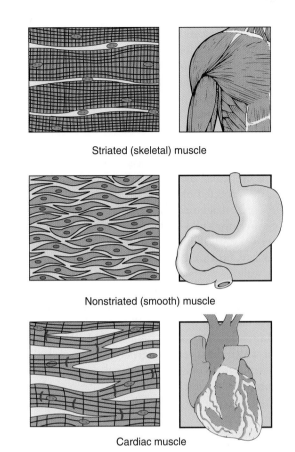

• **Figure 27-12** Types of muscles. (From Frazier MS, Drzymkowski JW. *Essentials of Human Diseases and Conditions.* 5th ed. St. Louis: Saunders; 2013.)

TABLE 27-2	**Laboratory Results for Joint Diseases**							
Disease	Comprehensive Metabolic Panel	HLA-B27	C-Reactive Protein	Rheumatoid Factor	Anti-CCP	Anti-MCV	Uric Acid	ESR
Osteoarthritis	Normal	Negative	Normal	Negative	Negative	Negative	Normal	Normal
Rheumatoid arthritis	Normal	Negative	Positive	Positive	Positive	Positive	Normal	Increased
Ankylosing spondylitis	Normal	Positive	Negative	Negative	Negative	Negative	Negative	Negative
Gout	Normal	Negative	Negative	Negative	Negative	Negative	Increased	Normal

anti-CCP, Anti–cyclic citrullinated peptide; *anti-MCV,* anti–mutated citrullinated vimentin; *ESR,* erythrocyte sedimentation rate; *HLA-B27,* human leukocyte antigen B27.

Muscle Diseases

Duchenne Muscular Dystrophy

The muscular dystrophies are a group of inherited, muscle-wasting diseases that affect skeletal and cardiac muscles. All types of muscular dystrophy produce progressive muscle weakness that eventually compromises the ability to walk, breathe, and pump blood. Progressive muscle weakness may also cause soft tissue contractures and spinal deformities. The disease compromises the ability to function and shortens life. After patients become wheelchair bound, they tend to rapidly develop progressive scoliosis, which reduces lung capacity and can be fatal.

Duchenne muscular dystrophy is the most common and most severe form of muscular dystrophy. It is an X-linked disease, and most of those who develop the disease are male. Individuals who inherit the defective gene cannot produce dystrophin, a protein normally found in muscles and some other tissues. Without dystrophin, muscle fibers atrophy and die.

The weakness of Duchenne muscular dystrophy occurs mainly in the pelvic and shoulder muscles. Infants with Duchenne muscular dystrophy appear to be normal and may not be suspected of having the disease unless a sibling was previously diagnosed with it. Muscle weakness is not apparent until the child begins to walk. Children with this disease may delay walking due to muscle weakness, and they may also have intellectual impairment that can affect the ability to walk. At age 5 years, children struggle with school-related activities such as climbing stairs and playing at recess (Fig. 27-13). As the disease progresses, children fall often and have a hard time getting up from a sitting or lying posture. Some children become wheelchair bound by 6 years of age, after which the disease progresses more rapidly. Duchenne muscular dystrophy is a terminal disease, and death usually occurs before the age of 30.

The most specific test available for diagnosing Duchenne muscular dystrophy is a creatine kinase (CK) assay. CK levels are elevated in muscle diseases, especially muscular dystrophy. CK levels are 50 to 300 times higher than reference ranges in the early stages of the disease. As muscle mass decreases, the CK level also decreases. Polymerase chain reaction (PCR) testing for the dystrophin gene helps in diagnosing the disease.

Becker Muscular Dystrophy

Becker muscular dystrophy, a milder form of the disease, was first described in 1955. Duchenne and Becker muscular dystrophies are caused by different mutations in the same gene *(DMD)* on the X chromosome that produces the protein dystrophin, which normally stabilizes and protects muscle fibers.

Those with Becker muscular dystrophy display symptoms later than individuals with Duchenne muscular dystrophy. Many men affected with Becker muscular dystrophy continue to walk after 15 to 20 years. Individuals with subclinical disease may have dilated cardiomyopathy, which may provide the first clue to the underlying disease.

Laboratory tests that may be helpful in diagnosing Becker muscular dystrophy include dystrophin gene deletion analysis, muscle biopsy, and assays of CK, aspartate aminotransferase (AST), and alanine aminotransferase (ALT). CK levels are moderately to severely elevated (i.e., 5 to 100 times the upper reference range value). The dystrophin gene analysis is positive for the mutation in about 98% of cases. AST and ALT levels can be elevated in this disease.

Rhabdomyolysis

Rhabdomyolysis causes rapid destruction of skeletal muscle cells. It often results from muscle injury and the consequent release of large quantities of myoglobin, which can be toxic. The disease was first described in World War II in victims of crush injuries. Other causes include medications, heatstroke, metabolic disorders, and alcohol and illicit drug use.

Symptoms include muscle weakness, muscle pain, and dark urine caused by excreted myoglobin. Life-threatening complications include renal failure and disseminated intravascular coagulation (DIC). Other complications include electrolyte abnormalities and hypoalbuminemia.

Laboratory tests that are helpful in diagnosing rhabdomyolysis include CK levels (i.e., elevations of 4 to 5 times the upper reference range values). Urine myoglobin detection can also be helpful.

Myasthenia Gravis

Myasthenia gravis is an autoimmune disease caused by the formation of antibodies against acetylcholine nicotinic postsynaptic receptors at the neuromuscular junction of skeletal muscles. This prohibits impulses from the brain from reaching muscles, causing the muscles to cease functioning.

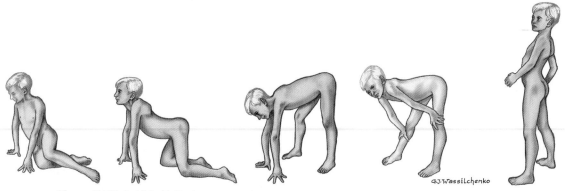

• **Figure 27-13** A child with Duchenne muscular dystrophy attains standing posture by kneeling and then gradually pushing his torso upright (with knees straight) by "walking" his hands up his legs (i.e., Gower sign). Notice the marked lordosis in an upright position. (From Hockenberry M, Wilson D. *Wong's Essentials of Pediatric Nursing.* 9th ed. St. Louis: Mosby; 2013.)

Symptoms include specific muscle weakness and extraocular muscle weakness. Muscle weakness tends to grow worse throughout the day. The weakness is progressive, and approximately 13 months after onset the disease becomes generalized. Symptoms are exacerbated by bright sunlight, surgery, immunization, emotional stress, menstruation, and medications.

Myasthenia gravis has five main classes and several subclasses. The anti-acetylcholine receptor test is used for diagnosing the disease. The test is 100% specific, and the result is positive for approximately 90% of individuals with the disease (Fig. 27-14 and Table 27-3).

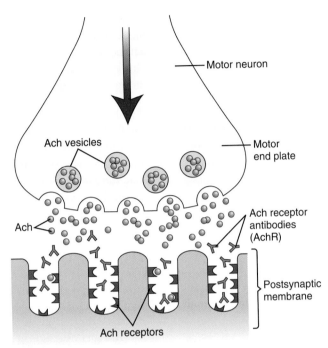

• **Figure 27-14** Antibodies in myasthenia gravis. Acetylcholine receptor antibodies block the acetylcholine receptor (AchR) and inhibit the stimulating effect of acetylcholine on the postsynaptic membrane. (Data from McCance KL, Huether SE. *Pathophysiology: The Biologic Basis for Disease in Adults and Children.* 7th ed. St. Louis: Mosby; 2015; Juel VC, Massey JM. Myasthenia gravis. *Orphanet J Rare Dis.* 200;2:44; Mahadeva B, Phillips LH 2nd, Juel VC. Autoimmune disorders of neuromuscular transmission. *Semin Neurol.* 2008;28:212-227; and Shigemoto K. Myasthenia gravis induced by autoantibodies against MuSK. *Acta Mycol.* 2007;26:185-191.)

TABLE 27-3 Laboratory Test Results for Muscle Diseases

Disease	Anti-acetylcholine Receptor	CK	AST	ALT	Dystrophin Gene Deletion	Myoglobin	Electrolytes	Albumin
Duchenne muscular dystrophy	Negative	50-300 × normal	Normal	Normal	Negative	Negative	Normal	Normal
Becker muscular dystrophy	Negative	5-100 × normal	Increased	Increased	Positive	Negative	Normal	Normal
Rhabdomyolysis	Negative	4-5 × normal	Normal	Normal	Negative	Positive	Abnormal	Decreased
Myasthenia gravis	Positive	Normal	Normal	Normal	Negative	Negative	Normal	Normal

ALT, Alanine aminotransferase; *AST,* aspartate aminotransferase; *CK,* creatine kinase.

Summary

Bones are metabolically active structures that support the body. Diseases that affect the bones include osteogenesis imperfecta, Paget disease, rickets, osteoarthritis, and rheumatoid arthritis. Osteogenesis imperfecta is a disease in which defective collagen is produced, causing fragile bones that easily deform and fracture. Paget disease is common among the elderly. It is characterized by areas of excessive bone resorption that are replaced by excessive, disordered bone that is susceptible to fracture. Rickets is a bone disease in which osteoid does not calcify, resulting in weak bones that are easily deformed. A similar disease diagnosed in adults is called osteomalacia.

Joints are the meeting places of two bones. They can contain a synovial membrane that produces fluid for lubrication. Joint diseases include osteoarthritis, rheumatoid arthritis, ankylosing spondylitis, and gout. Osteoarthritis, which is common among older people, results from the mechanical wear and tear of the joint. Rheumatoid arthritis is an inflammatory disorder of synovial joints. Ankylosing spondylitis is a chronic, systemic, inflammatory condition that affects the sacroiliac joint and axial skeleton before 40 years of age. Gout is an arthritic condition in which monosodium urate monohydrate crystals are deposited in a synovial joint, usually the big toe joint.

Muscles are groups of contractile fibers connected to motor nerves. This type of tissue cannot be regenerated. Healthy muscles require a good blood supply and healthy nerves. Muscle diseases include Duchenne muscular dystrophy, Becker muscular dystrophy, rhabdomyolysis, and myasthenia gravis. Duchenne muscular dystrophy affects children and produces muscle weakness that progresses until the individual is wheelchair bound. Death occurs before 30 years of age. Becker muscular dystrophy is a milder form of muscular dystrophy. Rhabdomyolysis causes rapid destruction of skeletal muscle cells, resulting in the release of large amounts of toxic substances, especially myoglobin, into the circulation. Myasthenia gravis is an autoimmune disease caused by antibodies against acetylcholine nicotinic postsynaptic receptors.

Review Questions

1. In Duchenne muscular dystrophy, which of the following enzymes is elevated to 50 to 300 times normal?
   a. Lactate dehydrogenase
   b. Creatine kinase
   c. AST
   d. Alkaline phosphatase
2. The level of which of the following enzymes is elevated in Paget disease?
   a. Alkaline phosphatase
   b. AST
   c. Creatine kinase
   d. Lactate dehydrogenase
3. Rickets is caused by a deficiency in which of the following compounds?
   a. Cholecalciferol
   b. Calcium
   c. Phosphate
   d. Lactate dehydrogenase
4. Symptoms of which of the following diseases include blue sclerae and brittle bones?
   a. Rickets
   b. Osteogenesis imperfect
   c. Paget disease
   d. Ankylosing spondylosis
5. Which of the following is the cause of neurogenic atrophy?
   a. Loss of blood supply
   b. Muscle wasting
   c. Loss of nerve supply
   d. Imperfect muscle formation
6. Which of the following diseases affects the sacroiliac joints and axial skeleton before age 40?
   a. Myasthenia gravis
   b. Paget disease
   c. Rhabdomyolysis
   d. Ankylosing spondylosis
7. Muscle wasting in which of the following diseases produces myoglobin, a protein that can be toxic to the body?
   a. Myasthenia gravis
   b. Ankylosing spondylosis
   c. Osteogenesis imperfecta
   d. Rhabdomyolysis
8. Which of the following is the cause of osteoarthritis?
   a. Mechanical wear and tear on joints
   b. Systemic inflammation
   c. Deposition of monosodium urate monohydrate crystals in synovial joints
   d. A genetic defect that affects collagen formation
9. Which of the following laboratory test is widely used to diagnose rheumatoid arthritis?
   a. LDH
   b. CK
   c. RF
   d. AST
10. The anti-acetylcholine receptor test is used to help diagnose which of the following diseases?
    a. Ankylosing spondylosis
    b. Myasthenia gravis
    c. Rhabdomyolysis
    d. Osteogenesis imperfecta

Critical Thinking Questions

1. Name the three types of calcium in the body, and describe the function of each type.
2. Which laboratory tests are used to diagnose rheumatoid arthritis, and how do the results correlate with the clinical picture?

3. How does Duchenne muscular dystrophy progress?

CASE STUDY

A 40-year-old woman complains to her provider of shortness of breath. She says that she has been unable to take deep breaths for the past 3 days and that it has been "very hard to breathe today." It seems to be worse later in the day than in the morning. About 5 years ago, she was diagnosed with a "lazy" eye.

The woman's oxygen saturation level is 75%. Her chest does not seem to be expanding well. While the provider is examining the woman, she collapses and stops breathing. She is rushed to the emergency department (ED) and put on oxygen. Because the ED physician is not successful in getting the woman to breathe regularly, she is put on a ventilator. The ED physician orders an anti–acetylcholine receptor test. What disease does the physician suspect this patient has?

Bibliography

Burtis CA, Bruns DE. Disorders of bone and mineral metabolism. In: Burtis CA, Bruns DE, eds. *Tietz Fundamentals of Clinical Chemistry and Molecular Diagnostics*. 7th ed. St. Louis: Saunders; 2015.

Engel AG, ed. *Myasthenia gravis and myasthenic disorders*. New York: Oxford University Press; 2012.

Gartner LM, Greer FR. Prevention of rickets and vitamin D deficiency: new guidelines for vitamin D intake. *Pediatrics*. 2003;111:908–910.

Lioté F, Terkeltaub R. Overview of gout therapy strategy and targets, and the management of refractory disease. In: *Gout and Other Crystal Arthropathies*. Philadelphia: Elsevier Saunders; 2011:194–208.

Mah JK, Korngut L, Dykeman J, et al. A systematic review and meta-analysis on the epidemiology of Duchenne and Becker muscular dystrophy. *Neuromuscul Disord*. 2014;24:482–491.

Niewold TB, Harrison MJ, Paget SA. Anti-CCP antibody testing as a diagnostic and prognostic tool in rheumatoid arthritis. *QJM*. 2007;100:193–201.

Rauch F, Glorieux FH. Osteogenesis imperfecta. *Lancet*. 2004; 363:1377–1385.

Roodman GD, Windle JJ. Paget disease of bone. *J Clin Invest*. 2005; 115:200.

Sieper J, Braun J, Rudwaleit M, Boonen A, Zink A. Ankylosing spondylitis: an overview. *Ann Rheum Dis*. 2002;61(suppl 3):iii8–iii18.

van Ruiten HA, Straub V, Bushby K, Guglieri M. Improving recognition of Duchenne muscular dystrophy: a retrospective case note review. *Arch Dis Child*. 2014;99:1074–1077.

Zutt R, van der Kooi AJ, Linthorst GE, Wanders RJ, de Visser M. Rhabdomyolysis: review of the literature. *Neuromuscul Disord*. 2014;24:651–659.

28

Nervous System Diseases

DONNA LARSON

CHAPTER OUTLINE

OBJECTIVES

After completion of this chapter, the reader will be able to:

1. Describe the central, peripheral, and autonomic nervous systems.
2. Diagram a neuron.
3. Describe developmental errors and the resulting nervous system diseases.
4. Compare and contrast subdural hematoma, epidural hematoma, and subarachnoid hemorrhage.
5. Explain the difference between meningitis and encephalitis.
6. Differentiate dementia, Alzheimer disease, and Parkinson disease.
7. Explain the difference between amyotropic lateral sclerosis and multiple sclerosis.
8. Describe peripheral neuropathy.
9. Describe Guillain-Barré syndrome.
10. Describe the collection and testing procedure for cerebrospinal fluid.
11. List the diseases and disorders that can be identified by CSF testing.

KEY TERMS

Alzheimer disease
Amyotrophic lateral sclerosis
Anencephaly
Cerebral palsy
Closed neural tube defects
Creutzfeldt-Jakob disease
Dementia

Encephalitis
Epidural hematoma
Guillain-Barré syndrome
Hydrocephalus
Meningitis
Multiple sclerosis
Neural tube defects

Open neural tube defects
Parkinson disease
Peripheral neuropathy
Spina bifida
Spongiform encephalopathy
Subarachnoid hemorrhage
Subdural hematoma

❖ Case in Point

A 25-year-old woman visits her provider because she has had blurred vision, fatigue, poor concentration, and speech issues spanning a 2-week period. It seems to be resolving but has not gone away. During the next 3 months, she has other unusual symptoms, including fatigue, weakness in her right arm, and muscles spasms in her fingers. Her provider treats the symptoms. When muscle weakness in her leg, spasms in her foot, and general weakness occur at 6 months, her provider decides to do an in-depth workup.

Her laboratory results are as follows: glucose, 98 g/dL; blood urea nitrogen (BUN), 20 mg/dL; creatinine, 0.72 mg/dL; sodium, 139 mEq/L; potassium, 4.5 mEq/L; chloride, 106 mEq/L; carbon dioxide, 26 mg/dL; phosphorus, 2.5 mg/dL; calcium, 9.8 mg/dL; total protein, 6.6 g/L; albumin, 4.2 g/L; alkaline phosphatase, 224 IU/L; lactate dehydrogenase, 178 IU/L; creatine kinase, 42 IU/L; aspartate aminotransferase, 16 IU/L; alanine aminotransferase, 16 IU/L; total cholesterol, 188 mg/dL; triglycerides, 167 mg/d; high-density lipoprotein cholesterol, 52 mg/dL.

Serum protein electrophoresis showed the following result:

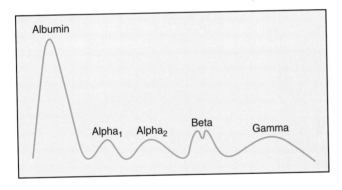

Cerebrospinal fluid (CSF) electrophoresis produced the following result:

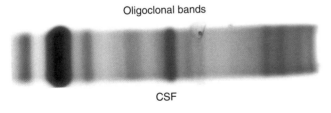

What disease is the provider probably looking for? What is the mechanism for this disease?

Points to Remember

- Nervous system diseases affect the central, peripheral, and autonomic nervous systems.
- Many nervous system diseases are progressive and chronic.
- Neural tube defects include spina bifida and hydrocephalus.
- Cerebral palsy results from a brain injury that occurs before age 2 years.
- An epidural hematoma is bleeding on the surface of the brain that is caused by a skull fracture that tears a meningeal artery
- A subdural hematoma is bleeding from a vein under the dura mater caused by a head injury that is not severe enough to cause a skull fracture.
- A subarachnoid hemorrhage is sudden, spontaneous bleeding into the subarachnoid space and usually is not associated with trauma.
- Meningitis is an infection of the meninges that usually is bacterial.
- Encephalitis is an infection of the brain caused by a virus in previously healthy individuals.
- Dementia is an abnormal, chronic, progressive disease caused by neurodegenerative and vascular diseases.
- Alzheimer disease is a form of dementia caused by amyloid deposits on the brain.
- Parkinson disease is characterized by a tremor and is caused by faulty nerve signal transmission due to a lack of dopamine, a neurotransmitter.
- Amyotrophic lateral sclerosis (ALS) is a degenerative condition affecting motor neurons. Lou Gehrig and Steven Hawking were diagnosed with this disease.
- Multiple sclerosis is a disease in which the myelin sheaths on axons are destroyed, preventing conduction of nerve impulses.
- Peripheral nerve disease is caused by other diseases, such as diabetes, that impair nerve function in the limbs.
- Guillain-Barré syndrome is a nervous system disorder that is usually temporary and is caused by the production of an autoantibody against nerve cells after immunization.
- Many nervous system diseases are diagnosed clinically, and laboratory test results are used for confirmation by ruling out other conditions.

Introduction

The nervous system is complex, and it controls many body functions. Nervous system disorders can result from impaired development, birth trauma, degenerative processes, deposition of abnormal proteins in the brain, ruptured arteries, infections, and routine immunizations. Many disorders affect the nervous system, including open neural tube defects, closed neural tube defects, spina bifida, cerebral palsy, hydrocephalus, epidural hematoma, subdural hematoma, subarachnoid hemorrhage, meningitis, encephalitis, Creutzfeldt-Jakob disease, spongiform encephalopathy, dementia, Alzheimer disease, Parkinson disease, amyotrophic lateral sclerosis, multiple sclerosis, peripheral neuropathy, and Guillain-Barré syndrome (GBS).

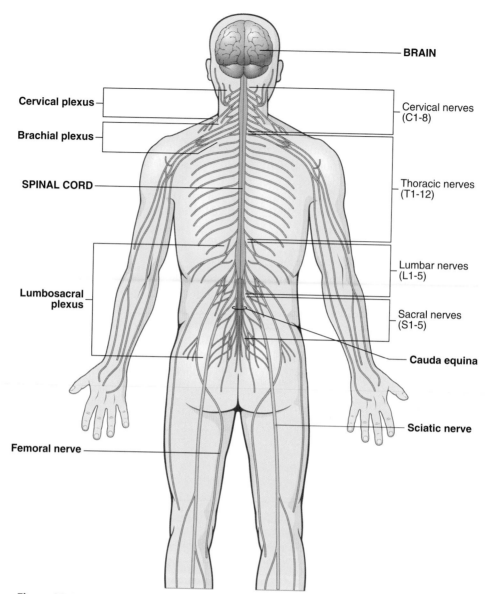

BRAIN

Cervical plexus

Brachial plexus

SPINAL CORD

Lumbosacral plexus

Femoral nerve

Cervical nerves (C1-8)

Thoracic nerves (T1-12)

Lumbar nerves (L1-5)

Sacral nerves (S1-5)

Cauda equina

Sciatic nerve

• **Figure 28-1** The human nervous system. (From Chabner DE. *The Language of Medicine.* 10th ed. St. Louis: Saunders; 2014.)

Nervous System Anatomy and Physiology

The human nervous system has three main parts, the central, peripheral, and autonomic nervous systems. The *central* nervous system (CNS) consists of the brain and the spinal cord. The *peripheral* nervous system consists of sensory neurons that carry signals (e.g., sight, smell) to the CNS and motor neurons that carry signals from the CNS to muscles and glands. The *autonomic* nervous system controls the heart, intestines, endocrine glands, and other involuntary functions (Fig. 28-1).

The brain and spinal cord are covered by three layers of membranes, called the *meninges* (Fig. 28-2). The outer layer is the dura mater, the middle layer is the arachnoid, and the inner layer (closest to nerve tissue) is the pia mater. The dura mater is thick, fibrous tissue that lines the skull and surrounds the spinal cord. In the CNS, the subarachnoid space is the interval

between the arachnoid membrane and pia mater. It contains major arteries and channels with cerebrospinal fluid (CSF).

CSF is found throughout the CNS, including the ventricles of the brain. The normal adult has 150 mL of CSF in the brain and spinal cord and produces approximately 500 mL per day. CSF functions as a cushion for the brain while maintaining a controlled chemical environment. It contains the nutrients needed by and transports waste products away from the CNS. The various CNS coverings selectively allow substances to cross the blood–brain barrier. The blood–brain barrier keeps most harmful substances away from the brain. Abnormal findings in CSF analysis reflect damage to the blood–brain barrier. Neurons and nodular collections of neurons (i.e., ganglia) are found in the gray matter of the brain. Bundles of axons make up the brain's white matter.

The peripheral nervous system is composed of 12 pairs of cranial nerves and 31 pairs of spinal nerves. The nerves carry

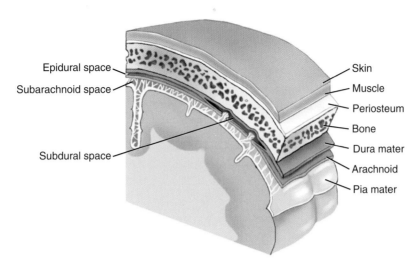

• **Figure 28-2** The brain and the spinal cord are covered by three protective membranes, collectively called meninges. The outer membrane is the dura mater, the middle layer is the arachnoid, and the inner membrane is the pia mater. (From VanMeter K, Hubert R. *Microbiology for the Healthcare Professional*, St. Louis: Elsevier; 2010.)

incoming sensory and outgoing motor signals between the CNS and tissues.

The autonomic nervous system contains nerves that control involuntary processes of cardiac muscle, smooth muscle, and glands. The sympathetic and parasympathetic nervous systems are subdivisions of the autonomic system. The sympathetic nervous system originates in the thoracic and lumbar spinal nerves. It stimulates the adrenal medulla to produce epinephrine and norepinephrine (i.e., fight or flight response). The parasympathetic system originates in the brain and sacral spinal cord. It releases acetylcholine, which reverses the fight or flight response.

Neurons, which conduct impulses throughout the body, consist of an axon, a body, and dendrites. Nerve fibers are insulated by a sheath of myelin, a mixture of proteins and phospholipids that increase the speed of impulse conduction (Fig. 28-3). Neurons are sensitive to very low oxygen and glucose levels.

Nervous System Diseases

Diseases can involve the CNS, peripheral nervous system, and autonomic nervous system. Disorders include neural tube defects, cerebral palsy, hydrocephalus, epidural hematoma, subdural hematoma, subarachnoid hemorrhage, meningitis, brain abscess, encephalitis, Creutzfeldt-Jakob, dementia, Alzheimer disease, Parkinson disease, amyotrophic lateral sclerosis, multiple sclerosis, cretinism, neuronal storage diseases, and GBS.

Neural Tube Defects

Neural tube defects occur in utero and are the result of defective closure of neuropores. Because the anterior and posterior neuropores close last, they are most likely to be affected by defects, and most neural tube defects occur in these areas.

The most severe neural tube defect is anencephaly, in which the skull fails to develop, and the exposed brain dies in utero.

Neural tube defects can be open or closed. Open neural tube defects, such as hydrocephalus, usually involve the entire CNS. In these disorders, the neural tissue is exposed, and CSF leaks out. Open neural tube defects are usually apparent at birth.

Closed neural tube defects are confined to one area and usually involve only the spine. Spinal presentations include spina bifida. Closed neural tube defects commonly manifest as an abnormality along the spine, such as a fluid-filled cyst, area of hypopigmentation or hyperpigmentation, capillary telangiectasia or hemangioma, hairy patch, skin appendage, or an asymmetric gluteal cleft (Fig. 28-4). The neural tube is not visible at birth.

An α-fetoprotein measurement is performed at 15 to 20 weeks' gestation to detect neural tube defects. The procedure and the interpretation of the test results are discussed in Chapter 26.

Cerebral Palsy

Cerebral palsy is characterized by permanent motor dysfunction such as uncontrollable movements, lack of coordination, spasticity, and paralysis. It is usually caused by a brain injury before 2 years of age. Brain injuries result from prenatal conditions, birth trauma, premature birth, low birth weight, intrauterine growth retardation, and postnatal injuries.

Symptoms include motor development delay during the first year of life. The most common symptom in children is abnormal muscle tone. They have difficulty crawling and fail to thrive.

Laboratory tests are ordered to rule out other diagnoses. The diagnosis of cerebral palsy is usually based on the clinical picture.

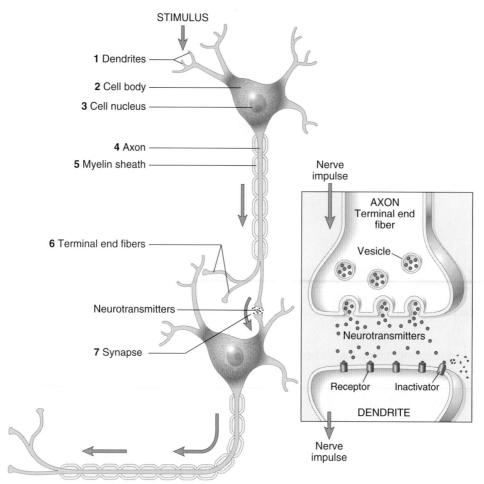

• **Figure 28-3** Structure of a typical neuron. Neurons are the parenchymal (essential) cells of the nervous system. The inset shows what happens in a synapse: Vesicles store neurotransmitters in the terminal end fibers of axons. Receptors on the dendrites bind the neurotransmitters released across the synapse. Inactivators end the activity of neurotransmitters after they have finished their job. (From Chabner DE. *The Language of Medicine.* 10th ed. St. Louis: Saunders; 2014.)

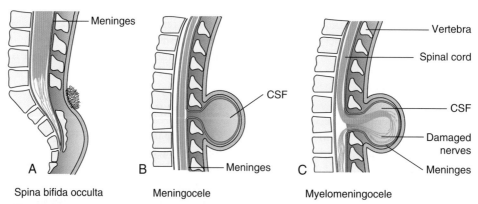

• **Figure 28-4** Closed neural tube defects. **A,** Spina bifida. **B,** Meningocele. **C,** Myelomeningocele. *CSF,* Cerebrospinal fluid. (From VanMeter K, Hubert R. *Gould's Pathophysiology for the Health Professions.* 5th ed. St. Louis: Saunders; 2015.)

Hydrocephalus

Hydrocephalus is a hydrodynamic disorder characterized by disturbance of CSF flow, formation, or absorption (Fig. 28-5). Defective CSF distribution leads to increased volume occupied by the CSF in the CNS. Symptoms in infants include poor feeding, irritability, reduced activity, and vomiting. Symptoms seen in children and adults include cognitive deterioration, headaches, neck pain, vomiting, blurred vision, drowsiness, and difficulty walking. A

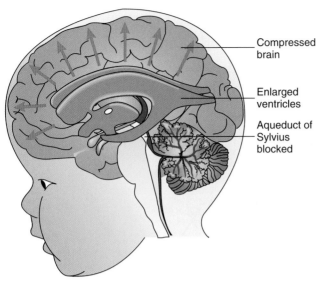

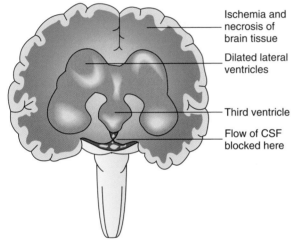

Compressed brain

Enlarged ventricles

Aqueduct of Sylvius blocked

Ischemia and necrosis of brain tissue

Dilated lateral ventricles

Third ventricle

Flow of CSF blocked here

• **Figure 28-5** Hydrocephalus. *CSF,* Cerebrospinal fluid. (From Van-Meter K, Hubert R. *Gould's Pathophysiology for the Health Professions.* 5th ed. St. Louis: Saunders; 2015.)

characteristic symptom is magnetic gait, in which the feet remain "stuck to the floor" despite the individual's efforts to lift them off the ground. Dementia can also be a symptom of this disorder. No specific blood tests are recommended for diagnosis.

Epidural Hematoma

Epidural hematoma is an accumulation of blood in the space between the dura mater and the bone. Intracranial epidural hematoma occurs in individuals with head injuries, and it is considered a medical emergency that requires immediate surgery. Epidural hematomas can also occur in the spinal cord.

Clinical chemistry tests ordered for this condition include assays for electrolytes, blood urea nitrogen (BUN), creatinine, and glucose; a toxicology screen; and a serum alcohol level. Other diagnostic laboratory tests include a complete blood count, prothrombin time, activated partial thromboplastin time, and type and hold of an appropriate number of units of blood.

Subdural Hematoma

A subdural hematoma is bleeding into the space beneath the dura mater and above the arachnoid membrane. It is the most common type of traumatic lesion. It usually results from a trauma that is not severe enough to cause a skull fracture. Bleeding is very slow, and individuals can lapse into a coma. The condition can lead to delayed brain damage.

The diagnosis is usually accomplished with a computed tomography (CT) scan. Blood tests are useful for detecting electrolyte abnormalities, coagulopathies, and low platelet counts. Identifying electrolyte abnormalities is important because hyponatremia can exacerbate brain edema and cause seizures.

Subarachnoid Hemorrhage

A subarachnoid hemorrhage is bleeding into the subarachnoid space in the brain. It can be caused by trauma, a ruptured cerebral aneurysm, or an arteriovenous malformation. Symptoms are nonspecific and include headache, dizziness, orbital pain, diplopia, visual loss, sensory or motor disturbance, seizures, and dysphasia. Symptom onset may be sudden.

The condition is diagnosed clinically and confirmed with a CT scan or lumbar puncture, or both. Useful laboratory tests include a chemistry panel, complete blood count, prothrombin time, activated partial thromboplastin time, type and screen of blood, assay of cardiac enzymes (especially troponin), and arterial blood gas determination. Troponin levels in individuals with a subarachnoid hemorrhage correlate well with neurologic complications and outcomes (Fig. 28-6).

Meningitis

Meningitis is a clinical syndrome involving inflammation of the meninges caused by an infection (Fig. 28-7). Bacterial meningitis is caused by bacteria such as *Escherichia coli, Haemophilus influenza, Streptococcus pneumoniae,* and *Neisseria meningitidis.* It is usually purulent, producing pus on the surface of the brain and in the CSF. Viruses can also cause meningitis, but no pus is produced in viral meningitis, which is sometimes called aseptic meningitis. Other causative organisms include acid-fast bacilli (AFB), spirochete bacteria (e.g., syphilis), parasites, and fungi.

Classic symptoms of meningitis include fever, headache, and neck stiffness. Other symptoms include nausea, vomiting, sleepiness, confusion, irritability, delirium, and coma. Routine clinical chemistry tests for suspected meningitis include electrolyte levels, glucose level, BUN, creatinine level, and a liver profile. Additional tests include serum syphilis testing (e.g., fluorescent treponemal antibody absorption test [FTA-ABS]; *Treponema pallidum* hemagglutination assay [TPHA]; microhemagglutination assay for *T. pallidum* [MHA-TP]) and CSF analysis.

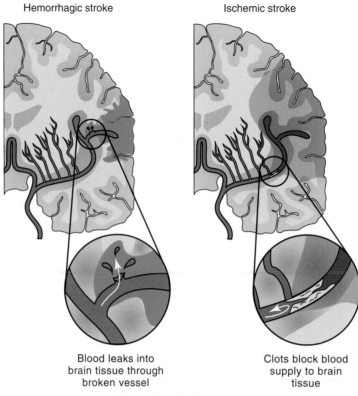

Hemorrhagic stroke

Ischemic stroke

Blood leaks into
brain tissue through
broken vessel

Clots block blood
supply to brain
tissue

• **Figure 28-6** Effects of a stroke.

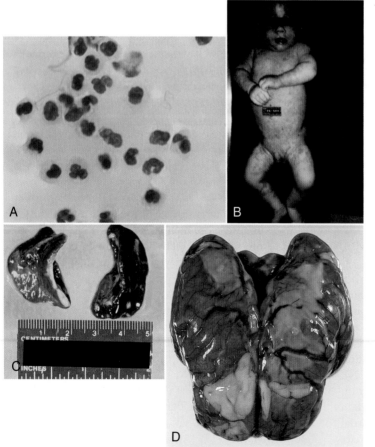

• **Figure 28-7 A,** Slide preparation of cerebrospinal fluid
shows many neutrophils in a case of bacterial meningitis.
B, Petechial rash associated with meningococcemia. **C,**
Hemorrhage *(dark areas)* in the adrenal glands in Water-
house-Friderichsen syndrome. **D,** Meningitis due to coliform
microorganisms. The meninges are reddened from vascular
congestion. Thick, greenish pus fills the subarachnoid space
over both hemispheres. (A, From Stevens ML. *Fundamentals of Clinical Hematology,* Philadelphia: Saunders; 1997; B
and C, from Mahon CR, Manuselis G. *Textbook of Diagnostic
Microbiology.* 2nd ed. Philadelphia: Saunders; 2000; D, from
Cooke RA, Stewart B: *Colour Atlas of Anatomical Pathology.*
3rd ed. Sydney: Churchill Livingstone, 2004.)

Encephalitis

Encephalitis is a viral infection of the brain. Causes include varicella-zoster, Epstein-Barr, cytomegalovirus, measles, mumps, St. Louis, Western equine, Eastern equine, and West Nile viruses. The classic presentation includes fever, headache, neck pain, nausea, vomiting, behavioral and personality changes, lethargy, seizures, movement disorders, and flaccid paralysis.

Routine laboratory tests are performed, including determination of urine electrolyte levels and a urine or serum toxicology screen. Suspected cases of encephalitis should have a CSF analysis performed. CSF glucose and protein concentrations are helpful in diagnosing this disease. Brain biopsy is the definitive diagnostic tool.

Creutzfeldt-Jakob Disease

Creutzfeldt-Jakob disease is a rare CNS disease caused by prions. It is a transmissible **spongiform encephalopathy**. Prion infection creates large, open spaces (i.e., holes) in infected brains, causing the brain to resemble a sponge. Characteristic symptoms include rapidly progressive dementia. Initially, individuals infected with this disease experience muscular coordination problems, impaired memory, impaired vision, insomnia, and depression. As the disease progresses, severe mental impairment ensues, and many people develop involuntary muscle jerks and blindness. Infected individuals become unable to move or speak and go into a coma. Death is usually caused by an infection such as pneumonia.

There is no single diagnostic test for this disease. Providers usually perform laboratory tests to rule out other conditions such as encephalitis or meningitis. Magnetic resonance imaging (MRI) of the brain helps to identify the characteristic signs of brain degeneration. Brain biopsy is the only way to confirm the diagnosis.

Dementia

Dementia is a chronic disorder of mental processes caused by a brain disease that results in memory loss, shortened attention span, and decreased reasoning abilities. Causes include neurodegenerative and vascular diseases. Dementia usually occurs in elderly individuals and increases with advancing age. Vascular brain injury can cause cognitive impairment that can lead to dementia. Vascular dementia is the second most common form of dementia.

Routine laboratory tests can rule out other causes of dementia. They include a complete blood count, glucose level, renal and liver function tests, syphilis serology tests, vitamin B_{12} level, and thyroid function tests. Some patients require specialized studies, such as tests for lupus anticoagulant, antiphospholipid antibody, and antinuclear antibody.

Alzheimer Disease

Alzheimer disease is the number one cause of neurodegenerative dementia. Progressive atrophy (wasting) of the brain starts in the hippocampus and mesial temporal lobe, spreads to the frontal and parietal lobes, and then encompasses the occipital lobe. The disease is characterized by amyloid deposits (i.e., plaques) in the brain and intraneuronal deposits of tau protein. Individuals with preclinical Alzheimer disease appear completely normal. Some regions of the brain (e.g., hippocampus) are affected approximately 10 to 20 years before visible symptoms appear.

Mild Alzheimer disease is associated with memory loss, confusion about the location of familiar places, longer times to accomplish daily tasks, compromised judgment, loss of spontaneity, increased anxiety, and mood and personality changes. Moderate Alzheimer disease is associated with memory loss and confusion, shortened attention span, problems recognizing friends and family members, difficulty with language, difficulty organizing thoughts, inability to learn new things, restlessness, tearfulness, hallucinations, suspiciousness, and loss of impulse control. Severe Alzheimer disease is associated with loss of communication, no recognition of family or loved ones, and complete dependence on others for care; all sense of self vanishes. People with severe Alzheimer disease spend much or all of their time in bed. Death is usually caused by other illnesses, especially infections such as pneumonia.

Laboratory tests are not used to diagnose Alzheimer disease. It is a clinical diagnosis (Fig. 28-8).

Parkinson Disease

Parkinson disease is a common neurologic disease that affects approximately 1% of individuals 60 years or older. The degenerative disease involves the basal ganglia, leading to a lack of dopamine (i.e., neurotransmitter) and faulty nerve transmission. Disease onset is slow. Symptoms include tremor, difficulty walking, rigidity, shuffling gait,

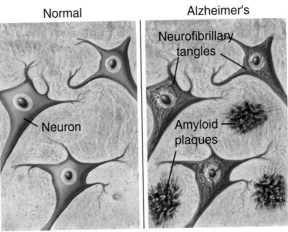

• **Figure 28-8** The formation of amyloid plaques and neurofibrillary tangles is thought to contribute to the degradation of the neurons (nerve cells) in the brain and the subsequent symptoms of Alzheimer disease. (From Monahan FD, Sands JK, Neighbors M, Marek JF, Green-Nigro CJ: *Phipps' Medical-Surgical Nursing.* 8th ed. St. Louis: Mosby; 2007.)

slurred speech, sleep disturbances, and a wooden, emotionless facial expression (Fig. 28-9).

There are no laboratory biomarkers to diagnose this disease. The diagnosis is based on a clinical evaluation. Symptomatic and disease-modifying therapies are available, but there is no cure for this disease.

Amyotrophic Lateral Sclerosis

Amyotrophic lateral sclerosis (ALS), also known as Lou Gehrig disease, is the most common degenerative disease of the motor neuron system. It was named after the New York Yankee baseball player who played in the 1920s and 1930s. The disease is incurable, and the median survival time is 3 years after diagnosis. Stephen Hawking, the famous British theoretical physicist, has ALS, but he has survived more than 50 years after his diagnosis.

Initial symptoms of ALS include tripping, stumbling, awkwardness when running, footdrop, reduced finger dexterity, cramping, wristdrop that interferes with work, slurred speech, hoarseness, choking during a meal, depression, and maladaptive social behavior. Symptoms of advanced disease include muscle atrophy, spasticity, muscle cramps, painful joint contractures, lost speech, swallowing difficulties, and drooling.

The diagnosis of early ALS takes several months. Individuals initially have upper and lower motor neuron signs. Providers must ensure the disease is progressive and rule out many other possible diagnoses. One form of hereditary ALS is linked to a genetic mutation on chromosome 21. Laboratory test results are used to rule out other possible diagnoses because most laboratory test results for patients with ALS are within reference ranges.

Multiple Sclerosis

Multiple sclerosis (MS) is an autoimmune disease that destroys the myelin sheaths on motor and sensory nerves in the CNS. It affects young adults between the ages of 18 and 40 years, and women are affected twice as often as men. Each case of MS is different because the pattern of myelin destruction varies.

Thirty percent of MS patients develop a significant physical disability during the 20- to 25-year course of the disease. Because MS affects the optic nerve, initial symptoms often include blurred vision or scotomata (i.e., spots). Other symptoms include tingling, numbness, minor gait irregularities, pain, trigeminal neuralgia, optic neuritis, fatigue, dizziness, cognitive difficulties (e.g., concentration, memory, judgment), depression, spasticity, and speech problems. For most individuals, the course of the disease involves neurologic deficits that occur and then resolve completely or almost completely. These episodes are separated by years or months and affect different anatomic areas.

Diagnosing MS is a complicated process and is based on a series of documented episodes. A single episode is not diagnostic because nerve demyelination is a chronic process. Laboratory test results are usually normal in MS, but they can be used to rule out other conditions with symptoms similar to MS. MRI is the diagnostic test of choice. When MRI is unavailable or nondiagnostic, CSF is analyzed for oligoclonal bands, which can aid in the diagnosis (Figs. 28-10 and 28-11).

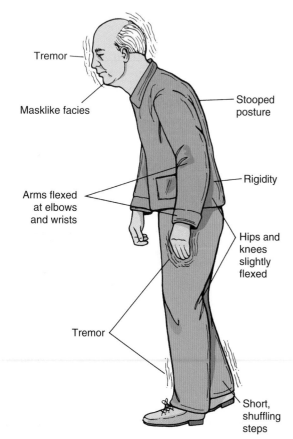

Tremor

Masklike facies

Arms flexed at elbows and wrists

Tremor

Stooped posture

Rigidity

Hips and knees slightly flexed

Short, shuffling steps

• **Figure 28-9** Clinical characteristics of Parkinson disease. (From Monahan FD, Drake T, Neighbors M. *Nursing Care of Adults.* Philadelphia: Saunders; 1994.)

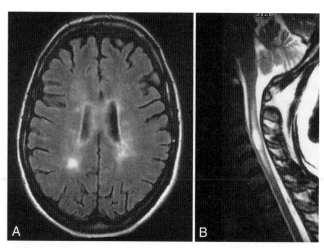

A   B

• **Figure 28-10 A,** Magnetic resonance imaging shows the typical white matter changes around the ventricles in multiple sclerosis. **B,** Changes in the spinal cord. (From Perkin GD. *Mosby's Color Atlas and Text of Neurology.* 2nd ed. London: Mosby; 2002.)

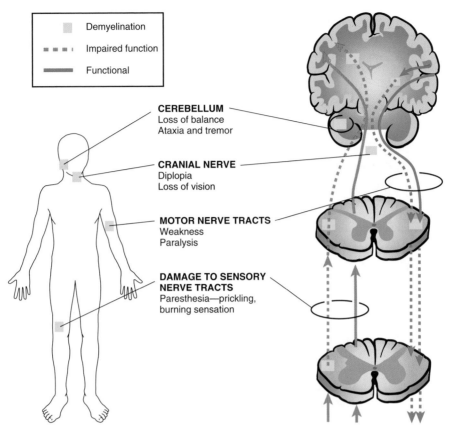

• Figure 28-11 Distribution of lesions in multiple sclerosis. (From VanMeter K, Hubert R. *Gould's Pathophysiology for the Health Professions.* 5th ed. St. Louis: Saunders; 2015.)

Peripheral Neuropathy

Peripheral neuropathy is a malfunction of sensory or motor nerves. The signal is disrupted by a disease process, causing weakness, paralysis, numbness, tingling, pain, or other sensations. Many diseases cause peripheral neuropathy, including diabetes, acquired immunodeficiency syndrome (AIDS), renal failure, lead poisoning, and alcoholism.

Guillain-Barré Syndrome

Guillain-Barré syndrome (GBS) is an acute autoimmune disorder that involves an anti-myelin antibody. It is an excessive immune response to immunization or an infection. If the syndrome is not treated, it can be fatal because it can lead to respiratory muscle paralysis. The motor nerve dysfunction causes weakness that begins in the legs and arms and then moves upward to the respiratory muscles in a few days to a few weeks.

No laboratory tests are used for the diagnosis, and patients usually recover very slowly. Most individuals recover fully, but some continue to experience muscle weakness.

Cerebrospinal Fluid Analysis

CSF is collected by a lumbar puncture that is usually performed between the L3 and L4 vertebrae (Fig. 28-12).

Using aseptic technique, a physician inserts a needle into the L3-L4 space and punctures the spinal cord to obtain fluid. Four tubes are collected with approximately 2 to 4 mL of fluid in each tube. The physician also measures the CSF pressure when beginning and completing the puncture. Conditions that increase brain pressure or obstruct CSF flow (e.g., tumors, infection, hydrocephalus, bleeding) can also increase CSF pressure. Dehydration, shock, or CSF leakage due to a sinus fracture can decrease CSF pressure.

Each tube is delivered to a particular department for analysis: tube 1, microbiology; tube 2, cytology; tube 3, chemistry; and tube 4, hematology. When the four tubes arrive in each department, the appearance of the CSF is usually compared with a sample of water because CSF is usually clear and colorless. Although the color changes are not diagnostic, they do indicate an abnormal condition with other substances in the CSF. For example, yellow, orange, or pink CSF may indicate lysed red blood cells from bleeding or bilirubin in the blood. Green CSF is indicative of infection or bilirubin in CSF. CSF turbidity is also observed. The CSF can appear cloudy due to the presence of red or white blood cells, microorganisms, or increased protein levels. CSF viscosity is observed. Usually, CSF has the consistency of water, but thicker CSF can indicate cancer or meningitis.

CSF specimens are considered STAT specimens and are analyzed immediately after delivery to the laboratory.

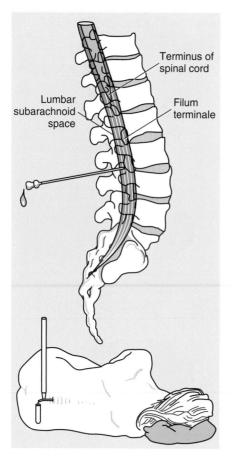

• **Figure 28-12** Lumbar puncture. Cerebrospinal fluid is obtained by inserting a needle into the subarachnoid space in the lumbar region. (From Mahon CR, Manuselis G. *Textbook of Diagnostic Microbiology.* 2nd ed. Philadelphia: Saunders; 2000.)

A few routine tests are performed on CSF specimens. In microbiology, a routine culture and Gram stain are done for CSF specimens. The CSF sample is centrifuged to concentrate the organisms, a drop is placed on a slide for a Gram stain, and culture media are inoculated. CSF should contain no microorganisms, and their presence indicates bacterial or fungal meningitis or encephalitis. Culture findings indicate the best choices for antimicrobial therapy for the affected individual and prophylaxis for close contacts. In some cases, the Gram stain and culture may have negative results although the individual has meningitis. Causes include prior antibiotic treatment or a small number of organisms in the CSF. If there are abnormal test results from other laboratory departments or the physician suspects a CNS infection, additional tests may be ordered:

- Polymerase chain reaction tests for herpesviruses and enteroviruses
- Viral antigen tests
- Viral cultures that may indicate viral meningitis or encephalitis
- Increased viral antibodies in initial and subsequent samples over time, indicating recent viral infection (e.g., a twofold increase in the West Nile virus antibody in two samples drawn weeks apart)

- CSF cryptococcal antigen (i.e., detects *Cryptococcus neoformans* infection)

Other tests that can be performed on CSF for less common pathogens include an AFB smear and culture, CSF molecular tests for AFB, and CSF syphilis testing (e.g., Venereal Disease Research Laboratory [VDRL] test).

In cytology testing, a cytocentrifuged sample is stained and examined for malignant cells. This test is ordered when a CNS tumor or metastatic cancer is suspected. Glucose and chemistry tests are initially performed on the CSF specimen. CSF glucose levels are two thirds of plasma blood glucose levels, and reference ranges are 45 to 75 mg/dL. CSF glucose levels are decreased when bacteria, white blood cells, or tumor cells, which are not normally found in CSF, use glucose. The CSF protein concentration is usually low because the blood–brain barrier prevents these large molecules from crossing into CSF. The reference range for CSF protein is 15 to 45 mg/dL. Increased CSF protein levels occur in cases of meningitis, brain abscess, brain or spinal cord tumors, multiple sclerosis, GBS, and syphilis. If either test result is abnormal, additional tests may be ordered:

- CSF protein electrophoresis: Multiple sclerosis and Lyme disease may produce oligoclonal bands.
- CSF immunoglobulin G (IgG): Levels can be increased in multiple sclerosis, herpesvirus infection, encephalitis, and connective tissue disease.
- Myelin basic protein: Demyelinization of nerves, as occurs in multiple sclerosis, produces a positive result.
- CSF lactic acid: Bacterial and fungal meningitis produce an increased level, and viral meningitis produces a slightly increased or normal level.
- CSF lactate dehydrogenase: Results are used to differentiate bacterial (i.e., elevated level) from viral (i.e., normal level) meningitis. Elevated levels are also found in leukemia and stroke.
- CSF glutamine: Elevated levels occur in liver disease, hepatic encephalopathy, and Reye syndrome.
- CSF C-reactive protein (CRP): The acute phase reactant is elevated in inflammatory conditions. Extremely high levels are found in bacterial meningitis, and low levels are found in viral meningitis. CRP is a sensitive marker of early bacterial meningitis.
- Tumor markers: Carcinoembryonic antigen (CEA), α-fetoprotein (AFP), and human chorionic gonadotropin (hCG) are tumor markers that can be found in the CSF of patients with metastatic cancer.

A complete blood cell count is performed on the fourth tube. Normal CSF contains few or no cells. If the CSF sample is clear, a drop is placed on a hemocytometer, and cells are counted manually. If five or fewer cells are counted, a white cell differential count may or may not be performed. If many cells are counted, the sample is centrifuged, a drop of the sediment is placed on a slide and stained with Wright's stain, and 100 cells are evaluated. Neutrophil numbers are increased in bacterial infections, lymphocyte numbers are

TABLE 28-1   Cerebrospinal Fluid

Characteristic	Normal Values
Appearance	Clear and colorless
Pressure	9-14 mm Hg or 150 mm H$_2$O
Red blood cells	None
White blood cells	Occasional
Protein	15-45 mg/dL
Glucose	45-75 mg/dL
Sodium	140 mEq/L
Potassium	3 mEq/L
Specific gravity	1.007
pH	7.32-7.35
Volume in the system at one time	125-150 mL
Volume formed in 24 hours	500-800 mL

From VanMeter K, Hubert R. *Gould's Pathophysiology for the Health Professions*. 5th ed. St. Louis: Saunders; 2015.

increased in viral or fungal infections, and eosinophils may be found in parasitic infections. Leukemia in the CNS produces abnormal and normal white blood cells in the CSF. Malignant cells from solid CNS tumors may also appear in CSF. Multiple sclerosis can produce an increase in the number of lymphocytes.

Many red blood cells may indicate bleeding into the CSF or a traumatic spinal tap. During a traumatic tap, blood is introduced into the CSF tube during specimen collection. There are normally five or fewer white blood cells in a sample of CSF. Infection or inflammation markedly increases the number of white blood cells in the CSF. The number of white blood cells found may be increased by brain abscess, seizures or bleeding within the brain or skull, metastatic tumor, GBS, and sarcoidosis (Table 28-1).

Summary

Nervous system diseases affect the central, peripheral, and autonomic nervous systems. Many nervous system diseases are progressive, chronic diseases, whereas others are acute. Some such as neural tube defects (including spina bifida and hydrocephalus) result from developmental errors in the embryo. Cerebral palsy results from a brain injury that occurs before the age of 2 years. The injury produces permanent motor problems (i.e., paralysis and spasticity).

Three types of brain bleeding are epidural hematoma, subdural hematoma, and subarachnoid hemorrhage. Epidural hematoma results from a skull fracture that tears a meningeal artery. Subdural hematoma occurs from head trauma that is not severe enough to cause a skull fracture but severe enough to damage a vein. Subarachnoid hemorrhage is a sudden, spontaneous type of bleeding that occurs as the result of a brain aneurysm or congenital malformation.

Two main types of infection occur in the brain: meningitis and encephalitis. Meningitis is an infection of the meninges that is usually caused by bacteria, and encephalitis is caused by a viral infection in previously healthy individuals.

Chronic, progressive neurologic diseases (e.g., Alzheimer disease, Parkinson disease) cause dementia. Alzheimer disease is caused by amyloid deposits in the brain, and Parkinson disease is a neurodegenerative disease resulting from a lack of dopamine, which inhibits nerve impulse transmission.

Amyotrophic lateral sclerosis is a degenerative disease that destroys motor neurons. Multiple sclerosis is a progressive, degenerative disease that destroys the myelin sheaths of neurons, short-circuiting nerve impulse conduction. Peripheral neuropathy results from diseases such as diabetes mellitus. Peripheral neuropathy affects sensory or motor neurons. GBS is a temporary immune reaction to a viral infection or immunization.

Review Questions

1. Which of the following is considered an acute nervous system disease?
   a. Spina bifida
   b. Epidural hematoma
   c. Dementia
   d. Alzheimer disease

2. Which of the following diseases results from a brain injury before 2 years of age, results in permanent damage, and causes motor problems such as paralysis and spasticity?
   a. Cerebral palsy
   b. Hydrocephalus
   c. Anencephaly
   d. Encephalitis

3. Which type of brain bleed results from a traumatic skull fracture that damages a meningeal artery?
   a. Subdural hematoma
   b. Epidural hematoma
   c. Subarachnoid hemorrhage
   d. Cerebral palsy

4. Which type of brain bleed results from trauma that damages a vein?
   a. Epidural hematoma
   b. Subarachnoid hemorrhage
   c. Subdural hematoma
   d. Guillain-Barré syndrome

5. Encephalitis is
   a. A bacterial infection produced in immunocompromised individuals
   b. A condition that results from the deposit of abnormal proteins in the brain
   c. An inflamed brain resulting from a skull fracture
   d. A viral infection produced in otherwise healthy individuals

6. All of the following statements about Alzheimer disease are true EXCEPT
   a. It is present for 10 to 20 years before the individual becomes symptomatic.
   b. It is a neurodegenerative disease that affects the motor neurons, causing a tremor.
   c. It is a progressive disease that results from amyloid deposits in the brain.
   d. Individuals affected by this disease may have difficulty recognizing loved ones.

7. Parkinson disease is a neurodegenerative disease with this characteristic symptom:
   a. Tremor
   b. Hearing difficulties
   c. Difficulty recognizing loved ones
   d. Decreased level of acetylcholine

8. What two famous people were diagnosed with amyotrophic lateral sclerosis?
   a. Mickey Mantle and Enrico Fermi
   b. Sandy Koufax and Louis Pasteur
   c. Lou Gehrig and Stephen Hawking
   d. Joe Green and Sheldon Cooper

9. Many individuals diagnosed with diabetes mellitus suffer from which of the following nervous system diseases?
   a. Guillain-Barré syndrome
   b. Dementia
   c. Multiple sclerosis
   d. Peripheral neuropathy

10. Multiple sclerosis results from which of the following?
    a. Lack of the neurotransmitter dopamine
    b. Amyloid deposits in the brain
    c. Destruction of motor neurons
    d. Destruction of the myelin sheath on neurons

Critical Thinking Questions

1. What tests are routinely performed on a sample of cerebrospinal fluid (CSF)? For each test performed, indicate the reference ranges, and describe what abnormal laboratory results indicate.

2. Describe the CSF protein test method, and explain why CSF protein tests cannot be performed with a routine chemistry panel using the biuret test method.

3. What are the clinical features of spina bifida, and how are clinical chemistry tests used to detect this disease?

CASE STUDY

A 30-year-old man has a flu shot after work on Wednesday. On Thursday morning, he notices motor weakness in his legs. He goes to his provider. What disease does this man have? Are there laboratory tests for the diagnosis of this disease?

Bibliography

Burtis CA, Bruns DE. *Tietz Fundamentals of Clinical Chemistry and Molecular Diagnostics*. 7th ed. St. Louis: Saunders; 2015.

Coyle PK. Overview of acute and chronic meningitis. *Neurol Clin*. 1999;17:691–710.

Furukawa K, Ishiki A, Tomita N, Arai H. Diagnosis and treatment of dementia: overview. *Clin Neurol*. 2014;54:1171–1173.

Heldner MR, Arnold M, Nedeltchev K, et al. Vascular diseases of the spinal cord: a review. *Curr Treat Options Neurol*. 2012;14:509–520.

Kaplan LA, Pesce AJ, eds. *Clinical Chemistry: Theory, Analysis, Correlation*. 5th ed. St. Louis: Mosby; 2010.

Kellner CP, Scully BF, Connolly Jr ES. Subdural and epidural hemorrhage. In: Colosimo C, Gil-Nagel A, Gilhus NE, et al., eds. *Handbook of Neurological Therapy*. Oxford, UK: Oxford University Press; 2015.

Kiernan MC, Vucic S, Cheah BC, et al. Amyotrophic lateral sclerosis. *Lancet*. 2011;377:942–955.

Levitt S. *Treatment of Cerebral Palsy and Motor Delay*. New York: John Wiley & Sons; 2013.

Lew M. Overview of Parkinson's disease. *Pharmacotherapy*. 2007;27(Pt 2):155S–160S.

McCance KL, Huether SE. *Pathophysiology: The Biologic Basis for Disease in Adults and Children*. St. Louis: Elsevier Health Sciences; 2014.

McConnell TH. Disorders of the nervous system. In: *The Nature of Disease: Pathology for the Health Professions*. 2nd ed. Philadelphia: Lippincott Williams & Wilkins; 2007.

Patton KT, Thibodeau GA. *Anatomy and Physiology*. 8th ed. St. Louis: Elsevier Health Sciences; 2014.

Piaceri I, Nacmias B, Sorbi S. Genetics of familial and sporadic Alzheimer's disease. *Front Biosci (Elite Ed)*. 2013;5:167–177.

Stagno V, Navarrete EA, Mirone G, Esposito F. Management of hydrocephalus around the world. *World Neurosurg*. 2013;79(suppl):S23.e17–S23.e20.

Stoeck K, Sanchez-Juan P, Gawinecka J, et al. Cerebrospinal fluid biomarker supported diagnosis of Creutzfeldt-Jakob disease and rapid dementias: a longitudinal multicentre study over 10 years. *Brain*. 2012;135(Pt 10):3051–3061.

Wallingford JB, Niswander LA, Shaw GM, Finnell RH. The continuing challenge of understanding, preventing, and treating neural tube defects. *Science*. 2013;339:1222002.

Zhong W, Chen H, You C, et al. Spontaneous spinal epidural hematoma. *J Clin Neurosci*. 2011;18:1490–1494.

29

Skin, Hair, and Nail Diseases

DONNA LARSON

CHAPTER OUTLINE

Introduction

Skin Diseases

 Albinism

 Scleroderma

 Malignant Melanoma

Effects of Systemic Disease on Skin

 Diabetes

 Thyroid Disease

 Blood Lipid Abnormalities

 Addison Disease

 Systemic Lupus Erythematosus

Hair Diseases

 Menkes Disease

 Hirsutism

Nail Diseases

 Yellow Nail Syndrome

 Nail Clubbing

 Koilonychia

 Terry's Nails

 Beau's Lines

 Onycholysis

Summary

OBJECTIVES

After completion of this chapter, the reader will be able to:

1. Define albinism.
2. Describe the disease mechanism for scleroderma.
3. List the tests used to diagnose scleroderma.
4. Describe malignant melanoma.
5. Describe diabetic ulcers.
6. Describe the dermal manifestations of systemic lupus erythematosus.
7. Describe how thyroid diseases can cause changes in the skin.
8. Define xanthoma, and describe how the irregular yellow patches occur.
9. Describe the dermal manifestations of Addison disease.
10. Describe Menkes syndrome.
11. Describe hirsutism.
12. Describe yellow nails, nail clubbing, koilonychia, Terry's nails, Beau's lines, and onycholysis and explain what produces these conditions.

KEY TERMS

Addison disease
Albinism
Beau's lines
Diabetic neuropathy
Diabetic ulcers
Discoid lupus
Hirsutism
Hypopigmentation

Koilonychia
Malar rash
Malignant melanoma
Melanocyte
Menkes disease
Nail clubbing
Onycholysis
Photosensitivity

Scleroderma
Systemic lupus erythematosus
Terry's nails
Xanthomas
Yellow nail syndrome

❖ Case in Point

A medical laboratory technician student walked into the phlebotomy room and prepared to draw blood from a patient. The student was taken aback by the patient's appearance when she entered the room. The young woman had long white hair and pink eyes. What condition did this woman have, and what caused it?

Points to Remember

- Hair, skin, and nails protect the body from the environment.
- Albinism is a general term for various types of hypopigmentation.
- Hypopigmentation disorders are caused by mutations of genes responsible for melanin synthesis, distribution of pigment by the melanocyte, and melanosome biogenesis.
- Scleroderma produces thick, leather-like skin.
- Forms of scleroderma include limited skin involvement, diffuse skin sclerosis, severe and progressive organ involvement, and fulminant systemic sclerosis.
- Malignant melanoma involves the transformation of normal melanocytes.
- Melanoma is treated with surgery, immunotherapy, and chemotherapy.
- Diabetics are prone to *Candida* infections, diabetic ulcers, and diabetic neuropathy.
- Hyperthyroidism causes the skin to become warm, moist, velvety, and more pigmented.
- Hypothyroidism causes the skin to become dry, coarse, and yellowish.
- Hereditary blood lipid diseases cause lipid deposition in the skin in formations call xanthomas.
- People with Addison disease have hyperpigmented skin.
- Systemic lupus erythematosus causes a malar rash over the cheeks and nasal bridge.
- Infants with Menkes disease have fine, wiry, silver hair.
- Women with hirsutism grow thick, dark hair in a male pattern (especially facial hair).
- Nail diseases can separate the nail from its base, turn the nail yellow, cause clubbing of the ends of fingers, turn the nail sides and top upward from the nail bed, turn the nail bed white, and cause white marks in response to trauma.

Introduction

Most skin, hair, and nail disorders result from systemic diseases. Systemic diseases affect all body systems. This chapter examines the effects of systemic diseases on the skin, hair, and nails and considers diseases that originate in the skin.

The skin, hair, and nails protect the body from the environment. The skin provides a barrier that preserves bodily fluids and maintains normal temperatures. The skin is the largest organ in the body, and its thickness varies. The thinnest layers of skin are over the eyes and genitals, and the thickest layers are on the back, the palms, and the soles of the feet (Fig. 29-1). Hair protects the body (especially the scalp) from the sun and insulates the body by trapping air between the skin and hair. Nails protect the fingertips from injury and enable precise manipulation of the fingers and hand.

Skin Diseases

Albinism

Albinism is a general term used to describe several types of hypopigmentation disorders, such as oculocutaneous albinism (types 1 through 4) and ocular albinism. These disorders are caused by mutations in genes responsible for melanin synthesis, distribution of pigment by the melanocyte, and melanosome biogenesis. The symptoms are complete or partial loss of pigment in the skin, hair, and eyes. With complete pigment loss, the hair is white and the eyes pink (Fig. 29-2). The laboratory workup does not involve common laboratory tests.

Scleroderma

Scleroderma means "hard skin" (Fig. 29-3). Also called *systemic sclerosis,* it is an autoimmune disease of connective tissue that can produce thick, leather-like skin. It is a progressive disease that affects many other systems in addition to the skin. Different forms of the disease can be characterized by limited skin involvement, diffuse skin sclerosis, severe and progressive organ involvement, or fulminant systemic sclerosis. The form with limited skin involvement affects areas above the elbows and knees, the face, and the neck. The diffuse cutaneous form causes skin thickening of the trunk and areas below the elbows and knees; the face is also involved. Involvement of the heart, lungs, or kidneys can be life-threatening. Systemic sclerosis is most obvious in the skin and in the gastrointestinal, respiratory, renal, cardiovascular, musculoskeletal, endocrine, and genitourinary tracts. Loss of range of joint motion is caused by skin tightening. Thickening of the skin is caused by chronic inflammation leading to fibrosis of tissue. The trigger for this autoimmune reaction is unknown.

Useful diagnostic laboratory tests include a complete blood count, erythrocyte sedimentation rate, and assays of creatine kinase (CK), aldolase, the CXC chemokine ligand 4 (CXCL4), N-terminal pro–brain natriuretic peptide, antinuclear antibodies (ANAs), anti-SCL-70, and anti-centromere antibodies. CK and aldolase levels are elevated due to muscle inflammation. The CK determination is performed as part of a routine chemistry panel, and aldolase is quantitated with the use of an immunoassay. CXCL4 is an anti-angiogenesis cytokine, and elevated levels indicate pulmonary fibrosis and progression of pulmonary hypertension. The concentration of N-terminal pro–brain natriuretic peptide is elevated in early pulmonary hypertension.

ANAs are detected in a speckled or centromere pattern in 90% to 95% of patients. ANA results indicate that antibodies are being produced against tissue cells. Topoisomerase

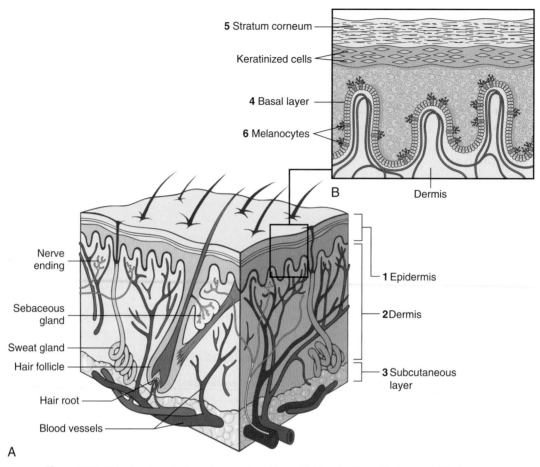

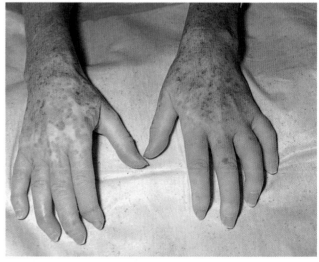

• **Figure 29-1** Skin structure. **A,** Three layers of the skin. **B,** Epidermis. (From Chabner DE. *The Language of Medicine.* 10th ed. St. Louis: Saunders; 2014.)

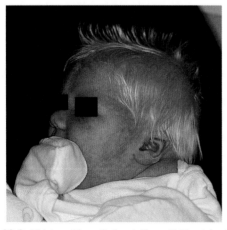

• **Figure 29-2** Albinism. (From Callen J, Greer K, Hood A, et al. *Color Atlas of Dermatology.* 2nd ed. Philadelphia: Saunders; 2000. Courtesy of Jeffrey P. Callen, MD.)

• **Figure 29-3** Scleroderma of the hands. (From Swartz MH. *Textbook of Physical Diagnosis: History and Examination.* 7th ed. Philadelphia: Saunders; 2014.)

I antibody (i.e., anti-SCL-70) is present in 30% of individuals with diffuse disease. Anticentromere antibodies are identified in 45% to 50% of patients with limited scleroderma. ANA, anti-SCL-70, and anticentromere antibodies can be quantitated by immunoassays and immunofluorescent methods.

Malignant Melanoma

Malignant melanoma is caused by the malignant transformation of melanocytes. Melanoma remains confined to the skin during the early stages (Fig. 29-4). Normal

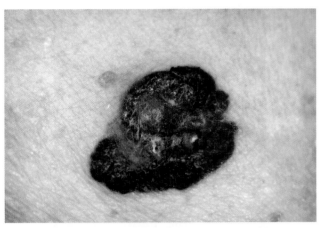

• **Figure 29-4** Malignant melanoma. (From Waugh A, Grant A. *Ross and Wilson Anatomy and Physiology in Health and Illness.* 12th ed. Edinburgh: Churchill Livingstone; 2014.)

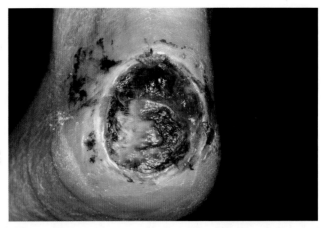

• **Figure 29-5** Diabetic foot ulcer. (From Waugh A, Grant A. *Ross and Wilson Anatomy and Physiology in Health and Illness.* 12th ed. Edinburgh: Churchill Livingstone; 2014.)

physiology is affected after melanoma invades the subcutaneous tissue.

Treatment for malignant melanoma can include surgery (particularly in the early stages), radiation therapy, targeted therapy with monoclonal antibodies, and chemotherapy. Chemistry test results can be altered for patients undergoing chemotherapy, and serial test results may be monitored during treatment. Common chemistry tests are not useful for the diagnosis of malignant melanoma.

Effects of Systemic Disease on Skin

Skin often shows the first signs of an internal disease. The following sections discuss some of the common diseases that affect the skin.

Diabetes

Diabetes affects every part of the body. Two skin conditions are particularly common in diabetics: *Candida* spp. infections and diabetic ulcers. *Candida* infections occur in warm, moist, dark places such as skin folds. The fungal infection commonly occurs on the genitals or in skin folds around the genitals or buttocks.

Diabetic ulcers usually occur on the foot and are caused by decreased blood flow and decreased pain sensation (Fig. 29-5). Diabetics have decreased blood flow because their blood becomes thicker due to increased glucose levels. Less blood reaches the outer surface of the skin, leading to breakdown of the skin in that area.

Diabetics experience less pain in their extremities due to diabetic neuropathy, which impairs sensory nerves. As a result, a person may suffer repeated trauma to an area of skin without realizing it.

Thyroid Disease

Thyroid function affects dermal and epidermal cell growth. As a result of overproduction of thyroid hormones (see

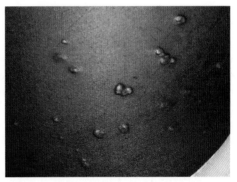

• **Figure 29-6** Eruptive xanthomas. Notice the yellowish hue and clustering of some lesions. (From Bolognia JL, Schaffer JV, Duncan KO, Ko CJ. *Dermatology Essentials.* London: Saunders; 2014.)

Chapter 23), the skin becomes warm, moist, velvety, and more pigmented. Changes occur in the color, shape, texture, and thickness of fingernails and toenails, and waxy, translucent plaques can appear over the lower part of the leg. Insufficient thyroid hormone production causes dry, coarse, and yellowish skin and loss of scalp and eyebrow hair.

Blood Lipid Abnormalities

Abnormally high blood lipid levels can cause lipid deposition in skin (see Chapter 17). When the triglyceride level is greater than 2000 mg/dL, eruptive xanthomas (i.e., dozens of small, yellow-red papules) can be deposited on the back of forearms, shins, and pressure points (e.g., elbows, feet, buttocks) (Fig. 29-6). When the cholesterol level is greater than 300 mg/dL, nodular xanthomas (i.e., nodular cholesterol deposits) can occur on the elbow, palms, soles, or Achilles tendon. Flat, bright yellow cholesterol xanthomas can appear on the eyelids or the nose.

Addison Disease

Addison disease is characterized by chronically decreased levels of glucocorticoids and mineralocorticoids (see Chapter 23)

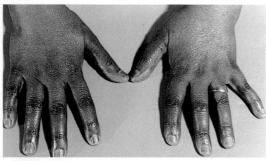

• **Figure 29-7** Hyperpigmentation typically seen in Addison disease. (From Lewis SL, Dirksen SR, Heitkemper MM, Bucher L. *Medical-Surgical Nursing: Assessment and Management of Clinical Problems.* 9th ed. St. Louis: Mosby; 2014.)

(Fig. 29-7). Individuals with Addison disease have hyperpigmented skin on sun-exposed areas, in skin creases, inside the cheek, at sites of friction (e.g., elbow, knee), in recent scars, and on the vermilion border of the lips.

Addison disease is diagnosed by measuring glucocorticoid and mineralocorticoid levels with the adrenocorticotropic hormone (ACTH) stimulation test. The ACTH test involves injecting an individual with ACTH and then measuring the levels of the glucocorticoids and mineralocorticoids at a specific time after injection. Decreased levels are diagnostic of Addison disease. Other abnormal laboratory test results for untreated Addison disease include metabolic acidosis and increased calcium, low glucose, low sodium, and increased potassium levels.

Systemic Lupus Erythematosus

Individuals with systemic lupus erythematosus (SLE) may have a malar rash, photosensitivity, and discoid lupus lesions (see Chapter 32). The malar rash (i.e., butterfly rash), a hallmark of SLE, is a red rash over the cheeks and nasal bridge that does not extend into the nasolabial folds (Fig. 29-8). Photosensitivity in SLE patients can produce a new rash or cause the malar rash to worsen. Discoid lupus consists of plaques on sun-exposed areas with follicular plugging and scarring.

SLE skin conditions are not diagnosed with routine clinical chemistry tests. SLE is diagnosed with ANA assays.

Hair Diseases

Menkes Disease

Menkes disease is an X-linked, recessive, multisystem disorder of copper metabolism. The disease occurs in male infants, who usually die by the age of 2 to 3 years. They have wiry, silver hair; connective tissue disorders; and neurologic deterioration (Fig. 29-9). Because of a defect in the transport of copper in the body, the serum copper level of Menkes patients is low, as is the ceruloplasmin level.

Early screening tests include a urine homovanillic acid/vanillylmandelic acid ratio. A ratio greater than 4 strongly

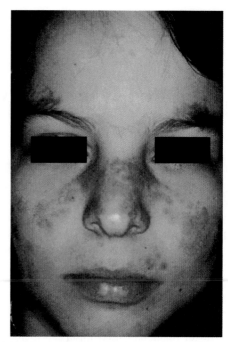

• **Figure 29-8** Butterfly (malar) rash in systemic lupus erythematosus. (From Klatt EC. *Robbins and Cotran Atlas of Pathology.* 3rd ed. Philadelphia: Saunders; 2015.)

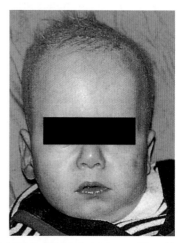

• **Figure 29-9** Menkes kinky hair syndrome. (From Newton RW. *Color Atlas of Pediatric Neurology.* London: Times Mirror International; 1995.)

suggests that the infant has Menkes disease. Individuals with Menkes disease also have hypercalciuria, albuminuria, and aminoaciduria.

Hirsutism

Women with hirsutism grow thick, dark hair in a male pattern (e.g., moustache) (Fig. 29-10). Chapter 25 discusses reproductive hormone diseases. Hirsutism is commonly caused by excess androgen production in females, but it can have an idiopathic origin with normal androgen levels.

The diagnosis depends on clinical chemistry test results. Testosterone levels are determined in a screening test. If the total testosterone concentration is not elevated, the free

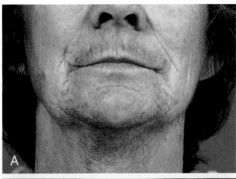

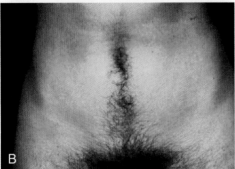

• **Figure 29-10 A,** Hirsutism. The woman has excess hair above the lip and on the chin. **B,** Virilization. The woman has a male distribution of hair from the mons pubis to the umbilicus. (From Goljian EF. *Rapid Review Pathology.* 4th ed. Philadelphia: Saunders; 2014.)

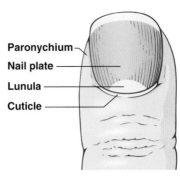

• **Figure 29-11** Structure of nails. (From Chabner DE. *The Language of Medicine.* 10th ed. St. Louis: Saunders; 2014.)

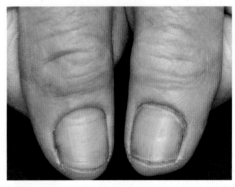

• **Figure 29-12** Yellow nail syndrome. (Courtesy Karynne O. Duncan, MD.)

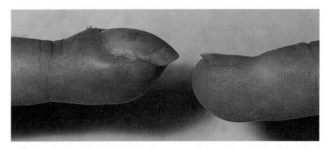

• **Figure 29-13** Nail clubbing. (From Swartz MH. *Textbook of Physical Diagnosis: History and Examination.* 7th ed. Philadelphia: Saunders; 2014.)

testosterone level should be obtained. Extremely high testosterone levels point to an adrenal or ovarian tumor that produces the hormones. Dehydroepiandrosterone sulfate (DHEAS) should also be measured. If the testosterone and DHEAS levels are both elevated, the cause is adrenal hyperplasia. If only testosterone is elevated, the likely cause is polycystic ovary syndrome. Other helpful tests include prolactin and follicle-stimulating hormone determinations, which can point to prolactinoma or ovarian failure, respectively.

Nail Diseases

Nail diseases are usually outward manifestations of systemic diseases. Emergency responders usually look at a person's nails to determine whether blood perfusion is adequate. Although it is not a precise indication of an adult's state of health, this evaluation allows first responders to quickly triage patients. Blue fingernail beds indicate cyanosis (i.e., lack of oxygen) due to poor lung function (Fig. 29-11). Common nail diseases include yellow nail syndrome, nail clubbing, koilonychia, Terry's nails, Beau's lines, and onycholysis.

Yellow Nail Syndrome

Yellow nail syndrome (Fig. 29-12) produces yellow nails that lack a cuticle, grow slowly, and can be detached (as in onycholysis). This rare condition usually occurs in people with lung disease and lymphedema. Lung diseases are diagnosed with a variety of laboratory tests.

Nail Clubbing

Nail clubbing (Fig. 29-13) is a condition in which the nails are curved and appear to bulge, similar to the bottom of an upside-down spoon. The most common cause of nail clubbing is lung cancer. Others are cystic fibrosis, endocarditis, celiac disease, cirrhosis, Graves disease, Wilson disease, and Hodgkin lymphoma. Common clinical chemistry tests are not used to diagnose lung cancer or other diseases thought to cause nail clubbing.

Koilonychia

Koilonychia, also known as spoon nails, is a nail disease that can be a sign of anemia, hyperthyroidism, and hemochromatosis (Fig. 29-14). Clinical chemistry tests

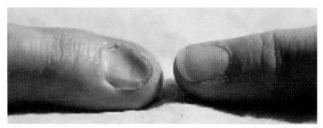

• **Figure 29-14** Koilonychia. (From Swartz MH. *Textbook of Physical Diagnosis: History and Examination.* 7th ed. Philadelphia: Saunders; 2014.)

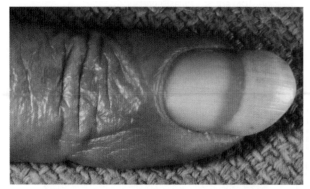

• **Figure 29-15** Terry's nails. (From Swartz MH. *Textbook of Physical Diagnosis: History and Examination.* 7th ed. Philadelphia: Saunders; 2014.)

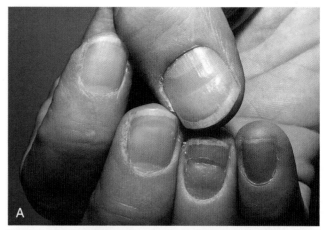

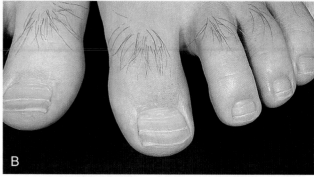

• **Figure 29-16** Beau's lines. **A,** Fingernails. **B,** Toenails. (From Swartz MH. *Textbook of Physical Diagnosis: History and Examination.* 7th ed. Philadelphia: Saunders; 2014.)

may be helpful for diagnosing hyperthyroidism and hemochromatosis.

Terry's Nails

Individuals with Terry's nails have a nail bed that is white and opaque, obscuring the lunula (Fig. 29-15). This condition occurs most often in individuals with cirrhosis, but it is also found in patients who are hospitalized for long periods. Cirrhosis can be diagnosed with the help of liver function tests.

Beau's Lines

Beau's lines are horizontal ridges and indentations in the nail plate (Fig. 29-16). They are found in individuals with previous severe illness, infection, or trauma, or with prolonged exposure to cold temperature in patients with Raynaud's syndrome.

Onycholysis

Onycholysis is a painless separation of the nail from the nail bed (Fig. 29-17). A yeast infection in the space under

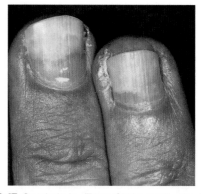

• **Figure 29-17** Onycholysis. (From Chabner DE. *The Language of Medicine.* 10th ed. St Louis: Saunders; 2014.)

the nail may result in a white area. The most common cause is local trauma, but it may also occur in cases of onychomycosis and periungual warts. Because the condition occurs in patients with hyperthyroidism, thyroid function tests are helpful for the diagnosis.

Summary

The status of skin, hair, and nails can be an indication of overall health. Few diseases that originate in these areas are diagnosed with clinical chemistry tests; most are diagnosed clinically. Many of the conditions described result from systemic diseases such as diabetes, systemic lupus erythematosus, and thyroid disease.

Review Questions

1. Hirsutism is
   a. Fast growth of hair
   b. Slow growth of hair
   c. Growth of terminal hair in a male pattern
   d. Growth of fine vellus hair in place of a beard or terminal hair
2. Menkes disease is
   a. A disorder of copper metabolism
   b. A lipid storage disease that causes lipid deposition on the hands as xanthomas
   c. The result of a genetic mutation that causes hair to become thin and silvery
   d. Caused by a genetic mutation that causes loss of all body hair
3. Diagnostic hallmarks of systemic lupus erythematosus include all of the following EXCEPT
   a. Kinky hair
   b. Malar rash
   c. Photosensitivity
   d. Discoid lupus
4. A triglyceride level greater than 2000 mg/dL may cause
   a. Xanthomas
   b. Discoid lupus
   c. Malar rash
   d. Koilonychias
5. Effects of hypothyroidism on the skin include all the following EXCEPT
   a. Velvety skin
   b. Dry skin
   c. Hair loss
   d. Coarse skin
6. Diabetic ulcers are caused by
   a. Decreased blood flow to an extremity
   b. Ketones in the blood
   c. Acid blood pH breaking down skin and tissue
   d. Patient inactivity
7. All of the following laboratory tests are useful in diagnosing scleroderma EXCEPT
   a. Glucocorticoids and mineralocorticoids
   b. Anti-SCL-70
   c. Anticentromere antibodies
   d. Aldolase
8. Common causes for nail clubbing include all of the following EXCEPT
   a. Melanoma
   b. Endocarditis
   c. Wilson disease
   d. Cirrhosis
9. Hyperthyroidism or hemochromatosis can cause this nail condition:
   a. Koilonychias
   b. Terry's nails
   c. Beau's lines
   d. Yellow nails
10. What test is used to screen for hirsutism?
    a. Testosterone
    b. Estrogen
    c. Melatonin
    d. Triglycerides

Critical Thinking Questions

1. Why are diabetics more susceptible to *Candida* infections and diabetic ulcers?
2. How do the different forms of scleroderma affect the body and the skin?
3. Why do some albinos have pink eyes?

CASE STUDY

A 68-year-old man bought a new pair of walking shoes. He wore socks with the new shoes and went out for a 30-minute walk. He developed a blister on the bottom of his foot. He put antibiotic ointment on his foot and bandaged it so it would heal.

Two weeks later, the blister turned into a diabetic foot ulcer. How are diabetic foot ulcers formed? What keeps them from healing?

Bibliography

Barnhill RL, Piepkorn M, Busam KJ. *Pathology of Melanocytic Nevi and Melanoma*. 3rd ed. New York: Springer-Verlag; 2014.

Blume–Peytavi U. An overview of unwanted female hair. *Br J Dermatol*. 2011;165(suppl 3):19–23.

Bode D, Seehusen DA, Baird D. Hirsutism in women. *Am Fam Physician*. 2012;85:373–380.

Burtis CA, Bruns DE. *Tietz Fundamentals of Clinical Chemistry and Molecular Diagnostics*. 7th ed. St. Louis: Elsevier Health Sciences; 2014.

Fawcett RS, Linford S, Stulberg DL. Nail abnormalities: clues to systemic disease. *Am Fam Physician*. 2004;69:1417–1424.

Lipsker D. Palpable lesions: overview. In: Lipsker D, *Clinical Examination and Differential Diagnosis of Skin Lesions*. Paris: Springer; 2013:183–184.

Mayes MD. *Brief Overview of Scleroderma: Localized Scleroderma and Systemic Sclerosis (SSc)*. New York: Springer; 2014.

Napier C, Pearce SH. Autoimmune Addison's disease. *Presse Med.* 2012;41:e626–e635.

Piraccini BM. Clubbing. In: Piraccini BM, *Nail Disorders: A Practical Guide to Diagnosis and Management*. New York: Springer; 2014.

Piraccini BM. Yellow nail syndrome. In: Piraccini BM, ed. *Nail Disorders: A Practical Guide to Diagnosis and Management*. New York: Springer; 2014.

Schrieber L, O'Neill S. Systemic lupus erythematosus: an overview for GPs [in Korean]. *Med Today.* 2004;5(6):28–39.

Seshadri R, Bindu PS, Gupta AK. Teaching neuroimages: Menkes kinky hair syndrome. *Neurology.* 2013;81:e12–e13.

Suzuki T. Genetics of hypopigmentary disorders. *J Dermatol.* 2013;40:309.

30

Eye and Ear Diseases

DONNA LARSON

CHAPTER OUTLINE

Introduction

Eyes
Eye Anatomy
Eye Disorders

Ears
Ear Anatomy
Ear Disorders

Summary

OBJECTIVES

After completion of this chapter, the reader will be able to:

1. Describe the pathological effect of systemic diseases on the eye.
2. List three eye conditions that are caused by systemic diseases.

3. Describe the effect of ear diseases on other bodily functions.
4. List the drugs that are considered to be ototoxic.

KEY TERMS

Arcus senilis
Cataract
Diabetic retinopathy

Hypertensive retinopathy
Meniere disease
Ototoxicity

Vertigo
Vestibular neuronitis

 Case in Point

As you attempt to get out of bed one morning, the room starts spinning. You lie down again, but the room continues to spin. This constant motion begins to make you motion sick, and you vomit. What is making you sick? Can the condition be detected using clinical chemistry tests? Can it cause temporary changes in your clinical chemistry test results? If yes, which tests?

Points to Remember

- Eye diseases can be caused by systemic conditions such as hypertension and lipidemia.
- Arcus senilis is the deposition of lipids in the outer edge of the cornea.
- Juveniles with abnormally high lipid levels can have lipids deposits in the outer edges of the cornea.

- Cataracts usually result from degradation of the lens fibers, and they typically occur in older individuals.
- Hypertension affects the coronary and eye arteries and can cause extensive damage to the retina if the condition is not controlled.
- Diabetic retinopathy occurs in uncontrolled diabetes and is the leading cause of blindness among diabetics.
- Vertigo is caused by an inner ear condition that can alter a person's physiologic state because it can cause vomiting.

Introduction

Systemic diseases affect the entire body. Some diseases of the eye and ear are extensions of systemic diseases. This chapter summarizes the main eye and ear conditions that a laboratory technician may encounter.

Eyes

Many eye diseases are diagnosed or monitored with clinical chemistry tests. In this section, a review of eye anatomy is followed by a discussion about eye disorders that are associated with abnormal chemistry processes.

Eye Anatomy

The eye is a small sensory organ that is approximately 1.5 inches in diameter. Despite its small size, it provides much of the information we gather about our environment. Movement is controlled by six muscles that allow the eye to move up, down, and side to side. The eyeball is filled with vitreous humor.

The front one third of the eye, called the anterior segment, contains the lens, pupil, iris, and cornea. The iris is a thin, colored, contractile membrane behind the cornea with an adjustable circular opening in the center called the pupil. Together with the iris, the pupil is responsible for regulating the amount of light entering the eye by constricting or dilating. The lens is a biconvex, oval, transparent body suspended behind the iris and pupil. Along with the cornea, it focuses light from near and far objects on the retina. The cornea is a domed structure located in front of the iris and pupil, and it has more light-bending power than the lens. The lens and the cornea lack blood vessels and lymphatics.

The retina is a layer at the back of the eyeball containing cells that are sensitive to light. The cells receive the light that passes through the pupil and lens, triggering nerve impulses that are sent through the optic nerve to the brain for interpretation (Fig. 30-1).

Eye Disorders

Arcus Senilis

Arcus senilis is a narrow, opaque, gray to white band of lipid deposited around the edge of the cornea, and it is common

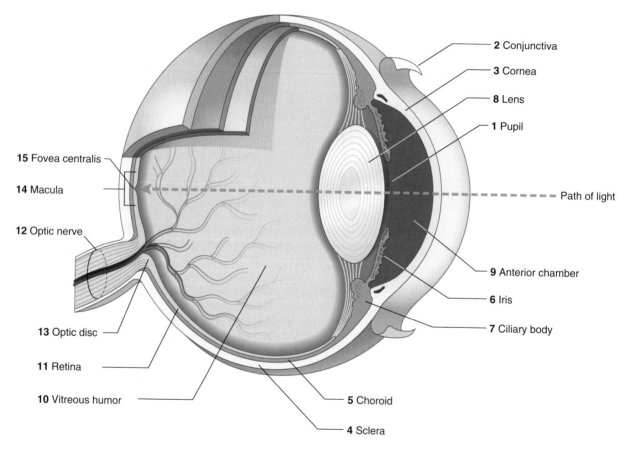

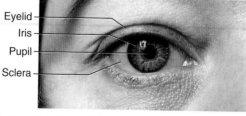

• **Figure 30-1** Normal eye anatomy. (From Chabner DE. *The Language of Medicine.* 10th ed. St. Louis: Saunders; 2014.)

in elderly people (Fig. 30-2). It is usually not caused by high cholesterol levels, and treatment is unnecessary because it does not impair vision.

Younger people with genetic conditions that cause abnormally high lipid levels can have a lipid arc around the cornea. Their triglyceride levels usually exceed 4000 mg/dL, and cholesterol levels exceed 1200 mg/dL.

Tangier disease, an inherited disorder characterized by abnormally low blood levels of high-density lipoprotein (HDL) cholesterol (<5 mg/dL), results in diffuse opacity of the cornea due to deposition of cholesterol.

Cataracts

A **cataract** is a condition in which the lens of the eye becomes progressively cloudy, usually due to deterioration of the lens fibers and protein clumping (Fig. 30-3). Cataracts are a major cause of blindness throughout the world. There are several types of cataracts (Box 30-1). Most are age-related, but cataracts can also be congenital, caused by a traumatic incident, or the result of a systemic disease such as hypertension-related glaucoma, chronic steroid use, genetic disorders, or congenital rubella.

In cataracts, the lens fibers degrade into small molecules that increase osmotic pressure in the eye by attracting water into the lens, which causes the characteristic clouding. In

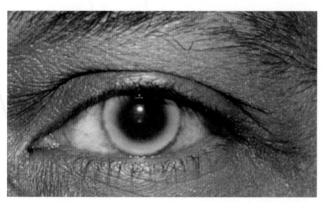

• **Figure 30-2** Arcus senilis. (Swartz MH. *Textbook of Physical Diagnosis: History and Examination*. 7th ed. Philadelphia: Saunders; 2014.)

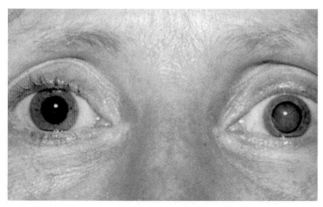

• **Figure 30-3** Cataract of the left eye. (Swartz MH. *Textbook of Physical Diagnosis: History and Examination*. 7th ed. Philadelphia: Saunders; 2014.)

uncontrolled diabetes, a large amount of glucose enters the lens, where it is converted to sorbitol by the enzyme aldose reductase. Sorbitol accumulates and attracts water, increasing the osmotic pressure and causing epithelial apoptosis, which clouds the lens and impairs function.

Hypertensive Retinopathy

Hypertensive retinopathy is caused by two common diseases: diabetes and hypertension (Fig. 30-4). Hypertensive individuals have high blood pressure in all arteries, including the eye arteries. Atherosclerosis (i.e., hardening of the arteries) also involves the eye arteries. Atherosclerosis causes small aneurysms (i.e., blood-filled bulges) in the arterial walls. Untreated hypertension can cause aneurysms in the small arteries to rupture, similar to the small arteries in the brain that rupture in a cerebrovascular accident. This damages the retina and affects eyesight due to a reduction in blood supply. Atherosclerosis also causes the arteries to become less flexible, which can affect their ability to deliver oxygenated blood to the eye. This causes damage to the retina and leads to impaired vision.

Diabetic Retinopathy

Diabetic retinopathy is progressive loss of vision as a consequence of diabetes (Fig. 30-5). Cataracts, glaucoma, and retinal detachment are complications of diabetic retinopathy. The condition is widespread among diabetics, and most newly diagnosed diabetic patients already show signs of early diabetic retinopathy due to persistently elevated blood sugar levels.

Chronically high blood sugar levels cause hypertension, increasing the microaneurysms and oxidative damage in retinal arteries. Microaneurysms burst, leaking plasma or blood and causing hemorrhages and retinal exudates. This is considered the early phase of the disease, which can progress. Later phases of diabetic retinopathy often involve proliferative vascular changes, including growth of new blood vessels in the retina that are delicate, bleed easily, and hinder vision. Scarring can occur, eventually leading to blindness. Monitoring of hemoglobin A_{1C} levels of diabetic patients is key to assessing the risk of developing diabetic retinopathy and for following progression of the disease in diagnosed patients.

• BOX 30-1 Types of Cataracts

- *Nuclear:* slowly progressive. Patients often have a temporary improvement in near vision ("second sight"), color-related vision problems, and reduced far vision.
- *Cortical:* usually stationary. Cataracts create a problem only if they are in the visual field. Patients may have areas of blurred or blocked vision.
- *Posterior subcapsular:* spotty opacities in the central posterior cortex. Patients have problems with glare and near vision.

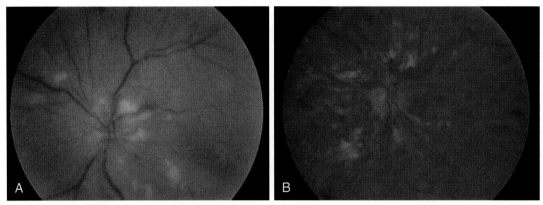

• **Figure 30-4** Retinal changes caused by systemic hypertension. **A,** Grade 4 hypertensive retinopathy, showing a swollen optic disc, retinal hemorrhages, and multiple cotton-wool spots (i.e., infarcts). **B,** Central retinal vein thrombosis, showing a swollen optic disc and widespread fundal hemorrhage. (From Walker BR, Colledge NR, Ralston SH, Penman I. *Davidson's Principles and Practice of Medicine.* 22nd ed. London: Churchill Livingstone; 2014.)

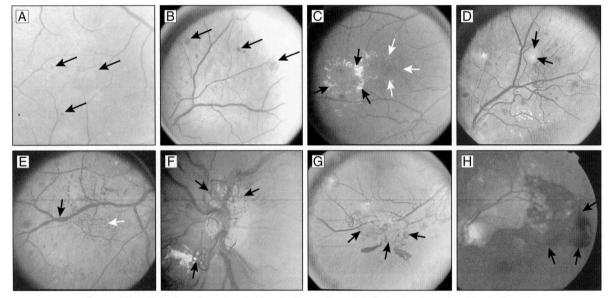

• **Figure 30-5** Diabetic retinopathy. **A,** Usually the earliest clinical abnormality, microaneurysms arise mainly from the venous end of capillaries and appear as discrete, circular, dark red dots near to but separate from the retinal vessels and no wider than a vessel at the optic disc margin *(arrows)*. **B,** Larger than a microaneurysm and with indistinct margins and at least as wide as a vessel at the optic disc margin, hemorrhages occur in deeper layers of the retina *(arrows)*. They result from microaneurysms that have burst or from leaky capillaries. Superficial flame-shaped hemorrhages in the nerve fiber layer may also occur, particularly if the patient is hypertensive. **C,** Hard exudates are irregularly shaped lesions that are formed from leakage of cholesterol, often through microaneurysms *(black arrows)*. They can be associated with retinal edema. If the exudate affects the center of the macula, it can cause clinically significant macular edema *(white arrows)*, which is sight-threatening. **D,** Cotton-wool spots are white, feathery, fluffy lesions that indicate capillary infarcts within the nerve fiber layer *(arrows)*. They are most often seen in rapidly advancing retinopathy or in association with uncontrolled hypertension. **E,** Venous beading occurs in cases of extensive retinal ischemia. Walls of veins develop saccular bulges, looking like a string of sausages *(black arrow)*. Intraretinal microvascular anomalies are spidery vessels that often have sharp corners, which indicate dilations of preexisting capillaries *(white arrow)*. **F** and **G,** Neovascularization is new vessel formation in response to widespread retinal ischemia. It may arise from the venous circulation on the optic disc *(arrows in* **F***)* or elsewhere in the retina *(arrows in* **G***)*. Initially, fine tufts of delicate vessels form arcades on the surface of the retina; later, they may extend forward onto the posterior surface of the vitreous. Serous products leaking from new vessels stimulate a connective tissue reaction with gliosis and fibrosis that first appears as a white, cloudy haze among the network of new vessels and later extends to obliterate the area with a dense white sheet. **H,** New vessels are fragile and liable to rupture during vitreous movement, causing a preretinal (i.e., subhyaloid) or vitreous hemorrhage *(arrows)*, which may lead to sudden visual loss. (From Walker BR, Colledge NR, Ralston SH, Penman I. *Davidson's Principles and Practice of Medicine.* 22nd ed. London: Churchill Livingstone; 2014.)

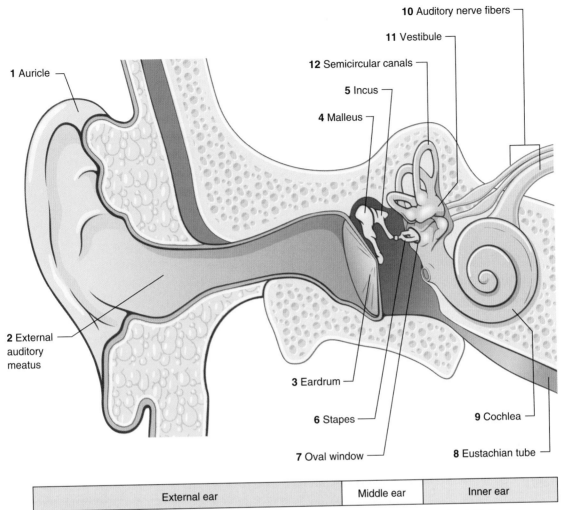

10 Auditory nerve fibers

11 Vestibule

12 Semicircular canals

5 Incus

4 Malleus

1 Auricle

2 External auditory meatus

3 Eardrum

6 Stapes

7 Oval window

9 Cochlea

8 Eustachian tube

External ear	Middle ear	Inner ear

• **Figure 30-6** Structures of the ear. (From Chabner DE. *The Language of Medicine.* 10th ed. St. Louis: Saunders; 2014.)

Ears

Ear Anatomy

The ear is divided into the outer ear, the middle ear, and the inner ear. The outer ear consists of the auricle, which is made of cartilage. The middle ear consists of the tympanic membrane and three bones: malleus, incus, and stapes. The inner ear consists of the labyrinth, which includes the cochlea and the vestibular apparatus (Fig. 30-6).

Ear Disorders

Disorders involving the inner ear can affect hearing and balance. Drugs such as aminoglycosides (e.g., streptomycin, gentamicin), vancomycin, furosemide, quinine, and related compounds cause ototoxicity and can damage the auditory nerve. Large doses of aspirin can also cause tinnitus (i.e., ringing in the ears) and temporary hearing loss. Several conditions that affect the ear, including vertigo, Meniere disease, and vestibular neuronitis, can alter clinical chemistry test results by causing vomiting.

Vertigo is usually caused by a buildup of inner ear fluid or by infection or inflammation of the inner ear. The fluid buildup creates the erroneous sensation that the environment is moving (i.e., illusory movement). It can cause balance problems, nausea, and vomiting.

Meniere disease is a chronic condition caused by an imbalance of fluid in the inner ear, which creates increased pressure and volume in the area. Symptoms include episodic vertigo, tinnitus, and hearing loss (Fig. 30-7).

Vestibular neuronitis is an inflammatory condition that results in severe, limited episodes of nausea and vertigo, usually after an infection. These conditions do not significantly alter clinical chemistry test results unless the patient has been vomiting.

Healthy inner ear

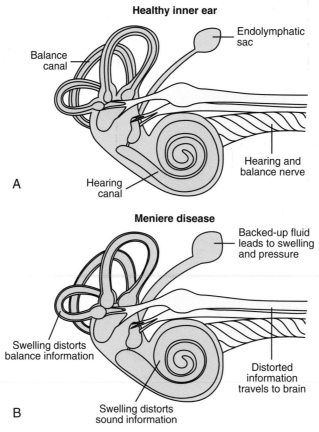

• **Figure 30-7** **A,** Healthy inner ear. **B,** Meniere disease.

Summary

Eye diseases may result from systemic diseases, as indicated by abnormal clinical chemistry test results. Eye diseases include arcus senilis, cataracts, hypertensive retinopathy, and diabetic retinopathy. Symptoms include lipid deposition in the cornea, clouding of the lens, and damage to the retina. Ear diseases that affect balance can cause nausea and vomiting, which can affect electrolyte profiles and acid-base balance. Ear diseases include vertigo, Meniere disease, and vestibular neuronitis.

Review Questions

1. Which of the following parts of the eye senses light?
   a. Retina
   b. Pupil
   c. Iris
   d. Cornea
2. Which of the following parts of the eye allows light to enter?
   a. Iris
   b. Lens
   c. Pupil
   d. Cornea
3. Which of the following eye structures lack blood vessels and lymphatics?
   a. Iris and pupil
   b. Iris and cornea
   c. Lens and pupil
   d. Lens and cornea

4. Which of the following eye diseases does hypertension lead to if it is uncontrolled?
   a. Hypertensive retinopathy
   b. Hypertensive cataracts
   c. Diabetic retinopathy
   d. Arcus senilis
5. Triglyceride levels greater than 4000 mg/dL and cholesterol levels greater than 1200 mg/dL can cause which of the following conditions?
   a. Deposition of lipids in the iris
   b. Deposition of lipids in the cornea
   c. Diabetic retinopathy
   d. Hypertensive cataracts
6. In Tangier disease, lipid is deposited in the eye due to
   a. Abnormally high HDL
   b. Very low or absent HDL
   c. Abnormally low LDL
   d. Abnormally high LDL

7. Diabetic cataracts develop because
   a. Glucose transported to the eye is converted to sorbitol, which attracts water into the lens.
   b. Glucose in the blood makes it much thicker, and when the thick blood circulates through the eye, it causes cloudiness in the cornea.
   c. Thick blood in the diabetic creates mini-aneurysms in the eye, causing damage to the retina and cataracts.
   d. Diabetics have a decreased amount of lipoprotein lipase, and lipids deposit in the eye.
8. Diabetic retinopathy is
   a. A reversible process
   b. Found only in diabetics who have blood sugar levels greater than 240 mg/dL

   c. A process that may cause damage in the eye but does not cause blindness
   d. Found in all diabetics
9. Ototoxic drugs include all of the following EXCEPT
   a. Streptomycin
   b. Gentamicin
   c. Clindamycin
   d. Vancomycin
10. Vertigo is
   a. Inflammation of the anvil bone
   b. Fluid in the middle ear causing the tympanum to bulge
   c. Ringing in the ear
   d. A condition of the inner ear that makes it seem as though the environment is moving

Critical Thinking Questions

1. What disease processes in diabetic retinopathy can lead to blindness?
2. How does atherosclerosis affect the eye?

3. What drugs affect hearing, and how do they cause problems?

CASE STUDY

A 17-year-old boy visited his physician because he was concerned about a white line around the outer portion of the cornea. He had been diagnosed 5 years earlier with Tangier disease. His physician performed laboratory tests with the following results: glucose, 95 mg/dL; creatinine, 1.0 mg/dL; calcium, 9.3 mg/dL; cholesterol, 1500 mg/dL; triglycerides, 5000 mg/dL; HDL, 4 mg/dL. What condition did the boy have? What caused the condition?

Bibliography

Burtis CA, Bruns DE. *Tietz Fundamentals of Clinical Chemistry and Molecular Diagnostics.* 7th ed. St. Louis: Saunders; 2015.

Cooper CW. Vestibular neuronitis: a review of a common cause of vertigo in general practice. *Br J Gen Pract.* 1993;43:164–167.

Grossniklaus HE, Nickerson JM, Edelhauser HF, Bergman LA, Berglin L. Anatomic alterations in aging and age-related diseases of the eye. *Invest Ophthalmol Vis Sci.* 2013;54: ORSF23-ORSF27.

Linton AD, Lach HW. *Matteson and McConnell's Gerontological Nursing: Concepts and Practice.* 3rd ed. St. Louis: Saunders; 2007.

Marill KA. Vestibular neuronitis. In: *Vestibular Neuronitis Updated.* Boston: Massachusetts General Hospital. 2013. <http://emedicine.medscape.com/article/794489-overview> Accessed 30.10.15.

McConnell TH. Diseases of the eye and ear. In: *The Nature of Disease: Pathology for the Health Professions.* 2nd ed. Philadelphia: Lippincott Williams & Wilkins; 2007.

Quaranta N, Coppola F, Casulli M, et al. Epidemiology of age related hearing loss: a review. *Hearing Balance Commun.* 2015;13(2): 77–81.

Riga M, Bibas A, Xenellis J, Korres S. Inner ear disease and benign paroxysmal positional vertigo: a critical review of incidence, clinical characteristics, and management. *Int J Otolaryngol.* 2011;2011:1.

Rothrock JC, Alexander SA. *Alexander's Surgical Procedures.* St. Louis: Mosby; 2012.

Ryan W, Sachin D. Drug induced ototoxicity. *Clin Exp Pharmacol.* 2014;4:e132.

Sharma K, Kanaujia V, Mishra P, Agarwal R, Tripathi A. Hypertensive retinopathy. *Clinical Queries: Nephrology.* 2013;2(3):136–139.

Syed I, Aldren C. Meniere's disease: an evidence based approach to assessment and management. *Int J Clin Pract.* 2012;66:166–170.

Yau JW, Rogers SL, Kawasaki R, et al. Global prevalence and major risk factors of diabetic retinopathy. *Diabetes Care.* 2012;35:556–564.

31

Nutritional and Metabolic Diseases

DONNA LARSON

CHAPTER OUTLINE

OBJECTIVES

After completion of this chapter, the reader will be able to:

1. Describe cold injuries and their significance to clinical chemistry.
2. Describe heat injuries and their significance to clinical chemistry.
3. Describe the hormonal effects of food.
4. Define eicosanoid and give four examples.
5. Describe eicosanoid synthesis and function.
6. Differentiate between dietary sources, functions, and nutritional requirements for macronutrients.
7. Identify laboratory methods to measure vitamins.
8. Compare and contrast the properties and functions of vitamins.
9. Describe the vitamin deficiency conditions.
10. Identify the laboratory methods commonly used to measure trace elements.
11. Describe the clinical significance of each trace element.
12. Identify the deficiency conditions associated with trace metals and the symptoms and laboratory results.
13. Discuss malnutrition worldwide, in the United States, and in institutionalized populations.
14. Describe neonatal screening for aminoacidurias.
15. Identify methods for performing screening tests for aminoacidurias.
16. Compare and contrast phenylketonuria, tyrosinemia, alkaptonuria, homocystinuria, maple syrup disease, cystinuria, and Hartnup disease.
17. Compare and contrast Tay-Sachs disease, Niemann-Pick disease, Gaucher disease, Krabbe disease, and Hurler syndrome.

KEY TERMS

Alkaptonuria
Cystinuria
Eicosanoid
Essential fatty acid
Folic acid
Frostbite
Frostnip
Gaucher disease

Health
Heat cramp
Heat exhaustion
Heat stroke
Homocystinuria
Hurler syndrome
Hyperthermia
Hypothermia

Kashin-Beck disease
Keshan disease
Krabbe disease
Kwashiorkor
Leukotriene
Linoleic acid
Linolenic acid
Lipolysis

KEY TERMS—cont'd

Lipoxin	Nutrition	Vitamin B$_2$
Macronutrient	Obesity	Vitamin B$_6$
Malnutrition	Phenylketonuria	Vitamin B$_{12}$
Maple syrup disease	Prostaglandin	Vitamin C
Marasmus	Rhabdomyolysis	Vitamin D
Menkes disease	Tachycardia	Vitamin E
Metabolic syndrome	Tay-Sachs disease	Vitamin H
Micronutrient	Thromboxane	Vitamin K
Niacin	Tyrosinemia	Wilson disease
Niemann-Pick disease	Vitamin A	
Nutrient	Vitamin B$_1$	

❖ Case in Point

A 40-year-old woman is experiencing fatigue and depression. Her physician also diagnoses osteomalacia. She lives on the coast in the Pacific Northwest where there are more than 200 days of clouds and rain every year. Her routine chemistry test results are within normal limits:

Glucose, 105 mg/dL
Blood urea nitrogen (BUN), 30 mg/dL
Creatinine, 1.2 mg/dL
Na, 142 mEq/L
K, 4.3 mEq/L
Cl, 107 mEq/L
CO$_2$, 32 mg/dL
Phosphorus, 3.7 mg/dL
Calcium, 8.4 mg/dL
Alkaline phosphatase (ALP), 101 IU/L

What test would the physician order next? Why? What would the results of that test be expected to show? How would this woman be treated?

Points to Remember

- People are more susceptible to cold injuries when hungry, dehydrated, or abusing substances or when an underlying condition impairs cardiovascular function.
- Potassium levels correlate well with recovery from a cold-related injury; a value greater than 10 mEq/L indicates a very low likelihood of recovery.
- As with blood gas testing, coagulation testing is performed on samples that are heated to 37° C, and this may not reflect the patient's actual condition. Results of laboratory tests must be interpreted carefully because reference ranges and test results assume that the patient's body temperature is 37° C.
- Symptoms of heat exhaustion include pale, moist skin; fever between 34° C and 40° C; nausea; vomiting; diarrhea; headache; fatigue; weakness; anxiety; and faint feeling.
- Heat stroke is a medical emergency and can lead to death if not treated immediately.

- Symptoms of heat stroke include a body temperature greater than 41° C, neurologic dysfunction, tachycardia, hyperventilation, gastrointestinal hemorrhage, hepatic injury, rhabdomyolysis, and acute kidney injury.
- All humans require common macronutrients and micronutrients to perform physiologic body processes. Diseases and chronic conditions can result from too much or too little of each of these nutrients.
- Laboratory testing in nutritional assessment is focused on the protein concentration in the body.
- Hormones are produced when food enters the body, and these hormones help regulate digestion and absorption of nutrients.
- Two hormones are exceptionally important in maintaining optimal function of the body: insulin and glucagon.
- Insulin is a storage hormone; it takes carbohydrates and stores them as fat. Insulin is also released when excess amino acids or calories are consumed.
- Glucagon is a mobilization hormone; it releases stored glucose (glycogen and fat) to increase blood glucose levels. Glucagon secretion is also stimulated by the presence of protein in the blood.
- Amino acids that are not produced by the body but must be ingested to build and maintain tissues are called essential amino acids. Essential amino acids include isoleucine, leucine, lysine, methionine, phenylalanine, threonine, tryptophan, valine, histidine, arginine, and taurine.
- The essential fatty acids include both ω-6 (linoleic acid) and ω-3 (linolenic acid) fatty acids, and both classes are used to make eicosanoids.
- The eicosanoids consist of prostaglandins (PG), thromboxanes (TX), leukotrienes (LT), and lipoxins (LX). The PGs and TXs are called prostanoids.
- Eicosanoids have a short half-life, are extremely potent, and cause profound physiologic effects at very dilute concentrations.
- The eicosanoids made from arachidonic acid (series 2 PGs and TXs and series 4 LTs) increase the inflammatory response, increase vasoconstriction, induce labor, and activate platelet aggregation and thrombosis.
- The other biologically important eicosanoids (i.e., PG$_1$ and TX$_1$) are made from dihomo-γ-linolenic acid

(DGLA); they inhibit gastric acid secretion, increase vasodilation, decrease the inflammatory response, and inhibit platelet aggregation and thrombosis.

- If there is more DLGA, more favorable eicosanoids will be produced; if there is more arachidonic acid, more unfavorable eicosanoids will be produced. This is an important nutritional metabolic pathway because it demonstrates that eating the right foods can prevent the inflammation that may lead to atherosclerosis, diabetes, and other chronic diseases.
- Micronutrients are substances that are needed by the body in very small amounts but are essential for good health; deficiency of a micronutrient may cause disease. Vitamins are considered micronutrients, as are trace metals.
- Vitamin A has a role in reproduction, growth and embryonic development, and immune function. Retinol and its metabolites can also protect against certain types of cancer.
- Vitamin E is a potent antioxidant that halts the production of molecular oxygen and free radicals during fat oxidation.
- Vitamin E is needed for neurologic and reproductive functions, red cell membrane protection, and inhibition of reactive oxygen species production during lipid metabolism. Vitamin E is also believed to decrease cardiovascular disease and cancer.
- The function of vitamin D is to maintain the calcium and phosphate concentrations in serum. This compound is regulated by parathyroid hormone and blood levels of calcium and phosphate.
- Vitamin K consists of two types—K_1 (phylloquinone) and K_2 (menaquinone). This vitamin is required for the production of several clotting factors, including factor II (prothrombin), factor VII (proconvertin), factor IX (plasma thromboplastin component), and factor X (Stuart factor). It may also be involved in bone metabolism.
- Biotin participates in chemical reactions leading to the synthesis of fatty acids and citrate and in the metabolism of odd-numbered fatty acids and branched-chain fatty acids.
- Vitamin B_1, also known as thiamine, is required for decarboxylation reactions.
- Vitamin B_2, also known as riboflavin, is an essential part of coenzymes (e.g., flavin adenine dinucleotide, or FAD) that are involved in redox reactions.
- Vitamin B_6, also called pyridoxine, is used in the synthesis, catabolism, and interconversion of amino acids.
- Vitamin B_{12} is a coenzyme in many enzyme systems and is primarily responsible for amino acid metabolism.
- Niacin (nicotinic acid) is converted to the redox coenzymes, NAD and NADP, which participate in reactions that convert alcohols to aldehydes or ketones, aldehydes to acids, and certain amino acids to keto acids.
- Folic acid is involved in the synthesis of thymidine, purines, DNA, RNA, hormones, neurotransmitters, and membrane lipids and proteins as well as the metabolism of homocysteine.

- Vitamin C functions as a cofactor for synthesis of adrenal hormones, corticosteroids, aldosterone, bile acids, and folate metabolism. Vitamin C is the most effective water-soluble antioxidant because it binds to reactive oxygen and nitrogen species in the body.
- Chromium (trivalent) is used by the body to enhance the action of insulin.
- Copper is an important component in ceruloplasmin. Ceruloplasmin is an acute phase reactant that is increased in infection and tissue injury. Copper also serves as a component of enzymes such as cytochrome *c* oxidase and other proteins.
- Fluoride is used extensively in public health to prevent tooth caries. Small studies indicate that it may be useful in reducing bone fracturing in individuals with osteoporosis.
- Manganese is associated with the formation of connective tissue, growth, reproduction, and carbohydrate and lipid metabolism.
- Selenium is a component of compounds that act as antioxidants in the body and of many enzymes.
- Zinc plays a key role in growth and wound healing and in regulating synthesis of steroids, thyroid hormones, and other hormones. In addition, large amounts of zinc are required to maintain an antibacterial and vital environment in the prostate so that sperm maintain their function.
- An individual with metabolic syndrome is twice as likely to develop heart disease and five times as likely to develop diabetes as a healthy person.
- Malnutrition occurs when a person does not ingest the macronutrients and micronutrients necessary to maintain good health.
- Inborn errors of metabolism are caused by single-gene mutations that result in a blocked metabolic pathway.
- Tay-Sachs disease is a fatal genetic lipid storage disorder in which gangliosides build up in the tissues and in the brain.
- Niemann-Pick disease is a genetic disease that affects the production of sphingomyelinase, an enzyme that is used in the breakdown, transport, and metabolism of fats and cholesterol in the body.
- Gaucher disease is a genetic disease that produces serious neurologic problems including hydrops fetalis.
- Krabbe disease is a genetic disease that impairs the growth and maintenance of myelin, resulting in irritability, muscle weakness, feeding difficulties, and slowed mental and physical development.
- Hurler syndrome is a genetic disease that allows mucopolysaccharides to build up in organs, causing damage.
- Phenylketonuria is a genetic disease that results in the accumulation of phenylalanine, phenylketones, and phenylamines, which can lead to brain damage and severe mental retardation.
- Tyrosinemia is a genetic disease that leads to the buildup of tyrosine in the body, resulting in failure to thrive, diarrhea, vomiting, jaundice, and increased nosebleeds.

- Alkaptonuria is a genetic condition that results in increased levels of homogentisic acid. This acid deposits dark pigment in the connective tissue and causes heart problems and arthritis in early adulthood.
- Homocystinuria is a mild genetic disease that may cause myopia, osteoporosis, dislocation of the lens at the front of the eye, and possible developmental delay.
- Maple syrup disease is a genetic disorder that produces sweet-smelling urine, poor feeding of infants, vomiting, lethargy, and developmental delay. Death can result if the disease is not treated.
- Cystinuria is a genetic condition that causes cysteine crystals or stones to develop in the kidney or bladder.

Introduction

This chapter examines disorders that result from daily activities involving exposure to air, water, work, recreation, food, drink, and behavior. It is important to know when a disorder will affect clinical chemistry test results and which disorders do not affect clinical chemistry test results. Physical trauma is a condition that affects many individuals; depending on the severity of the trauma, clinical chemistry test results may or may not be affected. Trauma can be caused by temperature extremes, pollution, occupational environments, toxic substances, radiation, inhalation, or ingestion. Nutrition can also affect the health of an individual, and many clinical laboratories perform nutritional assessments.

General Concepts of Health and Disease

Over the years, the definition of "health" has changed. In the past, health was defined merely as the absence of disease. As medical science advanced and researchers learned more about the human body, this definition did not adequately describe health. The World Health Organization defines **health** as "a state of complete physical, mental, and social well-being and not merely the absence of disease or infirmity." This differentiation is important when one examines how environment can affect health. The environment is filled with pollutants, animals, chemicals, plants, foods, drinks, machines, radiation (i.e., from the sun), tools, and weather, all of which have effects on the body and can even injure or kill under certain circumstances (Table 31-1).

The first section of the chapter discusses physical threats to health. The second section discusses **nutrition** and its role in health, and the final section discusses a group of diseases called inborn errors of metabolism.

Cold Injuries

Cold injuries occur when a person's body is exposed to cold temperatures for a period that reduces body temperature below 37° C (**hypothermia**) or when, in subfreezing temperatures, body tissue freezes. People are more susceptible to these types of injuries when they are hungry, dehydrated, abusing substances, and have an underlying

TABLE 31-1 Components of Health

Component	Aspect	Examples
Diet	Carbohydrates Fats Proteins	Whole grains Fiber Vitamins Variety of foods Fruits Vegetables Dairy products Meats Vegetable protein
Sleep	Consequences of inadequate sleep Insomnia 33% of one's life	Making mistakes Stress Difficulty concentrating Tips: comfortable mattress, regular sleeping hours, regular exercise
Exercise	Flexibility Stretching Warmup Strength training Toning	Bicycling Treadmill Stair climber Smooth, slow movements No pain
Stress	Causes Effects Solutions Relaxation	Examinations Work Relationships Crying Diarrhea Insomnia Anxiety Avoid smoking, alcohol, caffeine Exercise Set goals Deep breathing Meditation Yoga

condition that impairs cardiovascular function. Hypothermia causes all physiologic functions to slow down. A person loses consciousness when the body temperature falls below 32° C and cardiac arrest follows. Hypothermia can manifest with wide fluctuations in electrolyte levels (Fig. 31-1).

Potassium levels correlate well with recovery: A value greater than 10 mEq/L indicates a very low likelihood of recovery. Blood gas measurements in hypothermic patients are not accurate. Oxygen and carbon dioxide are less soluble in hypothermic blood, and the partial pressure of oxygen (pO_2) and partial pressure of carbon dioxide (pCO_2) test results can be higher than actual patient values because the instrument warms specimens to 37° C before measuring the gases. The pH of the patient's blood appears lower than the actual value. In addition, a person's coagulation system may be disrupted due to protein denaturation of enzymes vital to the processes. Disseminated intravascular coagulation may be present. Results of laboratory tests must be interpreted carefully because reference ranges and test results assume that the person's body temperature is 37° C.

Extended exposure of body tissue to subfreezing temperatures can cause tissue to turn white and begin the freezing process (frostnip) or totally freeze (frostbite) when the blood supply is cut off, ice crystals form in the tissue, and the tissue turns black (Fig. 31-2). Frostnip and frostbite are diagnosed clinically, and laboratory tests do not provide any useful or clinically important information for diagnosis. Laboratory tests can be used to identify delayed systemic complications such as wound infection and sepsis. Initial testing may include complete blood count (CBC), electrolytes, blood urea nitrogen (BUN), creatinine, glucose, and liver function tests. Individuals suffering from frostbite may experience myoglobinuria, which can be detected by urinalysis.

Heat Illnesses

Heat cramps are the mildest form of heat illness. They are painful muscle cramps that occur when an individual

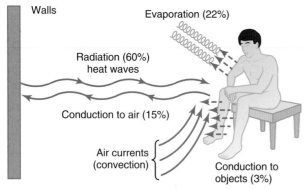

• **Figure 31-1** Mechanisms of heat loss from the body. (From Hall JE. *Guyton and Hall Textbook of Medical Physiology.* 12th ed. Philadelphia: Saunders; 2011.)

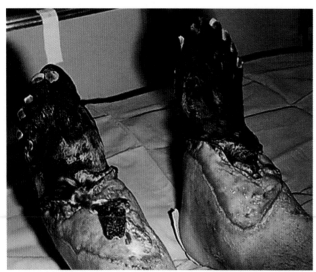

• **Figure 31-2** Frostbite. Gangrenous necrosis develops 6 weeks after the original injury. (From Lewis SL, Dirksen SR, Heitkemper MM, Bucher L. *Medical-Surgical Nursing: Assessment and Management of Clinical Problems.* 9th ed. St. Louis: Mosby; 2014.)

loses water and salt through excessive sweating. The condition usually abates after the water and salt lost in sweat are replenished.

Heat exhaustion is the next level of heat illness. If not treated, it can quickly turn into heat stroke, a medical emergency. Symptoms include pale, moist skin; fever between 34° C and 40° C; nausea; vomiting; diarrhea; headache; fatigue; weakness; anxiety; and faint feeling (Table 31-2). Heat exhaustion is usually diagnosed clinically, but glucose and troponin I and T tests are needed to rule out hypoglycemia and coronary disease. Electrolyte levels are measured to exclude severe hyponatremia in patients with excessive free water intake.

Heat Stroke

Heat stroke is a medical emergency that can lead to death if not treated immediately. In heat stroke, a person's heat gain overwhelms the body's ability to lose heat, thus increasing body temperature (hyperthermia). Symptoms of heat stroke include a body temperature higher than 41° C, neurologic dysfunction, tachycardia (rapid heartbeat), hyperventilation, gastrointestinal hemorrhage, hepatic injury, rhabdomyolysis (breakdown of muscle tissue with release of toxic substances), and acute kidney injury. Cardiovascular collapse can occur with a very high body temperature. The high temperature interferes with cellular processes and denatures proteins and cellular membranes. This combination of effects leads to the production of inflammatory cytokines, interleukins, and heat shock proteins. An individual can progress from heat exhaustion to heat stroke when there is a systemic inflammatory response and multiorgan dysfunction.

TABLE 31-2	Signs and Symptoms of Heat-Related Illnesses	
Observations	**Heat Exhaustion**	**Heat Stroke**
Skin	Profuse diaphoresis	Dry; no diaphoresis
Nausea	Present	Present
Headache	Present	Present
Breathing	Shallow, rapid	Labored
Pulse	Weak, rapid	Strong, rapid
Color	Pale	Flushed or changes to gray
Temperature	Normal or slightly elevated	Very elevated (106-110° F)
Behavior	Exhaustion, collapse	Exhaustion, collapse, convulsions
Consciousness	Unconscious	Unconscious
Eyes	Pupils normal	Pupils contract, then dilate

From Fairchild DL. *Pierson and Fairchild's Principles and& Techniques of Patient Care.* 5th ed. St. Louis: Saunders; 2013.

Laboratory test results in heat stroke are very abnormal. Arterial blood gas analysis may reveal respiratory alkalosis or metabolic acidosis or both due to lactic acidosis. Hypoglycemia may results from liver failure. Many patients are dehydrated, and this results in increased sodium levels with decreased potassium levels. Hypophosphatemia, hypocalcemia, and hypomagnesemia are also common. Liver damage leads to aspartate aminotransferase (AST) and alanine aminotransferase (ALT) levels tens of thousands of times greater than normal during the early phases of the disease. Jaundice may occur 36 to 72 hours after liver failure. Muscle necrosis leads to elevated creatinine kinase (CK), lactate dehydrogenase, aldolase, and myoglobin values. The CK levels can be greater than 100,000 IU/L. Patients who experience renal failure have elevations in uric acid, BUN, and creatinine levels.

Nutritional Conditions

Diet is associated with health and disease. Every culture has its own understanding of what foods produce a healthy body and health in general. People in Western, industrialized countries tend to consume a diet that is high in carbohydrates and processed foods but low in fiber. This type of diet can increase the risk of cardiovascular disease and cancer, as demonstrated by the disease statistics for these countries. All humans require common macronutrients and micronutrients to perform physiologic body processes. Diseases and chronic conditions can result from consuming too much or too little of each of these nutrients (Fig. 31-3).

Nutrition

Nutrition is the process by which organisms take in and utilize food for health and growth. Eating a healthy diet is not simple, and many people and groups have differing ideas on the composition of a healthy diet. The recommended daily allowances (RDAs) were created by the Food and Nutrition Board of the National Academy of Sciences in 1941 and have been updated 10 times since then. The Food Guide Pyramid was later developed by the federal government to

help Americans eat healthier, based on the RDAs. In June 2011, the Food Guide Pyramid was replaced by MyPlate as the primary food group symbol (Fig. 31-4).

The types and amounts of food that are eaten play a large part in health. Since the RDAs were created, Americans have, on average, gained weight, and excess weight negatively affects health. Obesity (excessive accumulation of body fat that adversely affects health) is at an all-time high in the United States and is related to diet and lifestyle. This section reviews the hormonal effects of food, macronutrients, micronutrients, trace metals, and toxic metals and how each of these affects the body.

Hormonal Effects of Food

Certain hormones are produced when food enters the body and help regulate digestion and absorption of nutrients. In this way, food controls the hormones produced in digestion and absorption (see Chapter 20 for further discussion). Two of these hormones are exceptionally important in maintaining optimal function of the body: insulin and glucagon. Insulin is the hormone produced when glucose levels in the blood rise, and glucagon is produced when blood glucose levels fall.

Macronutrients

Any compound that can be used for calories or energy is considered a nutrient. Nutrients that are required by the body in large amounts are called macronutrients. This section focuses on the specific digestion of the macronutrients—carbohydrates, proteins, and fats—and how they affect normal body function.

Carbohydrates

Carbohydrates are classified as monosaccharides (glucose, fructose, and galactose), disaccharides (lactose, sucrose, maltose, and trehalose), oligosaccharides (dextrins), and polysaccharides

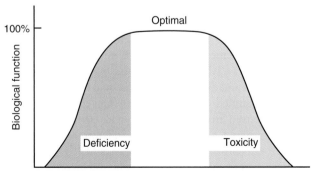

• **Figure 31-3** Essential nutrient balance curve. (From Burtis CA, Bruns DE. *Tietz Fundamentals of Clinical Chemistry and Molecular Diagnostics.* 7th ed. St. Louis: Saunders; 2015.)

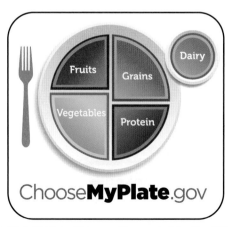

• **Figure 31-4** MyPlate. This graphic, created by the U.S. Department of Agriculture, represents the proper serving size of various food groups. (From the U.S. Department of Agriculture. *Getting started with MyPlate.* Revised August 2012. <www.choosemyplate.gov> Accessed 22.06.15.)

(cellulose) (Box 31-1). Dietary carbohydrates are digested and broken down into glucose to fuel the body (see Fig. 21-2 in Chapter 21). The glucose level in blood increases, causing insulin to be released into the bloodstream to decrease the blood glucose level. Insulin is a storage hormone: It takes carbohydrates and stores them as fat. Insulin is also released when excessive amounts of amino acids or calories are consumed. Glucagon secretion is also stimulated by the presence of protein in the blood; this is referred to as the insulin–glucagon axis. Glucagon is a mobilization hormone: It releases stored glucose (glycogen and fat) to increase blood glucose levels.

Proteins

Proteins are large, folded chains of amino acids (Box 31-2). Most Americans ingest more protein than is needed by their bodies. In addition to dietary protein, protein enters the digestive tract in gastrointestinal secretions and from sloughed mucosal cells. Protein digestion begins in the stomach when the enzyme pepsin and stomach acid begin denaturing the protein (see Fig. 21-3 in Chapter 21). Digestive enzymes work more effectively when the protein is reduced to its primary structure (a long chain of amino acids). The pancreas produces enzymes that continue protein digestion in the intestines: trypsin, chymotrypsin, and elastase. Proteins are catabolized into single amino acids and then absorbed in the intestines. These amino acid macronutrients are used to synthesize other proteins that are required for functions throughout the body.

Amino acids that are not produced by the body and must be ingested for the body to build and maintain tissues are called *essential amino acids*. Essential amino acids include isoleucine, leucine, lysine, methionine, phenylalanine,

threonine, tryptophan, valine, histidine, arginine, and taurine. *Protein quality* is based on the amount of essential amino acids contained in the protein. Infants and children require a higher percentage of essential amino acids (43% and 36%, respectively) in their food compared with adults (10%).

Additional protein intake is required by the body when protein losses are greater than normal, as with fevers, burns, surgical trauma, or fractures. Too much protein also can be detrimental to health in some disease states. Protein intake is restricted in patients with acute liver failure or end-stage renal disease.

Fats

Dietary fat consists of cholesterol, triglycerides, and fatty acids (see Chapter 17 for coverage of cholesterol and triglyceride metabolism). Essential fatty acids are those that must be ingested because the body cannot produce them. They are split by enzymes called *lipases* but do not require complete lipolysis to be absorbed into the blood. There are two types of essential fatty acids: the ω-6 fatty acids and the ω-3 fatty acids. Both classes are used to make eicosanoids. Linoleic acid, an ω-6 fatty acid, is found in vegetable oils, especially borage oil, evening primrose oil, and black current oil; it is processed in the body to γ-linolenic acid (GLA). The best dietary sources for α-linolenic acid (ALA), an important member of the ω-3 fatty acid (linolenic acid) family, are seed oils, especially chia, perilla, flaxseed, canola, and soy oils.

Eicosanoids control the production of hormones and physiologic functions. They consist of prostaglandins (PGs), thromboxanes (TXs), leukotrienes (LTs), and lipoxins (LXs). The PGs and TXs are called *prostanoids*. The naming convention for eicosanoids involves use of a subscript digit indicating the number of carbon–carbon double bonds in the molecule. Most of the biologically active PGs (e.g., PGE$_2$) and TXs are series 2 molecules because they have two double bonds; some are series 1. Biologically active LTs are series 4 molecules. LXs are potent antiinflammatory molecules that are created through lipoxygenase interactions (hence the name).

All mammalian cells except erythrocytes produce eicosanoids. These molecules have a short half-life, are extremely potent, and cause profound physiologic effects at very dilute concentrations. They use receptor-mediated signaling pathways in the cell to produce a local effect. Some biologically important eicosanoids are derived from the ω-6 fatty acid, *arachidonic acid*, which is synthesized from dietary linoleic acid via GLA and dihomo-γ-linolenic acid (DGLA) and can also be consumed directly in meats (Fig. 31-5). The eicosanoids derived from arachidonic acid (series 2 PGs and TXs and series 4 LTs) increase the inflammatory response, increase vasoconstriction, induce labor, and activate platelet aggregation and thrombosis. The other biologically important eicosanoids (series 1 PGs and TXs) are made from DGLA via a different pathway. They inhibit gastric acid secretion, increase vasodilation, decrease the inflammatory response, and inhibit platelet aggregation and thrombosis.

• BOX 31-1 Common Carbohydrates

Corn	Candy
Potatoes	Cake
Bread	Pies
Sugar	Pasta
Rice	Chips
Cereal	Pretzels
Fruits	Soda
Tomatoes	Fruit juice
Honey	Muffins
Vegetables	Cookies
Ice cream	

• BOX 31-2 Common Proteins

Dairy (e.g., milk, cheese, cottage cheese)
Eggs
Meat (e.g., beef, pork)
Poultry (e.g., chicken, turkey)
Seafood (e.g., fish, lobster, shrimp, crab, scallops)
Beans
Soy products (e.g., tofu)

(One of these products, PGE₁, is such a powerful vasodilator that it is used to treat erectile dysfunction.)

Ingested linoleic acid is first converted to GLA. This reaction is catalyzed by an enzyme, Δ-6-desaturase, but the process is very slow. GLA can also be introduced directly in certain foods. The GLA undergoes elongation into DGLA (see Fig. 31-5). The cyclooxygenase (COX) enzyme can act on DGLA, resulting in synthesis of the series 1 PGs and TXs. These molecules produce favorable responses in the body—vasodilation and antiinflammatory effects. If the enzyme Δ-5-desaturase acts on DGLA, arachidonic acid is produced. Other enzymes then act on the arachidonic acid: a COX-mediated pathway produces series 2 PGs and TXs, and the action of 5-lipoxygenase (5-LOX) produces series 4 LTs. These molecules cause unfavorable responses in the body—vasoconstriction and inflammation. The activities of both Δ-6-desaturase and Δ-5-desaturase can be affected by nutritional deficiencies as well as inflammation and other environmental conditions.

Notice in Figure 31-5 that Δ-5-desaturase is inhibited by glucagon and activated by insulin. Consumption of proteins releases glucagon, thus inhibiting this enzyme and the production of arachidonic acid. Carbohydrate consumption, on the other hand, releases insulin, activating Δ-5-desaturase and producing more arachidonic acid. Because DGLA and arachidonic acid compete for the same positions in cell membrane phospholipids, diets rich in GLA can lead to an increased ratio of DGLA to arachidonic acid in cell membranes and thus to greater production of favorable versus unfavorable eicosanoids. This demonstrates one way that eating the right foods helps prevent the inflammation that can lead to atherosclerosis, diabetes, and other chronic diseases.

As mentioned earlier, linoleic acid is converted to GLA by Δ-6-desaturase in a very slow process. Alcohol use, smoking,

intake of saturated fats and *trans*-fats, and deficiencies of magnesium, vitamin B₆, and zinc can all further reduce the speed of this reaction. Chronic conditions such as hypertension, arthritis, psoriasis, and diabetes also slow the reaction. If proinflammatory and antiinflammatory eicosanoids are not balanced (i.e., if arachidonic acid derivatives predominate), disease may ensue, including heart disease, arthritis, and cancer. The series 2 PGs and TXs and series 4 LTs are some of the most powerful hormones produced in the body by a macronutrient—fat.

Assessing Macronutrients

Poor nutritional status can lead to increased morbidity and mortality during acute illness. A nutritional assessment is a comprehensive evaluation that includes a tailored history, physical examination, laboratory assessment, body composition analysis, and functional status. Laboratory testing in a nutritional assessment is focused on the protein concentration in the body. Albumin, transferrin, prealbumin, and retinol-binding protein are measured. Low concentrations of these proteins in the body correlate well with **malnutrition.** Specific vitamin and metal levels may also be measured to rule out or rule in particular diseases.

Micronutrients

In addition to macronutrients, many micronutrients play a large part in keeping the human body healthy. **Micronutrients** are substances that are needed by the body in very small amounts but are essential for good health and may cause disease if deficient. Vitamins are considered micronutrients, as are trace metals. These substances are important reactants in many physiologic reactions. Vitamins important for good health include vitamins A, E, D, K, H, B₁, B₂, B₆, B₁₂, and niacin (Table 31-3).

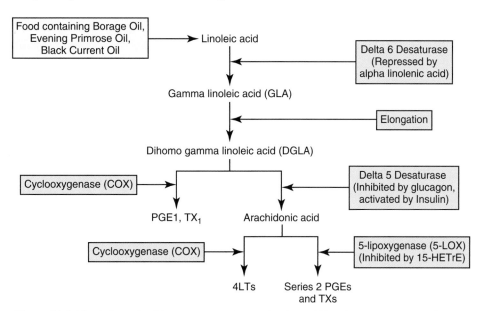

• **Figure 31-5** Metabolism of ω-6 fatty acids to series 4 leukotrienes (*LT*), series 2 thromboxanes (*TX*), and series 1 and series 2 prostaglandin E (*PGE*). 15-Hydroxyeicosatetrienoic acid (*15-HETrE*) is derived from dihomo-γ-linolenic acid (*DGLA*) via a 15-LOX–mediated pathway.

TABLE 31-3 **Human Vitamin Requirements and Reference Ranges**

Common Name	Trivial Chemical Names	General Roles	Reference Range	Symptoms of Deficiency or Disease	Direct and Indirect Assays
Fat Soluble					
Vitamin A	Retinol, retinal, retinoic acid	Vision, growth reproduction	30-80 µg/dL adult	Nyctalopia, xerophthalmia, keratomalacia	Photometric, HPLC, fluorometric, RIA
Vitamins D_2, D_3	Ergocalciferol, cholecalciferol	Modulation of Ca^{2+} metabolism, calcification of bones and teeth	15-60 pg/mL	Rickets (young), osteomalacia (adult)	CPB, HPLC, RIA
Vitamin E	Tocopherols, tocotrienols	Antioxidant for unsaturated lipids, neurologic and reproductive functions	0.5-1.8 mg/dL adult (plasma)	Lipid peroxidation, including red blood cell fragility, hemolytic anemia (premature, newborn)	Photometric, HPLC, erythrocyte hemolysis
Vitamins K_1, K_2	Phylloquinones, menaquinones	Blood clotting, osteocalcins	0.13-1.19 ng/mL (plasma)	Increased clotting time, RIA time; hemorrhagic disease (infant)	HPLC, prothrombin (abnormal prothrombin, PIVKA test)
Water Soluble					
Vitamin B_1	Thiamine	Carbohydrate metabolism, nervous function	90-140 nmol/L whole-blood (thiamine pyrophosphate)	Beriberi, Wenicke-Korsakoff syndrome	Fluorometric, HPLC
Vitamin B_2	Riboflavin	Oxidation-reduction reactions	4-24 µg/dL plasma	Angular stomatitis, dermatitis, photophobia	Fluorometric, HPLC, glutathione reductase
Vitamin B_6	Pyridoxine, pyridoxal, pyridoxamine	Amino acid, phospholipid, and glycogen metabolism	5-30 mg/dL plasma (pyridoxal-5′-phosphate)	Epileptiform convulsions, dermatitis, hypochromic anemia	HPLC, aspartate transaminase, urine pyridoxic acid
Niacin	Nicotinic acid, nicotinamide	Oxidation-reduction reactions	2.4-6.4 mg/day urine (excretion rate)	Pellagra	Fluorometric, HPLC, niacinamide nicotinamide coenzymes
Folic acid	Pteroylglutamic acid	Nucleic acid and amino acid biosynthesis	2.6-12.2 µg/L serum	Megaloblastic anemia, neural tube defects	Microbiological, homocysteine, CPB
Vitamin B_{12}	Cyanocobalamin	Amino acid and branched-chain keto acid metabolism	>201 ng/L serum	Pernicious and megaloblastic anemia, neuropathy	Microbiological, RIA, CPB, methylmalonate
Biotin (Vitamin H)		Carboxylation reactions	0.5-2.20 nmol/L whole blood	Dermatitis	Microbiological, carboxylases, avidin binding, CPB
Pantothenic acid		General metabolism, acetyl transfer	344-583 µg/L serum or whole blood	Burning feet syndrome	Microbiological, RIA, HPLC, CPB
Vitamin C	Ascorbic acid	Connective formation, antioxidant	0.4-1.5 mg/dL	Scurvy	Photometric, HPLC, enzymatic

Adapted from Burtis CA, Bruns DE. *Tietz Fundamentals of Clinical Chemistry and Molecular Diagnostics*. 7th ed. St. Louis: Saunders; 2015.
CPB, Competitive protein binding; *HPLC,* high-performance liquid chromatography; *PIVKA,* proteins induced by or involved in vitamin K antagonism or absence; *RIA,* radioimmunoassay.

Vitamin A

Vitamin A contains retinol and plays an important role in vision. This vitamin is ingested as dietary β-carotene in organ meats, fish oils, full-cream milk, butter, pumpkin, carrots, tomatoes, apricots, grapefruit, lettuce, and most green vegetables. Vitamin A is oil soluble and is insoluble in water. Once ingested, β-carotene is emulsified with bile salts in the intestines, packaged into chylomicrons, and released into the blood. As retinol circulates through the liver, it undergoes chemical reactions; as it gets to the eye, it forms photosensitive pigments. Vitamin A also has roles in reproduction, growth and embryonic development, and immune function. Retinol and its metabolites can protect against certain types of cancer. The RDA for vitamin A is 700 to 900 μg/day for adults. Vitamin A deficiency can be caused by celiac disease, chronic pancreatitis, protein–energy malnutrition, or liver disease. Vitamin A deficiency can lead to anemia.

Clinical signs and symptoms of a deficiency state include degenerative changes in the eyes and skin. Eye conditions include nyctalopia (night blindness), xerophthalmia (dry conjunctiva with small gray spots), and keratomalacia (ulceration and necrosis of the cornea). Associated skin conditions are dryness, papular eruptions, and follicular hyperkeratosis.

Even though vitamin A metabolism is tightly controlled, excess ingestion of vitamin A can occur. The liver can store retinol and its metabolites at levels up to 3000 μg/g of liver tissue. To reach this level, a person would need to ingest 30,000 μg/day for months or years. Symptoms of chronic toxicity include bone and joint pain, hair loss, dryness and fissures of the lips, anorexia, benign intracranial hypertension, weight loss, and hepatomegaly.

Laboratory Procedures and Limitations

Vitamin A status is assessed by measurement of serum vitamin A levels. However, the liver stores much vitamin A, and critical blood levels will occur only after liver stores are depleted. Vitamin A is detected through normal-phase and reverse-phase high-performance liquid chromatography (HPLC) using photometric, electrochemical, or mass spectrometric detectors. Reference ranges are 20 to 40 μg/dL for children aged 1 to 6 years, 26 to 49 μg/dL for ages 7 to 12 years, 26 to 72 μg/dL for ages 13 to 19 years, and 30 to 80 μg/dL for adults (see Table 31-3).

Vitamin E

Vitamin E is a complex consisting of 10 lipid-soluble substances, with tocopherol being the most common form of the vitamin in American diets. Vitamin E is a potent antioxidant that halts the production of molecular oxygen and free radicals during fat oxidation. Dietary vitamin E can be found in oils and fats (particularly wheat germ oil and sunflower oil), grains, and nuts. α-Tocopherol is the major form of vitamin E in the blood. Vitamin E is absorbed through the small intestine when bile is present. The absorbed vitamin E is packaged in chylomicrons, then metabolized by the liver into very-low-density lipoproteins (VLDL).

Vitamin E is needed for neurologic and reproductive functions, for red cell membrane protection, and for inhibition of reactive oxygen species production during lipid metabolism. It is also believed to decrease the risks of cardiovascular disease and cancer. The RDA for adults is 3 to 4 mg/day.

Signs and symptoms of vitamin E deficiency (<3 μg/mL in adults; <1.5 μg/mL in infants) include irritability, edema, and hemolytic anemia. Fat malabsorption states (e.g., cystic fibrosis) can cause neuropathy and hemolytic anemia.

Vitamin E toxicity (>40 μg/mL) can be accomplished only by taking supplements, and Vitamin E has been found to be safe at 3000 mg/day. Reversible signs and symptoms of toxicity include gastrointestinal symptoms, impaired immunity, heart failure, and blood coagulation abnormalities.

Laboratory Procedures and Limitations

Vitamin E is measured in serum specimens, and HPLC is the method of choice. The reference range for adults is 0.5 to 1.8 μg/mL (see Table 31-3). Patients should be fasting, and the specimen needs to be collected in a light-protective container.

Vitamin D

Vitamin D_3 (cholecalciferol) is the major form of vitamin D produced by exposure of skin to sunlight and absorption from dietary sources. Dietary sources for vitamin D include fish liver oils, fatty fish, egg yolks, and liver in addition to vitamin D–fortified foods such as cereals, bread, and milk. Cholecalciferol is metabolized in the liver into the biologically active compound, 1,25-dihydroxyvitamin D_3 (1,25[OH]$_2D_3$) or calcitriol, then transported to the kidneys, where the metabolites are transformed into active forms of the vitamin. The function of vitamin D is to maintain the calcium and phosphate concentrations in serum. This compound is regulated by parathyroid hormone and the blood levels of calcium and phosphate. The RDA is 400 IU/day.

Deficiency of vitamin D results in impaired formation of bone, leading to rickets in children and osteomalacia in adults. Causes of vitamin D deficiency include breastfeeding in infants; strict vegetarianism (no milk or eggs); elderly age; inadequate exposure to sunlight; dietary deficiency; certain conditions such as malabsorption syndromes, gastric or small bowel resection, severe hepatocellular disease, and nephrotic syndrome; and drugs such as phenytoin, phenobarbital, or rifampin. The most common use for this test is to rule out a diagnosis of hypocalcemia.

Laboratory Procedures and Limitations

Vitamin D is measured in the serum. Test methods used include competitive protein binding assay, immunoassay, ultraviolet (UV) light absorbance after HPLC separation, and liquid chromatography–tandem mass spectrometry (LC-MS/MS). The reference range for 1,25(OH)$_2D_3$ is 15 to 60 pg/mL (see Table 31-3).

Vitamin K

Vitamin K is composed of two types: K_1 (phylloquinone) and K_2 (menaquinone). This vitamin is required for the production of several clotting factors, including factor II (prothrombin), factor VII (proconvertin), factor IX (plasma thromboplastin component), and factor X (Stuart factor), and it may also be involved in bone metabolism. Vitamin K is produced by the bacteria that inhabit the intestines. Dietary sources include green vegetables, margarines, cheese and milk products, eggs, and plant oils. Between 15% and 65% of ingested vitamin K is absorbed through the intestines with the help of bile. Once absorbed, it is transported in chylomicrons to the liver, where it is incorporated into β-lipoproteins for transport to other areas of the body. RDAs for vitamin K are 120 µg/dL for men and 90 µg/dL for women.

Because bacteria produce much of the vitamin K utilized in the body, deficiencies of this vitamin are rare. Vitamin K deficiency states can result from malabsorption syndromes such as bile duct obstruction, cystic fibrosis, and chronic pancreatitis. Drugs that interfere with vitamin K metabolism, such as Coumadin anticoagulants and certain antibiotics (cephalosporins), can also cause deficiency states. Vitamin K deficiency is characterized by defective blood coagulation. Consumption of high doses of vitamin K appears to have no harmful effects.

Laboratory Procedures and Limitations

Vitamin K is present in the blood in very small amounts—1000 times lower than vitamins A or E. This factor presents a challenge for measuring the concentration of vitamin K in the blood. Measurement of plasma phylloquinone by HPLC after a protein and lipid extraction produces accurate results. The reference range is 0.13 to 1.19 ng/mL (see Table 31-3).

Vitamin H (Biotin)

Vitamin H, also known as biotin, is a member of the B-vitamin complex. Good dietary sources of biotin include liver, kidney, pancreas, eggs, yeast, and milk. Biotin is usually bound to protein and must be released by the action of gastrointestinal hormones so that it can be absorbed from the intestines and transported to the liver, kidneys, and peripheral tissues. Biotin participates in chemical reactions leading to the synthesis of fatty acids and citrate, as well as the metabolism of odd-numbered fatty acids and branched-chain fatty acids. The RDA is 30 µg/day. Biotin deficiency is rare but can be seen in patients who are undergoing total parenteral nutrition or who have certain genetic conditions. Symptoms include anorexia, nausea, vomiting, glossitis, pallor, depression, and dermatitis. No toxic conditions are described.

Laboratory Procedures and Limitations

Biotin is usually measured through immunoassays. Reference ranges are 0.5 to 2.2 nmol/L (see Table 31-3).

Vitamin B₁ (Thiamine)

Vitamin B₁, also known as thiamine, is required for decarboxylation reactions. Large amounts of thiamine are found in unrefined cereal grains, plant tissue, and animal tissue. Most flours and cereals on the market today are enriched with this vitamin. Thiamine is absorbed through the small intestine and carried to the liver. It is stored in skeletal muscle, heart, liver, kidneys, and nervous tissue. The form used by the body is thiamine pyrophosphate (TPP). TPP is required for the production of acyl-coenzyme A (acyl-CoA), which is used in the Krebs citric acid cycle. The RDAs in adults are 1.2 mg/day for males and 1.1 mg/day for females.

Thiamine deficiency leads to a disease called *beriberi*. Clinical signs of thiamine deficiency include mental confusion, anorexia, muscular weakness, ataxia, peripheral paralysis, ophthalmoplegia, edema, muscle wasting, tachycardia, and an enlarged heart. Thiamine deficiency can occur in individuals who ingest a diet of nonenriched grains, are chronic alcoholics, ingest raw fish, receive total parenteral nutrition, or undergo dialysis. No adverse effects from large doses of thiamine are reported.

Laboratory Procedures and Limitations

Thiamine levels in the body are usually measured by HPLC using erythrocytes as the specimen. Reference intervals are 90 to 140 nmol/L (see Table 31-3).

Vitamin B₂

Vitamin B₂, also known as riboflavin, is an essential part of coenzymes that are involved in redox reactions, such as flavin adenine dinucleotide (FAD). Dietary sources of riboflavin include organ meats, vegetables, and milk. Cereals are naturally low in riboflavin, but fortification and enrichment processes make them a good source of the vitamin as well. Riboflavin is absorbed in the small intestine with the help of bile salts. It is absorbed into the blood until a blood level of 27 mg/day is reached, after which any excess is excreted in urine. Riboflavin participates in many redox reactions in the body and also lowers homocysteine levels in the blood. The RDAs for riboflavin are 1.3 mg/day for men and 1.1 mg/day for women. Riboflavin deficiency is characterized by sore throat, hyperemia, edema of the pharyngeal and oral mucous membranes, glossitis, seborrheic dermatitis, and normocytic normochromic anemia. No toxic effects are described.

Laboratory Procedures and Limitations

Riboflavin levels are usually measured by HPLC using fluorometric detection. Reference intervals are 4 to 24 µg/dL (see Table 31-3).

Vitamin B₆

Vitamin B₆ is also called pyridoxine; it is used for the synthesis, catabolism, and interconversion of amino acids. Pyridoxine can be found in meat, poultry, fish, yeast, certain seeds, bran, and bananas. This is another vitamin that is fortified in breakfast cereals. The vitamin diffuses into the blood through the mucosal cells of the intestines. Pyridoxine directly enters the cell and the cell's organelles. It is involved in many reactions dealing with the metabolism of macronutrients as well as the biosynthesis of heme. RDAs for pyridoxine are 1.3 to 1.7 mg/day for men and 1.3 to 1.5 mg/day for women. Vitamin B_6 deficiency is uncommon, but a few drugs (isoniazid, penicillamine, benserazide, carbidopa, and theophilline) can cause a deficiency. The only cases of toxicity with this vitamin were caused by high levels of oral supplements and resulted in neurotoxicity and photosensitivity.

Laboratory Procedures and Limitations

Vitamin B_6 is most commonly measured in blood by HPLC with fluorescence detection. The reference interval is 5 to 30 mg/dL (see Table 31-3).

Vitamin B_{12}

Vitamin B_{12} is commonly known as cyanocobalamin. Vitamin B_{12} is produced by bacteria; plants do not use this compound. The main dietary sources of Vitamin B_{12} are meat and meat products, dairy products, fish, shellfish, and fortified ready-to-eat cereals. Vitamin B_{12} absorption is a complex process. Vitamin B_{12} is attached to a carrier protein as it enters the stomach. The stomach's acidity disconnects the carrier protein, and the vitamin B_{12} molecule binds to intrinsic factor. The intrinsic factor carries the vitamin to the intestines, where the complex enters the mucosal cells. The intrinsic factor is dissociated, and another carrier protein transports the vitamin into the blood. The blood carries the vitamin to the liver where it is stored until needed. Vitamin B_{12} is a coenzyme in many enzyme systems and is primarily responsible for amino acid metabolism. The RDA is 2.4 µg/day.

Vitamin B_{12} deficiency is associated with megaloblastic anemia and neuropathy. The most common cause of this deficiency is pernicious anemia, in which an autoimmune process prevents production of intrinsic factor. Other causes include age older than 65 years, malabsorption syndromes, vegan diet, autoimmune conditions, medication interference with absorption (e.g., phenytoin, nitrous oxide), gastrectomy, ileum resections, tropical sprue, and human immunodeficiency virus (HIV) infection. High doses of vitamin B_{12} are not associated with toxicity.

Laboratory Procedures and Limitations

Vitamin B_{12} is measured through immunoassays and chemiluminescence. Reference ranges are 201 ng/L or higher (see Table 31-3).

Niacin

Niacin, another water-soluble B vitamin, is also known as nicotinic acid; in the body, it is converted to niacinamide (nicotinamide), a structure with the same vitamin functions but a different pharmacological profile. Dietary sources include yeast, lean meats, liver, poultry, milk, canned salmon, leafy green vegetables, and fortified cereals. Niacin is hydrolyzed by enzymes in the intestinal mucosa, then rapidly absorbed into the blood. The blood transports the hydrolyzed forms of nicotinic acid and nicotinamide to the tissues, where both species are converted to the important redox coenzymes, nicotinamide adenine dinucleotide (NAD$^+$) and nicotinamide adenine dinucleotide phosphate (NADP$^+$). NAD and NADP participate in reactions that convert alcohols to aldehydes or ketones, aldehydes to acids, and certain amino acids to keto acids. The RDAs for niacin are 16 mg/day for men and 14 mg/day for women.

Pellagra is the disease caused by a deficiency of niacin. This condition is found among peoples who rely mainly on corn for their subsistence. Pellagra can also be a secondary condition associated with carcinoid syndrome, Hartnup disease, and isoniazid treatment. Large amounts of niacin are not thought to be toxic but can produce adverse effects such as flushing (a burning or tingling sensation of the face, arms, and chest), pruritus, nausea, vomiting, and diarrhea.

Laboratory Procedures and Limitations

No assays for the direct measurement of niacin in blood are available; however, HPLC methods are available to measure two metabolites in urine specimens (see Table 31-3).

Folic Acid

Folic acid (folate) is a coenzyme. Dietary sources of folic acid include liver, spinach, dark green leafy vegetables, legumes, orange juice, and fortified ready-to-eat cereals. Folate is ingested, is absorbed and participates in various chemical reactions in the intestines, then enters the blood. Because folic acid and vitamin B_{12} metabolism are linked by a single reaction, deficiency of vitamin B_{12} can cause folate to become trapped and unavailable for the body to use. Folic acid is involved in the synthesis of thymidine, purines, DNA, RNA, hormones, neurotransmitters, and membrane lipids and proteins as well as the metabolism of homocysteine. The RDA is 400 µg/day for adults.

Causes for folic acid deficiency include gut sterilization, poor intestinal absorption, insufficient dietary intake, cancer, liver disease, antifolate drugs, and anticonvulsant therapy. The deficiency is characterized by megaloblastic anemia, sensory loss, and neurologic changes. Toxic states are usually caused by ingesting too much supplemental folate. The main symptom in folate toxicity is neuropathy.

Laboratory Procedures and Limitations

Folate is measured directly in blood specimens. Reference ranges are 2.6 to 12.2 µg/L for serum samples (see Table 31-3).

Vitamin C

Vitamin C, otherwise known as ascorbic acid, is a water-soluble vitamin. Dietary sources for vitamin C include citrus fruits, berries, melons, tomatoes, green peppers, broccoli, Brussels sprouts, and leafy green vegetables. Vitamin C is absorbed through the intestinal wall into the blood through facilitated diffusion. From the blood, it is further absorbed into tissue. Tissues with the highest concentrations of vitamin C include the pituitary gland, adrenal cortex, corpus luteum, and thymus. The retina contains 20 to 30 times as much vitamin C as in the blood. Vitamin C functions as a cofactor for synthesis of adrenal hormones, corticosteroids, aldosterone, and bile acids and for folate metabolism. Vitamin C is the most effective water-soluble antioxidant because it binds to reactive oxygen and nitrogen species in the body. The RDAs are 90 mg/day for men and 75 mg/day for women.

Scurvy is caused by a long-standing vitamin C deficiency. Symptoms include swollen, bleeding, or bruised joints; anemia; osteoporosis; and heart failure. This disease is common in elderly men, individuals with alcohol addiction, smokers, people with unbalanced diets, mentally ill individuals, patients undergoing peritoneal dialysis, and patients with cancer. Individuals taking large supplements (2 to 4 g/day) commonly experience diarrhea. Other, rare adverse effects include kidney stones, increased uric acid excretion, excess iron absorption, and low vitamin B_{12} levels.

Laboratory Procedures and Limitations
Vitamin C is measured directly by photometric or fluorometric methods. Reference ranges are 0.4 to 1.5 mg/dL (see Table 31-3).

Trace Elements

The term *trace* is used to indicate that only a miniscule amount of the substance needed for a physiologic process (Table 31-4).

Chromium
Chromium (Cr), in its trivalent form, is used by the body to enhance the action of insulin. Dietary sources of chromium include processed meats, whole grain products, green beans, broccoli, and spices. The RDAs are 25 µg/day for women and 35 µg/day for men. Chromium is ingested and absorbed through the small intestine. Once it enters the blood, it binds with transferrin for transport to the liver, spleen, soft tissue, and bone. Unabsorbed dietary chromium is excreted in feces and urine. The function of chromium is to activate insulin receptors on cell membranes to enhance the uptake of glucose from the blood. Chromium deficiency is reported in patients receiving long-term parenteral nutrition. The symptoms include insulin-resistant glucose intolerance, weight loss, and neurologic deficits.

Chromium in its hexavalent form is a recognized industrial carcinogen that causes lung cancer, dermatitis, and skin

---

TABLE 31-4	**Trace Elements**			
Trace Element	**General Role**	**Reference Range (µg/L)**	**Symptoms of Deficiency**	**Laboratory Methods**
Chromium	Enhances the action of insulin	0.1-0.2 (serum)	Insulin-resistant glucose intolerance, weight loss, neurologic deficits	Spectrophotometric methods and atomic absorption
Copper	Component of ceruloplasmin and cytochrome *c* oxidase	70-140 (plasma)	Menkes disease, malabsorption syndromes (cystic fibrosis, celiac disease, sprue, short bowel syndrome), premature birth; seen in individuals receiving parenteral nutrition and those with cardiovascular disease	Atomic absorption spectrophotometry
Fluoride	Prevents tooth caries	0.2-0.32 (urine)	None	Fluoride-specific electrode
Manganese	Formation of connective tissue, growth, reproduction, carbohydrate and lipid metabolism	0.5-1.3 (serum)	None	Atomic spectrophotometry
Selenium	Component of compounds that act as antioxidants and many enzymes	63-160 (plasma)	*Severe deficiency states:* Keshan disease (cardiac myopathy), Kashin-Beck disease (severe arthritis) *Marginal deficiency states:* thyroid disease, impaired cell-mediated immunity and B-cell function, mood disorders, inflammatory conditions	Carbon furnace atomic absorption spectroscopy
Zinc	Plays a key role in growth and wound healing; regulates synthesis of steroid, thyroid, and other hormones	80-120 (plasma)	Depressed growth with stunting, increased infections, diarrhea, skin lesions, alopecia	Atomic absorption spectrophotometry

ulcers. Chromium (trivalent) molecules are considered nontoxic because they are poorly absorbed and rapidly excreted in urine. However, chromium picolinate, a widely used dietary supplement, can cause renal and hepatic damage at high doses.

Laboratory Procedures and Limitations

Laboratory assays for chromium can be conducted only if great care is taken to prevent contact with stainless steel, which would contaminate the sample. Detection of chromium in the urine is easier. Spectrophotometric methods can be used, as can atomic absorption. Reference values are 0.1 to 0.2 µg/L for serum and less than 0.2 µg/L for urine (see Table 31-4).

Copper

Copper (Cu) is used by the body in many functions. Dietary sources include organ meats, shellfish, nuts, whole-grain cereals, and cocoa-containing products. Copper is absorbed directly through the gastrointestinal system and into the blood. Once in the blood, copper binds with albumin and is transported to the liver. Copper is an important component in ceruloplasmin. Ceruloplasmin is an acute phase reactant that is increased in infection and tissue injury. Copper also serves as a component of enzymes such as cytochrome *c* oxidase and other proteins.

The RDA for copper is 0.9 mg/day. Copper deficiency conditions include Menkes disease, malabsorption syndromes (cystic fibrosis, celiac disease, sprue, short bowel syndrome), prematurity in infants, parenteral nutrition, and cardiovascular disease. Due to the role copper plays in red and white blood cell production, individuals with copper deficiency may be misdiagnosed with myelodysplastic syndrome.

Menkes disease is a disease of the regulation of copper metabolism caused by a genetic defect (see Fig. 29-9 in Chapter 29). Wilson disease is another genetic disease involving the metabolism of copper; it leads to accumulations of the metal in liver, brain, kidney, cornea, and body tissue that can cause copper toxicity. Copper is deposited in the eye (Kayser-Fleischer rings) and in the liver. Liver function tests (especially transaminase levels) are elevated in patients with liver disease, and acute liver failure due to Wilson disease is difficult to diagnose. In these individuals, the serum copper level is elevated but the ceruloplasmin level is normal. Individuals with Wilson disease also excrete increased levels of copper in their urine (>500 µg/L). Copper toxicity can also occur through copper contamination of food and water supplies.

Laboratory Procedures and Limitations

Copper is assayed in the laboratory by atomic absorption spectrophotometry. Reference ranges are 70 to 140 µg/dL (see Table 31-4).

Fluoride

Fluoride (F) is used extensively in public health to prevent tooth caries. Small studies indicate that it may be useful in reducing bone fracturing in individuals with osteoporosis. Fluoride is absorbed from the stomach and the small intestine. Ninety-five percent of the body's fluoride is located in bones and teeth.

Laboratory Procedures and Limitations

Because excess fluoride is immediately excreted in the urine, fluoride determinations in blood are not clinically significant. Urine analysis is more practical. Fluoride is measured directly with the use of a fluoride-specific electrode. Reference ranges for urine fluoride are 0.2. to 3.2 mg/L (see Table 31-4).

Manganese

Manganese (Mn) is associated with the formation of connective tissue, growth, reproduction, and carbohydrate and lipid metabolism. Dietary sources include whole-grain foods, nuts, leafy vegetables, soy products, and teas. Manganese is absorbed from the small intestine, then transported to the liver by the blood. In the liver, it attaches to proteins, then travels to other tissues. It is usually excreted through the feces. Manganese is an integral part of metalloenzymes, and it also acts as a nonspecific enzyme activator. RDAs are 2.3 mg/day for men and 1.8 mg/day for women. No manganese-deficient conditions are described.

Prolonged exposure to manganese-containing dust or fumes in an industrial setting can cause manganese toxicity. Neurologic symptoms develop over months and years that resemble Parkinson disease. Patients receiving parenteral nutrition can also develop these symptoms.

Laboratory Procedures and Limitations

Whole-blood assays for manganese with atomic spectrophotometry are the ideal method for quantitating this metal. Reference intervals are 0.5 to 1.3 µg/L (see Table 31-4).

Selenium

Selenium (Se) is an essential element for humans that works with vitamin E. Dietary sources for selenium include wheat and other cereal products. Selenium is efficiently absorbed from the intestines, and any excess is excreted in the urine. Selenium is a component of compounds that act as antioxidants in the body as well as many enzymes. The RDA is set at 55 µg/day for adults. Severe selenium deficiency states include Keshan disease (cardiac myopathy) and Kashin-Beck disease (severe arthritis). Marginal deficiency states include thyroid disease, impaired cell-mediated immunity and B-cell function, mood disorders, and inflammatory conditions. A deficiency in selenium has been shown to protect against cancer. Carbon furnace atomic absorption spectroscopy is used to measure serum selenium. Reference intervals are 63 to 160 µg/L (see Table 31-4).

Zinc

Zinc (Zn) is the second most abundant trace element (after iron) in the human body. Dietary sources include red meat, fish, wheat germ, and whole bran. Zinc is absorbed through the intestines and transported to the liver, where it is attached to enzymes and proteins. Zinc is excreted through the feces.

Zinc is attached to important enzymes such as carbonic anhydrase, alkaline phosphatase, RNA and DNA polymerases, alcohol dehydrogenase, and thymidine kinase carboxypeptidases. It plays a key role in growth and wound healing and in regulating the synthesis of steroid, thyroid, and other hormones. In addition, large amounts of zinc are required to sustain an antibacterial and vital environment in the prostate so that sperm maintain their function. RDAs are 11 mg/day for men and 8 mg/day for women. Zinc deficiency is varied, nonspecific, and related to the degree of zinc depletion. Signs and symptoms of zinc deficiency include depressed growth with stunting, increased infections, diarrhea, skin lesions, and alopecia.

Zinc toxicity is characterized by abdominal pain, diarrhea, nausea, and vomiting. Zinc is measured in the laboratory by atomic absorption spectrophotometry. Reference intervals are 80 to 120 µg/dL (see Table 31-4).

Metabolic Diseases

Obesity

Millions of Americans are obese. Obesity is a condition in which there is excess body fat that leads to potential health risks (Table 31-5). Excess body fat is a risk factor for coronary heart disease, high blood pressure, type 2 diabetes, gallstones, breathing problems, and cancer. Weight is a result of environment, family history, genetics, metabolism, behavior, and habits. The advent of "junk food" and ubiquitous access to grains, starches, bread, and pasta have all contributed to weight gain in Americans. The popularity of television, computers, and video games also contribute by enticing Americans to sit and be entertained. Obsession with cutting fats has led to the consumption of large amounts of carbohydrates (which are fat free). An individual's diet should be balanced, which means eating macronutrients in moderation. Obesity does not lead to changes in

TABLE 31-5	Body Mass Index (BMI)
BMI*	**NIH Classification**
<18.5	Underweight
18.5-24.9	Normal weight
25-29.9	Overweight
30-34.9	Obesity I
35-39.9	Obesity II
>40	Extreme obesity

Data from U.S. Department of Health and Human Services. <https://www.nhlbi.nih.gov/health/educational/lose_wt/BMI/bmi_dis.htm> Accessed 01.11.15.
NIH, National Institutes of Health.
*BMI is equal to the weight (in kilograms) divided by the square of the height (in meters); alternatively, BMI = 203 × weight (in pounds) ÷ height (in inches) squared.

analytes, but when an obese individual develops one of the diseases discussed here, specific analytes can be measured to diagnose that disease (Fig. 31-6).

Metabolic Syndrome

The term metabolic syndrome describes factors that increase an individual's risk for heart disease and other diseases, such as stroke (Box 31-3). To be diagnosed with metabolic syndrome, one must have at least three of the following risk factors:

- Abdominal obesity
- High triglyceride levels
- Low levels of high-density lipoprotein (HDL)
- Hypertension
- High fasting blood sugar

The greater the number of risk factors, the greater the risk for heart disease, diabetes, and stroke. An individual with metabolic syndrome is twice as likely to develop heart disease and five times as likely to develop diabetes as a healthy person. People with metabolic syndrome also seem to have excessive blood clotting and constant, low-grade inflammation.

People who are overweight or obese and also lack physical activity are more likely to develop metabolic syndrome. Elevated triglycerides, decreased HDL levels, and elevated fasting blood sugar values are the three laboratory test results used to diagnose metabolic syndrome. Triglycerides are measured spectrophotometrically by the Trinder methodology. HDL is measured directly by a two-step method in which low-density lipoproteins (LDL), VLDL, and chylomicrons are removed from the sample, after which HDL is dissolved and the resulting blue color complex is measured. The blood glucose concentration is commonly measured by glucose hexokinase or glucose oxidase test methods.

Malnutrition

Malnutrition occurs when a person does not ingest the macronutrients and micronutrients necessary to maintain good health (Fig. 31-7). Although malnutrition can be very mild, producing no symptoms, common symptoms include weight loss, fatigue, and dizziness. Sometimes, malnutrition can be so severe as to cause lasting damage. Signs and symptoms in more severe cases include swollen or bleeding gums, tooth decay, osteoporosis, muscle loss and weakness, heart

• BOX 31-3	Diseases Associated with the Metabolic Syndrome

Heart disease
Lipid problems
Hypertension
Type 2 diabetes
Dementia
Cancer
Polycystic ovarian syndrome (PCOS)
Stroke

problems, decreased liver function, kidney failure, decreased lung capacity, intestinal problems, stomach irregularities, abnormal menstrual cycles in women, ascites, and dry skin. Even in the 21st century, malnutrition continues to be a significant worldwide problem, particularly in children. The problem exists in the United States and other developed countries as well as in developing countries. Poverty, natural disasters, political problems, and war are factors that contribute to continuing starvation and malnutrition in the world.

Kwashiorkor and Marasmus

Kwashiorkor is a particular type of malnutrition involving low protein intake that occurs in regions with famine, limited food supplies, and low levels of education. **Marasmus** is inadequate intake of both protein and calories; it is characterized by emaciation. Kwashiorkor is described as a maladaptive response to starvation, whereas marasmus is an adaptive response.

Kwashiorkor is very rare in children in the United States. Symptoms include decreased muscle mass, changes in skin pigment, diarrhea, failure to gain weight and grow, fatigue, large protruding belly, lethargy, rash, and swelling (Fig. 31-8). In kwashiorkor, the body is no longer dependent on gluconeogenesis for energy. Instead, it begins to rely on ketone bodies, an end product of lipid metabolism, for energy. Long-term starvation results in depressed insulin levels, and increased glucagon, cortisone, epinephrine, and growth hormones to induce lipolysis in adipose tissue. The fatty acids from lipid metabolism sustain the heart and skeletal muscles, and the ketone bodies sustain the brain tissue. Once the body has used all the stored lipids, it begins to break down muscles so that it can use protein for energy. This is a progressive process. After all possible stores

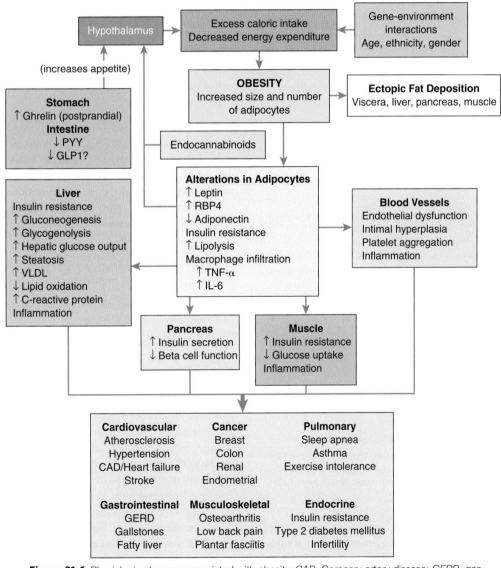

• **Figure 31-6** Physiologic changes associated with obesity. *CAD,* Coronary artery disease; *GERD,* gastroesophageal reflux disease; *GLP1,* glucagon-like peptide-1; *IL-6,* interleukin-6; *PYY,* peptide YY; *RBP4,* retinol binding protein 4; *TNF-α,* tumor necrosis factor-α; *VLDL,* very-low-density lipoprotein. (From McCance KL, Huether SE. *Pathophysiology: The Biologic Basis for Disease in Adults and Children.* 7th ed. St. Louis: Mosby; 2015.)

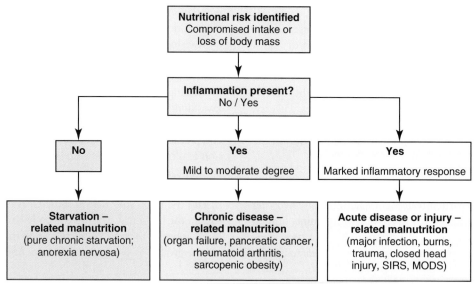

• **Figure 31-7** Malnutrition characteristics. *MODS,* Multiple organ dysfunction syndrome; *SIRS,* systemic inflammatory response syndrome. (Modified from Mahan LK, Raymond JL, Escott-Stump S. *Krause's Food and the Nutrition Care Process.* 13th ed. St. Louis: Saunders; 2012. Data from Jensen GL, Bistrian B, Roubenoff R, Heimburger DC. Malnutrition syndromes: a conundrum versus continuum. *JPEN J Parenter Enteral Nutr.* 2009;33:710; and Jensen GL, Mirtallo J, Compher C, et al. Adult starvation and disease-related malnutrition: a proposal for etiology-based diagnosis in the clinical practice setting from the International Consensus Guideline Committee. *JPEN J Parenter Enteral Nutr.* 2010;34:156.)

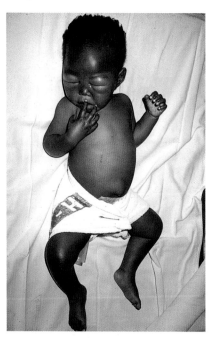

• **Figure 31-8** Kwashiorkor, a protein-energy malnutrition. The infant shows generalized edema, which is seen in the form of puffiness of the face, arms, and legs. (From Nix S. *Williams' Basic Nutrition and Diet Therapy.* 14th ed. St. Louis; Mosby; 2013.)

for energy-containing compounds are exhausted, death results from severe alterations in acid-base balance and shutdown of renal, cardiac, and respiratory systems.

The World Health Organization recommends the following laboratory tests for assessing individuals for kwashiorkor: glucose, hemoglobin, urinalysis, urine culture, ova and parasites, HIV, and electrolytes. Significant findings include hypoalbuminemia (10 to 25 g/L), hypoproteinemia, hypoglycemia, low insulin levels, low potassium, low magnesium, low lipid levels, decreased BUN, and low iron levels. Most often, iron deficiency anemia and metabolic acidosis are present.

In marasmus, laboratory values are usually within the reference range, even though muscle wasting and other physical changes are present.

Changes in Nutritional Markers in Institutionalized Individuals

Individuals in hospital and long-term care facilities can suffer from malnutrition. Between 20% and 30% of patients in these facilities show signs of malnutrition, and the rate for elderly patients is 23% to 85%. Some individuals enter these facilities with chronic conditions such as acquired immunodeficiency syndrome (AIDS) or cancer, and some become acutely ill during their stay due to trauma, surgery, or burns. Medical complications from being malnourished while institutionalized include delayed wound healing, increased risk for postoperative complications, decreased immune function, and even increased death rate. Medical complications lead to increased length of stay for patients and increased use of medical resources. Hospitals and long-term care facilities recognize the impact of malnutrition on the health of patients and establish policies to detect malnutrition early, effectively treat the condition, and monitor treatment.

Inborn Errors of Metabolism

Abnormalities in the synthesis or metabolism of proteins, carbohydrates, or fats can be caused by single-gene

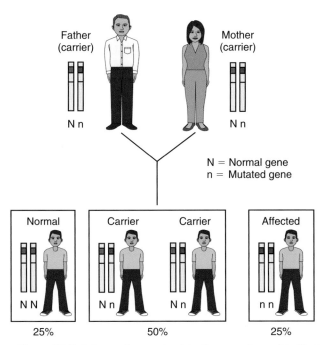

● **Figure 31-9** Autosomal recessive inheritance pattern. (Modified from Burtis CA, Bruns DE. *Tietz Fundamentals of Clinical Chemistry and Molecular Diagnostics.* 7th ed. St. Louis: Saunders; 2015.)

mutations. Many of these disorders are inherited in an autosomal recessive manner, meaning that males and females are equally affected because the mutation occurs in both alleles that code for an enzyme. Parents of affected individuals do not exhibit symptoms and are silent carriers—that is, they carry one normal allele and one mutant allele. If both parents are carriers, there is a 25% probability that the child will have two mutant alleles and clinical signs of the condition (Fig. 31-9).

When one of these mutations results in a blocked metabolic pathway, accumulation of the substrates in that pathway have toxic effects on the surrounding tissues. These diseases vary in age at onset (several occur in newborns), type of genetic inheritance, and clinical severity. Some of the most common inborn errors of metabolism include Tay-Sachs disease, Niemann-Pick disease, Gaucher disease, Krabbe, Hurler syndrome, phenylketonuria, tyrosinemia, alkaptonuria, homocystinuria, maple syrup disease, cystinuria, and Hartnup disease (Table 31-6).

Laboratory Methods

Laboratory testing for biochemical diseases (i.e., diseases present at birth that disrupt a key metabolic pathway) usually examine proteins instead of genes. The laboratory tests measure enzyme activity, metabolites (as an indirect measurement of enzyme activity), and protein structure. Tests can be performed on blood, urine, amniotic fluid, or cerebrospinal fluid. Because of the instability of the enzymes or proteins, all specimens should be collected, properly stored and handled, and shipped promptly to the testing laboratory.

Technologies used to detect the enzyme or protein include HPLC, gas chromatography/mass spectrometry (GC/MS), tandem mass spectrometry (MS/MS), fluorometry, and thin-layer chromatography.

If the gene sequence of interest is known, then DNA analysis is the test of choice. This test can be performed on an extremely small tissue sample. Polymerase chain reaction is used to amplify the DNA in the sample, after which comparative genome hybridization is used to identify the gains or losses in the sample.

Lipid Defects

Tay-Sachs Disease

Tay-Sachs disease is a fatal genetic lipid storage disorder in which gangliosides build up in the tissues and in the brain. This is caused by decreased activity of the enzyme, β-hexosaminidase A. Infants progress well during the first few months of life, then get progressively worse as the gangliosides destroy neurons in the brain and spinal cord. Children usually die before 4 years of age. This disease is found in people of Ashkenazi Jewish heritage.

The frequency of this disease in newborns is 1 in 320,000. One of every 25 to 30 adults of Ashkenazi Jewish descent is a symptom-free, heterozygous carrier. At this time, only 36 laboratories are certified testing centers for Tay-Sachs disease (Fig. 31-10).

Laboratory Procedures and Limitations

Tay-Sachs disease is diagnosed through enzyme assays and mutation analysis. The enzyme assays detect low levels of β-hexosaminidase A (phenotype), and the mutation analysis detects mutations in the DNA (genotype). The two methods are used together because the enzyme assay detects altered levels of enzymes regardless of the cause (inclusive for diagnosis), whereas the mutation analysis shows only known mutations.

Niemann–Pick Disease

Niemann-Pick disease is a rare disorder that is most common in people of Ashkenazi Jewish descent. It is a genetic disease that affects the production of sphingomyelinase, an enzyme required in the breakdown, transport, and use of fats and cholesterol in the body. Lipids accumulate in the spleen, liver, lungs, bone marrow, and brain (Fig. 31-11).

There are four major classifications of this disease. Niemann-Pick A is the neurologic disease that affects mainly children. Patients do not survive past early childhood. Niemann-Pick disease type B usually affects the liver and spleen, produces frequent lung infections, and slows growth. This is the non-neurologic type of the disease, and individuals survive into adulthood. Niemann-Pick disease type C is subclassified as type C1 and C2—each caused by a different gene mutation. Although this disease usually appears in childhood, infants and adults can also become symptomatic. Symptoms include seizures, feeding problems, breathing difficulties, severe liver disease, eye movement problems

TABLE 31-6 **Selected Inborn Errors of Metabolism**

Error	Deficient Enzyme	Accumulated Substrate(s)	Comments
Alkaptonuria	Homogentisate oxidase	Homogentisate (black pigment); binds to collagen (connective tissue, tendons, cartilage)	Black urine (undergoes oxidation when exposed to light); black pigmentation nose, ears, cheeks; black cartilage in joint and intervertebral disc producing degenerative arthritis
Homocystinuria	Cystathionine synthase	Homocysteine and methionine	Mental retardation, vessel thrombosis (homocysteine); lens dislocation, arachnodactyly (similar to Marfan syndrome)
Maple syrup urine disease	Branched-chain α-ketoacid dehydrogenase	Leucine, valine, isoleucine, and their ketoacids	Mental retardation, seizures, feeding problems, sweet-smelling urine
Phenylketonuria	Phenylalanine hydroxylase	Phenylalanine Neurotoxic byproducts	Mental retardation, microcephaly, mousy odor (phenylalanine converted into phenylacids), ↓pigmentation (melanin derives from tyrosine) Must be exposed to phenylalanine (milk) *before* phenylalanine is increased. Restrict phenylalanine; avoid sweeteners containing phenylalanine (e.g., Nutra Sweet). Add tyrosine to diet. Pregnant women with PKU must be on a phenylalanine-free diet or newborns will be mentally retarded at birth.
"Malignant" phenylketonuria	Dihydropterin reductase	Phenylalanine Neurotoxic byproducts	Similar to PKU Inability to metabolize tryptophan or tyrosine, which both require BH_4; this causes ↓synthesis of neurotransmitters (serotonin and dopamine, respectively). Neurologic problems occur despite adequate dietary therapy. Restrict phenylalanine in diet. Administer L-dopa and 5-hydroxytryptophan to replace neurotransmitters. Administer BH_4.
McArdle disease	Muscle phosphorylase	Glycogen	Glycogenosis with muscle fatigue and a propensity for rhabdomyolysis with myoglobinuria *No* lactic acid increase with exercise due to lack of glucose in muscle and a corresponding lack in anaerobic glycolysis (lactic acid is the end product)
Pompe disease	α-1,4-Glucosidase (lysosomal enzyme)	Glycogen	Glycogenosis, cardiomegaly with early death from heart failure (restrictive cardiomyopathy)
Von Gierke disease	Glucose-6-phosphatase (gluconeogenic enzyme)	Glucose 6-phosphate	Glycogenosis, enlarged liver and kidneys (both contain gluconeogenic enzymes), fasting hypoglycemia (no response to glucagon or other gluconeogenesis stimulators)

Modified from Goljian EF. *Rapid Review Pathology*. 4th ed. Philadelphia: Saunders; 2014.

AcAc, Acetoacetate; *AcCoA*, acetyl CoA; *BH₄*, tetrahydrobiopterin; *CoA*, coenzyme A; *DHAP*, dihydroxyacetone phosphate; *PKU*, phenylketonuria.

Normal - β-N-acetylhexosaminidase present

Tay-Sachs disease - β-N-acetylhexosaminidase
not present or deficient

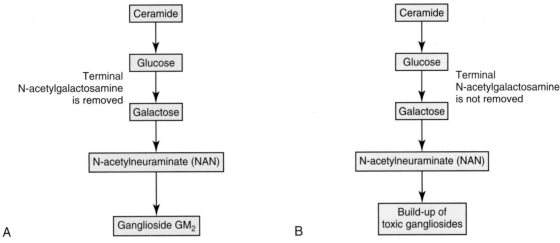

A

Terminal
N-acetylgalactosamine
is removed

Ceramide → Glucose → Galactose → N-acetylneuraminate (NAN) → Ganglioside GM$_2$

B

Terminal
N-acetylgalactosamine
is not removed

Ceramide → Glucose → Galactose → N-acetylneuraminate (NAN) → Build-up of toxic gangliosides

• **Figure 31-10 A,** Normal metabolism. **B,** Tay-Sachs disease. (Modified from Kierszenbaum AL, Tres LL. *Histology and Cell Biology: An Introduction to Pathology.* 3rd ed. Philadelphia: Mosby; 2012.)

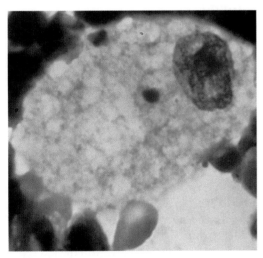

• **Figure 31-11** Niemann-Pick disease (BM ×1000).This bone marrow cell is filled with accumulated sphingolipids. These are the light-colored areas in the cell's cytoplasm. *BM,* Bone marrow. (From Carr JH, Rodak BF. *Clinical Hematology Atlas.* 4th ed. St. Louis: Saunders; 2013.)

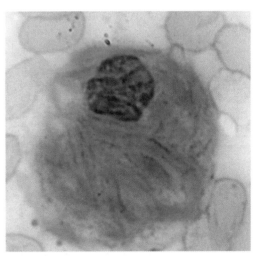

• **Figure 31-12** Gaucher cell (BM ×1000). The cell in this photograph is a classic Gaucher cell. What appear to be strands in the cytoplasm of the macrophage are actually glycolipid molecules. This is the classic crumpled-tissue-paper appearance of a Gaucher cell. *BM,* Bone marrow. (From Carr JH, Rodak BF. *Clinical Hematology Atlas.* 4th ed. St. Louis: Saunders, 2013.)

(especially vertically), poor muscle tone, and developmental delay. Affected individuals can survive into adulthood.

Laboratory Procedures and Limitations

Niemann-Pick disease is diagnosed by measuring acid sphingomyelinase (ASM) activity in white blood cells. ASM activity is low in individuals with the disease. Carriers can be identified by performing genetic tests for the *SMPD1* gene, which codes for ASM.

Gaucher Disease

Gaucher disease is a rare genetic disorder that affects production of the enzyme, β-glucocerebrosidase. There are several types: perinatal, type 1, type 2, and type 3 (Fig. 31-12). The perinatal type is the most lethal form of the disease.

It produces serious neurologic problems including hydrops fetalis. Infants with this type of Gaucher disease live for only a few days.

Type 1 is the most common type of Gaucher disease. Symptoms include hepatosplenomegaly, anemia, thrombocytopenia, lung disease, and bone abnormalities. Types 2 and 3 Gaucher disease have the same symptoms as type 1 but include in addition abnormal eye movements, seizures, and brain damage. The differentiating factor for types 2 and 3 is the rate of progression of the disease: Type 2 causes life-threatening medical problems in infancy, whereas type 3 progresses more slowly. Gaucher disease is most common in Jewish people of Eastern European descent, among whom 1 in 855 people are affected.

Laboratory Procedures and Limitations

Gaucher disease can be diagnosed by measuring glucocerebrosidase activity in leukocytes. A diagnosis can be made when less than 15% of mean normal activity of the enzyme is present. Molecular diagnostic tests for mutations of the *GBA* gene have limited value in predicting disease progression. CBCs are performed to discover the extent of cytopenia in a patient. Coagulation and liver function tests are performed to assess the degree of liver involvement in this disease. Other enzymes that are elevated and can aid in diagnosis include angiotensin-converting enzyme, acid phosphatase, and ferritin. Chitotriosidase measurements are useful for monitoring disease progression in most individuals.

Krabbe Disease

Krabbe disease is a genetic disorder that causes a deficiency of the enzyme, galactosylceramidase. This deficiency impairs the growth and maintenance of myelin, the insulating material that covers neurons (Fig. 31-13). Without this enzyme, nerves demyelinate, causing erratic processing of nerve impulses. Infants with this disease exhibit irritability, muscle weakness, feeding difficulties, fevers of unknown origin, and slowed mental and physical development. As the child ages, muscles continue to weaken, causing problems with moving, eating, and breathing. The demyelinization of the nerves also leads to seizures and vision loss. Late-onset cases of this disease also occur in childhood, adolescence, and adulthood. Individuals with late onset usually have visual problems and walking difficulties. The incidence of Krabbe disease is 1 case per 100,000 population. Most reported cases have occurred in people of European ancestry.

Laboratory Procedures and Limitations

Routine chemistry tests do not provide any abnormal results that would help diagnose Krabbe disease. Measurement of galactosylceramide β-galactosidase (GALC) activity can help confirm a diagnosis of Krabbe disease when the GALC activity levels are 5% or less of reference values in leukocytes, cultured fibroblasts, cultured aminocytes, and chorionic villi. Molecular testing for parents and newborns with the disease is helpful to identify heterozygous carriers. CSF from individuals with this disease shows elevated protein levels and an abnormal protein electrophoresis pattern: elevated albumin, elevated α_2-globulin levels, decreased β_1-globulin, and decreased γ-globulin levels. The cell count is normal.

Hurler Syndrome

Hurler syndrome is also called mucopolysaccharidosis type I. People with this disease do not form the enzyme lysosomal α-L-iduronidase. As a result, glycosaminoglycans (formerly called mucopolysaccharides) build up in organs, causing damage.

The severe form of this disorder appears during the first year of life, whereas the less severe form becomes symptomatic later in childhood. Symptoms of the severe form include macrocephaly, hydrocephalus, heart valve abnormalities, hepatosplenomegaly, macroglossia, sleep apnea, and frequent respiratory infections. These individuals can also develop cataracts, hearing loss, recurrent ear infections, and many skeletal deformities (Fig. 31-14).

Individuals with the severe form of Hurler syndrome usually die in late childhood; those with the less severe form can reach adulthood. The frequency of Hurler disease is 1 case in 16,000 to 30,000 births. Most reported cases have occurred among Israeli Jews or French Canadians.

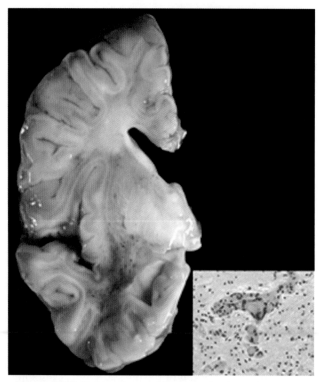

• **Figure 31-13** Krabbe disease. This image is of a brain of an individual with Krabbe disease. Much of the white matter is gray-yellow because of the loss of myelin. *Inset,* "Globoid" cells are the hallmark of the disease. (From Kumar V, Abbas AK, Aster JC. *Robbins and Cotran Pathologic Basis for Disease.* 9th ed. Philadelphia: Saunders; 2015.)

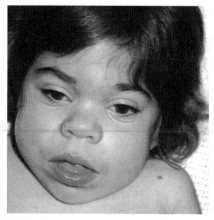

• **Figure 31-14** Patient with Hurler syndrome. (From Ansell BM. *Color Atlas of Pediatric Rheumatology.* London: Mosby-Wolfe; 1992.)

Laboratory Procedures and Limitations

Diagnostic tests for Hurler syndrome include genetic mutation analysis and urine tests for glycosaminoglycans. Enzyme assays are available to test for lysosomal α-L-iduronidase enzyme activity.

Aminoacidurias

Phenylketonuria

Phenylketonuria (PKU) is a genetic disease that causes a deficiency in the phenylalanine hydroxylase enzyme (Fig. 31-15). This deficiency results in accumulation of phenylalanine, phenylketones, and phenylamines which, in turn, impair brain development. Infants affected by this condition are asymptomatic at birth and develop symptoms at several months of life when brain damage occurs. This condition produces microcephaly and severe mental retardation.

Laboratory Procedures and Limitations

All newborns in the United States are tested for PKU. In the original test developed by Guthrie in the 1960s, a sample of blood from a newborn was collected on filter paper and transferred to a bacterial culture to determine whether it contained high levels of phenylalanine. Today, most states use MS/MS to test for more than 30 substances.

Tyrosinemia

Tyrosinemia is an inherited disease that leads to elevated blood levels of tyrosine (Fig. 31-16). The three types of tyrosinemia (types I, II, and III) are classified according to the specific enzyme deficiency. Type I tyrosinemia, the most severe form, is caused by a deficiency of fumarylacetoacetate hydrolase. Infants are asymptomatic at birth, and the symptoms appear during the first few months of life. Symptoms include failure to thrive, diarrhea, vomiting, jaundice, a cabbage-like odor, and increased nosebleeds. This disease can lead to liver and kidney failure.

Type II tyrosinemia is caused by a deficiency in tyrosine aminotransferase. Type II symptoms include excessive tearing, photophobia, eye pain and redness, and painful skin lesions on the palms and soles. Affected individuals are also developmentally delayed. Type III tyrosinemia is caused by a deficiency of 4-hydroxyphenylpyruvate dioxygenase. Type III symptoms include developmental delay, seizures, and intermittent ataxia.

Laboratory Procedures and Limitations

Tyrosinemia is diagnosed based on the results of enzyme assays and mutation analysis. Elevated tyrosine and succinylacetone levels are determined by MS/MS.

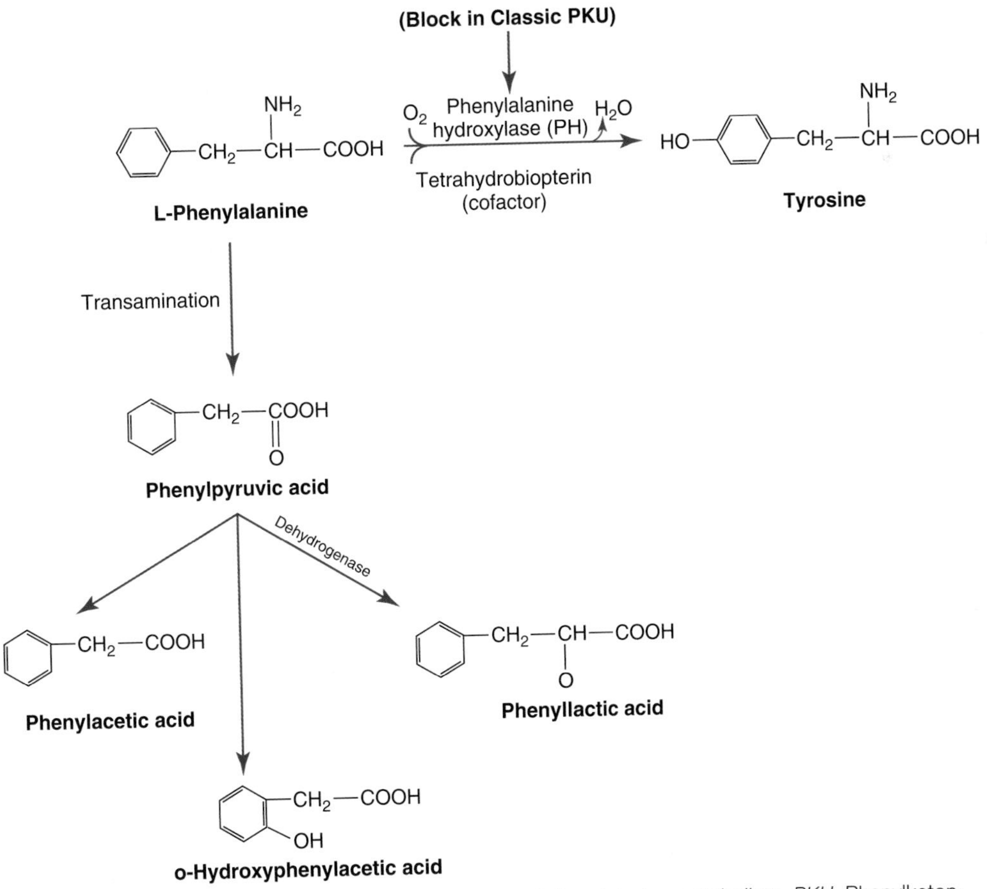

• **Figure 31-15** Major (tyrosine) and minor pathways of phenylalanine metabolism. *PKU,* Phenylketonuria. (From Brunzel NA. *Fundamentals of Urine and Body Fluid Analysis.* 3rd ed. St. Louis: Saunders; 2013.)

Alkaptonuria

Alkaptonuria is a genetic condition that results in a deficiency of the enzyme, homogentisate oxidase. Urine that is exposed to air turns black due to the presence of homogentisic acid. Individuals with alkaptonuria also experience a buildup of dark pigment (homogentisic acid) in connective tissue (cartilage and skin) which appears after age 30 years. Other symptoms of this disease include heart problems, kidney stones, prostate stones, and arthritis (in the spine and large joints in early adulthood).

Laboratory Procedures and Limitations

Diagnosis of alkaptonuria is confirmed by the presence of a significant amount of homogentisate acid in urine based on gas chromatography-mass spectrometry analysis.

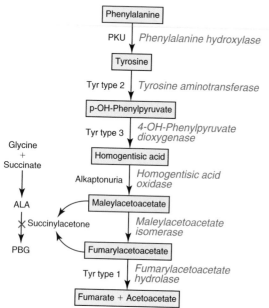

• **Figure 31-16** Disorders of inborn errors of metabolism resulting from deficiency of key enzymes required in the metabolic catabolism of phenylalanine. Specific deficiencies are shown on the right (*red letters*) and resulting disorders on the left. *ALA*, Alanine; *PBG*, porphobilinogen; *Tyr*, tyrosinemia (Modified from Burtis CA, Bruns DE. *Tietz Fundamentals of Clinical Chemistry and Molecular Diagnostics*. 7th ed. St. Louis: Saunders; 2015.)

Homocystinuria

Homocystinuria is a genetic disease with multiple forms that produces a deficiency in cystathionine β-synthase (Fig. 31-17). As a result, amino acids and toxic byproducts build up in the blood and produce symptoms. Homocystinuria, in its most common form, produces myopia, osteoporosis, an increased risk of abnormal blood clotting, dislocation of the lens at the front of the eye, and possible developmental delay. Usually, the symptoms appear during the first year of life. Some patients survive into adulthood.

Laboratory Procedures and Limitations

Homocystinuria can be detected with the use of the Guthrie test or MS/MS. Newborns in the United States are routinely tested for this disease. It can also be diagnosed on the basis of mutation analysis.

Maple Syrup Disease

Maple syrup disease (branched-chain ketoacidosis) is a genetic disorder that prevents the body from processing certain amino acids properly. The name refers to the sweet odor of the urine produced by affected infants. Symptoms include poor feeding, vomiting, lethargy, and developmental delay. Seizures, coma, and death can result if the disease is not treated. Milder versions manifest later in infancy or childhood, but all involve developmental delay and other medical problems. There are four genes that make proteins work together as a complex. This protein complex breaks down leucine, isoleucine, and valine. Mutations in any of the genes can reduce or eliminate a functioning protein complex, preventing the normal breakdown of these three amino acids. The buildup of these amino acids and their byproducts are toxic to the brain and other organs.

Laboratory Procedures and Limitations

Maple syrup disease can be detected with the use of MS/MS.

Cystinuria

Cystinuria is a genetic condition that leads to the development of cystine crystals or stones in the kidneys or bladder. Mutations in genes that encode for the cystine

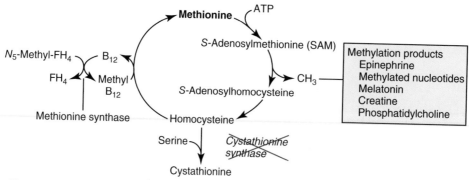

• **Figure 31-17** Homocystinuria. In this inborn error of metabolism, cystathione synthase is deficient, causing an increase in homocysteine and methionine. Increased homocysteine produces vessel thrombosis. *ATP*, Adenosine triphosphate; *FH₄*, tetrahydrofolate. (From Pelley JW, Goljan EF. *Rapid Review Biochemistry*. 2nd ed. Philadelphia: Mosby; 2007.)

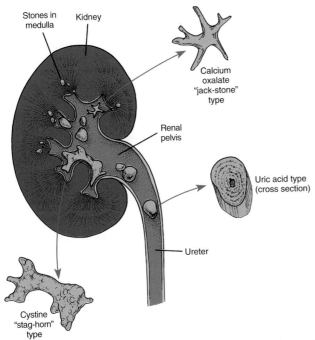

• Figure 31-18 Cystinuria prevents the reabsorption of cystine and other amino acids. This causes stones of cystine to develop in the urinary tract. (Grodner M, Roth SL, Walkingshaw BC. *Nutritional Foundations and Clinical Applications: A Nursing Approach.* 5th ed. St. Louis: Mosby; 2012.)

transport protein lead to this condition. Without a transport protein to provide a vehicle for reabsorption, cystine remains in the urine, and the excess cystine forms crystals (Fig. 31-18). These stones can become very large and create blockages and infections in the urinary tract and kidneys.

Laboratory Procedures and Limitations

Cystinuria can be diagnosed by analysis of a 24-hour urine collection and a random urine sample to determine levels of cystine in the urine. Cystinuria is also diagnosed through an analysis of kidney stones to determine whether they contain cystine.

Summary

Health is a complex concept that has changed over the years. Temperature, macronutrients, micronutrients, and genetic mutations all affect a person's health. Cold temperatures can cause tissue injury and tissue death (frostbite). High temperatures can cause heat illnesses including heat stroke, which is a medical emergency. Diet is associated with health and disease. Macronutrients (carbohydrates, proteins, and fats) and micronutrients (vitamins and trace metals) play a large part in maintaining health. A shortage of any of the macronutrients or micronutrients results in disease.

In addition to heat, cold, and diet, genetic mutations can also cause disease states. Genetic mutations can produce a group of conditions called inborn errors of metabolism. Inborn errors of metabolism usually involve the toxic accumulation of substrates in tissues or disorders of energy production and utilization. Inborn errors of metabolism usually appear in neonates but can manifest in adulthood. Mortality can be very high for inborn errors of metabolism, especially those that manifest in neonates. Early detection and careful management of the disorder are essential for a positive outcome.

Review Questions

1. Which of the following essential fatty acids is the basis for synthesis of antiinflammatory and proinflammatory eicosanoids?
   a. Arachidonic acid
   b. Linolenic acid
   c. ω-3 fatty acid
   d. Hydroxylated fatty acids
2. Symptoms of heat stroke include all the following EXCEPT:
   a. Acute kidney injury
   b. Myocardial infarction
   c. Tachycardia
   d. Rhabdomyolysis

3. A lack of homogentisate oxidase produces homogentisic acid in urine. A urine specimen that will turn black when exposed to air. What condition does this describe?
   a. Cystinuria
   b. Phenylketonuria
   c. Alkaptonuria
   d. Hartnup's disease
4. High triglycerides, low levels of low-density lipoproteins, and a high fasting blood glucose concentration are three test results used to diagnosis which of the following?
   a. Metabolic syndrome
   b. Lead poisoning
   c. Vitamin E deficiency
   d. Zinc toxicity

5. Common symptoms of malnutrition include all of the following EXCEPT:
   a. Night blindness
   b. Weight loss
   c. Fatigue
   d. Dizziness

6. Individuals with copper deficiency may be misdiagnosed with
   a. Weight loss
   b. Encephalopathy
   c. Nephropathy
   d. Myelodysplastic syndrome

7. What is the second most abundant trace element in the body?
   a. Copper
   b. Selenium
   c. Zinc
   d. Manganese

8. Dietary sources of vitamin K include all of the following EXCEPT:
   a. Eggs
   b. Plant oils
   c. Grains
   d. Green vegetables

9. Which of the following vitamins causes flushing—a burning or tingling sensation of the face, arms, and chest—when consumed in large amounts?
   a. B_6
   b. B_{12}
   c. Vitamin E
   d. Niacin

10. Vitamin C functions as a cofactor for synthesis of which of the following?
   a. Insulin
   b. Glucagon
   c. Biotin metabolism
   d. Adrenal hormones

Critical Thinking Questions

1. Why are vitamins and trace metals required for good health?
2. How does the ingestion of particular types of fats increase or decrease inflammation?

3. Why is a PKU test performed on all newborns?

CASE STUDY

A 38-year-old man comes to his physician with visual field constriction and hearing loss. He is an avid fisherman. He fishes every weekend and enjoys eating the fish he catches. His physician performs a chemistry panel with the following results:

Glucose, 95 mg/dL
BUN, 15 mg/dL
Creatinine, 1.0 mg/dL
Calcium, 9.8 mg/dL
Phosphate, 3.9 mg/dL
Sodium, 141 mEq/L

Potassium, 4.0 mEq/L
Chloride, 102 mEq/L
CO_2, 23 mEq/L
AST, 24 IU/L
ALT, 22 IU/L
Cholesterol, 180 mg/dL

The physician sends him home, and he returns 1 week later with worsening symptoms. What test should the physician order next and why? What is causing his symptoms?

Bibliography

Ahuja S, Caldwell JD, Shanks BC, Flores R. Effects of macronutrient composition and meal frequency on cortisol levels in humans. *Agro Food Industry Hi Tech.* 2012;23(2):4–5.

Burtis CA, Bruns DE. *Tietz Fundamentals of Clinical Chemistry and Molecular Diagnostics.* 7th ed. St. Louis: Elsevier Health Sciences; 2014.

Casas JS, Couce MD, Sordo J. Coordination chemistry of vitamin B6 and derivatives: a structural overview. *Coord Chem Rev.* 2012;256(23):3036–3062.

Center for Nutrition Policy and Promotion, U.S. Department of Agriculture. *MyPlate and Historical Food Pyramid Resources.* Last modified June 15, 2015. <http://fnic.nal.usda.gov/dietary-guidance/myplate-and-historical-food-pyramid-resources> Accessed 22.06.15.

Danzl DF. Hypothermia and frostbite. In: Longo DL, Fauce AS, Kasper DL, et al., eds. *Harrison's Principles of Internal Medicine.* 18th ed. New York: McGraw-Hill; 2012. Chapter 19.

Fischer R, Konkel A, Mehling H, et al. Dietary omega-3 fatty acids modulate the eicosanoid profile in man primarily via the CYP-epoxygenase pathway. *J Lipid Res.* 2014;55(6):1150–1164.

Garrett WS. Kwashiorkor and the gut microbiota. *N Engl J Med.* 2013;368(18):1746–1747.

Kaplan LA, Pesce JA, eds. *Clinical Chemistry: Theory, Analysis, and Correlation.* 3rd ed. St. Louis: Mosby; 1996.

Laumbach R, Kipen H. Mechanistic data support protecting non-smokers from the lethal effects of second-hand smoke. *Int J Public Health.* 2014;59(4):575–576.

McCance K, Huether S. *Pathophysiology: The Biologic Basis for Disease in Adults and Children.* 7th ed. St. Louis: Elsevier; 2014.

National Academy of Sciences, Institute of Medicine, Food and Nutrition Board. *Dietary Reference Intakes (DRIs): Recommended Dietary Allowances and Adequate Intakes, Vitamins and Elements.* Last modified June 15, 2015. <http://www.nal.usda.gov/fnic/DRI/DRI_Tables/RDA_AI_vitamins_elements.pdf> Accessed 22.06.15.

Zabrocki LA, Shellington DK, Bratton SL. Heat illness and hypothermia. In: Wheeler DS, Vong HR, Shanley TP, eds. *Pediatric Critical Care Medicine.* London: Springer; 2014:677–693.

32

Immune System Diseases

SHERYL BERMAN

CHAPTER OUTLINE

OBJECTIVES

After completion of this chapter, the reader will be able to:

1. Recognize the primary and secondary immune organs and tissues.
2. Compare and contrast humoral immunity and cell-mediated immunity
3. Provide an overview of a normal immune response.
4. Differentiate hypersensitivity reaction types I, II, III, and IV.
5. Describe a typical allergic response and the laboratory tests used for its diagnosis.
6. Describe the disease mechanisms of systemic lupus erythematosus and the laboratory tests used for its diagnosis and monitoring.
7. Describe the disease mechanisms of rheumatoid arthritis and the laboratory tests used for its diagnosis.
8. Differentiate between primary and secondary Sjögren syndrome and identify the laboratory tests used in its diagnosis.
9. Discuss why the lungs and kidneys are the two primary sites affected by Goodpasture syndrome and what laboratory tests are used in its diagnosis.
10. Describe how Wiskott-Aldrich syndrome manifests, its underlying genetic mutations, and the laboratory tests used for its diagnosis.

11. Describe ataxia telangiectasia, the abnormalities caused by the mutated *ATM* gene, and the laboratory tests used for its diagnosis.
12. Describe an amyloid protein and explain why amyloidosis may include more than 60 different proteins.
13. Compare the disease mechanisms and diagnostic laboratory tests for DiGeorge syndrome and severe combined immunodeficiency (SCID).
14. Discuss similarities and differences between Bruton X-linked agammaglobulinemia and common variable immune deficiency.
15. Explain the role of the complement cascade in innate immunity and how deficiencies affect susceptibility to disease.
16. Differentiate human immunodeficiency virus (HIV) infection and acquired immunodeficiency syndrome (AIDS).
17. Describe the tests used for diagnosis of HIV infection and monitoring of disease progression.
18. Define monoclonal and polyclonal gammopathies.

KEY TERMS

Acquired immunodeficiency syndrome
Adaptive immunity
Alloimmunity
Amyloidosis
Anaphylaxis
Anti–cyclic citrullinated peptide antibody
Anti–double-stranded DNA antibody
Antinuclear antibody
Anti-Smith antibody
Anti-SSA/Ro autoantibody
Anti-SSB/La autoantibody
Anti-U1RNP antibody

Ataxia telangiectasia
Autoimmune diseases
Autoimmunity
Bruton agammaglobulinemia
CH_{50} assay
Citrullination
Cytokines
Delayed hypersensitivity reactions
DiGeorge syndrome
Goodpasture syndrome
Hypersensitivity
Immediate hypersensitivity reactions

Membrane attack complex
Peyer patches
Pinocytosis
Raynaud syndrome
Scleroderma
Sensitization
Severe combined immunodeficiency
Sjögren syndrome
Systemic lupus erythematosus
Waldenström macroglobulinemia
Wiskott-Aldrich syndrome

Case in Point

An 8-month-old boy was brought to the emergency department because he was listless and had a fever and cough. This was the child's fourth respiratory infection in 4 months. The provider ordered a complete blood count, metabolic panel, and urinalysis, with the following results:

Complete Blood Count	Metabolic Panel	Urinalysis
White blood cells: 2000/L	Glucose; 100 mg/dL	Color: straw yellow
Red blood cells: 4.24 × 10⁶/L	Blood urea nitrogen: 25 mg/dL	Specific gravity: 1.015
Hemoglobin: 15.8 g/dL	Sodium: 142 mEq/L	Glucose: negative
Hematocrit: 48.2%	Potassium: 4.5 mEq/L	Ketones: 1+
Mean corpuscular volume: 102 µm³	Chloride: 102 mEq/L	Microscopic findings: negative
Platelet count: 250,000/L	Calcium: 9.4 mg/dL	

Are any of the laboratory results abnormal? What is the likely cause of these results? What follow-up test is needed to diagnose the child's condition? What is the most probable diagnosis?

Points to Remember

- One function of the immune system is to differentiate self from non-self antigens.
- Innate immunity involves no memory cells and therefore reacts the same way every time an antigen is encountered.
- Because adaptive immunity includes memory cells, exposure to an antigenic stimulus or foreign antigen results in an ability to respond to a foreign cell or tissue with increased strength and efficiency after each exposure.
- The humoral arm of the immune system is controlled by B cells; its primary purpose is to produce antibodies in response to antigenic stimulation.
- The cell-mediated arm of the immune system is controlled by T cells; its primary purpose is to create killer cytotoxic T cells that destroy infected cells.
- Hypersensitivity reactions can be categorized according to the antigen that is attacked by the immune system (i.e., allergy, autoimmunity, and alloimmunity) or the mechanism of the attack (i.e., types I, II, III, and IV).
- Symptoms of systemic anaphylaxis include itching, erythema, headaches, vomiting, abdominal cramps, diarrhea, and breathing difficulties. Severe anaphylaxis leads to contraction of bronchial smooth muscle, laryngeal edema (throat swelling), vascular collapse leading to respiratory distress, decreased blood pressure, shock, and death.

- Histamine release contracts bronchial smooth muscle, increases vascular permeability, and dilates blood vessels.
- In the first mechanism of type II hypersensitivity, the classical complement pathway is activated, resulting in membrane damage and cell lysis.
- In the second mechanism of type II hypersensitivity, antibodies bind to the cell, and the cell is then phagocytized by macrophages.
- In the third mechanism of type II hypersensitivity, antibodies bind to the cell and attract complement.
- In the fourth mechanism of type II hypersensitivity, natural killer cells, which are part of the innate arm of the immune system, recognize and kill aberrant cells by releasing cytotoxic molecules.
- In the fifth mechanism of type II hypersensitivity, antibodies bind to antigens on cell surfaces and cause cellular malfunction and destruction.
- Type IV hypersensitivity differs from other hypersensitivity reactions in that it is mediated by T lymphocytes instead of antibodies.
- Although most allergies are type I hypersensitivity reactions, type II, III, and IV reactions also produce allergies.
- When type I hypersensitivity reactions are responsible for an allergic reaction, high titers of immunoglobulin E (IgE) are formed after exposure to normally harmless substances. IgE binds to and initiates degranulation of mast cells, releasing histamine and other chemicals.
- Because the body cannot differentiate between self and non-self antigens in autoimmune disorders, it views self antigens as foreign and produces antibodies against them.
- Systemic lupus erythematosus (SLE) involves type II and type III hypersensitivity reactions in which antibodies attack antigens on cells and antibody–antigen complexes are deposited in tissues, causing inflammation.
- Useful laboratory tests for diagnosis of SLE include assays of antinuclear antibodies (ANAs) (>1:160), antibodies to native double-stranded DNA (dsDNA), anti-Smith (Sm) antibodies, anticardiolipin IgG or IgM antibodies, lupus anticoagulant, anti-SSA/Ro antibodies, anti-SSB/La antibodies, and anti-ribonucleoprotein (anti-RNP).
- Rheumatoid arthritis is a progressive, disabling disease that causes pain, deformity, and loss of mobility and function. Damage spreads from the synovial to the articular cartilage, the fibrous joint capsule, and surrounding ligaments and tendons.
- Useful laboratory tests for rheumatoid arthritis include those that detect inflammation (i.e., C-reactive protein and erythrocyte sedimentation rate), hematologic parameters (i.e., complete blood count), and specific antibodies (i.e., rheumatoid factor, antinuclear antibodies, and anticitrullinated protein antibodies).
- In Sjögren syndrome, inflammation produces lymphocytes that infiltrate exocrine glands. This infiltration is especially pronounced in parotid glands.

- Goodpasture syndrome is a type II hypersensitivity reaction in which antibodies are made against collagen type IV in glomerular basement membranes. These membranes are found primarily in the kidneys and in smaller amounts in the lungs.
- Diagnosis of Wiskott-Aldrich syndrome is based on clinical findings and results of laboratory tests such as complete blood count, total immunoglobulin levels, Wiskott-Aldrich syndrome protein (WASP) detection, and genetic analysis.
- Children with ataxia telangiectasia have an increased susceptibility to infection, increased incidence of certain cancers (e.g., leukemia, lymphoma), problems with movement and coordination (i.e., ataxia), and oculomotor apraxia (i.e., inability of the eyes to track objects with head motion).
- Immunodeficiencies are caused by malfunction of the self-defense portion of the immune system and are classified as primary or secondary.
- Immunodeficiencies often lead to recurrent, severe infections (e.g., pneumonia, otitis media, sinusitis, bronchitis, septicemia, meningitis) or infections with opportunistic or unusual pathogens (e.g., *Pneumocystis jirovecii,* cytomegalovirus).
- In DiGeorge syndrome, gene deletions cause various abnormalities, including a small thymus or absent thymus, small or absent parathyroid glands, structural defects of the heart and aorta, underdeveloped chin, low-set ears, and cleft palate. The structural defects can usually be repaired, but the thymus and parathyroid abnormalities have devastating functional effects on the immune system and the ability to fight infection.
- Individuals with X-linked agammaglobulinemia (XLA) have decreased or abolished antibody production capabilities, making them susceptible especially to bacterial infections.
- Common variable immune deficiency (CVID) is a collection of various B-cell and immunoglobulin disorders and is the most commonly diagnosed immunodeficiency disease. Diagnostic tests include total serum immunoglobulin levels (which decrease over time) and B- and T-cell phenotyping.
- The most severe and rare form of severe combined immunodeficiency (SCID) is reticular dysgenesis, a genetic disorder that results in no T cells, B cells, or phagocytic cells developing in the bone marrow; as a result, neither the adaptive nor the innate immune system functions properly.
- Deficiencies of the lectin complement pathway are common. Complement pathway deficiencies increase the likelihood of microbial infections, particularly bacterial infections.
- Human immunodeficiency virus (HIV) selectively infects and destroys helper T cells. When the level of helper T cells is less than 200 cells/μL, infected individuals cannot fight off opportunistic infections and cancer.
- Progression of HIV infection is monitored by measuring viral load, usually as viral particles per milliliter.
- Monoclonal gammopathies are caused by proliferation of a single clone of B cells and are characterized by monoclonal immunoglobulins in serum or urine.
- In polyclonal gammopathies, clones of multiple cell lines are involved, producing an increase in many types of immunoglobulins.

Introduction

This chapter reviews the physiology of the immune system, immunologic response mechanisms, and the symptoms and laboratory tests used to diagnose immune diseases. The three major categories of immune system diseases are allergies, autoimmune diseases, and immunodeficiencies.

Many immune system diseases are inherited, including Bruton agammaglobulinemia, complement deficiency, Wiskott-Aldrich syndrome, severe combined immunodeficiency (SCID), common variable immunodeficiency, ataxia telangiectasia, and polyclonal and monoclonal gammopathies. Some diseases are acquired, including human immunodeficiency virus (HIV) infection, which produces acquired immunodeficiency syndrome (AIDS). Other diseases have an inherited component but may also have environmental factors (i.e., triggers) that influence their expression. They include multiple myeloma, systemic lupus erythematosus, rheumatoid arthritis, Sjögren syndrome, Goodpasture syndrome, and Waldenström macroglobulinemia.

Normal Immune System

The immune system is the body's third level of response to external threats. First-line defenses are physical barriers such as the skin and mucosa. The second line of defense is inflammation. After physical barriers are breached, the inflammatory response is initiated. Acute inflammation is the short-lived, nonspecific, and rapid response of the innate immune system. The adaptive immune system provides a slower, specific, and long-lived response that prevents reinfection and provides long-term security (e.g., memory cells). Both arms of the immune system work together to provide a robust, layered defense of the body. When these systems fail, pathological conditions result.

The immune system normally protects the body by differentiating self from non-self antigens and responding to harmful antigens. Antigens are molecules (usually proteins) on the surfaces of cells, viruses, fungi, and bacteria; nonliving substances (e.g., toxins, soot particles) can also be antigens. Antigens that are perceived by the body as non-self induce an immune response (e.g., antibody production).

The immune system is composed of organs and tissues classified as primary lymphoid organs or secondary lymphoid organs (Fig. 32-1). The organs and tissues are connected by the blood and lymphatic systems. The primary organs of the immune system that produce lymphocytes are the thymus and bone marrow. The secondary organs that house these cells after they are produced include the lymph nodes, spleen, appendix, tonsils, and tissues throughout the body that are loosely categorized as mucosa-associated lymphoid tissue (MALT).

Lymphocytes are the major cell mediators of the immune response because they produce antibodies. Lymphocytes are divided into two major categories: T cells and B cells. T cells originate in the thymus (a lymphoid organ located in the neck), and B cells originate in the bone marrow. Lymphocytes enter the blood as immature cells that react with antigens. The cells migrate to secondary lymphoid organs such as the spleen or the lymph nodes, where they lie in wait for antigens to be presented to them (Table 32-1).

To generate an immune response, antigens must be processed and presented to immune cells in a specific way. Antigen-presenting cells carry peptide antigens on their surface; this activates Helper T cells, which work with the antigen-presenting cells to present the antigens to immunocompetent B or T cells. B cells that are presented with antigens differentiate and become active antibody-producing cells (i.e., plasma cells). T cells that are presented with antigens can become cytotoxic T cells that destroy virus-infected cells and tumor cells.

Innate Immunity and Adaptive Immunity

The immune system has two primary divisions, the nonspecific innate immune system and the specific acquired or adaptive immune system. Innate immunity exists at birth or shortly after birth. Adaptive immunity develops in response to antigen exposures throughout a lifetime.

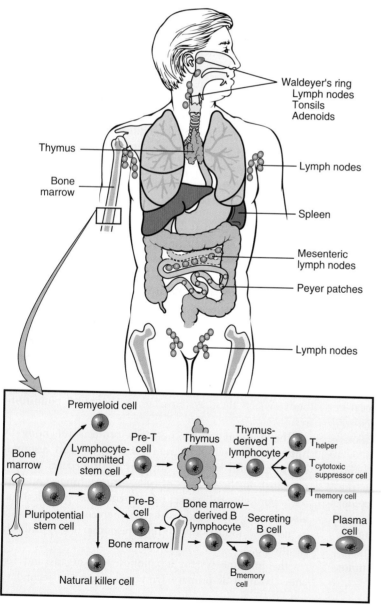

Major lymphoid organs

Waldeyer's ring
Lymph nodes
Tonsils
Adenoids

Thymus

Bone marrow

Lymph nodes

Spleen

Mesenteric lymph nodes

Peyer patches

Lymph nodes

Premyeloid cell

Bone marrow

Lymphocyte-committed stem cell

Pre-T cell

Thymus

Thymus-derived T lymphocyte

T_{helper}

$T_{cytotoxic}$ suppressor cell

$T_{memory cell}$

Pluripotential stem cell

Pre-B cell

Bone marrow

Bone marrow–derived B lymphocyte

Secreting B cell

Plasma cell

Natural killer cell

B_{memory} cell

• **Figure 32-1** Location of immune organs and tissues in the human body. (From Damjanov I. *Pathology for the Health Professions.* 4th ed. St. Louis: Saunders; 2012.)

Innate Immunity

The cells of the innate immune system recognize and respond to antigens in a generic way. With every exposure, the components of innate immunity behave in the same manner. Innate immunity does not involve immunologic memory.

Examples of innate immunity include the layers of the skin, which prevent most foreign antigens from entering the body; the complement system (including plasma proteins), which helps destroy microbes; macrophages and dendritic cells, which engulf and present antigens to T cells; and natural killer (NK) cells, which kill tumor cells and other abnormal cells.

Adaptive Immunity

In adaptive immunity, some T and B cells become memory cells after an initial encounter with a specific antigenic stimulus (e.g., vaccination, exposure to a virus). Subsequent encounters with the same agent prompt much stronger and faster immune reactions than occurred with the initial exposure The immune memory results in an ability to respond with increased strength and efficiency after each exposure (Fig. 32-2).

Humoral and Cell-Mediated Immunity

Like the innate system, the adaptive system includes humoral and cell-mediated immunity components (Fig. 32-3). Humoral immunity is mediated by molecules such as complement proteins and secreted antibodies. It is controlled by B cells, which produce antibodies in response to antigenic stimulation. On exposure to a new antigen and with the help of helper T cells, B cells mature into plasma cells and produce antibodies called immunoglobulins. There are five types of immunoglobulins: IgG, IgA, IgM, IgE, and IgD (see Chapter 15). Immunoglobulins play a key role in removing foreign antigens from the body.

Cell-mediated immunity is controlled by T cells and involves the activation of phagocytes and antigen-specific T lymphocytes in response to an antigen. Its primary purpose is to create cytotoxic T cells that destroy infected cells (e.g., virus-infected cells) and cancer cells.

The humoral and cell-mediated components are controlled by helper T cells through secretion of chemical messengers called cytokines. The cell-mediated component also regulates immune reactions so that they do not become excessive and harm normal tissues. The goal of the immune response is to mount a defense against pathogens and then return the system to homeostasis.

Immune System Mechanisms
Activation of T and B Cells

The immune system protects the body against non-self pathogens and cells, including infectious agents, as well as cancer cells. An invading organism must bypass the skin,

TABLE 32-1	Functions of Immune System Organs and Tissues
Organ or Tissue	**Functions**
Bone marrow	• The bone marrow is a primary immune organ because it produces all blood cells, especially the lymphocytes that mount the specific immune response. • The bone marrow provides the physical support for hematopoiesis and the growth factors (e.g., cytokines) necessary for the maturation of B cells.
Thymus	• The thymus is a primary immune organ and is found in the anterior mediastinum (i.e., upper center of the chest). The base of the thymus rests on the surface of the heart. • The thymus grows until puberty and then ceases functioning and shrivels up. • By middle adulthood, the thymus is primarily adipose tissue with only small amounts of lymphoid tissue remaining. • The thymus is the site of T-cell development until puberty. • As the thymus shrinks, its role in T-cell development is taken over by lymphoid tissues throughout the body.
Spleen	• The spleen acts as an early site of hematopoiesis before the bone marrow in the long bones has fully developed. • In the adult, the spleen is a site for the breakdown of dying blood cells. • The spleen removes opsonized microbes. • At any time, approximately 25% of blood cells may be circulating through the spleen.
Lymph nodes	• Lymph nodes are kidney bean–shaped structures that are usually clustered in groups around the body. They are often found where blood and lymph vessels meet. • The function of lymph nodes is to filter, concentrate, and prepare antigens for presentation to helper T cells. • Lymph nodes contain lymph, which is predominantly extracellular fluid. • During a response to an infection or inflammation, B and T cells in the lymph node are activated. • Fluid and cells accumulate in the node during the activation, causing nodes to swell (i.e., lymphadenopathy).
Mucosa-associated lymphoid tissue (MALT)	• The mucosal immune system is composed of lymphoid tissue in the respiratory, gastrointestinal, and genitourinary tracts. Tissues contain specialized epithelial cells (i.e., M cells) that by pinocytosis take up inhaled or ingested antigens. • Antigens are then presented to T cells to initiate immune reactions.

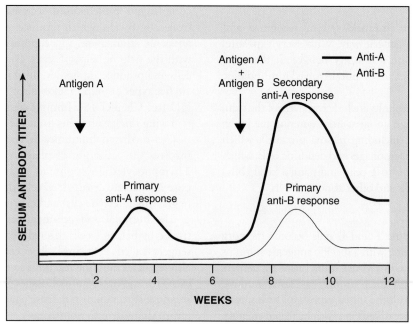

• **Figure 32-2** Illustration of the primary and secondary (memory) adaptive immune responses. (Adapted from Abbas AK, Lichtman AH. *Cellular and Molecular Immunology.* 5th ed. Philadelphia: Saunders; 2003.)

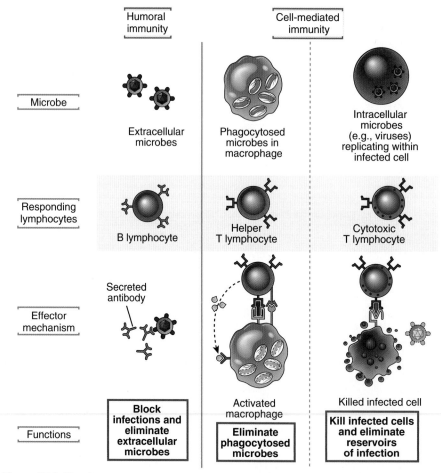

• **Figure 32-3** The effector cell of humoral immunity is the antibody-producing B cell. The effector cell of cell-mediated immunity is the cytotoxic T cell. (From Abbas AK, Lichtman AH, Pillai S. *Basic Immunology.* 4th ed. Philadelphia: Saunders; 2014.)

TABLE 32-2 Hypersensitivity Mechanisms of Tissue Destruction

Type	Name	Rate of Development	Antibody Class	Principal Effector Cells	Complement Participation	Examples
I	IgE mediated	Immediate	IgE	Mast cells	No	Seasonal allergic rhinitis, asthma, allergic conjunctivitis, food allergies, skin reactions
II	Tissue specific	Immediate	IgG, IgM	Tissue macrophages	Frequently	Autoimmune thrombocytopenic purpura, autoimmune hemolytic anemia, Graves disease
III	Immune complex–mediated	Immediate	IgG, IgM	Neutrophils	Yes	Systemic lupus erythematosus
IV	Cell mediated	Delayed	None	Lymphocytes, macrophages	No	Contact sensitivity to poison ivy and metals (e.g., jewelry)

From McCance KL, Huether SE. *Pathophysiology: The Biologic Basis for Disease in Adults and Children.* 7th ed. St. Louis: Mosby; 2015.
Ig, Immunoglobulin.

tears, and various enzymes in fluids to enter the body. After it enters through the nasopharynx, mouth, urogenital tract, or a break in the skin, the organism is engulfed and processed by dendritic cells or macrophages. Foreign antigens are displayed on the surfaces of these antigen-presenting cells and presented to helper T cells. Antigen recognition begins the adaptive immunity process. Helper T cells secrete cytokines that activate B cells, cytotoxic T cells, and regulatory T cells. Activated B cells replicate and form plasma cells, which produce immunoglobulins specific to the invading organism. Activated cytotoxic T cells destroy abnormal cells such as fungus-infected cells, parasites, and cancer cells. Regulatory T cells help to stop the immune response before it damages normal cells.

Hypersensitivity

Hypersensitivity is an exaggerated immune response that leads to tissue damage. Abnormal or impaired cells, signaling, or immune processes can result from genetic or environmental factors. Hypersensitivity reactions may be categorized by the antigen that is attacked by the immune system (i.e., allergy, autoimmunity, and alloimmunity) or by the attack mechanism (i.e., types I, II, III, and IV).

Allergy refers to a hypersensitivity response to external antigens, whereas autoimmunity refers to a defect in recognizing self antigens and the resulting hypersensitivity reaction to them. Alloimmunity occurs when an individual mounts a hypersensitivity response to the antigens of another individual (e.g., blood transfusion).

Hypersensitivity diseases are classified as hypersensitivity type I (IgE mediated), hypersensitivity type II (tissue specific), hypersensitivity type III (immune complex–mediated), or hypersensitivity type IV (cell mediated) according to the mechanism that causes the disease. This classification was developed to provide a better understanding of immune responses, but it is not a true picture

of clinical situations. Most immune responses have characteristics of some or all of the categories of hypersensitivity mechanisms.

Hypersensitivity reactions are preceded by sensitization, which results from the initial exposure to an antigen. Some hypersensitivity reactions occur within minutes or hours after antigen exposure and are called immediate hypersensitivity reactions. Hypersensitivity reactions that do not manifest for hours or days are called delayed hypersensitivity reactions.

Anaphylaxis is a life-threatening immediate hypersensitivity reaction. It can manifest systemically or cutaneously. Systemic symptoms of anaphylaxis include itching, erythema, headache, vomiting, abdominal cramps, diarrhea, and breathing difficulties. Severe anaphylaxis leads to contraction of bronchial smooth muscle, laryngeal edema (throat swelling), vascular collapse resulting in respiratory distress, decreased blood pressure, shock, and death. Certain individuals who are allergic to bee stings, peanuts, or fish may carry a self-injector filled with epinephrine (e.g., EpiPen) that can be used to prevent severe anaphylaxis if they are stung by a bee or ingest food that contains peanuts or fish (Table 32-2).

Type I Hypersensitivity

Type I hypersensitivity is also known as immediate hypersensitivity because it occurs within minutes after exposure to an antigen. In a type I hypersensitivity response, IgE binds to mast cell receptors. When two antibodies bound to two separate receptors on the same cell crosslink, the mast cells release the contents of their cytoplasmic granules. Chemicals released by mast cells include histamine, proteases, and chemotactic factors. Histamine is the most powerful mediator. It contracts bronchial smooth muscle, increases vascular permeability, and dilates blood vessels. These chemicals modulate the inflammatory response and cause a range of symptoms

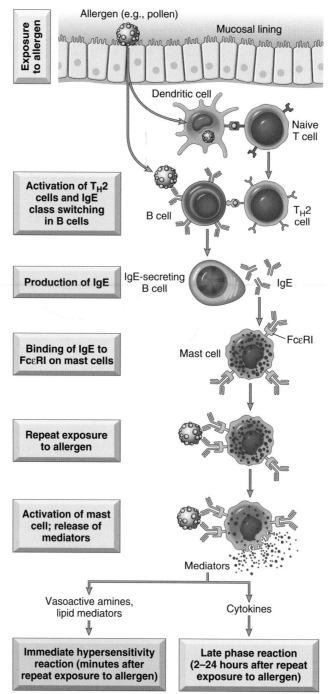

Allergen (e.g., pollen)

Mucosal lining

Exposure to allergen

Dendritic cell

Naive T cell

Activation of T$_H$2 cells and IgE class switching in B cells

B cell

T$_H$2 cell

Production of IgE

IgE-secreting B cell

IgE

Binding of IgE to FcɛRI on mast cells

FcɛRI

Mast cell

Repeat exposure to allergen

Activation of mast cell; release of mediators

Mediators

Vasoactive amines, lipid mediators

Cytokines

Immediate hypersensitivity reaction (minutes after repeat exposure to allergen)

Late phase reaction (2–24 hours after repeat exposure to allergen)

• **Figure 32-4** Type I hypersensitivity reaction. Type 2 helper T-cell (T$_H$2) responses and immunoglobulin E (IgE) production are stimulated in genetically susceptible individuals. IgE binds to Fc receptors (FcɛRI) on mast cells, and subsequent exposure to the allergen activates the mast cells to secrete the mediators that are responsible for the pathologic manifestations of immediate hypersensitivity. (From Kumar V, Abbas AK, Aster JC. *Robbins and Cotran Pathologic Basis for Disease*. 9th ed. Philadelphia: Saunders; 2015.)

that can be life-threatening in some cases (Fig. 32-4). In addition to these chemicals, cytokines are produced, and membrane phospholipids are released. Cytokines are small proteins that carry messages between cells. The cytokines released in this reaction are proinflammatory, meaning that they send signals to maintain or increase inflammation.

Type II Hypersensitivity

Type II or cytotoxic hypersensitivity reactions can affect cells by five different mechanisms. To initiate a type II hypersensitivity reaction, certain antibodies (i.e., IgG or IgM) bind to tissue-specific antigens on cells in the body or to external antigens that are bound to a specific tissue. These reactions

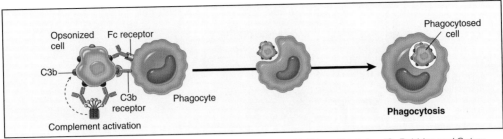

• **Figure 32-5** Opsonization and phagocytosis. (From Kumar V, Abbas AK, Aster JC. *Robbins and Cotran Pathologic Basis for Disease.* 9th ed. Philadelphia: Saunders; 2015.)

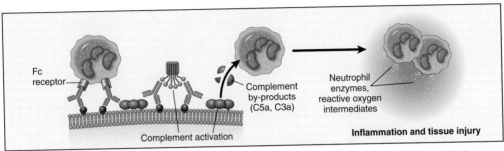

• **Figure 32-6** Complement and Fc receptor-mediated inflammation. (From Kumar V, Abbas AK, Aster JC. *Robbins and Cotran Pathologic Basis for Disease.* 9th ed. Philadelphia: Saunders; 2015.)

usually occur in the lungs, skin, cardiovascular system, nervous system, and thyroid gland.

The first mechanism of type II hypersensitivity involves activation of the classical complement pathway that results in membrane damage and cell lysis. Examples include transfusion reactions (e.g., receipt of the wrong ABO type of blood) and hemolytic disease of the newborn.

In the second mechanism, antibodies bind to the cell, and the cell is phagocytized by macrophages (Fig. 32-5). An example is autoimmune thrombocytopenic purpura.

In the third mechanism, antibodies bound to the abnormal cell attract complement. Complement components C3a and C5a attract neutrophils. After the complement cascade begins, neutrophils come to the area and attempt to phagocytize abnormal cells (Fig. 32-6). Because the cells are part of a tissue, cellular phagocytosis does not occur, but the neutrophils damage the tissue. Examples of disorders resulting from this mechanism are Goodpasture syndrome and pemphigus vulgaris.

In the fourth mechanism, NK cells recognize the antibody attached to a cell and release a toxic chemical that kills the cell (Fig. 32-7). Macrophages, neutrophils, and eosinophils can also mediate this response. For example, IgE can attach to helminths, and eosinophils can kill the worms.

In the fifth mechanism, an antibody binds to the cell and causes it to malfunction. An example of this mechanism is the binding of antibodies to thyroid cells in Graves disease, which causes excess thyroxine to be produced. The antibody renders the thyroid cells unresponsive to the normal feedback loop by which increased thyroxine in the blood signals the body to decrease the amount of thyroid-stimulating hormone (and therefore

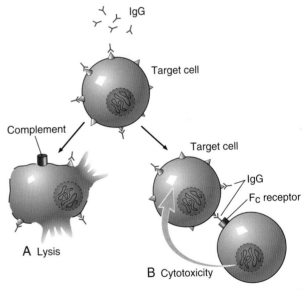

• **Figure 32-7** Type II hypersensitivity reaction involves cell lysis **(A)** and antibody-dependent cell-mediated cytotoxicity **(B).** (From Damjanov I. *Pathology for the Health Professions.* 4th ed. St. Louis: Saunders; 2012.)

thyroxine) that is produced. The antibody attached to the cells allows them to continue producing thyroxine even without thyroid-stimulating hormone (Fig. 32-8).

Type III Hypersensitivity

Type III or immune complex hypersensitivity occurs when antibody–antigen complexes are formed, circulate in the blood, and deposit in vessel walls or extravascular tissues (Fig. 32-9). This type of hypersensitivity is not

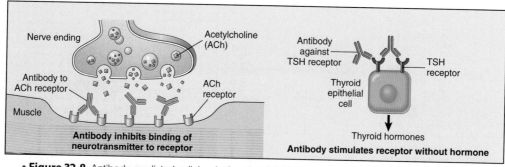

• **Figure 32-8** Antibody-mediated cellular dysfunction. *TSH,* Thyroid-stimulating hormone. (From Kumar V, Abbas AK, Aster JC. *Robbins and Cotran Pathologic Basis for Disease.* 9th ed. Philadelphia: Saunders; 2015.)

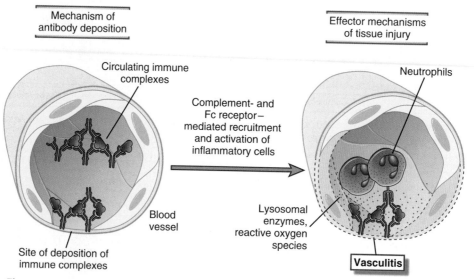

• **Figure 32-9** Type III hypersensitivity reactions in blood vessels. (From Abbas AK, Lichtman AH, Pillai S. *Cellular and Molecular Immunology.* 8th ed. Philadelphia: Saunders; 2015.)

tissue specific. The affected tissue is damaged because the immune complexes activate C3b, which attracts neutrophils that try to ingest the complexes. The surrounding tissues are damaged in the process, mostly due to release of lysosomal enzymes from the cells. Examples of type III hypersensitivity include rheumatoid arthritis (in which immune complexes settle in joints) and poststreptococcal glomerulonephritis (in which immune complexes settle in the glomerular basement membrane of the kidney) (Fig. 32-10 and Table 32-3).

Type IV Hypersensitivity

Type IV hypersensitivity is also called delayed hypersensitivity because it may take 48 to 72 hours before symptoms appear. Type IV hypersensitivity is mediated by T lymphocytes, not antibodies (Fig. 32-11). The NK cells target and destroy aberrant cells by using cytotoxic molecules stored in secretory lysosomes. Examples of type IV hypersensitivity include contact dermatitis associated with sensitivity to jewelry, allergy to poison oak or ivy, and graft rejection.

Type IV hypersensitivity mechanisms may play a part in autoimmune conditions. T cells destroy collagen and joints in rheumatoid arthritis, T cells destroy thyroid tissue in Hashimoto disease (autoimmune thyroiditis), and T cells destroy beta cells in the islets of Langerhans of the pancreas in type 1 diabetes.

This type of mechanism can also be used to detect exposure to a particular antigen. For example, in the tuberculosis skin test, a small amount of tuberculin antigen is injected under the skin. The test is read in 2 days because it takes 48 to 72 hours for the hypersensitivity reaction to occur. If the individual has previously been exposed to tuberculosis, the area of skin where the tuberculin was injected will become red, swollen, and hard (Table 32-4).

Disease States

There are many overlaps between hypersensitivity and autoimmune disease. Many conditions result from excessive immune reactions or immunodeficiencies, which can be classified as genetic or acquired.

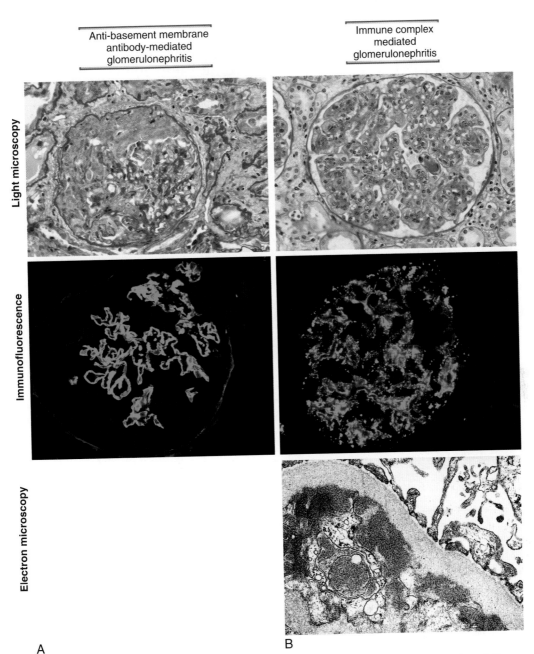

Anti-basement membrane antibody-mediated glomerulonephritis

Immune complex mediated glomerulonephritis

Light microscopy

Immunofluorescence

Electron microscopy

A

B

• **Figure 32-10** Pathologic features of antibody-mediated glomerulonephritis. **A,** Glomerulonephritis induced by an antibody against the glomerular basement membrane (i.e., Goodpasture syndrome). The light micrograph shows glomerular inflammation and severe damage, and immunofluorescence shows smooth (linear) deposits of antibody along the basement membrane. **B,** Glomerulonephritis induced by deposition of immune complexes (i.e., systemic lupus erythematosus). The light micrograph shows neutrophilic inflammation, and the immunofluorescence and electron micrograph show coarse (granular) deposits of antigen–antibody complexes along the basement membrane. (From Abbas AK, Lichtman AH, Pillai S. *Cellular and Molecular Immunology.* 8th ed. Philadelphia: Saunders; 2015.)

Allergies

Millions of people suffer from allergies to pollen, molds, fungi, food, animals (e.g., dog dander), cigarette smoke, latex, or other external antigens. *Allergy* is a common term most often used to describe type I hypersensitivity reactions, but type II, III, and IV reactions can also produce allergies. Type II and III reactions are uncommon but may be induced when antibiotics (e.g., penicillin, sulfonamides) or soluble antigens produced by hepatitis B infection are encountered. External antigens that can cause type IV reactions include plant resins (e.g., poison ivy, poison oak), metals (e.g., nickel, chromium), acetylated proteins, rubber, cosmetics, detergents, and topical antibiotics such as neomycin. Type IV reactions usually occur after prior exposure to antigens.

When type I hypersensitivity reactions are responsible for an allergic reaction, large amounts of IgE are formed after exposure to normally harmless substances. The IgE binds to mast cells and initiates their degranulation, which releases histamine and other chemicals. Histamine produces runny nose, itchy eyes, tissue swelling, vasodilation, and bronchoconstriction. If the allergies are mild (e.g., hay fever), symptoms can be troublesome but are rarely debilitating. However, some type I hypersensitivity reactions to external antigens can be extreme, as in anaphylaxis. In these cases, bronchoconstriction leads to asphyxia, and excessive vasodilation leads to a dangerous drop in blood pressure, either of which can be life-threatening. Allergies to peanuts, shellfish,

TABLE 32-3 Conditions With Circulating Immune Complexes

Classification	Condition
Autoimmune diseases	Systemic lupus erythematosus (lupus nephritis) Rheumatoid arthritis
Drug reactions	Allergies to penicillin and sulfonamides
Infectious diseases	Poststreptococcoal glomerulonephritis Meningitis Hepatitis Mononucleosis Malaria Trypanosomiasis

TABLE 32-4 Intracellular Pathogens and Contact Antigens That Induce Type IV (Delayed) Hypersensitivity

Pathogens and Contact Antigens	Examples
Intracellular bacteria	*Mycobacterium tuberculosis* *Mycobacterium leprae* *Brucella abortus* *Listeria monocytogenes*
Intracellular fungi	*Pneumocystis jirovecii* *Candida albicans* *Histoplasma capsulatum* *Cryptococcus neoformans*
Intracellular parasites	*Leishmania* sp.
Intracellular viruses	Herpes simplex virus Variola (smallpox) Measles virus
Contact antigens	Picryl chloride Hair dyes Nickel salts Poison ivy Poison oak

From Owen JA, Punt J, Stranford SA. *Kuby Immunology*. 7th ed. New York: WH Freeman; 2012.

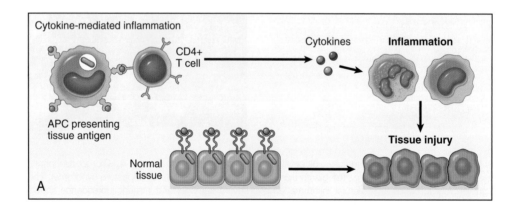

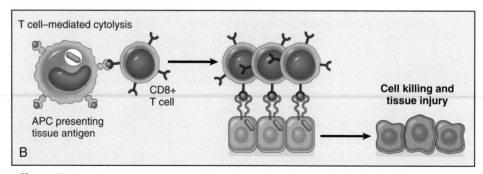

• **Figure 32-11 A,** Delayed-type hypersensitivity. **B,** T-cell-mediated cytolysis. *APC,* Antigen-presenting cell. (From Kumar V, Abbas AK, Aster JC. *Robbins and Cotran Pathologic Basis for Disease.* 9th ed. Philadelphia: Saunders; 2015.)

and insect stings may lead to anaphylaxis in susceptible individuals.

Allergies resulting from type I (IgE-mediated) hypersensitivity reactions can be identified by measuring total IgE levels and by antigen-specific IgE blood test, skin scratch tests, and intradermal testing. Antigen-specific IgE levels are most often detected by enzyme immunoassay (EIA). In a scratch test, a drop of a potential allergen is placed on the skin, and the outer layer of skin is pricked or scratched to allow entry of the antigen. In intradermal testing, small amounts of antigens are injected into the skin. An immediate wheal-and-flare reaction to the antigen indicates an allergy.

Autoimmune Diseases

Immune cells in the body differentiate between self and non-self antigens. When presented with a non-self antigen, an immune response is initiated to destroy the foreign antigen.

In autoimmune diseases, the body loses its ability to differentiate between self and non-self antigens. The body views self antigens as foreign and produces antibodies against them. The mechanisms for most autoimmune disorders are unknown. In a few, antigens from infectious agents are known to mimic self antigens, and haptens (small molecules that elicit an immune response when attached to a large carrier molecule such as a protein) bind to the self antigens and become immunogenic. Autoreactive lymphocytes survive the maturation process and attack self antigens, leading to further dysregulation of the immune response and clinical manifestations of an autoimmune disease. Polymorphisms of many genes are involved in conferring a predisposition to or protection from autoimmune diseases. Therapy for autoimmune diseases includes treating the symptoms, eliminating triggers, and preventing further organ damage, especially by reducing inflammation.

Systemic Lupus Erythematosus

Systemic lupus erythematosus (SLE) is a chronic, inflammatory, autoimmune disease in which the body produces antibodies to nucleic acids, red blood cells, coagulation proteins, phospholipids, lymphocytes, and platelets. SLE is a type II and a type III hypersensitivity reaction in which bound antibodies attack antigens on cells and antibody–antigen complexes are deposited in tissues, causing inflammation. Complexes that contain anti-DNA antibodies usually settle in glomerular basement membranes in the kidneys, which are often damaged by the disease. The circulating immune complexes also cause damage in the brain, heart, spleen, lung, gastrointestinal tract, skin, and peritoneum. The course of the disease is unpredictable. SLE occurs nine times more often in women than in men, and most commonly affects women between the ages of 15 and 35 years.

The classical manifestations of SLE include fever, joint pain (i.e., arthritis and arthralgia), malar rash, malaise, renal disease, myalgia, fatigue, anemia, and cardiovascular disease (Fig. 32-12). Autoantibody production causes progressive damage, which can begin as long as 10 years before clinical signs are apparent. SLE affects many organs simultaneously, providing a confusing list of symptoms and making diagnosis difficult. Patients experience symptomatic and asymptomatic periods, further complicating the diagnosis. The diagnosis of SLE is usually based on clinical findings, and eleven common findings were compiled to help health care providers establish a diagnosis earlier in the disease. The presence of four of these common clinical findings yields a sensitivity of 85% and a specificity of 95% for the diagnosis (Box 32-1).

Laboratory tests are also useful in the diagnosis of SLE. Laboratory tests are available for antinuclear antibodies (ANAs) (>1:160), antibodies to native double-stranded DNA (dsDNA), anti-Smith (Sm) antibodies, anticardiolipin IgG or IgM, lupus anticoagulant, anti-SSA antibodies, anti-SSB/La antibodies, and anti-ribonucleoprotein (anti-RNP), anti–β_2-glycoprotein antibodies, leukopenia, lymphopenia, thrombocytopenia, low hemoglobin and hematocrit levels, proteinuria (>0.5 g/day), creatinine, urinalysis, complement levels (low levels suggest consumption by the immune system), electrolytes, liver function, erythrocyte sedimentation rate (ESR), C-reactive protein (CRP), and renal function, which is disturbed if the kidney is involved.

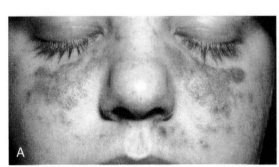
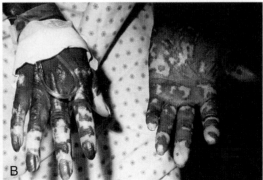

• **Figure 32-12** Symptoms of systemic lupus erythematosus (SLE). **A,** Typical butterfly rash of SLE. **B,** SLE in black skin. (From Frazier MS, Drzymkowski JW. *Essentials of Human Diseases and Conditions.* 5th ed. St. Louis: Saunders; 2013.)

1. *Malar rash:* butterfly-shaped rash across the cheeks and nose
2. *Discoid rash:* raised red patches on the skin
3. *Photosensitivity:* rash as result of an unusual reaction to sunlight
4. Mouth or nose ulcers, usually painless
5. Arthritis (nonerosive) in two or more joints, along with tenderness, swelling, or effusion; with nonerosive arthritis, the bones around joints are not destroyed
6. *Cardiopulmonary involvement:* inflammation of the lining around the heart (i.e., pericarditis) and/or the lungs (i.e., pleuritis)
7. *Neurologic disorder:* seizures and/or psychosis
8. *Kidney disorder:* excessive protein in the urine or cellular casts in the urine
9. *Blood disorder:* hemolytic anemia, low white blood cell count, or low platelet count
10. *Immunologic disorder:* antibodies to double-stranded DNA, antibodies to Sm, or antibodies to cardiolipin
11. *Antinuclear antibodies (ANAs):* positive test result in the absence of drugs known to induce it

<http://www.lupusresearchinstitute.org/lupus-facts/lupus-diagnosis> Accessed 01.11.15.

TABLE 32-5 **Fluorescence Patterns of Serum Antinuclear Antibodies and Disease Associations**

Fluorescence Pattern	Molecular Target	Disease Association
Homogenous	dsDNA	95% SLE
Homogenous	Histones	SLE
Nucleolar	hnRNP	SLE
Speckled, fine	SSA/Ro, SSB/La	40% SLE
Speckled, course	snRNP	SLE. SLE overlap syndrome

dsDNA, Double-stranded DNA; *RNP,* ribonucleoprotein; *SLE,* systemic lupus erythematosus; *SSA/Ro,* type of autoantibody; *SSB/La,* type of autoantibody.

ANA testing is the primary screening test used to diagnose SLE. The most common test method used to detect antinuclear antibodies is indirect immunofluorescence. Microscope slides are coated with a HEp-2 cell substrate, and the patient's serum is incubated with the cells for a specified period, then washed off. Substrate with fluorescent-conjugated anti-human antibody is then applied and incubated for a specified time, after which the slide is washed again. After the slide dries, the staining pattern is observed with the use of a fluorescent microscope. If antibodies are present, they bind to the antigens on the cells and produce five major staining patterns: homogenous, rim, speckled, nucleolar, and centromere. The pattern of fluorescence suggests the types of ANAs present in the patient's serum. ANAs that may be associated with SLE include anti-Smith antibodies, anti–double-stranded DNA antibodies, antihistone antibodies, anti-U1RNP antibodies, anti-SSA/Ro autoantibodies, and anti-SSB/La autoantibodies. Each is associated with a distinct pattern of fluorescence (Table 32-5).

Total complement levels are measured by the CH_{50} assay, which measures the complement proteins of the classical pathway, and the APH_{50} assay, which measures the complement proteins of the alternative pathway. Both tests measure the reciprocal dilution of a serum that is required to produce 50% hemolysis of a standard preparation of antibody-sensitized red blood cells. Enzyme immunoassays are used to measure levels of specific complement proteins, including C1, C2, C3, C4, and C1q.

Kidney and liver function tests are commonly used to diagnose and monitor individuals with SLE, in which kidney damage with nephrotic syndrome typically progresses to renal failure in advanced disease. Sodium, potassium, and chloride levels and renal function measurements such as blood urea nitrogen (BUN) and creatinine are affected in active disease. As the disease continues to damage organs, the liver may become inflamed, resulting in elevated levels of liver enzymes such as alanine aminotransferase (ALT) and aspartate aminotransferase (AST).

In most SLE patients, anemia accompanies the other clinical findings. It is usually a moderate anemia (i.e., anemia of inflammation or chronic disease), indicated by a low hemoglobin level (not lower than 9 g/dL), hematocrit, and red blood cell count (Table 32-6).

Rheumatoid Arthritis

In rheumatoid arthritis, the immune system produces antibodies against the synovial lining of the joints, resulting in a chronic, systemic, autoimmune inflammatory disease. The antibodies induce joint swelling and tenderness and eventually destroy the joints. During the course of the disease, damage spreads from the synovial to the articular cartilage, the fibrous joint capsule, and surrounding ligaments and tendons. Rheumatoid arthritis frequently affects the fingers, feet, wrists, elbows, ankles, and knees; it less frequently affects the shoulders, hips, and cervical spine (Fig. 32-13). Pain, deformity, and loss of mobility and function disable the patient. In addition to attacks on synovial joints, individuals with rheumatoid arthritis may experience fever, malaise, rash, lymph node or spleen enlargement, and Raynaud phenomenon.

Rheumatoid arthritis is thought to result from a combination of genetic susceptibility (e.g., *HLA-DRB1*) and exposure to an appropriate environmental trigger. The autoimmune antibodies, usually IgM or IgG, produced against host tissues during disease progression are called rheumatoid factors. The disease mechanism that produces rheumatoid arthritis is well understood. In the setting of chronic inflammation, arginine, an amino acid, is transformed into citrulline, another amino acid. The process, called citrullination,

TABLE 32-6   Autoantibody Tests for Systemic Lupus Erythematosus

Test	Description
ANA	Used as a screening test because it is 95% sensitive; must be used in conjunction with clinical findings
Anti-dsDNA	High specificity, low sensitivity (70%); levels can vary with disease activity
Anti-Sm	Most specific antibody for SLE, but only 30-40% sensitive
Anti-SSA/Ro or Anti-SSB/La	15% of SLE patients have these antibodies
Anti-RNP	May indicate connective-tissue disease; overlaps with scleroderma and myositis
Anticardiolipin	Used to screen for antiphospholipid antibody syndrome, important in SLE diagnosis
Lupus anticoagulant	Screen for inhibitors in the clotting system in the antiphospholipid antibody syndrome seen in SLE

Adapted from Elkon KB. Systemic lupus erythematosus: autoantibodies in SLE. In: Klippel JH, Dieppe PA, eds. *Rheumatology*. 2nd ed. St. Louis: Mosby; 1998.
ANA, Antinuclear antibody; *dsDNA,* double-stranded DNA; *RNP,* ribonucleoprotein; *SLE,* systemic lupus erythematosus; *SSA/Ro,* type of autoantibody; *SSB/La,* type of autoantibody.

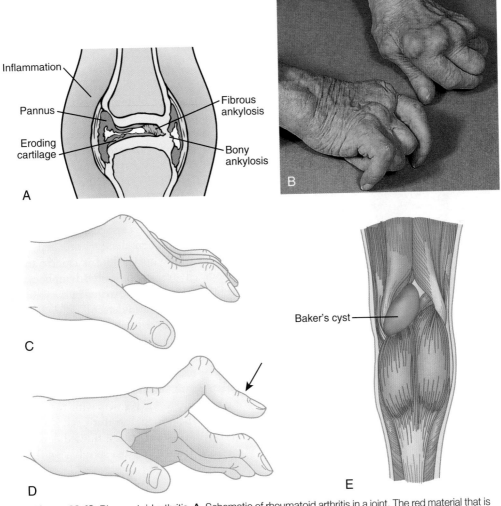

• **Figure 32-13** Rheumatoid arthritis. **A,** Schematic of rheumatoid arthritis in a joint. The red material that is growing over the articular cartilage and destroying it is pannus (i.e., granulation tissue, a precursor to scar tissue). Notice that fibrous ankylosis is beginning at the margin of the joint. **B,** Patient with rheumatoid arthritis has bilateral ulnar deviation of the hands and prominent swelling of the second and third metacarpophalangeal joints. **C,** Swan neck deformity of the fingers: flexion of the distal interphalangeal (DIP) joint and extension of the proximal interphalangeal (PIP) joint. **D,** Boutonnière deformity of the index finger: extension of the DIP joint and flexion of PIP joint and index finger with a swan neck deformity of the third through fifth fingers. **E,** Baker cyst is an is an extension of the semimembranosus bursa posteriorly. This bursa is often connected to a joint cavity. (A, From Kumar V, Abbas AK, Fausto N, Mitchell RN: *Robbins Basic Pathology.* 8th ed. Philadelphia: Saunders Elsevier, 2007:820. B, From Forbes C, Jackson W: *Color Atlas and Text of Clinical Medicine.* 2nd ed. London: Mosby; 2002:121. C to E, From Marx J: *Rosen's Emergency Medicine Concepts and Clinical Practice.* 7th ed. Philadelphia: Mosby Elsevier; 2010:514, 664.)

usually affects other proteins (e.g., fibrin) during cell death. The immune system considers proteins that undergo this process to be foreign antigens and mounts an immune response against them. The antibodies produced against the antigens form immune complexes that settle on the synovial tissue and articular cartilage, which are then damaged by phagocytosis of the antigens by macrophages and neutrophils and subsequent release of enzymes (Fig. 32-14). Most of the tissue damage that occurs in rheumatoid arthritis is associated with the mistaken inflammatory response to host tissues. Because the inflammatory response is not specific, it is not unusual for the lung pleura, pericardial sac, and subcutaneous tissues to be affected as well.

Rheumatoid arthritis is diagnosed on the basis of symptoms, physical examination, imaging tests, and laboratory

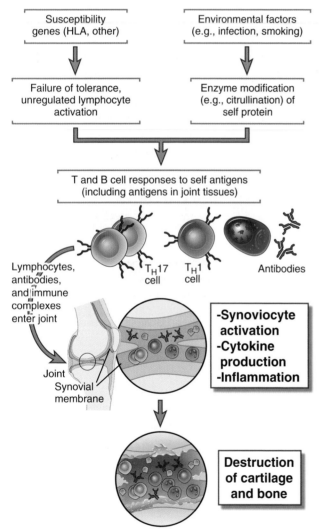

• **Figure 32-14** According to this model for the pathogenesis of rheumatoid arthritis, citrullinated proteins induced by environmental stimuli elicit T-cell and antibody responses in genetically susceptible individuals. The T cells and antibodies enter joints, respond to the self proteins, and cause tissue injury mainly by cytokine secretion and by antibody-dependent effector mechanisms. Protein modifications other than citrullination may lead to the same result. (From Abbas AK, Lichtman AH, Pillai S. *Cellular and Molecular Immunology.* 8th ed. Philadelphia: Saunders; 2015.)

tests. As with most autoimmune diseases, the first symptoms are mild and may not be noticeable. However, in some cases of acute onset, the symptoms appear abruptly. The first noticeable symptoms are fever, fatigue, weakness, anorexia, weight loss, aching, and stiffness. Over the course of the disease, the joints of the fingers, hands, and wrists begin to swell and become painful, tender, and stiff. The larger joints of the body (e.g., hip) become involved as the disease progresses. On examination, the swollen finger joints feel warm and soft due to the fluid accumulation, and the skin looks red and shiny. Inflammation of the synovial joint weakens the joint's ligaments and tendons, resulting in deformities of the hands, fingers, feet, and toes (see Fig. 32-13). Useful tests for diagnosis of rheumatoid arthritis include those that detect inflammation (i.e., CRP and ESR), hematologic parameters (i.e., complete blood count), and specific antibodies (i.e., rheumatoid factor, ANAs, and anti-citrullinated protein antibodies).

The most useful laboratory assay for diagnosing rheumatoid arthritis is a blood test for anti-citrullinated protein antibodies (ACPAs). When the result is combined with clinical findings, a diagnosis of rheumatoid arthritis can be made. Criteria used to diagnose rheumatoid arthritis include two or more swollen joints, morning stiffness lasting longer than 1 hour for at least 6 weeks, and a positive ACPA test result. The ACPA tests are moderately sensitive but very specific. The most commonly ordered one is the anti–cyclic citrullinated peptide antibody (anti-CCP) test. It is an immunoassay that uses serum to test for the antibodies. Results are interpreted as shown in Box 32-2.

Synovial fluid analysis is a good tool for detecting rheumatoid arthritis. Infections and autoimmune diseases have different disease processes occurring in joints and are easily distinguished when the data are analyzed. In rheumatoid arthritis, the synovial fluid is cloudy and has many white blood cells (mostly T and B lymphocytes and NK cells). In infections, there are many leukocytes and bacteria in the fluid. Ultrasound can detect fluid in the synovial joints, and radiographs can detect erosion of bone in the joints.

The CRP measurement is a sensitive but nonspecific test. Levels usually are extremely elevated in rheumatoid arthritis. The test is performed with the use of direct immunoturbidimetric or immunonephelometric assays in which an antibody to CRP reacts with the protein in the patient sample. The normal level for CRP is less than 5 mg/dL.

The ESR ("sed rate") is used less frequently than in the past. It measures the speed at which red blood cells in

---

• BOX 32-2 **Anti–Cyclic Citrullinated Peptide Antibody Test Results for the Detection of Rheumatoid Arthritis**

Negative: <20 EU/mL
Weak positive: 20-39 EU/mL
Moderate/strong positive: 40-59 EU/mL
Strong positive: >59 EU/mL

anticoagulated blood fall in a tube over a specified period (usually 1 hour). If inflammatory proteins are present in the blood, the cells fall much faster than in normal samples. Because of the inflammatory nature of rheumatoid arthritis, it is associated with very elevated ESRs. The normal range for an ESR is 20 to 30 mm/hr.

Rheumatoid factor is an abnormal immunoglobulin that is seen in approximately 85% of individuals with rheumatoid arthritis. Because the rheumatoid factor concentration can be very low early in the disease course, it may not be detected. Rheumatoid factor is measured by immunoturbidimetry, and the reference range is less than 14 IU/mL. The rheumatoid factor assay cannot be used alone to diagnose rheumatoid arthritis because it is not specific for the disease. Rheumatoid factor is not found in all individuals with rheumatoid arthritis, and it may be found in individuals with other connective tissue diseases, infections, or other autoimmune disorders.

Sjögren Syndrome

Sjögren syndrome is an autoimmune disease which damages the exocrine glands that produce saliva, tears, and other secretions. Primary Sjögren syndrome occurs by itself. In approximately 50% of those affected, secondary Sjögren syndrome occurs in conjunction with other autoimmune diseases such as SLE, scleroderma (i.e., local or extensive hardening and contraction of the skin and connective tissue), and rheumatoid arthritis.

In Sjögren syndrome, inflammation produces lymphocytes that infiltrate exocrine glands. This infiltration is especially pronounced in the parotid glands. The disease begins as a localized condition, but as it progresses, the inflammation damages the lungs, gastrointestinal tract, and kidneys. Myalgia (i.e., muscle pain), arthritis, and Raynaud syndrome (i.e., vasoconstriction of capillaries in the fingers and toes) may also occur.

Because no single laboratory test is diagnostic for Sjögren syndrome, clinical criteria are important. Laboratory tests (including ANAs, anti-SSA/Ro antibodies, anti-SSB/La antibodies, rheumatoid factor, cryoglobulins, and serum protein electrophoresis), ocular tests, saliva tests, imaging techniques, and labial biopsy are used to diagnose the condition. ANAs are a good indicator of an autoimmune process. Specific ANAs such as anti-SSA/Ro and anti-SSB/La are associated with Sjögren syndrome. They are most often detected with the use of an immunofluorescence antibody assay.

A rheumatoid factor assay is done because many individuals with Sjögren syndrome have positive test results. It is not a diagnostic test for Sjögren syndrome, but it can provide an important piece of the puzzle. The same is true for the cryoglobulin and serum protein electrophoresis tests. Cryoglobulins are proteins that precipitate from the serum at low temperatures. Serum protein electrophoresis tests are discussed in Chapter 15.

The Schirmer test is helpful in diagnosing Sjögren syndrome because it measures tear production, which is decreased in the disease. Sjögren syndrome is diagnosed clinically, and four of the following six criteria must be met:

- *Ocular symptoms:* dry eyes for longer than 3 months, foreign body sensation, use of tear substitutes more than three times daily
- *Oral symptoms:* dry mouth, recurrently swollen salivary glands, frequent use of liquids to aid swallowing
- *Ocular signs:* results of the Schirmer test performed without anesthesia (<5 mm in 5 minutes), positive vital dye staining result
- *Oral signs:* abnormal salivary scintigraphy findings, abnormal parotid sialography findings, abnormal sialometry findings (unstimulated salivary flow <1.5 mL in 15 minutes)
- Positive minor salivary gland biopsy findings
- Positive anti-SSA/Ro or anti-SSB/La antibody results

Goodpasture Syndrome

Goodpasture syndrome is a rare, autoimmune, pulmonary-renal syndrome characterized by bleeding in the lungs and kidney failure. Goodpasture syndrome is a type II hypersensitivity reaction in which antibodies are made against collagen type IV in the glomerular basement membrane. The glomerular basement membrane is found primarily in the kidney, with a small amount in the lungs, which explains why the effects are manifested in the lungs and kidneys (Fig. 32-15).

Although the diagnosis of Goodpasture syndrome is not easy due to the vagueness of early signs of the disease, an accurate and timely diagnosis is required because the disease progresses rapidly. Useful laboratory studies are a urinalysis, measurement of anti-glomerular basement membrane (anti-GBM) antibodies, and chest radiographs. Individuals with Goodpasture disease have hematuria, proteinuria, and red blood cell casts in the urine. Anti-GBM antibodies in the blood are usually diagnostic of Goodpasture syndrome

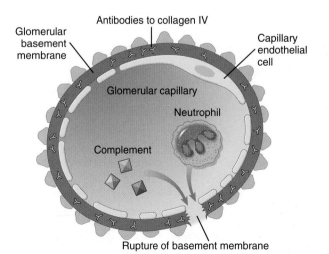

• **Figure 32-15** In Goodpasture syndrome, antibodies to collagen type IV activate complement and attract polymorphonuclear neutrophils that contribute to the damage and rupture the glomerular basement membrane. (From Damjanov I. *Pathology for the Health Professions.* 4th ed. St. Louis: Saunders; 2012.)

along with confirmation from a kidney biopsy. The biopsy detects the lymphocytic infiltration and antibody-induced damage to the glomeruli and basement membranes.

Amyloidosis

Amyloidosis is a condition in which abnormal, insoluble amyloid fibrils are deposited in organs or tissues and interfere with normal function. Approximately 23 proteins in the human body can form amyloid fibrils. Most amyloid fibrils are the result of defective folding of a protein.

Genetic mutations transform proteins into amyloid fibrils. Amyloidosis causes damage to the heart, liver, spleen, central nervous system, kidneys, and gastrointestinal tract. The diagnosis of amyloidosis is based on serum and urine electrophoresis and a biopsy of the affected organ.

Immunodeficiencies

Immunodeficiencies are caused by malfunction of the self-defense portion of the immune system and are classified as primary or secondary. Primary (congenital) immunodeficiencies are caused by a genetic mutation (Table 32-7). Examples are Bruton agammaglobulinemia and SCID. Secondary immunodeficiencies are those caused by another illness or by aging. When an individual has recurrent, severe infections (e.g., pneumonia, otitis media, sinusitis, bronchitis, septicemia, meningitis) or infection with an opportunistic or unusual pathogen (e.g., *Pneumocystis jirovecii,* cytomegalovirus), immune

deficiencies should be considered. Oral antibiotics usually do not work, and intravenous antibiotics are required to end the infection.

The nature of the infecting organism may point to a particular immunodeficiency. Viral and fungal infections may indicate a deficient T-cell response, and infections with *Streptococcus pneumoniae* or other encapsulated organisms may indicate B-cell or phagocytosis deficiencies.

Wiskott-Aldrich Syndrome

Wiskott-Aldrich syndrome is a rare, X-linked, recessive disease characterized by eczema, thrombocytopenia, bloody diarrhea, and immune deficiency. In Wiskott-Aldrich syndrome, a mutated gene *(WAS)* encodes a defective protein (WASP). This protein is involved in signaling and organizing the cytoskeletal structure of blood cells. *WAS* mutations result in thrombocytopenia, immunodeficiency, eczema, and a high susceptibility for developing tumors and autoimmune disease.

Diagnosis of Wiskott-Aldrich syndrome is based on clinical findings and the results of laboratory tests (i.e., complete blood count, total immunoglobulin levels, WASP levels, and genetic analysis). In Wiskott-Aldrich syndrome, a complete blood count reveals low values for red and white blood cells and for platelets, which have abnormal sizes and shapes. Total levels of immunoglobulin are usually low, as are levels of IgM and IgA. Low levels of WASP are usually seen, and a genetic analysis of the X chromosome demonstrates *WAS* mutations.

TABLE 32-7	Common Congenital Immunodeficiencies		
Disease	**Functional Deficiencies**	**Disease Mechanism**
Severe Combined Immunodeficiency (SCID)		
X-linked SCID	Markedly decreased T cells; normal or increased B cells; reduced serum Ig levels	Cytokine receptor common γ-chain gene mutations, defective T-cell maturation due to lack of IL-7 signals
Autosomal recessive SCID due to ADA, PNP deficiency	Progressive decreased in T and B cells (mostly T); reduced serum Ig in ADA deficiency, normal B cells and serum Ig in PNP deficiency	ADA or PNP deficiency leads to accumulation of toxic metabolites in lymphocytes
Autosomal recessive SCID due to other causes	Decreased T and B cells; reduced serum Ig levels	Defective maturation of T and B cells; may be mutations in *RAG* genes and other genes involved in VDJ recombination of IL-7R signaling
B-Cell Immunodeficiencies		
X-linked agammaglobulinemia	Decrease in all serum Ig isotypes; reduced B-cell numbers	Block in maturation beyond pre-B cells because of mutation in BTK
Ig heavy-chain deletions	IgG1, IgG2, or IgG4 absent; sometimes associated with absent IgA or IgE	Chromosomal deletion involving Ig heavy-chain locus at 14q32
T-Cell Immunodeficiences		
DiGeorge syndrome	Deceased T cells; normal B cells; normal or deceased serum Ig levels	Anomalous development of third and fourth brachial pouches, leaving to thymic hypoplasia

From Abbas AK, Lichtman AH, Pillai S: *Basic Immunology.* 4th ed. Philadelphia: Saunders; 2014.
ADA, Adenosine deaminase; *BTK,* Bruton tyrosine kinase; *Ig,* immunoglobulin; *IL,* interleukin; *PNP,* purine nucleoside phosphorylase.

Ataxia Telangiectasia

Ataxia telangiectasia is a rare, autosomal recessive, neuro-degenerative immune disorder that causes severe disability. The term *ataxia* refers to a defect in balance and coordination, and the term *telangiectasia* refers to dilated blood vessels. It is usually detected in children who are having difficulty learning to walk.

Ataxia telangiectasia is caused by many sporadic mutations in the ataxia telangiectasia gene *(ATM)*. The genetic defect prevents repair of damaged or broken DNA and causes dilation of capillaries in the eyes and skin of the ears, neck, and extremities. This leads to cell death in many areas of the body, including the cerebellum, cerebrum, and immune system. Children with this disease have an increased susceptibility to infection, increased incidence of malignancies (e.g., leukemia, lymphoma), problems with movement and coordination (i.e., ataxia), and oculomotor apraxia (i.e., inability of the eyes to track objects during head motion).

Diagnosis of ataxia telangiectasia uses clinical findings supported by laboratory tests such as total immunoglobulin levels, cancer markers such as carcinoembryonic antigen and α-fetoprotein, and genetic analysis. Total immunoglobulin levels are decreased, as are individual levels of IgM, IgG, and IgA. Determining the mutations in the *ATM* gene provides a definitive diagnosis.

DiGeorge Syndrome

DiGeorge syndrome (i.e., congenital thymic aplasia or hypoplasia) is a rare congenital disease that affects T-cell maturation. It is caused by the deletion of several genes on chromosome 22. The deletions cause various abnormalities, including a small or absent thymus, small or absent parathyroid glands, structural defects of the heart and aorta, underdeveloped chin, low-set ears, and cleft palate. The structural defects can usually be repaired, but the thymus and parathyroid abnormalities have devastating functional effects on the immune system and the ability of the body to fight infection.

The thymus is essential for the normal development of T cells. Without T lymphocytes, every part of the mature immune system is crippled, including antibody formation. The defects leave the body unprotected against infectious agents and unable to perform cancer surveillance.

Diagnosis of DiGeorge syndrome is based on clinical findings and confirmed with chromosomal analysis. Laboratory tests can offer supportive information, such as calcium levels that indicate hypocalcemia, total immunoglobulin tests that show low levels of antibodies, and immunophenotyping to determine T- and B-cell counts.

Bruton Agammaglobulinemia

Bruton agammaglobulinemia is also called X-linked agammaglobulinemia (XLA) because the mutated gene occurs on the X chromosome. As a result, boys (who have only one X chromosome) with the mutated gene have the disease, girls with one mutated gene are carriers, and girls with two copies of the mutated gene have the disease.

Bruton tyrosine kinase (BTK) is necessary for the development and maturation of B-cell precursors into mature B cells. Without BTK, there are no plasma cells and no antibody production. T-cell production and function are normal. The organs and tissues that normally house B cells (i.e., tonsils, adenoids, Peyer patches, lymph nodes, and spleen) are absent or smaller than normal. Individuals with XLA have decreased immune responses, especially to bacterial infections (Fig. 32-16).

Laboratory testing for this disease in infants and children begins after maternal antibodies disappear from fetal circulation (about 6 months after birth). The child has an increased rate and severity of infections, which is especially noticeable with bacterial infections of the respiratory and gastrointestinal tracts. A complete blood count (white counts may be low or low normal), B-cell count (very low or absent), and analysis of the BTK protein or BTK RNA constitute the definitive test for XLA.

Common Variable Immunodeficiency Disease

Common variable immune deficiency (CVID), a collection of B-cell and immunoglobulin disorders, is the most commonly diagnosed immunodeficiency disease. Because the clinical picture varies, it is often difficult to recognize. Whereas most inherited diseases are apparent within 2 years after birth, CVID usually manifests after 2 years of age and can occur as late as the 20s.

A constant finding is hypogammaglobulinemia. Most patients have low IgG levels, but IgA or IgM or both may also be decreased, and some individuals have normal numbers of B cells. In addition to the immune defects, affected individuals can have arthritis, gastrointestinal symptoms (e.g., malabsorption, chronic diarrhea), autoimmune disease, and cancer. Diagnosis of CVID includes measurements of total serum immunoglobulin levels (which decrease with disease progression) and B- and T-cell phenotyping.

Severe Combined Immunodeficiency

Severe combined immunodeficiency (SCID) is a spectrum of disorders. The most severe and uncommon form is reticular dysgenesis, which is a genetic disorder that results in no T cells, B cells, or phagocytes developing in the bone marrow. Although most individuals with SCID do not have lymphocytes, they do have other white blood cells. The thymus, spleen, and lymph nodes are very small because of the absence of lymphocytes.

Children with this disease usually die in utero or before their first birthday because they are unable to fend off even the most benign infectious agents. Chromosomal analysis confirms the diagnosis.

Complement Deficiencies

The complement system is a part of the innate immune system. It consists of more than 30 proteins that are activated by several triggers, resulting in a chain or cascade of events in the tissues (see Chapter 11). The end products of the complement cascade are the membrane attack complex (MAC),

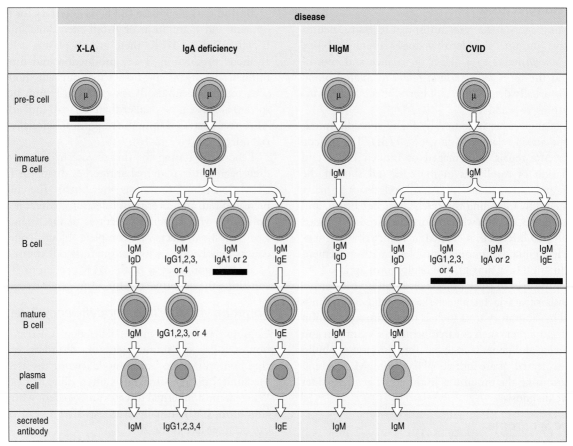

• **Figure 32-16** B-cell maturation in X-linked immunodeficiencies. *Ig,* Immunoglobulin. (From Male D, Brostoff J, Roth D, Roitt I: *Immunology.* 8th ed. Philadelphia: Saunders; 2013.)

which lyses infected or abnormal cells, and the various chemicals that increase the efficiency and effectiveness of the innate and adaptive immune systems. Examples of enhanced actions include phagocytosis of microbes and trafficking or chemotaxis of white cells to the site of infection.

There are at least three ways to activate the complement cascade. The three major pathways are called the classical pathway, the alternative pathway, and the lectin pathway. Deficiencies of components of the classical and alternative pathways of the complement system are rare, but deficiencies of the lectin complement pathway are common. Deficiencies of the complement pathways result in increased microbial infections, particularly bacterial infections.

Blood samples are used to measure total complement levels based on the degree of cell lysis in the CH_{50} and APH_{50} tests. Enzyme immunoassays are used to measure levels of specific complement proteins. These tests were described earlier.

Human Immunodeficiency Virus Infection

Human immunodeficiency virus (HIV) is a retrovirus that causes a profound immune deficiency. It is transmitted through sexual intercourse, shared intravenous drug paraphernalia, and in utero exposure. HIV selectively attacks helper T cells and destroys them. When the population of helper T cells (i.e., CD4+ T cells) reaches a level of less than

200 cells/μL, infected individuals are unable to fight off opportunistic infections and cancer.

The helper T cell is the most important cell in the immune system because it secretes the cytokines necessary for stimulating antibody production by B cells, killing infected cells, monitoring and killing cancer cells, and controlling the immune system. When the population of helper T cells is low or nonexistent, all phases of the immune response are compromised. HIV-infected persons have increased numbers and severity of bacterial, viral, fungal, and parasitic infections, some of which can be life-threatening. Because cancer surveillance is compromised, the incidence of certain cancers increases. Due to a lack of immune regulation, the likelihood of autoimmune conditions in individuals with advanced HIV infection increases (Fig. 32-17).

Initially, HIV infection may produce no signs or symptoms. When seroconversion occurs (i.e., antibodies against the virus begin to be produced), the individual may have a flulike illness with fever, malaise, and a rash. He or she may also have swollen lymph nodes. After seroconversion, the number of CD4 T cells begins to decrease. When the count falls to less than 200 cells/μL, the diagnosis changes to acquired immunodeficiency syndrome (AIDS).

The screening tests for detecting HIV antibodies use serum or saliva specimens and enzyme-linked

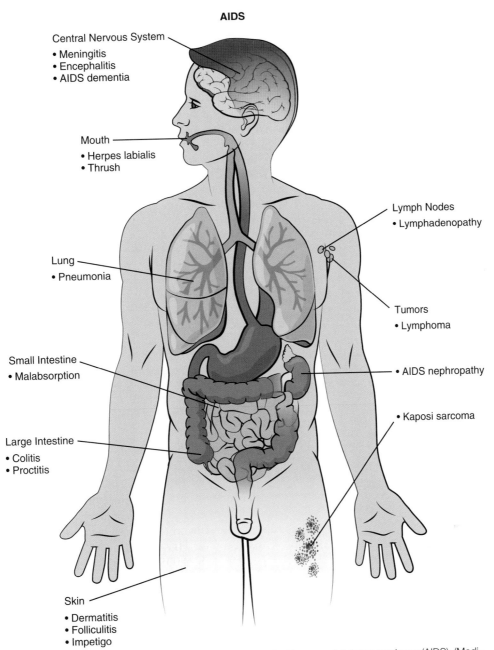

AIDS

Central Nervous System
- Meningitis
- Encephalitis
- AIDS dementia

Mouth
- Herpes labialis
- Thrush

Lymph Nodes
- Lymphadenopathy

Lung
- Pneumonia

Tumors
- Lymphoma

Small Intestine
- Malabsorption

- AIDS nephropathy

- Kaposi sarcoma

Large Intestine
- Colitis
- Proctitis

Skin
- Dermatitis
- Folliculitis
- Impetigo

• **Figure 32-17** Pathologic changes associated with acquired immune deficiency syndrome (AIDS). (Modified from Damjanov I. *Pathology for the Health Professions.* 4th ed. St. Louis: Saunders; 2012.)

immunosorbent assay (ELISA) techniques. The Western blot test (see Chapter 15) is used to confirm the diagnosis of HIV infection. The most common test used to monitor progression or infectivity of HIV infection is viral load. Viral load is a quantitative test that uses nucleic acid sequence–based amplification or reverse transcription–polymerase chain reaction.

Monoclonal and Polyclonal Gammopathies

Monoclonal and polyclonal gammopathies are disorders in which B cells secrete excessive levels of immunoglobulins. In monoclonal gammopathies, one B-cell clone produces a single line of immunoglobulins. In polyclonal gammopathies, multiple clones produce increased numbers of many types of immunoglobulins. In some cases, only light or heavy chains are secreted by the B-cell clone.

Rheumatoid arthritis and SLE are examples of polyclonal gammopathies. Monoclonal gammopathies include multiple myeloma (a blood malignancy that develops in the bone marrow) and Waldenström macroglobulinemia (a type of non-Hodgkin lymphoma that produces large amounts of an abnormal protein). Monoclonal gammopathies, polyclonal gammopathies, multiple myeloma, and Waldenström macroglobulinemia are discussed in Chapter 15.

Summary

Immune disorders include allergy, immune deficiencies, and autoimmune diseases. Type I through IV hypersensitivity reactions underlie the cell damage that occurs in allergies and autoimmune diseases. Immunodeficiencies include congenital diseases such as Bruton agammaglobulinemia, complement deficiencies, and inherited and acquired immunodeficiencies such as SCID and AIDS. Immune disorders also include autoimmune diseases such as SLE, rheumatoid arthritis, and Sjögren syndrome, as well as polyclonal and monoclonal gammopathies such as multiple myeloma and Waldenström macroglobulinemia.

Review Questions

1. Which of the following is considered a primary organ of the immune system?
   a. MALT
   b. Spleen
   c. Bone marrow
   d. Peyer patches
2. Which of the following are *not* directly associated with the functions of T cells?
   a. Regulation
   b. Help and secretion of cytokines
   c. Killing infected cells
   d. Production of immunoglobulin
3. Helper T cells are considered key components in
   a. Innate immunity
   b. Adaptive or cell-mediated immunity
   c. Transforming B cells
   d. The complement system
4. Which of the following is the preferred method of diagnosis for rheumatoid arthritis, systemic lupus erythematosus, and Sjögren syndrome?
   a. Antinuclear antibodies
   b. Clinical criteria
   c. Rheumatoid factor
   d. Serum electrophoresis
5. Labial biopsy and the Schirmer test are part of the diagnosis for
   a. Systemic lupus erythematosus
   b. Sjögren syndrome
   c. Waldenström's macroglobulinemia
   d. Scleroderma
6. All of the following diseases are considered primary immune deficiencies in which cells of the immune system do not develop into mature cells EXCEPT

   a. Bruton agammaglobulinemia
   b. Waldenström macroglobulinemia
   c. Nezelof syndrome
   d. Severe combined immunodeficiency
7. If a patient has a deficiency in a complement protein that prevents synthesis of the membrane attack complex, which of the following essential functions is likely to be decreased?
   a. Helper T-cell function
   b. Lysis of infected cells
   c. Antibody production
   d. Phagocytosis of viruses
8. Anti-citrullinated protein antibody assay results are used to diagnose which of the following autoimmune diseases?
   a. Rheumatoid arthritis
   b. Sjögren syndrome
   c. Goodpasture syndrome
   d. Wiskott-Aldrich syndrome
9. Which of the following disorders is a type II hypersensitivity reaction that coats a cell with an antibody so that the cell can be phagocytized.
   a. HIV infection
   b. AIDS
   c. Wiskott-Aldrich syndrome
   d. Autoimmune thrombocytic purpura
10. All of the following tests are useful for detecting the presence or progression of HIV infection EXCEPT
    a. Enzyme immunoassay detecting antiviral antibodies
    b. Chest radiograph
    c. Western blot
    d. Viral genome detection by polymerase chain reaction

Critical Thinking Questions

1. Please discuss the cell-mediated and humoral components of the immune system and their roles in adaptive immunity. Explain how the slow destruction of the helper T-cell population in HIV infection can affect antibody production, production of cytotoxic T cells, and the regulation of the immune system in general.

2. Compare and contrast types I, II, III, and IV hypersensitivity. Please explain the tremendous crossover between hypersensitivity and autoimmune disease with examples.

3. What is the mechanism for rheumatoid arthritis, and how are deformities of the hands and feet produced?

CASE STUDY

Ms. F, a 24-year-old woman, reported to her physician with exhaustion, nausea, and swollen lymph nodes lasting 3 months. A careful history revealed many recent infections, including pneumonia, and multiple sexual partners with unprotected sex. Her physician ordered a test to detect the human immunodeficiency virus (HIV). The test result was positive. Describe the difference between HIV infection and AIDS. What tests are used for the diagnosis of HIV, and what tests are used to track progression of the disease?

Bibliography

Abbas AK, Lichtman AH, Pillai S. *Basic Immunology: Functions and Disorders of the Immune System*. St. Louis: Elsevier Health Sciences; 2012.

Ballanti E, Perricone C, Greco E, et al. Complement and autoimmunity. *Immunol Res*. 2013;56:477–491.

Bossuyt X. Advances in serum protein electrophoresis. *Adv Clin Chem*. 2006;42:43–80.

Buchbinder D, Nugent DJ, Fillipovich AH. Wiskott-Aldrich syndrome: diagnosis, current management, and emerging treatments. *Appl Clini Genet*. 2014;7:55.

Burton OT, Oettgen HC. Beyond immediate hypersensitivity: evolving roles for IgE antibodies in immune homeostasis and allergic diseases. *Immunol Rev*. 2011;242:128–143.

Cohen MS, Shaw GM, McMichael AJ, Haynes BF. Acute HIV-1 infection. *New Engl J Med*. 2011;364:1943–1954.

Deane S, Slemi C, Naguwa SM, Teuber SS, Gershwin ME. Common variable immunodeficiency: etiological and treatment issues. *Int Arch Allergy Immunol*. 2009;150:311–324.

Gibofsky A. Overview of epidemiology, pathophysiology, and diagnosis of rheumatoid arthritis. *Am J Manag Care*. 2012;18(Suppl):S295–S302.

Haynes BF, Eisenbarth GS. Use of monoclonal antibodies to identify cell-surface antigens of human neuroendocrine thymic epithelium. In: *Monoclonal Antibodies: Probes for the Study of Autoimmunity and Immunodeficiency*. Orlando, FL: Academic Press, Inc.; 1983.

Havlicekova Z, Jesenak M, Freiberger T, Banovcin P. X-linked agammaglobulinemia caused by new mutation in BTK gene: a case report. *Biomed Papers*. 2014;158:470–473.

Hellmark T, Segelmark M. Diagnosis and classification of Goodpasture's disease (anti-GBM). *J Autoimmun*. 2014;48:108–112.

Janeway Jr CA, Travers P, Walport M, Shlomchik M. *Immunobiology: The Immune System in Health and Disease*. 6th ed. New York: Garland Science; 2005.

Jarvis JN, Percival A, Bauman S, et al. Evaluation of a novel point-of-care cryptococcal antigen test on serum, plasma, and urine from patients with HIV-associated cryptococcal meningitis. *Clin Infect Dis*. 2011;53:1019–1023.

Katzmann JA, Snyder MR, Rajkumar SV, et al. Long-term biological variation of serum protein electrophoresis M-spike, urine M-spike, and monoclonal serum free light chain quantification: implications for monitoring monoclonal gammopathies. *Clin Chem*. 2011;57:1687–1692.

Keren DF, Alexanian R, Goeken JA, et al. Guidelines for clinical and laboratory evaluation of patients with monoclonal gammopathies. *Arch Pathol Lab Med*. 1999;123:106–107.

Kivity S, Arango MT, Ehrenfeld M, Tehori O, et al. Infection and autoimmunity in Sjogren's syndrome: a clinical study and comprehensive review. *J Autoimmun*. 2014;51:17–22.

Kono S. Aceruloplasminemia: an update. *Int Rev Neurobiol*. 2013;110:51–125.

Kyriakidis NC, Kapsogeorgou EK, Tzioufas AG. A comprehensive review of autoantibodies in primary Sjögren's syndrome: clinical phenotypes and regulatory mechanisms. *J Autoimmun*. 2014;51:67–74.

Landgren O, Kyle RA, Pfeiffer RM, et al. Monoclonal gammopathy of undetermined significance (MGUS) consistently precedes multiple myeloma: a prospective study. *Blood*. 2009;113:5412–5417.

Leleu X, Koulieris E, Maltezas D, et al. Novel M-component based biomarkers in Waldenström's macroglobulinemia. *Clin Lymphoma Myeloma Leuk*. 2011;11:164–167.

Lennon P, Crotty M, Fenton JE. Infectious mononucleosis. *BMJ*. 2015;350:h1825.

Mackay IR, Rose NR, eds. *The Autoimmune Diseases II*. St. Louis: Elsevier; 2012.

Manjunath R, Nandi D, Karande P. Cells and organs of the immune system, part 1. In: *Essentials in Immunology*. 2012. <http://nptel.iitm.ac.in/courses/104108055/2> Accessed 01.11.15.

National Institute of Neurological Disorders and Stroke, National Institutes of Health: *Ataxia Telangiectasia Information*. <www.ninds.nih.gov/disorders/a_t/a-t.htm> Accessed 20.09.15.

National Institutes of Health: *Learning about Severe Combined Immunodeficiency (SCID)*. <http://www.genome.gov/13014325> Accessed 20.09.15.

Nilsson B, Ekdahl KN. Complement diagnostics: concepts, indications, and practical guidelines. *Clin Dev Immunol*. 2012;2012:962702.

Nuvolone M, Palladini G, Merlini G. Amyloid diseases at the molecular level: general overview and focus on AL amyloidosis. In: *Amyloid and Related Disorders*. New York: Humana Press; 2012:9–29.

Ochs HD, Puck JM, eds. *Primary Immunodeficiency Diseases: A Molecular and Genetic Approach*. New York: Oxford University Press; 2013.

Petri M, Orbai AM, Alarcón GS, et al. Derivation and validation of the Systemic Lupus International Collaborating Clinics classification criteria for systemic lupus erythematosus. *Arthritis Rheum*. 2012;64:2677–2686.

Puck JM. Laboratory technology for population-based screening for severe combined immunodeficiency in neonates: the winner is T-cell receptor excision circles. *J Allergy Clin Immunol*. 2012;129:607–616.

Siddique A, Kowdley KV. Review article: the iron overload syndromes. *Aliment Pharmacol Ther*. 2012;35:876–893.

Welch K, Resnick ES. DiGeorge syndrome. In: Sampson HA, ed. *Allergy and Clinical Immunology*. Chichester, UK: John Wiley & Sons, Ltd; 2005:368–374. doi: 10.1002/9781118609125.ch44.

Yu C, Gershwin ME, Chang C. Diagnostic criteria for systemic lupus erythematosus: a critical review. *J Autoimmun*. 2014;48:10–13.

33

Therapeutic Drug Monitoring

LAIRD C. SHELDAHL AND DONNA LARSON

CHAPTER OUTLINE

OBJECTIVES

After completion of this chapter, the reader will be able to:

1. State two reasons for measuring drug levels in body fluids.
2. Describe the mechanism of action of a drug.
3. Define clinical pharmacokinetics.
4. Describe five factors that affect drug disposition.
5. Identify the carrier proteins that transport drugs in the blood.
6. Discuss the importance of free drug in relation to cellular uptake and excretion by the kidneys.
7. Describe the formation of metabolites from the parent drug and the importance of these metabolites.
8. Explain how a change in serum protein levels affects free drug concentration and tissue uptake.
9. Explain the effects of decreased renal output on drug levels.
10. List three major routes for drug administration.
11. Define generic drug, steady state, subtherapeutic range, therapeutic range, toxic range, and half-life.
12. Discuss the importance of knowing the time and specifics of drug administration for properly determining sample times.
13. Describe the trough level and peak level.
14. Discuss the effects of aging and pregnancy on drug metabolism and excretion.
15. List the physiologic effects and examples of drugs for the following categories: cardiovascular, antibiotics, antiepileptic, psychoactive, bronchodilators, immunosuppressive, and protease inhibitor.
16. Describe the techniques for measuring prescription drugs.

KEY TERMS

Adverse drug reaction
Antineoplastic drug
Bacteriocidal drug
Bacteriostatic drug
Bioavailability
Biotransformation
Bound drug
Broad-spectrum antibiotic
Drug concentration

Drug–drug interaction
Free drug
Half-life
Induction
Inhibition
Loading dose
Maintenance dose
Mechanism of action
Narrow-spectrum antibiotic

Peak level
Pharmacodynamics
Pharmacokinetics
Steady state
Subtherapeutic dose
Sympathomimetics
Therapeutic index
Therapeutic range
Trough level

 ### Case in Point

A 15-year-old girl arrives at the emergency department with severe shortness of breath. She has a history of asthma. She has been using her rescue inhaler, but it is not helping her to breathe easier. The emergency department physician administers theophylline intravenously to open her airways. After about an hour, the patient begins to feel better, but she then becomes nauseated and vomits. She continues vomiting as the physician comes in, reexamines her, and orders a theophylline level determination and a metabolic panel. The test results show a theophylline level of 30 μg/mL; calcium, 7.9 mg/dL; and potassium, 2.9 mEq/L. What condition is revealed by the test results? Why does the physician treat the girl with this drug?

Points to Remember

- Therapeutic drug monitoring is based on the assumption that the size of the pharmacologic effect is directly proportional to the amount of drug at the target area.
- Pharmacokinetics is the study of the rate of absorption, distribution, biotransformation, and excretion of drugs.
- After a drug is absorbed from the gastrointestinal system, it is transported by the hepatic portal venous system for processing in the liver.

- Bioavailability is the fraction of an administered dose that reaches the systemic circulation.
- Drug distribution is the process of moving the substance from the site of absorption to other areas of the body.
- The blood–brain barrier limits chemicals in the general circulation from entering into the cerebrospinal fluid.
- In the liver, enzymes metabolize the drug and convert it to other compounds, which then move into the systemic circulation.
- Biotransformation occurs when the liver converts lipophilic, nonpolar molecules to more polar, water-soluble molecules.
- Water-soluble metabolites usually are excreted by the kidneys in urine, lipid-soluble metabolites are excreted in bile and feces, and volatile metabolites are excreted by the lungs.
- The route of drug administration can affect the amount of the drug that reaches target cells.
- The metabolic process affects how much active drug enters the blood.
- The goal of drug administration is to reach and maintain a concentration that is within the therapeutic range, which is the span of concentrations within which the drug effectively treats a disease with minimal toxicity for most patients.
- The peak level is the highest concentration of a drug in the patient's bloodstream. Peak level samples are usually

drawn 2 hours after oral administration, 30 minutes at the end of intravenous administration, and 60 minutes after intramuscular administration.

- The trough level is the lowest concentration in the patient's bloodstream. The specimen should be collected just before the next dose of a drug is administered (30 minutes for intravenous or oral administration).
- Many drugs are used to modify heart activity, including digoxin, lidocaine, quinidine, procainamide, disopyramide, flecainide, propranolol, amiodarone, mexiletine, and verapamil.
- Antibiotics with serious side effects, such as amikacin, gentamicin, kanamycin, tobramycin, vancomycin, and chloramphenicol, require monitoring.
- Antiepileptic or anticonvulsant drugs, which are used in the treatment of seizure disorders (e.g., grand mal, petit mal, psychomotor) and trigeminal neuralgia (i.e., tic douloureux), include phenobarbital, phenytoin, carbamazepine, clonazepam, ethosuximide, gabapentin, lamotrigine, levetiracetam, oxcarbazepine, primidone, topiramate, valproic acid, and zonisamide.
- Psychiatrists use many drugs whose levels must be monitored to ensure that they remain within the therapeutic ranges. These drugs include lithium, amitriptyline, nortriptyline, desipramine, imipramine, and diazepam.
- Most bronchodilators target the lungs, causing bronchodilation without also increasing the heart rate or elevating blood pressure. They include theophylline and aminophylline.
- Common drugs used to prevent organ transplant rejection include cyclosporine, mycophenolic acid, sirolimus, tacrolimus, and cyclophosphamide.

Introduction

Therapeutic drug monitoring (TDM) is used to measure medication levels in the blood and maintain the right amount of drug in a patient's system. Too little drug in the blood may not effectively treat the disease or symptoms, and too much may cause toxic side effects. TDM and commonly monitored drugs are discussed in this chapter.

Individuals respond differently to the same dose of the same drug. Providers use clinical data and the patient's history to individualize drug doses. TDM is a multidisciplinary science that uses laboratory test results and clinical information to select the best drug at an appropriate dosage for an individual. TDM is also used to assess treatment results, toxic effects, and drug interactions. TDM has been transformed by the assessment of biomarkers and genetic mutations that can affect drug responses.

Drug Disposition

A drug's mechanism of action is the manner in which it produces a pharmacologic effect in the target area. The mechanisms of action for many drugs are not clear, but theoretical models have been developed to help explain them.

The pharmacologic effect initially increases with rising drug levels, but it stabilizes as target sites become saturated with the drug. TDM is based on the assumption that the size of the pharmacologic effect is directly proportional to the amount of drug at the target area. For example, the pharmacologic effect of digoxin is directly proportional to the amount of drug that reaches the heart. The concentration in the blood may not equal the concentration of the drug at the target area, but the concentration in the blood reflects the pharmacologic effect.

The therapeutic range of a drug reflects the minimum effective concentration and the minimum toxic concentration. The lower level in the therapeutic range is the lowest amount of drug in the blood that produces a pharmacologic effect. The larger number reflects the highest level that produces a pharmacologic effect and the lowest level at which toxic symptoms begin to occur.

Pharmacodynamics is the study of the biochemical and physiologic effects of drugs and their mechanisms of action (Fig. 33-1). Pharmacokinetics assesses the rate of absorption, distribution, biotransformation, and excretion of drugs. Mathematical models exist that describe drug disposition.

Absorption

Drugs that are administered orally are absorbed through the gastrointestinal tract. The drug first dissociates from its dosing form and then dissolves in gastrointestinal juices before entering the blood. After absorption from the gastrointestinal tract, it is carried through the hepatic portal vein into

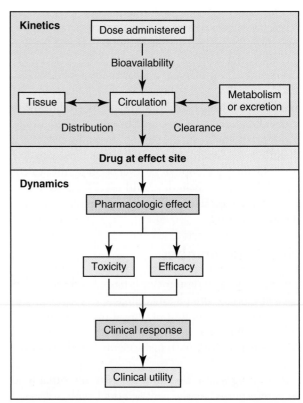

• **Figure 33-1** Pharmacokinetics and pharmacodynamics.

the liver. The drug is extensively metabolized in the liver (i.e., first-pass effect) before entering the systemic circulation.

The absorption rate is influenced by the drug formulation. Drug absorbance is also affected by abnormal gastrointestinal motility, diseases of the stomach and small and large intestines, gastrointestinal infections, irradiation, food, and interactions with other substances in the gastrointestinal tract. These variables should be taken into consideration when performing TDM and management.

Bioavailability

Bioavailability is the fraction of the dose administered that reaches the systemic circulation. For intravenous and inhalation drugs, absorption is much less of a factor, and bioavailability is 100%. Because not all ingested substances are absorbed, the bioavailability of most orally administered drugs is less than 100%. For some drugs, the rate at which the chemical is liberated from its formulation may play a significant role in availability (e.g., slow-release forms) (Fig. 33-2).

Distribution

Drug distribution is the process of moving the substance from the site of absorption to other areas throughout the body. Larger individuals may need higher drug doses to reach the same concentration in the blood than smaller individuals, and other factors may affect distribution.

After a drug enters the systemic circulation, it interacts with other substances in the blood (mostly proteins) as it is distributed throughout the body. Factors that affect the distribution pattern include binding to blood components, binding to cell surface receptors, passing through cellular membranes, and dissolving in structural or storage lipids (Fig. 33-3). In the circulation, drugs may be unbound or bound to plasma proteins. Typically, an equilibrium is maintained between unbound drug (i.e., free drug) and bound drug. The free drug is available for distribution, transport across cellular membranes, interaction with drug receptors,

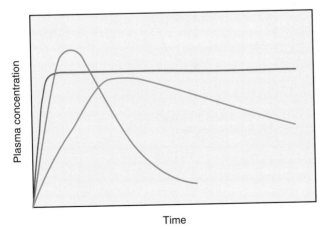

■ Zero-order release ■ Sustained release ■ Immediate release

• **Figure 33-2** The dose–effect relationship for zero-order, immediate-release, and sustained-release drugs.

and elimination (Fig. 33-4). Acidic drugs bind to albumin, and basic drugs bind to globulins (primarily α_1-acid glycoprotein) (Fig. 33-5).

Diseases and changes in physiologic status affect the free drug concentration. Despite a steady total drug concentration measured in blood, the drug may be released from plasma proteins, resulting in an elevated free drug level. This can lead to toxicity. In elderly individuals, an early sign of drug intoxication is confusion.

Distribution of drugs in the brain and spinal cord (i.e., central nervous system [CNS]) requires special consideration. The blood–brain barrier limits many chemicals in the general circulation from entering the cerebrospinal fluid (CSF). For instance, common antibiotics cannot be used to treat meningitis because the drugs cannot diffuse into the CSF to kill the infecting bacteria. Transporter proteins also affect distribution of drugs across the placenta.

Metabolism and Biotransformation

When drugs arrive at the liver and before they move into the systemic circulation, liver enzymes convert a drug to other compounds or metabolize the drug. Most drugs are metabolized through first-order kinetics (i.e., metabolism is proportional to drug concentration). Some drugs, such as phenytoin, salicylate, ethanol, and theophylline, have a nonlinear rate of metabolism. In nonlinear metabolism, metabolism of the drug changes with concentration. The liver converts potentially harmful chemicals into inactive metabolites through a process called biotransformation. Lipophilic, nonpolar molecules are converted to more polar, water-soluble molecules (Table 33-1).

Drug metabolism involves a large number of enzymes in liver cells. The most important are those in the cytochrome P-450 (CYP) enzyme family (Table 33-2). Most drugs are cleared by these CYP proteins, which share key features that can affect drug metabolism and contribute to food–drug and drug–drug interactions (Table 33-3). A single CYP enzyme can metabolize many different chemicals. If two or more drugs are present, they can compete for the enzyme's active site. This slows the rate of metabolism of each drug, an effect called inhibition. For instance, a dose of morphine may not reach toxic levels in the blood because the liver is metabolizing the drug at a constant rate. However, if the patient has both alcohol and morphine in his system, the drugs can compete for the CYP enzyme's active site. If the enzymes are metabolizing more alcohol than morphine, blood levels of morphine can become elevated. Even a so-called safe dose of morphine can lead to toxic blood levels when the drug must compete with other drugs such as alcohol.

One drug can also boost the metabolism of a second drug. Some drugs, for example, increase the amount of CYP enzyme by increasing its synthesis rate (i.e., induction) or reducing its degradation rate. For instance, phenobarbital can induce the liver's metabolism of some antibiotics. When liver enzymes break down phenobarbital, induction leads to increased amounts of enzymes. Subsequently, when the patient takes an antibiotic, more enzymes are available to break down the second drug, which reduces the blood levels of the antibiotic to

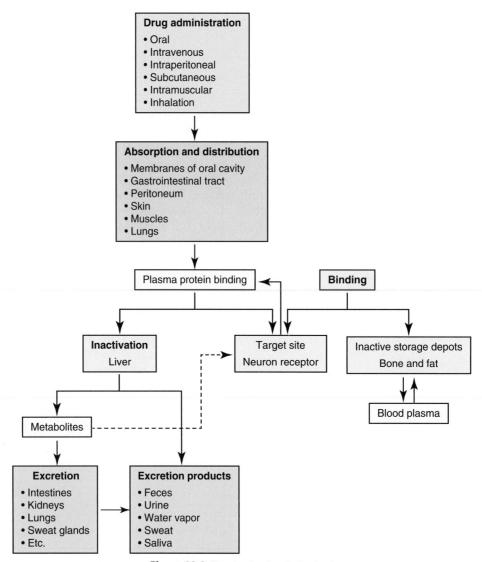

• **Figure 33-3** Travels of a drug in the body.

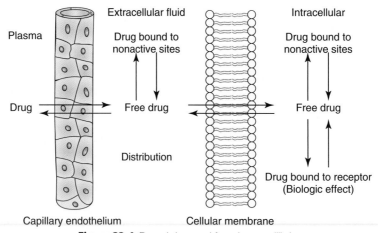

• **Figure 33-4** Bound drug and free drug equilibrium.

subtherapeutic levels. Induction is not permanent, nor does it occur instantaneously. Phenobarbital and theophylline are two drugs that induce more enzymes when they are metabolized.

For some drugs, the inactive form that is administered must first pass through the liver, where it is acted on by liver enzymes and converted into an active form. These drugs require a well-functioning liver for bioactivation. When primidone or procainamide is metabolized by the liver, for example, active metabolites are produced that enhance the action of the drug.

TABLE 33-1 Mechanisms of Biotransformation

Type of Biotransformation	Mechanism	Result
Oxidation, reduction, hydrolysis	Chemical reactions	Increases polarity of chemical, making it more water soluble and more easily excreted; often results in a loss of pharmacologic activity
Conjugation (e.g., glucuronidation, glycination, sulfation, methylation, alkylation)	Combination with another substance (e.g., glucuronide, glycine, sulfate, methyl groups, alkyl groups)	Forms a less toxic product with less activity

From Lilley LL, Rainforth Collins VS, Snyder JS: *Pharmacology and the Nursing Process*. 7th ed. St. Louis: Mosby.

TABLE 33-2 Common Liver Cytochrome P-450 Enzymes and Corresponding Drug Substrates

Enzyme	Common Drug Substrates
CYP1A2	Acetaminophen, caffeine, theophylline, warfarin
CYP2C9	Ibuprofen, phenytoin
CYP2C19	Diazepam, naproxen, omeprazole, propranolol
CYP2D6	Codeine, fluoxetine, hydrocodone, metoprolol, oxycodone, paroxetine, risperidone, tricyclic antidepressants
CYP2E1	Acetaminophen, ethanol
CYP3A4	Acetaminophen, amiodarone, cyclosporine, diltiazem, ethinyl estradiol, indinavir, lidocaine, macrolides, progesterone, spironolactone, sulfamethoxazole, testosterone, verapamil

From Lilley LL, Rainforth Collins VS, Snyder JS. *Pharmacology and the Nursing Process*. 7th ed. St. Louis: Mosby; 2014.

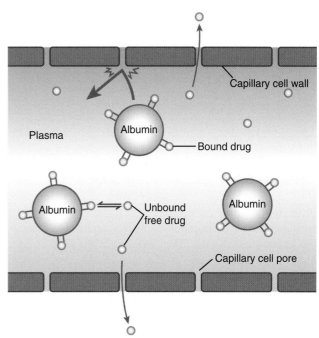

• **Figure 33-5** Protein binding of drugs. Albumin is the most prevalent protein in plasma and the most important of the proteins to which drugs bind. Only unbound (free) drug molecules can leave the vascular system. Bound molecules are too large to fit through the pores in the capillary wall. (From Lilley LL, Rainforth Collins VS, Snyder JS. *Pharmacology and the Nursing Process*. 7th ed. St. Louis: Mosby; 2014.)

TABLE 33-3 Factors That Affect Drug Metabolism

Factor	Examples	Increased Metabolism	Decreased Metabolism
Diseases	Cardiovascular dysfunction		×
	Renal insufficiency		×
Conditions	Starvation		×
	Obstructive jaundice		×
	Genetic constitution	×	×
	Fast acetylator	×	
	Slow acetylator		×
Drugs	Barbiturates	×	
	Rifampin (P-450 inducer)	×	
	Phenytoin (P-450 inducer)	×	
	Ketoconazole (P-450 inhibitor)		×

From Lilley LL, Rainforth Collins VS, Snyder JS. *Pharmacology and the Nursing Process*. 7th ed. St. Louis: Mosby; 2014.

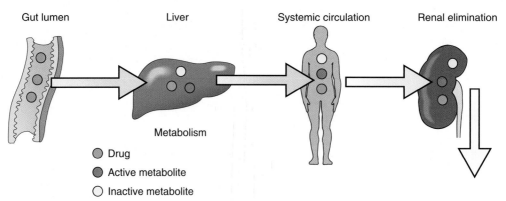

• **Figure 33-6** Passage of drugs through the body, including unchanged drugs, active metabolites, and inactive metabolites. (From McKenry L, Tessier E, Hogan MA. *Mosby's Pharmacology in Nursing.* 22nd ed. St. Louis: Mosby; 2006.)

Excretion

Some drugs are totally cleared by the liver. Their clearance is affected by free drug concentration, hepatic function, enzyme inducers, and enzyme inhibitors. After a drug is metabolized by the liver, metabolites are often excreted from the body. Water-soluble metabolites usually are excreted by the kidneys in urine (Figs. 33-6 and 33-7), lipid-soluble metabolites are excreted in the bile and feces, and volatile metabolites are excreted by the lungs. Like liver metabolism, increased excretion through the kidneys lowers the amount of drug in the bloodstream. Conditions such as kidney failure must be taken into account when administering drugs to a patient. Decreased renal function leads to increased drug levels in the blood.

Excretion through tears, sweat, saliva, or other routes typically is unimportant pharmacologically, but the trace amounts of drugs detected in these excretions or even in hair can be clinically relevant. Similarly, the excretion of chemicals into breast milk can have significant consequences for the newborn, even if it does not significantly affect the plasma drug concentrations of the mother.

Administration of Drugs

Most medications bind to the surface of cells or enter cells to assert their effect. The route of drug administration can affect the amount of the drug that reaches the target cells. For instance, morphine can be administered orally or intravenously. The route affects the amount of time it takes for the drug to reach the target cells. Dose adjustments often must be made to maintain the correct effective blood concentration or therapeutic range. For example, the drug dose needed to attain the therapeutic level may be 10 times higher for the oral route than for the intravenous route. Administering the oral dose intravenously could easily exceed the effective dose and instead deliver a lethal dose.

Oral Route

Oral administration can be achieved by ingestion of tablets, capsules, or drops. Drugs in these forms must be able to survive the acidic contents of the stomach and digestive

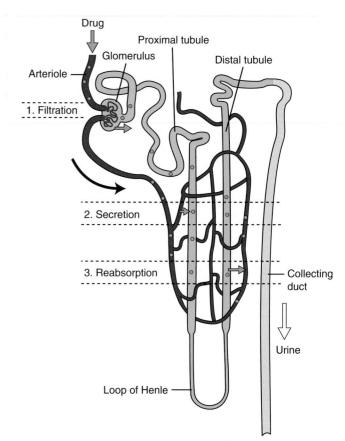

• **Figure 33-7** Drug excretion process. (From McKenry L, Tessier E, Hogan MA. *Mosby's Pharmacology in Nursing.* 22nd ed. St. Louis: Mosby; 2006.)

enzymes of the intestines before being absorbed across the lining of the intestines. Many drugs (e.g., insulin) cannot be given orally because the stomach acid destroys them. Other drugs may irritate the gastrointestinal tract (e.g., chemotherapeutic drugs) and cause diarrhea or vomiting, excluding this route of administration.

Some drugs cannot be absorbed across the epithelial lining of the intestines. After a drug is absorbed from the gastrointestinal system into the bloodstream, it travels to the liver, where it

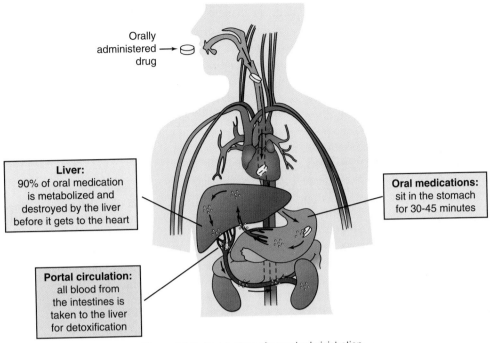

Orally administered → drug

Liver:
90% of oral medication is metabolized and destroyed by the liver before it gets to the heart

Oral medications:
sit in the stomach for 30-45 minutes

Portal circulation:
all blood from the intestines is taken to the liver for detoxification

• **Figure 33-8** Metabolism after oral administration.

is metabolized. The metabolic process affects how much active drug becomes available to the body (Fig. 33-8).

Intravenous Route

Intravenous injections or drips directly deliver a drug into the bloodstream, bypassing the challenges of the gastrointestinal tract. Because intravenous administration directly delivers the drug into the bloodstream, the dosage is lower, and the therapeutic effects occur rapidly, sometimes in less than a minute (Fig. 33-9). Drugs may be given as single (bolus) doses or administered continuously with a saline drip.

Intramuscular Route

Intramuscular injection administers a drug directly into a muscle, such as the deltoid (shoulder), vastus lateralis (thigh), or gluteal (buttock) muscle. Like intravenous administration, this route bypasses the gastrointestinal tract, and drugs are not degraded by stomach acid or digestive enzymes. A drug injected into muscle and connective tissue enters the blood more gradually than by the intravenous route. There is a delay between when the drug is injected and when it takes effect.

Subcutaneous injection delivers the drug below the skin. The time required for the drug to enter the bloodstream is similar to that for intramuscular delivery. A comparison of blood concentrations of a drug delivered by different delivery systems is found in Figure 33-10. The effective concentration is the concentration at which the drug exerts its effects.

Other Routes

Other routes of administration (e.g., suppository, inhalation, intraperitoneal, topical) may be used, depending

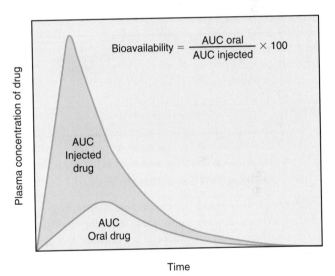

$$\text{Bioavailability} = \frac{\text{AUC oral}}{\text{AUC injected}} \times 100$$

Plasma concentration of drug

AUC Injected drug

AUC Oral drug

Time

• **Figure 33-9** Bioavailability of drugs: oral versus intravenous administration. *AUC*, Area under the curve.

on the target tissue in which the drug takes effect. By limiting the exposure of a drug to the area of the body that needs it, side effects are reduced. For instance, topical application delivers a drug to the surface of the body, but administering the same drug by a different route (e.g., intramuscular injection) can elicit a different effect. Topically administered lidocaine can reduce the pain of sunburn, but when injected into gums during a dental operation, it causes loss of sensation around the teeth. Inhaled drugs (i.e., inhalants) effectively deliver medication to the lungs (e.g., asthma medication) or the brain (e.g., anesthetics). Inhalants are absorbed quickly and exert their effects quickly.

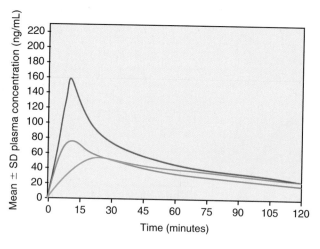

Figure 33-10 Blood concentration of a drug according to the method of administration. *SD*, Standard deviation.

5 mg intravenous   5 mg intramuscular   5 mg intranasal

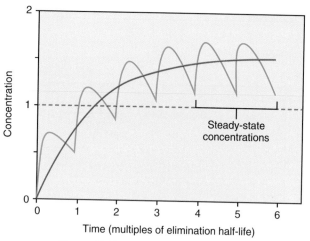

Figure 33-11 Steady-state concentrations.

Drugs can be injected into the peritoneal cavity (e.g., when treating cervical cancer) rather than into the bloodstream. Intraperitoneal injection can help concentrate the drug in target organs while limiting exposure to the rest of the body.

Drug Levels

Drug doses usually are measured in milligrams or milliliters. The drug concentration in blood or other target tissue determines its effectiveness. A large loading dose of a drug may be administered initially to achieve the desired blood concentration quickly. After the therapeutic concentration is reached, the remaining drug doses are lower (i.e., maintenance dose) to maintain the desired therapeutic level. When the amount of drug entering the body is equal to the amount of drug being eliminated, a steady state is reached (Fig. 33-11). In pharmacologic terms, the maintenance dose (minus the amount that is not absorbed or distributed properly) is equal to the amount of drug that is cleared by liver metabolism, kidney excretion, or biotransformation in tissues. The rate at which a drug is cleared from the body is measured by its half-life, which is the time it takes for the drug's concentration to decrease by one half.

> **• BOX 33-1 Information Required to Interpret Drug Concentration**
>
> Time the blood sample was taken
> Time the dose was given
> Dose regimen (e.g., dose, duration, form)
> Patient demographics
> Comedications
> Indication for monitoring
> Pharmacokinetics and therapeutic range

The goal is to reach and maintain a drug concentration that is within the therapeutic range—the range of concentrations at which a drug effectively treats a disease with minimal toxicity for most patients. Anything lower is a subtherapeutic dose, which is undesirable for treating disease. Subtherapeutic doses may have additional drawbacks, such as promoting the spread of antibiotic-resistant bacteria. However, subtherapeutic doses of a drug can be used off-label—that is, to treat alternative conditions for which it is not approved by the U.S. Food and Drug Administration (FDA)—especially for prophylactic or preventative therapy.

Activity of the Parent Drug and Metabolites

The parent drug is the chemical found in a formulation. In some cases, it is the compound that is active in the patient, and its levels are monitored.

In some cases, the levels of the parent drug are of less concern than its metabolites. Some drugs must first be metabolized by liver enzymes (or enzymes in other tissues) before having any effects in the individual. These effects may be desirable, but in some instances, metabolites can cause adverse drug reactions. In either case, providers monitor levels of the metabolites in the blood in addition to or instead of levels of the parent drug.

Therapeutic Drug Monitoring

The aim of TDM is to inform the provider about drug levels in a patient. TDM ensures that a patient's drug levels remain within the therapeutic range and do not reach toxic levels. For some drugs, the difference between a functional dose and a lethal dose is very small; these are said to have a low therapeutic index, and their levels must be monitored closely.

Sample Collection

Drugs are usually monitored in venous blood, serum, or plasma. Plasma and serum concentrations are comparable, but the tube used to collect blood samples can affect drug concentrations. Lipophilic drugs bind to the walls of certain collection tubes, altering measured drug levels. It is important to follow standard operating procedures and use the specified tube for collecting a specimen. The information required to interpret a drug level test result is given in Box 33-1.

TABLE 33-4 Effects of Age and Pregnancy on Pharmacodynamics

Physiologic Changes	Effects on Pharmacodynamics
Age	
Body fat increases 20-40%.	Increased half-life for lipid-soluble drugs
Body water decreases 10-15% as with aging.	Increased concentration of water-soluble drugs
Arterial hepatic blood flow declines with age, but venous blood flow does not change. Arteries become stiffer, systolic blood pressure increases, and liver function declines.	Decreased blood flow affects drugs that are metabolized by oxidation. May cause 30-40% reduction in elimination of drugs metabolized in liver. Bioavailability of drugs with high first-pass elimination increases with decreased activity of drug-metabolizing enzymes.
Renal blood flow and glomerular filtration decrease.	Increased half-life of drugs eliminated by kidneys Increased levels of drugs and active metabolites, causing increased potential for toxicity
Movement through the gastrointestinal track slows down.	Slows absorption of continuous-release drugs into the blood, leading to a lengthened effect
Pregnancy	
Nausea affects absorption.	Decreased absorption of drugs
Plasma volume increases by 30%.	Lower drug concentrations in the blood
Renal flow increases.	Increased removal of water-soluble drugs from the system
Levels of hepatic enzymes increase.	Increased metabolism of drugs
Placental transfer occurs.	Avoid teratogenic drugs. Water-soluble drugs usually do not cross the placenta. Lipid-soluble drugs cross the placenta easily.

Timing

When toxicity is a concern, specimens are collected and tested for peak and trough levels. The trough level is the lowest concentration in the patient's bloodstream, and the specimen should be collected just before the next dose of the drug is administered (i.e., 30 minutes for intravenous or oral administration). The peak level is the highest concentration of a drug in the patient's bloodstream. Peak level samples are usually drawn 2 hours after oral administration, 30 minutes after the end of intravenous administration, and 60 minutes after intramuscular administration.

For drugs that have a wider therapeutic index, samples for monitoring the therapeutic dose may be taken when the level has reached the steady state (i.e., 4 to 5 half-lives after starting therapy). For drugs with a long half-life, a randomly collected sample often suffices.

Effects of Age and Pregnancy on Drug Distribution

Age

Physiologic changes in the elderly must be taken into consideration when considering drug dosage (Table 33-4). Lower drug doses may produce the desired serum drug concentrations due to reduced function of the liver and kidneys and the lower amount of fluid in the body.

Absorption

Overall function of the gastrointestinal tract decreases during aging. Reduction in the absorptive capabilities of the gastrointestinal tract may reduce the amount of drug absorbed, lowering the amount of drug in the blood. This is much less likely to be a concern in healthy elderly patients than in those with gastrointestinal disorders.

Distribution

Aging produces changes throughout the body, including a reduction in body fluids. This change tends to increase plasma concentrations of water-soluble drugs for a given dose.

Clearance

Renal mass decreases with age, which reduces the speed at which the kidneys clear drugs from the blood. Similarly, aging is associated with reduced liver size and hepatic blood flow, lowering the rate at which the liver metabolizes drugs. Reduced renal and hepatic clearance tends to increase blood levels for most drugs at a given concentration and increase their half-life.

Pregnancy

Most effects of pregnancy on drug distribution are the opposite of those encountered in elderly individuals (see Table 33-4). For example, higher drug doses may need to be used to obtain therapeutic results. The effects of a drug on the fetus (if the drug can cross the placental blood–blood barrier) are always a concern. A drug's effects on the pregnancy itself must also be considered.

Absorption

Nausea may interfere with the absorption of oral medications during pregnancy.

Distribution

To meet the increased nutritional demands of a growing fetus, a pregnant woman experiences an increase in plasma volume (about 30%). This lowers the blood concentration of a drug at a given dose.

Waste produced by the fetus must be removed by the mother's kidneys. Renal flow during pregnancy increases by about 100%. This causes faster removal of water-soluble drugs from the bloodstream than in a nonpregnant woman. Similarly, the increased number of hepatic enzymes during pregnancy helps to protect the developing fetus and increase the metabolism of many drugs.

Placental Transfer

The teratogenic effects of drugs (i.e., their ability to cause birth defects) must be considered when dealing with pregnant patients. Normally, there is no direct mixing of fetal and maternal blood. To cross from the maternal blood supply to that of the fetus, drugs must cross the membranes of the placenta. As with the blood–brain barrier, large water-soluble drugs may be prevented from entering the fetal blood supply, but lipid-soluble drugs may cross more easily. Taking fetal blood samples is possible, but because of the risks and complicated nature of the procedure, it usually is done only if severe blood disorders are suspected (e.g., erythroblastosis fetalis).

Cardiovascular Drugs

There are many causes of arrhythmias. Any drug that increases the duration of action potentials or increases the absolute or relative refractory period of cardiac muscle cells can prevent heart muscle cells from contracting rapidly. Many antiarrhythmics and other cardiovascular drugs target the sodium-potassium pump (Na^+/K^+-ATPase) and the sodium or calcium ion channels in cardiac cells to keep them open longer.

Digoxin
Mechanism of Action

Digoxin (proprietary name: Lanoxin) is a glycoside that is extracted from the foxglove plant *Digitalis lanata* (Table 33-5). Digoxin binds to and inhibits the function of Na^+/K^+-ATPase in cardiac muscle cells. This increases the duration of each cardiac action potential, which increases the time between heartbeats and lowers the heart rate. Digoxin also increases vagal nerve activity, slowing activity of the atrioventricular (AV) node, which also reduces the heart rate. Digoxin and other cardiac glycosides are used to treat atrial flutter and atrial fibrillation.

TABLE 33-5	Digoxin
Characteristics	**Specifications**
Purpose	Treatment of congestive heart failure and atrial fibrillation or atrial flutter
Usual bioavailability	Approximately 60-85% for tablet or elixir, 90-100% for liquid-filled capsules
Half-life	Approximately 35-40 hr but prolonged in patients with decreased renal function
General therapeutic range	0.5-2.0 mg/dL
General toxic level	>2 mg/dL, but somewhat variable
Transport	Approximately 20-25% plasma protein bound
Metabolism	Generally, only small amounts are metabolized (liver, lumen of large intestine)
Elimination	Approximately 50-75% unchanged in urine
Steady state	Approximately 7 days in undigitalized patients with normal renal function
Mechanism of action	Causes release of calcium ions in the T-tubule system of myocardium, shows atrioventricular node conduction
Toxic effects	Gastric disturbances, nausea, vomiting, atrial and ventricular arrhythmias, irregular pulse

From McPherson RA, Pincus MR. *Henry's Clinical Diagnosis and Management by Laboratory Methods.* 22nd ed. Philadelphia: Elsevier: 2012.

Dosing and Drug Actions

Digoxin can manage the symptoms of cardiac insufficiency, arrhythmias, and heart failure. It may be taken orally. Digoxin starts working within 1 to 2 hours after oral administration. Approximately 50% to 75% of a dose is excreted unchanged in the urine.

Toxic Effects

Digoxin has a narrow therapeutic range (0.5 to 2.0 µg/L). The toxic concentration for this drug is greater than 2.0 µg/L. Symptoms of toxicity include gastrointestinal disturbances, nausea, vomiting, ventricular tachycardia, ventricular fibrillation, atrial and ventricular arrhythmias, irregular pulse, and heart block.

Lidocaine
Mechanism of Action

Lidocaine (proprietary name: Xylocaine) is used as a local anesthetic and antiarrhythmic (Table 33-6). It is a fast-acting anesthetic that can be administered topically or intravenously. Topical application of lidocaine is common in many over-the-counter burn creams. Lidocaine can also

TABLE 33-6	Lidocaine
Characteristics	**Specifications**
Purpose	Acute control and prevention of ventricular arrhythmias after acute myocardial infarction and local anesthetic
Usual bioavailability	Not highly protein bound nor stored in body tissues
Half-life	Approximately 2 hr
General therapeutic range	1.5-5 mg/dL
General toxic level	>6 mg/dL
Transport	None
Metabolism	90% metabolized in liver
Elimination	10% excreted in urine
Steady state	5-8 hr
Mechanism of action	Blocks sodium channels mainly in ventricular but not atrial tissue
Toxic effects	Convulsions, coma, respiratory depression, bradycardia, and hypotension

TABLE 33-7	Quinidine
Characteristics	**Specifications**
Purpose	Prevents ventricular tachycardia or frequent premature ventricular contractions and cardioversion or chronic therapy for atrial flutter or atrial fibrillation
Usual bioavailability	90-100%, with 85% of drug bound to plasma protein
Half-life	5-12 hr
General therapeutic range	2-5 mg/dL
General toxic level	>8 mg/dL
Transport	Protein bound
Metabolism	60-85% metabolized in the liver with some active metabolites
Elimination	20% excreted in urine
Steady state	1-3 hr
Mechanism of action	Blocks sodium channels and outward potassium currents, resulting in prolong action potentials
Toxic effects	Vertigo, tinnitus, headache, visual disturbances, disorientation, fever, hepatitis, blood dyscrasias, ventricular arrhythmias, atrioventricular block, ventricular fibrillation, death

be injected (commonly in conjunction with epinephrine to reduce blood loss) as a local anesthetic. Lidocaine is used after acute myocardial infarction to control and prevent ventricular arrhythmias.

Lidocaine binds to and blocks voltage-gated sodium channels, which can block or reduce the transmission of action potentials. For instance, blocking the activity of peripheral nociceptors can block pain signals from reaching the CNS. Lidocaine is thought to treat arrhythmias by altering the conduction of action potentials in the heart.

Dosing and Drug Actions

Administration of lidocaine hydrochloride depends on the desired effect. For treating acute myocardial infarctions, a loading dose is usually administered intravenously over 2 to 3 minutes. Additional doses may be administered in 5- to 10-minute intervals. Additional doses may then be administered until the desired clinical effect is achieved. When the intravenous route is not possible, endotracheal administration can be given at roughly double the intravenous dose.

For use as an anesthetic, the dosage depends on the degree of anesthesia desired. The therapeutic range for lidocaine is 1.5 to 5 mg/dL.

Toxic Effects

Correct use of lidocaine normally causes few adverse drug effects. Up to 90% of a lidocaine dose is metabolized in

the liver, and the remaining 10% is excreted in the urine. Accidental overdoses can depress CNS function, leading to headache, dizziness, drowsiness, confusion, convulsions, coma, respiratory depression, bradycardia, arrhythmia, cardiac arrest, and hypotension.

Quinidine

Mechanism of Action

Quinidine is used to treat supraventricular and ventricular arrhythmias and tachyarrhythmias (Table 33-7). It is used to prevent ventricular tachycardia or frequent premature ventricular contractions and for cardioversion or chronic therapy for atrial flutter or atrial fibrillation. Quinidine blocks several molecular targets to inhibit the influx of sodium ions into cardiac cells. This prolongs the duration of action potentials in cardiac muscle cells, and slowing the rate of action potentials reduces arrhythmias. Off-label uses for this drug include treatment of malaria and paroxysmal supraventricular tachycardia.

Dosing and Drug Actions

Quinidine comes in two forms, quinidine sulfate and quinidine gluconate, which are dosed differently. With quinidine sulfate, a test dose is administered orally several hours before

TABLE 33-8 Procainamide

Characteristics	Specifications
Purpose	Treatment of supraventricular or ventricular arrhythmias
Usual bioavailability	75-95%
Half-life	Approximately 3.5 hr in patients with normal renal function
General therapeutic range	4-8 mg/dL
General toxic level	>12 mg/dL
Transport	Approximately 15% plasma bound
Metabolism	Hepatic: *N*-acetylprocainamide (active metabolite) has a half-life of approximately 7 hr in patients with normal renal function
Elimination	50-60% unchanged in urine
Steady state	Minimum of 12 hr
Mechanism of action	By blocking the influx of sodium ions into cardiac muscle cells, the drug prolongs the duration of cardiac action potentials, increasing the maximum frequency the heart can beat.
Toxic effects	Reversible lupus erythematosus-like syndrome, irregular, hypotension, rash, agranulocytosis

From McPherson RA, Pincus MR. *Henry's Clinical Diagnosis and Management by Laboratory Methods*. 22nd ed. Philadelphia: Elsevier: 2012.

the full dose. If there is no reaction, a dose is administered orally every 6 hours for atrial fibrillation. For premature atrial or ventricular contractions, a dose is administered orally three to four times daily. Quinidine can also be used to treat malaria. Quinidine sulfate can be administered orally every 8 to 12 hours for 5 to 7 days. Quinidine gluconate is also used to treat malaria and uses the same dosing schedule as quinidine sulfate.

Quinidine reduces the chance that an arrhythmia will be triggered, but it can lead to an elevated heart rate by blocking activity of the vagus nerve and can lower blood pressure by inhibiting the force of contraction of the heart. Between 65% and 85% of administered quinidine is metabolized in the liver, and 20% is excreted in urine.

Toxic Effects

Symptoms of toxicity include vertigo, tinnitus, headache, visual disturbances, disorientation, fever, hepatitis, and blood dyscrasias. Syncope and sudden death may occur when ventricular arrhythmias, AV block, or ventricular fibrillation occurs as a side effect. Quinidine inhibits a type

of CYP in the liver, and it can elevate levels of other drugs normally metabolized by the liver, such as lidocaine, antidepressants, β-blockers, and opioids.

Procainamide
Mechanism of Action

Procainamide (proprietary name: Pronestyl) is a sodium channel blocker used to treat supraventricular or ventricular arrhythmias (Table 33-8). By blocking the influx of sodium ions into cardiac muscle cells, the drug prolongs the duration of cardiac action potentials, increasing the maximum frequency the heart can beat.

Dosing and Drug Actions

Procainamide can be administered intravenously (i.e., loading and maintenance doses), intramuscularly, or orally. Dosage is usually increased until the dysrhythmia is suppressed. An increase in the QT interval on an electrocardiogram may be observed. The therapeutic range is 4 to 8 mg/dL. Fifty percent of procainamide is excreted by the kidneys.

Toxic Effects

The toxic level of procainamide is greater than 12 mg/dL. Overdoses can depress the activity of the heart to dangerous levels, resulting in hypotension and bradycardia. This effect is more common in patients with renal insufficiency.

Disopyramide
Mechanism of Action

Disopyramide (proprietary name: Norpace) is similar to quinidine in that it blocks the inward sodium current, reducing the excitability of heart muscle cells and increasing the duration of action potentials (Table 33-9). Disopyramide is used in place of quinidine when the side effects of quinidine become intolerable.

Disopyramide is almost completely absorbed from the gastrointestinal tract. A small amount is metabolized by the liver, but 45% to 70% of the drug enters the blood and binds to plasma proteins. Most disopyramide is excreted through the kidneys.

Dosing and Drug Actions

Disopyramide is usually administered orally, and it comes in immediate- and slow-release forms. Immediate-release forms are taken orally every 6 hours. Slow-release forms are taken orally every 12 hours. At the therapeutic dose, cessation of the dysrhythmia should be observed.

Toxic Effects

Because sodium ion channels are not specific to the heart, disopyramide at higher doses may also inhibit neurons, especially cholinergic neurons, and produce anticholinergic effects. Like quinidine, the most serious adverse reactions are hypotension and congestive heart failure. The most common adverse reactions of disopyramide are associated with anticholinergic properties of the drug.

TABLE 33-9 Disopyramide

Characteristics	Specifications
Purpose	Treatment of atrial flutter and atrial fibrillation and prevention of ventricular arrhythmias
Usual bioavailability	60-83%, with 50%-65% protein bound
Half-life	4-10 hr
General therapeutic range	2-5 mg/dL
General toxic level	>5 mg/dL
Transport	Protein bound
Metabolism	45% in liver and 16% in intestinal wall
Elimination	40-80% in urine, 15% in feces
Steady state	1-2.5 hr
Mechanism of action	Directly depresses the nerve membrane to decrease conduction velocity, slowing heart rate; also reduces repolarization abnormalities
Toxic effects	Dry mouth, urinary hesitancy, constipation, atrioventricular node blockage, bradycardia, and heart failure

TABLE 33-10 Flecainide

Characteristics	Specifications
Purpose	Treatment of paroxysmal atrial fibrillation, paroxysmal supraventricular tachycardia (PSVT), and sustained ventricular tachycardia
Usual bioavailability	85-90%
Half-life	12-27 hr
General therapeutic range	0.2-1 mg/dL
General toxic level	>1 mg/dL
Transport	40-50% protein bound
Metabolism	Undergoes extensive biotransformation to two major and several minor metabolites
Elimination	80-90% excreted in the urine
Steady state	2-3 hr
Mechanism of action	Sodium channel blocker, slows conduction in cardiac tissue by altering transport of ions across membranes
Toxic effects	Excessive depression of the heart, including hypotension and bradycardia

Flecainide

Mechanism of Action

Flecainide (proprietary name: Tambocor) blocks sodium channels in cardiac cells, prolonging the duration of action potentials and slowing their transmission within the heart (Table 33-10). Flecainide is used to treat paroxysmal supraventricular tachycardia, paroxysmal atrial fibrillation, and sustained ventricular tachycardia. The drug is not widely used due to toxicity in individuals with myocardial infarctions. It can be used as a drug of last resort for patients who fail to respond to other sodium channel blockers.

Dosing and Drug Actions

Individuals with paroxysmal supraventricular tachycardia and paroxysmal atrial fibrillation take flecainide orally twice a day. A higher dose is needed to treat sustained ventricular tachycardia, but it is still taken orally twice a day. At the therapeutic range, control of the arrhythmia should be achieved. Gender may be taken into account for dosing because men may clear the drug faster than women.

Toxic Effects

Because flecainide has a narrow therapeutic range, toxicity can be significant for myocardial infarction patients. Toxicity may involve excessive depression of the heart, including hypotension and bradycardia.

Propranolol

Mechanism of Action

Propranolol (proprietary name: Inderal) is a β-blocker (Table 33-11). β-Blockers bind and inhibit β-adrenergic receptors, which are found primarily on heart muscle cells. Propranolol reduces sympathetic activation of the heart, opposing the effects of adrenaline. It lowers the heart rate and decreases the force of contraction. It is used to treat of hypertension, certain arrhythmias, migraine, angina, symptomatic coronary artery disease, pheochromocytoma, supraventricular arrhythmias, and other conditions related to sympathetic stimulation (e.g., panic disorder, aggressive behavior). Treatment of angina, hypertension, and symptomatic coronary artery disease (particularly after a myocardial infarction) depends on the drug's vasodilation effects.

Dosing and Drug Actions

Because propranolol can be used to treat a wide range of conditions, dosing varies widely. Dosing for hypertension, migraine, angina, pheochromocytoma, and supraventricular arrhythmia varies widely.

Toxic Effects

Side effects of propranolol result from excessive inhibition of the sympathetic nervous system, including bradycardia, hypotension, and cardiac failure. Propranolol can cross

TABLE 33-11	Propranolol
Characteristics	**Specifications**
Purpose	Treatment of hypertension, certain arrhythmias, migraine, angina, symptomatic coronary artery disease, pheochromocytoma, supraventricular arrhythmias, other conditions related to sympathetic stimulation (e.g., to alleviate panic disorder or aggressive behavior)
Usual bioavailability	30%
Half-life	3 hr
General therapeutic range	50-100 ng/mL
General toxic level	>1 g
Transport	93% is protein bound
Metabolism	Metabolized in the liver
Elimination	0.5% excreted in the urine unchanged
Steady state	6 hr
Mechanism of action	β-Blocker binds to and inhibits β-adrenergic receptors; lowers heart rate and decreases the force of contraction, opposing the effects of adrenaline
Toxic effects	Bradycardia, arterial insufficiency (Raynaud type), hypotension, atrioventricular block, nausea, vomiting, pharyngitis, bronchospasm, thrombotic thrombocytopenic purpura, and marrow suppression (rare)

TABLE 33-12	Amiodarone
Characteristics	**Specifications**
Purpose	Indicated only for life-threatening arrhythmias because of risk for substantial toxicity; poses major management problems that could be life threatening in patients at risk for sudden death
Usual bioavailability	35-65%
Half-life	3-10 days for rapid component, 25-110 days for slow component
General therapeutic range	0.5-2 mg/dL
General toxic level	>2 mg/dL
Transport	96% plasma protein bound
Metabolism	Metabolized by liver; extensive distribution in body because it is lipid-based
Elimination	Slow; occurs through skin, biliary tract, and lacrimal glands
Steady state	24 hr
Mechanism of action	Blocks potassium channels in cardiac muscle, prolonging the action potential, but also has weak calcium channel-blocking effects and some antiadrenaline effects
Toxic effects	Symptomatic bradycardia, heart block, fatal pulmonary fibrosis, fatal pulmonary toxicity, fatal hepatotoxicity, visual field disturbances, photodermatitis, hypothyroidism, and sometimes hyperthyroidism

the blood–brain barrier readily to cause a number of CNS effects, and it can significantly disrupt blood flow across the placenta in pregnant women.

Amiodarone

Mechanism of Action

Amiodarone (proprietary name: Cordarone) is an antiarrhythmic drug and is a structural analog of thyroid hormone (Table 33-12). The drug blocks potassium channels in cardiac muscle cells, which prolongs action potentials, and it has weak calcium channel blocking effects and some antiadrenaline effects. This drug is used for life-threatening ventricular arrhythmias and advanced cardiac life support.

Dosing and Drug Actions

Amiodarone is administered orally. A test dose is given for the first 3 weeks and if the clinical effect is achieved, then the same dosing continues. If the clinical effect is not achieved, dosing will be varied until the clinical effect is achieved.

For pulseless ventricular fibrillation or ventricular tachycardia, amiodarone is administered intravenously or injected directly into bone marrow (i.e., used as a noncollapsible entry point into the systemic venous system) after a dose of epinephrine if there is no initial response to defibrillation. Rapid intravenous push can be used if the patient is pulseless or has no blood pressure.

The therapeutic range for amiodarone is 0.5 to 2.0 mg/dL. Toxicity occurs with doses greater than 2 mg/dL.

Toxic Effects

Toxic doses can make arrhythmias worse or more difficult to reverse. Pulmonary and liver toxicities also can be fatal. Other toxic effects include acute myocardial infarction, AV block, bradycardia, hypertension, and cardiomegaly. Amiodarone also increases the risk for pulmonary fibrosis, liver disease, hyperthyroidism, optic neuropathy, pleural effusion, pneumonitis, and eosinophilic pneumonia.

TABLE 33-13	Mexiletine
Characteristics	**Specifications**
Purpose	Treatment of life-threatening ventricular arrhythmias
Usual bioavailability	80-90%
Half-life	6-17 hr
General therapeutic range	0.5-2 mg/dL
General toxic level	>2 mg/dL
Transport	50-70% protein bound
Metabolism	Metabolized in the liver
Elimination	8-15% excreted in the urine
Steady state	1-4 hr
Mechanism of action	Combines with fast sodium ion channels, resulting in decreased myocardial excitability and conduction velocity
Toxic effects	Tremor, dizziness, ataxia, dysarthria, diplopia, nystagmus, confusion, and hypotension

TABLE 33-14	Verapamil
Characteristics	**Specifications**
Purpose	Treatment of angina, hypertension, and supraventricular arrhythmias
Usual bioavailability	10-20%
Half-life	2-8 hr
General therapeutic range	50-250 ng/mL
General toxic level	>250 ng/dL
Transport	90% bound to plasma proteins
Metabolism	Extensive metabolism in the liver
Elimination	75% of active components excreted in the urine, remainder through the gastrointestinal tract
Steady state	2 hr
Mechanism of action	Calcium channel blocker; blocks activated and inactivated calcium channels in the atrioventricular node
Toxic effects	Hypotension, ventricular fibrillation, constipation, and peripheral edema

Mexiletine

Mechanism of Action

Mexiletine (proprietary name: Mexitil) is used for life-threatening ventricular arrhythmias and prophylaxis for ventricular arrhythmias in acute phase myocardial infarction (Table 33-13). It occupies sodium fast channels, inhibiting recovery after repolarization and resulting in decreasing myocardial excitability and conduction velocity.

Dosing and Drug Actions

Mexiletine is usually taken orally three times a day for life-threatening ventricular arrhythmias. The drug can also be used for prophylaxis of ventricular arrhythmias in acute phase myocardial infarction.

Toxic Effects

Toxic effects include cardiogenic shock, AV block, tremor, dizziness, ataxia, dysarthria, diplopia, nystagmus, confusion, and hypotension.

Verapamil

Mechanism of Action

Verapamil (proprietary name: Calan) is an antiarrhythmic drug (Table 33-14). It blocks activated and inactivated calcium channels in the AV node. Verapamil is used to treat angina, hypertension, and supraventricular arrhythmias. Calcium channel blockers such as verapamil do not reduce the mortality rate after myocardial infarction.

Dosing and Drug Actions

Verapamil is usually given orally in three or four divided doses per day.

Toxic Effects

Toxicity is characterized by hypotension, ventricular fibrillation, constipation, and peripheral edema.

Antibiotics

Antibiotics with serious side effects, such as amikacin, gentamicin, kanamycin, tobramycin, vancomycin, and chloramphenicol, require monitoring. They are indicated for use when infection-causing bacteria are resistant to other drugs or when less toxic antibiotics are not effective in killing the bacteria.

Antibiotics are classified as bacteriostatic drugs, which slow or stop bacterial cell division, or as bacteriocidal drugs, which directly kill bacteria. Bacteriostatic antibiotics work in conjunction with the immune system to eradicate infections and are less useful than bacteriocidal compounds when treating immunosuppressed patients.

Antibiotics may be further classified as broad-spectrum antibiotics, which are useful against a range of gram-positive and gram-negative bacteria, or as narrow-spectrum antibiotics, which may be useful only against a few types of bacteria. Broad-spectrum antibiotics are more likely to kill the enteric bacteria normally found in the gastrointestinal

TABLE 33-15	Amikacin
Characteristics	**Specifications**
Purpose	Treatment of bacterial infections that are resistant to less toxic drugs—usually those resistant to gentamicin and tobramycin; penetrates blood–brain barrier when meninges are inflamed; crosses placenta
Usual bioavailability	Zero—must be administered IV or IM
Half-life	2-3 hr
General therapeutic range	25-35 mg/dL
General toxic level	>35 mg/dL
Trough levels	1-8 mg/dL
Peak levels	25-35 mg/dL
Transport	0-11% bound to protein
Metabolism	0-2% in liver
Elimination	94-98% excreted in urine
Steady state	45-120 min
Mechanism of action	Binds to the 30S subunit of bacterial ribosomes, effectively stopping bacterial protein synthesis
Toxic effects	Neurotoxicity—bilateral auditory and vestibular ototoxicity, vertigo, nephrotoxicity, neuromuscular blockade, respiratory paralysis

TABLE 33-16	Gentamicin
Characteristics	**Specifications**
Purpose	Usually a first-line aminoglycoside against infections with gram-negative organisms such as *Pseudomonas aeruginosa*, *Escherichia coli*, *Proteus*, *Klebsiella*, *Enterobacter*, *Serratia*, and *Citrobacter* as well as *Staphylococcus* (gram-positive); minimally penetrates blood–brain barrier when meninges are inflamed; crosses placenta
Usual bioavailability	Zero—must be administered IV or IM
Half-life	2-3 hr
General therapeutic range	1-5 mg/dL
General toxic level	>10 mg/dL
Trough levels	1-2 mg/dL
Peak levels	5-8 mg/dL
Transport	<30 % bound to protein
Metabolism	30% in liver
Elimination	70% excreted in urine
Steady state	30-90 min
Mechanism of action	Binds to the 30S subunit of bacterial ribosomes, effectively stopping bacterial protein synthesis
Toxic effects	Neurotoxicity—bilateral auditory and vestibular ototoxicity, vertigo, nephrotoxic, neuromuscular blockade, respiratory paralysis

tract, which can lead to side effects such as nausea, diarrhea, and opportunistic infections.

Aminoglycosides

Aminoglycosides are a class of antibiotics that bind to bacterial ribosomes (particularly the 30S subunit, which is smaller than the eukaryotic small subunit found in humans) and inhibit bacterial protein synthesis, preventing bacteria from replicating or producing bacterial toxins. Most aminoglycosides are not absorbed by the gastrointestinal tract lining, and they must be given through intravenous or intramuscular routes.

Amikacin

Mechanism of Action
Amikacin (proprietary name: Amikin) binds to the prokaryotic 30S ribosome and inhibits bacterial protein synthesis, preventing bacterial growth and replication (Table 33-15). It is often used to treat multidrug-resistant, gram-negative bacterial infections.

Dosing and Drug Actions
Amikacin is administered intravenously or intramuscularly in divided doses every 8 to 12 hours. For urinary tract infections, amikacin is administered intravenously or intramuscularly in divided doses every 12 hours. At the therapeutic dose, infectious bacteria are eradicated. Loss of enteric bacteria can also occur, which can lead to nausea and diarrhea.

Toxic Effects
Amikacin can accumulate in the kidneys and cause nephrotoxicity, which can be monitored by a creatinine clearance test. Nephrotoxicity is reversible with removal of the drug. Prolonged exposure causes ototoxicity. Damage to inner ear cells leads to hearing loss, starting with the upper frequency ranges.

Gentamicin

Mechanism of Action
Gentamicin is a broad-spectrum aminoglycoside antibiotic (Table 33-16). Like amikacin, it binds to and inhibits the bacterial 30S ribosomal subunit, preventing bacterial protein synthesis and growth.

TABLE 33-17	Kanamycin
Characteristics	**Specifications**
Purpose	For use against infections with gram-negative organisms such as *Pseudomonas aeruginosa*, *Escherichia coli*, *Proteus*, *Klebsiella*, *Enterobacter*, *Serratia*, and *Citrobacter* as well as *Staphylococcus* (gram-positive); minimally penetrates blood–brain barrier when meninges are inflamed; crosses placenta
Usual bioavailability	Zero—must be administered IV or IM
Half-life	Not available
General therapeutic range	25-35 mg/dL
General toxic level	>35 mg/dL
Trough levels	4-8 mg/dL
Peak levels	25-35 mg/dL
Transport	Not available
Metabolism	Not available
Elimination	Urine
Steady state	Not available
Mechanism of action	Binds to the 30S subunit of bacterial ribosomes, effectively stopping bacterial protein synthesis
Toxic effects	Neurotoxicity—bilateral auditory and vestibular ototoxicity, vertigo, nephrotoxic, neuromuscular blockade, respiratory paralysis

TABLE 33-18	Tobramycin
Characteristics	**Specifications**
Purpose	Used against infections with gram-negative organisms such as *Pseudomonas aeruginosa*, *Escherichia coli*, *Proteus*, *Providencia*, *Klebsiella*, *Enterobacter*, *Serratia*, and *Citrobacter* as well as *Staphylococcus* (gram-positive); minimally penetrates blood–brain barrier when meninges inflamed; crosses placenta
Usual bioavailability	Zero—must be administered IV or IM
Half-life	2-3 hr
General therapeutic range	5-8 mg/dL
General toxic level	>10 mg/dL
Trough levels	1-2 mg/dL
Peak levels	5-8 mg/dL
Transport	<30% bound to plasma proteins
Metabolism	Not available
Elimination	90-95% in urine within 24 hr
Steady state	30-60 min
Mechanism of action	Binds to the 30S subunit of bacterial ribosomes, effectively stopping bacterial protein synthesis
Toxic effects	Neurotoxicity—bilateral auditory and vestibular ototoxicity, vertigo, nephrotoxic, neuromuscular blockade, respiratory paralysis

Dosing and Drug Actions

Gentamicin can be given intravenously, intramuscularly, or topically. Conventional dosing by either route is given in divided doses every 8 hours. The many dosage regimens are adjusted according to baseline creatinine clearance test results. At the therapeutic dose, infectious bacteria should be eradicated. Because gentamicin can kill all bacteria in the body, loss of enteric bacteria leads to nausea and diarrhea.

Toxic Effects

Similar to amikacin, gentamicin can accumulate in the kidneys and cause nephrotoxicity, which can be monitored by a creatinine clearance test. Nephrotoxicity is usually reversible with removal of the drug. Prolonged exposure can lead to ototoxicity; damage to inner ear cells leads to hearing loss, starting with the upper frequency ranges. Gentamicin also can cause vertigo, neuromuscular blockade, and respiratory paralysis.

Kanamycin

Mechanism of Action

Kanamycin (proprietary name: Kantrex) is made of kanamycin A, the major chemical produced by the bacterium *Streptomyces*

kanamyceticus. The minor chemicals are kanamycin B and C (Table 33-17). Like other aminoglycoside antibiotics, kanamycin binds to and inhibits the bacterial 30S ribosomal subunit, preventing bacterial protein synthesis and growth.

Dosing and Drug Actions

Kanamycin can be administered orally, intravenously, or intramuscularly. At therapeutic doses, infectious bacteria should be killed.

Toxic Effects

Kanamycin can cause nephrotoxicity, which is reversible with removal of the drug. Prolonged exposure can lead to ototoxicity; damage to inner ear cells leads to hearing loss, starting with the upper frequency ranges.

Tobramycin

Mechanism of Action

Tobramycin (proprietary name: Nebcin) is an aminoglycoside antibiotic, especially useful against gram-negative infections such as pseudomonas (Table 33-18). It is in the same class as amikacin, gentamicin, and kanamycin.

TABLE 33-19	Vancomycin
Characteristics	**Specifications**
Purpose	Because of serious side effects, typically used only as a last resort in the treatment of drug-resistant bacterial strains such as methicillin-resistant *Staphylococcus aureus* (MRSA) and infections such as pseudomembranous colitis or staphylococcal enterocolitis and endocarditis
Usual bioavailability	Poor absorption when administered orally
Half-life	5-11 hr
General therapeutic range	20-40 mg/dL
General toxic level	>80 mg/dL
Trough levels	5-10 mg/dL
Peak levels	20-40 mg/dL
Transport	50% protein bound
Metabolism	Not available
Elimination	80-90% excreted unchanged in urine
Steady state	30 min
Mechanism of action	Inhibits cell wall biosynthesis; blocks polymerization of glycopeptides by binding tightly to D-alanyl-D-alanine portion of cell wall precursor
Toxic effects	Fever, phlebitis, and pain at infusion site

These antibiotics kill gram-negative bacteria, especially those that are resistant to most other broad-spectrum oral drugs.

Like other aminoglycoside antibiotics, tobramycin binds to and inhibits the bacterial 30S ribosomal subunit, preventing bacterial protein synthesis and bacterial growth. This drug is used to treat infections with *Citrobacter* spp., *Escherichia coli*, *Pseudomonas aeruginosa*, *Proteus* spp., members of the Enterobacteriaceae family (including *Providencia*, *Klebsiella*, *Enterobacter*, and *Serratia*), and *Staphylococcus aureus* (coagulase positive and negative).

Dosing and Drug Actions

Tobramycin may be administered intravenously or intramuscularly. A nebulized (inhaled) form is used for treating respiratory infections with *Pseudomonas* spp. Due to neurotoxicity and nephrotoxicity, blood concentrations must be monitored through peak and trough concentrations. The peak levels for life-threatening infections should be 8 to 10 mg/dL; for a serious infection, peak levels should be 6 to 8 mg/dL; and for urinary tract infections, peak levels should be 6 to 8 mg/dL.

Toxic Effects

Like other aminoglycosides, tobramycin is ototoxic. This effect usually is irreversible. Other signs of neurotoxicity include vertigo, nephrotoxicity, neuromuscular blockade, and respiratory paralysis. Overdose of the inhaled form may lead to difficulty breathing.

Vancomycin

Mechanism of Action

Vancomycin (proprietary name: Vancocin) is an older antibiotic that typically is used only as a last resort due to its serious side effects. It may be used in the treatment of drug-resistant bacterial strains such as methicillin-resistant *Staphylococcus aureus* (MRSA). The Centers for Disease Control and Prevention (CDC) has issued guidelines for the use of vancomycin due to the emergence of vancomycin-resistant *Enterococcus* spp. It is used to treat infections such as pseudomembranous colitis, staphylococcal enterocolitis, and endocarditis (Table 33-19).

Vancomycin crosses into inflamed meninges with only a 20% to 30% blood level. The drug inhibits cell wall synthesis. It blocks glycopeptides polymerization by binding tightly to the D-alanyl-D-alanine portion of cell wall precursor.

Dosing and Drug Actions

Vancomycin is normally given intravenously, but it also comes in a nebulized (inhaled) form. At the therapeutic dose, infectious bacteria should be killed.

Toxic Effects

Monitoring of the vancomycin plasma level is necessary due to the potential for ototoxicity and nephrotoxicity, especially in those with reduced renal function or an increased propensity for bacterial infection.

Chloramphenicol

Mechanism of Action

Chloramphenicol (proprietary name: Chloromycetin) is an inexpensive, broad-spectrum antibiotic often used in Third World countries (Table 33-20). Because of safety concerns, it is not typically used as a first-line treatment in developed countries. Before this drug is used, its toxicity for the target organism is compared with that for the host. If the drug is more likely to kill the bacteria than damage the host, it is used to treat the infection.

Chloramphenicol is bacteriostatic and binds to the large (50S) subunit of bacterial ribosomes, inhibiting protein synthesis. This drug readily crosses the placenta, enters breast milk, and enters the CSF. The blood level ratio in normal or inflamed meninges is at least 66%

Dosing and Drug Actions

Chloramphenicol may be administered orally, intravenously, intramuscularly, or topically (for eye infections). Chloramphenicol is usually administered intravenously in divided doses every 6 hours for serious infections with susceptible bacteria.

TABLE 33-20 Chloramphenicol

Characteristics	Specifications
Purpose	Used at a concentration of 6 µg/mL to treat infections with *Haemophilus influenza, Neisseria meningitidis, Neisseria gonorrhoeae, Salmonella typhi, Brucella* spp., *Bordetella pertussis, Vibrio cholera,* and *Shigella* spp.; used at a concentration of 12 µg/mL to treat infections with *Escherichia coli, Klebsiella pneumonia, Pseudomonas pseudomallei, Chlamydia,* and *Mycoplasma*
Usual bioavailability	Good
Half-life	1.6-3.3 hr
General therapeutic range	10-25 mg/dL
General toxic level	>25 mg/dL
Trough levels	10 mg/dL
Peak levels	10-25 mg/dL
Transport	60% protein bound
Metabolism	Extensively (90%) metabolized in liver to inactive metabolites
Elimination	5-15% excreted in urine, 4% in feces
Steady state	4-6 hr
Mechanism of action	Binds to the large 50S subunit of bacterial ribosomes, inhibiting protein synthesis
Toxic effects	Blood dyscrasias, cardiovascular collapse, aplastic anemia

TABLE 33-21 Phenobarbital

Characteristics	Specifications
Purpose	Treatment of generalized tonic-clonic seizures, simple partial seizures, anxiety, insomnia
Usual bioavailability	90-100%
Half-life	5-6 days
General therapeutic range	10-40 mg/dL
General toxic level	>40 mg/dL
Transport	40-60% bound to protein
Metabolism	75% in inactive metabolites
Elimination	25% unchanged in urine
Steady state	14-21 days
Mechanism of action	Stabilizes damaged neuron membranes and raises threshold for neuronal membrane depolarization
Toxic effects	Drowsiness, depression of many body systems, respiratory depression, coma, sedation, hypotension

Chloramphenicol is used to treat infections with *Haemophilus influenzae, Neisseria meningitidis, Neisseria gonorrhoeae, Salmonella typhi, Brucella* spp., *Bordetella pertussis, Vibrio cholera,* and *Shigella* spp. It is used to treat *E. coli, Klebsiella pneumonia, Pseudomonas pseudomallei, Chlamydia,* and *Mycoplasma.*

Toxic Effects

Chloramphenicol is toxic to bone marrow and can cause aplastic anemia. This serious side effect is rare and usually fatal. There is no treatment or any way of predicting who may develop the side effect. Other adverse effects include blood dyscrasias and cardiovascular collapse.

Antiepileptic Drugs

Antiepileptic (anticonvulsant) drugs are used in the treatment of seizure disorders, such as grand mal, petit mal, and psychomotor seizures, and for treating trigeminal neuralgia (i.e., tic douloureux). Although these disorders are poorly understood, epileptic seizures are characterized by neurotransmission feedback loops within the brain. Most antiepileptic drugs block sodium influx into neurons with damaged membranes. This slows rapid firing in these cells.

Phenobarbital

Mechanism of Action

Phenobarbital (proprietary names: Luminol, Solfoton) is a common barbiturate with anticonvulsant, sedative, and hypnotic properties. It is a long-acting barbiturate used to treat grand mal tonic-clonic seizures, simple partial seizures with motor or somatosensory symptoms, anxiety, and insomnia (Table 33-21). It should not be used for petit mal seizures because phenobarbital can worsen them. It may also be used as a sedative before surgery or in the treatment of alcohol and benzodiazepine withdrawal symptoms.

Phenobarbital and other barbiturates bind to and activate γ-aminobutyric acid (GABA) receptors in the CNS. These stimulated receptors normally hyperpolarize neurons, inhibiting neuronal activity. Phenobarbital depresses the sensory and motor cortex and the cerebellum, and it raises the seizure threshold and inhibits the spread of discharges from seizure foci. The sedative-hypnotic effects of phenobarbital inhibit the reticular formation (i.e., reticular activating system [RAS]), which controls CNS arousal.

Dosing and Drug Actions

Phenobarbital may be administered orally, rectally, or parenterally. The dose is then adjusted to maintain therapeutic

TABLE 33-22	Phenytoin	
Characteristics	Specifications	
Purpose	Treatment of generalized tonic-clonic seizures, simple partial seizures, complex partial seizures	
Usual bioavailability	Variable (30-95%)	
Half-life	12-36 hr	
General therapeutic range	10-20 mg/dL	
General toxic level	>20 mg/dL	
Transport	90-95% protein bound	
Metabolism	Hepatic; inactive metabolites produced	
Elimination	5% unchanged in urine	
Steady state	7-8 days	
Mechanism of action	Inhibits Na^+ channels found along all axons in the nervous system, leading to reduced ability of the neuron to respond at high frequency	
Toxic effects	Nystagmus, ataxia, diplopia, drowsiness, coma; rapid intravenous administration may produce cardiovascular collapse and/or central nervous system depression	

TABLE 33-23	Valproic Acid	
Characteristics	Specifications	
Purpose	Treatment of absence seizures; can be used to treat tonic-clonic and partial seizures in conjunction with phenobarbital or phenytoin	
Usual bioavailability	81-89%	
Half-life	8-15 hr	
General therapeutic range	50-100 mg/dL	
General toxic level	>100 mg/dL	
Transport	90% protein bound	
Metabolism	90-100% metabolized in the liver	
Elimination	30-50% excreted in urine	
Steady state	1-4 days	
Mechanism of action	Reduces the ability of the neuron to respond at high frequency by inhibiting γ-aminobutyric acid (GABA) transaminase	
Toxic effects	Produces birth defects; sedation, gastric disturbances, hematologic reactions, ataxia, somnolence, and coma	

concentrations. Oral doses of 30 to 120 mg/day are used for anxiety, and doses of 100 to 320 mg orally are used for sleep induction. Individuals who use barbiturates on a long-term basis have a tendency to develop dependence and tolerance.

Toxic Effects

Symptoms of phenobarbital toxicity typically include depression of many body systems, which can cause sluggishness, lack of coordination, foggy thinking, slow speech, drowsiness, shallow breathing, coma, and death. The lethal dose of barbiturates varies greatly, as does tolerance to the drug.

Phenytoin

Mechanism of Action

Phenytoin (proprietary name: Dilantin) is used to treat primary and secondary tonic-clonic seizures, partial or complex partial seizures, and status epilepticus (Table 33-22). This drug is not used for absence seizures. Phenytoin inhibits sodium ion channels found along all axons in the nervous system, which reduces the ability of neurons to respond at a rapid rate. It does not have the sedative properties of phenobarbital. It can also be used to treat trigeminal neuralgia, a disease of the fifth cranial nerve (trigeminal nerve) that is characterized by intense pain.

Dosing and Drug Actions

Phenytoin may be administered orally or intravenously. The average daily maintenance dose should be tailored to the individual's response. It reduces activity of brain stem centers responsible for the tonic-clonic (grand mal) seizures. It dampens the runaway brain activity seen in seizures by reducing electrical conductance among neurons.

Toxic Effects

Phenytoin overdose causes depression of many body systems by severely depressing the CNS, which can lead to coma, difficulty in pronouncing words, involuntary eye movement, lack of muscle coordination, low blood pressure, nausea, sluggishness, slurred speech, tremors, and vomiting.

Valproic Acid

Mechanism of Action

Valproic acid (proprietary names: Depakene, Depakote) is used to treat absence seizures (Table 33-23). It is used to treat tonic-clonic and partial seizures when used in conjunction with phenobarbital or phenytoin. Valproic acid reduces the ability of the neuron to respond at high frequency by inhibiting GABA transaminase.

Dosing and Drug Actions

Valproic acid may be administered orally. At therapeutic doses, valproic acid can manage seizure disorders and mania.

TABLE 33-24	Carbamazepine
Characteristics	**Specifications**
Purpose	Treatment of tonic-clonic seizures, simple partial and complex partial seizures, and combinations of these types of seizures; may exacerbate absence, myoclonic, and atonic seizures
Usual bioavailability	70%
Half-life	8-20 hr
General therapeutic range	4-12 mg/dL
General toxic level	>12 mg/dL
Transport	60-70% protein bound
Metabolism	Hepatic
Elimination	1-2% unchanged in urine
Steady state	3-7 days
Mechanism of action	Carbamazepine keeps voltage-gated Na+ channels in their inactivated state, blocking action potentials and making neurons less excitable
Toxic effects	Mild symptoms: vomiting, drowsiness, ataxia, slurred speech, jaundice, hepatitis, nystagmus, and hallucinations Severe intoxications: seizures, respiratory depression, hypotension aplastic anemia, agranulocytosis, and coma Fatal dermatologic reactions (toxic epidermal necrolysis and Stevens-Johnson syndrome) have been reported

TABLE 33-25	Ethosuximide
Characteristics	**Specifications**
Purpose	Drug of choice for absence (petit mal) seizures
Usual bioavailability	85%
Half-life	60 hr
General therapeutic range	40-100 mg/dL
General toxic level	>100 mg/dL
Transport	None protein bound
Metabolism	60-90% metabolized in the liver
Elimination	72% excreted in urine, 28% in feces
Steady state	8-10 hr
Mechanism of action	Calcium channel blocker; stabilizes inactivated state of Na+ channels, making neurons less excitable
Toxic effects	Nausea, vomiting, gastric distress, drowsiness, ataxia, aplastic anemia, systemic lupus erythematosus, and pancytopenia

Toxic Effects

Mild symptoms may include vomiting, drowsiness, ataxia, slurred speech, jaundice, hepatitis, nystagmus, and hallucinations. Severe intoxications may produce seizures, respiratory depression, hypotension aplastic anemia, agranulocytosis, and coma. Fatal dermatologic reactions (i.e., toxic epidermal necrolysis and Stevens-Johnson syndrome) have been reported with carbamazepine use.

Ethosuximide

Mechanism of Action

Ethosuximide (proprietary name: Zarontin) is the drug of choice for absence (petit mal) seizures in which there is a brief loss of consciousness (Table 33-25). Ethosuximide is a calcium channel blocker. It stabilizes the inactivated state of sodium channels, making neurons less excitable.

Dosing and Drug Actions

Ethosuximide is taken orally in divided doses.

Toxic Effects

Ethosuximide overdose may produce nausea, vomiting, and coma with respiratory depression.

Primidone

Mechanism of Action

Primidone (proprietary name: Mysoline) is used to treat tonic-clinic, simple partial, and complex partial seizures

Toxic Effects

Symptoms of valproic acid overdose may include coma, extreme drowsiness, and heart irregularities.

Carbamazepine

Mechanism of Action

Carbamazepine (proprietary name: Tegretol) is a primary antiepileptic drug that is used to treat tonic-clonic seizures, simple partial and complex partial seizures, and combinations of these types of seizures (Table 33-24). Taking carbamazepine may exacerbate absence, myoclonic, and atonic seizures. The drug is also used to treat trigeminal neuralgia and glossopharyngeal neuralgia.

Carbamazepine keeps voltage-gated sodium ion channels in their inactivated state, blocking action potentials and making neurons less excitable.

Dosing and Drug Actions

The dose for seizure maintenance and trigeminal neuralgia is taken orally in divided doses.

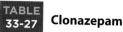

TABLE 33-26 Primidone	
Characteristics	**Specifications**
Purpose	Treatment of tonic-clinic, simple partial, and complex partial seizures
Usual bioavailability	60-80%
Half-life	10-12 hr
General therapeutic range	5-10 mg/dL
General toxic level	>12 mg/dL
Transport	20% protein bound
Metabolism	Metabolized in the liver to phenobarbital and phenylethylmalonamide
Elimination	15-25% excreted in the urine
Steady state	4-7 days
Mechanism of action	Phenobarbital inhibits neuronal activity by binding to and activating γ-aminobutyric acid (GABA) receptors in the central nervous system that normally hyperpolarize neurons
Toxic effects	Sluggishness, fogginess, slowness of speech, drowsiness or coma, shallow breathing, staggering; in severe cases, coma and death

TABLE 33-27 Clonazepam	
Characteristics	**Specifications**
Purpose	Treatment of panic disorders, absence seizures, infantile spasms, akinetic seizures, and Lennox-Gastaut syndrome
Usual bioavailability	90%
Half-life	17-60 hr
General therapeutic range	0.02-0.07 mg/dL
General toxic level	0.06 mg/dL
Transport	85% protein bound
Metabolism	Metabolized in the liver
Elimination	Excreted in the urine
Steady state	5-7 days
Mechanism of action	Increases the duration of chloride flow into a synapse; this raises the seizure threshold and stops the spread of discharges from epileptic foci
Toxic effects	Drowsiness and ataxia

(Table 33-26). The chemical structure of primidone is similar to the basic structure of barbiturates. When primidone is metabolized in the liver, one of its metabolites is phenobarbital. Primidone and phenobarbital levels should be measured when monitoring the clinical effectiveness of primidone.

Primidone binds to and activates GABA receptors in the CNS. These receptors normally hyperpolarize neurons, inhibiting neuronal activity. The phenobarbital metabolite of primidone has the same mechanism. Primidone may also increase the threshold for membrane depolarization in CNS neurons, which prevents seizures.

Dosing and Drug Actions

Primidone is started with a low dose and builds to the maintenance dose.

Individuals taking primidone should have a complete blood count and a metabolic panel every 6 months. If the drug is discontinued abruptly, status epilepticus may result. Individuals may need to be followed for several weeks to evaluate the therapeutic efficacy of the dosing regimen.

Toxic Effects

Symptoms of toxicity include sluggishness, fogginess, slow speech, drowsiness, shallow breathing, staggering, and in severe cases, coma and death.

Clonazepam
Mechanism of Action

Clonazepam (proprietary name: Klonopin) is a long-acting drug used to treat panic disorders, absence seizures, infantile spasms, akinetic seizures, and Lennox-Gastaut syndrome (Table 33-27). It is a benzodiazepine closely related to diazepam (Valium). Benzodiazepines increase the duration of chloride ion flow into synapses. This raises the seizure threshold and stops the spread of discharges from epileptic foci. It decreases the spike and wave discharge in absence seizures by depressing nerve transmission. Tolerance for clonazepam does not develop as quickly as for diazepam.

Dosing and Drug Actions

Initially, individuals with panic disorders take clonazepam orally, which can increase after several days. For seizure disorders, individuals initially take clonazepam orally in divided doses, usually more frequently than for panic disorders. The dosage increases until the desired effect is achieved.

Toxic Effects

Symptoms of clonazepam toxicity include drowsiness and ataxia.

Gabapentin
Mechanism of Action

Gabapentin (proprietary name: Neurontin) is used to treat drug-resistant partial seizures (Table 33-28). Gabapentin is a chemical analog of GABA that promotes the release of

TABLE 33-28 Gabapentin

Characteristics	Specifications
Purpose	Treatment of drug-resistant partial seizures
Usual bioavailability	90%
Half-life	5-9 hr
General therapeutic range	2-12 mg/dL
General toxic level	>12 mg/dL
Transport	10% protein bound
Metabolism	0%
Elimination	Excreted in urine
Steady state	5-7 hr
Mechanism of action	Chemical analog of γ-aminobutyric acid (GABA) that promotes the release of GABA; mechanism for analgesic and anticonvulsant activity is unknown
Toxic effects	Somnolence, ataxia, dizziness, fatigue

TABLE 33-29 Lamotrigine

Characteristics	Specifications
Purpose	Adjunct therapy for partial seizures
Usual bioavailability	98%
Half-life	25-33 hr
General therapeutic range	5-8 mg/dL
General toxic level	>8 mg/dL
Transport	55% protein bound
Metabolism	Metabolized in the liver
Elimination	Excreted in urine
Steady state	1-1.5 hr
Mechanism of action	Considered to be a γ-aminobutyric acid (GABA) antagonist; blocks repetitive nerve firings created by depolarization of spinal cord neurons
Toxic effects	Dizziness, ataxia, diplopia, blurred vision, nausea, vomiting

TABLE 33-30 Levetiracetam

Characteristics	Specifications
Purpose	Adjunctive therapy for the treatment of partial onset seizures in adults with epilepsy
Usual bioavailability	100%
Half-life	6-8 hr
General therapeutic range	10-63 mg/dL
General toxic level	>63 mg/dL
Transport	<10% protein bound
Metabolism	24% metabolized in the liver
Elimination	Almost all is excreted in urine
Steady state	1-8 hr
Mechanism of action	Unknown
Toxic effects	Decreased red blood cell count, decreased hematocrit, decreased neutrophil count, somnolence, asthenia, and dizziness

GABA. The mechanism for analgesic and anticonvulsant properties is unknown.

Dosing and Drug Actions

Initial dosing of gabapentin is taken orally several times a day. The dosage may increase at a standard interval, depending on when the desired state is reached.

Toxic Effects

Toxic symptoms of gabapentin include somnolence, ataxia, dizziness, and fatigue.

Lamotrigine

Mechanism of Action

Lamotrigine (proprietary name: Lamictal) is used as an adjunct therapy for partial seizures (Table 33-29). It is considered a GABA antagonist. It blocks repetitive nerve firings created by depolarization of spinal cord neurons. It prevents rapid firing of neurons during a seizure.

Dosing and Drug Actions

Initial dosing of lamotrigine is taken orally for 2 weeks; it then increases and is taken orally in divided doses for 2 weeks. At the fifth week and beyond, the dose is increased and is taken orally in divided doses at a standard interval.

Toxic Effects

Toxic effects of lamotrigine include dizziness, ataxia, diplopia, blurred vision, nausea, and vomiting.

Levetiracetam

Mechanism of Action

Levetiracetam (proprietary name: Keppra) is used as adjunctive therapy for the treatment of partial seizures in adults with epilepsy (Table 33-30). Its precise mechanism of action is unknown.

TABLE 33-31	Oxcarbazepine	
Characteristics	**Specifications**	
Purpose	Treatment of partial seizures with and without secondarily generalized seizures in adults	
Usual bioavailability	100%	
Half-life	1-2.5 hr	
General therapeutic range	3-35 mg/dL	
General toxic level	Not well established	
Transport	40% bound to protein	
Metabolism	100% in the liver	
Elimination	>95% excreted in urine	
Steady state	8-12 hr	
Mechanism of action	Stabilizes neuronal membranes by blocking sodium channels; inhibits repetitive firing including from epileptic loci	
Toxic effects	Hyponatremia, dizziness, somnolence, diplopia, fatigue, nausea, vomiting, ataxia, abnormal vision, abnormal pain, tremor, dyspepsia, and abnormal gait	

TABLE 33-32	Lithium	
Categories	**Specifications**	
Purpose	Treatment of bipolar disorder	
Usual bioavailability	100%	
Half-life	12-27 hr	
General therapeutic range	0.6-1.2 mEq/L	
General toxic level	>2 mEq/L	
Transport	<10% protein bound	
Metabolism	Not metabolized in the liver	
Elimination	Excreted through the kidneys	
Steady state	Not available	
Mechanism of action	Unknown, although it may affect ion movements across the excitatory glutamate receptors in the central nervous system	
Toxic effects	Acute toxicity: tremulousness, dystonia, hyperreflexia, ataxia, cardiac dysrhythmias Renal toxicity: renal tubular acidosis, chronic tubulointerstitial nephritis, nephrotic syndrome Chronic toxicity: altered mental status, coma, seizures, cognitive impairment, sensorimotor peripheral neuropathy, cerebellar dysfunction, hypothyroidism, aplastic anemia	

Dosing and Drug Actions

Dosing and Drug Actions

Adults take levetiracetam twice daily to achieve the desired end state.

Toxic Effects

Toxic Effects

Toxic symptoms of levetiracetam include decreased red blood cell count, decreased hematocrit, decreased neutrophil count, somnolence, asthenia, and dizziness.

Oxcarbazepine

Mechanism of Action

Mechanism of Action

Oxcarbazepine (proprietary names: Trileptal, Oxtellar) is used to treat partial seizures with and without secondary generalized seizures in adults (Table 33-31). This drug is immediately metabolized to 10-hydroxy-10,11-dihydrocarbamazepine, the active metabolite. Oxcarbazepine stabilizes neuronal membranes by blocking sodium ion channels and inhibiting repetitive firing, including signals from epileptic loci.

Dosing and Drug Actions

Dosing and Drug Actions

Patients are treated with oxcarbazepine taken orally twice a day. The dose may be increased at weekly intervals, up to a maximum dosage.

Toxic Effects

Toxic Effects

Toxic symptoms of oxcarbazepine include hyponatremia, dizziness, somnolence, diplopia, fatigue, nausea, vomiting, ataxia, abnormal vision, abnormal pain, tremor, dyspepsia, and abnormal gait.

Psychoactive Drugs

Psychiatrists use drugs such as lithium, amitriptyline, nortriptyline, desipramine, imipramine, and diazepam. The drug levels must be monitored to ensure they remain within the therapeutic ranges.

Lithium

Mechanism of Action

Mechanism of Action

Lithium (proprietary name: Eskalith) has been used since the 19th century. It is currently used as a mood stabilizer in the treatment of bipolar disorder (Table 33-32). The FDA banned it during the 1940s but lifted the ban in 1970. Lithium can counteract mania and depression. Noticeable effects of lithium treatment usually require months, which suggests that lithium triggers some sort of negative-feedback homeostatic response in the body.

The precise mechanism of action of lithium as a mood-stabilizing agent is unknown, although it may affect ion movements across the excitatory glutamate receptors in the CNS.

TABLE 33-33   Amitriptyline

Characteristics	Specifications
Purpose	Treatment of depression, migraines, chronic pain, irritable bowel, diabetic neuropathy, schizophrenia; control of aggressive behavior
Usual bioavailability	95-100%
Half-life	9-27 hr
General therapeutic range	80-200 µg/L
General toxic level	>300 µg/L (including the concentration of nortriptyline in the blood)
Transport	Unknown
Metabolism	Metabolized in the liver to nortriptyline
Elimination	18% excreted in the urine
Steady state	Not available
Mechanism of action	Inhibits reuptake of norepinephrine (NE) and serotonin (5-HT) equally; boosts NE and 5-HT signaling in synapses in the central nervous system and in some peripheral tissues
Toxic effects	Hypotension, confusion, convulsions, drowsiness, hallucinations, rapid or irregular heartbeat, reduced body temperature, stupor, coma

Dosing and Drug Actions

Lithium is available only orally, and it comes in a variety of forms. Effects may take months to become established. It can control the adverse symptoms of bipolar disorder, including depression and mania.

Toxic Effects

Because lithium salts have a narrow therapeutic index, plasma concentrations should be monitored. Lithium may adversely affect those with thyroid or kidney disorders. Acute toxicity (i.e., lithium plasma concentrations greater than 1.5 mmol/L) may be fatal. Symptoms of acute toxicity include tremulousness, dystonia, hyperreflexia, ataxia, cardiac dysrhythmias, and renal toxicity, including renal tubular acidosis, chronic tubulointerstitial nephritis, and nephrotic syndrome. Symptoms of chronic toxicity include altered mental status, coma, seizures, cognitive impairment, sensorimotor peripheral neuropathy, cerebellar dysfunction, hypothyroidism, and aplastic anemia.

Tricyclic Antidepressants

Amitriptyline

Mechanism of Action

Amitriptyline (proprietary name: Elavil) is the most widely used tricyclic antidepressant (TCA) (Table 33-33). It is also used to treat migraines, chronic pain, irritable bowel, diabetic neuropathy, and schizophrenia and to control aggressive behavior.

There is little consensus on the exact mechanism of action. The active metabolite of amitriptyline (i.e., nortriptyline) inhibits the reuptake of norepinephrine and serotonin equally. This boosts levels of norepinephrine and serotonin signaling found in synapses in the CNS and in some peripheral tissues. This mechanism is thought to underlie the antidepressant effects of the drug; however, it is more likely to be a short-term effect of TCAs. Long-term treatment may reduce norepinephrine and serotonin signaling by inducing a negative-feedback homeostatic response, and some think this may be the mechanism by which TCAs ameliorate the symptoms of depression.

TCAs also block histamine, α-adrenergic, and muscarinic receptors, which accounts for their sedative, hypotensive, and anticholinergic effects (e.g., blurred vision, dry mouth, constipation, urinary retention).

Dosing and Drug Actions

Individuals are initially treated with oral doses of amitriptyline usually taken at bedtime. The dose is then increased every 5 to 7 days to reach maximum dosage for the patient. The doses may be divided throughout the day, or the total dose may be taken at bedtime.

Toxic Effects

Amitriptyline can be particularly dangerous in overdose, and it and other TCAs are no longer recommended as first-line therapy for depression. Symptoms of overdose include hypotension, confusion, convulsions, drowsiness, hallucinations, rapid or irregular heartbeat, reduced body temperature, stupor, and coma.

Nortriptyline

Mechanism of Action

Nortriptyline (proprietary names: Pamelor, Aventyl) is a second-generation TCA and a metabolite of amitriptyline. It is used to treat major depression and childhood bedwetting. It is sometimes used for chronic illnesses such as chronic fatigue syndrome and chronic pain.

Nortriptyline inhibits reuptake of norepinephrine and serotonin (to a lesser extent), thereby boosting levels of these neurotransmitters within synapses. Nortriptyline also has antagonistic effects on histamine, muscarinic, and serotonin receptors.

Dosing and Drug Actions

Individuals treated with nortriptyline take doses orally at standard intervals or take the total dose before bedtime.

TABLE 33-34	Desipramine
Characteristics	**Specifications**
Purpose	Second-line antidepressant; treatment of attention-deficit/hyperactivity disorder, irritable bowel syndrome
Usual bioavailability	Unknown
Half-life	15-24 hr
General therapeutic range	100-300 µg/L
General toxic level	>500 µg/L
Transport	Unknown
Metabolism	Highly metabolized—produces 2-hydroxydesipramine (active metabolite)
Elimination	70% excreted in urine
Steady state	2-5 days
Mechanism of action	Selectively blocks reuptake of norepinephrine from the neuronal synapse
Toxic effects	Sedation, hypertension or hypotension, cardiotoxicity, tachycardia, congestive heart failure, impaired memory, and delirium

TABLE 33-35	Imipramine
Characteristics	**Specifications**
Purpose	Treatment of depression
Usual bioavailability	100%
Half-life	6-18 hr
General therapeutic range	175-300 µg/L
General toxic level	>300 µg/L (including desipramine concentration)
Transport	90% protein bound
Metabolism	Metabolized in the liver into desipramine
Elimination	Excreted in the urine
Steady state	Unknown
Mechanism of action	More potent at boosting norepinephrine (NE) levels compared with serotonin (5-HT) levels
Toxic effects	Sedation, hypertension or hypotension, cardiotoxicity, tachycardia, congestive heart failure, impaired memory, and delirium

Toxic Effects

The symptoms of a nortriptyline overdose are largely the same as for amitriptyline.

Desipramine

Mechanism of Action

Along with its use as a second-line antidepressant, desipramine (proprietary name: Norpramin) may be used to treat symptoms of attention-deficit/hyperactivity disorder (ADHD) and irritable bowel syndrome (Table 33-34).

Desipramine, like other TCAs, selectively blocks reuptake of norepinephrine from the neuronal synapse. It inhibits serotonin reuptake to a lesser extent compared with other TCAs. Like other TCAs, inhibition boosts levels of norepinephrine found in synapses, which may lead to reduction in the symptoms of depression.

Dosing and Drug Actions

The dosage for desipramine is taken orally before bed or taken in divided doses twice a day.

Toxic Effects

Effects of a desipramine overdose may include sedation, hypertension or hypotension, cardiotoxicity, tachycardia, congestive heart failure, impaired memory, and delirium.

Imipramine

Mechanism of Action

Imipramine (proprietary name: Tofranil) is the prototypical TCA (Table 33-35). The mechanism of action of imipramine is similar to that of amitriptyline and other TCAs. Imipramine is more potent at boosting norepinephrine levels than serotonin levels.

Dosing and Drug Actions

Dosing of imipramine is taken orally, and it may gradually be increased. The total dose may be given before bedtime, or the drug can be given in divided doses. It may require more than 2 weeks for maximum effects.

Toxic Effects

Toxic effects of imipramine may include sedation, hypertension or hypotension, cardiotoxicity, tachycardia, congestive heart failure, impaired memory, and delirium.

Diazepam

Mechanism of Action

Diazepam (proprietary name: Valium) is in a class of drugs called benzodiazepines, which are sedative-hypnotics. Diazepam is mainly used to treat anxiety disorders, insomnia, muscle spasms, and symptoms of acute alcohol withdrawal (Table 33-36). It is also used as a premedication for inducing sedation or reducing anxiety before certain medical procedures.

TABLE 33-36 Diazepam

Characteristics	Specifications
Purpose	Treatment of anxiety disorders, insomnia, muscle spasms, and symptoms of acute alcohol withdrawal; preoperative sedation
Usual bioavailability	90%
Half-life	20-70 hr
General therapeutic range	200-1000 µg/L
General toxic level	>5000 µg/L
Transport	98% protein bound
Metabolism	Highly metabolized into active metabolites (nordiazepam)
Elimination	Excreted in the urine
Steady state	Unknown
Mechanism of action	Modulates effects of γ-aminobutyric acid (GABA) transmission, producing presynaptic inhibition; produces a calming effect
Toxic effects	Somnolence, confusion, coma, and diminished reflexes

TABLE 33-37 Theophylline

Characteristics	Specifications
Purpose	Treatment and prevention of moderate to serve asthma
Usual bioavailability	Varies, but 100% for oral formulations
Half-life	8-9 hr
General therapeutic range	10-20 µg/mL
General toxic level	>20 µg/mL
Transport	60% protein bound
Metabolism	Metabolized in the liver
Elimination	85-90% by the liver and 10-15% excreted in urine
Steady state	Unknown
Mechanism of action	Relaxes smooth muscle cells surrounding bronchioles
Toxic effects	Nausea, vomiting (severe and protracted), abdominal pain, mild metabolic acidosis, hypokalemia, hypophosphatemia, hypomagnesemia, hypocalcemia/hypercalcemia, hyperglycemia, tachycardia.

Diazepam and other benzodiazepines modulate the effects of GAGA transmission, producing presynaptic inhibition. The drug produces a calming effect.

Dosing and Drug Actions

Dosing of diazepam for anxiety is given orally or administered intravenously or intramuscularly two to four times a day. Dosing for alcohol withdrawal is given orally up to eight times during the first 24 hours; the dosage is then reduced and given orally two to four times a day as needed. Dosing for preoperative sedation is administered intramuscularly before surgery.

Toxic Effects

Toxic symptoms of diazepam include somnolence, confusion, coma, and diminished reflexes.

Bronchodilators

Activation of the sympathetic nervous system (SNS) generates several responses throughout the body, including bronchodilation, elevated heart rate and force of contraction, pupil dilation, and vasoconstriction. Each is mediated by activation of adrenergic receptors by the neurotransmitter norepinephrine or by the hormone epinephrine (i.e., adrenaline).

Most bronchodilators target the lungs, causing bronchodilation without also increasing the heart rate or elevating blood pressure. These drugs are said to be **sympathomimetics**

because of their ability to mimic the effects of the sympathetic nervous system.

Theophylline
Mechanism of Action

Theophylline (proprietary name: Theo-Dur) is used to treat moderate or severe asthma. It can prevent attacks and treat acute attacks (Table 33-37). Theophylline relaxes smooth muscle cells surrounding bronchioles. It also blocks adenosine-mediated bronchoconstriction.

Dosing and Drug Actions

Theophylline may be administered orally, intravenously, or intramuscularly. Dosing is individualized for each patient and depends route of administration and the age, body weight, and condition of the patient.

Toxic Effects

Symptoms of theophylline overdose include seizures, arrhythmias, and gastrointestinal disturbances.

Aminophylline
Mechanism of Action

Aminophylline (proprietary names: Norphyl, Phyllocontin, Truphylline) is a combination of theophylline (a bronchodilator) and ethylenediamine, which improves solubility. It is most commonly used in the treatment of bronchial asthma. It has the same mechanism of action as theophylline.

Dosing and Drug Actions

Aminophylline can be taken orally or administered intravenously. When it is given intravenously, there is a loading dose. A maintenance dose is then given by continuous intravenous infusion or given orally to maintain therapeutic levels.

Toxic Effects

Aminophylline has the same toxic effects as theophylline.

Immunosuppressant Drugs

Immunosuppressant drugs repress immune system responses. They are mainly used to treat organ transplant rejection but can also treat autoimmune conditions such as rheumatoid arthritis. Humoral and cell-mediated forms of immunity are essential to protect the body from infectious microorganisms. However, the responses sometimes cause more harm than good, as in organ transplant rejection, autoimmune diseases, allergies, multiple myeloma, and chronic nephritis.

Cell-mediated immunity must be suppressed to prevent organ transplant rejections. Cell-mediated immunity is responsible for graft-versus-host disease, which is caused by the activation of CD4+ T cells. Activation unleashes a cascade of events that result in the ultimate destruction of the foreign antigen or organ. Common drugs used to prevent organ transplant rejection include cyclosporine, mycophenolic acid, sirolimus, tacrolimus, and cyclophosphamide.

Cyclosporine
Mechanism of Action

Cyclosporine (proprietary names: Neoral, Sandimmune, Gengraf) is an immunosuppressant used to treat transplant rejection, rheumatoid arthritis, and severe psoriasis. It is also used prophylactically to prevent rejection of kidney, liver, and heart allogenic transplants.

Cyclosporine inhibits the production of the cytokine interleukin-2. Interleukin-2 is responsible for activating T cells to differentiate, proliferate, and produce antibodies, eventually causing antigen destruction.

Dosing and Drug Actions

Cyclosporine is administered before transplantation in a single oral dose. It is then taken orally after transplantation given in divided doses. The doses are reduced each week until a daily maintenance dose is achieved. Cyclosporine is also indicated for severe active rheumatoid arthritis and for kidney, heart, and liver transplantation.

Toxic Effects

Therapeutic doses of cyclosporine may be associated with potentially serious adverse drug reactions, such as gingival hyperplasia, convulsions, pancreatitis, infections, fever, vomiting, myelosuppression, malignancies, cerebral hemorrhage, diarrhea, confusion, hypertension, hyperkalemia, and kidney and liver dysfunction.

Mycophenolic Acid
Mechanism of Action

Mycophenolate mofetil (proprietary name: CellCept) is the most used immunosuppressant for transplantation of solid organs. Mycophenolic acid inhibits T- and B-cell proliferation and antibody production. Mycophenolate mofetil inhibits the synthesis of DNA nucleotides and affects rapidly dividing cells such as bone marrow stem cells.

Dosing and Drug Actions

For kidney, heart, or liver transplantations, mycophenolate mofetil is used in conjunction with cyclosporine and corticosteroids, taken orally or administered intravenously via infusion.

Toxic Effects

Mycophenolate mofetil is less toxic than azathioprine. Possible adverse effects include leukopenia, abdominal pain, diarrhea, nausea, vomiting, and dyspepsia.

Sirolimus
Mechanism of Action

Sirolimus (proprietary name: Rapamune) is used to prevent rejection of renal transplants. Sirolimus is a macrolide antibiotic that also suppresses the immune system. It is produced by *Streptomyces hygroscopicus*. The drug suppresses cytokine-driven T-cell proliferation, inhibiting the cell-mediated immune response.

Dosing and Drug Actions

Sirolimus is taken orally. The solution usually contains 1 mg/mL of sirolimus and other chemicals such as propylene glycols, monoglycerides, and fatty acids. Sirolimus is absorbed quickly from the gastrointestinal tract and is metabolized by the liver. Testing is done to confirm the drug is in the therapeutic range determined for the patient.

Toxic Effects

Toxic effects of sirolimus include thrombocytopenia, anemia, gastrointestinal symptoms, leukopenia, and hypertriglyceridemia.

Tacrolimus
Mechanism of Action

Tacrolimus (proprietary name: Prograf) is used to prevent rejection of heart, allogenic liver and kidney transplants. It may also be used for other solid organ transplants and for preventing graft-versus-host disease after transplantation of allogenic stem cells and pancreatic islet cells.

Tacrolimus is a macrolide antibiotic and a potent immunosuppressant. It is isolated from *Streptomyces tsukubaensis* and is metabolized in the liver. Tacrolimus suppresses cytokine and inflammatory mediator synthesis, similar to the mechanism of cyclosporine.

Dosing and Drug Actions

For heart transplantation, tacrolimus is used with aza-thioprine or mycophenolate mofetil. It is administered by continuous infusion or given in divided doses twice a day initially. The initial dose is administered no sooner than 6 hours after transplantation.

For liver transplantation, the dose of tacrolimus is administered by continuous infusion or given in divided doses twice a day. Providers adjust the dosage according to the clinical response.

For kidney transplantation, tacrolimus is used with azathioprine, mycophenolate mofetil, or an interleukin-2 receptor antagonist and corticosteroids. With azathioprine, the dose of tacrolimus is taken orally in divided doses twice a day initially. With mycophenolate mofetil or an interleu-kin-2 receptor antagonist, the dose of tacrolimus is admin-istered by continuous infusion in divided doses twice a day initially and then reduced to daily doses.

Toxic Effects

Toxic effects of tacrolimus include nephrotoxicity, tremors, headache, high blood pressure, nausea, vomiting, and elec-trolyte disturbances such as hyperkalemia.

Cyclophosphamide

Mechanism of Action

Cyclophosphamide (proprietary name: Cytoxan) is used to treat nephrotic syndrome and malignancies such as non-Hodgkin lymphoma and breast cancer.

Cyclophosphamide binds to and alters DNA, preventing the synthesis of new DNA. Rapidly dividing malignant cells cannot undergo mitosis, and they undergo programmed death or apoptosis. This drug is also a potent immunosuppressant.

Dosing and Drug Actions

Cyclophosphamide can be taken orally in divided doses over 4 to 5 days.

Toxic Effects

Common adverse effects include nausea, vomiting, and alo-pecia. Other toxic effects of cyclophosphamide are suscepti-bility to infection, immunosuppression, and cardiac toxicity.

Azathioprine

Mechanism of Action

Azathioprine (proprietary name: Imuran) is an immunosup-pressive drug used in kidney transplantation and for autoim-mune diseases such as rheumatoid arthritis and Crohn disease.

Azathioprine is a purine analog that inhibits an enzyme required for the synthesis of DNA, RNA, and proteins. It interferes with cellular metabolism and inhibits mitosis. It therefore most strongly affects rapidly proliferating cells such as T cells or B cells.

Dosing and Drug Actions

Azathioprine is administered orally. A larger dose is given initially, dropping to a lower maintenance dose after several

days. Therapeutic doses lead to immunosuppression, which is used to prevent organ transplant rejection and treat auto-immune diseases.

Toxic Effects

Toxic effects include symptoms of marrow suppression, including bleeding, mouth ulcers, infection, and death.

Methotrexate

Mechanism of Action

Methotrexate (proprietary name: Rheumatrex) is an anti-metabolite used to treat acute lymphatic leukemia, Hodg-kin lymphoma, mesothelioma, refractory non–small cell carcinoma of the lung, and rheumatoid arthritis.

Methotrexate is a folic acid antagonist. It mimics DNA nucleotides and inhibits the formation of new strands of DNA. It affects rapidly dividing cells, such as bone marrow stem cells and tumor cells.

Dosing and Drug Actions

Methotrexate may be taken orally or intravenously. At low doses, it acts as an immunosuppressant, decreases inflam-mation, and slows progress of rheumatoid arthritis, which can improve physical activity. At much higher doses, metho-trexate acts as an antineoplastic drug for the control and eradication of cancer.

Toxic Effects

Because of the drug's lack of specificity, many adverse reac-tions may occur. At higher doses of methotrexate, adverse reactions are common and include ulcerative colitis and a low white blood cell count. Other toxic effects include bone marrow suppression (e.g., leukopenia, thrombocy-topenia), oral and gastrointestinal effects (e.g., ulceration, glossitis, stomatitis, nausea, vomiting), cirrhosis, pulmo-nary fibrosis, leukoencephalopathy, and increased CSF pressure.

Leflunomide

Mechanism of Action

Leflunomide (proprietary name: Arava) is used to treat rheumatoid arthritis and psoriatic arthritis. Although the exact mechanism of action is not well understood, leflunomide inhibits the formation of DNA nucleotides, interfering with progression of white blood cells through the development cycle.

Dosing and Drug Actions

Leflunomide may be taken orally; initially, a large dose is given every day for several days. A lower maintenance dose is then taken orally every day. At therapeutic doses, leflu-nomide decreases inflammation and slows the progress of rheumatoid arthritis, which can improve the physical activi-ty of patients.

Toxic Effects

A leflunomide overdose may lead to hepatotoxicity.

Chlorambucil

Mechanism of Action

Chlorambucil (proprietary name: Leukeran) is an antineoplastic alkylating agent. It is used to treat chronic lymphocytic leukemia and Hodgkin lymphoma. The drug works by crosslinking DNA and interfering with DNA replication and RNA transcription.

Dosing and Drug Actions

Chlorambucil is taken orally for 3 to 6 weeks for treatment of chronic lymphocytic leukemia and Hodgkin lymphoma.

Toxic Effects

Chlorambucil overdose may lead to infection, polyneuropathy, immunosuppression, and hepatotoxicity.

Summary

TDM measures patients' drug levels to ensure they are receiving enough of a drug for effective treatment but not an amount that could cause harm. Drugs behave differently in different patients, so personalization of drug dosing is important. Therapeutic ranges are the levels at which particular drugs are effective at reducing clinical symptoms.

Many drugs are metabolized by the liver. Factors that affect blood drug levels include absorption from the gastrointestinal tract, availability of the drug after it reaches the systemic circulation, distribution of the drug throughout the body, extent of drug metabolism, and excretion. Drugs can be administered orally, intravenously, intramuscularly, intraperitoneally, topically, or by suppository or inhalation.

It is important to collect samples in the correct tubes to ensure an accurate analysis. Peak and trough levels are determined at specific times before and after the drug is administered. Adherence to these time frames is critical for TDM. Age and pregnancy have an effect on the effective dose of drugs and drug levels.

Review Questions

1. Therapeutic drug monitoring is based on the assumption that
   a. The size of the pharmacologic effect is directly proportional to the amount of drug in the target area.
   b. All drugs are toxic and therefore must be monitored.
   c. The size of the pharmacologic effect is inversely proportional to the amount of drug in the target area.
   d. The drug concentration in blood equals the concentration of the drug in the liver.
2. Pharmacokinetics is the study of
   a. The rate of absorbance, half-life of drugs, steady-state mode, and maintenance doses
   b. Drug administration
   c. The rate of absorbance, distribution, biotransformation, and excretion of a drug
   d. The rate of target activation
3. When a drug is absorbed from the gastrointestinal tract, it goes directly
   a. Into the systemic circulation
   b. To the portal vein
   c. To the target area
   d. Into the urine
4. All the following are involved in determining a drug's distribution pattern EXCEPT
   a. The drug's ability to dissolve in storage lipids
   b. Drug binding to fixed receptors
   c. Drug passing through membranes
   d. Drug resistance to metabolism
5. When is a steady state for a drug reached?
   a. 4 hours
   b. After 4 half-lives

   c. 8 hours
   d. 12 hours
6. Cardiovascular drugs that are monitored by therapeutic drug monitoring include all the following EXCEPT
   a. Tacrolimus
   b. Digoxin
   c. Procainamide
   d. Verapamil
7. Antibiotics that are monitored by therapeutic drug monitoring include all the following EXCEPT
   a. Chloramphenicol
   b. Gentamicin
   c. Tobramycin
   d. Valproic acid
8. Antiepileptic drugs that are monitored by therapeutic drug monitoring include all the following EXCEPT
   a. Phenytoin
   b. Theophylline
   c. Carbamazepine
   d. Ethosuximide
9. Psychoactive drugs that are monitored by therapeutic drug monitoring include all the following EXCEPT
   a. Amitriptyline
   b. Lithium
   c. Primidone
   d. Desipramine
10. Immunosuppressant drugs that are monitored by therapeutic drug monitoring include all the following EXCEPT
    a. Diazepam
    b. Cyclosporine
    c. Tacrolimus
    d. Sirolimus

Critical Thinking Questions

1. Explain the concept of therapeutic drug monitoring and why it is important.
2. How does absorption of a drug play a role in therapeutic drug monitoring?
3. What are toxic effects, and why do they occur?

CASE STUDY

A 62-year-old man is admitted to the hospital with a *Klebsiella pneumoniae* infection. The infection started more than 3 weeks ago. He began to recover and then relapsed 2 days ago with a high fever, lethargy, and a fulminant pneumonia. He went to his physician 2.5 weeks ago and received antibiotics to treat the infection. Because the infection did not get better, he returned to his physician yesterday.

His temperature was 102.5° F, he was coughing up much sputum, and he had severe muscle aches. His physician started him on gentamicin on admission. His trough and peak drug levels were 0.5 mg/dL and 3 mg/dL, respectively. His trough level was determined 1 hour before he received his intravenous dose, and his peak level was determined 2 hours after the drug finished infusing.

What is the therapeutic range for this antibiotic? Are the peak and trough levels accurate? What might the physician do to determine the patient's true peak and trough levels? Are the values within the accepted ranges for trough and peak values? Why or why not?

Bibliography

Beaumont C, Young GC, Cavalier T, Young MA. Human absorption, distribution, metabolism and excretion properties of drug molecules: a plethora of approaches. *Br J Clin Pharm*. 2014;78:1185–1200.

Brill MJ, Diepstraten J, van Rongen A, et al. Impact of obesity on drug metabolism and elimination in adults and children. *Clin Pharm*. 2012;51:277–304.

Costantine MM. Physiologic and pharmacokinetic changes in pregnancy. *Front Pharm*. 2014;5:65.

Estudante M, Morais JG, Soveral G, Benet LZ. Intestinal drug transporters: an overview. *Adv Drug Deliv Rev*. 2013;65:1340–1356.

Gaulton A, Bellis LJ, Bento AP, et al. ChEMBL: a large-scale bioactivity database for drug discovery. *Nucl Acids Res*. 2012;40:D1100–D1107.

Goodman DJ, Rossen RM, Cannom DS, Rider AK, Harrison DC. Effect of digoxin on atrioventricular conduction: studies in patients with and without cardiac autonomic innervation. *Circulation*. 1975;51:251–256.

Gross AS. Best practice in therapeutic drug monitoring. *Br J Clin Pharmacol*. 1998;46:95–99.

Lee WM. Acetaminophen and the U.S. Acute Liver Failure Study Group: lowering the risks of hepatic failure. *Hepatology*. 2004;40:6–9.

Libretto SE. A review of the toxicology of salbutamol (albuterol). *Arch Toxicol*. 1994;68:213–216.

Loebstein R, Lakin A, Koren G. Pharmacokinetic changes during pregnancy and their clinical relevance. *Clin Pharmacokinet*. 1997;33:328–343.

Petrovic M, van der Cammen T, Onder G. Adverse drug reactions in older people. *Drugs Aging*. 2012;29:453–462.

Roberts DJ, Hall RI. Drug absorption, distribution, metabolism and excretion considerations in critically ill adults. *Expert Opin Drug Metab Toxicol*. 2013;9:1067–1084.

Shipkova M, Petrova DT, Rosler AE, et al. Comparability and imprecision of 8 frequently used commercially available immunoassays for therapeutic drug monitoring. *Ther Drug Monit*. 2014;36:433–441.

Soldin OP, Chung SH, Mattison DR. Sex differences in drug disposition. *J Biomed Biotechnol*. 2011;2011:187103.

Stachulski AV, Baillie TA, Kevin Park B, et al. The generation, detection, and effects of reactive drug metabolites. *Med Res Rev*. 2013;33:985–1080.

Welzl K, Kern G, Mayer G, et al. Effect of different immunosuppressive drugs on immune cells from young and old healthy persons. *Gerontology*. 2014;60:229–238.

Wiley 2nd JF, Spiller HA, Krezel EP, Borys DJ. Unintentional albuterol ingestion in children. *Pediatr Emerg Care*. 1994;10:193–196.

Wood DM, Dargan PI. Understanding how data triangulation identifies acute toxicity of novel psychoactive drugs. *J Med Toxicol*. 2012;8:300–303.

Yasiry Z, Shorvon SD. The relative effectiveness of five antiepileptic drugs in treatment of benzodiazepine-resistant convulsive status epilepticus: a meta-analysis of published studies. *Seizure*. 2014;23:167–174.

34

Toxicology

LAIRD C. SHELDAHL AND DONNA LARSON

CHAPTER OUTLINE

OBJECTIVES

After completion of this chapter, the reader will be able to:

1. Compare and contrast the routes of exposure for toxic substances in this chapter.
2. Describe the dose-response relationship.
3. Differentiate acute and chronic toxicity.
4. Differentiate conditions caused by pollutants: secondhand smoke, cigarette smoking, and radiation.
5. Describe the mechanisms of injury for the toxic substances covered in this chapter.
6. Construct a table for the drugs of abuse that contains the name, mechanism of action, health effects, and two methods of analysis for each drug.
7. Describe how drugs and toxic substances are metabolized in the liver.
8. Describe the proper blood collection procedures for legal and medical alcohol analysis.
9. Identify the major active ingredients of marijuana, oxycodone, morphine, barbiturates, methamphetamine, and phencyclidine (PCP).
10. Explain the term *designer drug*.
11. Discuss the importance of properly maintaining the chain of evidence when handling specimens for drug analysis.
12. Discuss the use of immunoassays and mass spectrometry for identifying and quantifying drugs of abuse.
13. Discuss the role of drugs in sexual assaults.

KEY TERMS

Addiction
Bioaccumulation
Chain of custody
Designer drug
Detection window
Dose-response curve
Forensic specimen
Gas chromatography with mass spectrometry

Lethal dose
Lowest observed effect level
Median lethal dose
Methylenedioxymethamphetamine
Neonatal drug testing
No observable effect level
Poison
Postmortem sample
Secondhand smoke

Substance Abuse and Mental Health Services Administration
Tolerance
Toxic dose
Toxicity

◆ Case in Point

A 65-year-old man was found unconscious in his home on a cold, snowy day. He was unconscious but alive and was brought to the emergency department. His laboratory results were as follows: sodium, 142 mEq/L; potassium, 4.2 mEq/L; chloride, 102 mEq/L; total carbon dioxide, 32 mg/dL; calcium, 9.6 mg/dL; phosphorus, 3.7 mg/dL; pH, 7.40; Pco_2, 32 mm Hg, Po_2, 95 mm Hg, bicarbonate (HCO_3^-), 25 mEq/L, and carboxyhemoglobin, 20%. What condition does this man have? What is the likely cause? How could it have been prevented? Why does this condition lead to death?

Points to Remember

- Among the thousands of chemicals that have toxic effects on the body, approximately 24 common drugs or toxins account for 80% of emergency department visits each year.
- Anticholinergic, cholinergic, opioid, sedative-hypnotic, and sympathomimetic toxidromes are common.
- A chemical's physical state (i.e., solid, liquid, or gas) and the route of exposure influence toxicity.

- Injection is a common route for introduction of toxic substances into blood.
- Most drugs and toxins exhibit a dose-response curve; low doses produce no observable effects, but the effects increase as the dose increases.
- Blood and urine are the most commonly analyzed specimens in toxicology. More information about drug and alcohol levels can be obtained from them than from other specimen types.
- A negative screening test result reliably indicates that there are no drugs in the specimen, but a positive test result should be considered presumptive until a confirmatory test (i.e., more specific test method) is performed.
- Gas chromatography with mass spectrometry (GC-MS) is often used to confirm and quantitate positive screening test results.
- Chemicals that increase the osmol gap include ethanol, methanol, isopropanol, acetone, and ethylene glycol.
- According to the U.S. Surgeon General's report, people who inhale secondhand smoke increase their risk of arthrosclerosis, myocardial infarction, cerebrovascular accidents, and lung cancer.

TABLE 34-1	Comparison of Pharmacology and Toxicology
Pharmacology	**Toxicology**
Pharmacology is the study of the origin, nature, chemistry, effects, and use of drugs.	*Toxicology* is the study of the adverse effects of chemicals on health.
Dose is the amount of a drug absorbed from an administration.	*Dose* is the amount of a chemical absorbed from a chemical exposure.
A drug can be administered one time or on a short-term or long-term basis.	*Exposure* is contact with a chemical. Exposure can be one time or occur on a short-term or long-term basis.
A *dose-response curve* graphically represents the relationship between the dose of a drug and the response elicited.	A *dose-response curve* describes the relationship of the body's response to different amounts of an agent such as a drug or toxin.
Routes of administration include oral, intramuscular, intravenous, dermal, or topical.	*Routes of entry* are ingestion, inhalation, or dermal absorption.
Drugs have therapeutic responses (desirable effects) and side effects (undesirable effects). Beyond the therapeutic dose, a drug may become toxic.	Only toxic effects are of concern. *Toxicity* is the degree to which a chemical damages an organ system, disrupts a biochemical process, or disturbs an enzyme system.
Potency is the amount of drug required to produce the desired response.	*Potency* of a toxic chemical is the amount it takes to elicit a toxic effect compared with other chemicals.
Biologic monitoring is done for some drugs. Clotting time is monitored in patients taking anticoagulants such as warfarin. Drug levels are measured for some drugs such as digoxin.	*Biologic monitoring* is done for some toxic exposures, such as blood lead levels or metabolites of chemicals such as cotinine found in tobacco smoke.

Courtesy B. Sattler, Environmental Health Education Center, University of Maryland School of Nursing, 1998.

- According to the U.S. Surgeon General, cigarette smoking is linked to chronic obstructive pulmonary disease, lung cancer, colorectal cancer, acute myeloid leukemia, liver cancer, chronic lung infections, kidney cancer, and lip cancer.
- Ionizing radiation causes the most damage to tissues undergoing rapid cell division (e.g., bone marrow, lymphoid tissues, gastrointestinal tract, skin).
- Accumulation of toxic methanol metabolites (e.g., formic acid, lactic acid) causes metabolic acidosis, blindness, and respiratory failure.
- Isopropanol and its metabolite acetone are central nervous system depressants.
- Ethylene glycol is a parent compound that exerts most of its toxicity by conversion to metabolites such as glycolaldehyde, glycolic acid, and glyoxylic acid.
- Carbon monoxide is called the *silent killer*. It is odorless, tasteless, and colorless. It binds tightly to hemoglobin, preventing oxygen from being carried throughout the body to nourish organs, and the person dies.
- Since the advent of the industrial age, workers have become exposed to toxic metals such as aluminum, arsenic, chromium, cadmium, lead, mercury, and beryllium. Exposure injures tissues.
- Legal and illegal drugs are abused to provide a desired effect. In addition to acute toxic effects, many drugs of abuse have a high potential for addiction and tolerance. The major drugs of abuse used recreationally are amphetamine, methamphetamine, methylenedioxymethamphetamine (MDMA), cocaine, marijuana, phencyclidine, codeine, morphine, methadone, propoxyphene, barbiturates, benzodiazepines, ethanol, hydromorphone, hydrocodone, and oxycodone.
- Drug-facilitated sexual assault occurs when alcohol and drugs are used to incapacitate the victim. Associated drugs include benzodiazepines (e.g., flunitrazepam, diazepam, triazolam, temazepam, clonazepam), choral hydrate, sedative-hypnotics (e.g., zopiclone, eszopiclone, zolpidem, zaleplon), γ-hydroxybutyric acid (GHB), dextromethorphan, and phencyclidine.

Introduction

Toxicology is the study of the adverse effects of chemicals on the body and includes the symptoms, mechanisms, detection methods, and treatment of poisons (Table 34-1). Of the thousands of chemicals that can cause toxic effects, approximately 24 common drugs or toxins account for 80% of emergency department visits each year.

Each laboratory chooses its own drug-testing menu based on the local pattern of drug use and the laboratory's resources. Drug testing is valuable in the workplace, in competitive sports, during pregnancy, for drug exposure and withdrawal in newborns, for pain management and drug rehabilitation programs, and in situations that require a prompt diagnosis of toxicity so that proper treatment or an antidote can be given.

When an individual arrives in the emergency department, clinical information can help guide test selection and interpretation. Useful clinical information includes time and date of suspected exposure, time and date of specimen

TABLE 34-2	Symptoms of Important Toxidromes
Toxidrome	**Symptoms**
Anticholinergic	Agitation, blurred vision, decreased bowel sounds, dry skin, fever, flushing, hallucinations, ileus, lethargy, coma, mydriasis, myoclonus, psychosis, seizures, tachycardia, urinary retention
Cholinergic	Diarrhea, meiosis, bradycardia, bronchorrhea, emesis, lacrimation, salivation, urination
Opioid	Bradycardia, decreased bowel sounds, hypotension, hypothermia, lethargy, coma, meiosis, shallow respirations, slow respiratory rate
Sedative-hypnotic	Ataxia, blurred vision, confusion, diplopia, dysesthesias, hypotension, lethargy, coma, nystagmus, respiratory depression, sedation, slurred speech
Sympathomimetic	Agitation, diaphoresis, excessive motor activity, excessive speech, hallucinations, hypertension, hyperthermia, insomnia, restlessness, tachycardia, tremor

collection, collection procedures, patient history, and evaluation of the patient's current physical condition.

The patient's physical condition and symptoms can aid identification of the drug or toxin. Each substance produces a specific toxic syndrome (i.e., toxidrome) when a large amount of the chemical is introduced into the body. Symptoms may overlap, making identification difficult. Anticholinergic, cholinergic, opioid, sedative-hypnotic, and sympathomimetic toxidromes are common (Table 34-2).

Routes of Exposure

A chemical's physical state (i.e., solid, liquid, or gas) and the route of exposure influence toxicity. The chemical's state often determines the route of exposure. For example, gases are usually absorbed by the lungs or eyes, not the intestines. For many chemicals, the toxic effects occur at the site of absorption. The site of exposure may also affect the dose of the chemical that enters the body. Toxins enter the body through the skin, gastrointestinal tract, and lungs (Box 34-1).

Skin

Toxins enter the body through the skin (i.e., transdermal absorption). The epithelial (outer or epidermal) layer of the skin, unlike the lungs or gastrointestinal tract, is specialized to provide protection, and it often proves to be an adequate barrier to toxic chemicals. The skin is more permeable to fat-soluble chemicals (e.g., organic solvents) than water-soluble ones. Chemicals in contact with the skin can cause local effects, and they may enter the circulation through broken or intact skin and cause effects throughout the body. Skin exposure can have delayed-onset systemic effects compared with entry through the lungs, which rapidly produces systemic effects due to quick entry of toxins into the bloodstream. Broken skin (e.g., a cut) allows toxic substances to penetrate the epidermis and quickly enter the bloodstream.

• BOX 34-1 Toxin Exposure Routes

Dermal (skin)
Ingestion (stomach, digestive tract)
Inhalation (respiratory tract)

Gastrointestinal Tract

Toxic substances are ingested deliberately or accidentally. Many physical factors affect their absorption. After a chemical is absorbed, its effects depend on its concentration in target organs, chemical and physical form, distribution, metabolism, and length of time in the target tissue.

Lungs

Gases, vapors, airborne particulates, and aerosols are inhaled. Toxic gases damage the respiratory mucosa, causing burning pain, irritation, and increased secretions.

Inhalation, which is the fastest route for toxins to enter the systemic circulation, produces toxic effects throughout the body. The alveolar epithelium is highly specialized for absorption of gases into and out of the blood. Damage caused by a toxic gas is determined by the concentration of toxic gas in the air, size of gas molecules, solubility of gas in the blood, respiratory rate, condition of the respiratory tract (i.e., healthy person or chronic smoker), and length of exposure.

Other Routes

Injections can introduce toxic substances into the blood. Methods include intravenous injections (i.e., into a vein), intramuscular injections (i.e., into a muscle), intraperitoneal injections (i.e., into the abdominal cavity), intradermal injections (i.e., into the skin), and subcutaneous injections (i.e., under the skin). These routes are commonly used for drugs of abuse.

The eye, especially the cornea, is a common point of contact for toxic substances. Toxic substances can be splashed into the eye, or toxic gases can come in contact with the eye. Acids and bases can damage eye tissue after being splashed into the eye. Small amounts of damage are repaired by the epithelial cells of the cornea, but higher amounts may lead to blindness and a need for tissue transplantation. Because eye tissue is exposed to the environment (e.g., in an office, outdoors), toxic gases in the air may come in contact with the eye.

Dose-Response Relationship

Any chemical, even water, is toxic at a high enough dose (i.e., hyponatremia). Most drugs and toxins exhibit a **dose-response curve.** Low doses may produce no observable effect, but the effects increase as the dose increases. This curve is different for each drug or toxin. A generic dose-response curve is provided in Figure 34-1.

Studying the dose-response relationship and building models to better visualize it are essential for defining safe and hazardous drug dosages. Curve construction considers the exposure time and exposure route. The curve is plotted with the logarithm of the drug concentration on the x axis and response effect on the y axis.

When the U.S. Food and Drug Administration (FDA) sets guidelines for safe levels of exposure, absolute values are used. The values, which depend on many variables, are used for risk assessment. If the measured effect is death, the safe level may be set to the **no observable effect level** (NOEL), which is the highest dose of a drug or chemical at which no response is measured (Fig. 34-2). For less serious outcomes, the **lowest observed effect level** (LOEL) may be of interest; it is the dose at which an effect is first measured. For measurement of adverse effects, the terms *no observable adverse effect level* (NOAEL) and *low observed adverse effect level* (NOAEL) are used. For a given substance, the levels are estimates based on limited human exposure data or calculations based on experimental trials involving rats or mice.

A few chemicals have no well-defined safe level of exposure and are treated with special care. For instance, for some people with peanut allergies, any level of exposure above zero triggers a life-threatening allergic reaction. These particularly toxic chemicals are often referred to as **poisons,** which means that they have very serious effects at very low levels. These substances are discussed in terms of their **toxicity,** which is the degree to which they cause damage in the body.

Some chemicals exhibit **bioaccumulation** (i.e., they are stored rather than excreted from the body), and they receive special consideration. For some chemicals, particularly endocrine disruptors (i.e., chemicals that mimic or inhibit hormones), the classic dose-response relationship is not seen. Instead, small doses may have the opposite effect, or a more intense effect, than higher doses.

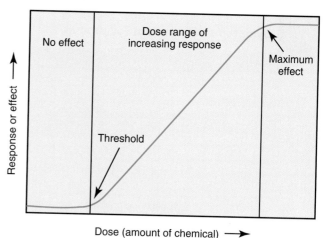

• **Figure 34-1** Dose-response curve.

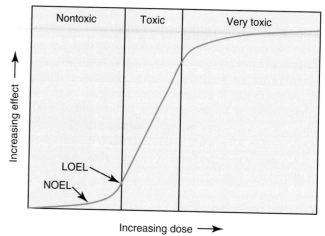

• **Figure 34-2** Dose-response curve shows the no observable effect level (NOEL), lowest observed effect level (LOEL), and the nontoxic, toxic, and very toxic levels for a particular drug.

Acute and Chronic Toxicity

The **toxic dose** (TD) of a chemical is the amount of the chemical that produces a toxic effect. The **lethal dose** (LD) is the amount of the chemical or agent that causes death.

The acute toxicity of a substance is expressed as the **median lethal dose** (LD_{50}). The LD_{50} is the amount of a chemical capable of killing one half of the members of a tested population. Because human testing is rarely possible or desirable, most LD_{50} values are determined using animals and extrapolated to humans.

Acute Toxicity

Acute toxicity is the term used to describe the adverse effects of a chemical that result from a single exposure or from multiple exposures in a short amount of time (<24 hours). Adverse effects usually occur within 14 days after exposure.

Chronic Toxicity

Chronic toxicity is continuous or repeated exposure that produces toxic effects. An example is continuous exposure of individuals to lead in a plant that makes batteries. The workers are exposed to lead vapor and possibly to lead oxide (a solid). Inhaling lead vapor or ingesting lead oxide can lead to chronic lead toxicity (discussed later).

Specimen Collecting and Handling

Blood and urine are the most commonly analyzed specimens in toxicology. The detection window is the time in which a drug or chemical can be detected in fluids after acute exposure. Drugs are detected in blood on a scale of hours, whereas they can be detected in urine on a scale of days.

Routine Collection Procedures

More information about drug and alcohol levels is derived from blood and urine samples than other sources. Postmortem samples, which are samples collected after death (i.e., forensic toxicology), may involve other fluids, including the vitreous humor of the eye, stomach contents, or cerebrospinal fluid. Tissues, especially liver, kidney, brain, and lung tissue, also may be sampled.

Urine is the specimen of choice for screening for drugs of abuse. A single urine specimen typically is used for drug testing. Many methods may be used to mask or adulterate specimens to avoid detection, such as substituting urine from a drug-free person, diluting urine by drinking lots of water or using a diuretic before providing a sample, and directly adding water to a sample to dilute it. Other substances, such as detergent, bleach, salt, alkali, ammonia, tetrahydrozoline, acid, nitrite, chromate, peroxide, peroxidase, and glutaraldehyde, may be added to a specimen to interfere with testing.

To ensure an unadulterated specimen, many measures are put in place. Another person often accompanies the individual submitting a urine sample to observe the specimen collection. A coloring agent (usually blue) is added to toilet water. There are limitations on clothing allowed in the specimen collection area. Temperature strips are applied to specimens immediately after collection to record their temperature, and hot water faucets are inactivated in the collection room.

The U.S. Department of Transportation (DOT) has set rules for specimen collection, processing, transportation, testing, and storage for drug testing their employees and prospective employees. Testing programs for athletes are usually more extensive than those for the DOT.

The first test ordered when an overdose is suspected is a screening test. Screening tests have good clinical sensitivity but lack specificity. A negative test result means that there is a good probability that no drugs are in the specimen, but a positive test result should be considered presumptive until a confirmatory test (i.e., more specific method) is performed.

Gas chromatography with mass spectrometry (GC-MS) is often used to confirm and quantitate the results of

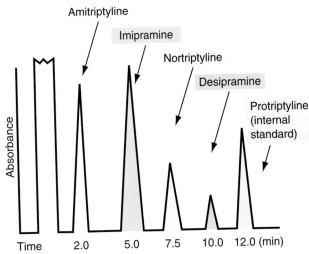

• **Figure 34-3** Typical separation of the major tricyclic antidepressants on high-performance liquid chromatography. Complete separation can be effected in 12 minutes. The concentration of each drug is on the order of 100 μg/mL. (From McPherson RA, Pincus MR: *Henry's Clinical Diagnosis and Management by Laboratory Methods.* 22nd ed. Philadelphia: Elsevier; 2012.)

• **BOX 34-2 MUDPILES Mnemonic for Remembering Causes of an Increased Anion Gap**

Methanol
Uremia
Diabetic ketoacidosis
Paraldehyde
Iron, inhalants (e.g., carbon monoxide, cyanide, toluene), isoniazid, ibuprofen
Lactic acidosis
Ethylene glycol, ethanol ketoacidosis
Salicylates, starvation ketoacidosis, sympathomimetics

From Burtis CA, Bruns DE. *Tietz Fundamentals of Clinical Chemistry and Molecular Diagnostics.* 7th ed. St. Louis: Saunders; 2015.

---

a positive screening test result. The GC separates chemicals based on their volatility, or ease with which they evaporate. MS is used to identify chemicals based on their mass-to-charge ratio. GC-MS is more time-consuming and costly than immunoassays, but it is quantitatively much more accurate. High-pressure liquid chromatography (HPLC) can also be used to confirm and quantitate drugs of abuse after a positive screening test result (Fig. 34-3).

The anion gap test is useful for investigating the cause of a toxidrome. An increased anion gap indicates an increase in unmeasured anions in the specimen. The acronym MUDPILES is used to remember the drugs that produce an increased anion gap (Box 34-2). The calculated osmolality is often compared with the measured osmolality in toxicology. The main ions and substances measured in serum and urine specimens are sodium (Na+), chloride (Cl−), bicarbonate

(HCO_3^-), glucose, and urea. The following equation is used to calculate osmolality:

$$\text{Osmolality (Osm/kg)} = \\ 2\,[Na^+]\,(mEq/L) + \text{glucose (mg/dL)} / \\ 18 + \text{urea (mg/dL)} / 2.8$$

The osmol gap is the difference between observed osmolality and calculated osmolality. Chemicals that increase the osmol gap include ethanol, methanol, isopropanol, acetone, and ethylene glycol. Because alcohols are volatile, freezing point depression is the method of choice for measuring osmolality.

Forensic specimens are used in civil or criminal cases, and they require highly standardized protocols for specimen collection. Similarly, federal workplace drug testing requirements mandate strict technical protocols, which are published by the U.S. Department of Health and Human Services (HHS), for the collection of specimens. In both situations, collectors must ensure the integrity of samples and strictly adhere to collection protocols for samples to be considered as evidence. Forensic testing also details procedures for the proper handling and sampling of debris and clothing from the donor.

Neonatal drug testing may be called for when mothers are suspected of abusing drugs during pregnancy. Fetal exposure to drugs can cause low birth weight, premature birth, and impaired neurologic functioning. Drug-addicted mothers are more likely to abuse or neglect children. Specimens are collected within 24 hours after the birth.

Chain of Custody

The chain of custody is a process for maintaining control of and accountability for each specimen from the point of collection to its final destination. This requires documentation of every individual handling the sample using a chain of custody form. Specimens must be placed in a permanently sealed, tamper-evident container. Some laboratories use tamper-proof tape on the containers. The tape is colored, and if the tape is removed, the color coating stays on the container, and the tape becomes clear. Every individual who handles a sample must sign the chain of custody form. Without these forms, later allegations of tampering or misconduct may compromise prosecution toward acquittal or overturn a guilty verdict on appeal.

Conditions Caused by Pollutants

Pollutants are substances in air or water that injure people on exposure. Pollutants can produce short-term, acute effects or long-term, chronic effects. Outdoor air pollutants are usually produced by industrial plants, waste incinerators, or facilities that burn fossil fuels. Air pollutants can manifest as smog (i.e., smoky fog), especially in large cities with vehicle emissions and industrial plants. Some chemicals released into the atmosphere undergo photochemical and other reactions to produce more hazardous substances (e.g., ozone).

Indoor pollutants can produce similar health results. Indoor pollutants include secondhand smoke, cigarette smoke, radon, carbon monoxide, radiation, and common household products (Table 34-3).

TABLE 34-3	Sources of Home Pollution	
Agent	**Description**	**Sources in Home**
Radon	Colorless, odorless, radioactive gas from the natural breakdown (radioactive decay) of uranium; radon may cause up to 36,000 lung cancer deaths per year	Soil or rock under the home, well water, building materials
Asbestos	Mineral fiber used extensively in building materials for insulation and as a fire retardant; deteriorated asbestos should be removed by professionals; exposure to asbestos fibers can cause irreversible and often fatal lung diseases, including cancer	Sprayed-on acoustical ceilings or textured paint, pipe and furnace insulation materials, floor tiles, automobile brakes and clutches
Biologic contaminants	Bacteria, mold and mildew, viruses, animal dander and saliva, dust mites, and pollen can cause infectious diseases or allergic reactions; moisture and dust levels in the home should be kept as low as possible	Mold and mildew, standing water or water-damaged materials, humidifiers, house plants, household pets, ventilation systems, household dust
Indoor combustion	Produces harmful gases (carbon monoxide, nitrogen dioxide), particles, and organic compounds (benzene); health effects range from irritation to the eyes, nose, and throat to lung cancer; outdoor ventilation of gas appliances minimizes risks	Tobacco smoke, unvented kerosene or gas space heaters, unvented kitchen gas stoves, wood stoves or fireplaces, leaking exhaust flues from gas furnaces and clothes dryers, car exhaust from an attached garage
Household products	Can contain potentially harmful organic compounds; health effects vary greatly; elimination of household chemicals by use of nontoxic alternatives or by using only in well-ventilated rooms or outside minimizes risks	Cleaning products, paint supplies, stored fuels, hobby products, personal care products, mothballs, air fresheners, dry-cleaned clothes

TABLE 34-3	Sources of Home Pollution—cont'd	
Agent	**Description**	**Sources in Home**
Formaldehyde	Released into the air as a colorless gas; can cause eye, nose, throat, and respiratory system irritation, headaches, nausea, and fatigue; may be central nervous system depressant and causes cancer in laboratory animals; remove sources of formaldehyde from the home if health effects occur	Widely used in particleboard, plywood, and fiberboard in cabinets, furniture, subflooring, and paneling; carpeting, durable-press drapes, other textiles; urea-formaldehyde insulation; glues and adhesives
Pesticides	Insecticides, termiticides, rodenticides, and fungicides contain toxic organic compounds; exposure to high levels of pesticides can damage the liver and central nervous system and increase cancer risks; when possible, nonchemical methods of pest control should be used; if the use of pesticides is unavoidable they should be used strictly according to the manufacturer's directions	Contaminated soil or dust that is tracked in from outside; stored pesticide containers; residue if used inside
Lead	A long-recognized harmful environmental pollutant; fetuses, infants, and children are more vulnerable to toxic effects; if the community health nurse suspects that a home has lead paint, it should be tested	Lead-based paint that is peeling, sanded, or burned; automobile exhaust; lead in drinking water; contaminated soil; food contaminated by lead from lead-based ceramic cookware or pottery; lead-related hobbies or occupations; folk remedies

From Maurer FA, Smith CM. *Community/Public Health Nursing*. 5th ed. St. Louis: Saunders; 2013.

Secondhand Smoke

Secondhand smoke is produced by lit cigarettes and exhaled by smokers. According to the U.S. Surgeon General's report, people who inhale secondhand smoke increase their risk of arthrosclerosis, myocardial infarction, cerebrovascular accidents (CVAs), and lung cancer (Fig. 34-4). Clinical chemistry tests aid in the detection of arthrosclerosis, myocardial infarction, and CVAs. Lipid measurements are important for the detection of arthrosclerosis (see Chapter 17). Myocardial infarction is diagnosed with tests for creatine kinase isoenzymes (e.g., CK-MB), troponin I, and troponin T levels (see Chapter 18). CVAs are usually diagnosed with computed tomography (CT) or magnetic resonance imaging (MRI). Clinical chemistry tests are not used for diagnosing CVAs.

Cigarette Smoke

Since 1964, the U.S. Surgeon General has been warning individuals that smoking is hazardous to their health. Cigarette smoking is linked to chronic obstructive pulmonary disease (COPD), lung cancer, colorectal cancer, acute myeloid leukemia, liver cancer, chronic lung infections, kidney cancer, and lip cancer. Cancer is definitively diagnosed with a biopsy, and clinical chemistry tests are not used for this purpose.

COPD occurs when the toxic chemicals in cigarette smoke damage the bronchi and lung tissue (see Chapter 19). The damage impairs uptake of oxygen and discharge of carbon dioxide by the lungs. Blood gas results for these individuals show a chronic respiratory acidosis because their lungs retain carbon dioxide.

Radiation

Radiation, which is the emission of energy as electromagnetic waves or as high-energy particles that cause ionization, is encountered by the human body in the environment and in medical settings (Fig. 34-5). Three types of radiation are alpha particles, beta particles, and gamma rays. Radiation is emitted in many forms, such as sunlight and radio waves. High-energy radiation poses the most risk to tissue. Ionizing radiation consists of particles, x-rays, or gamma rays with sufficient energy to cause damage to tissues, especially those undergoing rapid cell division (e.g., bone marrow, lymphoid tissues, gastrointestinal tract, skin).

The short, high-frequency wavelengths in the ultraviolet portion of the spectrum have the most energy and the highest ionization potential. Because sunlight can cause skin damage and cancer, sunscreens containing chemicals that block ultraviolet rays are applied.

Gamma rays penetrate deep into the body and can injure tissues. Radiation sickness results from intense exposure to gamma rays and is characterized by bone marrow and lymphoid failure, severe diarrhea, and skin blisters. Survivors of the atomic bomb blasts of Hiroshima and Nagasaki in 1945, the Chernobyl nuclear plant disaster in 1986, and the Fukushima power plant disaster in 2011 suffered from exposure to high doses of radiation and radiation sickness. This disease is usually diagnosed clinically, and clinical chemistry tests are not used.

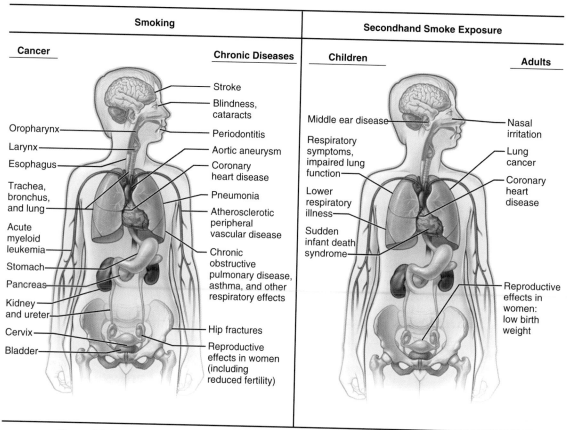

Smoking		Secondhand Smoke Exposure	
Cancer	**Chronic Diseases**	**Children**	**Adults**

Smoking – Cancer:
Oropharynx
Larynx
Esophagus
Trachea, bronchus, and lung
Acute myeloid leukemia
Stomach
Pancreas
Kidney and ureter
Cervix
Bladder

Smoking – Chronic Diseases:
Stroke
Blindness, cataracts
Periodontitis
Aortic aneurysm
Coronary heart disease
Pneumonia
Atherosclerotic peripheral vascular disease
Chronic obstructive pulmonary disease, asthma, and other respiratory effects
Hip fractures
Reproductive effects in women (including reduced fertility)

Secondhand Smoke Exposure – Children:
Middle ear disease
Respiratory symptoms, impaired lung function
Lower respiratory illness
Sudden infant death syndrome

Secondhand Smoke Exposure – Adults:
Nasal irritation
Lung cancer
Coronary heart disease
Reproductive effects in women: low birth weight

• **Figure 34-4** Adverse effects of tobacco smoking and exposure to secondhand smoke. (From U.S. Department of Health and Human Services: *How Tobacco Smoke Causes Disease: The Biology and Behavioral Basis for Smoking-Attributable Disease: A Report of the Surgeon General.* Atlanta: U.S. Department of Health and Human Services, Centers for Disease Control and Prevention, National Center for Chronic Disease Prevention and Health Promotion, Office on Smoking and Health; 2010. <http://www.surgeongeneral.gov/library/reports/tobaccosmoke/executivesummary.pdf> Accessed 27.08.15.)

Toxic Agents

Methanol

Methanol (i.e., methyl alcohol or wood alcohol) is a colorless liquid and is a common household solvent. It is also found in antifreeze, paints, illegal moonshine, and as a denaturant in ethyl alcohol and diesel fuel. Laboratory tests that are useful for detecting methanol intoxication include renal tests (including anion gap) and measurements of serum osmolality, serum amylase, and serum methanol.

Exposure Routes

Methanol may be ingested (accidentally or intentionally when mixed with ethanol), absorbed through the skin, or inhaled. Methanol usually is not used for suicide attempts. Instead, accidental overdoses are seen in children who ingest antifreeze (which tastes sweet), perfumes, paint solvents, and windshield-washing fluids; in alcoholics who substitute it for ethanol or drink moonshine; and in industrial workers who inhale it.

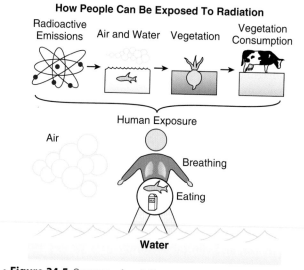

How People Can Be Exposed To Radiation

Radioactive Emissions → Air and Water → Vegetation → Vegetation Consumption

Human Exposure

Air
Breathing
Eating
Water

• **Figure 34-5** Sources of radiation exposure. (Modified from Centers for Disease Control and Prevention/National Center for Environmental Health. *Radiation Studies.* Atlanta: U.S. Department of Health and Human Services, Centers for Disease Control and Prevention; 1993.)

Mechanism of Action

Methanol is quickly absorbed after ingestion and is metabolized in the liver into formaldehyde. Formaldehyde has a half-life of 1 to 2 minutes and is then is metabolized to formic acid. Formic acid is further metabolized to carbon dioxide and water. The metabolism of formic acid is a slow process, which allows it to accumulate in the body and produce metabolic acidosis. People who ingest methanol develop blindness as a result of the buildup of formic acid in the optic nerve.

Methanol has two primary mechanisms of action. First, it acts as a central nervous system (CNS) depressant similar to ethyl alcohol. Second, methanol is converted by liver enzymes to the toxic metabolites formaldehyde and formic acid. Pharmacologic blockade of the liver enzyme alcohol dehydrogenase may slow or reduce the toxic effects of methanol.

Health Effects

Symptoms usually appear 12 to 24 hours after ingestion, even though methanol levels peak 30 to 90 minutes after ingestion. Initial effects are similar to those of ethanol intoxication (e.g., disinhibition, ataxia). Later effects of methanol ingestion or inhalation include blurred vision, headache, dizziness, tachycardia, and confusion, followed by unconsciousness and death at significant doses. The accumulation of toxic metabolites (e.g., formic acid, lactic acid) causes metabolic acidosis, blindness, and respiratory failure. More than 90% of patients have died or survived with permanent damage when formic acid levels were greater than 17.5 mmol/L, lactic acid levels were greater than 7 mmol/L, or the pH was less than 6.87. Injury to the eyes occurs when serum methanol levels exceed 20 mg/dL. Some long-term survivors of methanol poisoning have developed parkinsonian motor impairment.

Toxic Levels

As little as 4 mL (20 mg/dL) of methanol can cause permanent blindness. The toxic level for humans varies with age, size, liver function, and ethanol tolerance. For infants, 15 mL is a lethal dose. For adults, the minimum lethal dose is 1 mg/kg of body weight.

Methanol poisoning depends on the amount of methanol consumed and the degree of metabolic acidosis that results. The more severe the acidosis, the worse the prognosis. The prognosis also depends on the concentration of formic acid in the blood. The blood level of formic acid correlates directly with morbidity and mortality. Long-term improvement is not expected in patients with neurologic symptoms.

Analytical Methods

The patient may supply an accurate history to identify methanol intoxication. Otherwise, plasma methanol levels are determined with GC-MS.

Isopropanol

Isopropanol is commonly used as a solvent and disinfectant. It is also found in mouthwashes, skin lotions, rubbing alcohol, and hand sanitizers. It can be used as an ethanol substitute.

Exposure Routes

After isopropanol is ingested, it is rapidly absorbed through the gastrointestinal tract and reaches peak serum levels in 30 to 120 minutes. It is metabolized in the liver to acetone, which reaches peak levels approximately 4 hours after ingestion. Because acetone is slowly eliminated, it tends to accumulate in the body.

Mechanism of Action

Isopropanol and its metabolite acetone are CNS depressants.

Health Effects

Isopropanol has twice the CNS depressant action of ethanol. Fatality from isolated isopropyl alcohol toxicity is rare. Acute inhalation of isopropanol can produce CNS depression. Although fatality from isopropanol is rare, it has been implicated in the deaths of some adults, particularly alcoholics.

Toxic Levels

The estimated lethal dose of isopropanol for humans is 250 mL. Children and adults who consumed much larger doses have survived with treatment.

Analytical Methods

Plasma isopropanol levels and urine acetone levels may be measured to determine a patient's status. HPLC and GC-MS can be used to quantitate isopropanol and acetone levels.

Ethylene Glycol

Ethylene glycol is an organic solvent widely used in antifreeze and as a precursor molecule for polymers. Its sweet taste makes it a danger to accidental ingestion by children and animals.

Exposure Routes

Ethylene glycol is primarily ingested, often as an erroneous substitute for ethyl alcohol. It is readily absorbed by the gastrointestinal tract.

Mechanism of Action

Ethylene glycol itself is nontoxic. The major toxicities result from its metabolites glycolaldehyde, glycolic acid, and glyoxylic acid and from the small amounts of oxalic acid and formic acid produced. Oxalic acid precipitates in urine as calcium oxalate crystals. Finding these crystals in the urine of an overdose patient can provide an important clue about the toxin. Glycolic acid has the highest blood level of any metabolite, and its concentration correlates directly with symptoms and mortality rates. The high anion gap seen in ethylene glycol poisoning and metabolic acidosis mostly result from glycolic acid.

Health Effects

The main symptoms of acute ethylene glycol poisoning are anuria and necrosis that leads to kidney failure. Other symptoms are nausea, vomiting, myoclonus, seizures, convulsions, depressed reflexes, and coma. Acute effects start with CNS depression (including dizziness, respiratory depression, and unconsciousness), which can be mistaken for ethanol intoxication, followed by depression of heart function and kidney failure. Ingestion of sufficient amounts can be fatal if untreated.

Toxic Levels

The oral lethal dose is 786 mg/kg for humans. This equates to approximately 100 g of ethylene glycol.

Analytical Methods

Ethylene glycol poisoning is diagnosed by measuring ethylene glycol and glycolic acid by HPLC.

Formaldehyde

Formaldehyde is a colorless, water-soluble gas. It is a byproduct of combustion. It has been widely used commercially as a disinfectant (i.e., as a mixture of water and formaldehyde known as formalin) and as a fixative for tissue specimens. The use of formaldehyde has decreased because it is a known carcinogen. It is still used commercially to produce building materials and some household products and in histology and pathology laboratories.

Exposure Routes

Formaldehyde gas may be inhaled, causing toxic or carcinogenic effects, or be absorbed by the skin, producing sensitivity reactions.

Mechanism of Action

Formaldehyde is chemically reactive and can cause immediate damage to mucous membranes or skin. Its reactivity and ability to permeate the skin allow formaldehyde to come into contact with cells and readily interact with DNA, causing mutations and carcinogenesis.

Health Effects

Exposure to formaldehyde gas causes burning of the eyes and irritates mucous membranes. Its pungent odor is detectable in trace amounts, which can limit accidental acute exposure. Large acute exposures can damage mucous membranes of the respiratory and gastrointestinal tracts.

Chronic exposure can produce hypersensitivity reactions. It is listed by the U.S. Environmental Protection Agency (EPA) as a probable carcinogen, which means that there is limited but very good evidence that it causes cancer in humans.

Toxic Levels

Formaldehyde is listed as a class B carcinogen by the EPA. Toxic oral doses are not described.

Analytical Methods

Plasma formaldehyde levels are quantitated by HPLC or GC-MS

Benzene

Benzene is a colorless liquid. It is an aromatic hydrocarbon that is a natural constituent of crude oil and most other petrochemicals (e.g., gasoline). It is a ubiquitous component of automobile engine exhaust and tobacco smoke.

Exposure Routes

Exposure of the general population occurs mainly through inhaling benzene fumes. Benzene is a colorless to light yellow liquid with an aromatic odor. Liquid benzene can be ingested or absorbed through the skin or eyes.

Mechanism of Action

Benzene is metabolized to phenolic compounds, which are transported to the bone marrow and converted to reactive oxygen species. The reactive oxygen species cause DNA strand breaks, mitotic recombinations, chromosome translocations, and aneuploidy (i.e., abnormal number of chromosomes in a cell). These changes foster development of a leukemic clone or destroy precursor cells, leading to aplastic anemia.

Health Effects

Benzene is not generally regarded as an acutely toxic material. Acute exposure results in irritated eyes, skin, nose, and respiratory system; dizziness, headache, and a staggered gait; nausea, anorexia, weakness, and exhaustion; and dermatitis and bone marrow depression. With petrochemicals such as gasoline, the primary acute danger is aspiration (i.e., entry into the lungs). Vomiting should not be induced after accidental ingestion of petrochemicals because it can increase the chance of aspiration.

Benzene is a potent human carcinogen. Chronic exposure can lead to several malignancies, especially leukemia. Chronic benzene exposure may also lead to aplastic anemia.

Toxic Levels

Oral toxicity occurs at a concentration of 0.03 mg/m^3. The U.S. Occupational Safety and Health Administration (OSHA) and EPA have set limits on benzene exposure in the workplace and drinking water, respectively, to limit chronic exposure.

Analytical Methods

Benzene can be measured in breath, blood, or urine, but testing is usually limited to the first 24 hours after exposure due to rapid removal through biotransformation in tissues and by the respiratory system. It is more common to monitor airborne benzene levels. Benzene is measured using GC-MS.

Xylene

Xylene is a liquid aromatic hydrocarbon that is created along with benzene and toluene by extraction during petroleum refining. Xylene is one of the top 30 chemicals produced in the United States in terms of volume. It is used as a solvent in many industries and laboratories (e.g., for removal of immersion oil from microscope slides). It may leak into and contaminate groundwater and soil, and it is a component of automobile pollution.

Exposure Routes

Xylene is likely to be inhaled from contaminated air, paint fumes, and cigarette smoke. Xylene exposure may also be dermal, especially if the skin comes in contact with gasoline. Due to xylene's highly lipophilic nature, it is readily absorbed across biologic membranes.

Mechanism of Action

Acute reactions result from to xylene's ability to dissolve lipid membranes, irritating eyes, mucous membranes, and skin. The lipophilicity of xylene is also responsible for its narcotic and anesthetic properties, although the exact mechanism is poorly understood. The chemical may also inhibit cellular antioxidant enzymes, contributing to the chronic toxic effects of xylene exposure.

Health Effects

Short-term exposure of people to high levels of xylene can cause irritation of the skin, eyes, nose, and throat; difficulty in breathing; impaired function of the lungs; delayed response to a visual stimulus; impaired memory; stomach discomfort; and possible changes in the liver and kidneys (Table 34-4).

Short-term and long-term exposure to high concentrations of xylene can cause several CNS effects, including headaches, lack of muscle coordination, dizziness, confusion, and impaired balance. Some people (e.g., industry workers) exposed to very high levels of xylene for a short period have died.

Toxic Levels

The LD_{50} of xylene for animals ranges from 200 to 4000 mg/kg. OSHA and the EPA have set maximum levels for xylene exposure in the workplace and drinking water, respectively.

Analytical Methods

Xylene metabolites can be measured in the urine. However, a urine sample must be provided within hours after exposure because xylene is quickly eliminated. Because the blood concentration of xylene does not correlate with the clinical symptoms, available tests can only indicate exposure to xylene.

Carbon Monoxide

Carbon monoxide (CO) is an odorless, colorless gas. It is toxic at higher levels but is produced at low levels by many cells in the body. Normal circulating CO levels in blood are between 0% and 3%. It is a ubiquitous constituent of air pollution and cigarette smoking.

Exposure Routes

CO is produced by the incomplete combustion of fuels. The gasoline engines of automobiles produce 5% carbon monoxide in exhaust emissions. Other sources of CO include gas water heaters, kerosene space heaters, charcoal grills, and propane heaters and stoves. CO is called the *silent killer* because it is odorless, tasteless, and colorless. It has more affinity for hemoglobin than oxygen does. After CO binds to hemoglobin, it cannot be removed easily; oxygen cannot be delivered to nourish organs, and the body dies.

Symptoms of CO poisoning include headache, nausea, and fatigue (Box 34-3). These vague symptoms usually do not prompt an individual to go to the hospital for an examination.

Toxic acute doses of CO can be attained by deliberately or accidentally (e.g., inadequate ventilation) inhaling a significant amount of the exhaust fumes of a running car engine. Modern catalytic converters have reduced the amount of CO produced by automobile exhaust, but toxic levels can be reached in enclosed spaces. CO can be produced by gas appliances (i.e., gas water heaters), some heating systems, and other household devices.

Mechanism of Action

CO intoxication results in tissue hypoxia due to decreased oxygen transport. CO binds irreversibly to hemoglobin, producing carboxyhemoglobin, which does not bind or transport oxygen. The reduced oxygen carrying capacity of the bloodstream prompts new red blood cells to be produced. CO also binds to myoglobin, damaging skeletal and cardiac muscles. CO causes cerebral vasodilation, leading to unconsciousness. CO induces nitric oxide synthesis, which decreases systemic blood pressure. Elevated levels of nitric

TABLE 34-4	Effect of Xylene on the Nervous System

Level (ppm)	Effects
100-200	Nausea, headache
200-500	Feeling "high," dizziness, weakness, irritability, vomiting, slowed reaction time
800-10,000	Giddiness, confusion, clumsiness, slurred speech, loss of balance, ringing in the ears
>10,000	Sleepiness, loss of consciousness, death

BOX 34-3 Symptoms of Carbon Monoxide Poisoning

Headache
Nausea
Dizziness
Breathlessness
Collapse
Loss of consciousness

oxide free radicals cause oxidative brain damage and delayed neurologic sequelae such as mental deterioration, mutism, memory impairment, gait disturbance, and urinary and fecal incontinence.

Health Effects

The brain and heart are areas affected most by CO intoxication. Common symptoms include dyspnea, headache, visual disturbances, tachycardia, syncope, tachypnea, coma, convulsions, and death.

Toxic Levels

Exposures to CO at 100 ppm or greater can be dangerous to human health. Toxic CO levels in the blood have been reported for 3% to 70% carboxyhemoglobin levels.

Analytical Methods

CO poisoning is diagnosed using carboxyhemoglobin levels. The tests are sometimes performed in the hematology department, or they may be performed in the clinical chemistry department. Carboxyhemoglobin levels are measured using its spectral absorption properties. Automated instruments read specimen absorbances at several wavelengths and then calculate the amount of deoxyhemoglobin, oxyhemoglobin, carboxyhemoglobin, and methemoglobin. Reference ranges are less than 2.3% for adults, 2.1% to 4.2% for smokers, 8% to 9% for heavy smokers (>2 packs/day), and greater than 15% for toxicity.

Cyanide

Cyanide is a chemical that contains the cyano group ($-C \equiv N$). Cyanides can occur naturally (e.g., apple seeds) or be synthesized. Many are powerful and rapid-acting poisons. The gas hydrogen cyanide (HCN) and simple cyanide salts (i.e., sodium cyanide and potassium cyanide) are examples of common cyanide compounds. Cyanides are used in pest control and mining.

Exposure Routes

Cyanide can be inhaled or ingested. Dermal exposure and absorption may occur in people who work in cyanide-related industries without adequate protective gear.

Mechanism of Action

Cyanide binds to iron in the ferric state, forming a stable cyanoferric complex. This complex inactivates iron-containing enzymes and keeps iron in the ferric state. Heme iron in hemoglobin is usually in the ferrous state, and when it is converted to the ferric state, methemoglobin is formed. Methemoglobin does not bind or transport oxygen. Normally, less than 1.5% of total hemoglobin is methemoglobin.

Cyanide also binds to a cytochrome, inhibiting the electron transport system and blocking oxygen use and aerobic respiration. Reliance on anaerobic instead of aerobic respiration produces a large amount of lactic acid and metabolic acidosis.

Health Effects

Cyanide overdose first causes tachypnea (i.e., rapid breathing) and then respiratory depression, cyanosis, hypotension, convulsions, and coma. Cyanide is a fast-acting toxin, and it can cause death in minutes.

Diagnosis is difficult, and a good history or high index of suspicion can speed the diagnosis. Symptoms specific to cyanide overdose that may help to pinpoint the diagnosis include the odor of bitter almonds, an altered mental state, tachypnea without cyanosis, unexplained metabolic acidosis, and an increased anion gap.

Tissues that depend highly on aerobic respiration, such as the CNS and heart, are particularly affected. At lower doses, loss of consciousness may be preceded by general weakness, giddiness, headaches, vertigo, and confusion. Difficulty breathing progresses to a deep coma, sometimes accompanied by pulmonary edema, and then to cardiac arrest. Skin color turns pink from the formation of cyanide-hemoglobin complexes.

Toxic Levels

Many cyanide compounds are highly toxic. Harmful effects can occur when blood levels of cyanide are higher than 0.05 ppm or 1.5 mg/kg of body weight.

Analytical Methods

After cyanide poisoning, blood and urine levels of cyanide and thiocyanate are detectable. Whole blood cyanide levels are measured by spectrophotometry or GC. Routine arterial blood gas (ABG) measurements can rapidly and easily detect low oxygenation of the blood. Methemoglobin levels are determined by a co-oximeter, which measures the absorbance of whole blood at multiple wavelengths. Because methemoglobin is not stable at room temperature, the specimen must be refrigerated or kept on ice until analyzed. Specimens should not be frozen.

Organophosphates

Organophosphates are found mainly in insecticides. They kill insects by inactivating the acetylcholinesterase found at nerve junctions. This allows acetylcholine to accumulate at the nerve junctions, which causes the signs and symptoms described by the acronym SLUDGE (i.e., salivation, lacrimation, defecation, gastrointestinal distress, and emesis) or DUMBBELS (i.e., diarrhea, urination, meiosis, bradycardia, bronchorrhea, bronchoconstriction, emesis, lacrimation, sweating, and salivation). Other symptoms include muscle twitching, cramping, weakness, and respiratory muscle paralysis. Atropine is administered as an antidote.

Radon

Radon is a naturally occurring radioactive gas that is odorless and tasteless. It is formed from the radioactive decay of uranium, which is found in small amounts in most rocks and soil. Radon is responsible for most public exposure to

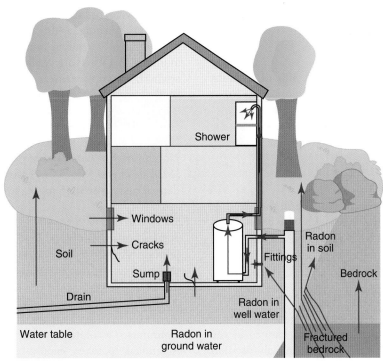

• **Figure 34-6** Routes by which radon enters and exits a home.

ionizing radiation, and it is often the single largest contributor to an individual's background radiation dose. Since the accidental discovery of radon contamination in homes in 1985, environmental radon testing and abatement have become common practices.

Exposure Routes

Radon gas can diffuse through soil and accumulate in houses due to negative-pressure flow (Fig. 34-6).

Mechanism of Action

Radon gas emits alpha radiation (i.e., 2 neutrons plus 2 protons), a high-energy radiation capable of inducing DNA damage and mutations.

Health Effects

Radon 222 (^{222}Rn) is a known human carcinogen. Indoor radon exposure may cause 7000 to 30,000 lung cancer deaths annually in the United States.

Toxic Levels

Due to the long latency period of most carcinogens, toxic levels are difficult to define. For a lifetime exposure at the recommended guideline of 4 pCi/L, the EPA estimates that the risk of developing lung cancer is 1% to 5%.

Analytical Methods

Radon exposure is assessed using a short-term or long-term devices placed in a home or other location and then sent to a clinical laboratory for analysis. Neither radon nor the alpha particles it emits accumulate in the body. Patients suspected of radon exposure may be tested for several cancers,

including lung cancer and blood malignancies. Previous data, such as chest radiographs, can be useful.

Household Products

Bleach

Bleach refers to a number of chemicals that remove color or disinfect by oxidation. They may come in liquid or powder form. Some bleaches contain peroxide instead of chlorine. If bleach is mixed with ammonia, chlorine gas is produced.

Exposure Routes

Individuals can be exposed to small amounts of bleach in household products, but workers in occupations that use these chemicals have the highest risk. Liquid bleach may be ingested or deposited on skin. Inhalation of chlorine gas from bleach solutions (especially when mixed with cleaners containing ammonia) may be a route of exposure.

Mechanism of Action

The toxic effects of bleach primarily result from the corrosive properties of hypochlorite. Hypochlorite reacts with and destroys proteins and fats, resulting in deep tissue destruction and liquefaction necrosis.

Health Effects

Ingestion of a small amount of household bleaches (3% to 6% hypochlorite) may cause gastrointestinal irritation. Concentrated commercial bleach (≥10%) causes severe corrosive injuries to the mouth, throat, esophagus, and stomach, causing bleeding, perforation, and eventual death.

Permanent scars and narrowing of the esophagus may occur in survivors of severe bleach intoxication.

Toxic Levels

Ingestion of large amounts (approximately 300 mL in adults and 100 mL in children) of sodium hypochlorite (<10%) or more concentrated sodium hypochlorite (>10%) may cause severe damage to exposed tissues. Higher amounts may cause perforation of the gastrointestinal mucosa, leading to shock or death.

Analytical Methods

Sodium hypochlorite does not accumulate in the blood or other tissues because it reacts very quickly with cellular proteins and fats. Exposure levels are based on the amount of damage visible and patient testimony if possible.

Paint

Most homes built before 1960 contain lead-based paint (see "Lead"). Use of lead-based paint was banned in the United States in 1977. Other toxic chemicals used in older paints include chromates, arsenic, and antimony. These chemicals were used as paint pigments, which were designed to last, and they pose dangers long after their use. This is especially true for children younger than 6 years of age, who are most likely to ingest paint chips, can have the longest exposure times, and can suffer from developmental defects that do not affect adults. Signs and symptoms of lead-based paint ingestion are similar to those of other toxic metals.

Bug Repellants

Most bug repellents contain *N,N*-diethyl-*m*-toluamide (DEET) in concentrations of 14% to 95%. DEET was developed by the U.S. Army in 1946 for protection of military personnel in insect-infested areas.

Exposure Routes

Exposure is normally dermal, and between 5% and 17% of the applied dose of DEET can be absorbed into the bloodstream. Toxic exposure usually involves accidental ingestion, although about a dozen pediatric deaths due to extreme dermal exposure have been reported, as has exposure through the eyes or by inhalation.

Mechanism of Action

DEET works as an insect repellant because most insects intensely dislike the odor, which makes it hard for biting bugs to smell humans. Human toxicity likely results from inhibition of the CNS enzyme acetylcholinesterase, boosting acetylcholine levels in the brain.

Health Effects

DEET is neurotoxic. Use of high concentrations of DEET on the skin over a long period, such as by military personnel or game wardens, may cause severe skin reactions, including blistering, burning, and scarring. Exposure to the eyes or mucous membranes may cause severe irritation. When small amounts of DEET are swallowed, symptoms may include stomach irritation, nausea, and vomiting. Hypotension and bradycardia may occur if large amounts are ingested.

Toxic Levels

DEET is classified as slightly toxic (class III) by the EPA. No chronic toxicity has been observed. The probable oral lethal dose is 0.5 to 5.0 g/kg of body weight. The lowest dermal toxic dose is 35 mg/kg over 5 days.

Analytical Methods

Analysis of human blood for DEET levels is not routinely performed. DEET exposure is diagnosed using patient testimony, and it is treated based on the clinical symptoms.

Ammonia

Ammonia is a colorless, water-soluble gas. Its distinct odor is familiar to many people because ammonia is used in smelling salts, household and industrial cleaners, and window-cleaning products. It is also used in fertilizers and other nitrogenous compounds.

Exposure Routes

Ammonia is most dangerous when inhaled, which causes nasopharyngeal and tracheal burns, bronchiolar and alveolar edema, and airway destruction resulting in respiratory failure. Ammonia is produced routinely in the body during amino acid deamination reactions, and the liver and kidneys are well equipped to metabolize and excrete ammonia very quickly from the blood. Exposure can cause burns of the skin, eyes, and gastrointestinal tract.

Mechanism of Action

Ammonia is very alkaline, and when it combines with moisture of mucous membranes, it forms ammonium hydroxide. Ammonium hydroxide destroys tissues by disrupting cell membrane lipids. The disrupted membrane releases proteins and water, which elicits an inflammatory response. The inflammatory response causes more damage.

Health Effects

Exposure to high levels of ammonia in air can irritate the skin, eyes, throat, and lungs and cause coughing and burns. Exposure to very high concentrations of gaseous ammonia can result in lung damage and death. Swallowing concentrated solutions of ammonia can cause burns of the mouth, throat, and stomach. Ammonia splashed into eyes can cause burns and blindness.

Toxic Levels

A blood ammonium concentration of 200 μmol/L is associated with coma and convulsions.

Analytical Methods

Laboratory tests to measure ammonia in blood and urine are available, but they cannot be used to treat a medical emergency because ammonia is normally found in blood.

Toxic Metals

Some metals are essential for body function, and some metals are toxic to the body. Toxic metals such as arsenic and mercury have been used as poisons. Since the advent of the industrial age, many workers have been chronically exposed to a variety of metals that injure tissues. Toxic metals include aluminum, arsenic, chromium, cadmium, lead, mercury, and beryllium (Table 34-5).

Aluminum

Over-the-counter antacids can contain aluminum, and frequent use can cause aluminum toxicity. Because individuals with renal failure are unable to excrete aluminum in urine, it is retained in the body and can reach toxic levels over time. Normal levels of aluminum in the blood are less than 6 μg/L.

Signs and symptoms of aluminum toxicity include osteomalacia and encephalopathy. Although aluminum is not cited as a cause of Alzheimer disease, increased levels are found in the brains of people with the disease. Blood specimens for aluminum assays must be collected in special aluminum-free tubes because the stoppers in evacuated tubes contain aluminum silicate. Aluminum is measured by MS.

Lead

Lead is one of the heavy metals (metals that have high atomic weights). Other heavy metals are arsenic, cadmium, and mercury. Lead is a soft and malleable metal that can accumulate in soft tissues, causing several adverse health effects. Lead is an environmental toxin that is found in lead-based paint manufactured before 1978, crystal, artisan bowls and dishes, and soil. Soil is contaminated from vehicles using lead-based fuels before it was discontinued in 1978. Lead is excreted in the feces and urine.

Exposure Routes

Lead may be ingested, inhaled, or absorbed through the skin. When ingested, lead is absorbed from the gastrointestinal tract and accumulates in red blood cells, bones, and the CNS. Lead-based paints are a common source of ingested lead, and industrial pollution is a common source of inhaled lead. Some folk remedies and traditional medicines may contain lead.

Mechanism of Action

Lead turnover in soft tissues occurs in 120 days. Lead disrupts the production of heme and can inhibit the release of neurotransmitters in the CNS, disrupting neuronal function. Because the formation of neuronal connections is activity dependent, lead poisoning can irreversibly inhibit childhood mental development.

Health Effects

Lead accumulates in blood, soft tissues, and bone tissues, where it exerts toxic effects. Because lead in the bones, teeth, hair, and nails is bound tightly and not available to other tissues, it is thought not to be harmful. Children with high levels of lead in their bodies can suffer CNS damage leading to behavioral and learning problems, slowed growth, hearing problems, and anemia. Symptoms of lead toxicity include anemia, encephalopathy, nephropathy, severe abdominal pain, peripheral neuropathy, infertility, hypertension, and decreased hearing.

Toxic Levels

The Centers for Disease Control and Prevention (CDC) states that lead levels above 5 μg/dL are a concern, although levels below that also can impair development.

Analytical Methods

Blood lead levels are measured using atomic absorption spectroscopy and MS. Hair can also be used as a specimen to determine lead levels.

Chromium

Hexavalent chromium (Cr^{6+}) refers to chromium in the +6 oxidation state; chromium may also exist stably in 0 and +3 states. Trivalent chromium (Cr^{3+}) is an essential nutrient in small amounts and is found in many foods. Cr^{6+} is used in the production of stainless steel, chrome plating, dyes for textile manufacturing, and in solutions used for wood

TABLE 34-5	Conditions Resulting From Metal Toxicities
Metal	**Condition**
Aluminum	Dialysis, encephalopathy, dementia
Arsenic	Bilateral pain radiating from feet to legs, peripheral neuropathy, unexplained impaired renal function
Cadmium	Impaired renal function in aerosol painters
Lead	Children younger than 2 years living in older homes, unexplained gastric upset, anemia, impaired renal function at any age
Mercury	Acute changes in behavior, impaired speech, visual field constriction, hearing loss, somatosensory disorders
Beryllium	Hypersensitivity to the metal; chronic scarring lung disorder characterized by cough, shortness of breath, chest pains, night sweats, and fatigue

From Burtis CA, Bruns DE. *Tietz Fundamentals of Clinical Chemistry and Molecular Diagnostics.* 7th ed. Philadelphia: Saunders; 2015.

preservation, cleaning, leather tanning, and anticorrosion coatings.

Exposure Routes

Cr^{6+} exposure may occur through inhalation or ingestion of contaminated foods and water.

Mechanism of Action

Cr^{6+} is a rare valence state for chromium, and it is produced in a strong oxidizing environment. When Cr^{6+} is inhaled, it is lipid soluble and can cross cell membranes and erode nasal passages. It has been implicated in squamous cell cancers of the lung.

Health Effects

Cr^{6+} is a known human carcinogen according to the EPA. Acute toxic effects include hemolysis (i.e., destruction of blood cells) and renal and liver failure.

Toxic Levels

The LD_{50} for Cr^{6+} is between 50 and 150 mg/kg of body weight.

Analytical Methods

Analyzing blood and urine specimens for Cr^{6+} is not practical or useful for detecting chromium toxicity because Cr^{6+} is converted to Cr^{3+} when it enters a cell. Cr^{3+} is nontoxic to cells. A better way to detect Cr^{6+} is to monitor the air for its presence.

Arsenic

Arsenic can be found in medicines, rodenticides, weed killers, insecticides, paints, pressure-treated lumber, livestock feed, tanning agents, and metal alloys. Toxic forms of arsenic include sodium arsenate, lead arsenite, copper arsenite, carbarsone, tryparsamide, and arsine gas.

Exposure Routes

Exposure to arsenic usually happens through the gastrointestinal system. Arsenic is absorbed quickly through the gastrointestinal tract and the lungs but more slowly through the skin. Within 24 hours of ingestion, all body tissues contain arsenic. The main elimination route for arsenic is through the kidneys. Systemic poisoning from arsenic ingestion occurs when arsenic reacts with enzyme sulfhydryl groups and disrupts metabolic processes.

Arsine gas is the most dangerous form of arsenic. It irreversibly binds to the sulfhydryl groups on hemoglobin, causing intravascular hemolysis, hemoglobinemia, and nephrotoxicity leading to acute renal failure. Children who eat soil are at higher risk, especially soil near former smelting or mining facilities. Many foods, especially fish, contain organic forms of arsenic, which are much less toxic than inorganic forms from industrial pollution. Contact with pressure-treated wood (e.g., children's play structures) is not thought to be a significant route of exposure.

Mechanism of Action

Arsenic disrupts metabolic processes by reversibly interacting with multiple enzyme sulfhydryl groups. Arsine gas irreversibly binds to the sulfhydryl groups of hemoglobin.

Health Effects

In acute poisoning, symptoms appear within the first hour after ingestion. The most common initial symptoms are burning and dryness of the mouth and throat, difficulty swallowing, vomiting, and watery or bloody diarrhea. As the poisoning continues, cyanosis, hypotension, tachycardia, and ventricular arrhythmias develop; 1 to 2 weeks later, neuropathy develops. Hypovolemic shock and acute renal tubular necrosis lead to death from circulatory failure. Arsenic poisoning also produces the characteristic cutaneous symptoms of hyperpigmentation of the skin and keratosis.

Symptoms for exposure to arsine gas start 2 to 24 hours after exposure and include nausea, vomiting, headache, anorexia, bloody vomit, abdominal pain, acute renal failure, cardiac damage, anemia, hemolysis, and pulmonary edema. Chronic arsenic poisoning is difficult to diagnose without a clear cause, but individuals with gastrointestinal symptoms; neuropathy; and cutaneous, cardiovascular, and renal symptoms should be tested for arsenic.

Toxic Levels

Acute fatal doses are 120 mg for arsenic trioxide, 30 ppm for arsine gas, and 0.1 to 0.5 g/kg of body weight for organic arsenicals.

Analytical Methods

Ion emission spectroscopy is used to measure arsenic levels in blood, urine, hair, or fingernails to determine exposure to arsenic.

Beryllium

Beryllium is an alkaline earth metal. It is not needed to sustain human life, but it has many commercial uses. It is used in dental appliances, golf clubs, nonsparking tools, wheelchairs, satellite and spacecraft manufacturing, circuit board production, and for producing nuclear power. Beryllium exposure occurs from inhaling and ingesting contaminated dust in industrial settings.

Exposure Routes

Most cases of beryllium toxicity occur when the metal is inhaled. Inhaled beryllium compounds take a long time to clear from the lungs. When the metal is ingested, it is usually absorbed from the gastrointestinal tract as beryllium salts, which are strongly acidic when dissolved in water. Absorbed beryllium accumulates in the skeleton, and elimination through the kidneys is slow.

Mechanism of Action

The mechanism of action for beryllium is not fully understood. Acute exposure may involve destruction of the integrity of the lysosomal membrane, releasing lysosomal enzymes that injure the cell. Lung inflammation may result from excess activation of alveolar macrophages. Chronic beryllium disease likely involves beryllium interacting with cell surface proteins to generate antigens (i.e., beryllium is a hapten), triggering chronic autoimmune reactions. Enzymes inhibited by beryllium include alkaline phosphatase, acid phosphatase, phosphoglycerate mutase, hexokinase, and lactate dehydrogenase.

Health Effects

Acute exposure to beryllium is rare. Chronic exposure through inhalation can damage the lungs, causing pneumonia-like symptoms (i.e., acute beryllium disease). Some people may become hypersensitive to beryllium after 10 to 15 years of exposure (i.e., chronic beryllium disease [CBD]). CBD is characterized by anorexia, granulomas in the lungs, weight loss, and blue discoloration of hands and feet. Acute and chronic beryllium disease can be fatal.

Toxic Levels

Exposure to relatively low concentrations ($0.5 \ \mu g/m^3$) of soluble or insoluble beryllium compounds can result in CBD. CBD does not correlate with duration of exposure and can have a long latency period. Acute beryllium disease has been reported in workers exposed to high concentrations of soluble beryllium compounds, although no reliable NOAEL or LOAEL has been identified.

Analytical Methods

Beryllium levels can be measured in urine and blood, but levels in urine vary, making it difficult to use them to assess total exposure. The beryllium lymphocyte proliferation test (BeLPT) is used to measure chronic exposure and hypersensitivity. It is the method of choice for diagnosing CBD.

Cadmium

Cadmium is a product of zinc and lead smelting. It is used in electroplating, nickel batteries, organic-based paints, and tobacco products. Breathing cadmium can lead to nasal epithelial deterioration and pulmonary congestion. The most common route of exposure is through spray painting. Respirators are required for automotive industry workers who spray paint cars and trucks.

Exposure Routes

The most dangerous form of occupational exposure to cadmium is inhalation of fine dust or ingestion of soluble cadmium compounds. Tobacco smoke is the most common source of cadmium exposure in the general population. Smokers have four to five times higher blood cadmium concentrations and two to three times higher kidney cadmium concentrations than nonsmokers.

Cadmium is an environmental hazard, especially near mining facilities, and it can be ingested when it contaminates water supplies or food sources. A common source of chronic exposure is spray painting using organic paints without a respirator. Auto repair technicians run a great risk of chronic exposure to cadmium.

Mechanism of Action

The mechanism of cadmium toxicity is not fully understood but probably involves cadmium's anionic state (+2 charge). Accumulation in the kidneys may disrupt ion concentrations and lead to dehydration of cells in nephrons, ultimately causing kidney failure. Acute lung toxicity may involve cadmium's ability to alter zinc-protein complexes, disrupt DNA transcription, and trigger apoptosis.

Health Effects

Cadmium accumulates in the kidneys, where it can generate reactive oxygen species and activate cell death pathways. Clinically overt kidney damage takes years to develop. Inhalation of cadmium can result initially in metal fume fever, but it may progress to pneumonitis, pulmonary edema, and death. Chronic inhalation of lower doses can cause cadmium to build up in the kidneys over time, leading to kidney failure. Cadmium exposure is a risk factor for atherosclerosis, hypertension, and cardiovascular disease.

Toxic Levels

The normal blood cadmium level is less than $5 \ \mu g/mL$. Moderately increased cadmium levels (3 to $7 \ \mu g/mL$) can be found in smokers.

Analytical Methods

Urine is the specimen of choice for laboratory tests, but care must be taken when collecting specimens. Rubber catheters and brightly colored urine specimen containers should not be used because they may contain cadmium. Cadmium can be measured in blood, urine, hair, or nails by atomic absorption spectroscopy or by inductively coupled plasma mass spectrometry (ICP-MS).

Mercury

Elemental mercury (i.e., quicksilver) is a dense liquid that vaporizes easily at room temperature. Mercury is an environmental toxin produced by natural outgassing of rock. It is used in industry (e.g., electrolysis, electrical switches, fungicides) and dental amalgams (i.e., fillings). Mercury combines with elements such as chlorine, sulfur, and oxygen to form toxic inorganic mercury compounds (i.e., salts), which are usually white powders or crystals. Mercury is most toxic when it combines with methanol to make methylmercury (CH_3Hg^+): Hg^0 (nontoxic) $\ll Hg^{2+} \lll CH_3Hg^+$ (most toxic).

In the past, it was used in many devices such as thermometers and sphygmomanometers, but its toxicity led to the use of alcohols instead. It was also used in many pigments and paints. Although there is significant fear about mercury compounds such as thimerosal, which was previously used in vaccinations, there are no data to support its toxicity and ample evidence to the contrary.

Exposure Routes

Mercury can be inhaled and absorbed through the skin and mucous membranes. Fish and shellfish have a tendency to accumulate methylmercury, which can subsequently be ingested. Methylmercury and metallic mercury vapors are more harmful than other forms because more mercury reaches the brain.

After inhalation or ingestion, mercury and mercury compounds are quickly distributed through the bloodstream. They are toxic to the CNS if they cross the blood–brain barrier, as elemental mercury and methylmercury do.

Mechanism of Action

Ions of metal mercury (Hg^{2+}) react with the sulfhydryl groups of proteins, denaturing their tertiary structure and eliminating their biologic functions. Mercury concentrates in the kidneys, causing much damage before being excreted. When mercury denatures proteins, some become immunogenic and elicit an immune response, which increases the tissue damage. Methylmercury is partially lipophilic, and it settles in lipid-rich tissue such as myelin around neurons.

Health Effects

Mercury pollution of waterways greatly increases mercury levels in fish. People who ingest the fish can develop mercury toxicity. Symptoms of methyl mercury poisoning include ataxia, impaired speech, visual field constriction, hearing loss, somatosensory changes, and cerebral cortex necrosis. Short-term exposure to high levels of metallic mercury vapors may cause lung damage, nausea, vomiting, diarrhea, increased blood pressure or heart rate, rashes, and eye irritation.

Mercury alters the tertiary structure of proteins and concentrates in kidneys before excretion. Denatured proteins become immunogenic and signal the body to produce autoantibodies against collagen tissue. Mercury binds to nervous tissue, causing injury.

Long-term exposure to mercury or methylmercury is toxic to the CNS, causing irritability, tremors, vision or hearing changes, and memory problems. Mercury poisoning can result in infantile acrodynia (i.e., pink disease), Hunter-Russell syndrome, and Minamata disease. Bile is the main route of mercury excretion.

Toxic Levels

Normal whole blood mercury concentrations are less than 10 µg/L. Mild exposure is indicated by levels up to 15 µg/L. In severe exposure, methylmercury levels are greater than 50 µg/L, or Hg^{2+} levels are greater than 200 µg/L.

Analytical Methods

Mercury can be detected in blood, urine, and hair samples. A 24-hour urine specimen can be diagnostic for acute mercury toxicity. Hair analysis can be used to identify chronic mercury exposure. Reference values are less than 10 µg/L. Mercury is measured using mass spectroscopy and atomic absorption spectroscopy.

Drugs of Abuse

Drugs of abuse are legal and illegal drugs that provide the user a desired effect. For example, many individuals take cocaine because it provides a euphoric state. Aside from acute toxic effects, many drugs of abuse have a high potential for addiction and tolerance. Addiction occurs when an individual continues to use a drug despite adverse effects, and it usually includes drug-seeking behaviors. Tolerance reduces the body's reaction to the drug, and addicts require escalating doses to produce the same effect as the lower initial dose. As tolerance increases, higher drug doses also become necessary to alleviate withdrawal symptoms.

Drugs of abuse may be purely recreational drugs that are classified as schedule 1 or 2 drugs by the Federal Controlled Substances Act. Some pharmaceuticals also may be abused, especially opiate analgesics such as morphine. Some drugs of abuse are designer drugs, which are slightly modified versions of known narcotics or pharmaceuticals that are not regulated by the FDA. They may be sold to the general public under coded labels (e.g., bath salts, plant food, herbal supplements) with the intention of being used as recreational drugs.

The major drugs of abuse covered in this chapter include amphetamine, methamphetamine, methylenedioxymethamphetamine (MDMA), cocaine, marijuana, phencyclidine, codeine, morphine, methadone, propoxyphene, barbiturates, benzodiazepines, ethanol, hydromorphone, hydrocodone, and oxycodone, which are taken illegally to induce euphoric states. Measurements are performed during routine drug screening and in cases of overdose.

The federal government guidelines set by the Substance Abuse and Mental Health Services Administration (SAMHSA) apply to many employees, such as the transportation industry and truck drivers in particular. Employees must pass a standardized urine drug screen (i.e., National Institute on Drug Abuse drug screen) for five categories of drugs of abuse: amphetamines, cannabinoids, opiates, phencyclidine, and cocaine. Expanded screening tests may detect additional drugs of abuse or use other tissue samples such as blood or hair. These tests often involve a preliminary immunoassay as a screening test and a GC-MS assay for confirmation. Figure 34-7 shows the results of several drug screens.

Amphetamine and Methamphetamine

Amphetamines are a class of psychostimulant drugs that increase wakefulness and focus and decrease fatigue and appetite. The effects last for hours. Amphetamines are frequently used recreationally or as performance-enhancing drugs. An estimated 13 million Americans use amphetamines

Toxi-lab A Worksheet

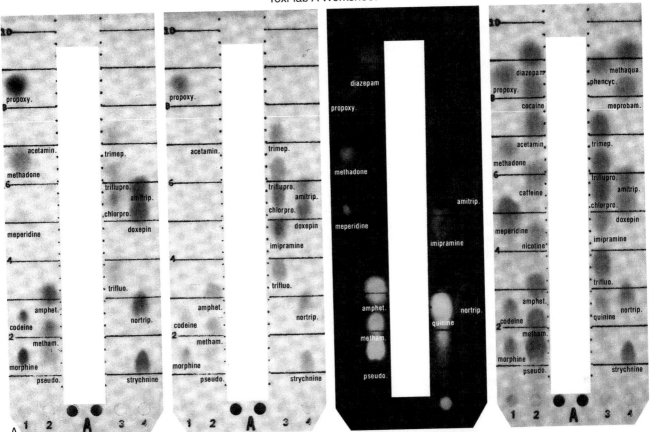

Toxi-lab B Worksheet

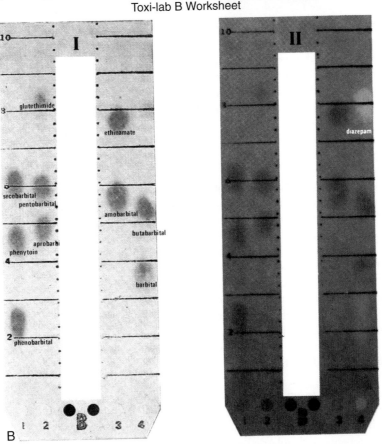

• **Figure 34-7** Typical separations of the major drugs of abuse and some therapeutic drugs on Toxi-Lab thin-layer chromatography. The Toxi-Lab **A** worksheet shows the typical separation of basic drugs on the **A** strip and the characteristic color changes. The third Toxi-Lab **A** strip shows the characteristic fluorescence of various drugs. Notice that amphetamine and methamphetamine on the lower left are fluorescent. The Toxi-Lab **B** worksheet shows the typical separation of the more acidic drugs on the **B** strip and characteristic color changes *(left)*. The major use of the **B** strip is to identify the presence of the barbiturates. Fluorescence patterns of the drugs are shown on the **B** strip *(right)*. (From McPherson RA, Pincus MR: *Henry's Clinical Diagnosis and Management by Laboratory Methods.* 22nd ed. Philadelphia: Elsevier, 2012.)

without medical supervision. Methamphetamine is easily synthesized from readily available products, including some flammable and corrosive chemicals. In addition to producing euphoria, methamphetamine also enhances self-esteem and increases libido.

Exposure Routes

Intravenous injection is the fastest route of drug administration, followed by smoking, anal or vaginal suppository insertion, insufflations (i.e., snorting), and ingestion.

Mechanism of Action

Amphetamines are structurally related to epinephrine, norepinephrine, and dopamine. Amphetamines boost the secretion of the neurotransmitters norepinephrine and dopamine (i.e., catecholamines) and serotonin throughout the CNS and PNS.

Health Effects

Amphetamines exert sympathomimetic and dopaminergic effects. Elevated epinephrine levels in the CNS increase arousal and decrease fatigue. In the peripheral nervous system (PNS), these effects can cause tachycardia and arrhythmias. Increased dopamine signaling is responsible for movement disorders, schizophrenia, and euphoria. Serotonergic signals may play a role in hallucinations and appetite suppression.

Individuals take amphetamines because they cause euphoria and increase mental alertness, but amphetamines also increase the heart rate and blood pressure and cause palpitations, bronchodilation, anxiety, pallor, and tremulousness. Stimulation of the heart, kidneys, and nerves can lead to serious side effects, such as heart attacks in young people. Weight loss is another side effect of amphetamines. Long-term use of the drugs can lead to necrosis of the heart, dilated cardiomyopathy, hypertension, and psychosis resembling paranoid schizophrenia.

Tolerance rapidly develops when abusing amphetamines. Withdrawal symptoms include mental fatigue, depression, and increased appetite. These symptoms may last for days after occasional use and months after chronic use.

Initial symptoms of an overdose include flushing, pallor, tachypnea, palpitations, tremors, hypertension, hypotension, cardiac arrhythmia, heart block, and circulatory collapse. Neurologic symptoms that may accompany the initial symptoms include delirium, confusion, delusions, disorientation, hallucinations, restlessness, homicidal or suicidal tendencies, panic state, paranoid ideation, and combativeness. If the overdose is severe enough, death from cardiovascular collapse occurs.

Chronic use of amphetamines leads to emotional lability, somnolence, loss of appetite, mental impairment, and social withdrawal. Prolonged high-dosage use leads to paranoid schizophrenia. Rarely, pancytopenia and aplastic anemia can lead to death.

With chronic or high doses of methamphetamine, convulsions, heart attack, stroke, and death may occur.

Methamphetamine is highly addictive. Because of methamphetamine-induced neurotoxicity to dopaminergic neurons, chronic abuse may lead to a syndrome that persists beyond the withdrawal period for months to years. Although withdrawal itself may not be dangerous, the symptoms are common with heavy use, and relapse is common. Methamphetamine users and addicts lose their teeth abnormally quickly, a condition known as *meth mouth*.

Toxic Levels

The amount of amphetamine that causes an overdose can vary significantly. It depends on whether the user has acquired a tolerance for the drug. A level teaspoon contains between 3 and 5 g of powder. Assuming the purity to be 8%, a teaspoon contains 240 to 400 mg of pure drug, or two to three times the maximum therapeutic dose. However, deaths have been reported at levels as low as 1.3 mg/kg. The LD_{50} for amphetamine in mice is between 55 and 125 mg/kg.

Analytical Methods

Amphetamines are detected using urine drug screens (usually an immunoassay method), with confirmation using GC-MS. Amphetamine levels may not be ordered, but laboratory tests for electrolytes, troponin I, and creatine kinase may be ordered, depending on the individual's symptoms. Methamphetamine stays in the system for 3 to 5 days. Hair and blood tests may also be performed; methamphetamine use can be detected in hair samples 90 days after exposure.

Methylenedioxymethamphetamine

Methylenedioxymethamphetamine (i.e., MDMA, ecstasy, E, or X) is a member of the amphetamine class of drugs. MDMA can induce euphoria, a sense of intimacy with others, and diminished anxiety, which makes it a popular nightclub drug. Studies have suggested that MDMA has therapeutic benefits for the treatment of posttraumatic stress disorder (PTSD) and some behavioral affective disorders.

Exposure Routes

MDMA is taken orally, usually as a capsule or tablet.

Mechanism of Action

MDMA binds to a serotonin transporter, which removes serotonin from the synapse. MDMA increases and prolongs serotonin signals. Some reports suggest that MDMA may be neurotoxic, but this has not been demonstrated in the absence of hyperthermia. MDMA's intimacy-inducing effects may be mediated by the release of the hormone oxytocin.

Health Effects

Few people die of an MDMA overdose each year. The major short-term physical health risk of MDMA consumption is hyperthermia (i.e., elevated body temperature). In conjunction with continuous activity and lack of rehydration, MDMA may cause body temperature to rise to dangerous levels. Alcohol and other diuretics exacerbate these risks. All of these effects are commonly seen in nightclubs, where MDMA use is popular.

Repeat recreational users of MDMA have increased rates of depression and anxiety, even after quitting the drug. However, studies of these effects and lowered cognitive ability among chronic MDMA users have been confounded by the test subjects' use of multiple drugs.

Ecstasy tablets are notoriously impure. Other chemicals frequently found in MDMA tablets include amphetamine, methamphetamine, ephedrine, and paramethoxyamphetamine, a potent neurotoxic hallucinogen. Kits to test the purity of MDMA tablets are commercially available in the United States. MDMA interactions with other drugs and medications can produce toxic effects.

Toxic Levels

The LD_{50} of MDMA ranges from 100 to 300 mg/kg for rodents. The LD_{50} for humans is estimated to be between 10 and 20 mg/kg (oral).

Analytical Methods

An expanded immunoassay drug screen can reveal MDMA in urine. Confirmation testing uses GC-MS technology.

Cocaine

Cocaine is a powerfully addictive stimulant drug obtained from the leaves of the coca plant. Early in the 20th century, Coca-Cola contained cocaine, but the formula was discontinued when people became addicted to the drink. Cocaine is currently abused by more than 5.3 million Americans. Cocaine also has legitimate medical uses. It is used as a local anesthetic and vasoconstrictor of mucous membranes for nasal surgery and for emergency nasotracheal intubation.

Exposure Routes

Cocaine is usually snorted or dissolved in water and injected. Crack, a potent form of cocaine, is the street name given to cocaine that has been processed to make a rock crystal, which when heated produces vapors that are smoked. Blood cocaine levels rise more sharply when crack is injected or smoked than when powder cocaine is snorted, producing a stronger high and greater potential for overdose. As a result of the popularity of crack cocaine, emergency department admissions related to cocaine overdoses have increased.

Smugglers who use the gastrointestinal tract as a hiding place for large quantities of carefully wrapped packages of cocaine (i.e., body packers) may become exposed to high levels of cocaine when packages rupture.

Mechanism of Action

Cocaine produces a quick, short-lived euphoric state and enhanced mental alertness after it is inhaled, ingested, or injected. It is a potent CNS stimulant and produces effects similar to those of amphetamines, but the effects of cocaine last for only 1 to 2 hours, whereas the effects of amphetamines last much longer.

Cocaine crosses the blood–brain barrier and blocks dopamine reuptake at the synapses to prolong the effect of dopamine on the CNS. Dopamine is used in many brain regions, including the brain's reward circuit (i.e., nucleus accumbens) and in risk analysis (i.e., prefrontal cortex). Norepinephrine is used throughout the CNS for tasks such as in maintaining alertness. Cocaine blocks the reuptake of norepinephrine at the presynaptic terminals, producing a sympathomimetic response (i.e., increased blood pressure, heart rate, and body temperature) (Fig. 34-8).

Health Effects

Cocaine is a powerful nervous system stimulant that causes euphoria and increased alertness and boosts energy and motor activity. Anxiety, paranoia, and restlessness are frequent symptoms. With excessive dosage, tremors, convulsions, and hyperthermia may occur.

Acute cardiovascular or cerebrovascular emergencies (i.e., heart attack or stroke) can occur at high doses and may cause sudden death. Cocaine-related deaths are often a result of cardiac arrest or a seizure followed by respiratory arrest.

Acute cocaine toxicity produces a sympathomimetic response that may include dilated pupils, unusually heavy perspiration (i.e., diaphoresis), hyperactive bowel sounds, tachycardia, hypertension, increased body temperature, hyperactivity, agitation, seizures, and coma. Cocaine users can experience cardiotoxicity leading to sudden death.

Unfortunately, cocaine passes through the placenta and into the lactating mammary gland, and fetuses and nursing infants can be exposed to the drug. Cocaine can cause mental retardation, delayed development, and drug addiction in newborns.

Toxic Levels

Among deaths caused by drugs of abuse in the United States, cocaine-related deaths are the most common. However, the doses and cause of death vary significantly between new users and chronic users. Autopsies in cases of cocaine-related deaths have suggested that preexisting heart conditions may be a factor in the susceptibility to overdose. Roughly 600 mg/kg is considered a fatal dose.

The use of cocaine and ethanol increases toxicity significantly. When coadministered, the liver produces cocaethylene, which boosts cocaine's euphoric effects and greatly increases the risk of overdose. Between 30% and 60% of cocaine users regularly mix cocaine and alcohol. Combining cocaine and heroin into a speedball causes frequent complications, which accounts for 12% to 15% of cocaine-related episodes among patients admitted to emergency departments in the United States.

Analytical Methods

Immunoassay urine drug screening tests are designed to detect cocaine metabolites. The cutoff for these tests is 300 ng/mL, and they can detect metabolites for 1 to

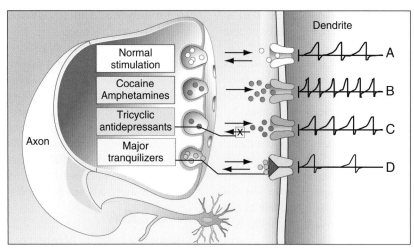

• **Figure 34-8** Possible mechanisms of action of drugs of abuse and some therapeutic drugs on sympathomimetic amine (dopamine and norepinephrine) pathways. **A,** Normal neural transmission. A nerve impulse is conducted down the axon to the terminal boutons at the nerve ending. Vesicles, represented by the round, gray structure, release their neurotransmitter (i.e., dopamine) contents *(white circles)*. Dopamine molecules traverse the synaptic cleft and bind to dendritic receptors, initiating action potentials in the dendrites. The arrows indicate that dopamine is released and taken up by the vesicles. **B,** In the presence of cocaine or amphetamines, release of the neurotransmitter *(red circles)* from vesicles is enhanced, increasing the rate of firing of the dendrites. **C,** Tricyclic antidepressants block *(X in yellow box)* reuptake of the neurotransmitter *(purple circles),* in this case norepinephrine and, less specifically, dopamine, causing more neurotransmitter to recycle to the dendritic receptors, resulting in increased firing. **D,** Some neuroleptics act by blocking *(black wedge)* postsynaptic dendritic receptors for dopamine *(blue circles),* decreasing firing. (From McPherson RA, Pincus MR. *Henry's Clinical Diagnosis and Management by Laboratory Methods.* 22nd ed. Philadelphia: Elsevier; 2012.)

3 days after use. For chronic users, the time of detection is extended to 10 to 22 days after use because tissue stores cocaine. Positive screening test results are confirmed with GC-MS.

Marijuana

Marijuana (i.e., cannabis) is the most commonly abused illicit drug in the United States. It is a dry, shredded, green and brown mix of flowers, stems, seeds, and leaves derived from the hemp plant *Cannabis sativa.* Hashish is more potent and is produced by extracting resin from the plant. Marijuana is also used for some religious ceremonies. A number of states have legalized the use of marijuana for medicinal purposes, although the federal government considers marijuana a schedule 1 narcotic (i.e., high potential for abuse with no medical benefit).

Tetrahydrocannabinol (THC) is the principal psychoactive agent in marijuana. Synthetic derivatives of THC are manufactured for therapeutic use and can be found in pill form.

Exposure Routes

All forms of marijuana must be heated to activate the psychoactive effects of THC. Marijuana is usually smoked as a cigarette (i.e., joint) or in a pipe. Marijuana can also be mixed in cooked food or brewed as a tea. The concentrated, resinous form is called *hashish,* and the sticky black liquid is called *hash oil.*

Mechanism of Action

THC acts on specific sites in the brain called *cannabinoid receptors.* This mimics the effects of endocannabinoid neurotransmitters and ultimately leads to the "high" that users experience. The major effects of THC include euphoria, relaxation, and a sense of well-being.

Health Effects

Marijuana intoxication can cause distorted perceptions, impaired coordination, difficulty with thinking and problem solving, and problems with learning and memory. Research has shown that marijuana's adverse impact on learning and memory in chronic users can last for days or weeks after the acute effects of the drug wear off.

Medicinal uses of marijuana in a prescribed medication (i.e., Dronabinol) include reduction of nausea and stimulation of hunger in chemotherapy and AIDS patients, lowered intraocular eye pressure for treating glaucoma, and analgesic effects that are particularly useful in the treatment of chronic pain disorders.

Marijuana can be habit forming, which may lead to reduced intelligence and memory. A possible relationship between cannabis use and mental disorders (e.g., depression, schizophrenia) is the subject of current study.

Marijuana smoke contains higher doses of carcinogens than tobacco smoke. Similar to tobacco, chronic marijuana use can lead to lung problems other than cancer, such as irritation and inflammation.

Toxic Levels

There have been no documented human fatalities from overdosing on THC or cannabis in its natural form.

Analytical Methods

THC and its major (inactive) metabolite (i.e., hydroxy-THC [11-COOH-THC]), can be measured in blood, urine, hair, saliva, or sweat. The most common screening test is an immunoassay test. Confirmation of a positive screening test result is accomplished using GC-MS.

Phencyclidine

Phencyclidine (i.e., PCP or angel dust) is a recreational dissociative drug. It distorts perceptions of sight and sound and produces feelings of detachment. Functional dissociation of pain perception, consciousness, movement, and memory result from PCP use. PCP causes severe psychological disturbances (i.e., hallucinogenic and neurotoxic). PCP is used recreationally for a mind-altering or "out-of-body" experience. It is a potent veterinary analgesic and anesthetic.

Exposure Routes

PCP may be ingested, smoked, or inhaled.

Mechanism of Action

PCP blocks *N*-methyl-D-aspartate (NMDA) receptors and binds the chloride channels of neurons, resulting in bizarre and paradoxical symptoms.

Health Effects

Effects can vary and are unpredictable. They include euphoria, dysphoria, ataxia, nystagmus, agitation, anxiety, paranoia, amnesia, seizures, muscle rigidity, hostility, delirium, delusions of grandeur, and hallucinations. People on PCP may believe they have superhuman strength, and coupled with a reduced pain threshold, that can lead to excessive physical exertion, causing accidental or intentional trauma. High doses of PCP can also cause suicidal thoughts, seizures, coma, and death, although death most often results from accidental injury or suicide during PCP intoxication. Most emergency department visits by PCP abusers are because of the severe psychological, not physical, effects of the drug.

Chronic PCP users have reported memory loss, difficulties with speech and thinking, depression, and weight loss. Due to the extremely variable symptoms, diagnosis must depend on the results of a drug screen.

Toxic Levels

The oral LD_{50} in mice is 75 mg/kg.

Analytical Methods

Determining the serum level of PCP is not helpful because there is no correlation between the amount of PCP in blood and the drug's effects. Qualitative identification of PCP in urine helps to diagnose PCP toxicity. Urine drug screens use immunoassay techniques to identify PCP in samples.

GC-MS is used to confirm and quantitate a positive qualitative test result. PCP is detectable in the urine 3 to 30 days after use. Blood testing and hair testing may detect PCP use 5 days or 90 days after use, respectively. Because PCP accumulates in fatty tissue, chronic users with high body fat levels may test positive after even longer periods.

Lysergic Diethylamine

Lysergic diethylamine (LSD) is an extremely potent psychedelic and hallucinogenic drug. It is synthesized from an ergot alkaloid produced by the fungus *Claviceps purpurea,* which grows on grains. It is the most commonly abused drug in this class. Users believe it provides great insights and new ways of solving problems.

Exposure Routes

LSD is ingested in powder, gelatin capsules, or LSD-impregnated sugar cubes, filter paper, or postage stamps. The drug is rapidly absorbed through the gastrointestinal tract, and effects are felt 40 to 60 minutes after ingestion. The effects peak at 2 to 4 hours and subside within 6 to 8 hours.

Mechanism of Action

LSD's structure is similar to the structure of serotonin. It is thought to work in multiple sites in the CNS in complex ways, and it affects the sympathetic and parasympathetic nervous systems. It is excreted mainly in bile.

Health Effects

LSD is a hallucinogenic drug that produces perceptual distortions of colors, sound, distance, and shape; depersonalization and loss of body image; and rapidly changing emotions from ecstasy to depression or paranoia. The physiologic effects of the drug include dilated pupils, tachycardia, increased body temperature, excessive sweating, and hypertension. At higher doses, salivation, lacrimation, nausea, and vomiting occur.

Toxic Levels

The clinical effects of LSD usually run their course, and no medical intervention is needed. However, panic attacks and psychosis may need to be treated with therapeutic drugs. Massive overdoses (rare) lead to life-threatening hyperthermia, rhabdomyolysis, acute renal failure, hepatic failure, disseminated intravascular coagulation, respiratory arrest, and coma. Death occurs as a result of an individual's poor judgment while taking the drug.

Analytical Methods

LSD identification is challenging because the detection window is only 12 to 24 hours. Methods used to detect LSD include radioimmunoassay (RIA), cloned enzyme donor immunoassay (CEDIA), enzyme multiplied immunoassay technology (EMIT), and enzyme-linked immunosorbent assay (ELISA). Confirmation is accomplished using GC-MS.

Codeine

Codeine is an opiate narcotic that is used to relieve mild to moderate pain. It is also used in combination with other medications to reduce coughing (i.e., antitussive). Although not as potent as most other opiates, codeine's use in over-the-counter cold medications has made it a commonly abused drug, usually by taking a higher than recommended dose.

Exposure Routes

Codeine is usually ingested in pill or liquid form, but it can also be injected.

Mechanism of Action

Codeine is a μ opioid receptor agonist. It activates numerous CNS regions, including those responsible for the transmission of pain to higher brain centers, respiratory control, and the reward system.

Health Effects

Respiratory depression is the main risk of acute codeine toxicity. The characteristic triad of opiate poisoning is coma, pinpoint pupils, and respiratory depression. Most fatalities occur after intravenous administration by drug abusers who have taken codeine in association with other depressant drugs or alcohol, although deaths can also occur after an oral overdose.

Toxic Levels

The adult lethal blood and urine levels are 2.8 mg/L and 103.8 mg/L, respectively. Tolerance to opiates can significantly alter susceptibility.

Analytical Methods

The initial screening test for codeine is an immunoassay, and confirmatory testing is performed with GC-MS. Cutoff values for codeine in the immunoassay test for medical purposes is 300 ng/mL. The SAMHSA test for workplace drug screening has a cutoff value of 2000 ng/mL. Individuals test positive on the urine test for 1 to 3 days with a cutoff of 300 ng/mL but test positive 12 to 24 hours using the higher cutoff (2000 ng/mL).

Morphine

Morphine is the most abundant alkaloid found in opium, the milky liquid found in unripe poppy seeds. Morphine has been used in the treatment of pain as long as humans have had written language. Opium also contains small amounts of codeine. Morphine is a powerful opiate analgesic used to relieve severe pain, and it can be used to treat the pain of myocardial infarction and labor pains. It is the clinical benchmark for opiate pain relievers. Morphine has a high potential for addiction and tolerance.

Semisynthetic derivatives of morphine have similar mechanisms of action and produce effects similar to morphine. These compounds include heroin, oxycodone, hydrocodone, oxymorphone, hydromorphone, and levorphanol. Heroin crosses the blood–brain barrier and is then converted to morphine, causing CNS effects. Morphine produces PNS and CNS effects.

Exposure Routes

Morphine may be administered orally or intravenously. Heroin can be injected, snorted, sniffed, and smoked.

Mechanism of Action

Morphine is a μ opioid receptor agonist with a mechanism of action similar to that of codeine. It binds to opioid receptors in the CNS and PNS. It can also bind and activate κ and δ opioid receptors.

Heroin is converted to morphine only after it crosses the blood–brain barrier. It has the same effects as morphine in the CNS, but it is more rapid and intense.

Health Effects

Morphine stimulates μ receptors, causing sedation, euphoria, analgesia, respiratory depression, and gastrointestinal dysmotility (i.e., constipation). As a κ receptor stimulator, morphine produces spinal analgesia, miosis (i.e., pinpoint pupils), diuresis, and depression.

Overdose or toxic symptoms include coma, miosis, respiratory depression, pulmonary edema, and death from cardiopulmonary arrest. Morphine and heroin have a high potential for addiction and tolerance and can produce severe withdrawal symptoms on cessation, including stroke, heart attack, and death. Withdrawal can be dangerous. Other withdrawal symptoms are usually the opposite of the drug's effects, such as dysphoria (i.e., intense depression) and hyperalgesia (i.e., chronic pain).

Toxic Levels

The human lethal dose by ingestion is 120 to 250 mg of morphine sulfate, although lethal doses can vary significantly with tolerance. An added danger of morphine or heroin withdrawal is that tolerance levels wear off faster than addiction, and relapsed addicts who return to their last used dose often overdose.

Analytical Methods

The initial screening test for morphine is an immunoassay, and confirmatory testing is performed using GC-MS. Cutoff values for morphine in the immunoassay test for urine specimens is 300 ng/mL. The SAMHSA test for workplace drug screening has a cutoff value of 2000 ng/mL.

There is no separate test for heroin because it is rapidly converted to morphine in the CNS.

Methadone

Methadone is a synthetic analog of morphine and heroin. It is used medically as an analgesic and in the treatment of opioid dependency. It can bind to the same receptors as morphine and produce the same analgesic effects. Methadone is more active and more toxic than morphine, and duration of action in the body is more prolonged. Methadone withdrawal is also more prolonged, but symptoms are less severe than those of morphine withdrawal, making it a useful substitute drug in the treatment of opiate dependency. Methadone has other pharmacologic properties that allow it to block some of the withdrawal symptoms of opiate addiction.

Exposure Routes

Methadone is usually administered orally, but it may also be injected or delivered intravenously.

Mechanism of Action

Methadone is a μ opioid receptor agonist, similar to codeine and morphine. Methadone also reduces opiate cravings and withdrawal symptoms. It has a much longer half-life than other opiates.

Health Effects

Methadone produces analgesia, sedation, respiratory depression, miosis, antitussive effects, and constipation after ingestion. Methadone users also develop tolerance, but it takes much longer than developing tolerance to morphine. Discontinuing methadone use produces a withdrawal syndrome, but it is much less intense and more prolonged than that of other opiates. Withdrawal symptoms include weakness, anxiety, insomnia, abdominal discomfort, sweating, and hot and cold flashes.

Symptoms of overdose include CNS and respiratory system depression, miosis, bradycardia, hypotension, circulatory collapse, hypothermia, coma, seizures, and pulmonary edema. Apnea, respiratory depression, circulatory collapse, cardiac arrest, and death may occur from acute overdose.

Toxic Levels

Methadone toxicity in humans is difficult to quantify because opiate tolerance has profound effects. Methadone intoxication deaths are often complicated by the victim's opiate withdrawal symptoms and dangerous drug-seeking behaviors.

Analytical Methods

Methadone and its metabolite 2-ethylidene-1,5-dimethyl-3,3-diphenylpyrrolidine (EDDP) are often measured in urine as part of drug abuse testing programs. It may also be detected in blood to confirm a diagnosis of poisoning in hospitalized victims or to assist in a forensic investigation. A history of methadone use is considered in interpreting the results because a chronic user can develop tolerance to doses that would be fatal to an opioid-naïve individual.

Dextropropoxyphene

Dextropropoxyphene (Darvon) was used commonly in combination with acetaminophen to treat mild pain. It has antitussive and local anesthetic effects. An FDA-directed recall in 2009 took dextropropoxyphene off the market in the United States, and it was removed in Europe due to concerns about fatal overdoses and arrhythmias. Deaths were most often caused by intentional overdose (i.e., suicide) or multiple-drug toxicity, especially when it was mixed with alcohol.

Exposure Routes

Dextropropoxyphene was taken orally.

Mechanism of Action

Dextropropoxyphene is a μ opioid receptor agonist, similar to codeine.

Health Effects

Overdose is commonly considered in two categories: liver damage from acetaminophen toxicity and dextropropoxyphene overdose. Dextropropoxyphene poisoning causes excessive opioid receptor stimulation, which is responsible for CNS depression, respiratory depression, aspiration pneumonia, and gastrointestinal disturbances.

Toxic Levels

Opiate tolerance can significantly alter lethal dose levels.

Analytical Methods

Dextropropoxyphene and its major metabolite norpropoxyphene can be measured in blood, urine, or hair samples. However, numerous technical difficulties, such as an overlap in the therapeutic and lethal doses, make interpretation of the results difficult.

Barbiturates

Barbiturates are a class of CNS depressants used for their mild sedative, anesthetic, anxiolytic, hypnotic, and anticonvulsant properties. Their effects are felt quickly, and they have a short duration of action. Barbiturates such as phenobarbital have largely been replaced by benzodiazepines in medical practice. When used recreationally, barbiturates produce effects similar to those of ethanol intoxication.

Exposure Routes

Barbiturates are commonly administered orally or intravenously.

Mechanism of Action

Barbiturates enhance γ-aminobutyric acid (GABA) signaling in the CNS. GABA is the predominant inhibitory neurotransmitter, and barbiturates cause widespread CNS depression.

Health Effects

Symptoms of barbiturate intoxication include respiratory depression, hypotension, fatigue, fever, irritability, dizziness, sedation, confusion, impaired coordination, and impaired judgment. Overdose may cause respiratory arrest and death.

Barbiturates are addictive. CNS tolerance builds more quickly than PNS tolerance, increasing the risk of overdose among addicts.

Toxic Levels

One gram of phenobarbital (oral) can be highly poisonous, and dosages of 2 to 10 g (or 95 mg/mL in blood) usually are fatal. Because of the reduced capacity for metabolizing barbiturates in older people, those older than 65 years of age are at higher risk for the harmful effects, including drug dependence and accidental overdose.

Analytical Methods

Barbiturates can be measured in blood or urine samples. Semiquantitative immunoassays for serum samples are available, as are capillary GC methods. Barbiturates can be detected in urine samples using screening tests such as thin-layer chromatography and immunoassays or confirmatory tests such as GC-MS. Immunoassay methods used to detect barbiturates include EMIT, fluorescence polarization immunoassay (FPIA), Siemens Healthcare Diagnostics (formerly DPC) RIA, and CEDIA.

Benzodiazepines

Benzodiazepines (e.g., Valium, Xanax) are used as sedative-hypnotics (i.e., sleep-inducing drugs), anxiolytics (i.e., antianxiety drugs), anticonvulsants, and muscle relaxants. They are much less toxic than barbiturates, and death rarely results when used alone. However, when combined with other CNS depressants (e.g., alcohol, opiates), toxicity increases.

Exposure Routes

Benzodiazepines are usually administered orally or intravenously.

Mechanism of Action

After absorption, benzodiazepines are rapidly distributed in the CNS. They are metabolized by the liver, and many form active metabolites. Like barbiturates, benzodiazepines enhance the effect of the neurotransmitter GABA.

Health Effects

A classic benzodiazepine overdose manifests as coma with normal vital signs. Other symptoms include drowsiness, slurred speech, ataxia, blurred vision, hypotonia (i.e., loss of muscle tone), amnesia, and hallucinations. Chronic use of benzodiazepines leads to tolerance and dependence.

Toxic Levels

Death from oral benzodiazepine overdose is rare. Because it usually occurs in conjunction with the use of alcohol or other sedative-hypnotics, toxic doses vary.

Analytical Methods

Benzodiazepines may be analyzed from blood or urine samples by immunoassay and GC.

Ethyl Alcohol

Ethyl alcohol (i.e., ethanol, alcohol, grain alcohol, or drinking alcohol) is widely used and abused. It is the primary intoxicant in beer, wine, and liquor and one of the oldest recreational drugs. In the CNS, it acts as a depressant, intoxicant, and psychoactive substance.

Analysis of specimens for ethanol is a common test in laboratories. Although ethanol use is legal, driving automobiles while intoxicated is illegal and strictly enforced. Tests for blood alcohol content (e.g., breathalyzer) are routinely performed by police because ethanol intoxication reduces reaction time and inhibits good decision making.

Exposure Routes

Individuals usually ingest ethanol to become intoxicated. Ethanol is rapidly absorbed from the gastrointestinal tract, with a peak concentration occurring 20 to 60 minutes after ingestion. Ethanol is metabolized in the liver by alcohol dehydrogenase. The elimination rate varies among individuals, but the usual rate for men is between 15 and 18 mg/dL/hr. Alcoholics have a higher elimination rate than normal individuals because they have high levels of enzymes in the liver.

Mechanism of Action

Ethanol's mechanism of action is poorly understood, although the CNS depressant effects are thought to result from modification of GABA signals. The adverse effects of ethanol intoxication (e.g., hangover) and its addictive properties are thought to be primarily mediated by the metabolite acetaldehyde.

Heath Effects

The effects of ethanol depend on the amount ingested. Euphoria and decreased inhibition occur at blood levels of less than 50 mg/dL; increased disorientation and incoordination occur at levels between 100 and 300 mg/dL; coma and death at occur at levels greater than 400 mg/dL. The federal statutory limit for operating a motor vehicle is 80 mg/dL. The effects of ethanol are greater when the blood concentration is increasing rather than decreasing. Heavy alcohol use leads to tolerance and addiction.

When combined with other drugs, ethanol creates a synergistic depressant effect. Combinations of ethanol and drugs can result in death. When a pregnant women abuses ethanol during pregnancy, the baby can be born with fetal alcohol spectrum disorder (FASD). FASD includes physical, mental, behavioral, and learning disabilities. FASD can be prevented by refraining from ethanol consumption during pregnancy.

Toxic Levels

Alcohol tolerance varies with use and ethnicity. The levels of the liver enzymes alcohol dehydrogenase and acetaldehyde dehydrogenase can vary significantly. In children, blood concentrations of alcohol above 50 to 100 mg/dL cause dangerous levels of intoxication (Table 34-6).

TABLE 34-6   Effect of Acute Ethanol Ingestion on Blood Levels and Behavior

Ounces Ingested	Blood Concentration (mg/dL)	Behavior
1-2	10-50	None to mild euphoria
3-4	50-100	Mild influence on stereoscopic vision and dark adaptation
4-6	100-150	Euphoria, disappearance of inhibition, prolonged reaction time
6-7	150-200	Moderately severe poisoning, reaction time greatly prolonged, loss of inhibition and slight disturbances in equilibrium and coordination
8-9	200-250	Severe degree of poisoning, disturbances of equilibrium and coordination, retardation of the thought processes and clouding of consciousness
10-15	250-400	Deep coma, possibly fatal

From McPherson RA, Pincus MR. *Henry's Clinical Diagnosis and Management by Laboratory Methods*. 22nd ed. Philadelphia: Elsevier; 2012.

Analytical Methods

Blood alcohol content is routinely determined by breathalyzer or other portable devices, and the result is expressed as a percentage. Alcohol may also be analyzed clinically from blood or urine samples.

Enzymatic methods are used for ethanol analysis. Ethanol is oxidized to acetaldehyde by alcohol dehydrogenase, and NAD$^+$ is converted to NADH. The amount of NADH produced is directly proportional to the amount of ethanol in the sample. Drawing a blood sample is a cumbersome process for determining the blood alcohol level of an impaired driver. Instead, devices that detect the amount of alcohol in a person's breath have been developed.

Breathalyzers measure the concentration of alcohol (a volatile substance) in the air exhaled by a suspect. The device then calculates the concentration of alcohol in the blood, based on the principle that the ratio of alcohol in capillary blood to that in alveolar air is about 2100:1. The breath alcohol expressed as g/L is therefore approximately equal to blood alcohol concentration in g/dL. In practice, a low breath alcohol value produces a low blood alcohol result. Because the difference favors the person being tested, the courts have ruled that this is permissible evidence.

An alcohol test has been developed for saliva specimens, which are easy to collect. Saliva is absorbed by a swab, which is inserted into a test cartridge. The test for saliva alcohol content involves an alcohol dehydrogenase method coupled with a chromophore to produce a visual end point. This method is also used on card or strip tests.

To monitor sobriety in recovering alcoholics, ethyl glucuronide is measured. It is a metabolite of ethanol and can indicate alcohol use within the previous 3 to 4 days.

The person who is having blood drawn to determine the blood alcohol level must give consent. Usually, a police officer accompanies the suspect and provides the kit to be used for collecting the sample. When collecting blood samples, Betadine or another disinfectant is used prepare the site instead of alcohol. The blood alcohol kit should include a sticky label for the tube of blood. The label must be completed, including the patient's name, date of collection, time of collection, and name of the phlebotomist. The phlebotomist may be subpoenaed to testify about the collection of the specimen. A chain of custody form must be completed when drawing a blood alcohol specimen for legal purposes.

Hydromorphone

Hydromorphone (Dilaudid) is a morphine derivative and a potent centrally acting analgesic. It is used as an alternative to morphine for the treatment of pain and occasionally as an antitussive. It is used recreationally because it produces euphoria and relieves stress. Like many other opiates, it is addictive and causes severe withdrawal symptoms.

Exposure Routes

Hydromorphone is most often administered orally and sometimes intravenously or by suppository. It may be insufflated when used recreationally.

Mechanism of Action

Hydromorphone is a μ receptor agonist with a mechanism of action similar to that of codeine and morphine. It penetrates the blood–brain barrier more effectively than morphine, generating more CNS than peripheral effects.

Health Effects

Hydromorphone stimulates μ receptors and causes sedation, euphoria, analgesia, respiratory depression, and gastrointestinal dysmotility (i.e., constipation). As a κ receptor stimulator, hydromorphone produces spinal analgesia, miosis, diuresis, and a dysphoric response (i.e., depression). Overdose or toxic symptoms include coma, miosis, respiratory depression, pulmonary edema, and death from cardiopulmonary arrest.

Toxic Levels

The LD$_{50}$ for hydromorphone is similar to that for heroin or morphine. Like morphine, when hydromorphone is combined with alcohol or other CNS depressants, lethal doses can be much lower.

Analytical Methods

Hydromorphone and other synthetic opiates are not detected by standard drug screens. It can be detected in the urine or blood using more specific tests.

Hydrocodone and Oxycodone

Hydrocodone (Vicodin) and oxycodone (OxyContin) are synthetic opioids similar to hydromorphone. They can be used medically as analgesics or used recreationally. Hydrocodone and oxycodone are the most commonly abused pharmaceuticals and the top two causes of pharmaceutical-related emergency department visits. They are combined with weaker analgesics such as ibuprofen or acetaminophen to discourage recreational use, but these compounds have their own toxic effects.

Exposure Routes

Hydromorphone and oxycodone are most often administered orally, and they can be given intravenously or by suppository if oral administration is not possible. They may be insufflated when used recreationally.

Mechanism of Action

Hydrocodone and oxycodone are μ receptor agonists, making their mechanism of action similar to morphine and codeine. They bind to opioid receptors in the CNS and PNS. It can also bind and activate δ and κ opioid receptors.

Health Effects

Hydrocodone and oxycodone stimulate μ receptors and cause sedation, euphoria, analgesia, respiratory depression, and gastrointestinal dysmotility. As κ receptor stimulators, they produce spinal analgesia, miosis, diuresis, and depression. Overdose or toxic symptoms include coma, miosis, respiratory depression, pulmonary edema, and death from cardiopulmonary arrest.

Toxic Levels

There are no pure hydrocodone or oxycodone pills. Toxicity usually results from other drugs (e.g., acetaminophen) that are added to hydrocodone or oxycodone preparations.

Analytical Methods

Hydrocodone, oxycodone, and other synthetic opiates are not detected by routine drug tests. They can be detected in urine or blood using an expanded test.

Drugs Used for Sexual Assault

Drug-facilitated sexual assault occurs when alcohol and other drugs are used to incapacitate and sexually assault an individual. Some of the drugs used for this purpose include benzodiazepines (e.g., flunitrazepam, diazepam, triazolam, temazepam, clonazepam), choral hydrate, sedative-hypnotics (e.g., zopiclone, eszopiclone, zolpidem, zaleplon), γ-hydroxybutyric acid (GHB), dextromethorphan, and phencyclidine.

These drugs are fast acting, colorless, and tasteless and can be obtained easily. Clinical effects include impaired judgment, reduced inhibitions, sedation, a hypnotic state, loss of muscle coordination, and anterograde amnesia. A person with anterograde amnesia (i.e., true amnesia) cannot form new memories after an incident. Effects are enhanced when drugs are coadministered.

The drugs are commonly administered without the victim's knowledge or permission. Victims who suffer from amnesia may not report the sexual assault for several days. If a long period of time passes before a victim reports the sexual assault, sensitive techniques are required to detect the drugs. Alternative biologic specimens such as hair are being investigated for use in drug detection in these cases.

Benzodiazepines

Benzodiazepines used for incapacitating victims in sexual assaults include diazepam, triazolam, temazepam, and clonazepam. The most common benzodiazepine used is flunitrazepam (Rohypnol). The drug is more potent than diazepam and is not detected in routine immunoassay-based drug screens. It is rapidly absorbed and distributed, taking only 20 to 30 minutes to exert its effects. The drugged individual experiences sedation, amnesia, and hypnosis and loses his or her inhibitions.

Rohypnol's long half-life (25 hours) provides an extended window for detecting the drug. A specific immunoassay is available for detection of the drug. It must be ordered as a specific test, not a drug screen.

Chloral Hydrate

Chloral hydrate can be used for incapacitating an individual. This drug has sedative and hypnotic effects, and it is not detected in a routine drug screen.

Sedative-Hypnotics

Sedative-hypnotics used to incapacitate an individual before a sexual assault are drugs that are normally prescribed as sleep aids, such as zopiclone, eszopiclone (Lunesta), zolpidem (Ambien), and zaleplon (Sonata). These drugs cause individuals to lose their inhibitions and become more passive. They produce retrograde amnesia, which is loss of memory of events that happened before amnesia set in. ELISAs are available to identify and quantitate these drugs.

γ-Hydroxybutyrate

GHB is a chemical that is normally found in the brain. When it is taken orally, it produces sedation and hypnosis. It is detected with GC-MS.

Dextromethorphan

Dextromethorphan is a cough suppressant related to opiate drugs. It is found in over-the-counter cough medicines. High doses lead to respiratory depression, CNS depression, lethargy, agitation, ataxia, nystagmus, diaphoresis, and hypertension. Because dextromethorphan contains bromine, large doses may result in bromine poisoning.

TABLE 34-7   **Drugs Used in Sexual Assault**

Drugs	Effects	Detection
Diazepams: diazepam, triazolam, temazepam, clonazepam and flunitrazepam (Rohypnol)	Rapidly absorbed and distributed, amnesia, sedative-hypnotic effects, disinhibition	Not on routine drug screen, immunoassay test available
Choral hydrate	Sedative and hypnotic	Not on routine drug screen
Sedative-hypnotics: zopiclone, eszopiclone (Lunesta), zolpidem (Ambien), and zaleplon (Sonata)	Disinhibition, passivity, retrograde amnesia	Not on routine drug screen, ELISA available
γ-Hydroxybutyric acid (GHB)	Sedation and hypnosis	GC-MS
Dextromethorphan	Respiratory and CNS depression, lethargy, agitation, ataxia, nystagmus, diaphoresis, hypertension	GC-MS
Phencyclidine (PCP)	Dissociation of perception, consciousness, movement, and memory; awake but incapacitated; limited arm and leg movement	Routine drug screen

CNS, Central nervous system; *ELISA*, enzyme-linked immunosorbent assay; *GC-MS*, gas chromatography with mass spectrometry.

Phencyclidine

Phencyclidine (PCP) is not approved by the FDA for use in humans. It is a potent analgesic and general anesthetic. It is a fast-acting drug that produces dissociation of perception, consciousness, movement, and memory. Used as an anesthetic, it produces a patient who is awake but incapacitated, with limited arm and leg movement. PCP is detected in routine drug screens (Table 34-7).

Summary

Chemical toxicology focuses on the adverse effects of chemicals on the body. Chemicals can be absorbed through the skin, gastrointestinal tract, lungs, nose, and rectum. Low doses of drugs may have no observable effects, but the effects increase with increasing doses to a designated dose. After that point, all receptor sites are full, and no further effects occur with increasing doses. Acute toxic effects result from a single exposure to a chemical. Chronic toxic effects occur after repeated exposure to a chemical over a long period of time.

Collecting specimens for toxicologic analysis must proceed with attention to details of emergencies and legal issues. Toxic conditions can result from pollutants such as secondhand smoke, cigarette smoking, and radiation. Tests are used to determine exposure to alcohols, ethylene glycol, formaldehyde, benzene, xylene, carbon monoxide, cyanide, radon, harmful household products, toxic metals, and drugs of abuse, including those used for sexual assault.

Review Questions

1. Exposure to toxins may result from any of the following routes EXCEPT
   a. Intravenous administration
   b. Inhalation
   c. Transdermal absorption
   d. Ingestion
2. Toxic effects of methanol include all the following EXCEPT
   a. Confusion
   b. Severe metabolic acidosis
   c. Blindness
   d. Death
3. Carbon monoxide is toxic because
   a. Exposure occurs by inhalation and transdermal absorption.
   b. It binds very tightly to hemoglobin and does not allow oxygen to attach to hemoglobin.
   c. It binds very tightly to tissue cells and does not allow carbon dioxide to be released into the lungs.
   d. It binds very tightly to the myoglobin and does not allow oxygen to attach to the myoglobin.
4. Acute toxic effects of cocaine include all the following EXCEPT
   a. Sedation
   b. Seizures
   c. Myocardial infarction
   d. Hypertension
5. Damage caused by a toxic gas is affected by
   a. Other drugs taken by an individual
   b. Body temperature
   c. Solubility of the gas in the blood

d. Partial pressure of gas in the air

6. What is LD_{50}?

  a. It is the median lethal dose.

  b. The lethal dose is 50 mg/dL.

  c. The lethal dose is 50% of the toxin's concentration.

  d. It is determined using human subjects.

7. All of the following measures are taken to ensure a good-quality urine specimen for drug testing EXCEPT

  a. Adding a blue color to toilet water

  b. Having someone accompany the person providing the specimen to observe the collection process

  c. Wearing excess clothing in the collection room

  d. Inactivation of the hot water faucet

8. Most drugs of abuse are detected using an immunoassay-based drug screen and confirmed using

  a. GC-MS

  b. Ion-sensitive electrodes

  c. Colorimetric enzymatic assays

  d. Capillary electrophoresis

9. The most serious effect of methanol ingestion is

  a. Hallucinations

  b. Blindness

  c. Psychosis

  d. Liver damage

10. Common drugs used in sexual assault include all the following EXCEPT

  a. Flunitrazepam

  b. Dextromethorphan

  c. Methamphetamine

  d. Diazepam

Critical Thinking Questions

1. What is the relationship between the dose of a toxic substance and the body's response?

2. What are the analytical methods used to detect ethanol, and how are blood alcohol specimens collected?

3. What features of opiate drugs (e.g., morphine, codeine, hydromorphone, hydrocodone, oxycodone) make them attractive for abuse, and what factors make it difficult to stop taking this class of drugs?

CASE STUDY

A 35-year-old woman was brought to the emergency department at about 2 PM. She was experiencing blurred vision, headache, and dizziness. Initial examination revealed tachycardia and confusion. Family members accompanying the patient indicated that she was drinking illegal altered alcohol with friends late into the night. Test results for the laboratory studies ordered by the physician included the following: sodium, 140 mEq/L; potassium, 3.5 mEq/L; chloride, 100 mEq/L; total carbon dioxide, 15 mEq/L; glucose, 100 mg/dL; blood urea nitrogen (BUN), 25 mg/dL; creatinine, 1.3 mg/dL; calcium, 9.2 mg/dL; phosphorus, 3.4 mg/dL; alkaline phosphate, 85 IU/L; creatine kinase, 98 IU/L; osmolality, 230 mOsm/kg; pH, 7.10, P_{CO_2}, 40 mm Hg; P_{O_2}, 95 mm Hg; and bicarbonate (HCO_3^-), 15 mEq/L.

What is the anion gap for this patient? Is the anion gap normal? Why or why not? How does the calculated osmolality compare with the measured osmolality? What accounts for the difference? What additional test should be ordered? What is the most probable diagnosis?

Bibliography

Agency for Toxic Substances and Disease Registry (ATSDR). *Medical Management Guidelines for Hydrochloric Acid.* Atlanta: U.S. Department of Health and Human Services, Public Health Service; March 2011.

Agency for Toxic Substances and Disease Registry (ATSDR). *Toxicological Profile for Ammonia.* Atlanta: U.S. Department of Health and Human Services, Public Health Service; September 2004.

Agency for Toxic Substances and Disease Registry (ATSDR). *Toxicological Profile for Arsenic.* Atlanta: U.S. Department of Health and Human Services, Public Health Service; August 2007.

Agency for Toxic Substances and Disease Registry (ATSDR). *Toxicological Profile for Beryllium.* Atlanta: U.S. Department of Health and Human Services, Public Health Service; September 2002.

Agency for Toxic Substances and Disease Registry (ATSDR). *Toxicological Profile for Cadmium.* Atlanta: U.S. Department of Health and Human Services, Public Health Service; September 2002.

Agency for Toxic Substances and Disease Registry (ATSDR). *Toxicological Profile for Carbon Monoxide.* Atlanta: U.S. Department of Health and Human Services, Public Health Service; June 2012.

Agency for Toxic Substances and Disease Registry (ATSDR). *Toxicological Profile for Chromium.* Atlanta: U.S. Department of Health and Human Services, Public Health Service; September 2008.

Agency for Toxic Substances and Disease Registry (ATSDR). *Toxicological Profile for Cyanide.* Atlanta, GA: U.S. Department of Health and Human Services, Public Health Service; September 2004.

Agency for Toxic Substances and Disease Registry (ATSDR). *Toxicological Profile for DEET.* Atlanta: U.S. Department of Health and Human Services, Public Health Service; December 2004.

Agency for Toxic Substances and Disease Registry (ATSDR). *Toxicological Profile for Lead (Update).* Atlanta: U.S. Department of Health and Human Services, Public Health Service; August 2007.

Agency for Toxic Substances and Disease Registry (ATSDR). *Toxicological Profile for Mercury.* Atlanta, GA: U.S. Department of Health and Human Services, Public Health Service; March 1999.

Agency for Toxic Substances and Disease Registry (ATSDR). *Toxicological Profile for Nitrates and Nitrites.* Atlanta: U.S. Department of Health and Human Services, Public Health Service; January 2011.

Agency for Toxic Substances and Disease Registry (ATSDR). *Toxicological Profile for Radon.* Atlanta: U.S. Department of Health and Human Services, Public Health Service; June 2003.

Agency for Toxic Substances and Disease Registry (ATSDR). *Toxicological Profile for Sodium Hydroxide.* Atlanta: U.S. Department of Health and Human Services, Public Health Service; September 2004.

Agency for Toxic Substances and Disease Registry (ATSDR). *Toxicological Profile for Sodium Hypochlorite.* Atlanta: U.S. Department of Health and Human Services, Public Health Service; April 2002.

Agency for Toxic Substances and Disease Registry (ATSDR). *Toxicological Profile for 1,1,1-Trichloroethane*. Atlanta: U.S. Department of Health and Human Services, Public Health Service; July 2006.

Agency for Toxic Substances and Disease Registry (ATSDR). *Toxicological Profile for Xylene*. Atlanta: U.S. Department of Health and Human Services, Public Health Service; January 2011.

Environmental Protection Agency. *Isopropanol Final Test Rule*; October 23, 1989. <http://www.epa.gov/oppt/chemtest/pubs/sun70.pdf> Accessed 27.08.15.

Environmental Protection Agency. *Toxicological Review of Ethylene Glycol Monobutyl Ether (EGBE)*; March 2010. <http://www.epa.gov/iris/toxreviews/0500tr.pdf> Accessed 27.08.15.

Environmental Protection Agency. *Formaldehyde Hazard Summary*; January 2000. <http://www.epa.gov/airtoxics/hlthef/formalde.html> Accessed 27.08.15.

Kruse JA. Methanol poisoning. *Intensive Care Med*. 1992;18:391–397.

National Institute on Drug Abuse. *Drug Facts: Cocaine*. Atlanta: U.S. Department of Health and Human Services, Public Health Service; March 2010.

National Institute on Drug Abuse. *Drug Facts: Hallucinogens—LSD, Peyote, Psilocybin and PCP*. Atlanta: U.S. Department of Health and Human Services, Public Health Service; June 2009.

National Institute on Drug Abuse. *Drug Facts: Marijuana*. Atlanta: U.S. Department of Health and Human Services, Public Health Service; November 2010.

National Institute on Drug Abuse. *Drug Facts: MDMA (Ecstasy)*. Atlanta: U.S. Department of Health and Human Services, Public Health Service; December 2010.

National Institute on Drug Abuse. *Drug Facts: Methamphetamine*. Atlanta: U.S. Department of Health and Human Services, Public Health Service; March 2010.

National Institute on Drug Abuse. *Prescription Drugs*. Atlanta: U.S. Department of Health and Human Services, Public Health Service; June 2009.

Riegel AC, Kalivas PW. Neuroscience: lack of inhibition leads to abuse. *Nature*. 2010;463:743–744.

U.S. Department of Health and Human Services *Chemical Hazards and Emergency Medical Management* <http://chemm.nlm.nih.gov/> Accessed 27.08.15

35

Transplantation

DANIELLE FORTUNA, LAURA J. MCCLOSKEY, ZI-XUAN WANG, DOUGLAS F. STICKLE

CHAPTER OUTLINE

Introduction

Overview of Transplantation
  Indications
  Evaluation of Candidates
  Contraindications
  Establishment of Priority and Organ Allocation

Role of Medical Laboratories in Transplantation

Overview of the Immune System
  Innate Immune System
  Adaptive Immune System
  Immune System Dysfunction

Role of the Immune System in Transplantation
  Genetics of the Major Histocompatibility Complex

Histocompatibility Matching

Human Leukocyte Antigen Laboratories and Testing
  Methods

Graft-Versus-Host Disease

Transplant Rejection

Immunosuppression
  Immunosuppressant Drugs
  Complications of Immunosuppression
  Monitoring Immunosuppression

Exceptional Cases in Transplantation

Future of Transplantation

OBJECTIVES

After completion of this chapter, the reader will be able to:

1. Describe transplantation.
2. Describe why pretransplantation screening is important, and list contraindications for transplantation.
3. Explain the purpose of psychosocial screening of organ transplant recipients.
4. Describe the role of immunosuppressants to control rejection of a transplanted organ.
5. List several immunosuppressants used in organ transplantation.
6. Describe laboratory assays, specimen timing, and test principles for measuring various immunosuppressants.
7. Discuss the different types of rejection of transplanted organs and physiologic changes that can be detected by laboratory tests to indicate rejection is occurring.
8. Explain graft-versus-host disease and the clinical chemistry tests used to diagnose the condition.
9. Describe the effects of transplantation on the recipient's kidneys.
10. Describe how the use of immunosuppressants can lead to cancer in transplant recipients.

KEY TERMS

ABO-Rh typing
Biopsy
Blood spots
Cancer
Creatinine
Crossmatch
Cyclosporine
Cystatin C
Donor testing
Everolimus

Expert systems
Flow cytometry
Graft-versus-host disease
Hematopoietic stem cell
Human leukocyte antigens
Immunofixation
Immunosuppressants
Immunosuppression
Major histocompatibility complex
Medical ethics

Mycophenolic acid
Next-generation sequencing
Psychological assessment
Rejection
Renal insufficiency
Serologic typing
Sirolimus
Tacrolimus
Tissue typing
Transplantation

❖ Case in Point

K.T. is a 55-year-old man with history of type 2 diabetes mellitus diagnosed 10 years earlier. His diabetes has not been well controlled, with measured hemoglobin A_{1c} consistently in the range of 11% to 12%. Over the past several years, he has experienced a progressive decline in renal function caused by diabetic nephropathy, a complication of diabetes involving renal vascular damage and scarring. His creatinine level is greatly elevated (>20 mg/dL). K.T. is currently receiving hemodialysis three times each week. It is a last-resort method used for end-stage renal disease to eliminate waste products from blood. KT is awaiting a renal transplant. What is the process to determine if he is a good candidate for a transplant? If he is a good candidate, what tests would be performed to find a suitable donor?

Points to Remember

- Transplantation can involve solid organs or hematopoietic cells from donor bone marrow or cord blood.
- The most common solid organ transplants are the heart, lung, kidney, liver, pancreas, and intestines.
- The need for solid organ transplants exceeds the availability of organs.
- The many reasons for transplantation include congenital defects, acute poisoning, and progressive disease.
- Candidates for transplantation undergo psychosocial testing.
- Donor testing includes blood typing (i.e., ABO-Rh typing) and screening for infectious disease.
- Testing for immune system compatibility between donor and recipient is especially important for hematopoietic stem cell transplantation.
- Compatibility testing involves characterization of human leukocyte antigens (HLAs) for the donor and the recipient.
- HLA testing involves flow cytometry, DNA sequence analysis, and crossmatching.
- The natural response of the immune system to transplantation is rejection of foreign tissue.
- The immune system comprises innate, rapid, nonspecific response systems and adaptive, delayed, sustained, specific response systems.
- Success of transplantation depends on suppression of the immune system.
- A few drugs are used to promote immunosuppression.
- Immunosuppressants act largely to suppress the humoral response system by inhibiting proliferation of lymphocytes.
- Cyclosporine and tacrolimus are calcineurin inhibitors.
- Sirolimus and everolimus are inhibitors of the mammalian target of rapamycin (mTOR).
- Corticosteroids are potent inhibitors of inflammatory and immune responses, and their long-term use produces many adverse side effects.
- Lifelong immunosuppression therapy using various combinations of drugs and doses is needed by transplant recipients.
- The kidney is especially subject to the toxic side effects of immunosuppression.
- Concentrations of immunosuppressant drugs must be monitored to mitigate toxic side effects.
- Immunosuppressant drug monitoring is ideally performed by mass spectrometry.
- Immunosuppression is a risk factor for infectious diseases and some malignancies.
- Graft-versus-host disease (i.e., transplanted tissue promotes destruction of host tissue) is a common complication of hematopoietic stem cell transplantation.
- Laboratory monitoring of organ function after transplantation involves organ-specific profiles of analytes that indicate progression of disease.
- Organ rejection is most often assessed by a pathologist's review of biopsy specimens.
- Medical ethics are a consideration in many aspects of transplantation, such as how candidates are prioritized and how organs are allocated to regional waiting lists.
- Transplantation practices continue to evolve due to developments in basic science and technology.

Introduction

This chapter reviews transplantation and the role of the laboratory in management of the process. Successful transplantation depends on matching donor to recipient by pretransplantation testing and monitoring for posttransplantation disease, rejection, therapeutic drug levels, and unwanted side effects of immunosuppression. This describes current practices, delineate the immunology related to transplant rejection, and detail the extensive use of laboratory testing in all phases of transplantation.

Overview of Transplantation

Transplantation refers to the transfer of tissue, organs, or bone marrow cells from a donor to a recipient. The major categories for which laboratory involvement is an integral part are solid organ (e.g., heart, lung, kidney, liver, pancreas, intestines) and hematopoietic stem cell (e.g., bone marrow, umbilical cord blood) transplantation, although corneal, skin, and bone grafts are also used.

Extensive databases for transplantation are maintained by the Health Resource and Services Administration of the U.S. Department of Health and Human Services. In 2014, almost 29,000 solid organs were transplanted in the United States (Table 35-1) among 247 centers. Although most solid organ procedures involve organs from deceased donors, approximately 6000 involved living donors of kidneys (i.e., approximately 35% of kidney transplants).

Transplantation is most often a lifesaving procedure, and organ shortage is a major roadblock. In 2013, approximately 125,000 patients in the United States were on waiting lists for solid organ transplants, and approximately 20 patients die each day awaiting transplants. Hematopoietic stem cell transplantation (HSCT) occurs at a lower rate than solid

TABLE 35-1	Organ Transplantation Procedures in the United States, 2014
Transplanted Organ	**Number of Procedures**
Kidney	16,895
Liver	6455
Pancreas	256
Kidney and pancreas	762
Heart	2531
Lung	1923
Heart and lung	23
Intestine	109
Total	28,954

Data from Organ Procurement and Transplantation Network. Information database. <http://optn.transplant.hrsa.gov/converge/data/> Accessed 30.06.15.

organ transplantation, with about 18,000 HSCT procedures performed in 2012. Approximately 55% of HSCTs are autologous (i.e., using patient's own cells after in vitro modification to replace their own bone marrow). The highest level of involvement of laboratories in pretransplantation testing is for allogenic HSCTs (i.e., using a non-self donor).

Indications

Hundreds of conditions may require a solid organ transplant. Examples are given in Table 35-2. Indications are categorized as follows:

- Congenital structural abnormality of an organ (e.g., heart, liver)
- Congenital metabolic disease (e.g., inborn errors of metabolism) or other inherited disorders (e.g., cystic fibrosis)
- Medical conditions that lead to acute or progressive organ failure (e.g., renal disease due to diabetes or hypertension, liver disease due to infection or toxin exposure)

There are more than 100 diseases for which HSCT is recognized as an appropriate treatment, although it is primarily used for leukemias and lymphomas. Major categories of disorders associated with HSCT are summarized in Box 35-1.

Numerous criteria are used to determine whether an individual with organ failure can be considered a candidate for transplantation, including the following indications:

- A condition for which transplantation is considered an effective treatment
- Severe and progressive disease that no longer responds to medical treatment and may be fatal
- Willingness to accept the risks of surgery and subsequent medical treatment
- Physically and emotionally capable of undergoing surgery and subsequent medical treatment

Evaluation of Candidates

Transplantation is a lifesaving but life-altering event. The transplant recipient must have significant commitment and motivation, dedication to medical compliance and lifestyle modifications, and a strong support system.

An important step in the pretransplantation workup is review of the patient's psychiatric history and current status and evaluation of his or her understanding of the entire process. The patient and patient's family must be prepared for transplantation and all that follows. A thorough psychological assessment helps to identify psychosocial or psychiatric barriers to a good outcome. Unfortunately, depression is not uncommon among transplant recipients.

Contraindications

A patient may not be considered a candidate for transplantation for numerous reasons despite organ failure. Contraindications reflect knowledge about factors known to negatively impact outcomes. The lists of contraindications are organ specific and not necessarily absolute or universal reasons for exclusion; they are instead dictated by the experience and criteria of individual transplantation centers.

Common contraindications are shown in Box 35-2. Most are comorbidities (i.e., coexisting disease) that may not be directly related to organ failure. For instance, metastatic cancer and positive human immunodeficiency virus (HIV) status may be reasons for exclusion. Psychosocial contraindications such as sustained drug abuse are often reasons for exclusion. Age of the patient alone may be reason for exclusion for some types of transplantation.

Establishment of Priority and Organ Allocation

Establishment of priority among patients awaiting transplantation is a highly complex process. A U.S. system of priority on waiting lists for organ allocation has been in place since 1998. Issues of medical ethics are paramount because rules must reflect acceptable conventions and judgments about the value of transplantation in diverse circumstances (e.g., relative value of saving the life of a child versus an adult). Because of their complexity and ethical implications, waiting list rules are continuously reviewed and reevaluated.

Organ allocation is not strictly fixed according to the national waiting list priority. It also depends on the location of the patient because a major factor is the limited allowable time between organ procurement and transplantation (Table 35-3). The likelihood of organ allocation among patients on the national waiting list is, therefore, based in part on the region of the country in which a patient is enlisted. When an organ and the associated organ donor data become available, a computer program operating at the national level generates a list of potential recipients who are ranked according to predetermined objective criteria, which include blood type, tissue type, size of the organ, medical urgency, time on the waiting list, and distance between donor and recipient.

TABLE 35-2 Conditions Leading to End-Stage Organ Failure and Requiring Solid Organ Transplantation

Organ	Condition	Organ	Condition
Kidney	Glomerular diseases	Lung	Congenital disease
	Diabetes		Emphysema, chronic obstructive pulmonary disease
	Polycystic kidneys		Cystic fibrosis
	Hypertensive nephrosclerosis		Idiopathic pulmonary fibrosis
	Renovascular and other vascular diseases		Primary pulmonary hypertension
	Congenital, rare familial, and metabolic disorders		α_1-Antitrypsin deficiency
	Tubular and interstitial diseases		Graft failure/repeat transplantation
	Neoplasms	Intestines	Short gut syndrome
	Graft failure/repeat transplantation		Intestinal atresia
Pancreas	Diabetes mellitus, type 1		Necrotizing enterocolitis
	Diabetes mellitus, type 2		Intestinal volvulus due to malrotation
	Diabetes due to chronic pancreatitis		Intestinal volvulus due to adhesions
	Diabetes due to cystic fibrosis		Intestinal volvulus due to persistent omphalomesenteric duct
	Pancreatic cancer		Gastroschisis
	Bile duct cancer		Massive resection due to inflammatory bowel disease (e.g., Crohn disease)
	Other cancers		Massive resection due to tumor
	Graft failure/repeat transplantation		Massive resection due to mesenteric arterial thrombosis or embolus
	Pancreatectomy		Massive resection due to mesenteric venous thrombosis
Liver	Noncholestatic cirrhosis		Functional bowel problem
	Cholestatic liver disease or cirrhosis		Hirschsprung disease
	Biliary atresia		Neuronal intestinal dysplasia
	Acute hepatic necrosis		Pseudo-obstruction, neuropathic or myopathic
	Metabolic diseases		Protein-losing enteropathy
	Malignant neoplasms		Microvillous inclusion disease
Heart	Cardiomyopathy		Graft failure/repeat transplantation
	Coronary artery disease		
	Congenital heart disease		
	Valvular heart disease		
	Graft failure/repeat transplantation		

Data from Organ Procurement and Transplantation Network. Organ datasource. <http://optn.transplant.hrsa.gov/converge/organDatasource/> Accessed 30.06.15.

Role of Medical Laboratories in Transplantation

Laboratory medicine plays a central role in the success of solid organ transplantation and HSCT. Responsibilities include testing the donor for infectious disease, pretransplantation testing for immunologic compatibility of donor and recipient, and posttransplantation monitoring of organ function, immunosuppressant therapy, and adverse effects of immunosuppression.

Overview of the Immune System

Progression of transplantation as a viable treatment option for patients with failing organs followed development of drugs for immunosuppression, beginning with the

---

• BOX 35-1 Diseases That Can Be Treated by Hematopoietic Stem Cell Transplantation

Acute lymphoblastic leukemia (ALL)
Acute myelogenous leukemia (AML)
Chronic lymphocytic leukemia (CLL)
Chronic myelogenous leukemia (CML)
Juvenile myelomonocytic leukemia
Hodgkin and non-Hodgkin lymphomas
Hemoglobinopathies (e.g., sickle cell anemia, thalassemia)
Inherited immune system disorders (e.g., severe combined immunodeficiency [SCID], Wiskott-Aldrich syndrome)
Inherited metabolic disorders (e.g., Hurler syndrome, leukodystrophies)
Marrow failure (e.g., severe aplastic anemia, Fanconi anemia)
Myelodysplastic syndromes
Myeloproliferative disorders
Plasma disorders (e.g., multiple myeloma)

Data from Health Resources and Services Administration, U.S. Department of Health and Human Services. Transplant frequently asked questions. <http://bloodcell.transplant.hrsa.gov/transplant/understanding_tx/transplant_faqs/> Accessed 30.06.15.

• BOX 35-2 Possible Contraindications for Solid Organ Transplantation

Age >65 years
Severe malnutrition
Severe disease of other organs
Previous surgery
Poor functional status
Poor medical compliance
Disseminated or untreated cancer
Severe psychiatric disease
Irresolvable psychosocial problems
Persistent substance abuse
Severe mental retardation
Human immunodeficiency virus (HIV) infection
Insulin-dependent diabetes mellitus (IDDM)
Life-threatening diseases that severely limit length or quality of life despite successful transplantation

Data from Transplant Center, University of Maryland Medical Center. Services. <http://umm.edu/programs/transplant/services> Accessed 30.06.15.

TABLE 35-3 Preservation Time between Procurement and Transplantation of Solid Organs

Harvested Organ	Time to Transplantation
Heart	4-6 hr
Liver	12-24 hr
Kidney	48-72 hr
Lung	4-6 hr

From Organ Procurement and Transplantation Network. Partnering with your transplant team: the patient's guide to transplantation. <http://optn.transplant.hrsa.gov/ContentDocuments/PartneringWithTransplantTeam_508v.pdf> Accessed 30.06.15.

---

introduction of cyclosporine in the 1970s. To understand the need for and the mechanism of immunosuppression, we begin with an overview of the immune system, which protects the body from pathogens. It distinguishes between the body's own cells (i.e., self) and foreign cells (i.e., non-self) and defends against non-self invaders. Successful transplantation requires suppression of this natural response to enable transplants to survive and function.

The human immune system involves coordination of cellular elements (e.g., leukocytes) and humoral elements (e.g., antibodies, complement proteins, enzymes) that recognize and eradicate foreign entities such as bacteria, viruses, and parasites. The immune system treats all non-self material as potential pathogens.

The first line of defense is the physical barrier between the body and the external environment: the skin and mucous membranes, including the epithelia lining the gastrointestinal, respiratory, and genitourinary-reproductive tracts. Although normal microbial flora exists on the skin and mucosa, physical properties (e.g., mucin production, cilia) of these tissues provide resistance to pathogen entry. Breaches in the physical barrier, such as a needlestick injury, skin wound, or sufficient inoculation of the pharynx by *Streptococcus pyogenes* (i.e., strep throat), enable pathogens to evade the first line of defense. They then encounter the innate and adaptive immune systems.

Innate Immune System

The innate system, also known as the nonspecific immune system, provides rapid but short-term responses to bacteria, viruses, and toxins. The innate immune system consists of preformed cellular and humoral elements that patrol the body's tissues, enabling an immediate response to a pathogen breach of the physical barrier. The major constituents include neutrophils, eosinophils, basophils, macrophages, natural killer cells, and soluble molecules such as complement and lysozyme. Human tissues provide an abundant supply of nutrients for a pathogen to survive, thrive, and proliferate. The goal of the nonspecific immune response is to neutralize or eliminate the pathogen quickly.

Mechanisms by which the cellular arm of the immune system respond to various types of pathogens include recognition of structurally conserved pathogen products (e.g., bacterial surface molecules, double-stranded RNA). Mechanisms of the humoral arm include components of the complement cascade, which may interact directly with pathogen biopolymers, and proinflammatory cytokines secreted by sentinel cells activated by products or antigens of infectious agents.

Macrophages and neutrophils recognize and engulf pathogens by phagocytosis. Inside the cell, the pathogen is digested by potent cytoplasmic enzymes such as lysozyme, which digests bacterial cell walls. Complement proteins kill pathogens indirectly by aiding in phagocytosis or directly by killing of the microorganism by cell membrane disruption.

The innate immune system also is responsible for alerting the adaptive immune system. The presence and nature of the threat is communicated by antigen presentation and major histocompatibility complex interactions.

Adaptive Immune System

The adaptive system, also known as the acquired immune system, provides long-term defense against pathogens through highly specific responses to foreign antigens. The adaptive immune system is primarily composed of lymphocytes (i.e., T and B cells) and antibodies (i.e., immunoglobulins), which are proteins secreted by specialized, differentiated B cells called plasma cells.

The adaptive system depends on **major histocompatibility complex** (MHC) proteins, also known as **human leukocyte antigens** (HLAs). The MHC class I and class II genes (discussed later) encode proteins with similar topology: a transmembrane anchor region and a cell surface domain with a structurally conserved peptide-binding fold (i.e., groove). MHC complexes are located on nucleated cells and are recognized by T cells. Class I MHC molecules are located on all nucleated cells, and class II MHC molecules are more concentrated on specialized antigen-presenting cells (APCs) such as macrophages, dendritic cells, and B cells. The class I and class II proteins present processed peptide antigens to T lymphocytes to stimulate an immune response.

For intracellular antigens, such as in viral infections, the proteasome degrades cytoplasmic proteins encoded by the virus to peptides, which are transferred to the endoplasmic reticulum by the transporter associated with antigen processing. In this compartment, the peptides bind to the class I complex, which is trafficked to the cell surface and presented to CD8 cytotoxic T lymphocytes. The viral peptides are recognized as foreign, and the cytotoxic T cells kill the infected cell.

For extracellular antigens, such as in bacterial infections, the pathogen is phagocytized by an APC and degraded intracellularly in lysosomes. Fusion of lysosomes with the Golgi apparatus results in binding of the bacterial peptides to class II proteins, and this complex is trafficked to the cell surface. The class II protein complexed with the foreign (bacterial) peptide then binds to a CD4 helper T lymphocyte, which subsequently stimulates expansion of CD8 cytotoxic T lymphocytes and differentiation of B lymphocytes to form plasma cells that secrete antibodies specific to pathogens. An example of these interactions is shown in Figure 35-1. Some of the activated B cells form memory B cells, which remember the antigen and become reactivated on reexposure.

HLAs present foreign material to be recognized by T cells, and because they are located on all cells, they serve as markers of self. T cells routinely assess whether HLAs are clean (i.e., not presenting antigen), present (i.e., loss is a sign of cell disruption or infection), and consistent with the MHC profile of the rest of the body (i.e., self). Even if a cell is not infected by a pathogen, it is recognized as non-self if it does not have the correct MHC profile and is targeted accordingly.

In a similar fashion, the immune system is responsible for the anticellular activity leading to transplant rejection. The immune system is also involved in the body's defenses against development of certain types of malignancy (i.e., cancer).

Immune System Dysfunction

Although the intended function of the immune system is to prevent disease, inherited or acquired errors and dysregulation of the system can produce disease. For example, severe combined immunodeficiency disease (SCID) is an inherited

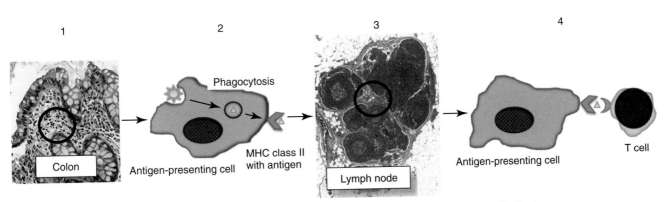

• **Figure 35-1** Interaction between antigen-presenting cells and T cells activates the adaptive immune response. In bacterial infections, antigen-presenting cells phagocytize the bacteria, as shown in the colon *(1)*. Bacteria are ingested and degraded intracellularly. Small peptide fragments of them are shuttled to the outer surface of the antigen-presenting cell, where they are held by class II major histocompatibility complex (MHC) molecules *(2)*. Each antigen-presenting cell travels through the lymphatic system to a lymph node *(3)*, where a CD4 helper T cell responds to the antigen-presenting molecule by stimulating clonal expansion of CD8 cytotoxic T cells, which kill the bacteria-infected population of cells *(4)*. After presentation of antigen to T cells by means of class II MHC molecules, B cells are stimulated by the T cells to differentiate into a special subpopulation of lymphocytes (i.e., plasma cells), which produce antibodies specific for the pathogen. Some activated B cells form memory B cells, which remember the antigen and become reactivated on reexposure to it. These interactions also involve costimulatory steps, such as cytokine production, which are necessary for the full immune response.

disease in which T and B cells are defective, and patients have recurrent infections caused by various types of microorganisms. Human immunodeficiency virus (HIV) infection causes an acquired form of immunodeficiency from viral infection of CD4 T cells, macrophages, and dendritic cells and causes progressive failure of cell-mediated immunity.

Hypersensitivity reactions result from an exaggerated response to environmental stimuli. Severe hypersensitivity reactions can result in anaphylaxis, a life-threatening condition involving multiple organ systems, especially the respiratory and cardiovascular systems. Autoimmune diseases occur as a result of the body perceiving self as non-self, which results in the production of autoantibodies that damage or destroy tissue.

Role of the Immune System in Transplantation

Although the immune system is essential to survival, the natural and expected responses of the immune system pose a significant challenge to transplantation. Typically, foreign organs or tissues (i.e., allografts) are transplanted into a patient. Because the immune system has a highly effective way of distinguishing self from non-self, pretransplantation and posttransplantation steps must be taken to ensure the best possible outcome for the patient and the transplanted organ. HLAs are matched as closely as possible between donor and recipient to mitigate the recipient's immune response to non-self tissue. Success also relies on effective pharmacologic intervention to suppress the immune response.

Genetics of the Major Histocompatibility Complex

Class I MHC proteins include HLA-A, HLA-B, and HLA-C; class II MHC proteins include HLA-DR, HLA-DQ, and HLA-DP. The genes that encode these six HLAs are located on the short arm of chromosome 6. Each HLA gene is highly polymorphic (i.e., has many variants). The HLA region is the most polymorphic region in the human genome. Table 35-4 shows the number of antigen group serotypes and the associated large number of gene alleles, demonstrating the complexity of this system.

HLA genes are located in a cluster and often are inherited as a unit, called a haplotype. Every individual has two haplotypes of these genes: one paternal haplotype and one maternal haplotype. The genes are expressed in a codominant fashion, meaning that both haplotypes are expressed. Consequently, as many as 12 different HLA proteins can be expressed. For example, because a macrophage is an APC, it expresses class I and class II MHC proteins. The macrophage therefore has paternal class I (i.e., HLA-A, HLA-B, HLA-C), paternal class II (i.e., HLA-DR, HLA-DQ, and HLA-DP), maternal class I (i.e., HLA-A, HLA-B, and HLA-C), and maternal class II (HLA-DR, HLA-DQ, and HLA-DP) protein expression.

Histocompatibility Matching

Histocompatibility matching (i.e., HLA matching or tissue typing) between the donor and recipient is a fundamental step in planning organ and tissue transplantation. The goal is to determine the MHC haplotypes of donors and recipients to find an optimal match. This work is most often performed by a specialized HLA laboratory.

A certain amount of donor testing precedes the work of the HLA laboratory. The donor undergoes testing equivalent to that associated with blood donation: tests to determine the blood type of the donor (i.e., ABO-Rh typing) and tests to ensure that the donor is free from a list of infectious diseases (Box 35-3). The HLA laboratory then conducts complex tests called tissue or antigen typing associated with phenotyping and genotyping of the donor and recipient. The tests determine compatibility of common classes of antigens that are primary factors in the initiation of immune response. Crossmatching is performed to identify preformed antibodies in the recipient that will react on exposure to the donor's antigens.

The extent of HLA matching required depends on the type of transplant. Characterization of HLA-A, -B, -Bw4, -Bw6, -C, -DR, and -DQB is required for kidney and pancreas transplants, although exact matching of all antigens

TABLE 35-4	Numbers of Serotypes and Alleles per Human Leukocyte Antigen Locus	
Locus	No. of Serotypes	No. of Alleles
A	28	2884
B	61	3589
C	10	2375
DRB1	24	1540
DQB1	9	664
DPB1	Not applicable	422

Data from Immuno Polymorphism Database (IPD). Statistics. <http://www.ebi.ac.uk/ipd/imgt/hla/stats.html> Accessed 30.06.15.

• BOX 35-3 Infectious Disease Tests Performed on Organ Donors

Anti-cytomegalovirus (CMV) antibody
Anti-human immunodeficiency virus (HIV) 1 and 2 antibodies
Epstein-Barr virus (EBV) antibody
Hepatitis B surface antigen (HBsAg)
Hepatitis B core antibody (HBcAb)
Anti-hepatitis C virus (HCV) antibody
Venereal Disease Research Laboratory (VDRL) or rapid plasma reagin (RPR)

From Organ Procurement and Transplantation Network. Policies. <http://optn.transplant.hrsa.gov/ContentDocuments/OPTN_Policies_PC_07-2012.pdf> Accessed 30.06.15.

is not a necessary condition for transplantation. For solid organ transplants, immunosuppression regimens appear to be more likely responsible for successful transplantation than exact HLA matching.

The requirements for HLA matching are much more extensive for HSCT. The greatest degree of HLA match between donor and recipient improves transplant survival and can reduce the incidence and severity of acute and chronic graft-versus-host disease (GVHD). The National Marrow Donor Program recommends that donors should be high-resolution typed at HLA-A, -B, -C, and -DRB1, and donors unrelated to the recipient should be mismatched by at most only a single locus.

A different strategy, called haploidentical stem cell transplantation, in which the donor and recipient share only one of the two sets of the HLA genes, is a relatively common practice in treating patients with hematologic malignancies such as acute myeloid leukemia. Donors are family members such as siblings, parents, or children of the patient. In this setting, the medical benefit is the graft's immunologic response against leukemic cells. T lymphocytes from the donor recognize leukemia cells as foreign (based on mismatched class I and class II molecules from the non-identical alleles between the donor and recipient) and kill the cells. The increased risk for GVHD is managed with immunosuppressants.

Human Leukocyte Antigen Laboratories and Testing Methods

HLA laboratories are accredited by the American Society for Histocompatibility and Immunogenetics (ASHI) and operate under strict regulations regarding methods, quality control, quality assurance, and proficiency. Testing is performed in accordance with international consensus guidelines.

HLA testing involves flow cytometry (i.e., measurement of suspended cells flowing singly through a detection system), DNA sequence analysis, and crossmatching methods. HLA testing comprises tissue (antigen) typing, which is used to identify donor and recipient antigens by serologic typing or gene alleles by DNA-based typing, and antibody screening, which is used to detect preformed antibodies in recipient serum.

Serologic typing uses a typing tray from a commercial source to identify antigen groups of a donor or recipient. Each typing tray consists of a panel of premixed alloantisera or monoclonal antibodies with known antibody specificities. Monoclonal antibodies more consistently generate accurate typing results than conventional antisera. T and B cells from the tested patient are purified, dispensed into the wells of the typing tray, and incubated with the antibodies and complement. Detection is based on complement-dependent cytotoxicity (CDC). Antibodies in the well bind with antigens on the surface of lymphocytes and activate the complement system, resulting in cell lysis and death that is revealed by staining with a dye. The result is low-resolution identification of antigen groups such as HLA-B27 or HLA-DQ2.

DNA-based HLA typing includes methods such as sequence-specific primer (SSP) polymerase chain reaction (PCR), sequence-specific oligonucleotide probe (SSOP), and sequence-based typing (SBT). Genomic DNA extracted from a patient's buccal swab or blood is used as the template for PCR or sequence reactions. SSP and SSOP are designed to resolve a specific nucleotide at a specific polymorphic location of a gene.

A set of SSP reactions can yield low- or high-resolution typing results, depending on what SSPs are used. Specific DNA sequences of the primer set are generated by SBT. When an entire gene, including all exons and introns, is sequenced without any ambiguity, the typing result reaches the allelic level, the highest possible level of resolution. When crucial exons such as exon 2 and 3 for class I and exon 2 for class II MHC genes are sequenced, the typing results are called high resolution because the antigens with the same genotype at this level have the same amino acid sequence. A high-resolution HLA genotype is sufficient for all types of transplantation according to current standards.

When Sanger DNA sequencing is used, some mixed nucleotides occur at certain positions because both alleles are sequenced together. This phase ambiguity may be further resolved by specific SSP or SSOP reactions. Another limitation of Sanger DNA sequencing reaching resolution at the allelic genotype level is the expense and intensity of labor required to sequence all exons and introns of HLA genes. The time constraint between organ procurement and transplantation can limit the choice of HLA testing method.

Technological developments are changing the way in which HLA testing is performed. In the future, the practice of HLA matching may move uniformly to testing at the level of high-resolution DNA sequencing, made possible by a technique known as next-generation sequencing (NGS). Desktop NGS sequencers such as MiSeq and Ion Torrent can generate millions of DNA sequences in one assay. Sequencing of all critical exons or even all exons of HLA genes to achieve high-resolution HLA genotyping is feasible. Each DNA strand is clonally sequenced in parallel to resolve the phase ambiguity encountered by Sanger sequencing. Currently, most workflow time for NGS is still long (approximately 3 days), and the process is cumbersome. An even bigger challenge is the ability to handle the volume and complexity of NGS data, which are often beyond the current data analysis capabilities of most clinical HLA laboratories.

Automation solutions for bench work and data analysis are being sought by industry and academic institutes in the field. HLA genotyping results from NGS will continue to increase the pace of allele discovery, further refining knowledge about HLA genes. How this high level of information can be used clinically to improve transplant outcomes is yet to be determined. Ultimately, high-resolution HLA genotyping results by NGS technology will allow identification of HLA genes at all loci, enabling more accurate matches between donor and recipient than can be achieved with current methods.

HLA antibody screening is also performed to identify preformed anti-HLA antibodies in transplant recipients.

The antibodies are formed in response to exposure to foreign antigens in the setting of transplantation, transfusion, or pregnancy. The CDC-based antibody screening assay uses cells from many individuals as target cells (described earlier). This method has largely been replaced by more sensitive techniques, such as solid-phase assays that use beads coated with antigens, and a flow cytometer or Luminex analyzer is used to detect the specific binding of antigens to antibodies in recipient serum. If HLA antibodies are detected, testing proceeds to identification of antibodies or antibody specificity. The type and titer of anti-HLA antibodies have clinical consequences for transplantation and transfusion.

The crossmatch is a critical assay in transplantation. It is used for testing the recipient's serum for preformed antibodies against the donor lymphocytes. The testing principle is the same as for CDC in serologic HLA typing. Crossmatching can also be performed by solid-phase assays for increased sensitivity. Along with ensuring ABO blood type compatibility, crossmatching helps to prevent hyperacute rejection (discussed later).

The terminology of crossmatch results is important. A negative crossmatch means that no immunoreactivity between donor and recipient is observed and that the donor and recipient are immunologically compatible at this level of testing. A positive crossmatch means that immunoreactivity is observed and that the donor and recipient are immunologically incompatible.

Graft-Versus-Host Disease

Graft-versus-host disease (GVHD) occurs when immunoreactive cells of a transplant begin to attack the tissues of the transplant recipient. This is a particular complication of HSCT, in which the graft replaces major components of the recipient's immune system. GVHD is a likely complication in most cases of HSCT.

Just as recipient T cells can recognize donor HLAs as foreign, donor (graft) T cells can recognize host tissues as foreign. Although GVHD most commonly occurs in the setting of bone marrow transplantation (i.e., HSCT), it can also be seen in the transplantation of organs rich in lymphocytes, such as the liver. In HSCT, the recipient's bone marrow is depleted to allow acceptance of the donor bone marrow. After transplantation, CD4 and CD8 T cells in the graft target host HLAs and react as previously described.

GVHD is a potentially fatal condition. The immune reaction can destroy liver, skin, and gastrointestinal tissues. The risk of developing GVHD is minimized by HLA matching, but it is not completely eliminated due to intact donor T cells in some grafts.

Transplant Rejection

Transplant rejection by the recipient's immune system is based on MHC incompatibility. Humoral (i.e., antibodies) or cellular (i.e., T-cell recognition of HLAs) mechanisms can be responsible. Hyperacute rejection occurs within minutes of graft placement—while the patient is still on the operating table—and is caused by preformed antibodies to donor HLAs or ABO blood type incompatibility. Surgeons see a rapid change from viable to nonviable organ soon after organ reperfusion. This type of rejection occurs in less than 0.4% of transplantations because crossmatching and ABO compatibility testing is part of pretransplantation practice.

Acute rejection occurs within days to weeks in an immunocompetent patient or months to years in an immunosuppressed patient. It is caused by T-cell recognition of donor organ HLAs (i.e., acute cellular rejection) or formation of antibodies to donor organ HLAs (i.e., acute humoral rejection). The patient has signs and symptoms of organ dysfunction with associated abnormal laboratory values (e.g., elevated creatinine level in the renal transplant recipient). Biopsy (i.e., examination of tissue removed from a living body to determine the existence, cause, or extent of disease) of the organ shows a combination of lymphocyte infiltration, tissue injury, and graft vasculature damage.

Chronic rejection occurs months to years after transplantation and involves T-cell reactions and nonimmune mechanisms. Biopsy of the organ shows tissue damage and scarring. Figure 35-2 is an example of a normal renal biopsy compared with a renal biopsy showing signs of organ rejection.

Histologic evaluation is important in assessing and grading rejection, but it is equally important to rule out other causes of organ damage or failure, including drug toxicity and recurrence of original disease. For example, histologic evaluation is necessary to distinguish between acute rejection and recurrent hepatitis C infection. In this case, the medication intensity typically used to treat acute rejection poses a risk of recurrence of infection, and caution is necessary to distinguish between the two events to treat the patient. Figure 35-3 compares a normal liver biopsy with a liver biopsy showing signs of recurrence of hepatitis C infection.

Immunosuppression

Immunosuppressant Drugs

Transplantation success depends on effective suppression of the immune system to prevent rejection of the transplanted organ. Many drug classes with different mechanisms of action are used with the same goal: dampen the ability of the immune system to recognize non-self. The primary immunosuppressants used to prevent organ rejection are drugs that target proliferation of lymphocytes in their central role in the adaptive immune response.

Usually more than one immunosuppressant drug is used during multiple drug therapy phases. The induction phase begins immediately postoperatively and consists of strong medication doses for at least 2 to 4 weeks after transplantation. The maintenance phase begins after the induction phase and is a lower-intensity, long-term, stable regimen. Acute rejection is an unpredictable phase occurring 1 week to 1 year after transplantation. It requires immediate intensification of immunosuppression therapy using high-dose corticosteroids.

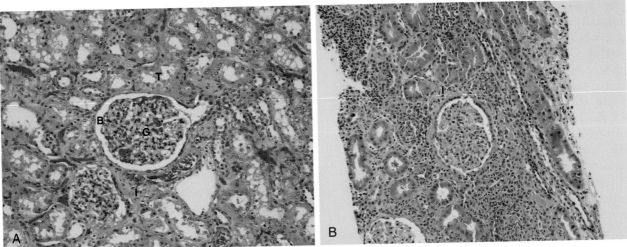

• **Figure 35-2** **A,** Normal kidney histology. The basic functional unit of the kidney is the nephron, which maintains homeostasis of electrolytes, acids, and water. The glomerulus (G) is a network of capillaries that filters blood plasma. The filtrate passes into the Bowman space (B) and into the tubules (T), where the filtrate is altered by reabsorption or secretion of various molecules. These structures are embedded within the renal interstitium (I), which is background supportive tissue. The filtrate passes farther through the collecting system to ultimately be excreted from the body as urine. **B,** The kidney biopsy shows acute cellular rejection. The overall appearance of the stained biopsy is blue because there is a significant infiltration of small, chronic inflammatory cells (i.e., lymphocytes and plasma cells) within the renal interstitium (I). There is also a loss of tubules.

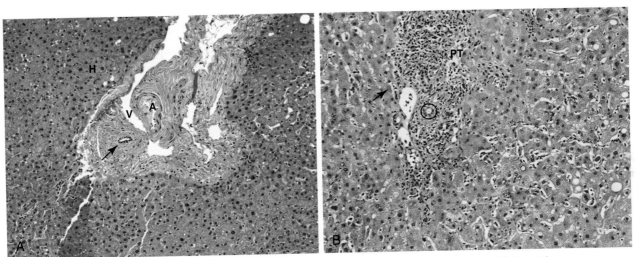

• **Figure 35-3** **A,** Normal liver histology. The liver is composed of plates of hepatocytes (H), the main functional cells in the liver; portal tracts; and hepatic or central veins (not shown). The portal tracts are composed of bile ducts *(arrow)*, which drain bile from the liver, and branches of the portal vein (V) and hepatic artery (A), which deliver blood to the liver. The liver is a multifaceted organ involved in metabolism of energy sources, detoxification of substances (e.g., drugs, toxins), storage of metabolic products, and production of bile. **B,** Liver biopsy shows recurrent hepatitis C infection after transplantation. The blue appearance of the portal tracts (PT) after staining results from significant infiltration of lymphocytes in the portal tract. Biopsies can be challenging because of overlap between the histologic features of recurrent hepatitis C infection and acute allograft rejection, especially when patients have both. Features that favor recurrence of hepatitis C infection are relative preservation of the bile ducts *(circle)* and evidence of death of individual cells, called apoptosis *(arrow)*.

The exact regimen and combinations of immunosuppressants for different transplant types remains an active area of research.

There are many immunosuppressants with different mechanisms of action. The primary drugs prescribed are corticosteroids, cyclosporine, tacrolimus (previously designated FK506), sirolimus (i.e., rapamycin), everolimus, and mycophenolic acid (MPA). Each drug has a mechanism of action that interferes with the proliferation of lymphocytes.

Corticosteroids

Corticosteroids (i.e., prednisolone and prednisone) are potent, broad-acting inhibitors of chemical pathways that are part of the inflammatory and immune responses.

Prednisolone is the active metabolite of prednisone. The compound binds to glucocorticoid receptors in the cytoplasm, which bind to glucocorticoid response elements (GREs) in the nucleus. GREs reside on the promoter sequences of genes. Corticosteroids stimulate promoter-enhanced transcription of genes (e.g., interleukin-1 receptor) that are involved in antiinflammatory responses and block the function of other factors that are required for transcription of proinflammatory mediators. Lymphocyte activity is diminished, and corticosteroids suppress antiinflammatory responses by macrophages and monocytes.

Adverse effects of corticosteroids include susceptibility to infection, impaired wound healing, growth suppression in children, osteoporosis, glucose intolerance, hypertension, hyperlipidemia, and emotional lability. Current immunosuppression regimens try to minimize the use of corticosteroids, but corticosteroids are regarded as essential in the initial stages after transplantation and in response to early signs of acute organ rejection.

Cyclosporine

Cyclosporine is a calcineurin inhibitor (CNI). Cyclosporine binds first to a cytoplasmic protein called cyclophilin. This complex then binds to and inhibits calcineurin, a regulated serine/threonine protein phosphatase that normally activates transcription factors necessary to produce the cytokines that are essential to lymphocyte proliferation.

The side effect of greatest concern from cyclosporine is nephrotoxicity. The kidney is susceptible to arterial vasoconstriction caused by cyclosporine. Hypertension, hyperlipidemia, and diabetes due to pancreatic effects are also unwanted consequences of cyclosporine.

Tacrolimus

Tacrolimus is a CNI. Combined cyclosporine and tacrolimus is a common regimen for maintenance of immunosuppression. Unlike cyclosporin, which first binds to cyclophilin, tacrolimus binds first to a cytoplasmic protein called FK506 binding protein 12 (FKBP12). Tacrolimus has less nephrotoxicity than cyclosporine; otherwise, long-term side effects of tacrolimus as a CNI are similar to those of cyclosporine.

Sirolimus and Everolimus

Sirolimus is an inhibitor of the mammalian target of rapamycin (mTOR). Like tacrolimus, sirolimus binds to an FK protein, but the complex then binds to mTOR. Inhibition of mTOR blocks the activation of interleukin-2 (IL-2) and prevents the G- to S-phase transition of T lymphocytes. Everolimus is a derivative of sirolimus with different pharmacokinetics. Side effects of sirolimus and everolimus include hyperlipidemia, anemia, edema, proteinuria, thrombosis, hyperlipidemia, and decreased glucose tolerance due to insulin resistance. They are also nephrotoxic in a way that is synergistic with CNIs.

Mycophenolic Acid

Mycophenolic acid (MPA) is the active form of the prodrug mycophenolate mofetil. Because its mode of action is different from those of CNIs and mTOR inhibitors, it can be prescribed in addition to them. MPA is an antimetabolite. It is a selective inhibitor of inosine monophosphate dehydrogenase (IMPD), which is found in activated lymphocytes and is necessary for purine synthesis and replication. The main adverse effects of MPA are on the gastrointestinal system (e.g., abdominal pain, nausea, diarrhea) and on hematologic parameters (e.g., anemia, leukopenia). MPA is regarded as safe for long-term immunosuppression.

Other Immunosuppressive Agents

Other immunosuppressants used in various stages of treatment are OKT3 (i.e., antibody that inactivates T lymphocytes); IL-2 receptor antagonists (i.e., anti-CD25 antibodies); polyclonal antibodies (i.e., Thymoglobulin and Atgam) that target T-lymphocyte markers; the monoclonal antibody alemtuzumab, which acts against the lymphocyte marker CD25; Janus kinase 3 (JAK3) inhibitors; protein kinase C–selective inhibitor AEB-071 (sotrastaurin); LEA29Y (Belatacept), an intravenously administered immunoglobulin that interferes with lymphocyte CD28 activity; and efalizumab, an anti-CD11a monoclonal antibody. Routine laboratory testing is not involved with the use of these agents.

Complications of Immunosuppression

Pharmacologic immunosuppression is critical in the post-transplantation period, but preservation of a functional graft comes at the cost of an intact immune system. With a suppressed immune system, the natural and expected ability to protect, recognize, and eliminate pathogens is compromised, posing a risk of infection to transplant recipients from usual, opportunistic, and atypical pathogens. This is especially true for HSCT patients because it is a rather severe undertaking. Preparation for transplantation involves chemical obliteration of existing bone marrow cells with or without whole-body radiation therapy. During this short-term form of immunosuppression, patients are highly susceptible to infection.

Complications resulting from immunosuppression are not limited to infections. Normally, HLAs reside on the cell surface and can be recognized by leukocytes. Tumor cells downregulate or decrease the MHC markers on their surface to evade the immune system and enhance survival. Despite evasion tactics, the immune system can respond to tumor cells under normal circumstances, but immunosuppression puts patients at increased risk for malignancies.

Monitoring Immunosuppression

Immunosuppression is essential for the success of transplantation, but long-term use of the drugs has unwanted side effects, including atherosclerosis, diabetes, and renal insufficiency. The kidney is particularly sensitive to the unintended effects of immunosuppressants. Monitoring for these effects is a routine part of posttransplantation patient care.

Drug concentrations must be maintained within the intended therapeutic range to protect the graft from rejection and to minimize or delay systemic toxicity. Drug levels are monitored beginning in the early phase after transplantation, and monitoring continues throughout the life of the graft.

Genetics plays a role in the variations of immunosuppressant metabolism observed among patients. Pharmacogenomics will increasingly influence the way in which immunosuppressants are prescribed and monitored.

For long-term monitoring, immunosuppressant drug concentrations are measured as trough levels (i.e., levels preceding the next dose), although absorption-phase measurements may be useful during the early phases of first-time administration. Immunosuppressants are most commonly measured by immunoassays or by mass spectrometry. Because it is not subject to cross-reactivity with metabolites and is highly specific for the compound of interest, mass spectrometry is the preferred method of measurement.

MPA and its active metabolite are measured using serum specimens, whereas cyclosporine, tacrolimus, sirolimus, and everolimus are measured in whole blood specimens. Cyclosporine, tacrolimus, sirolimus, and everolimus can be measured simultaneously by mass spectrometry using a single preparation and method. The method is commonly used for measurement of many analytes besides immunosuppressant drugs.

The liquid chromatography–tandem mass spectrometry (LC-MS/MS) analytical system is shown in Figure 35-4. It combines liquid chromatography with two (tandem) mass spectrometers in series. Beginning with whole blood, protein is precipitated and drug extracted by addition of an organic solvent. The supernatant sample is injected into the liquid chromatography system, in which the drug is captured in an organic column. Water-soluble electrolytes such as sodium and chloride pass through the column and are diverted to waste; they would otherwise interfere with drug measurement. After this step, the composition of the solvent of the liquid chromatography system is altered to elute the drugs from the column, and the flow is sent to the mass spectrometer. An electrical charge is imparted to the drug (i.e., drug becomes ionized) in the source. The first of two mass spectrometers then selects for and filters the known mass-to-charge ratio of the drug of choice. The selected molecule is then fragmented in a collision chamber using inert gas. Fragmentation occurs according to a known pattern for each drug, and the second mass spectrometer selects for and filters these fragments according to their mass-to-charge ratio. The molecules are then counted by the detector.

A drug is identified and its concentration measured according to the elution time from the column, the known masses of the drug and its characteristic fragments, the relative proportions of fragments, and the total count obtained for each fragment. Simultaneous measurement of multiple drugs in one assay is achieved by rapidly cycling the mass spectrometry system parameters through a list of specifications that are unique for each drug.

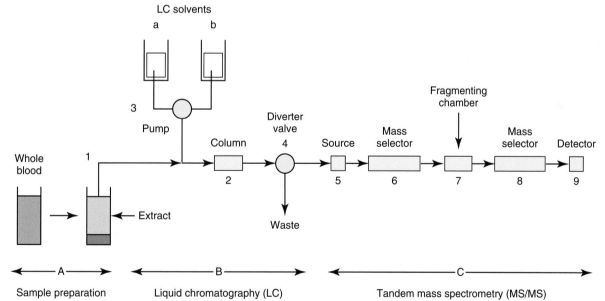

• **Figure 35-4** Schematic diagram of a liquid chromatography–tandem mass spectrometry (LC-MS/MS) system for measurement of immunosuppressants. **A,** In step 1, starting with whole blood, protein is precipitated, and drug is extracted by addition of an organic solvent. **B,** In step 2, the supernatant sample is injected into the LC system, which captures the drug in an organic column. In step 3, the composition of the solvents (a and b) of the LC system is altered to elute the drugs from the column. In step 4, water-soluble electrolytes such as sodium and chloride pass by the column and are diverted to waste, after which the flow is sent to the mass spectrometer. **C,** In step 5, an electrical charge is imparted to the drug (i.e., the drug becomes ionized) in the source. In step 6, the first of two tandem mass spectrometers selects for and filters ions according to the known mass-to-charge ratio of the drug of choice. In step 7, the selected molecule is fragmented in a collision chamber using inert gas. In step 8, fragmentation occurs according to a known pattern for each drug, and the second mass spectrometer selects for and filters these known fragments according to their mass-to-charge ratio. In step 9, molecules are counted by the detector.

Guidelines

Immunosuppressants have relatively long half-lives, typically on the order of 18 hours or more. This aspect of their pharmacology affects the relationship between monitoring and dosing intervention. If a drug level is too high, the next dose must be lowered or eliminated, but otherwise, the return to normal levels requires waiting.

Despite the long-standing use of immunosuppressants, guidelines and strategies for monitoring continue to evolve. Practices for obtaining immunosuppressant levels for inpatients often use a simple algorithm of ordering once per day rather than reliance on guidelines based on the principles of pharmacokinetics or pharmacodynamics. There is a psychological component to this practice from the caregiver's standpoint; physicians want to obtain as much information as possible to ensure they are providing the best possible care, despite the limited information obtained from orders placed at short intervals.

From a laboratory medicine perspective, it is likely that daily testing represents significant overuse of assays. Costs associated with overuse is one reason for the great interest in development and deployment of automated expert systems (i.e., computer algorithms) to guide test orders for therapeutic drug monitoring and for many other common inpatient test orders. In inpatient settings, expert systems may in the future be able to query and assess all relevant data and stipulate appropriate test orders and ordering intervals.

Methods

The need for immunosuppressive therapy is lifelong, although monitoring frequency becomes less as a patient progresses through years of stable life. One method for monitoring immunosuppressant therapy is evaluation of dried blood spots collected on filter paper, such as those used in newborn screening.

Blood spots can be advantageous for many patients, who can collect fingerprick blood samples at home without a visit to the hospital. Dried blood spots are analytically stable and can be sent to the laboratory by regular mail. Researchers have demonstrated a novel point-of-care method of analysis of drugs using blood spots that can aid availability of routine testing of immunosuppressants for patients in remote areas.

Continued Monitoring of Organ Function

Patients are monitored closely after transplantation for continued functioning of the graft. For certain organs, functional monitoring may include routine medical checkup procedures, such as blood pressure measurement, electrocardiography (i.e., heart function), and air exchange capacity (i.e., lung function). Medical imaging of the transplanted organ may also be routine.

Laboratory testing is a crucial component of monitoring. Measurement of immunosuppressants over time is essential, and because of the side effects of immunosuppressants, all patients are monitored for hyperlipidemia (i.e., lipid panel), diabetes (i.e., fasting plasma glucose and glycated

hemoglobin), and kidney function (i.e., serum creatinine or cystatin C, urine creatinine, and urine albumin). Creatinine or cystatin C is used to estimate the glomerular filtration rate (GFR). Urine creatinine and albumin levels are used to monitor for progressive development of proteinuria, which can signal disease progression or rejection. A complete blood count (CBC) and a comprehensive metabolic panel (CMP) are tests performed routinely for all transplant recipients.

Some tests specific to transplant type may be performed. Liver transplants are monitored by tests of liver enzymes, cholesterol, and bilirubin. Pancreatic transplants are monitored for pancreatic enzymes (i.e., amylase and lipase) or insulin production (i.e., C-peptide levels). Depending on the original indication for HSCT, serum protein electrophoresis or immunofixation, or both, may be performed to determine whether there is abnormal expression of monoclonal immunoglobulins. Identification of a monoclonal paraprotein by serum protein electrophoresis and immunofixation is shown in Figure 35-5.

If laboratory tests indicate a severe abnormality or progressive change in organ function, a biopsy of the transplanted organ is often performed. It enables the pathologist to evaluate tissue integrity and determine whether there is histologic evidence of disease or rejection.

Identification of biochemical markers for transplant rejection is an active area of biomedical research. Promising markers include circulating cell-free donor DNA, certain RNA markers, and inflammatory chemical markers. It is likely that routine posttransplantation monitoring will increasingly include measurement of a variety of these markers.

Exceptional Cases in Transplantation

Despite extensive pretransplantation donor testing, comprehensive testing is not available for all possible pathological conditions, especially infectious diseases. It is therefore important that the medical history and circumstances of death of a potential donor are fully investigated. In one case, transplantation of organs occurred from a person later determined to have been infected with rabies. Although such cases are rare, they prompt consideration of broader pretransplantation testing, and it is likely that the standard menu of pretransplantation testing will continue to grow as technology makes screening more rapid and more widely available.

Two other unusual circumstances of transplantation are worth consideration. Domino transplantation involves removal of a diseased organ from a primary recipient, which is then transplanted into a recipient who because of a low waiting list priority would otherwise not receive an organ. One case involved transplantation of a liver affected by an inborn error of metabolism. After removal from a pediatric patient during transplantation of a new donor organ, the affected liver was transplanted into an adult patient for whom the effects of the metabolic error were considered

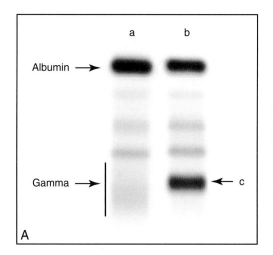
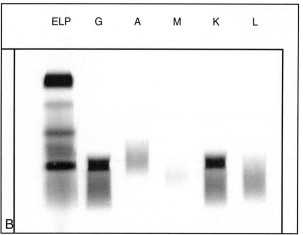

• **Figure 35-5** Identification of a monoclonal paraprotein by serum protein electrophoresis (ELP) and immunofixation. **A,** Compared with a normal control sample (a), the distinct protein band in the gamma region of a patient's serum protein electrophoresis (b) is patently abnormal (c). **B,** In this case, the paraprotein (i.e., abnormal protein) is a monoclonal immunoglobulin G with a kappa chain locus (IgGκ) identified by immunofixation. For a hematopoietic stem cell transplant recipients treated for multiple myeloma, this finding indicates a recurrence of disease.

manageable compared with the life-threatening state of the patient's prior condition. A second unusual circumstance is pregnancy planning to provide a source of HLA-matched hematopoietic cells for a sibling awaiting a transplant. One case involved preimplantation testing of HLA genes after in vitro fertilization to ensure a HLA match for HSCT. Both of these cases raise fundamental issues of medical ethics about which there is unlikely to be a society-wide consensus.

Future of Transplantation

The current level of success of transplantation is a medical marvel, with contributions ranging from the astounding technical feat of surgery itself to advances in basic biomedical sciences such as immunology and pharmacology. The art of transplantation continues to evolve. In the future, developments in medicine may make some fraction of transplantation cases preventable, particularly those resulting from infectious disease. Genetic engineering may be able to successfully treat or cure disorders such as hemoglobin S disease, thalassemia, and inborn errors of metabolism. Advances in organ preservation and transport techniques may mitigate the constraints on the time between organ procurement and transplantation and the geographic constraints on organ allocation procedures.

Advances in the basic sciences may greatly improve our ability to target immune suppression and limit the unwanted consequences of current immunosuppression regimens. Discoveries may promote the use of xenografts (i.e., organs transplanted from nonhuman species) and prevent deaths due to organ shortages. For some organs (e.g., heart, pancreas), mechanical devices may be able to provide permanent alternatives to transplantation. In the future, tissue engineering and three-dimensional printing may make possible the ex vivo production of replacement organs that are exactly matched to the genetics of the recipient. Many dramatic changes and improvements in the practice of transplantation are likely in the next few decades.

Review Questions

1. A kidney transplant recipient displays progressive increases in cystatin C levels, indicating a reduced glomerular filtration rate (GFR). Which of the following is the best test to investigate whether this finding is caused by immune response–mediated rejection?
   a. Alternative GFR as estimated by measurement of serum creatinine
   b. Continued monitoring of cystatin C
   c. Biopsy with review by a pathologist
   d. Ratio of urine protein to creatinine

2. Which of the following is the primary advantage of using of liquid chromatography–tandem mass spectrometry (LC-MS/MS) for measurement of immunosuppressants?
   a. The test is easy to perform.
   b. The test is not subject to cross-reactivity with metabolites.
   c. LC-MS/MS is inexpensive.
   d. The calibration curve for LC-MS/MS assays is linear.

3. High-resolution of human leukocyte antigen (HLA) matching between donor and recipient using DNA

analysis is especially important for transplantation of which of the following?

a. Heart
b. Kidney
c. Lung
d. Hematopoietic cells

4. Which of the following interpretations of the results of crossmatching is correct?
    a. Negative crossmatch: donor and patient are incompatible
    b. Positive crossmatch: donor and patient are compatible
    c. Negative crossmatch: donor and patient are compatible
    d. Positive crossmatch: further testing by DNA analysis is required

5. Which of the following descriptions of the mode of action of immunosuppressants is *incorrect*?
    a. Cyclosporine is an inhibitor of calcineurin.
    b. Tacrolimus is an inhibitor of mTOR.
    c. Sirolimus is an inhibitor of mTOR.
    d. Everolimus is an inhibitor of mTOR.

6. Which of the following is usually the preferred sample time for routine monitoring of immunosuppressants?
    a. Two hours after the drug dose
    b. Six hours after the drug dose
    c. Random time relative to the drug dose
    d. Trough, before the next drug dose

7. Graft-versus-host disease (GVHD) is most likely to occur in which of the following types of transplantation?
    a. Autologous (self donor) hematopoietic stem cell transplantation
    b. Allogenic (i.e., non-self donor) hematopoietic stem cell transplantation
    c. Liver transplantation
    d. Living donor kidney transplantation

8. T.I. is a 52-year-old man who received a heart transplant 6 months earlier for nonischemic cardiomyopathy. He went to his primary care physician because of fever, night sweats, and shortness of breath with a cough. These symptoms are most likely due to an infection. An infection at 6 months after transplantation can most likely be attributed to
    a. A postoperative surgical complication
    b. A side effect of immunosuppressive medications
    c. Allograft rejection
    d. Reemergence of long-standing lung disease

9. Two months after receiving a renal transplant, N.H. had a rapid elevation in creatinine level. Which of the following is the *least* likely cause of the patient's renal failure?
    a. Hyperacute allograft rejection
    b. Chronic allograft rejection
    c. An unwanted side effect of immunosuppressive medications
    d. A combination of chronic allograft rejection and side effects of medication

10. M.S. is a laboratory technician who receives a specimen with the request for measurement of the tacrolimus level. After reviewing the specimen and associated documentation, M.S. decides to reject the specimen and notify the ordering physician. Which of the following is a reason for rejecting this specimen?
    a. The specimen was not labeled.
    b. The specimen was stored improperly after collection.
    c. The specimen was collected in a syringe, and the needle is still attached.
    d. All of the above

Critical Thinking Questions

1. Describe the differences in pretransplantation testing for human leukocyte antigen (HLA) matching between solid organ transplantation and hematopoietic stem cell transplantation (HSCT). Describe why graft-versus-host disease (GVHD) is most common in HSCT.

2. Describe the mechanisms by which the natural response of the body seeks to destroy foreign tissue. Describe the mechanism by which immunosuppressant drugs block this response. Describe the common side effects of immunosuppressants.

CASE STUDY

LB is 3-year-old boy who recently underwent liver transplantation to correct for a homozygous deficiency of α_1-antitrypsin. What drugs are likely to be prescribed for this patient? What laboratory tests are likely to be ordered to monitor him over the next few months? Why are tests related to monitoring kidney function likely to be ordered? Is there a time after which transplantation can be declared successful enough that no further testing is required to monitor the patient? In the future, how may expert systems influence test orders?

Bibliography

Allison AC, Eugui EM. Mycophenolate mofetil and its mechanisms of action. *Immunopharmacology*. 2000;47:85–118.

Alqahtani SA, Larson AM. Adult liver transplantation in the USA. *Curr Opin Gastroenterol*. 2011;27:240–247.

American Society for Histocompatibility and Immunogenetics. ASHI website. <http://www.ashi-hla.org> Accessed 30.06.15.

Annesley TM, Clayton LT. Quantification of mycophenolic acid and glucuronide metabolite in human serum by HPLC-tandem mass spectrometry. *Clin Chem*. 2005;51:872–877.

Arpini J, Antunes MV, Pacheco LS, et al. Clinical evaluation of a dried blood spot method for determination of mycophenolic acid in renal transplant patients. *Clin Biochem*. 2013;46:1905–1908.

Atkinson K. Chronic graft-versus-host disease. *Bone Marrow Transplant*. 1990;5:69–82.

Badell IR, Hanish SI, Hughes CB, et al. Domino liver transplantation in maple syrup urine disease: a case report and review of the literature. *Transplant Proc*. 2013;45:806–809.

Ball LM, Egeler RM. EBMT Paediatric Working Party. Acute GvHD: pathogenesis and classification. *Bone Marrow Transplant*. 2008;41(suppl 2):S58–S64.

Batabyal P, Chapman JR, Wong G, Craig JC, Tong A. Clinical practice guidelines on wait-listing for kidney transplantation: consistent and equitable? *Transplantation*. 2012;94:703–713.

Becker LE, Susal C, Morath C. Kidney transplantation across HLA and ABO antibody barriers. *Curr Opin Organ Transplant*. 2013;18:445–454.

Bloom RD, Reese PP. Chronic kidney disease after nonrenal solid-organ transplantation. *J Am Soc Nephrol*. 2007;18:3031–3041.

Bray RA, Tarsitani C, Gebel HM, Lee JH. Clinical cytometry and progress in HLA antibody detection. *Methods Cell Biol*. 2011;103:285–310.

Buchwald A, Winkler K, Epting T. Validation of an LC-MS/MS method to determine five immunosuppressants with deuterated internal standards including MPA. *BMC Clin Pharmacol*. 2012;12:2.

Campbell P. Clinical relevance of human leukocyte antigen antibodies in liver, heart, lung and intestine transplantation. *Curr Opin Organ Transplant*. 2013;18:463–469.

Capitaine L, Van Assche K, Pennings G, Sterckx S. Pediatric priority in kidney allocation: challenging its acceptability. *Transpl Int*. 2014;27:533–540.

Carrion AF, Aye L, Martin P. Patient selection for liver transplantation. *Expert Rev Gastroenterol Hepatol*. 2013;7:571–579.

Center for Biologics Evaluation and Research. Guidance for industry: eligibility determination for donors of human cells, tissues, and cellular and tissue-based products. <http://www.fda.gov/biologicsbloodvaccines/guidancecomplianceregulatoryinformation/guidances/cellularandgenetherapy/ucm072929.htm> Accessed 30.06.15.

Colombo MB, Haworth SE, Poli F, et al. Luminex technology for anti-HLA antibody screening: evaluation of performance and of impact on laboratory routine. *Cytometry B Clin Cytom*. 2007;72:465–471.

Committee on Organ Procurement and Transplantation Policy, Institute of Medicine. *Organ Procurement and Transplantation: Assessing Current Policies and the Potential Impact of the DHHS Final Rule*. Washington, DC: National Academies Press; 1999.

Corbett C, Armstrong MJ, Parker R, Webb K, Neuberger JM. Mental health disorders and solid-organ transplant recipients. *Transplantation*. 2013;96:593–600.

Corthay A. Does the immune system naturally protect against cancer? *Front Immunol*. 2014;5:197.

Damewood MD. Ethical implications of a new application of preimplantation diagnosis. *JAMA*. 2001;285:3143–3144.

Dasgupta A. Impact of interferences including metabolite crossreactivity on therapeutic drug monitoring results. *Ther Drug Monit*. 2012;34:496–506.

De Vlaminck I, Valantine HA, Snyder TM, et al. Circulating cell-free DNA enables noninvasive diagnosis of heart transplant rejection. *Sci Transl Med*. 2014;6. 241ra77.

Deeg HJ, Henslee-Downey PJ. Management of acute graft-versus-host disease. *Bone Marrow Transplant*. 1990;6:1–8.

Delves PJ, Martin SJ, Burton DR. Innate immunity. In: *Roitt's Essential Immunology*. 12th ed. Chichester, UK: Wiley-Blackwell Publishing; 2011.

Delves PJ, Martin SJ, Burton DR. Specific acquired immunity. In: *Roitt's Essential Immunology*. 12th ed. Chichester, West Sussex, UK: Wiley-Blackwell Publishing; 2011.

Delves PJ, Martin SJ, Burton DR. Transplantation. In: *Roitt's Essential Immunology*. 12th ed. Chichester, UK: Wiley-Blackwell Publishing; 2011.

Deng MC, Elashoff B, Pham MX, et al. Utility of gene expression profiling score variability to predict clinical events in heart transplant recipients. *Transplantation*. 2014;97:708–714.

Deol A, Ratanatharathorn V, Uberti JP. Pathophysiology, prevention, and treatment of acute graft-versus-host disease. *Transplant Res Risk Manag*. 2011;3:31–44.

DiMartini AF, Dew MA, Trzepacz PT. Organ transplantation. *Focus*. 2005;3:280–303.

Duong Van Huyen JP, Tible M, et al. MicroRNAs as non-invasive biomarkers of heart transplant rejection. *Eur Heart J*. 2014;35:3194–3202.

Engels EA, Pfeiffer RM, Fraumeni Jr JF, et al. Spectrum of cancer risk among US solid organ transplant recipients. *JAMA*. 2011;306:1891–1901.

Fagoaga OR. Human leukocyte antigen: the major histocompatibility complex of man. In: Pincus M, McPherson R, eds. *Henry's Clinical Diagnosis and Management by Laboratory Methods*. 22nd ed Philadelphia: Elsevier/Saunders; 2011.

Filipponi F, Soubrane O, Labrousse F, et al. Liver transplantation for end-stage liver disease associated with alpha-1-antitrypsin deficiency in children: pretransplant natural history, timing and results of transplantation. *J Hepatol*. 1994;20:72–78.

Fuji S, Kapp M, Einsele H. Possible implication of bacterial infection in acute graft-versus-host disease after allogeneic hematopoietic stem cell transplantation. *Front Oncol*. 2014;4:89.

Gabriel C, Furst D, Fae I, et al. HLA typing by next-generation sequencing—getting closer to reality. *Tissue Antigens*. 2014;83:65–75.

Gebel HM, Liwski RS, Bray RA. Technical aspects of HLA antibody testing. *Curr Opin Organ Transplant*. 2013;18:455–462.

Ghosh A, Holland AM, van den Brink MR. Genetically engineered donor T cells to optimize graft-versus-tumor effects across MHC barriers. *Immunol Rev*. 2014;257:226–236.

Grubb A, Horio M, Hansson LO, et al. Generation of a new cystatin C-based estimating equation for glomerular filtration rate by use of 7 assays standardized to the international calibrator. *Clin Chem*. 2014;60:974–986.

Halloran PF. Molecular mechanisms of new immunosuppressants. *Clin Transplant*. 1996;10(Pt 2):118–123.

Hansen K, Horslen S. Metabolic liver disease in children. *Liver Transpl*. 2008;14:713–733.

Heeger PS, Dinavahi R. Transplant immunology for non-immunologist. *Mt Sinai J Med.* 2012;79:376–387.

Holt DW, Johnston A. Monitoring immunosuppressive drugs: has it a future? *Ther Drug Monit.* 2004;26:244–247.

Holtan SG, Pasquini M, Weisdorf DJ. Acute graft-versus-host disease: a bench-to-bedside update. *Blood.* 2014;124:363–373.

Hsu S. Human leukocyte antigens. In: Quinley ED, ed. *Immunohematology: Principles and Practice.* 3rd ed. Philadelphia: Wolters Kluwer/Lippincott Williams & Wilkins; 2010.

Humar A, Dunn DL. Transplantation. In: Brunicardi F, Andersen DK, Billiar TR, et al., eds. *Schwartz's Principles of Surgery.* 9th ed. New York: McGraw-Hill; 2010.

Iwama I, Baba Y, Kagimoto S, et al. Case report of a successful liver transplantation for acute liver failure due to mitochondrial respiratory chain complex III deficiency. *Transplant Proc.* 2011;43: 4025–4028.

Johnston A, Holt DW. Immunosuppressant drugs—the role of therapeutic drug monitoring. *Br J Clin Pharmacol.* 2001;52(suppl 1): 61S–73S.

Johnston A, Holt DW. Therapeutic drug monitoring of immunosuppressant drugs. *Br J Clin Pharmacol.* 1999;47:339–350.

Kahn JP, Mastroianni AC. Creating a stem cell donor: a case study in reproductive genetics. *Kennedy Inst Ethics J.* 2004;14:81–96.

Khurana A, Brennan DC. Current concepts of immunosuppression and side effects. In: Liapis H, Wang HL, eds. *Pathology of Solid Organ Transplantation.* Berlin: Springer-Verlag; 2011:11–30.

Kuo HH, Fan R, Dvorina N, Chiesa-Vottero A, Baldwin 3rd WM. Platelets in early antibody-mediated rejection of renal transplants. *J Am Soc Nephrol.* 2014;26:855–863.

Leffell MS, Zachary AA. Antiallograft antibodies: relevance, detection, and monitoring. *Curr Opin Organ Transplant.* 2010;15:2–7.

Levey AS, Fan L, Eckfeldt JH, Inker LA. Cystatin C for glomerular filtration rate estimation: coming of age. *Clin Chem.* 2014;60: 916–919.

Linden PK. History of solid organ transplantation and organ donation. *Crit Care Clin.* 2009;25:165–184. ix.

Mahalati K, Kahan BD. Clinical pharmacokinetics of sirolimus. *Clin Pharmacokinet.* 2001;40:573–585.

Markey KA, MacDonald KP, Hill GR. The biology of graft-versus-host disease: experimental systems instructing clinical practice. *Blood.* 2014;124:354–362.

Martinez OM, Rosen HR. Basic concepts in transplant immunology. *Liver Transpl.* 2005;11:370–381.

Martins L, Fonseca I, Sousa S, et al. The influence of HLA mismatches and immunosuppression on kidney graft survival: an analysis of more than 1300 patients. *Transplant Proc.* 2007;39:2489–2493.

Matsuda S, Koyasu S. Mechanisms of action of cyclosporine. *Immunopharmacology.* 2000;47:119–125.

McPherson R, Massey D. Overview of the immune system and immunologic disorders. In: Pincus M, McPherson R, eds. *Henry's Clinical Diagnosis and Management by Laboratory Methods.* Philadelphia: Elsevier/Saunders; 2011.

Millan O, Rafael-Valdivia L, San Segundo D, et al. Should IFN-gamma, IL-17 and IL-2 be considered predictive biomarkers of acute rejection in liver and kidney transplant? Results of a multicentric study. *Clin Immunol.* 2014;154:141–154.

Mjörnstedt L1, Schwartz Sørensen S, von Zur Mühlen B, et al. Renal function three years after early conversion from a calcineurin inhibitor to everolimus: results from a randomized trial in kidney transplantation. *Transpl Int.* 2014;28:42–51.

Mohan S, Hirsch J. Risk of malignancy after renal transplantation. *Transplantation.* 2013;95:17–18.

Nassiri N, Eslani M, Panahi N, et al. Ocular graft versus host disease following allogeneic stem cell transplantation: a review of current knowledge and recommendations. *J Ophthalmic Vis Res.* 2013;8:351–358.

National Marrow Donor Program. HLA typing and matching. <https://bethematchclinical.org/Transplant-Therapy-and-Donor-Matching/HLA-Typing-and-Matching/> Accessed 30.06.15.

Organ Procurement and Transplantation Network. History of organ transplantation. <http://optn.transplant.hrsa.gov/learn/about-transplantation/history/> Accessed 30.06.15.

Organ Procurement and Transplantation Network. How organ allocation works. <http://optn.transplant.hrsa.gov/about/transplantation/matchingProcess.asp> Accessed 30.06.15.

Organ Procurement and Transplantation Network. Members. <http://optn.transplant.hrsa.gov/members/> Accessed 30.06.15.

Organ Procurement and Transplantation Network. Policies and statistics. <http://optn.transplant.hrsa.gov/policiesAndBylaws/policies.asp> Accessed 30.06.15.

Organ Procurement and Transplantation Network. Public forum addresses equity in liver distribution. <http://optn.transplant.hrsa.gov/news/public-forum-addresses-equity-in-liver-distribution/> Accessed 05.11.15.

Paczesny S, Krijanovski OI, Braun TM, et al. A biomarker panel for acute graft-versus-host disease. *Blood.* 2009;113:273–278.

Petrini C. Ethical models in bioethics: theory and application in organ allocation policies. *Minerva Med.* 2010;101:445–456.

Price A, Whitwell S, Henderson M. Impact of psychotic disorder on transplant eligibility and outcomes. *Curr Opin Organ Transplant.* 2014;19:196–200.

Ratanatharathorn V, Ayash L, Lazarus HM, Fu J, Uberti JP. Chronic graft-versus-host disease: clinical manifestation and therapy. *Bone Marrow Transplant.* 2001;28:121–129.

Saito PK, Yamakawa RH, da Silva Pereira LC, da Silva Junior WV, Borelli SD. Complement-dependent cytotoxicity (CDC) to detect anti-HLA antibodies: old but gold. *J Clin Lab Anal.* 2014;28: 275–280.

Sallustio BC. LC-MS/MS for immunosuppressant therapeutic drug monitoring. *Bioanalysis.* 2010;2:1141–1153.

Scales DC, Granton JT. The transplant patient. In: Hall JB, Schmidt GA, Wood LH, eds. *Principles of Critical Care.* 3rd ed. New York: McGraw-Hill; 2005.

Sehgal SN. Sirolimus: its discovery, biological properties, and mechanism of action. *Transplant Proc.* 2003;35(suppl):7S–14S.

Shaw LM, Holt DW, Keown P, Venkataramanan R, Yatscoff RW. Current opinions on therapeutic drug monitoring of immunosuppressive drugs. *Clin Ther.* 1999;21:1632–1652. discussion 1631.

Snyder TM, Khush KK, Valantine HA, Quake SR. Universal noninvasive detection of solid organ transplant rejection. *Proc Natl Acad Sci U S A.* 2011;108:6229–6234.

Socie G, Ritz J. Current issues in chronic graft-versus-host disease. *Blood.* 2014;124:374–384.

Song GW, Lee SG. Living donor liver transplantation. *Curr Opin Organ Transplant.* 2014;19:217–222.

Starzl TE, Lakkis FG. The unfinished legacy of liver transplantation: emphasis on immunology. *Hepatology.* 2006;43(suppl 1):S151–S163.

Suthanthiran M, Morris RE, Strom TB. Immunosuppressants: cellular and molecular mechanisms of action. *Am J Kidney Dis.* 1996;28: 159–172.

Tait BD, Susal C, Gebel HM, et al. Consensus guidelines on the testing and clinical management issues associated with HLA and non-HLA antibodies in transplantation. *Transplantation.* 2013;95: 19–47.

Taylor PJ. Therapeutic drug monitoring of immunosuppressant drugs by high-performance liquid chromatography-mass spectrometry. *Ther Drug Monit*. 2004;26:215–219.

Thomson AW, Bonham CA, Zeevi A. Mode of action of tacrolimus (FK506): molecular and cellular mechanisms. *Ther Drug Monit*. 1995;17:584–591.

Transplant Australia. Why people need transplants: the facts. <http://transplant.org.au/the-facts/> Accessed 30.06.15.

U.S. Department of Health and Human Services. Information on organ and tissue donation and transplantation. <http://www.org andonor.gov/index.html> Accessed 30.06.15.

U.S. Department of Health and Human Services. U.S. transplant data by disease report. <http://bloodcell.transplant.hrsa.gov/rese arch/transplant_data/us_tx_data/data_by_disease/national.aspx> Accessed 30.06.15.

van Dijk G, Hilhorst M, Rings E. Liver, pancreas and small bowel transplantation: current ethical issues. *Best Pract Res Clin Gastroenterol*. 2014;28:281–292.

Van Meter CH. The organ allocation controversy: how did we arrive here? *Ochsner J*. 1999;1:6–11.

Vastag B. Merits of embryo screening debated. *JAMA*. 2004;291:927–929.

Verlinsky Y, Rechitsky S, Schoolcraft W, Strom C, Kuliev A. Preimplantation diagnosis for Fanconi anemia combined with HLA matching. *JAMA*. 2001;285:3130–3133.

Verlinsky Y, Rechitsky S, Sharapova T, et al. Preimplantation HLA testing. *JAMA*. 2004;291:2079–2085.

Vora NM, Basavaraju SV, Feldman KA, et al. Raccoon rabies virus variant transmission through solid organ transplantation. *JAMA*. 2013;310:398–407.

Whitington PF, Alonso EM, Boyle JT, et al. Liver transplantation for the treatment of urea cycle disorders. *J Inherit Metab Dis*. 1998;21(suppl 1):112–118.

Wilflingseder J, Reindl-Schwaighofer R, Sunzenauer J, et al. MicroRNAs in kidney transplantation. *Nephrol Dial Transplant*. 2015;30:910–917.

Wong SH. Therapeutic drug monitoring for immunosuppressants. *Clin Chim Acta*. 2001;313:241–253.

Wu AH, French D. Implementation of liquid chromatography/mass spectrometry into the clinical laboratory. *Clin Chim Acta*. 2013;420:4–10.

Yang Z, Wang S. Recent development in application of high performance liquid chromatography-tandem mass spectrometry in therapeutic drug monitoring of immunosuppressants. *J Immunol Methods*. 2008;336:98–103.

36

Emergency Preparedness

DONNA LARSON

CHAPTER OUTLINE

OBJECTIVES

After completion of this chapter, the reader will be able to:

1. Describe the three parts of emergency preparedness.
2. Discuss six considerations that should be included in an emergency preparedness plan.
3. Describe five hazards that may affect the functioning of a clinical laboratory.
4. Describe resource management.
5. Describe the importance of communication during an emergency response.
6. Discuss the aspects of training that allow an organization to maintain readiness for any hazard.
7. Define a chemical emergency.
8. Describe two occasions when chemical weapons were used to injure and kill people.
9. Describe blister agents, including their health effects and medical management.
10. Describe blood agents, including their health effects and medical management.
11. Describe caustics, including their health effects and medical management.
12. Describe choking or pulmonary agents, including their health effects and medical management.
13. Describe incapacitating agents, including their health effects and medical management.
14. Describe metals, including their health effects and medical management.
15. Describe nerve agents, including their health effects and medical management.
16. Describe riot control agents such as tear gas, including their health effects and medical management.
17. Describe toxic alcohols, including their health effects and medical management.
18. Describe vomiting agents, including their health effects and medical management.
19. Describe biological threats, including their health effects and medical management.
20. Construct a table describing all chemical and biological agents, including their health effects and medical management.
21. Describe nuclear and radiation threats, including their health effects and medical management.
22. Discuss the history and mission of the Laboratory Response Network (LRN).
23. Describe the composition of the LRN.
24. Compare and contrast the LRN response structure for biological and chemical emergencies.
25. List the proper procedure for specimen collection, packaging, and shipping.

KEY TERMS

Abrin
Adamsite
Arsine
Biological threats
Blister agents
Blood agents
Botulinum
Brevetoxin
British anti-lewisite
Business continuity
Caustics
Centers for Disease Control and
   Prevention
Chemical weapons
Chloroacetophenone
Chloropicrin
Defense Threat Reduction Agency
Department of Homeland Security

Dirty bombs
Drill
Emergency preparedness
Federal Emergency Management
   Agency
Fentanyl
Full-scale exercise
Incapacitating agents
Incident management
Laboratory Response Network
Level 1 laboratories
Level 2 laboratories
Level 3 laboratories
Lewisite
Mitigate
Mustard-lewisite mixture
National laboratories
Nerve agents

Nitrogen mustards
Phosgene oxime
QNB
Reference laboratories
Ricin
Sarin
Saxitoxin
Sentinel laboratory
Soman
Staphylococcal enterotoxin B
Strychnine
Sulfur mustard
Tabletop exercises
Tabun
Tetrodotoxin
Trichothecene mycotoxins
VX

 Case in Point

On March 20, 1995, at 8:15 AM local time, the Aum Shinri-kyo Cult attacked innocent civilians in Tokyo, Japan. During the morning commute, cult members boarded at least three separate subway trains carrying a lethal nerve gas in drink and other common containers. The containers leaked the nerve gas inside the train cars, exposing thousands of passengers. As the trains stopped at stations, passengers affected by the gas stumbled out onto the platforms and fell to the ground. Victims exhibited symptoms of nerve gas poisoning, such as excessive salivation characterized by bubbles coming from the mouth and blood running from their noses. Tokyo responded by setting up tents outside subway stations to house the victims and investigate the cause of the odd syndrome that was killing and injuring people. Approximately 5000 people were exposed to the nerve gas, hundreds were injured, and 12 people died. Officials later confirmed that the gas released in the subway trains was sarin.

If you were working at a clinical laboratory in a hospital that received victims in its emergency department, what specimens would you collect to help determine the cause of the patients' illness? How would you prepare the specimens for transport through the U.S. Postal Service or other shipping company? Where would you send the specimens? Why did you choose the facility in which to receive your specimens?

Points to Remember

- Emergency preparedness includes learning about potential threats to a community, identifying characteristics of specific emergency situations, and demonstrating response actions for each emergency.
- Preparedness consists of planning, training, and education.

- Because each hazard has its own set of challenges, planning a response to and making a contingency plan for each hazard is practical.
- Terrorist groups are not opposed to killing people but rely more on the resulting chaos and psychological effects of an attack to make an impact.
- By releasing chemical agents in a crowded area, terrorists produce a mass casualty scenario, with overwhelmed medical services, victims with impaired psychological and physical functioning, and required decontamination of people and the environment.
- Blister agents include mustards such as a mustard-lewisite (military designation: HL) mixture, nitrogen mustards (HN-1, HN-2, HN-3), sulfur mustard (H), lewisite (L-1, L-2, L-3), and phosgene oxime (CX). These chemicals produce blisters when they come in contact with the eyes, skin, and respiratory tract.
- Blood agents, which become poisonous after absorption into the blood, include arsine (SA) and cyanogen chloride (CK).
- Caustics include hydrofluoric acid, which can burn skin, eyes, and mucous membranes on contact or produce many other systemic symptoms, including weak bones.
- Choking or pulmonary agents, which cause severe irritation and swelling of the respiratory tract, include ammonia, chlorine, mercury, phosgene, diphosgene, and phosphorus.
- Benzene, fentanyl, and 3-quinuclidinyl benzilate (QNB) are incapacitating agents that cause unconsciousness and altered states of consciousness such as confusion, delusions, hallucinations, and disorientation.
- Heavy metals can be poisonous after they are absorbed into the blood, where they interfere with the production of hemoglobin.

- Sarin, soman, tabun, and VX are nerve agents that interfere with the conduction of nerve impulses in the body. They cause death in 1 to 2 minutes.
- Riot control agents such as chloroacetophenone (i.e., tear gas) and chloropicrin are chemicals that irritate the eye and mucous membranes on contact. They are used by law enforcement to control crowds.
- Ethylene glycol commonly causes blindness.
- Adamsite is a riot control agent that causes severe vomiting, abdominal cramps, and diarrhea.
- Biological threats include naturally occurring substances produced by animals, plants, or microbes such as bacteria, fungi, parasites, and viruses.
- Biological toxins include abrin (i.e., ricin), brevetoxin, colchicine, saxitoxin, staphylococcal enterotoxin B (SEB), strychnine, tetrodotoxin, botulinum, and trichothecene mycotoxins.
- Biological agents can cause anthrax, brucellosis, glanders, melioidosis, plague, Q fever, tularemia, smallpox, Venezuela equine encephalitis (VEE), and viral hemorrhagic fevers.
- Terrorists can employ unconventional tactics and weapons, including nuclear and radiologic threats.
- The Laboratory Response Network (LRN) includes federal, state and local public health, veterinary, military, and international laboratories.
- LRN laboratories receive federal funding through a governmental cooperative agreement for laboratory positions, renovations, and state-of-the-art technology.
- LRN laboratories are located all over the world. The most concentrated and strategically placed laboratories are located in the United States.
- Because chemical and biological attacks are out of the ordinary, special training and planning must take place at the local and state levels to ensure that one attack does not overwhelm the national public health infrastructure.

Introduction

The risk of a deadly outbreak or chemical release is unknown, but as technology changes the way diseases or chemicals are delivered, the probability for a covert release increases. Biological and chemical weapons have been used to intentionally harm a population, as in the delivery of anthrax spores through the United States Post Office in 2001.

The medical community must be prepared to minimize injuries associated with chemical or biological terrorism. Early detection of an agent is the key to minimizing its effects, and it is made possible through a flexible, well-trained, and well-practiced medical system. The Centers for Disease Control and Prevention (CDC) lead the Laboratory Response Network (LRN) when responding to biological or chemical attacks. Clinical laboratories are called on to perform many functions to help detect and monitor hazardous situations. This chapter familiarizes medical laboratory technicians with the basics of emergency preparedness, chemical and biological agents and their effects, the laboratory's role in response, and the role and mission of the LRN.

Emergency Preparedness

Emergency preparedness, a necessary component of any business operation, gained attention in the United States after the World Trade Center attacks in 2001 and Hurricane Katrina in 2005. These situations demonstrated that emergency preparedness could help businesses and individuals by improving survivability until essential services are restored. Emergency preparedness includes learning about potential threats for a particular community, identifying characteristics of specific emergency situations, and demonstrating response actions for each emergency. Preparedness consists of planning, training, and education (Fig. 36-1).

Planning

Every business and individual should have a customized emergency preparedness plan for specific hazards, resource management, communication, information technology, emergency response, training, incident management, and business continuity. Planning includes hazard identification, vulnerability assessment, and impact analysis. Hazard identification recognizes the natural and manmade hazards that can occur in a community. After hazards are identified, vulnerability assessment evaluates the susceptibility of individuals, community infrastructure, and resources to a particular hazard. Planning for business continuity assesses the likely impact of a hazard on individuals and businesses.

Hazard Identification

The Federal Emergency Management Agency (FEMA) and the Department of Homeland Security (DHS) provide advice about planning for all hazards. Many types of hazards can impact the function of a laboratory. Manmade hazards include chemical agents, biological agents, and hazmat situations. Hazards from nature include severe winter storms, hurricanes, tornadoes, volcanoes, wildfires, thunderstorms, and earthquakes. Each hazard demands a specific response and a contingency plan. Planning goals include keeping people safe, protecting infrastructure, and minimizing disruptions of business operations.

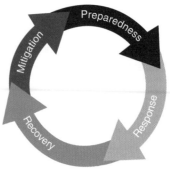

• **Figure 36-1** Preparedness cycle. (From Fuller JK. *Surgical Technology: Principles and Practice.* 6th ed. St. Louis: Saunders; 2013.)

Resource Management

An emergency presents very different circumstances from normal operations. This part of a plan tries to predict the resources that will be needed to respond to an emergency while keeping a business operating or minimizing interruptions. For example, electronic forms of payment may not be used during an emergency, and cash may be the only way to purchase needed items.

Communication and Information Technology

If the current technology is not usable after an incident, alternate methods for communicating with others will be needed. Employers need to communicate with employees and individuals with family members. Hospital laboratories need to communicate with other hospitals and with local and state officials. The blood bank and other medical departments may be critical in a regional or state response, especially in natural disasters such as earthquakes, volcanic eruptions, and tsunamis.

The Internet is a daily part of people's lives, and disruption of this valuable resource could cause chaos. Because an Internet disruption could severely disable businesses, an alternate plan for supplying services is important.

Response Planning and Training

Planning a response to a specific incident is critical for keeping people safe, saving infrastructure, and protecting the environment. Thinking through the entire situation before it occurs and planning for different scenarios (especially the lack of essential services for an extended period of time) can help build a resilient business capable of survival.

Training includes learning about chemical agents, biological agents, and natural and man-made threats to a community. Training involves learning how to mitigate or reduce the impact of the disaster, identifying signs and symptoms of chemical and biological agents, and communicating and coordinating response elements. Training can include simulations such as tabletop exercises, full-scale exercises, and drills. Tabletop exercises consider a plausible incident, and participants discuss its impact on buildings, businesses, and customers. They also discuss their response plan and how well the response plan promotes survivability. In a full-scale exercise, resources (i.e., people, equipment, and facilities) are mobilized in response to a planned incident. This type of exercise is usually conducted on a regional or statewide basis and can be quite expensive. A drill is another type of training that involves a specific aspect of the response. Fire and evacuation drills are common training scenarios.

Incident Management and Business Continuity

Incident management defines responsibilities for responder roles and coordination of activities involved in managing an incident. Business continuity involves actions that a business can take before an incident to ensure survivability and lessen the time a business is inoperable or partially operable after an incident. This usually is expressed in the form of a plan that details every step that will likely occur immediately after an incident.

Emergency Response

Every hospital has an emergency preparedness plan that details the responsibilities of its employees. Laboratories and the LRN play major roles in emergency responses.

Chemical Emergencies

A chemical emergency is an injury involving a chemical agent that is caused by an industrial accident, military stockpiling accident, war, or a terrorist attack. Chemical weapons or agents are highly toxic chemicals that can incapacitate or kill a large number of individuals after a single release. After exposure to a chemical agent, symptoms may not be apparent immediately. It may take hours to days before physicians and public health officials detect the chemical agent.

Chemical weapons were first used in World War I about 100 years ago. In 1993, many countries signed an agreement at the Paris Convention to cease production of chemical agents.

Terrorist groups continue to use these chemicals, which do not need to be lethal to be effective. Terrorist groups are not opposed to killing people, but they rely more on the resulting chaos and psychological effects to make an impact. By releasing chemical agents in a crowded area, terrorists create a mass casualty scenario, with overwhelmed medical services, people with impaired psychological and physical functioning, and required decontamination of people and the environment. Reports of chemical agents used by terrorists began around 1994, when sarin was released in a Tokyo subway by the Aum Shinrikyo cult. Chemical or biological agents may be used to pursue a political agenda because they can cover a large area, penetrate a defended area, focus on a specific target, and disorient, maim, or kill targeted individuals.

As a result of the use of chemical agents in international conflicts, the United States developed an arsenal of countermeasures for some agents. For example, deployed soldiers can use atropine injectors to offset the effects of a released nerve agent. The U.S. Department of Defense has an Army depot called the Defense Threat Reduction Agency to research, develop, and maintain effective countermeasures for military personnel.

Because many chemicals used in industry and by terrorists produce similar effects on people, the best way to discuss these chemicals is by categories (Table 36-1). Symptoms can also be grouped into clusters called case definitions, which include toxicity syndrome information. Medical management of exposed individuals is based on specific protocols, which may include decontamination as the initial response. The following sections discuss each category of potential chemical weapons.

TABLE 36-1	Chemical Agents	
Category	Examples	Comments
Nerve agents	Sarin, tabun, soman, VX, malathion, carbaryl (Sevin)	Interfere with transmission of signal from nerve to organ or muscle
Blood agents	Hydrogen cyanide, cyanogen chloride	Usually absorbed after inhalation; in the bloodstream, cause lethal damage by acting on the cytochrome oxidase enzyme responsible for cellular respiration; oxygen starvation occurs because cells are unable to use oxygen
Blister agents	Nitrogen and sulfur mustards, lewisite	Cause blistering of skin and internal organs; destroy tissue and cause massive numbers of mutations by crosslinking DNA and RNA
Heavy metals	Arsenic	Metallic elements form poisonous compounds, disrupting cellular metabolic processes
Pulmonary agents	Chlorine gas, phosgene	Damage membranes of the lungs, causing fluid buildup and oxygen deprivation and eventually suffocation
Dioxins	Tetrachlorodibenzodioxin	Associated with lymphomas, sarcomas, carcinomas, chloracne, and many other diseases; major long-term complication is type 2 diabetes
Incapacitating or psychotomimetic agents	Quinuclidinyl benzilate, phencyclidine	Cause pseudopsychotic disorders, affect ability to make decisions, and cause disorientation, any of which can incapacitate an individual; death due to respiratory arrest can occur with high doses
Corrosive acids and bases	Sulfuric acid, sodium hydroxide	Cause severe burning and destruction of tissue in exposed areas

From McPherson RA, Pincus MR. *Henry's Clinical Diagnosis and Management by Laboratory Methods*. 22nd ed. Philadelphia: Saunders; 2012.

Blister Agents

Blister agents are chemicals that produce blisters when they come in contact with the eyes, skin, and respiratory tract. Blister agents include mustards, including a mustard-lewisite mixture, nitrogen mustards, sulfur mustard, lewisite, and phosgene oxime. The nitrogen mustards, lewisite, and phosgene oxime are discussed as representatives of this category of chemical weapons.

Nitrogen Mustards

The nitrogen mustards (military designations: HN-1, HN-2, and HN-3) are oily, colorless to yellow liquids with distinctly different smells: HN-1 smells musty, HN-2 smells fruity, and HN-3 smells like butter almond. All of these compounds evaporate slowly, and as oil-based chemicals, the compounds do not dissolve in water.

Nitrogen mustards are vesicants (i.e., blister-producing agents) and DNA alkylating agents that damage cells within minutes of contact and may cause bone marrow suppression and neurologic toxicity. Acute exposure to nitrogen mustards affects many systems. In addition to damaging the skin on contact, the compounds can cause ocular damage when the eye is exposed, lung damage when inhaled, and gastrointestinal damage when ingested.

Victims exposed to nitrogen mustards may off-gas these compounds to emergency responders, if they are not decontaminated immediately. There is no antidote for nitrogen mustard toxicity.

Sulfur Mustard

Pure sulfur mustard (military designation: H) is a colorless, viscous liquid at room temperature. Impure forms, such as warfare agents, are usually yellow-brown. The gas, liquid, or solid forms smell like garlic, onions, or mustard or may have no odor. Sulfur mustard is considered a DNA alkylating agent that damages rapidly growing cells. It was used in World War I as a chemical warfare agent against the Allied Forces.

Exposure to sulfur mustard is not usually fatal. As with other chemical agents, adverse health effects depend on the route and amount of exposure. Symptoms do not usually occur for 2 to 24 hours after exposure. After skin exposure, redness and itching occur in 2 to 48 hours, eventually leading to yellow blisters. They constitute second- and third-degree burns, and extensive skin burns can be fatal. After the eyes are exposed, irritation, pain, swelling, and tearing occur 3 to 12 hours after a moderate exposure and 1 to 2 hours after a severe exposure. Severe exposure also produces photosensitivity, temporary blindness, and possibly permanent blindness. Runny nose, sneezing, bloody nose, sinus pain, shortness of breath, and cough occur 12 to 24 hours after a mild respiratory tract exposure and 2 to 4 hours after a severe exposure. Abdominal pain, diarrhea, fever, nausea, and vomiting occur after ingestion.

There is no antidote for sulfur mustard toxicity. Removal of clothing and decontamination by thorough washing of the skin with soap and water is essential to limit exposure.

Lewisite

Lewisite (military designations: L-1, L-2, and L-3) is an oily, arsenic-containing liquid ranging from colorless to violet-black, green, amber, or dark brown. It has the odor of geraniums, and it is extremely toxic. It was developed as a chemical weapon but has not been used in wartime.

Exposure to lewisite produces immediate pain and irritation and noticeable tissue destruction. If individuals are exposed to large amounts, it can cause death. Small concentrations that cannot be detected by smell can cause burning and tissue destruction in the lungs. When the eyes are exposed to lewisite for 15 to 30 minutes, redness and pain occur. The eyes swell shut due to fluid accumulation in the membranes and eyelids. Severe exposure can lead to scarring of the cornea, perforation of the eye, and blindness. When skin is exposed to lewisite, pain is immediate, redness occurs at 15 to 30 minutes, and pain and itching persist for 24 hours. Blisters appear within hours after exposure but do not reach their full extent for 12 to 18 hours. Pain lasts for 2 to 3 days.

Lewisite is completely absorbed by the skin within 3 to 5 minutes and can lead to shock. *Lewisite shock* is a term used to describe symptoms encountered after exposure to a large amount of lewisite. The capillaries are damaged, leading to leakage of proteins and plasma into surrounding tissues and hypovolemia. Hypovolemia may lead to kidney damage and hypotension.

Due to the reactive nature of this chemical, all victims need to be thoroughly decontaminated to stop the progression of cellular damage. The antidote, dimercaprol or British anti-lewisite (BAL), binds to the arsenic in lewisite to reduce its toxicity. BAL is usually injected and is not used to treat skin or eye damage. It has side effects, especially if individuals are allergic to peanuts. Exposure to BAL is clinically diagnosed, but electrolytes are monitored to ensure they are in balance.

Mustard-Lewisite Mixture

The mustard-lewisite mixture (military designation: HL) contains sulfur mustard and lewisite. It is a dark, oily liquid with a garlic odor. It is a blister agent and an alkylating agent that damages the DNA of rapidly dividing cells. The liquid has a low freezing temperature that allows better aerial spraying.

When a victim is exposed to this mixture, the lewisite produces effects immediately, and the sulfur mustard effects become apparent hours later (Table 36-2). As with lewisite alone, respiratory exposure produces burning and irritation of the upper respiratory tract, but the longer the exposure, the deeper into the respiratory tract the agent reaches and the more damage that results. Eye exposure produces immediate stinging, blinking, tearing, conjunctivitis, and temporary blindness. Permanent blindness can result from exposure to a large amount of this mixture. Because the mixture also possesses the properties of an alkylating agent, bone marrow suppression leading to fatal infections can result. Other systemic effects are weakness, restlessness, low

TABLE 36-2 Systemic Effects of Lewisite Exposure	
System	**Signs and Symptoms**
Central nervous system	Tremors, seizures, incoordination, ataxia, and coma
Respiratory system	Nasal and sinus pain or discomfort, pharyngitis, laryngitis, cough, dyspnea
Gastrointestinal system	Chemical burns of gastrointestinal tract, hemorrhagic diarrhea, nausea, vomiting
Eye	Intense conjunctival and sclera inflammation, pain, lacrimation, photophobia, corneal damage, blindness
Skin and mucous membranes	Erythema, blistering, second- and third-degree burns
Hematopoiesis	Bone marrow suppression leading to fatal complicating infections, hemorrhage, and anemia
Various, delayed	Menstrual irregularities, alopecia, hearing loss, tinnitus, jaundice, impaired spermatogenesis, generalized swelling, and hyperpigmentation; may cause chronic respiratory and eye conditions

body temperature, salivation, nausea, vomiting, diarrhea, hypotension, shock, and death.

To stop the damaging effects of the chemical, the victim is removed from the exposure. Clothing is then removed, and the skin is decontaminated. After eye exposure, eyes are washed for 10 to 15 minutes with clear water. No antidote exists for this mixture. BAL can be used for the lewisite in the mixture, but the sulfur mustard does not respond to that antidote. Supportive treatment is indicated for respiratory exposure, including oxygen, assisted ventilation, and artificial respiration. Electrolyte and fluid support may be indicated. Skin burns from this mixture should be treated with standard burn therapy.

Phosgene Oxime

Phosgene oxime (military designation: CX) is a colorless solid or yellow-brown liquid with a disagreeable, irritating odor. Phosgene oxime is a urticant (some sources consider it a corrosive), and when it contacts skin, it causes erythema and hives. It does not produce blistering like the other chemicals in this class.

The effect of this chemical is immediate when it touches skin; it produces extreme pain and tissue necrosis. Although it has never been used in wartime, tests show it penetrates rubber and protective clothing much quicker than other chemical agents. The potential exists for combining phosgene oxime with other chemical agents to allow skin penetration with the phosgene oxime and better access to tissue for the second agent. When phosgene oxime gets into the eyes, it causes severe pain, tearing, and temporary blindness. If it is inhaled, it may result in pulmonary edema with symptoms of shortness of breath and cough.

Decontamination is the most important part of the medical management of phosgene oxide. Because it is quickly absorbed into the skin and causes immediate symptoms, people exposed to this chemical need to take off all clothing and wash the chemical off the skin as quickly as possible. Exposed eyes are rinsed with plain water for 10 to 15 minutes. There is no antidote for this chemical, and medical care is supportive.

Blood Agents

Blood agents become poisonous after they are absorbed into the blood. They include arsine and cyanogen chloride.

Arsine

Arsine (military designation: SA) is a colorless, flammable, and highly toxic gas with a garlic or fish odor. Initial symptoms may develop up to several hours after exposure and include malaise, dizziness, nausea, abdominal pain, and dyspnea. Arsine binds to hemoglobin, preventing oxygen binding. Arsine also lyses red blood cells (RBCs) and converts Fe^{2+} to Fe^{3+} in hemoglobin, further reducing the oxygen carrying capacity. A significant sequela of arsine exposure is acute tubular necrosis with resulting kidney failure. Headache may be a symptom of early exposure. Several days after a severe exposure, victims demonstrate restlessness, memory loss, disorientation, and agitation.

After exposure to arsine, acute intravascular hemolysis develops and may continue for approximately 96 hours. Haptoglobin levels decline, free hemoglobin levels rise, and anemia develops. Examination of RBCs demonstrates anisocytosis, poikilocytosis, fragments, Heinz bodies, and ghost cells. The direct Coombs test, Ham acid hemolysis test, and RBC fragility test results are all negative. Urine specimens show large amounts of protein and free hemoglobin. Acute tubular necrosis and kidney failure may decrease urinary output. Elevated liver enzymes, prolonged prothrombin times, myoglobinuria, and elevated creatine kinase levels can be observed. There are no antidotes for arsine poisoning, so medical care is supportive.

Cyanogen Chloride

Cyanogen chloride (military designation: CK) is a colorless liquid or a highly volatile gas with irritating and choking vapors. Cyanogen chloride reacts with water to produce hydrogen cyanide, a toxic and corrosive chemical asphyxiant. Cyanide irreversibly attaches to RBCs and does not allow oxygen to attach. When oxygen does not attach to RBCs, the body is starved of oxygen, and metabolic end products (e.g., carbon dioxide) cannot be expelled.

Early symptoms of exposure include lightheadedness, giddiness, rapid breathing, nausea, vomiting, confusion, restlessness, and anxiety. Pulmonary edema occurs with severe exposure, which also can cause stupor, coma, muscle spasms (in which head, neck, and spine are arched backward), convulsions, fixed and dilated pupils, and death.

Cyanogen chloride poisoning can be quickly fatal. Cyanide levels in RBCs and urine can be analyzed in a laboratory, but obtaining the laboratory results takes a long time. Because empirical treatment must be rendered immediately after exposure, laboratory tests are not usually performed to confirm the diagnosis.

Caustics

Caustics are acids that produce chemical burns on the skin, eyes, and mucous membranes on contact. The only member of this group discussed here is hydrofluoric acid.

Hydrofluoric Acid

Hydrofluoric acid is a colorless liquid or a colorless gas. This agent produces hypocalcemia and hypokalemia. The fluoride ions also replace the calcium ions in the skeletal system, producing denser but weaker bones.

Hydrofluoric acid systemic poisoning can occur through ingestion, inhalation, and skin contact. Ingestion produces vomiting (possibly bloody), abdominal pain, and bloody diarrhea. If hydrofluoric acid is inhaled, symptoms include dyspnea, chest pain, stridor, and wheezing. After hydrofluoric acid contact with skin, it can initially look fine. Within hours, the skin may be pale and become painful. The skin then becomes necrotic. Systemic poisoning effects include hypocalcemia and hypokalemia, which can lead to dysrhythmias, seizures, and death.

Although no diagnostic test exists for hydrofluoric acid, serum fluoride levels can be determined. Calcium and potassium levels should be monitored because hypocalcemia and hypokalemia result from systemic poisoning with hydrofluoric acid.

Pulmonary Agents

Pulmonary agents are chemicals that cause severe irritation or swelling of the respiratory tract. Chemicals in this group include ammonia, chlorine, mercury, diphosgene, phosgene, and phosphorus (i.e., elemental, white, or yellow).

Ammonia

Ammonia is a colorless, irritating gas with a pungent, suffocating odor. In liquid form, it is clear and colorless.

Exposure to ammonia can occur through inhalation, skin or eye contact, and ingestion. Inhalation exposure causes nasopharyngeal and tracheal burns, bronchiolar and alveolar edema, and airway destruction. Damage results in dyspnea, pulmonary edema, and possible respiratory failure. The amount of ammonia and concentration of the solution contacting the skin or eyes determine the degree of damage. Eye and nose irritation appear first. Very concentrated solutions can cause skin burns, permanent eye damage, and blindness. Ingested ammonia causes mouth, throat, and stomach burns.

No specific test for ammonia exposure exists. Laboratory tests for victims include a complete blood count and glucose and electrolyte levels. If the victim was exposed through inhalation, pulse oximetry and arterial blood gas determinations may be necessary to monitor lung function.

Chlorine

Chlorine is a green-yellow gas and an amber liquid. Chlorine is caustic and causes burn injuries. The most likely route of exposure is inhalation.

Respiratory health effects are common after chlorine exposure and can occur immediately or after a delay. Symptoms from mild exposures usually resolve within a few hours, whereas symptoms from severe exposures can take several days or longer to resolve. Mild symptoms include eye, nose, and throat irritation and mild cough. Extensive exposure can cause corneal burns leading to tissue necrosis, pulmonary edema, and severe skin burns. Severe exposure can lead to death. No diagnostic tests are available to detect chlorine exposure.

Mercury

Mercury is a heavy, shiny, silver-white, liquid metal. The most toxic route of exposure to mercury is inhalation. Acute exposure begins with chemical pneumonitis, dyspnea, chest pain, and dry cough. Symptoms can progress to pulmonary edema, respiratory failure, and death. In addition to respiratory symptoms, mercury can cause tachycardia, heart attacks, kidney damage, and kidney failure.

Diagnostic tests for mercury can be used to determine systemic toxic exposure. Laboratory tests to diagnosis mercury are useful because chelation can be used to treat the condition. To be effective, however, chelation must begin as soon as possible after exposure. The effectiveness of chelation in reducing the effects of poisoning decreases as the time after exposure increases.

Phosgene

Phosgene (military designation: CG) is a colorless gas or liquid and is used most often in its gaseous state. Phosgene gas was released by the German army in World War I as a chemical weapon. Small amounts smell like newly mowed grass, but large amounts have a strong, suffocating, unpleasant odor. Diphosgene (military designation: DP) is related to phosgene and has comparable toxicity, but it is more conveniently handled because it is a liquid.

Victims exposed to phosgene gas may not realize they are being exposed. The gas may cause only mild irritation, and the victim continues to inhale the phosgene. There is a 30-minute to 72-hour period during which there are no symptoms. The more severe the exposure, the shorter the symptom-free period. If pulmonary edema appears within 6 to 8 hours, the exposure is considered severe. This agent disrupts protein synthesis. Severe exposure leads to shallow and rapid breaths, painful coughs, frothy sputum, laryngospasm, and possible cardiovascular collapse due to low blood oxygen levels. Victims exposed to phosgene are clinically diagnosed and treated.

Phosphorus

Phosphine, a combination of phosphorus with hydrogen, is a colorless, odorless, flammable gas. Inhalation is the main route of exposure. Exposure to phosphine gas produces symptoms within a few hours of exposure. Death may occur 12 to 72 hours after a severe exposure due to cardiovascular, kidney, or liver failure. Severe exposure results in death. Death is due to hypotension, ventricular dysrhythmias, peripheral vascular collapse, cardiac arrest, shock, convulsions, and coma.

Laboratory tests should be used to monitor the victim's liver and kidney functions. The victim's cardiac and respiratory functions need to be closely monitored for up to 72 hours.

Incapacitating Agents

Incapacitating agents are chemicals that impair brain function or cause an altered state of consciousness (e.g., unconsciousness). This group includes benzene (BZ), fentanyl, and 3-quinuclidinyl benzilate (QNB).

Benzene

Benzene is a clear to light yellow liquid with a sweet, aromatic, gasoline-like odor. Terrorists can expose people to liquid benzene through air, water, and food; air is the most desirable route of exposure.

Central nervous system function is depressed immediately after inhalation. When ingested, it takes 30 to 60 minutes to cause gastrointestinal irritation and central nervous system depression. Full recovery from benzene exposure takes 1 to 4 weeks.

Central nervous system depression manifests through drowsiness, dizziness, headache, lightheadedness, tremors, impaired gait, confusion, loss of consciousness, respiratory depression, coma, and death. Severe exposure to benzene can cause pulmonary edema, dermal edema, vesication, and dermatitis.

Fentanyl

Fentanyl is a synthetic opioid that is 80 times more potent than morphine and hundreds of times stronger than heroin. Fentanyl was used in October 2002 by the Russian army against a terrorist group holding hostages. The agent is a colorless, odorless gas.

Fentanyl causes respiratory depression and arrest. Intracranial hypertension, muscle rigidity, and spasms occur when exposed to fentanyl. Victims may also have hypotension, dysrhythmias, and pulmonary edema.

Laboratory tests can be helpful in determining mild or severe fentanyl exposure. The drug can be quantitated using gas chromatography with mass spectrometry.

3-Quinuclidinyl Benzilate

QNB is a white, crystalline solid and a very potent drug that incapacitates its victims. People can be exposed through air, water, and food routes.

In all types of exposure, the health effects are usually delayed. Signs and symptoms begin 30 minutes to 4 hours after exposure and peak 4 to 8 hours after exposure. Full recovery from exposure usually occurs within 3 to 4 days. QNB blocks the normal transmission of nerve signals at the receiving neuron. The resulting nervous system effects are called the *anticholinergic toxidrome*.

Signs and symptoms of the anticholinergic toxidrome include hyperthermia, dry mouth, dry skin, low urine output, flushing, dilated pupils, blurred vision, rapid heart rate, disorientation, delusions, hallucinations, poor judgment, distractibility, slurred speech, involuntary repetition of behaviors, ataxia, behavioral variability, and muscle weakness. Laboratory tests are not usually used to detect benzene in a person's system; however, a complete blood count and electrolyte determinations are used to monitor the victim's condition.

Metals

Heavy metals usually act as poisons after being absorbed into the body by interfering with the production of hemoglobin. The metallic poison group includes arsenic, barium, mercury, and thallium.

Thallium

Thallium is a blue-white metal that turns gray on exposure to air. It is tasteless and colorless and has been used to murder people because it is difficult to detect after the person dies. It was discovered in 1861, and the United States banned production in 1984.

Signs and symptoms of thallium poisoning are delayed, appearing 12 to 24 hours later and peaking 2 to 3 weeks after exposure. Initial symptoms include nausea and vomiting, followed by pain in the arms and legs after 1 to 5 days. Mild exposure can cause tachycardia, hypertension, dysrhythmias, respiratory failure, painful or burning sensations, muscle aches, weakness, headache, seizures, delirium, coma, loss of appetite, excessive salivation, green discoloration of urine shortly after exposure, kidney damage, RBC lysis, dry scaling of the skin, and inflammation of the mouth, lips, and gums. Severe exposure can lead to loss of muscle control in the head and the neck and respiratory failure. These symptoms manifest 2 to 3 weeks after exposure.

Prussian blue or activated charcoal should be administered to victims. Victims should have cardiac, renal, and hepatic function monitored along with calcium levels. Thallium is not normally present in urine, and levels above 5 μg/L are abnormal, but levels above 200 μg/L indicate poisoning. Similarly, thallium blood levels are usually below 2 μg/L, with concentrations greater than 200 μg/L indicating poisoning.

Nerve Agents

Nerve agents are highly poisonous. After they enter the body, they interfere with the conduction of nerve impulses. If nerve impulses do not reach the heart, it may stop beating and cause death. Nerve agents are considered to be G agents, including sarin (GB), soman (GD), and tabun (GA), or V agents such as VX. The adverse health effects of these agents are caused by the same mechanism.

Sarin is a clear, colorless, odorless, and tasteless liquid. Soman is also a clear, colorless liquid that smells like camphor or rotting fruit. Tabun is a clear, colorless to pale or dark amber liquid, which smells fruity like bitter almonds. VX is a clear, amber, oily, tasteless, and odorless liquid.

These chemicals are some of the most toxic chemical weapons. Nerve agents are potent acetylcholinesterase inhibitors, and exposure can cause death in minutes. A dose of 1 to 10 mL of sarin, soman, or tabun can be fatal. However, only 1 drop of VX can be fatal.

Excess acetylcholine produces a cholinogenic syndrome characterized by heavy respiratory and oral secretions, diarrhea and vomiting, sweating, altered mental status, autonomic instability, and generalized weakness that can lead to paralysis and respiratory failure. Table 36-3 lists the signs and symptoms for each system.

Laboratory tests can be helpful in diagnosing nerve agent poisoning. Although it results in decreased plasma or RBC cholinesterase activity, values must be interpreted with caution. A decreased RBC cholinesterase level should be determined using a baseline RBC cholinesterase level for each individual. Even though a decreased RBC level results from nerve agent poisoning, it is not possible to correlate the severity of the health effects with exposure. The particular nerve agent and the amount of exposure and time since exposure affect RBC cholinesterase inhibition. It is also important to monitor with a complete blood count, glucose level, and electrolyte determinations.

Organic Solvents

A chemical rule states that like dissolves like. Organic solvents dissolve fats and oils while disrupting and damaging living tissue by dissolving cell membranes and other organs made with fat and oils. One organic solvent is benzene. Benzene is discussed in the Incapacitating Agents section.

TABLE 36-3	Systemic Effects of Nerve Agents
System	**Signs and Symptoms**
Central nervous system	Miosis, headache, restlessness, convulsions, loss of consciousness, coma
Respiratory system	Perfuse watery nose, excessive bronchial secretions, wheezing, dyspnea, chest tightness, hyperpnea (early), bradypnea (late)
Cardiovascular system	Tachycardia, hypertension, bradycardia, hypotension, arrhythmias, dysrhythmias
Gastrointestinal system	Abdominal pain, nausea, vomiting, diarrhea, urinary incontinence
Musculoskeletal system	Weakness (may progress to paralysis), fasciculations
Skin and mucous membranes	Profuse sweating, lacrimation, and eye redness

Riot Control Agents

Riot control agents cause irritation to the eyes and mucous membranes on contact. The chemicals are used by law enforcement to control crowds and by individuals for protection. This group of chemicals includes bromobenzyl cyanide (military designation: CA), chloroacetophenone (CN), chlorobenzylidenemalononitrile (CS), chloropicrin (PS), and dibenzoxazepine (CR).

Chloroacetophenone

Chloroacetophenone is also known as tear gas. It is a colorless to gray or white crystalline solid. When released as a gas, it may appear to be a blue-white cloud. It has an irritating odor that has been described as apple blossoms.

Exposure to chloroacetophenone simultaneously affects the eyes, skin, and respiratory tract. Contact causes instant symptoms, especially in the eyes. Symptoms usually resolve 15 to 30 minutes after decontamination. Redness of the eyes and periorbital edema may take 1 to 2 days to resolve. Irritation of the respiratory tract may take 12 to 24 hours to manifest as pulmonary edema. Severe ocular exposure causes keratitis, conjunctivitis, chemical burns, loss of the corneal epithelium, photophobia, and blurred vision. Mild to moderate respiratory tract exposure results in rhinorrhea, coughing, sneezing, shortness of breath, wheezing, salivation, and vomiting. Severe exposure results in pulmonary edema, bronchospasm, and bronchopneumonia. Mild to moderate skin exposure results in irritation and pain, whereas severe exposure results in redness, blistering, and areas of dead skin.

Victims usually recover spontaneously in 1 to 3 days. Rare instances of hospitalization for burns, pulmonary edema, or damaged eyes occur after massive and prolonged exposure. Most victims are treated and released at the scene, and very few require hospitalization.

Chloropicrin

Chloropicrin is a colorless to faint yellow, oily liquid and is considered a lung-damaging agent. It is an irritant similar to tear gas and has a very irritating odor. Exposure routes include the eyes, skin, respiratory tract, and gastrointestinal tract.

Initial symptoms can resolve within 15 to 30 minutes after decontamination. However, gastrointestinal symptoms may last for weeks, and neurologic or muscular symptoms may last for months. Eye exposure results in tearing and possible eye damage. Exposure of the skin results in blisters, dyspnea, headache, and cyanosis. Mild to moderate exposure of the respiratory tract results in coughing, choking, dyspnea, chest tightness, pulmonary edema, nausea, vomiting, headache, dizziness, lethargy, fatigue, and cyanosis. Severe respiratory exposure results in severe inflammation of the lower respiratory tract leading to pulmonary edema, which can be fatal. Exposure of the gastrointestinal tract results in sore throat, nausea, vomiting, dyspnea, dizziness, cyanosis, and mouth, esophagus, and stomach burns.

Diagnosis of chloropicrin exposure is clinical. Immediate decontamination is necessary for a better outcome. Supportive treatment is used for respiratory function.

Toxic Alcohols

After absorption, alcohols produce toxic effects on the heart, kidney, and nervous system. The most common effect from this group of chemicals is blindness caused by ethylene glycol.

Ethylene Glycol

Ethylene glycol is a clear, colorless, viscous liquid at room temperature. It can be found in antifreeze, in which it is colored fluorescent yellow. Antifreeze has a sweet taste that can lead to accidental ingestion. The metabolic products of ethylene glycol are toxic to the central nervous system, heart, and kidneys. This chemical can be used to poison water and food because it is colorless and odorless, and victims do not know they were poisoned until they become symptomatic.

Ethylene glycol is absorbed 1 to 4 hours after ingestion, and 80% of the absorbed compound is converted to toxic metabolic products that affect three major systems: the central nervous system, cardiopulmonary system, and genitourinary system. Symptoms include central nervous system depression, intoxication (without the smell of alcohol on the victim's breath), euphoria, slurred speech, dizziness, disorientation, ataxia, stupor, loss of reflexes, and coma. The cardiopulmonary system is affected by the metabolic acidosis produced by metabolic products. Metabolic acidosis leads to increased rate and depth of breathing, heart damage, congestive heart failure, pulmonary edema, lung damage, adult respiratory distress syndrome (ARDS), and death. The genitourinary system is affected by metabolic acidosis, which can lead to reduced urinary output, no urinary output, and acute kidney failure, leading to death.

Because most of the damage from this chemical is caused by the metabolic products, serum ethylene glycol levels do not correlate with the clinical symptoms. Victims of ethylene glycol poisoning must be monitored closely. A complete blood count, lactate, osmolarity, arterial blood gas determination, urinalysis, and tests for glucose, electrolytes, magnesium, calcium, BUN, and creatinine should be performed on admission to the emergency department and often later to monitor the effects of the metabolic products. For severe exposures and patients in metabolic acidosis, hemodialysis is the most effective form of treatment.

Vomiting Agents

According to the CDC, adamsite is the only chemical classified as a vomiting agent. Exposure to it causes nausea and vomiting.

Adamsite

Adamsite is composed of light green to yellow crystals. Adamsite can be heated to form a gas that is canary yellow when concentrated but colorless when diluted in air. This riot control agent is usually delivered as an aerosol.

Mild exposure to adamsite causes self-limited symptoms that usually resolve within 30 minutes. Exposure to large concentrations or in an enclosed space can cause severe adverse health effects. Symptoms from short-term exposure include lacrimation, eye irritation and burning, spasmodic blinking, swelling of the blood vessels that supply the membranes lining the eye, and necrosis of corneal epithelium. Respiratory system symptoms include nose and throat irritation, increased nasal secretions, and uncontrollable and violent coughing. Severe exposure can produce nausea, vomiting, abdominal cramps, diarrhea, malaise, headache, and mental depression.

A clinical diagnosis is made. Laboratory tests are useful in monitoring system functions in victims suffering from severe exposure.

Biological Agents

Biological threats include naturally occurring chemicals produced by animals, plants, or microbes such as bacteria, fungi, parasites, and viruses. Advantages of using biological agents include their potent toxicity (i.e., more toxic than chemical weapons), minimal dermal activity (i.e., no damage to skin), no odor, no taste, and mode of delivery (i.e., aerosol or intradermal) (Table 36-4). However, they are more difficult and costly to produce. Ironically, some of the agents have a legitimate medical use.

Biological agents (i.e., microorganisms) include *Bacillus anthracis, Brucella* species, *Burkholderia mallei, Burkholderia pseudomallei, Yersinia pestis, Coxiella burnetii, Francisella tularensis,* and the viruses that cause smallpox, Venezuelan equine encephalitis, and viral hemorrhagic fevers. Biological agents also include toxins such as abrin (i.e., ricin), brevetoxin, colchicine, saxitoxin, staphylococcal enterotoxin B (SEB), strychnine, tetrodotoxin, botulinum, and trichothecene mycotoxins (Table 36-5).

Microorganisms

Biological agents can be bacterial, fungal, or viral. After World War II, the U.S. military actively researched offensive agents and defensive countermeasures in biological warfare. Offensive weapons research was suspended in 1969 (due to the Biological Weapons Convention), and research has concentrated on defensive countermeasures since then. The U.S. Department of Homeland Security awarded more than $8 billion since March 2003 to assist first responders and state and local governments to prevent, respond to, and recover from a bioterrorism event. The bioterrorism threat is more important now than at any other time in U.S. history because biological agents, production methods, and potential dissemination devices are available

TABLE 36-4	**Categories of Biological Agents**
Characteristics	**Agents**
Category A Agents*	
Easily disseminated and/or transmitted from person to person	Anthrax (*Bacillus anthracis*)
Can result in high mortality rates and major public health impact	Botulism (*Clostridium botulinum*)
May cause public panic	Plague (*Yersinia pestis*)
	Smallpox (variola major)
	Tularemia (*Francisella tularensis*)
	Viral hemorrhagic fevers, such as filoviruses (i.e., Ebola, Marburg) and arenaviruses (i.e., Lassa, Machupo)
Category B Agents	
Moderately easy to disseminate	Brucellosis (*Brucella* species)
Moderate morbidity and low mortality rates	Epsilon toxin of *Clostridium perfringens*
May require enhanced Centers for Disease Control and Prevention diagnostic capacity	Food safety threats (i.e., *Salmonella* sp., *Escherichia coli* 0157:H7, *Shigella*)
	Glanders (*Burkholderia mallei*)
	Melioidosis (*Burkholderia pseudomallei*)
	Psittacosis (*Chlamydia psittaci*)
	Q fever (*Coxiella burnetii*)
	Ricin toxin from *Ricinus communis* (i.e., castor beans)
	Staphylococcal enterotoxin B
	Typhus fever (*Rickettsia prowazekii*)
	Viral encephalitis (alphaviruses: Venezuelan equine encephalitis, Eastern and Western equine encephalitis)
	Water safety threats (e.g., *Vibrio cholerae, Cryptosporidium parvum*)
Category C Agents	
Availability	Hantavirus
Ease of production and dissemination	Nipah virus
Potential for high morbidity and mortality rates	Other emerging pathogens that could be engineered for mass dissemination
Potential major health impact	

Modified from McPherson RA, Pincus MR. *Henry's Clinical Diagnosis and Management by Laboratory Methods*. 22nd ed. Philadelphia: Saunders; 2012.
*Highest priority of agents that pose a national security risk.

TABLE 36-5 Bioterrorism Agents: Diagnosis and Treatment

Agent	Diagnosis	Tests and Specimens	Treatment
Anthrax	Clinical evaluation and laboratory findings	Culture: blood, CSF, wounds (definitive) Nasal culture: determines extent of spore spread in population IHC: tissue PCR: confirms diagnosis if culture is negative Serology: ELISA, IFA	Antibiotics, including penicillin, quinolones, tetracycline Treat inhalation anthrax for 60 days; can combine antibiotics (30 days) and vaccine (3 doses at 0, 14, and 28 days) Full vaccination regimen is 6 doses at 0, 2, and 4 weeks and 6, 12, and 18 months followed by yearly boosters
Plague	Clinical evaluation and laboratory findings	Culture: sputum, blood, lymph Direct FA: respiratory secretions Serology: F1-V fusion protein assay	Antibiotics, including tetracycline; quinolones, streptomycin, gentamicin, and chloramphenicol for 10-14 days Prophylaxis: medication for 7 days
Brucellosis	Difficult with many rule-outs; laboratory required	Culture: nasal, sputum, respiratory specimens (can also use PCR); blood culture is definitive test Serology: IFA, ELISA, and microagglutination (gold standard) to detect ABs	Combination antibiotics (6 weeks): doxycycline and rifampin or quinolone and rifampin Prophylaxis requires 3 weeks Numerous vaccines (killed or live attenuated) available with no proven success
Tularemia	Difficult with many rule-outs; laboratory required Key symptom: pneumonia with nonproductive cough	General laboratory tests not helpful Culture: bacterium does not grow on ordinary media, needs cysteine blood or chocolate agar Capsular AG detection or PCR: whole unclotted blood Direct FA and PCR: nasal, induced respiratory specimens IHC: tissue sometimes helpful Serology: ELISA, ABs	Treatment: antibiotics such as gentamicin, streptomycin, ciprofloxacin Prophylaxis: doxycycline Vaccine: live attenuated available
Botulism	Clinical evaluation; routine laboratory tests have no value; toxin assay may be useful if toxin present in serum	PCR and toxin assay: use nasal induced respiratory secretions and blood	Supportive treatment: trivalent and pentavalent antitoxin administered up to 24 hours after exposure Also available is a pentavalent toxoid vaccine
Smallpox	Clinical findings (exanthems)	Cell or chick embryo culture: skin lesions ideal; nasal swabs, respiratory secretions, serum specimens can also be cultured Electron microscopy: identifies virus PCR: use same specimens as for culture Agar gel precipitation: skin lesions Serology: tests are available	VIG used in conjunction with vaccinia vaccine if exposure occurs beyond 3-day time frame Within 3 days, only vaccinia vaccine given by scarification Cidofovir offers promise
VEE	Difficult with many rule-outs; laboratory required	PCR or culture in cells/suckling mice: nasal, induced respiratory secretions, and serum Serology: ELISA, IFA, and hemagglutination inhibition; detect ABs	Some drugs show promise but no specific therapy; treatment geared toward relieving symptoms Some vaccines show promise (e.g., C-84)
VHF	Clinical evaluation; key finding is vascular involvement (e.g., petechiae, bleeding, postural hypotension, edema)	General: leukopenia, thrombocytopenia; elevated AST Serology: ELISA, IFA, and PCR: detect different VHFs	Management of hypotension and fluid loss; aggressive supportive care needed Ribavirin and immune globulin therapy show promise Several vaccines under development

Modified from McPherson RA, Pincus MR: *Henry's Clinical Diagnosis and Management by Laboratory Methods.* 22nd ed. Philadelphia: Saunders; 2012.
ABs, Antibodies; *AG,* antigen; *AST,* aspartate aminotransferase; *CSF,* cerebrospinal fluid; *ELISA,* enzyme-linked immunosorbent assay; *FA,* fluorescent antibody; *IFA,* indirect fluorescent antibody; *IHC,* immunohistochemical; *PCR,* polymerase chain reaction; *VEE,* Venezuelan equine encephalitis; *VHF,* viral hemorrhagic fever; *VIG,* vaccinia immune globulin.

worldwide. The following sections address the most likely agents to be used in a bioterrorism attack, even though some of the organisms have never been weaponized.

Bacillus anthracis

Bacillus anthracis produces anthrax (Fig. 36-2). There are three types of anthrax infections: cutaneous (i.e., woolsorter's disease), gastrointestinal, and inhalation. Inhalation anthrax is the most deadly form of the disease and most likely to be used as a biological weapon. The infective form of the bacteria is the spore. It is readily weaponized (i.e., wet or dry forms) and usually released into the air. At the beginning of the respiratory infection, it causes flulike symptoms that lead to severe respiratory distress and death within 36 hours.

Infection can be treated with ciprofloxacin or doxycycline. The earlier antibiotics are administered, the better the patient outcome. The antibiotics can also be used to prevent the infection from occurring. A vaccine is available. The role of the level A laboratory is shown in Table 36-6.

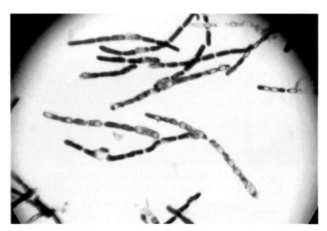

• Figure 36-2 The photomicrograph depicts several gram-positive, endospore-forming *Bacillus anthracis* bacteria. *B. anthracis* causes anthrax, an acute infectious disease that most commonly occurs in wild and domestic vertebrates such as cattle, sheep, goats, camels, antelopes, and other herbivores, but it can also occur in humans exposed to infected animals or tissue from them. (Courtesy Public Health Image Library, Centers for Disease Control and Prevention, Atlanta, GA.)

Brucella species

Brucella suis and *Brucella abortus* can be used as biological weapons. These organisms produce a disease called brucellosis (Fig. 36-3). Both species are readily weaponized and are usually released into the air. Infected individuals have headache, fever, chills, fatigue, back pain, and meningitis. The infections incapacitate people but usually do not kill them.

Both organisms can be treated with doxycycline. No vaccines are available to protect against infection with these organisms. The role of the level A laboratory is shown in Table 36-7.

Burkholderia mallei and Burkholderia pseudomallei

Burkholderia mallei and *Burkholderia pseudomallei* produce glanders and melioidosis, respectively. These diseases are typically found in animals, but they can also infect humans. Both bacteria are weaponized and released into the air. Glanders can be mistaken for smallpox in humans. It incapacitates people and can cause high mortality rates. Because the disease is found in animals, particularly horses, no antibiotics have been approved for use in humans.

Methylene blue or Wright stain of exudates reveals small bacilli with a bipolar safety-pin appearance. Culture, serology, polymerase chain reaction (PCR), and rapid immunoassay tests are used to confirm the diagnosis (Fig. 36-4). Aminoglycosides and macrolides can be used to treat infections. There is no vaccine for these bacteria.

Yersinia pestis

Yersinia pestis causes pneumonic and bubonic plague. Pneumonic plague can be transmitted from person to person. A presumptive diagnosis is made from a Gram stain showing gram-negative coccobacilli in sputum (Fig. 36-5). Definitive diagnosis requires identifying the bacterial from a culture.

Streptomycin or gentamicin is used to treat the infection. No vaccine is available. The role of the level A laboratory is shown in Table 36-8.

Coxiella burnetii

Coxiella burnetii causes Q fever, which is not a clinically distinctive disease. Because it is rare in humans, a high

TABLE 36-6	*Bacillus anthracis:* Level A Laboratory Role
Presumptively identify based on criteria below, and then submit culture to a level B or C laboratory for final identification.	
Direct smears	Samples such as blood, CSF, and skin (eschar) show encapsulated gram-positive rods, single or in chains. Spores usually are not seen.
Culture smears	Large gram-positive bacilli (1-1.5 × 3-5 µm) may be gram-variable after 72 hours. Spores can be found in culture, especially under non-CO_2 atmosphere but are not swollen and are terminal or subterminal.
Colonies on sheep blood agar plates	Rapidly growing 2-5 mm (overnight at 35° C), nonhemolytic, nonpigmented, dry ground-glass surface colonies with irregular edges have comma-shaped projections (i.e., Medusa head). The colony has a sticky (tenacious) consistency when teased with a loop.
Other criteria	Nonmotile, catalase-positive, urease-negative, nitrate-positive, encapsulated bacillus can be lysed by gamma phage; gamma phage typing is usually performed by a level B or C laboratory.

From McPherson RA, Pincus MR: *Henry's Clinical Diagnosis and Management by Laboratory Methods.* 22nd ed. Philadelphia: Saunders; 2012.
CO_2, Carbon dioxide; *CSF,* cerebrospinal fluid

degree of suspicion is needed to make the diagnosis. Diagnosis is usually made with indirect fluorescent antibody, enzyme-linked immunosorbent assay (ELISA), or PCR testing.

The organism is treated with tetracycline or doxycycline. No vaccine is available.

Francisella tularensis

Francisella tularensis causes tularemia, which is often thought of as a disease transmitted by rabbits. The physical findings are nonspecific. Diagnosis is usually established retrospectively by serology tests (Fig. 36-6).

The bacterium can be treated with streptomycin or gentamicin. A vaccine is available. The role of the level A laboratory is shown in Table 36-9.

Smallpox

Smallpox was declared eradicated from the world by the World Health Organization in 1979. There are still four known sets of living cultures in the world. They have not been destroyed so the organism can be further studied in case it is used as a biological warfare agent.

The viral disease is characterized by many pustular vesicles all over the body. PCR is able to differentiate smallpox from vaccinia, monkeypox, or cowpox (Fig. 36-7). Only supportive treatment is available for smallpox, and there is a vaccine for this disease. The role of the level A laboratory is shown in Table 36-10.

Venezuelan Equine Encephalitis

Venezuelan equine encephalitis (VEE) is a zoonosis with nonspecific physical findings. The disease manifests with

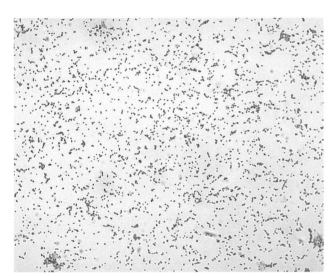

• **Figure 36-3** Gram stain of *Brucella* species. (Courtesy Public Health Image Library, Centers for Disease Control and Prevention, Atlanta, GA, and Larry Stauffer, Oregon State Public Health Laboratory, Hillsboro, OR.)

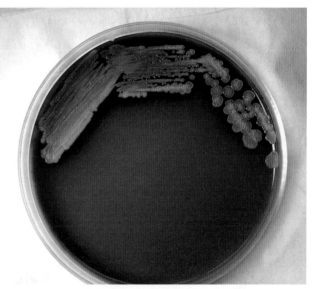

• **Figure 36-4** Colony of gram-negative *Burkholderia pseudomallei*. Bacteria were grown on a medium of chocolate agar for a 72 hours at 37° C. *B. pseudomallei* cause melioidosis. (Courtesy Todd Parker, PhD, and Audra Marsh, Public Health Image Library, Centers for Disease Control and Prevention, Atlanta, GA.)

TABLE 36-7	*Brucella* Species: Level A Laboratory Role
	Presumptively identify based on criteria below, and then submit culture to a level B or C laboratory for final identification and/or confirmation, although most level A laboratories can identify *Brucella*.
Direct smears	Blood and/or bone marrow most often submitted. *Brucella* appears as faintly staining, small, gram-negative coccobacilli (0.5-0.7 × 0.6-1.5 μm), mostly seen as single cells appearing like fine sand.
Culture smears	Similar to above.
Colonies on sheep blood (SBA) and chocolate (CA) agars	Usually not visible or are pinpoint at 24 hours; at 48 hours, colonies are tiny, nonpigmented, and smooth with an entire edge and are nonhemolytic on SBA. Growth of some strains is enhanced by carbon dioxide tension. Some strains grow on MacConkey agar; Thayer-Martin agar can be used as a selective medium. Blood cultures are held for 21 days for suspect cases.
Other criteria	The coccobacilli are catalase, urease, and oxidase positive (*B. canis* varies). They are nonmotile and do not require X and V factors. Brucellosis is one of the most commonly reported laboratory-acquired infections. Automated systems are not useful and not recommended for identification. Sniffing culture plates of *Brucella* can result in infection.

From McPherson RA, Pincus MR: *Henry's Clinical Diagnosis and Management by Laboratory Methods*. 22nd ed. Philadelphia: Saunders; 2012.

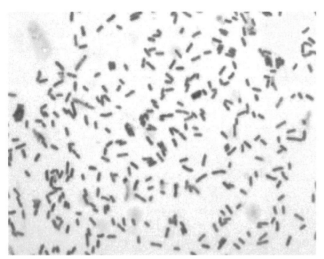

• **Figure 36-5** *Yersinia pestis* is a gram-negative bacillus (×1000). (Courtesy Public Health Image Library, Centers for Disease Control and Prevention, Atlanta, GA, and Larry Stauffer, Oregon State Public Health Laboratory, Hillsboro, OR.)

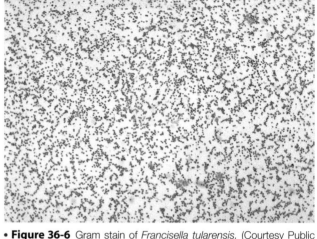

• **Figure 36-6** Gram stain of *Francisella tularensis*. (Courtesy Public Health Image Library, Centers for Disease Control and Prevention, Atlanta, GA, and Larry Stauffer, Oregon State Public Health Laboratory, Hillsboro, OR.)

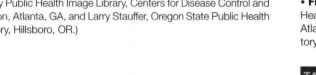

TABLE 36-8 *Yersinia pestis:* **Level A Laboratory Role**

Presumptively identify based on criteria below, and then submit culture to a level B or C laboratory for final identification.

Direct smears	More likely to see bipolar staining (safety pin) from clinical specimens (e.g., blood, sputum, aspirates) than from cultures. Bipolarity is better seen using Wayson or Wright-Giemsa stain. Bipolar staining is not always observed and is not unique to *Y. pestis*.
Culture smear	Plump gram-negative rods (1-2 × 0.5 μm), single or in short chains
Colonies on sheep blood agar plates	Grow at 35° C (faster at room temperature) as gray-white, nonhemolytic, translucent, pinpoint colonies at 24 hours, but by 48 hours, colonies are 1-2 mm in diameter, becoming yellowish with age. Growth occurs with or without carbon dioxide. Colonies can appear as fried egg or with hammered copper shiny surface. On MacConkey agar, grow as pinpoint, non–lactose-fermenting colonies after 24 hours; slightly larger at 48 hours.
Other criteria	The bacterium is nonmotile at 35° to 37° C and at room temperature (*Y. pestis* is the only *Yersinia* species that is nonmotile at room temperature). It is oxidase and urease negative and catalase positive. Growth in broth is flocculent and is described as stalactite; clumps seen at side and bottom of tube.

From McPherson RA, Pincus MR: *Henry's Clinical Diagnosis and Management by Laboratory Methods*. 22nd ed. Philadelphia: Saunders; 2012.

TABLE 36-9 *Francisella tularensis:* **Level A Laboratory Role**

Presumptively identify based on criteria below, and then submit culture to a level B or C laboratory for final identification.

Direct smears	Gram stain of blood, biopsy material, scrapings, or aspirates may be difficult to interpret because bacteria are tiny, pleomorphic, poorly staining, gram-negative coccobacilli seen mostly as single cells.
Culture smear	Very tiny (0.2-0.5 × 0.7-1.0 μm), poorly staining, pleomorphic, gram-negative coccobacilli. They are smaller than *Haemophilus influenzae* and *Brucella* spp. Their minuscule size should raise awareness.
Colonies on sheep blood agar (SBA), chocolate (CA), and blood cysteine (BCA) agars	Grow poorly and slowly on SBA as 1-2 mm, gray-white, nonhemolytic colonies after 48-72 hours. On CA and BCA, colonies are slightly larger, 1-3 mm, gray-white to bluish-gray, with an entire edge and smooth flat surface. Colonies do not subculture well to SBA (viability is usually lost). Subcultures should be made onto CA, BCA, or Thayer-Martin agar. Carbon dioxide is not required for growth. No growth occurs on MacConkey agar or eosin methylene blue agar.
Other criteria	*F. tularensis* is nonmotile and oxidase and urease negative; catalase results can be weakly positive or negative. X and V factors are not required. Slow growth in thioglycollate broth with a dense band near the top, which diffuses downward with time.

From McPherson RA, Pincus MR: *Henry's Clinical Diagnosis and Management by Laboratory Methods*. 22nd ed. Philadelphia: Saunders; 2012.

leukopenia and lymphopenia. Recent infection is indicated by paired sera with immunoglobulin G (IgG) for VEE or a single specimen with VEE-specific immunoglobulin M (IgM). No human-to-human or horse-to-human transmission has occurred.

PCR is used to confirm a VEE diagnosis (Fig. 36-8). Patients have an increased cerebrospinal fluid (CSF) pressure and up to 1000/mm^3 white blood cells and mild protein levels in their CSF. A vaccine is available for VEE. The role of the level A laboratory is shown in Table 36-11.

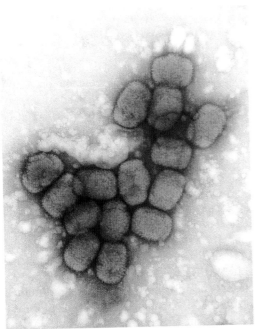

• **Figure 36-7** Transmission electron micrograph of smallpox virus using a negative staining technique. (Courtesy Dr. Fred Murphy, Public Health Image Library, Centers for Disease Control and Prevention, Atlanta, GA.)

Viral Hemorrhagic Fevers

More than one type of virus causes viral hemorrhagic fevers: Lassa fever, Argentine hemorrhagic fever, Bolivian hemorrhagic fever, Venezuelan hemorrhagic fever, Congo-Crimean hemorrhagic fever, Rift Valley fever, Ebola, Marburg, dengue, and yellow fever. The Junin virus causes Argentine hemorrhagic fever, the Machupo virus causes Bolivian hemorrhagic fever, the Sabia virus causes Venezuelan hemorrhagic fever, the Ebola virus causes Ebola (Fig. 36-9), the Marburg virus causes Marburg (Fig. 36-10), Lassa virus causes Lassa fever (Fig. 36-11), Hantaan viruses cause Congo-Crimean hemorrhagic fever and Rift Valley fever, and Flaviviridae viruses cause dengue and yellow fever. Some of these diseases are naturally spread through vectors such as mosquitos, but all can be transmitted through aerosols (Table 36-12).

The hemorrhagic characteristic of the diseases usually results from disseminated intravascular coagulation. Patients with hemorrhagic fevers (except Lassa) have thrombocytopenia, leukopenia, hematuria, and proteinuria. Lassa fever manifests with a high aspartate aminotransferase level.

There are no FDA-approved vaccines for these viruses. The role of the level A laboratory is shown in Table 36-13.

Biological Toxins

Biological toxins are poisonous substances produced by living organisms. They can be distinguished from chemical weapons because they are naturally occurring, nonvolatile, more toxic (by weight), and do not harm the skin (Table 36-14). Toxins are ideally suited for use as biological weapons if they are extremely toxic, stable, and easy to produce.

Even though terrorists are not opposed to killing people, incapacitating people can also meet their goals. Using biological toxins can lead to the medical infrastructure being overwhelmed if large numbers of ill people seek medical attention. This scenario can create panic and social disruption. According to the Department of Defense, the most likely toxins to be used as biological weapons are botulinum, ricin, staphylococcal enterotoxin B, and trichothecene (T-2) mycotoxins.

TABLE 36-10	**Smallpox: Level A Laboratory Role**			
Smallpox is highest-level emergency; submit specimens immediately to public health laboratory. Virus is highly infectious; avoid manipulation; if necessary use biological safety level 3 practices. Responsibility of level A laboratories is limited to advising medical staff on specimen selection, packing and shipping sample, and communicating with reference laboratory. Level A laboratories should not culture, sample, or perform assays on specimens suspected of containing the virus. Clinical diagnosis is confirmed by level D laboratory techniques.				
Specimen	**Technique**		**Transport**	**Storage**
Biopsy	Aseptically place two to four portions of tissue into sterile, leakproof, freezable containers.		≤6 hr at 4° C	−20° to −70° C
Scabs	Aseptically place scrapings/material into sterile, leakproof freezable container.		≤6 hr at 4° C	−20° to −70° C
Vesicular fluid	Collect fluid from separate lesions onto separate sterile swabs. Always include material from base of each vesicle.		≤6 hr at 4° C	−20° to −70° C

From McPherson RA, Pincus MR: *Henry's Clinical Diagnosis and Management by Laboratory Methods.* 22nd ed. Philadelphia: Saunders; 2012.

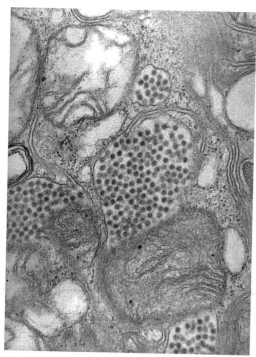

• **Figure 36-8** Electron micrograph of the Eastern equine encephalitis virus, an alphavirus, in a mosquito salivary gland. (Courtesy Dr. Fred Murphy and Sylvia Whitfield, Public Health Image Library, Centers for Disease Control and Prevention, Atlanta, GA.)

TABLE 36-11	Venezuelan Equine Encephalitis or Other Encephalitides: Level A Laboratory Role

Submit samples immediately to public health laboratory for evaluation and referral. Level A laboratory responsibility is limited to advising medical staff on specimen selection, packing and shipping sample, and communicating with reference laboratory.

Specimen	Use	Transport	Storage
Serum	For culture, PCR, or serologies (e.g., ELISA, FA)	<6 hr at 4° C	−20° to −70° C
CSF	For culture, PCR. or serologies	<6 hr at 4° C	−20° to −70° C
Nasal, respiratory (including induced samples)	For culture and PCR	<6 hr at 4° C	−20° to −70° C
Biopsy, autopsy, stool, other	For pathology, culture, hematology/chemistry analysis, other	<6 hr at 4° C	−20° to −70° C

From McPherson RA, Pincus MR: *Henry's Clinical Diagnosis and Management by Laboratory Methods.* 22nd ed. Philadelphia: Saunders; 2012.
CSF, Cerebrospinal fluid; *ELISA,* enzyme-linked immunosorbent assay; *FA,* fluorescent antibody (direct); *PCR,* polymerase chain reaction.

Ricin

Ricin, also called **abrin,** is a biological toxin made from castor beans. The toxin inhibits protein synthesis in the body. If ricin is ingested, profuse vomiting and diarrhea result, followed by multisystem failure and possible death within 36 to 72 hours. If ricin is inhaled, dyspnea, fever, and cough result, followed by pulmonary edema, hypotension, respiratory failure, and possible death within 36 to 72 hours. Inhalation of ricin causes symptoms that progress faster to severe symptoms than ingestion of ricin.

General laboratory results reveal metabolic acidosis, increased liver and renal function test results, hematuria, and leukocytosis (i.e., 2.5 times greater than normal). Ricin poisoning must be differentiated from staphylococcal enterotoxin B, ozone inhalation, enteric pathogens, mushrooms, caustics, or arsenic (see Table 36-14).

Brevetoxin

Brevetoxin is produced by a microscopic organism called *Karenia brevis.* It is a neurotoxin that binds to nerve cells and disrupts the normal neurologic processes in the body. In nature, the toxin is responsible for the neurotoxic shellfish poisoning that accompanies red tides.

When this agent is transmitted through oral ingestion, symptoms appear in 15 minutes to 18 hours. Gastrointestinal symptoms include abdominal pain, vomiting, and diarrhea, and neurologic symptoms include paresthesias, vertigo, ataxia, and reversal of hot and cold temperature sensations. If the toxin is transmitted through inhalation, symptoms include cough, dyspnea, and bronchospasm (see Table 36-14).

There are no U.S. Food and Drug Administration (FDA)–approved laboratory methods to confirm the diagnosis. However, an experimental ELISA test can detect brevetoxin in biological samples.

Saxitoxin

Saxitoxin is a neurotoxin produced by dinoflagellates of the genus *Gonyaulax.* This toxin is also produced by the blue ring octopus.

The toxin binds to sodium channels in nerve membranes, blocking transmission of nerve signals to muscles. It produces paralytic shellfish poisoning syndrome, which is a life-threatening illness. The onset of symptoms is usually quick (10 to 60 minutes) but depends on many factors (e.g., amount of toxin ingested). Symptoms include numbness or tingling in lips, tongue, and fingertips. Next, the neck and extremities become numb, accompanied by lack of coordination when moving. Other symptoms experienced by patients include lightheadedness, dizziness, weakness, aphasia, incoherence, memory loss, eyesight problems, and headaches. Often, cranial nerves are involved by paralysis.

Similar to other neurotoxins, fatalities result from respiratory failure, which can occur 2 to 12 hours after ingesting the toxins. No antidote or rapid diagnostic tests are available for this toxin (see Table 36-14).

Staphylococcal Enterotoxin B

Staphylococcal enterotoxin B (SEB) is one of many toxins produced by *Staphylococcus aureus*. The toxin is a cytotoxic toxin, meaning that it is toxic to cells. It is the primary cause of staphylococcal food poisoning. It is a stable toxin that requires small amounts to produce symptoms in victims.

The most effective route to release this agent as a biological weapon is an aerosol, enabling the toxin to be inhaled rather than ingested. After inhalation, symptoms

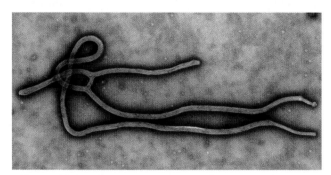

• **Figure 36-9** Colorized electron micrograph of the Ebola virus. (Courtesy Cynthia Goldsmith, Public Health Image Library, Centers for Disease Control and Prevention, Atlanta, GA.)

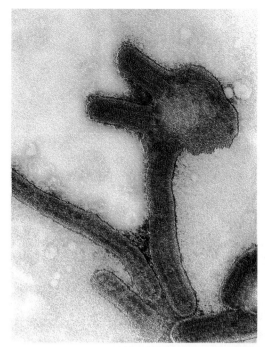

• **Figure 36-10** Colorized electron micrograph of the Marburg virus. (Courtesy Dr. Fred Murphy, Public Health Image Library, Centers for Disease Control and Prevention, Atlanta, GA.)

TABLE 36-12	Viral Hemorrhagic Fever Means of Transmission	
Viral Hemorrhagic Fever Agent	**Natural Means of Transmission**	
Ebola	Contact	
Marburg	Contact	
Lassa fever	Contact	
Argentine (Junin)	Contact and aerosol	
Bolivian (Machupo)	Contact and aerosol	
Crimean-Congo	Ticks and contact	
Hantavirus	Contact and aerosol	
Rift Valley fever	Mosquito and aerosol	
Dengue	Mosquito	
Yellow fever	Mosquito	

From McPherson RA, Pincus MR: *Henry's Clinical Diagnosis and Management by Laboratory Methods*. 22nd ed. Philadelphia: Saunders; 2012.

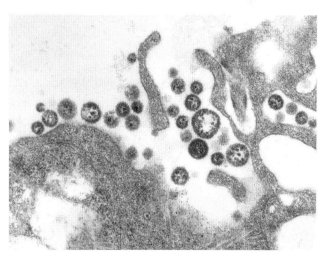

• **Figure 36-11** Transmission electron micrograph depicts Lassa virus virions adjacent to some cell debris. A member of the Arenaviridae family, the single-stranded RNA virus is a zoonotic (animal-borne) virus that can be transmitted to humans. (Courtesy C.S. Goldsmith, P. Rollin, and M. Bowen, Public Health Image Library, Centers for Disease Control and Prevention, Atlanta, GA.)

TABLE 36-13	Crimean-Congo and Other Hemorrhagic Fevers: Level A Laboratory Role		
Submit samples immediately to public health laboratory for evaluation and referral. Some viruses are highly infectious; avoid manipulation; if necessary, use biological safety level 3 practices. Level A laboratory responsibility is limited to advising medical staff on specimen selection, packing and shipping sample, and communicating with reference laboratory.			
Specimen	**Use**	**Transport**	**Storage**
Serum	For culture, PCR, or serologies (e.g., ELISA, HI, FA)	<6 hr at 4° C	−20° to −70° C
Biopsy, autopsy, stool, other	For pathology, culture, hematology/chemistry analysis, other	<6 hr at 4° C	−20° to −70° C

From McPherson RA, Pincus MR: *Henry's Clinical Diagnosis and Management by Laboratory Methods*. 22nd ed. Philadelphia: Saunders; 2012.
ELISA, Enzyme-linked immunosorbent assay; *FA,* fluorescent antibody (direct); *HI,* hemagglutination inhibition; *PCR,* polymerase chain reaction.

appear 1 to 6 hours later. Symptoms are vague and include fever, chills, headache, myalgia, and nonproductive cough. The fever can reach 102° to 106° F for 2 to 5 days. The cough may continue for 1 to 4 weeks. Victims have more severe symptoms from the toxin released as an aerosol than by ingesting it. However, the fatality rate is still less than 2%.

Staphylococcal enterotoxin B can produce severe symptoms in very small amounts, and contamination of food or water supplies would be difficult to detect. It can be identified using an ELISA test specific for the toxin (see Table 36-14).

Strychnine

Strychnine is naturally produced by the plant *Strychnos nux-vomica*, which is found in India, Sri Lanka, East Indies, and Australia. Strychnine is a strong poison that occurs as a white, odorless, bitter powder that can be administered through the gastrointestinal tract, respiratory tract, or venous tract.

Exposure to small amounts of this poison can cause severe adverse health effects or death. In the past, the toxin was used to treat human diseases, but it is now used as a pesticide and rat poison. The toxin competes with nerve inhibitors to produce an excitatory state in muscles. The muscles tire rapidly and fail.

Although strychnine is rapidly excreted in urine, no diagnostic tests are run because the only medical treatment available for victims of strychnine poisoning is supportive, such as administering intravenous fluid, performing gastric lavage, and providing painkillers for painful convulsions. Laboratory diagnosis is accomplished on urine or

TABLE 36-14	Biological Toxins, Their Actions, and Laboratory Support		
Biological Toxin	**Description**	**Health Effects**	**Laboratory Support**
Abrin or ricin	Biological toxin from castor beans	Inhibits protein synthesis; profuse vomiting and diarrhea leading to multisystem failure	Laboratory results reveal metabolic acidosis, increased liver function tests, increased BUN and creatinine levels; hematuria; and leukocytosis
Botulinum	Neurotoxin produced by *Clostridium botulinum* and considered the most lethal substance in the world	Progressive flaccid paralysis, moves to heart and diaphragm; person can die of asphyxiation	Specialized test available but can take days before the results are available
Brevetoxin	Neurotoxin produced by *Karenia brevis* (i.e., paralytic shellfish poisoning)	Abdominal pain, vomiting, diarrhea, paresthesias, vertigo, ataxia, reversal of hot and cold sensations	No FDA-approved tests to detect this toxin but experimental ELISA test is available
Saxitoxin	Neurotoxin produced by dinoflagellates and the blue ring octopus	Results in paralytic shellfish poisoning	Laboratory tests not useful in diagnosis but may be used to rule out other conditions
Staphylococcal enterotoxin B	Cytotoxin produced by *Staphylococcus*	Gastric symptoms (e.g., food poisoning), inhalation symptoms (e.g., fever, chills, headache, myalgia, non-productive cough)	Toxin can be identified using an existing ELISA test
Strychnine	Poison produced by the plant *Strychnos nux*-vomica	Toxin competes with nerve inhibitors to produce excitatory state in muscles, which tire rapidly and fail	Laboratory diagnosis using urine or gastric aspirations in a qualitative thin layer chromatography test
Tetrodotoxin	Neurotoxin secreted by pufferfish, porcupine fish, ocean sunfish, triggerfish, and blue ringed octopus	Gradual onset paralysis, starting with face and extremities, then headaches, epigastric pain, nausea, vomiting, then paralysis, accompanied by convulsions and cardiac arrhythmias	Existing ELISA test can detect toxin, but it is not FDA approved
Trichothecene mycotoxin	Toxins produced by *Fusarium, Myrothecium, Trichoderma, Acremonium (Cephalosporium), Verticimonosporium,* and *Stachybotrys* fungi	Inhibits protein synthesis in cells; causes eye pain, burning skin, weakness, dizziness, loss of coordination, tachycardia, hypothermia, hypotension, death	There is an extraction test which is performed on urine specimens available to detect this toxin

BUN, Blood urea nitrogen; *ELISA,* enzyme-linked immunosorbent assay; *FDA,* U.S. Food and Drug Administration.

gastric aspirates using a qualitative thin-layer chromatography test (see Table 36-14).

Tetrodotoxin

Tetrodotoxin is secreted by pufferfish, porcupinefish, ocean sunfish, triggerfish, certain bacterial species, and the blue-ringed octopus. This toxin is one of the oldest and strongest neurotoxins known. It is linked to severe adverse health effects and death.

After ingesting the toxin, slight numbness of the lips and tongue appear in 20 minutes to 3 hours, depending on the amount of toxin ingested. Next, the victim experiences increasing paraesthesia in the face and extremities, followed by a floating feeling. Soon, the victim experiences headache, epigastric pain, nausea, diarrhea, and vomiting. Increasing paralysis begins to set in after sufficient motor nerves are affected by the toxin. Victims may no longer be able to sit, and they experience increasing dyspnea and hypotension. Paralysis increases and is accompanied by convulsions and cardiac arrhythmias. The victim can become completely paralyzed but remain conscious and lucid until death occurs. From first symptoms to death can take 20 minutes to 8 hours.

An experimental diagnostic assay is available for research, but it is not FDA approved or commercially available (see Table 36-14).

Botulinum

Botulinum toxins are neurotoxins produced by the anaerobic bacterium *Clostridium botulinum.* The bacteria grow and multiply, producing toxin in the process. Botulinum toxins are considered the most lethal toxin substances in the world when ingested. Sixty percent of individuals who are untreated after ingestion of this toxin die.

Symptoms usually appear within 24 hours after ingestion. The toxin blocks acetylcholine release at the presynaptic muscular junctions of motor nerves. The resulting flaccid paralysis is progressive. It begins with drooping eyelids, dry mouth and throat, difficulty swallowing, and blurred vision. It progressively moves from the throat to the chest and extremities. When the diaphragm and chest muscles are affected, the person can die of asphyxiation unless placed on respiratory support (see Table 36-14).

Specialized laboratory tests can determine the botulinum toxin, but they can take days before results are available to clinicians. Clinical diagnosis is essential for early diagnosis and treatment. The role of the level A laboratory is shown in Table 36-15.

Trichothecene Mycotoxins

Trichothecene mycotoxins are biological poisons produced by fungi called molds: *Fusarium, Myrothecium, Trichoderma, Cephalosporium, Verticimonosporium,* and *Stachybotrys.* Trichothecene (T-2) mycotoxins were implicated in Soviet attacks from 1974 to 1981 in Laos, Cambodia, and Afghanistan. The Soviets produced aerosol and droplet clouds to deliver the toxins over a large area. The attacks in Laos were called *yellow rain* by the locals.

The toxins inhibit protein synthesis in cells. They also inhibit electron transport in the mitochondria. The toxins can enter the body through skin and epithelium in the mouth, throat, lungs, and gastrointestinal system. They are not very effective when delivered through the respiratory route. They are most effective when delivered through the skin. Symptoms start in minutes but can take up to hours:

- Eyes: eye pain, excessive, tearing, visual blurring, and scleral injections
- Respiratory tract: nasal itching and pain, epistaxis, runny nose, cough, difficulty breathing, and wheezing
- Integumentary system: burning skin, redness, blistering progressing to necrosis and skin sloughing
- Early systemic effects: weakness, loss of coordination, dizziness, ataxia, tachycardia, hypothermia, hypotension, death

TABLE 36-15	Botulinum Toxin Exposure: Level A Laboratory Role	
Submit specimens immediately to public health laboratory for evaluation and referral, even if criminal activity is not suspected. Level A laboratories should not manipulate specimens, culture, identify, or perform toxin assays. Level A laboratory responsibility* is limited to advising the medical staff on specimen selection, packing, shipping, and notifying the recipient laboratory about specimens from a suspected case.		
Specimen	Technique	Transport
Suspect food samples	Submit 25-50 g of food in original containers that have been placed in a leakproof sealed system.	4° C
Nasal swabs	If aerosolized release is suspected, collect nasal swabs for toxin testing and/or polymerase chain reaction analysis.	Room temperature
Stool, enema fluid	Collect 25-50 g of stool in sterile, leakproof containers.	4° C
Serum	Collect approximately 10 mL for serologic assays.	4° C
Other	Collect environmental and/or other samples on swabs.	4° C

From McPherson RA, Pincus MR: *Henry's Clinical Diagnosis and Management by Laboratory Methods.* 22nd ed. Philadelphia: Saunders; 2012.
*Level A laboratory responsibilities for other suspected toxins such as staphylococcal toxins, mycotoxin, saxitoxin, and ricin are similar.

- Late systemic effects (2 to 8 weeks after exposure): bone marrow suppression (i.e., severe neutropenia), hemorrhagic syndromes (i.e., petechiae, melena, hematuria, hematemesis, epistaxis, and vaginal bleeding), oral and gastrointestinal ulcers, and secondary sepsis.

Laboratory diagnosis involves a very complicated extraction test performed on urine specimens. No rapid diagnostic tests are available for these toxins (see Table 36-14).

Nuclear and Radiation Threats

In addition to chemical and biological threats, terrorists can employ unconventional tactics and weapons, including nuclear and radiologic threats. Possible scenarios include contamination of food or water with radioactive materials, radioactive materials placed in a public venue, dirty bombs (i.e., bombs that explode and introduce radioactive material over an area), and attacking nuclear power plants.

Radiation is colorless and odorless and comes in two forms that cause damage to humans: beta and gamma. Gamma radiation is the most destructive type of radiation because it is made up of energy rays that can penetrate walls, windows, and bodies. In an attack, people can be exposed to or contaminated with radiation. Exposure means that a person is irradiated by a high dose of gamma rays (i.e., penetrating radiation) in a short period of time (i.e., acute radiation syndrome).

Radiation exposure must be quickly and accurately assessed to ensure proper medical treatment (Table 36-16). There are four stages of the acute radiation syndrome:

1. Prodromal stage: symptoms include nausea, vomiting, anorexia, and diarrhea minutes to days after exposure
2. Latent stage: victim feels healthy for a few hours or up to a few weeks
3. Manifest illness stage: occurs in three forms
   - Bone marrow syndrome, in which bone marrow is destroyed and the patient dies of infection and hemorrhage
   - Gastrointestinal syndrome, in which irreparable changes in the gastrointestinal tract lead to dehydration and electrolyte imbalance
   - Cardiovascular and central nervous system syndrome, in which death occurs in 3 days due to circulatory system collapse and increased intracranial pressure
4. Recovery or death

A victim exposed to beta radiation or x-rays may develop cutaneous radiation syndrome. The basal cell layer of the skin that is exposed to radiation is damaged, resulting in inflammation, erythema, and dry or moist desquamation. Weeks later, intense reddening, blistering, and ulceration or necrosis of outer skin layers occurs. Most skin damage repairs itself naturally; however, large doses of radiation to the skin can lead to permanent damage of sebaceous and sweat glands, skin pigmentation, and atrophy.

Although devices such as a Geiger counter are available to assess the amount of radiation in the environment, assessing the radiation dose to an individual is difficult. Exposure is usually assessed using clinical signs and symptoms, but laboratory tests can help. Complete blood counts, with special attention to the lymphocyte counts, can help clinicians determine the extent of cellular damage due to gamma radiation (see Table 36-16).

Laboratory Response Network

History and Mission

The Laboratory Response Network (LRN) was created in 1999 by the CDC. It is a network of 150 laboratories that quickly respond to biological and chemical emergencies and to other public health emergencies. Federal, state, and local public health, veterinary, military, and international laboratories participate in the LRN (Table 36-17).

The LRN is composed of many laboratories working at different levels to respond to chemical and biological threats. For a laboratory to be included in the network, it must demonstrate specific capabilities and capacities to the CDC and meet agent-specific performance standards. Laboratories meeting these criteria must also be invited to participate by a state laboratory director. For continued inclusion in this network, laboratories must pass routine proficiency tests related to specific agents to prove continued competence.

The LRN is a CDC program funded by the federal government. LRN laboratories receive federal funds through a governmental cooperative agreement for laboratory positions, renovations, and state-of-the-art technology. The funds are distributed to the states, which then decide how to distribute the money to LRN laboratories.

Response to Biological and Chemical Emergencies

Bioterrorism

After a bioterrorism incident, the first laboratory to learn of the attack and collect patient specimens for testing is the sentinel laboratory (Fig. 36-12). Sentinel laboratories are the hospital laboratories on the front lines. Sentinel laboratories are closest to the patient and are responsible for wreferring suspicious specimens to the next level, called a reference laboratory. Reference laboratories perform tests to detect and confirm suspicious microbes. The laboratories perform confirmed testing instead of relying on the CDC, which allows local authorities to make decisions quickly. The third type of laboratory involved in the LRN response is the national laboratory. The national laboratories have unique resources for handling highly infectious agents. These laboratories can also identify specific microbe strains.

Complex laboratory instruments are necessary for a laboratory to perform confirmatory testing of chemical agents. On-site operation training is set up for laboratory personnel by the vendor as part of the purchase package. The CDC also provides hands-on training and computer-based training for level 1 and 2 laboratories on analytical methods. This type of instrumentation requires rigorous proficiency testing and quality assurance to guarantee precise,

TABLE 36-16   Acute Radiation Syndrome

Phase of Syndrome	Feature	Effects of Whole-Body, Irradiation, From External Radiation or Inter Absorption, by Dose Range in rad (1 rad = 1cGy; 100 = 1 Gy)					
		0-100	100-200	200-600	600-800	800-3000	>3000
Prodromal	Nausea, vomiting	None	5-50%	50-100%	75-100%	90-100%	100%
	Time of onset		3-6 hr	2-4 hr	1-2 hr	<1 hr	Minutes
	Duration		<24 hr	<24 hr	<48 hr	<48 hr	NA
	Lymphocyte count	Unaffected	Minimally decreased	<1000 at 24 hr	<500 at 24 hr	Decreases within hours	Decreases within hours
	CNS function	No impairment	No impairment	Routine task performance Cognitive impairment for 6-20 hr	Simple, routine task performance Cognitive impairment for >24 hr	Rapid incapacitation May have a lucid interval of several hours	
Latent	No symptoms	>2 wk	7-15 days	0-7 days	0-2 days	None	None
Manifest illness	Signs, symptoms	None	Moderate leukopenia	Severe leukopenia, purpura, hemorrhage, pneumonia, hair loss after 300 rad		Diarrhea, fever, electrolyte disturbance	Convulsions, ataxia, tremor, lethargy
	Time of onset		>2 wk	2 days-2 wk		1-3 days	1-48 hr
	Critical period		None	4-6 wk; greatest potential for effective medical intervention		2-14 days	
	Organ system	None		Hematopoietic, respiratory (mucosal) systems		GI tract Mucosal systems	CNS
	Hospitalization	0%	<5%	90%	100%	100%	100%
	duration	None	45-60 days	60-90 days	90+ days	Weeks to months	Days to weeks
	Mortality	None	Minimal	Low with aggressive therapy	High	Very high; significant neurologic symptoms indicate lethal dose	

CNS, Central nervous system; NA, not applicable.
*1 gray (Gy) = 100 rads; 1 centigray (cGy) = 1 rad.
From Military Medical Operations. *Medical Management of Radiological Casualties Handbook.* 2nd ed. Bethesda, MD: Armed Forces Radiobiology Research Institute; April 2003.

TABLE 36-17 Types of Laboratories

Laboratory Type	Designated Laboratories
Federal	CDC, USDA, FDA, others
State and local public health	Located in state and local areas, they test for category A biological agents, and some test for toxic chemical exposures
Military	Department of Defense laboratories, including the Naval Medical Research Center in Bethesda, MD
Food testing	FDA, USDA
Environmental	Test water and environmental samples
Veterinary	USDA laboratories that are part of the LRN perform tests on animals to look for biological and chemical threats
International	These LRN laboratories are located in Canada, United Kingdom, and Australia

CDC, Centers for Disease Control and Prevention; *FDA,* U.S. Food and Drug Administration; *LRN,* Laboratory Response Network; *USDA,* U.S. Department of Agriculture.

accurate, high-quality data. These laboratories can elect to send an individual (usually the chemical terrorism coordinator) to the CDC's Train the Trainer class; the individual then trains hospital staff and partners' staff in their area.

Chemical Emergencies

Different laboratories have different structures for responding to a chemical emergency (Fig. 36-13). As of 2010, 53 laboratories could provide a response to a chemical emergency.

Three levels of laboratories are involved in the LRN chemical emergency response. Level 3 laboratories are the lowest level of response, and all of the 53 laboratories in the LRN have level 3 capacity. Level 3 laboratories work with hospitals and first responders to ensure the quality of clinical specimen collection, storage, and shipment. The 34 level 2 laboratories in the LRN employ chemists trained to detect agents such as cyanide, nerve agents, and toxic metals. The 10 level 1 laboratories in the LRN are top-level laboratories that aid the CDC in a response. These laboratories have high-throughput analysis capabilities and can detect exposure to cyanide, nerve agents, toxic metals, mustard agents, and toxic industrial chemicals. These capabilities are vital during a chemical emergency, when hundreds or thousands of people may be exposed to a chemical agent.

LRN laboratories are located all over the world, with the most concentrated and strategically placed laboratories being located in the United States. The map in Figure 36-14 shows the locations of LRN laboratories.

Role of the Laboratory in Chemical Emergencies

Historically, chemical weapons were delivered through overt attacks because the agents were inhaled or absorbed through the skin. Overt attacks initiate an immediate response from first responders. Conversely, biological weapons are usually covertly delivered. Biological agents take time to cause symptoms, allowing more people to become infected with an agent before it is discovered. State and local health agencies must have a system in place to detect chemical and biological attacks. There also must be experts at the state and local levels with resources available to respond to these types of attacks.

Because these types of attacks are out of the ordinary, special training and planning must take place at the local and state

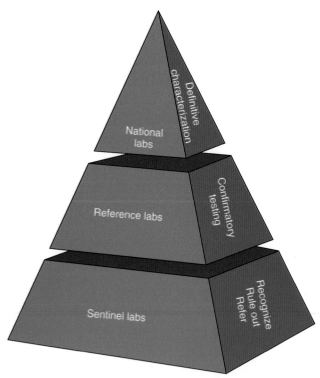

• **Figure 36-12** Structure of the Laboratory Response Network. *labs,* Laboratories. (From Mahon CR, Lehman DC, Manuselis G. *Textbook of Diagnostic Microbiology.* 5th ed. Philadelphia: Saunders; 2015.)

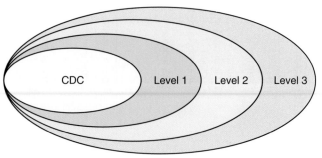

• **Figure 36-13** Laboratory levels in the Laboratory Response Network. *CDC,* Centers for Disease Control and Prevention. (Courtesy Centers for Disease Control and Prevention, Atlanta, GA.)

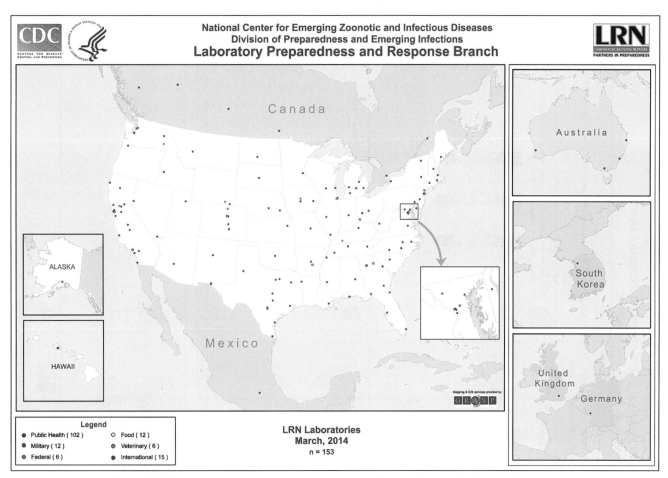

• **Figure 36-14** Laboratory Response Network branches. (Courtesy Centers for Disease Control and Prevention, Atlanta, GA.)

levels to ensure that one attack does not overwhelm the national public health infrastructure. Training in chemical and biological warfare focuses on the most probable agents because preparing for attacks with any possible agent would be impossible.

Good communication between the local health care agencies and state agencies is extremely important. If a local provider recognizes the symptoms of a possible chemical or biological agent, this information needs to be immediately communicated to the local public health system. If the public health system deems it a probable attack, a comprehensive response is initiated. The response involves an investigation to determine the source, medical diagnosis, treatment, and prophylaxis for victims and, if applicable, decontamination of the environment.

Level 3 laboratories are considered local health care facilities. Level 3 laboratories are responsible for early detection. They use clinical diagnosis to determine whether laboratory specimens from the victims need to be transported to a level 2 (i.e., state and local public health) laboratory for further testing. The technicians at the level 3 laboratory are trained in safe collection, packaging, labeling, and shipping of specimens.

Level 2 laboratories (i.e., state and local public health laboratories, academic research centers, federal facilities) receive specimens from the suspected victim and test for specific agents. These laboratories can perform confirmatory tests. If the level 2 laboratory is unable to identify the agent or there is a need for rapid identification, specimens are shipped to a level 1 laboratory.

Level 1 laboratories are specialized federal laboratories with unique experience in identifying exotic poisons. This laboratory is also responsible for developing or evaluating new tests.

Specimen Collection, Packaging, and Shipping

Clinical laboratory scientists and clinical laboratory technicians may be called on to collect, package, and ship specimens from chemical agent victims. Because the chemical agents are poisonous, special collection, handling, packing, and shipping procedures have been developed by CDC to ensure individuals packing and unpacking the specimens are safe. Handling these types of specimens requires a chain of custody to ensure fidelity of the specimens.

Collection

After a chemical event, blood and urine specimens are collected from adults, and urine specimens are collected from pediatric patients (Fig. 36-15). The CDC decides whether blood specimens will be drawn from pediatric patients

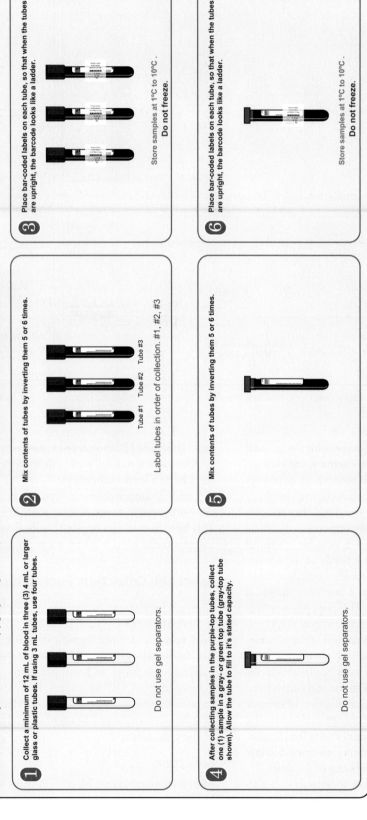

For detailed instructions see CDC's Shipping Instructions for Specimens Collected from People Who May Have Been Exposed to Chemical Agents.

Collect blood and urine samples for each person involved in the chemical exposure event.

Note: For children, collect only urine samples unless otherwise directed by CDC.

Blood-Sample Collection

For each person, collect blood in glass or plastics tubes in the following order: 1st: collect specimens in three (3) EDTA (purple-top) 4 mL or larger plastic or glass tubes; 2nd: collect another specimen in one (1) gray- or green-top tube. Collect the specimens by following the steps below:

1 Collect a minimum of 12 mL of blood in three (3) 4 mL or larger glass or plastic tubes. If using 3 mL tubes, use four tubes.

Do not use gel separators.

2 Mix contents of tubes by inverting them 5 or 6 times.

Tube #1　Tube #2　Tube #3

Label tubes in order of collection: #1, #2, #3

3 Place bar-coded labels on each tube, so that when the tubes are upright, the barcode looks like a ladder.

Store samples at 1°C to 10°C . Do not freeze.

4 After collecting samples in the purple-top tubes, collect one (1) sample in a gray- or green top tube (gray-top tube shown). Allow the tube to fill to it's stated capacity.

Do not use gel separators.

5 Mix contents of tubes by inverting them 5 or 6 times.

6 Place bar-coded labels on each tube, so that when the tubes are upright, the barcode looks like a ladder.

Store samples at 1°C to 10°C . Do not freeze.

Urine-Sample Collection

For each person, collect 40 mL- 60 mL of urine in a screw-cap urine cup.

Label the urine cup with the appropriate bar-coded label as shown. Indicate on the cup how the sample was collected if the method was other than "clean catch" (i.e., catheterization).

Freeze samples (optimally at -70°C).

Place bar-coded labels on all cups so that when the cup is upright, the barcode looks like a ladder.

Department of Health and Human Services
Centers for Disease Controland Prevention

CDC

• **Figure 36-15** Centers for Disease Control and Prevention (CDC) specimen collection protocol for a chemical exposure event. (Courtesy Centers for Disease Control and Prevention, Atlanta, GA.)

01 /2015

The technician collects 12 mL of blood in three 4-mL EDTA tubes or four 3-mL EDTA tubes. Using a permanent ink pen, the order of draw is marked on each tube (e.g., #1, #2) One green- or gray-top tube (at least 3 mL) is collected. For all draws, each vacuum tube is allowed to automatically fill.

Urine specimens (25 to 50 mL) are also needed from victims. Specimens are collected in a screw-capped container and frozen as soon as possible after collection. If specimens are collected through catheterization, collection method must be noted on the container. Two blanks from each lot of specimen containers and purple- and green-top tubes are needed to determine background contamination.

Labeling

All specimens should have labels generated by the responding health care facility. The labels should contain a unique patient identifier, initials of the collecting technician, and the date and time collected. If bar-coded labels are used, the bar codes are placed on the tube so they resemble the steps on a ladder. The submitting facility should keep a list of the names of victims, corresponding unique identifying numbers, date and time of collection, postmortem specimen, potential exposure time, and antidotes administered before collection.

Packaging

Packaging and shipping specimens from a suspected chemical event must follow strict guidelines, which are necessary so that evidence holds up in a court of law. One of the required documents is called a *chain of custody*, which records the names, times, and dates of individuals who handle a specimen. When a specimen is passed on to another individual, the individual must sign the form and indicate the time and date of specimen receipt. Every person who handles the specimen signs the form, including the technician performing the tests. The packages are shipped to the laboratory designated in the state's chemical terrorism response plan.

Summary

The CDC spearheaded the development of the LRN in 1999. The LRN is a network of local, state, and federal laboratories that are capable of responding to biological and chemical terrorist attacks. The most probable chemical agents that would be used in attacks include biotoxins, blister agents, blood agents, caustics, choking or pulmonary agents, incapacitating agents, metals, nerve agents, organic solvents, riot control agents, toxic alcohols, and vomiting agents. There may also be nuclear and radiation threats.

Review Questions

1. A customized emergency preparedness plan includes all the following EXCEPT
   a. Disaster recovery
   b. Hazard identification
   c. Vulnerability assessment
   d. Impact analysis

2. Training for emergency preparedness involves
   a. Vulnerability assessment
   b. Disaster recovery
   c. Protecting the environment
   d. Tabletop exercises

3. Terrorist groups are not opposed to killing people but rely more on
   a. Emotion and social unrest to cause a riot
   b. The resulting chaos and psychological effects to make an impact
   c. Covert release of the weapon to make a statement
   d. Sensationalism and shock to make a lasting impression

4. Which of the following U.S. agencies maintains effective countermeasures against chemical and biological agents?
   a. U.S. Army Medical Countermeasures Agency
   b. Defense Threat Reduction Agency
   c. Department of Defense Counterterrorism Agency
   d. Central Intelligence Agency

5. Which of the following chemical agents contains arsenic, smells like geraniums, and in large doses may be fatal?
   a. Sulfur mustard
   b. Nitrogen mustard
   c. Phosgene oxime
   d. Lewisite

6. Which of the following chemical weapons is delivered through air, food, and water routes and produces an anticholinergic toxidrome?
   a. Fentanyl
   b. Benzene
   c. QNB
   d. Hydrofluoric acid

7. All of the following are nerve agents EXCEPT
   a. Chloropicrin
   b. Sarin
   c. Soman
   d. VX

8. Which of the following biological agents commonly causes woolsorter disease but when released as an aerosol produces severe respiratory disease and death within 36 hours?
   a. *Burkholderia mallei*
   b. *Yersinia pestis*
   c. *Francisella tularensis*
   d. *Brucella anthracis*

9. The Junin, Machupo, Sabia, Lassa, and Marburg viruses are examples of viruses that cause which of the following groups of illnesses?
   a. Respiratory distress syndrome
   b. Viral hemorrhagic fevers
   c. Anticholinergic toxidrome
   d. Paralytic shellfish poisoning

10. Which of the following biological agents is a toxin that can be dispersed through aerosol and droplet clouds, resulting in yellow rain?
   a. T-2 mycotoxins
   b. SEB
   c. Botulinum
   d. Strychnine

Critical Thinking Questions

1. Discuss why a terrorist or a government would want to use chemical agents as an offensive weapon.
2. What is the role of a clinical laboratory in the response to a chemical weapon attack or a chemical emergency at a plant?

3. List the groups and characteristics of chemical agents.

CASE STUDY

A train derails about one-fourth mile from a college campus. The train cars contained hazardous materials. Police and fire fighters came to the campus and urged an evacuation. About 30 minutes after evacuating the campus, many people went to a nearby hospital complaining of red, itchy skin; some had blisters, and some had eye problems. What class of chemical agents most likely caused these symptoms? What other symptoms may be observed when people are exposed to these chemical agents? What types of special precautions must be taken when treating or drawing blood from these patients?

Bibliography

Agency for Toxic Substances and Disease Registry. *Arsine (AsH₃): medical management guidelines.* <http://www.atsdr.cdc.gov/MMG/MMG.asp?id=1199&tid=278> Accessed 07.07.15.

Agency for Toxic Substances and Disease Registry. *Benzene (C₆H₆).* <http://search.cdc.gov/search?utf8=%E2%9C%93&affiliate=cdc-main&sitelimit=www.atsdr.cdc.gov&;query=Benzene+%28C6H6%29&commit=Search> Accessed 07.07.15.

Agency for Toxic Substances and Disease Registry. *Blister agents.* <http://search.cdc.gov/search?query=Blister+Agents&searchButton.x=46&searchButton.y=8&action=search&sitelimit=www.atsdr.cdc.gov&utf8=%E2%9C%93&affiliate=cdc-main> Accessed 07.07.15.

Agency for Toxic Substances and Disease Registry. *Chlorine (Cl₂).* <http://search.cdc.gov/search?utf8=%E2%9C%93&affiliate=cdc-main&sitelimit=www.atsdr.cdc.gov&query=Chlorine+%28Cl2%29&commit=Search> Accessed 07.07.15.

Agency for Toxic Substances and Disease Registry. *Ethylene glycol (C₂H₆O₂).* <http://search.cdc.gov/search?utf8=%E2%9C%93&affiliate=cdc-main&sitelimit=www.atsdr.cdc.gov&query=Ethylene+Gglycol+%28C2H6O2%29&commit=Search> Accessed 09.07.15.

Agency for Toxic Substances and Disease Registry. *Nerve agents.* <http://search.cdc.gov/search?utf8=%E2%9C%93&affiliate=cdc-main&sitelimit=www.atsdr.cdc.gov&query=Nerve+Agents&commit=Search> Accessed 07.07.15.

Agency for Toxic Substances and Disease Registry. *Phosgene (COCL₂).* <http://search.cdc.gov/search?utf8=%E2%9C%93&affiliate=cdc-main&sitelimit=www.atsdr.cdc.gov&query=Phosgene+%28COCL2%29&commit=Search> Accessed 07.07.15.

Borron SW, Kazzi Z. Management of hazardous material emergencies. *Emerg Med Clin North Am.* 2015;33:xvii.

Craft DW, Lee PA, Rowlinson MC. Bioterrorism: a laboratory who does it? *J Clin Microbiol.* 2014;52:2290–2298.

Goans RE. *Medical Military Operations. Medical Management of Radiological Casualties.* 4th ed. Bethesda, MD: Armed Forces Radiobiology Research Institute, Uniformed Services University of the Health Sciences; July 2013.

Kman NE, Bachmann DJ. Biosurveillance: a review and update. *Adv Prevent Med.* 2012:301408. 2012.

Kost GJ, Curtis C, Sakaguchi RL, Sakaguchi A. Disaster point-of-care testing: fundamental concepts and new technologies. In: Arora R, Arora P, eds. *Disaster Management: Medical Preparedness, Response and Homeland Security.* Boston: CAB International; 2013:121.

Kost GJ, Mecozzi DM, Brock TK, Curtis CM. Assessing point-of-care device specifications and needs for pathogen detection in emergencies and disasters. *Point Care.* 2012;11:119–125.

Kost GJ, Sakaguchi A, Curtis C, et al. Enhancing crisis standards of care using innovative point-of-care testing. *Am J Disaster Med.* 2011;6:351–368.

Rambhia KJ, Waldhorn RE, Selck F, et al. A survey of hospitals to determine the prevalence and characteristics of healthcare coalitions for emergency preparedness and response. *Biosecur Bioterror.* 2012;10:304–313.

Stevens DA. Reflections on the approach to treatment of a mycologic disaster. *Antimicrob Agents Chemother.* 2013;57:1567–1572.

U.S. Army Medical Research Institute of Infectious Diseases. *Medical Management of Biological Casualties Handbook;* 2011. <http://www.usamriid.army.mil/education/instruct.htm> Accessed 08.07.15.

Zajtchuk R, Bellamy RF. *Medical Aspects of Chemical and Biological Warfare.* Falls Church, VA: Office of the Surgeon General of the United States Army; 1997.

Glossary

abnormal Not normal; contrary to the usual structure, position, condition, behavior, or rule.

ABO-Rh typing Assessing a person's blood type and Rh factor.

abrin Biological agent also known as ricin. See *ricin*.

accreditation Federal and state agencies impose standards that require laboratories to implement processes and procedures to ensure quality laboratory test results.

Accrediting Bureau of Health Education Schools ABHES; provides accreditation for health education programs.

accuracy How close a laboratory test result is to its true value.

acetoacetic acid One of three ketone bodies produced in the liver as a result of catabolism of fatty acids.

acetone One of three ketone bodies produced in the liver as a result of catabolism of fatty acids.

acid A substance that donates hydrogen atoms in a water solution.

acquired immunity See *adaptive immunity*.

acquired immunodeficiency syndrome AIDS; end-stage disease for an individual infected with the human immunodeficiency virus; diagnosed after the CD4+ T-cell count falls to less than 200/µL.

acromegaly A condition that occurs in adults with excessive amounts of growth hormone.

activation energy The change in Gibbs free energy needed to overcome the transition state and proceed to product formation; enzymes catalyze many physiologic reactions by lowering the activation energy.

activator A substance that combines with an enzyme to increase its catalytic activity.

active site Part of an enzyme where the substance that is acted on (i.e., the substrate) interacts and binds.

acute inflammation Inflammation, usually localized and of sudden onset and short duration (<2 weeks), characterized by the classical signs of heat, redness, pain, and swelling.

acute lymphocytic leukemia ALL, also called acute lymphoblastic leukemia; the most common type of leukemia among children and adolescents, but it can also affect adults. It is characterized by proliferation of early lymphoid precursors (i.e., lymphoblasts) that replace normal cells in bone marrow and peripheral blood.

acute myelogenous leukemia AML, also called acute myeloid leukemia; a malignant disease in which the bone marrow makes abnormal myeloid cell precursors that stop maturing in the early stages of development.

acute myocardial infarction Heart attack; occurs when part of a coronary artery is blocked and the heart tissue served by that artery becomes hypoxic due to ischemia.

acute pancreatitis Inflammation of the pancreas that occurs suddenly and can be life-threatening.

acute phase proteins Plasma proteins produced by the liver during the inflammatory response.

acute tubular necrosis Acute kidney disease characterized by damage to the tubule cells of the kidneys.

adamsite A vomiting agent that forms a gas when heated and is often used for riot control.

adaptive immunity Acquired immunity; immunity that develops in response to antigen exposure throughout a lifetime; reacts differently each time exposure to an antigenic stimulus or foreign antigen occurs.

addiction Occurs when an individual continues to use a drug despite adverse effects and usually includes drug-seeking behaviors.

Addison disease Primary adrenal insufficiency; a potentially fatal endocrine disorder characterized by chronically decreased levels of glucocorticoids (cortisol) and mineralocorticoids (aldosterone), usually from autoimmune mechanisms.

adenocarcinoma A malignant tumor originating from a gland.

adenoma A benign tumor originating from a gland.

adrenal cortex Outer portion of the adrenal gland; produces mineralocorticoids, glucocorticoids, and the adrenal androgens.

adrenal medulla Inner portion of the adrenal gland; secretes the catecholamines, epinephrine and norepinephrine.

adrenocorticotropic hormone ACTH; the pituitary hormone that is secreted in response to stress in the body and stimulates the adrenal cortex to produce glucocorticoids. It is also produced by pituitary and small cell lung tumors and is elevated in certain benign conditions.

adsorption chromatography Type of chromatography in which analytes are separated by the adsorption and desorption of solutes at the surface of a solid particle; uses physical forces such as electrostatic hydrogen bonding and dispersive interactions to separate and quantitate volatile compounds.

adverse drug reaction Unwanted or injurious effect of a drug; may occur after a single dose, after prolonged administration, or from the combination of two or more drugs.

affinity The strength of the bond between an antigen and an antibody.

affinity chromatography A liquid chromatographic technique for the separation and analysis of specific analytes within a sample. The method makes use of a biological interaction such as binding of an enzyme with a substrate, a hormone with its receptor, or an antibody with an antigen.

agarose The neutral fraction of agar obtained by separating it from agaropectin that is used in agarose gel electrophoresis (AGE). AGE has many applications including separation of proteins in serum, urine, and cerebrospinal fluid.

alanine transaminase (ALT) Formerly SGPT; an important enzyme that is released into the bloodstream after liver tissue damage.

albinism A general term for any of several hypopigmentation disorders caused by mutations in genes responsible for melanin synthesis, distribution of pigment by the melanocyte, and melanosome biogenesis.

albumin The most abundant protein in plasma; maintains colloidal osmotic pressure and transports calcium, fatty acids, drugs, hormones, and other molecules.

alcohol Compound that contains a hydrocarbon chain (R) and one or more hydroxyl (OH⁻) groups. Alcohols are extensively used in the clinical laboratory as preservatives or solvents, and they may be a component of stains and reagents.

aldehyde Functional group (—CHO) that consists of an oxygen atom double bonded to a carbon atom that also has a hydrogen atom attached. This group is attached to a hydrocarbon chain.

aldosterone Mineralocorticoid hormone secreted by the adrenal cortex; influences the kidneys to resorb sodium and accelerates the exchange of sodium and potassium ions across the cell membranes.

aldosteronism An electrolyte imbalance caused by excessive production of aldosterone.

alkaline phosphatase ALP; an enzyme that originates in liver, bone, and placenta; tumor marker for liver or bone cancer.

alloimmunity Hypersensitivity reaction to the antigens of another individual (e.g., blood transfusion).

allosteric site Alternative site on an enzyme molecule where a regulator molecule may bind and cause conformational changes that affect the active site and therefore the reaction rate.

alternative pathway One of the three activation methods for the complement cascade, using gram-negative bacterial and fungal cell wall polysaccharides.

Alzheimer disease Most common cause of neurodegenerative dementia; characterized by amyloid deposits (plaques) in the brain and intraneuronal deposits of tau protein.

American Society for Clinical Pathologists ASCP; provides registry board examinations to insure the competency of a graduate of an accredited laboratory training and educational program.

amine hormone Hormone derivative of the amino acid tyrosine. Amine hormones include triiodothyronine (T_3), thyroxine (T_4), and the catecholamines (epinephrine and norepinephrine).

amine Derivative of ammonia (NH_3). Amines are found in alkaloids, antihistamines, sulfa drugs, and barbiturates.

amino acid An organic compound that includes both a carboxyl group (—COOH) and an amino group (—NH_2). Amino acids form the building blocks of proteins.

amniocentesis A test usually performed between 15 and 20 weeks of gestation to screen for chromosomal abnormalities; involves a needle puncture of the amniotic sac and withdrawal of a few milliliters of amniotic fluid as a specimen.

amperometric Relating to amperometry, an electrolytic electrochemical process in which a fixed voltage (potential) is applied between two electrodes in a solution and the current is measured to detect the concentration of the analyte.

amperometry Based on the measurement of the current flowing through an electrochemical cell and the electrochemical potential between the two electrodes while a constant external voltage is applied.

amylase Enzyme that converts starch into sugar. Levels of amylase in serum rise significantly within hours after onset of acute pancreatitis.

amyloidosis A condition in which abnormal, insoluble amyloid fibrils are deposited in organs or tissues and interfere with normal function.

amyotrophic lateral sclerosis ALS, also known as Lou Gehrig disease; the most common degenerative disease of the motor neuron system.

analyte A chemical substance or biological component of the human body, such as a hormone, drug, or protein, that is measured, usually in a solute such as blood.

analytic run Automated testing of multiple specimens.

analytical phase Phase of the laboratory testing cycle that includes sample and reagent handling, the test measurement process, and calculation and interpretation of the results.

anaphylaxis Life-threatening immediate hypersensitivity; can manifest systemically or cutaneously.

anasarca Severe generalized edema.

anatomic pathology Medical specialty based on examination of all tissues, fluids, organs, and limbs removed from the body; includes surgical pathology, histology, and cytology.

androstenedione A hormone secreted by the adrenal cortex that has androgenic and estrogenic activity.

anemia of chronic renal and endocrine diseases A type of anemia that occurs in long-standing systemic disorders such as rheumatoid arthritis, diabetes mellitus, severe trauma, and heart disease.

anencephaly Severe neural tube defect in which the skull fails to develop and the exposed brain dies in utero.

angiogenesis Formation of new blood vessels to serve injured tissue or to facilitate tumor growth.

angiotensin I A chemical that is converted to angiotensin II in the kidney by the action of angiotensin-converting enzyme.

angiotensin II A powerful vasoconstrictor that causes a rise in blood pressure and stimulates release of aldosterone and antidiuretic hormone.

angiotensin II/III Peptide hormones that stimulate the production of aldosterone and function in the control of blood pressure.

angiotensin-converting enzyme ACE; acts on angiotensin I to produce angiotensin II.

angiotensinogen A precursor protein that is secreted by the liver and converted by renin to angiotensin I.

anion A negatively charged ion.

anion gap The difference between the unmeasured anions and the unmeasured cations after major electrolytes have been accounted for.

ankylosing spondylitis A chronic, systemic, inflammatory condition that affects the sacroiliac joints and the axial skeletal.

anneal To cause the association or reassociation of single-stranded nucleic acids so that double-stranded molecules are formed, often by heating followed by cooling.

anodic stripping voltammetry Method for detecting trace levels of toxic metals in clinical samples, used especially for the analysis of lead in whole blood.

anosmia Absent sense of smell.

anterior pituitary Adenohypophysis; the active, hormone-synthesizing portion of the pituitary gland; produces adrenocorticotropic hormone, growth hormone, prolactin, thyroid-stimulating hormone, luteinizing hormone, and follicle-stimulating hormone.

antibodies A protein (immunoglobin) produced by the body in response to exposure to a specific antigen epitope.

anti–cyclic citrullinated peptide Anti-CCP; antibody that forms the basis of a diagnostic test for rheumatoid arthritis.

antidiuretic hormone ADH, also called vasopressin; a hormone synthesized by the hypothalamus that helps the body retain water and thereby maintains the body's osmolarity.

anti–double-stranded DNA antibody Anti-dsDNA; an antinuclear antibody that targets double-stranded DNA and may be associated with systemic lupus erythematosus.

antigen Any material capable of reacting with an antibody without necessarily being capable of inducing antibody formation. These can be proteins, lipids, carbohydrates, or polysaccharides.

anti–mutated citrullinated vimentin Anti-MCV; antibody that forms the basis of a diagnostic test for rheumatoid arthritis.

antineoplastic drug A drug that restrains or prevents the development of neoplasms; used in chemotherapy to inhibit the maturation and proliferation of malignant cells.

antinuclear antibody ANA; any of a group of autoantibodies that target proteins within the cell nucleus and are measured as the primary screening test for systemic lupus erythematosus and other autoimmune disorders.

anti-Smith antibody Anti-Sm; an antinuclear antibody that targets core proteins of small nuclear ribonuclear particles; may be associated with systemic lupus erythematosus.

anti-SSA/Ro autoantibody An antinuclear antibody that targets ribonuclear proteins; may be associated with systemic lupus erythematosus or Sjögren syndrome.

anti-SSB/La autoantibody An antinuclear antibody that targets ribonuclear proteins; may be associated with systemic lupus erythematosus or Sjögren syndrome.

α_1-antitrypsin ATT; a serine protease inhibitor; deficiency may lead to lung or liver disease.

anti-U1RNP antibody Antinuclear antibody directed against the U1 ribonucleoprotein complex; may be associated with systemic lupus erythematosus or mixed connective tissue disease.

aplastic anemia A type of anemia that occurs when all cell lines fail to produce mature cells and the red, cell-producing bone marrow is replaced by fat and other tissues.

apolipoprotein Protein portion of a lipoprotein molecule. Apolipoproteins includes chylomicrons, very-low-density lipoprotein, low-density lipoprotein, and high-density lipoprotein; their structure is unique because they are soluble in plasma and bind to nonpolar lipids.

apolipoprotein A-I Apolipoprotein found on high-density lipoprotein molecules.

apolipoprotein B-100 Apolipoprotein found on low-density lipoprotein molecules.

apolipoprotein C-II Apolipoprotein found on all lipoproteins.

apoptosis Programmed cell death.

apotransferrin A glycoprotein that binds iron (Fe^{3+}) to form transferrin, which transports the iron to the liver and throughout the body.

arachidonic acid–derived hormone Any hormone derived from arachidonic acid, a degradation product of polyunsaturated fatty acids; see *eicosanoids*.

arcus senilis A narrow, opaque, gray to white band of lipid deposited around the edge of the cornea.

aromatic ring Refers to a hydrocarbon that contains one or more benzene rings. The smallest example, the benzene molecule, consists of six carbon atoms with alternating double bonds and single bonds.

arsine SA (military designation); a colorless, flammable, and highly toxic gas with a garlic or fish odor. It binds to hemoglobin, preventing oxygen binding, and lyses red blood cells.

ascites Abnormal accumulation of fluid in the abdominal cavity.

aspartate transaminase (AST) Formerly SGOT; an enzyme that is released into the bloodstream after liver tissue damage or damage to skeletal or cardiac muscle.

aspiration Refers to removal of a precise amount of a specimen or reagent, as by a peristaltic pump system, for use in a laboratory test.

assay A procedure for determining the amount of a particular constituent of a mixture or the biological or pharmacologic potency of a drug.

assayed control A control that comes with a predetermined target value established by the manufacturer.

assessment The gathering of data to measure a laboratory's performance against a standard or benchmark; one of the key essentials in a quality management system.

asthma Disorder in which the bronchial tree constricts, especially during exhalation, causing obstruction of air flow.

ataxia telangiectasia A rare, autosomal recessive, neurogenerative immune disorder causing severe disability.

atelactasis Partial collapse of a lung.

atherogenesis The formation of atheromas in arterial walls.

atheroma Abnormal deposit in the inner lining of an artery wall that contains primarily cholesterol, lipids, cellular debris, and, eventually, calcium and fibrous tissue.

atherosclerosis A disease that is characterized by the accumulation of plaques and inflammatory cells and the formation of thrombi in the arteries.

atherosclerotic plaque formation Progressive development of atheromas in the arteries due to the accumulation of foam cells and fibrofatty deposits.

atomic theory Scientific theory that states that all matter is made up of atoms.

atrial natriuretic peptide A peptide hormone secreted by heart muscle cells that causes the excretion of sodium.

atrial septal defect Congenital abnormal opening in the wall (i.e., septum) that divides the two upper chambers (atria) of the heart.

atrophy Decrease in cell size.

autoimmune disease A disease in which the body loses its ability to differentiate between self and nonself antigens. The body views self-antigens as foreign and produces antibodies against them.

automated pipettes Calibrated pipettes of fixed or variable volume that are used to draw up and dispense liquids; the amount aspirated and the time allowed for aspirating and dispensing liquids are usually under electronic, computerized control.

avidity The overall stability of an antibody–antigen complex.

azotemia The presence of excessive nitrogen products (e.g., urea) in the bloodstream.

B

bacteriocidal drug A drug that directly kills bacteria.

bacteriostatic drug A drug that slows or stops cell division in bacteria.

balance A device used to accurately weigh substances.

base A substance that donates hydroxide (OH⁻) ions in a water solution.

batch analyzer An analyzer that sequentially performs a test on each of a group of specimens.

Beau's lines Horizontal ridges and indentations in the nail plate; found in individuals with previous severe illness, infection, or trauma or with prolonged exposure to cold temperature in patients with Raynaud's syndrome.

Becker muscular dystrophy An X-linked form of muscular dystrophy first described in 1955; affects the same gene but is milder than Duchenne muscular dystrophy.

Beer's law The absorbance (A) of a colored solution is equal to the product of the concentration of the color-producing substance (C) times the depth of the solution through which the light must travel (L) times a constant (K).

Bence Jones protein A protein discovered in 1847 in the urine of patients with multiple myeloma. It was the first tumor marker discovered.

benign tumor A nonpathological tumor, usually well encapsulated. The cells retain their normal structure and do not metastasize.

β-human chorionic gonadotropin (β-HCG) See *human chorionic gonadotropin.*

bias The difference between the average value obtained from a large series of measurements and the true value based on the reference methodology for that test.

bicarbonate HCO_3^-; an anion that is present in large amounts in extracellular fluids.

bicarbonate buffer system The most important buffer system in the body. It is controlled by the lungs (releasing or retaining carbon dioxide) and the kidneys (increasing or decreasing bicarbonate absorption).

bile Released by the gallbladder to emulsify fats into smaller globules for further breakdown by lipid hydrolyzing enzymes.

bilirubin A breakdown product of hemoglobin that is conjugated in the liver.

bioaccumulation The accumulation of chemicals, especially toxic substances, in the body.

bioavailability The fraction of an administered dose of a drug that reaches the systemic circulation.

biochemistry Also called physiologic chemistry; the study of the chemistry of living organisms.

biohazard A biological or chemical substance that constitutes a threat to the health of humans or other living organisms; also, the danger posed by such an agent.

biohazardous waste Waste that contains infectious materials or otherwise poses a biohazard.

biological safety cabinet A space within a biosafety level 2 or higher laboratory where procedures that produce aerosols or involve pathogenic organisms can be conducted safely.

biological threat A naturally occurring chemical produced by an animal, plant, or microbe that can cause injury or disease.

bioluminescence Biochemical emission of light by living organisms.

biopsy Examination of tissue removed from a living body to determine the existence, cause, or extent of disease.

biosafety level 1 Laboratory that contains equipment, practices, and facilities used with organisms that do not consistently cause disease in healthy adults.

biosafety level 2 Laboratory that contains equipment, practices, and facilities used with moderate-risk agents derived from the community that cause disease in immunocompromised and immunocompetent people.

biosafety level 3 Laboratory that contains equipment, practices, and facilities used with organisms that cause severe or potentially lethal infections transmitted through inhalation.

biosafety level 4 Laboratory that contains equipment, practices, and facilities used with extremely hazardous infectious organisms that frequently cause fatal or incurable diseases or diseases with an unknown transmission mechanism.

biotransformation Chemical alterations of a compound occurring within the body, as when the liver converts lipophilic, nonpolar molecules to more polar, water-soluble molecules.

blister agent A chemical that produces blisters when it comes in contact with the eyes, skin, or respiratory tract.

blood agent A chemical agent that becomes poisonous after it is absorbed into the blood (e.g., arsine, cyanogen chloride).

blood bank Also known as the immunohematology department; tests red blood cells from donors for antigens and serum from recipients for antibodies.

blood gas analysis Performed to determine parameters such as the pH, oxygen content, and carbon dioxide content in arterial or venous blood.

blood glucose level Amount of glucose found in the blood.

blood spots Collected and dried on filter paper as a sample for monitoring of immunosuppressant therapy.

blood urea nitrogen The amount of nitrogen in the blood in the form of urea; measured as an important test of renal function.

bloodborne pathogen A microbiological pathogen that is carried in blood and body fluids.

Board of Registry Organization created in 1928 as part of the American Society of Clinical Pathologists to certify laboratory workers.

bone resorption Process by which osteoclasts break down bone, releasing calcium and other minerals into the blood.

botulinum Neurotoxin produced by the anaerobic bacterium *Clostridium botulinum.*

bound drug The amount of a drug that is bound to a chemical in the blood, usually a protein.

bradykinin Chemical mediator of chronic inflammation that dilates blood vessels, contracts smooth muscles, increases vascular permeability, and acts with E-series prostaglandins to induce pain.

BRCA1 A gene that, when mutated, serves as a DNA marker for breast and ovarian cancers; when normal, plays critical roles in DNA repair, cell cycle control, and maintenance of genomic stability.

BRCA2 A gene that, when mutated, serves as a DNA marker for breast and ovarian cancers; when normal, makes a protein that acts as a tumor suppressor.

brevetoxin A neurotoxin that binds to nerve cells and disrupts the normal neurologic processes in the body. In nature, it is responsible for the neurotoxic shellfish poisoning that accompanies red tides.

British anti-Lewisite BAL; antidote to lewisite; binds to the arsenic in lewisite to reduce its toxicity.

broad-spectrum antibiotic An antibiotic that is useful against a range of gram-positive and gram-negative bacteria.

Bruton agammaglobulinemia Also called X-linked agammaglobulinemia (XLA); an immunodeficiency disease caused by mutation of a gene on the X chromosome that encodes Bruton tyrosine kinase (BTK). Because BTK is necessary for the maturation of B lymphocytes, affected individuals produce no antibodies and have small or absent tonsils, adenoids, Peyer patches, lymph nodes, and spleen.

B-type natriuretic peptide A substance secreted from the ventricles of the heart in response to swelling of the ventricles; a sensitive and specific biomarker for heart damage in patients with congestive heart failure.

buffer A solution consisting of a weak acid and its conjugate base; when a strong base or strong acid is added to the solution, the pH changes very little.

business continuity One goal of an emergency preparedness plan; refers to actions that a clinical laboratory or other business can take to ensure survivability and a quicker return to operation after a hazardous incident.

C

CA 15-3 Tumor marker that is monitored to assess the progression of breast cancer.

CA 19-9 Tumor marker for colorectal and pancreatic carcinomas.

CA 27.29 Tumor marker that is monitored to assess the progression of breast cancer.

CA 72-4 Tumor marker associated with ovarian and gastrointestinal carcinomas.

CA 125 Tumor marker that is elevated in 50% of individuals with stage I ovarian cancer and in 90% of individuals with stage IV ovarian cancer.

CA 242 Tumor marker for pancreatic and colorectal cancers.

CA 549 Tumor marker that is monitored to assess recurrence; an increased CA 549 level after a decreased value indicates the recurrence of metastases and disease progression.

calcitonin A hormone that regulates serum calcium concentrations. Calcitonin is useful in detecting familial medullary carcinoma of the thyroid.

calcium oxalate crystals Normal crystals found in the urine.

calibrator A material, usually produced by an instrument manufacturer, that is used to align the signal strength of the instrument to a particular concentration of an analyte; often the analyte is contained in a different matrix from that used for controls and patient samples.

cancer A malignant neoplasm.

cap piercer A sturdy piece of metal with a sharp end that can easily pierce the rubber cap on a specimen tube.

capillary electrophoresis CE; a family of techniques in which fused silica capillary columns and high electric field strengths are used to separate a complex array of molecules based on differences in charge, size, and hydrophobicity.

capillary gel electrophoresis CGE; adaptation of traditional gel electrophoresis in which polymers in solution are used to create a molecular sieve also known as replaceable physical gel. This allows analytes having similar charge-to-mass ratios to be resolved by size.

capillary isoelectric focusing CIEF; technique that allows amphoteric molecules such as proteins to be separated by electrophoresis in a pH gradient generated between a cathode and an anode. A solute migrates to a point where its net charge is zero.

capillary zone electrophoresis CZE, also known as free-solution capillary electrophoresis (FSCE); the simplest form of CE. The separation mechanism is based on differences in the charge-to-mass ratio of the analytes.

carbohydrate A polyhydroxy aldehyde or polyhydroxy ketone substance with a general molecular formula of CH_2O; classified by the number of saccharide units in the molecule. Carbohydrates are the main food source used for energy by humans; they exist as sugars, starches, and cellulose.

carboxyhemoglobin Hemoglobin that is bound to carbon monoxide instead of oxygen. It is stable and therefore cannot absorb or transport oxygen.

carcinoembryonic antigen CEA; one of two major oncofetal antigens used as tumor markers. It is elevated in patients with colon cancer as well as in benign conditions.

carcinoma A type of tumor that originates in the epithelium.

carcinoma in situ A preinvasive epithelial malignant tumor of glands or squamous cells.

cardiac catheterization A test that involves passing a thin tube (catheter) into the right or left side of the heart, usually from the groin or the arm; used to detect cardiac blockage, to take biopsy samples, or to remove blockage from an artery.

cardiac tamponade Compression of the heart caused by fluid accumulation in the pericardium.

cardiomegaly Abnormally large heart, usually caused by compensation for poor efficiency of the heart.

cardiomyopathy Disease of the heart muscle.

cardiovascular disease Leading cause of illness and death in the United States; linked to levels of lipids and lipoproteins in the blood.

casts Microscopic structures in the urine formed primarily by precipitation of Tamm-Horsfall proteins that have remained in the kidney tubules for prolonged periods.

cataract A condition in which the lens of the eye becomes progressively cloudy, usually due to deterioration of the lens fibers and protein clumping.

catecholamine A type of neurotransmitter secreted by the adrenal medulla that is water soluble and does not require a carrier protein; includes epinephrine (also known as adrenaline) and norepinephrine. These hormones are responsible for the body's "fight or flight" response.

cation A positively charged ion

caustic An acid that produces chemical burns on the skin, eyes, and mucous membranes on contact.

celiac disease Also known as celiac sprue or nontropical sprue; an autoimmune disease associated with intestinal inflammation due to an intolerance to gluten products.

celiac sprue Gluten-sensitive enteropathy; see *celiac disease.*

cell death A process by which cells die in an orderly, programmed fashion after a specific life span. Cell death that occurs before the natural time alters body functions and can cause problems.

cell membrane A semipermeable barrier that surrounds each cell and keeps the cytoplasm, nucleus, and other parts of the cell isolated from the rest of the organism. See *plasma membrane.*

cell permeability Passage of solvents and solutes into and out of cells.

cellular adaptation Refers to changes made by a cell in response to adverse environmental conditions; examples are hyperplasia, metaplasia, neoplasia, and cancer.

Centers for Disease Control and Prevention CDC; government agency responsible for disease monitoring, disease control, and public safety related to infectious diseases.

central chemoreceptors Regulatory cells located in the ventral medulla of the brainstem. They trigger involuntarily changes in breathing rate and depth, as well as other factors.

centrifugal analyzer Automated instrument that uses the centrifugal force resulting from a spinning rotor to mix a specimen and a reagent, after which the reaction mixture is passed through a detector.

centrifuge A piece of motorized equipment that uses centrifugal force to separate a mixture such as clotted blood. There are four basic types of centrifuges: horizontal head or swinging bucket, angle-head or fixed angle, axial, and ultracentrifuge.

cerebral palsy A disease characterized by permanent motor dysfunction, usually caused by a brain injury before 2 years of age.

ceruloplasmin A protein that transports copper ions; accounts for 95% of the copper found in the plasma.

CH$_{50}$ assay Assay that measures the complement proteins of the classical pathway; based on the serum dilution required to produce 50% cell lysis.

chain of custody A process for maintaining control and accountability of each specimen from the point of collection to its final location. It requires documentation of every individual handling the sample.

chemical hygiene plan CHP; an OSHA-mandated plan to guide chemical usage in the laboratory. The plan must specify standard operating procedures, equipment, personal protective equipment, and laboratory practices to protect workers from chemical hazards.

chemical ionization An ionization method sometimes used in mass spectrometry in which gaseous molecules interact with ions. It is a lower-energy process than electron ionization, yielding less fragmentation and usually a simpler spectrum.

chemical symbol In the periodic chart of the elements, a letter or two letters that designate a specific chemical element.

chemical weapon A highly toxic chemical agent that can incapacitate or kill a large number of individuals after a single release.

chemiluminescence Emission of light during a chemical reaction; also, a reaction that produces light without producing heat.

chemiluminescent microparticle immunoassay CMIA; type of immunoassay that uses a chemiluminescent compound, which produces light when combined with a trigger reagent, to detect analytes.

chloroacetophenone Also known as tear gas or CN (military designation); a colorless to gray or white crystalline solid that irritates the eyes and mucous membranes on contact when released as a gas; may be used for crowd control.

chloropicrin PS (military designation); a colorless to faint yellow, oily liquid that is considered a lung-damaging agent. Exposure routes include the eyes, skin, respiratory tract, and gastrointestinal tract.

cholecalciferol Vitamin D$_3$

cholecystokinin A hormone secreted by the duodenal mucosa that regulates the release of bile by the gallbladder and the secretion of enzymes by the pancreas; also, a test used to assess the function of the gallbladder.

Cholesterol Reference Method Laboratory Network Organization created by the Centers for Disease Control and Prevention to help manufacturers develop a valid method that is traceable to the National Reference System for Cholesterol (NRS/CHOL).

cholesterol A sterol with ring compounds, an aliphatic chain, and a hydroxyl group that functions as a structural component in the body and a precursor for the synthesis of steroid hormones. It is the primary sterol in humans and is required for the production of bile acids, steroids, and cell membranes.

chorionic villi sampling A test usually performed between 10 and 12 weeks of gestation to screen for chromosomal abnormalities; involves a needle puncture and aspiration of cells from the fingerlike projections of the chorion that surround the developing fetus.

chromatography Collective term for a set of laboratory techniques for the physical separation and quantification of clinically important analytes. The sample mixture is dissolved in a fluid called the *mobile phase,* which carries it through a structure holding another material called the *stationary phase.*

chromogen In spectrophotometry, a substance such as a dye or analyte that absorbs light at a specific wavelength.

chronic bronchitis Obstructive lung disease characterized by enlargement of mucous cells, inflammation, and neutrophil infiltrations; diagnosed when a person has had a chronic productive cough for 3 months during each of 2 consecutive years.

chronic diarrhea Malabsorption condition that is diagnosed when an individual has passed liquid or loose stools more than three times a day for 4 weeks or longer.

chronic inflammation Inflammation that lasts longer than 2 weeks; may be a continuation of an acute form or a prolonged low-grade form.

chronic lymphocytic leukemia CLL; a slowly progressing malignant disease that is characterized by proliferation of a large number of small, nonfunctional lymphocytes; the most common form of leukemia among adults in Western countries.

chronic myelogenous leukemia CML; malignant disease in which the bone marrow produces increased numbers of mature myelocytes.

chronic obstructive pulmonary disease COPD; a group of diseases that obstruct the flow of air into and out of the lungs; includes chronic bronchitis, emphysema, and asthma.

chronic pancreatitis Inflammation of the pancreas that progresses over time and leads to permanent damage.

chronic pericarditis Prolonged inflammation or infection of the sac surrounding the heart.

chylomicron Category of lipoprotein; largest and least dense; used to transport triglycerides from the intestines to muscle and adipose tissue.

chyme Name for food that has been processed or digested in the stomach.

chymotrypsin One of the enzymes that directly breaks down proteins into oligopeptides.

circadian rhythm 24-hour biological clock that is influenced by light and dark periods in the day.

cirrhosis Liver disease characterized by loss of the normal microscopic lobular architecture with fibrosis and nodular regeneration.

citrullination A process by which arginine, an amino acid, is transformed into a different amino acid, citrulline; part of the disease mechanism of rheumatoid arthritis.

Clark electrode The pO₂ electrode on an amperometric sensor; consists of a platinum cathode surrounded by a tubular silver anode.

classical pathway One of the three activation methods for the complement cascade, using antibody-antigen complexes.

CLIA 67 See *Clinical Laboratory Improvement Act of 1967.*

CLIA 88 See *Clinical Laboratory Improvement Amendments of 1988.*

Clinical and Laboratory Standards Institute CLSI; international standards organization that produces many different standards for clinical laboratories.

clinical chemistry The medical discipline that uses various methods of analysis and instrumentation to determine values for chemical components in normal and diseased states, types and concentrations of blood toxins, and therapeutic drug levels.

Clinical Laboratory Improvement Act of 1967 CLIA 67; Act of Congress intended to regulate clinical laboratories involved in interstate commerce. Hospital and reference laboratories were the only clinical laboratories affected by this Act.

clinical laboratory scientists Also known as medical laboratory scientists; laboratory personnel who perform routine and specialized laboratory tests and troubleshoot problems with specimens, procedures, and instruments to ensure quality test results. They also perform microscopic analyses of blood and body fluids and communicate laboratory results to physicians and pathologists. This group of laboratory professionals have a bachelor's degree.

clinical laboratory technicians Also known as medical laboratory technicians; laboratory professionals who have 2-year associate degrees and perform all the routine testing in the clinical laboratory.

clinical pathology The largest portion of the work done in a clinical laboratory; composed of hematology, clinical chemistry, microbiology, immunohematology, toxicology, immunology and serology, urinalysis, specimen collection, and customer service. This also includes histology and cytology.

cloned enzyme donor immunoassay CEDIA; a competitive homogenous enzyme immunoassay used to measure therapeutic drugs and drugs of abuse. It was the first enzyme immunoassay designed with the use of genetic engineering techniques.

closed neural tube defect Congenital defect confined to one area and usually involving only the spine.

Clostridium difficile An opportunistic bacterial infectious agent associated with diarrhea.

coefficient of variation Ratio of the standard deviation of a set of sample values to their mean value, expressed as a percentage; measures the degree of variability or dispersion of the data points relative to the mean. It is used to determine the precision of the methods when a laboratory changes from one test method to another.

coenzyme An organic substance loosely bound to a protein that is required for enzyme function.

cofactor A nonprotein substance that is essential for enzyme activity and must bind to the enzyme before the reaction can take place.

College of American Pathologists CAP; an internationally known agency that accredits clinical laboratories.

colligative property Any physical property that depends on the ratio of the number of solute particles to the number of solvent molecules in a solution.

colloidal osmotic pressure Pressure that large proteins and other colloid molecules within a cell exert on the outer walls of adjoining blood vessels.

column chromatography Gas or liquid chromatography technique in which the stationary phase is coated onto the inner surface of the tube or chemically bonded to support particles that are then packed into the tube or capillary.

Commission on Accreditation of Allied Health Education Programs CAAHEP; organization that accredits short-term educational programs.

competency assessment A system for measuring and documenting the skills, knowledge, and experience of laboratory personnel in carrying out their duties; performed semiannually for new personnel and annually thereafter.

competency testing Minimal regulatory requirement for competency assessment required for each laboratory test an individual is approved to perform; includes direct observation, monitoring, and review of records and performance.

competitive immunoassay A type of immunoassay, such as a radioimmunoassay, that is based on competition between the unlabeled analyte in the sample and a labeled antigen. The analyte concentration is inversely proportional to the absorbance of the solution.

competitive inhibition Reaction in which an inhibitor binds to the active site of an enzyme, preventing the substrate from binding to the enzyme and thus inhibiting enzymatic function.

complement A set of molecules that function as part of the body's defense system against bacterial infection. The complement cascade can destroy pathogens directly or in conjunction with the clotting and kinin systems.

compression atelectasis Occurs when the lungs are compressed due to upward pressure on the diaphragm from any space-occupying lesion in the thorax.

conception Process by which a sperm fertilizes an ovum, marking the beginning of pregnancy.

conductometry Measurement of electrolytic conductivity to monitor the progress of a chemical reaction.

confidence interval Refers to the percentage of data points that can be expected to fall within a given distance from the mean when the data are set up on a normal curve; for example, the 95% confidence interval is the range of measured values that will lie within 2 standard deviations above or below the mean.

congenital hypothyroidism Cretinism; a treatable condition in which an inborn error of thyroid metabolism or iodine deficiency causes mental retardation in a child.

congenital idiopathic hypogonadotropic hypogonadism A condition in which the hypothalamus or pituitary fails to stimulate the gonads to produce sex hormones.

congestive heart failure A progressive disease in which the ability of the heart to pump efficiently gradually decreases over time.

conjugated bilirubin Direct bilirubin; bilirubin attached to glucuronic acid.

conjugated protein A protein that is attached to a non–amino acid chemical group.

constrictive pericarditis A condition in which the pericardium loses its elasticity because of the accumulation of scar tissue that keeps the heart from working properly.

continuous flow analyzer An analyzer in which reagent is continuously pumped while samples are injected into the system at regular intervals.

continuous process improvement program A system of quality management based on W. Edward Deming's fourteen quality points. Two of these points—"Create constancy of purpose for improvement" and "Improve constantly and forever"—are the mainstay of laboratory programs.

continuous quality improvement cycle CQI; refers to collaboration between departments and individuals that results in working together across organizational departments to improve shared processes; includes planning, corrective actions, monitoring, and evaluation.

contraction atelectasis Decreased lung volume caused by the contraction of scars in the lung.

control A material that is made with the same matrix as patient samples and contains a specific amount of an analyte. Controls are run along with patient specimens to help detect errors and instrument malfunctions.

control limits The acceptable range of measured values established for a given control in statistical process control methods; used to evaluate the accuracy and precision of an analytical system.

copper levels Blood levels of copper; low in Wilson disease.

coproporphyrin A porphyrin with four methyl and four propionic acid side chains attached to the tetrapyrrole backbone; elevated in certain types of porphyria.

coronary artery An artery that supplies oxygenated blood to the heart muscle.

corpus luteum Term for the follicle in the ovary after an ovum is released. As it disintegrates, the cells along its margin release estrogen.

correlation coefficient (r) A statistic that describes the strength of the relationship between two different methods; values range from –1 to +1. If $r = 0$, there is no relationship between the two values, whereas a value of 1 indicates a perfect relationship, and –1 indicates an inverse relationship. Values between –1 and +1 indicate varying degrees of relationship.

cortisol The major glucocorticoid secreted by the adrenal cortex; regulates the metabolism of carbohydrates, proteins, and lipids.

coulometry Measurement of the amount of charge (coulombs) passing between two electrodes at a fixed potential.

counterimmunoelectrophoresis CIE; a qualitative method used to evaluate antibody–antigen binding when the antibody and antigen have opposite charges; typically is used to identify antinuclear ribonucleoproteins. See *immunoelectrophoresis*.

covalent bond A chemical bond in which each atom donates one or more electrons that are subsequently shared between the two atoms.

C-reactive protein An acute phase protein synthesized by the liver that is used as a biomarker to detect inflammation and cardiac risk.

creatine kinase CK; an enzyme found in all muscles and the brain.

creatine kinase isoenzymes Multiple forms of the creatine kinase enzyme that can be measured to indicate cell damage in specific tissues.

creatine kinase MB CK-MB; isoenzyme of creatine kinase that is found in high concentrations in cardiac muscle; levels rise in the bloodstream usually 3 to 4 hours after a myocardial infarction and may return to the previous level within 36 hours.

creatinine A breakdown product of creatinine phosphate in muscle; its rate of clearance by the kidney is an indicator of renal function.

creatinine clearance A test used to measure the glomerular filtration rate.

cretinism See *congenital hypothyroidism*.

Creutzfeldt-Jakob disease A rare disease of the central nervous system in humans caused by prions.

critical value Also called panic value; a test value that indicates a life-threatening condition.

Crohn disease An inflammatory bowel disease associated with malabsorption, usually found in the small intestine but can occur anywhere in the gastrointestinal tract.

crossmatch A critical assay used in organ transplantation to determine whether a recipient's serum contains preformed antibodies against lymphocytes from a donor candidate. A negative test indicates compatibility for safe transplantation.

cross-reactivity The ability of an antibody to react with an unrelated antigen molecule.

Cushing syndrome A disease in which a pituitary adenoma causes excess secretion of ACTH, resulting in high circulating cortisol levels and Cushing syndrome. It is differentiated from an ACTH-producing adrenal or ectopic tumor by suppression of the excess ACTH after a high dose of dexamethasone.

customer service Meeting the customer's requirements.

cuvette A small vessel used to hold a liquid sample to be read in the light path of the spectrophotometer.

cyanosis A condition resulting from decreased oxygen saturation (sO_2) caused by a high concentration of nonfunctional hemoglobin.

cyclosporine An immunosuppressant drug that inhibits calcineurin signaling, which is essential to lymphocyte proliferation.

cystatin C A protein used mainly as a biomarker of kidney function; increased levels indicate a reduced glomerular filtration rate.

cysteine crystals A type of pathological crystals found in urine.

cystic duct Duct from the gallbladder that joins with the hepatic duct from the liver to empty bile into the small intestine.

cystinuria Genetic condition that leads to the development of cystine crystals of stones in the kidney or bladder.

cystitis Inflammation of the bladder that is caused by a bacterial infection.

cystolithiasis The presence of stones in the urinary bladder.

cytochrome P-450 Pathway of oxidation-reduction and hydrolysis that is catalyzed by specific enzymes found in hepatocyte membranes. This pathway is used to convert a toxic chemical to a less toxic form.

cytokines Small proteins that carry chemical messages between cells.

cytoplasm The material that is contained within the cell membrane; surrounds the nucleus and cell organelles.

D

Dalton's law Each gas in a mixture exerts the same pressure as if it were alone in solution.

data management Transcription and reporting of patients' test results.

deamination of amino acids Removal of the amino group from amino acids before their conversion into carbohydrates or fats; an important function of the liver in protein metabolism.

decontamination The removal of contaminating substances from an object.

Defense Threat Reduction Agency U.S. Department of Defense Army depot that researches, develops, and maintains effective countermeasures for military personnel against toxic chemicals.

degree of differentiation of a tumor The degree to which tumor cells resemble normal cells; normal tissues are 100% differentiated.

dehydration Presence of too little intravascular water (due to excessive water loss or decreased water intake).

dehydroepiandrosterone DHEA; an androgen secreted by the adrenal cortex.

dehydroepiandrosterone sulfate DHEA-S; an androgen secreted by the adrenal cortex.

delayed hypersensitivity reaction A hypersensitivity immune reaction that does not manifest until hours or days after exposure to an antigen.

delta check Comparison of the most recent patient test results with previously determined results for the same patient; used to detect mislabeled samples or other laboratory errors.

dementia Chronic disorder of mental processes caused by a brain disease that results in memory loss, shortened attention span, and decreased reasoning abilities.

denaturation Process that separates the strands of double-stranded DNA by breaking the hydrogen bonds between the nucleotides.

Department of Homeland Security U.S. government department that is responsible for immigration, border management, disaster preparedness, cyberspace security, and terrorism prevention.

designer drug A slightly modified version of a known narcotic or pharmaceutical agent that is not regulated by the U.S. Food and Drug Administration. These may be sold to the general public under coded labels—such as bath salts, plant food, or herbal supplements—with the intention of being used as recreational drugs.

detection Discovery of the presence or existence of something.

detection window The period during which a drug or chemical can be detected in body fluids after acute exposure.

detector Component of an instrument that detects the characteristics of light after it has passed through a sample being tested.

diabetes insipidus A condition associated with excessive thirst and the production of large amounts of dilute urine; caused by low levels of antidiuretic hormone due to excessive fluid intake (dipsogenic), deficient production (neurogenic), or insensitivity of the nephron (nephrogenic).

diabetes mellitus A group of diseases in which the pancreas fails to produce sufficient insulin due to autoimmune processes (type 1), or due to insulin resistance with or without a secretory defect (type 2), or as a complication of pregnancy (gestational). It is characterized by chronic hyperglycemia and over time can lead to diabetic retinopathy, nephropathy, neuropathy, and atherosclerosis.

diabetic ketoacidosis DKA; a complication of diabetes mellitus (primarily type 1) related to lack of circulating insulin; adipocytes (fat cells) release free fatty acids that stimulate the liver to produce more ketone bodies than can be used by the body, resulting in a metabolic acidosis.

diabetic nephropathy Diabetes-related damage to the glomerular basement membrane due to increased protein deposits that can lead to renal failure.

diabetic neuropathy Nerve damage related to diabetes; may lead diabetics not to realize that they have suffered trauma.

diabetic retinopathy Progressive loss of vision as a consequence of diabetes; can involve cataracts, glaucoma, and retinal detachments.

diabetic ulcer A type of ulcer found in diabetics; usually occurs on the foot and is caused by decreased blood flow and decreased pain sensation.

diagnostic sensitivity Ability of a test to detect the presence of a disease in an individual who actually has the disease. It is reported as the percentage of people with the disease who will have a positive result on the test.

diagnostic specificity Ability of a test to detect the absence of a disease in an individual who actually does not have the disease. It is reported as the percentage of people without the disease who will have a negative result on the test.

diarrhea Loose, watery, or frequent stools.

diastole Refilling of the heart with blood.

diastolic Second number of a blood pressure measurement; amount of pressure in the heart when it is at rest or refilling.

diffraction grating In a spectrophotometer, a device consisting of a glass plate with a thin metal coating containing many small parallel grooves to isolate the light beam and adjust the radiant energy reaching the photodetector.

DiGeorge syndrome Also called congenital thymic aplasia or hypoplasia; a rare congenital disease that affects T-cell maturation and is caused by the deletion of several genes from chromosome 22.

digestive enzymes Enzymes secreted by various organs in the gastrointestinal tract that help break down carbohydrates, proteins, and lipids into absorbable components.

1,25-dihydroxyvitamin D₃ Calcitriol; the active circulating form of vitamin D that is produced from cholecalciferol.

dipsogenic diabetes insipidus Condition in which excessive fluid intake lowers plasma osmolality to a level below the threshold for secretion of antidiuretic hormone.

dirty bomb A type of bomb that uses a conventional explosive to disperse radioactive material over a large area.

discoid lupus Skin condition observed in systemic lupus erythematosus; consists of plaques on sun-exposed areas with follicular plugging and scarring.

discrete analyzer An analyzer that allows laboratory technicians to select individual tests to be run on samples, each of which is contained in a separate reaction vessel.

disease Any deviation from or interruption of the normal structure or function of a part, organ, or system of the body as manifested by characteristic symptoms and signs.

disease mechanism An altered physiologic process or condition, such as inflammation, hyperplasia, or necrosis, that leads to disease.

diurnal variation Pattern of hormone secretion that is related to the sleep–wake cycle of an individual.

diverticulitis A condition in which inflammation is associated with diverticula; see *diverticulosis.*

diverticulosis Condition of having diverticula, which are outpouchings or weak areas in the large intestine.

DNA probe Small segments of DNA that are designed to attract other complementary pieces of DNA in a biological system. They are used to identify genes or specific DNA sequences in samples.

donor testing In transplantation medicine, the testing undergone by the donor that happens before histocompatibility matching and is equivalent to that associated with blood donation.

dose–response curve Graphical representation of the relationship between the dose of a drug and the response elicited; established to correlate signal values to known analyte concentrations.

Down syndrome (trisomy 21) A common and serious developmental disorder in which the affected individual has one extra copy of the long arm of chromosome 21. It is characterized clinically by moderate to severe mental retardation, hypotonia, congenital heart defects, and flat facial profile.

drill Type of training, such as a fire drill or evacuation drill, that involves practicing a specific aspect of the prepared response to an emergency.

drug concentration Relative amount of drug in the blood or other tissue that determines the drug's effectiveness.

drug–drug interaction Competition between drugs for attachment to the active site of an enzyme; can slow the rate of metabolism of each drug.

dry chemical extinguisher A type of extinguisher that can be used on class A, B, or C fires; uses a noncombustible dry chemical such as bicarbonate or monoammonium phosphate to smother the fire and prevent reignition.

Duchenne muscular dystrophy The most common and most severe form of muscular dystrophy. Individuals who develop this X-linked disease cannot produce dystrophin, a protein that normally stabilizes and protects muscle fibers.

dyspnea Shortness of breath.

E

eclampsia A life-threatening manifestation of preeclampsia in which a mother experiences grand mal seizures or falls into a coma; can lead to intracranial hemorrhage.

ectopic disease A disease of the endocrine system in which a hormone-secreting tumor is present in the body (other than in the target organ or in the hypothalamus or pituitary); see *primary disease* and *secondary disease.*

ectopic pregnancy Refers to the implantation of a fertilized egg somewhere outside the uterus.

edema Swelling.

Edwards syndrome (trisomy 18) A life-threatening disorder caused by an error in cell division that results in the presence of an extra copy of all or part of chromosome 18. It is characterized clinically by skeletal malformations; abnormalities of the heart, kidneys, and other internal organs; feeding and breathing difficulties; and developmental delays.

eicosanoid Any of a class of arachidonic acid–derived hormones that control the production of hormones and many physiologic functions. They consist of prostaglandins, thromboxanes, leukotrienes, and lipoxins.

elastase Enzyme that breaks down the elastic fibers in lung tissue.

electrocardiogram Test that measures the electrical conduction system of the heart.

electrochemiluminescence Type of luminescence in which the excitation event is caused by an electrochemical reaction rather than by photoillumination.

electrolytes Charged particles that sustain life by transmitting electrochemical impulses in nerves and muscles, playing a role in osmotic pressure, distributing water in the body, and controlling cell permeability.

electron ionization An ionization method widely used in mass spectrometry in which energetic electrons interact with gas phase atoms or molecules to produce ions.

electrophoresis Separation of analytes on an electrophoretic medium with the use of an electrical current.

electrospray ionization The ion source of choice to couple liquid chromatography with mass spectrometry.

elevated anion gap acidosis Acidosis that includes an increased anion gap.

embryo Term for a fertilized ovum from the time of implantation until the 10th week of pregnancy, after which it is termed a fetus.

emergency preparedness Planning, training, and education regarding any potential threats to a community; includes identifying the characteristics of specific emergency situations and demonstrating response actions for each emergency.

emphysema Disease in which the alveoli of the lungs are destroyed, leading to loss of elasticity and poor gas exchange. This results in hyperventilation, lowered cardiac output, and tissue hypoxia throughout the body.

encephalitis Term for a viral infection of the brain.

encephalocele A neural tube defect in which a sac containing brain tissue and membranes protrudes through an abnormal opening in the skull.

endocarditis Inflammation of the innermost lining of the heart.

endometrium The lining of the uterus.

endonuclease An enzyme that splits a nucleic acid by hydrolyzing an internal phosphodiester bond; used to produce DNA fragments of different lengths as part of the restriction fragment length polymorphism (RFLP) technique.

endothelial cell A cell in the inner lining of a blood or lymphatic vessel that can retract, allowing leukocytes and fluid to enter the interstitial space.

endotoxin A toxin produced by any of certain bacterial species that damages the body's cells. The cell walls of gram-negative organisms contain substances that become toxins when the bacteria die.

end-point or one-point method A method used to measure the catalytic activity of enzymes in which the reaction is started and allowed to continue for a fixed period of time and then stopped, after which the amount of product generated is measured.

engineering controls Devices, such as sharps disposal containers and self-sheathing needles, that remove, eliminate, or isolate the sharps hazard.

enzyme A biological catalyst that increases biochemical reaction rates without undergoing permanent changes or being consumed.

enzyme kinetics The rate of a chemical reaction under specific reaction conditions.

enzyme-linked immunosorbent assay ELISA; a type of immunoassay used to measure hormones, antibodies, biomarkers, drugs, and toxins; samples are incubated in wells onto which antibodies have been absorbed, and after enzymes and a substrate are added, the absorbance of the sample wells is measured. Sample absorbance is inversely proportional to the concentration of the analyte.

enzyme-multiplied immunoassay technique EMIT; a type of immunoassay used primarily for quantitation of therapeutic drugs and drugs of abuse; a sample is mixed with known concentrations of antibody and the analyte of interest bound to an enzyme; drug in the sample (if any) competes for antibody binding sites, and binding deactivates the enzyme. The remaining concentration of analyte-bound free enzyme produces greater enzyme activity in direct proportion to the amount of drug in the sample.

enzyme–substrate complex Also known as the ES complex or the adduct; formed by noncovalent binding forces between the enzyme molecule and the substrate molecule; an intermediate step in enzyme-catalyzed reactions.

epididymitis Inflammation of the epididymis, the tightly coiled portion of the sperm duct that connects each testicle to its vas deferens.

epidural hematoma An accumulation of blood in the space between the dura mater and the bone.

epinephrine Also known as adrenaline; one of the catecholamine hormones secreted by the adrenal medulla.

epitope The part of an antigen that is recognized by an antibody. Each antibody has an affinity and avidity for a specific epitope.

equipment maintenance program A component of quality management that requires documentation of the installation and calibration of a new instrument as well as all maintenance performed on it and any corrective actions. It also includes the preventive maintenance plan that guides troubleshooting and repair of the instrument.

ergonomic hazard The potential risk of injury that is inherent in tasks involving prolonged repetitive motion.

erythropoietin A hormone secreted by the kidney that increases the production of red blood cells.

essential fatty acid A fatty acid that is necessary for health but must be ingested because the body cannot synthesize it; includes α-linoleic acid and linolenic acid.

ester An alcohol derivative of carboxylic acid; found in many plants and in reagents used in chemical tests.

estrogen receptor Type of tumor marker; in a woman with breast cancer, the presence of estrogen and progesterone receptors leads to a better prognosis with hormone treatment.

euthyroid sick syndrome A condition, associated with hospitalized patients, in which the thyroid gland functions normally despite abnormal levels of thyroxine-binding globulin.

everolimus An inhibitor of the mammalian target of rapamycin (mTOR) that is derived from sirolimus and has different pharmacokinetics but similar side effects.

expert systems In transplantation medicine, computer algorithms for automated test ordering.

exposure control plan A required system to protect employees from exposure to blood, body fluids, and other potentially infectious materials; includes identifying and mitigating potential exposures through employee training, universal precautions, engineering and work practice controls, good housekeeping, and use of personal protective equipment, as well as documentation, evaluation, and follow-up after exposures.

external audit Systematic assessment of staff and equipment as well as all policies, processes, and procedures in the laboratory that is performed by an outside group such as an accrediting agency.

external respiration The exchange of oxygen and carbon dioxide between the alveoli and capillaries of the lungs.

extracellular Outside a cell's walls.

extracellular fluid The fluid located between cells in the body.

extravascular compartment The tissues of the body outside the lymph and blood vessels.

exudate A high-protein fluid with a high number of cells; it is produced by an inflammatory reaction or lymph system blockage.

exudation Oozing of fluid.

F

false negative Result that occurs when an individual has a condition but the test indicates that he or she does not have it.

false positive Result that occurs when an individual does not have a condition but the test indicates that the condition is present.

familial combined hyperlipidemia Also called familial combined hyperlipoproteinemia; refers to several conditions within families involving increased levels of lipoproteins—total cholesterol and low-density lipoprotein cholesterol (Fredrickson type IIa), triglycerides (type IV), or both (type IIb).

familial hypercholesterolemia Condition within families that is caused by a genetic mutation in the receptor gene for low-density lipoprotein; cholesterol is deposited in the skin, tendons, and arteries, with cutaneous xanthomas appearing before 30 years of age.

familial hypertriglyceridemia A fairly common disease within families that is inherited in an autosomal dominant pattern with delayed expression. The very-low-density lipoproteins in this condition are large and have an abnormally high triglyceride content.

familial hypocalciuric hypercalcemia A benign condition that occurs in families and is characterized by high blood calcium and low urinary calcium levels.

fat bodies Degenerated tubular cells containing abundant lipid; excreted in the urine in nephrotic syndrome.

fatty acid Carboxylic acid with long chains of carbon groups.

fecal fat The amount of fat in stool; also, a test used to detect malabsorption of dietary fat.

fecal fat test A nonspecific test used to determine whether there is increased fat in the stool.

fecal pancreatic elastase 1 A type of enzyme-linked immunosorbent assay used to evaluate exocrine pancreatic function.

Federal Emergency Management Agency FEMA; U.S. government agency responsible for disaster and emergency preparedness and response planning for natural and man-made disasters.

fentanyl A synthetic opioid that is eighty times more potent than morphine and hundreds of times stronger than heroin.

ferritin An iron-storage molecule that consists of an apoferritin shell surrounding an iron core complex of ferric oxyhydroxide.

ferrous protoporphyrin IX An immediate precursor of heme, the iron-containing constituent of hemoglobin and other respiratory pigments.

fetal hemoglobin Also known as hemoglobin F; the main type of hemoglobin present before birth; composed of two α-proteins and two γ-proteins, each of which contains a heme group. During the first year of life, it is slowly replaced by the normal adult hemoglobin A.

α-fetoprotein AFP; a small glycoprotein consisting of one peptide chain. It is a tumor marker associated with hepatocellular cancer that can be used for diagnosis and to assess the efficacy of treatment.

fetus Term that refers to a developing baby between 10 weeks of gestation and birth.

fiberoptics Also known as flexible light pipes; bundles of thin transparent fibers of glass, quartz, or plastic that are enclosed by a material with a lower index of refraction and transmit light through internal reflections.

fibrinogen An acute phase protein; in clot building, it is cleaved by thrombin to produce fibrin.

fibroma A benign tumor of fibrous tissue.

fibrosarcoma A malignant tumor originating from fibrous tissue.

fibrosis Scar tissue.

fight or flight response A coordinated effort of the nervous and endocrine systems that prepares the body for immediate strenuous activity.

filters Devices for spectral isolation that are used in spectrophotometers.

flag A label or note indicating that a result needs further action.

flammable Easy to ignite or set on fire.

flow cytometry A technique in which measurements are performed while cells or particles pass through a measuring device in a fluid stream in single file.

fluidics In automated instruments, the system by which specific fluids are moved to a particular location so they can react; includes pipetting and dispensing of specimens, reagents, and wash solutions.

fluorescence Occurs when a molecule absorbs light at one wavelength and reemits light at a longer wavelength.

fluorescence polarization A technique in which the rotational relaxation of a large fluorescent-labeled molecule (or of a small fluorophore attached to a large molecule such as an antibody) is slower than the fluorescence decay time of the molecule, causing the emitted light to become polarized; the intensity of the emitted light is measured in the vertical and horizontal planes, the polarization is calculated from an equation, and a standard curve is developed.

fluorescence polarization immunoassay FPIA; a homogeneous, competitive immunoassay in which labeled, antibody-bound antigen in the sample competes with labeled, free antigen for antibody binding sites; used to quantitate analytes according to the change in fluorescence polarization after an immunologic reaction. It provides accurate and sensitive quantitative measurements of therapeutic and abused drugs, toxic substances, and hormones.

fluorometer An instrument that uses filter monochrometers to isolate excitation and emission light.

fluorometry A technique for measuring emitted fluorescence; a method in which the analyte is complexed with a compound that fluoresces, and the amount of fluorescent light emitted in the final solution is directly proportional to the amount of analyte present.

fluorophore An atom or molecule that fluoresces.

foam cells Form when macrophages become engorged with cholesterol esters. The earliest indication of atherogenic lesions.

folate and vitamin B$_{12}$ deficiency anemia A type macrocytic anemia that occurs when the body does not get enough folate and vitamin B$_{12}$, resulting in enlarged red blood cells.

folic acid Also known as folate; a B vitamin that is involved in the production of red blood cells, among other functions. It is closely tied to vitamin B$_{12}$ and iron balance in the body.

follicle-stimulating hormone FSH; a hormone released from the anterior pituitary gland that stimulates testicular growth and the synthesis and release of testosterone in the male and ovulation in the female.

follicular cells Cells in the thyroid gland that secrete thyroid hormones.

forensic specimen A specimen used in a civil or criminal legal case. Highly standardized protocols must be followed for proper collection and handling.

Fredrickson classification of lipid disorders System developed to classify lipid disorders based on abnormal lipoprotein levels.

free drug The amount of a drug that is unbound in the circulation and therefore is available for distribution, activity within cells, and elimination.

free radicals Chemically unstable molecules that readily react with other molecules, resulting in chemical damage.

Friedewald formula Calculation used to estimate the concentration of low-density lipoprotein in the blood based on measured levels of total cholesterol, high-density lipoprotein, and triglycerides.

frostbite Freezing of body tissue caused by extended exposure to subfreezing temperatures.

frostnip Damage to body tissue caused by extended exposure to subfreezing temperatures; the tissue turns white and begins the freezing process.

fructosamine A laboratory test that reflects glucose control in a 3- to 6-week window; the test is affected by levels of protein in the blood.

full-scale exercise Part of planning and training for emergency or hazardous situations, usually conducted on a regional or statewide basis; resources are mobilized to practice the response to a planned incident.

fume hood A ventilation device in the clinical laboratory that limits toxic or hazardous fumes, dust, and particles by enclosing the work area and pulling air out of the area via a duct or other filtration system.

G

gas chromatography Type of chromatography in which a gaseous mobile phase is used to carry a mixture of volatile solutes through a column containing the stationary phase; it cannot be reused.

gas chromatography with mass spectrometry GC-MS; an analytical method that combines the features of gas chromatography and mass spectrometry; often used to confirm and quantitate a positive screening test result.

gastrin A hormone that stimulates secretion of gastric acid (i.e., hydrochloric acid) by the parietal cells of the stomach; secreted by the stomach in response to neurogenic brain impulses as food enters the stomach.

gastrinoma A benign, non–β-islet cell, gastrin-secreting tumor.

Gaucher disease Rare genetic disorder that affects the production of β-glucocerebrosidase; there are three types of this disease.

Gaussian curve Also known as a normal or Gaussian distribution; a bell-shaped distribution curve that includes the small percentage of errors, such as random errors in laboratory testing; it is symmetrical about the mean, which is at the center of the curve.

gestational diabetes mellitus A variable degree of carbohydrate intolerance with onset during pregnancy.

giantism Produced by an excessive amount of growth hormone in a child or adolescent.

Gilbert syndrome Also called Gilbert cholemia; a common genetic condition in which an abnormal liver enzyme affects the breakdown of hemoglobin, leading to mild elevations of bilirubin without other consequences.

globulin Any of a group of simple proteins that are insoluble in water but soluble in salt solutions. Globulins form a large fraction of blood serum proteins.

glomerular filtration rate The amount of blood that is filtered through the kidney per minute.

glomerular filtration The primary filtering action of the kidney; wastes and excess fluid are removed from the blood and passed into the kidney tubules to form urine.

glomerulonephritis Inflammation of the glomerulus.

glucagon Regulates blood glucose by stimulating the breakdown of glycogen to glucose.

glucocorticoids A class of hormones produced in the adrenal cortex; includes cortisol, cortisone, and corticosterone.

gluconeogenesis See *glyconeogenesis*.

glucuronyl transferase An enzyme that conjugates bilirubin to a water-soluble form.

glucose oxidase method Common method for measuring glucose in body fluids including cerebrospinal fluid; a coupled enzyme assay in which glucose oxidase first catalyzes the reaction of glucose, water, and oxygen into gluconic acid and hydrogen peroxide, after which a chemical reaction step (indicator reaction) produces a measurable chromagen.

glucose-6-phosphate dehydrogenase (G6PD) deficiency An inherited X-linked disorder that is one of the most common disease-producing enzyme deficiencies; leads to early red blood cell destruction and anemia, decreases the haptoglobin level, and increases the concentration of indirect (unconjugated) bilirubin.

γ-glutamyl transferase GGT, also known as γ-glutamyl transpeptidase; a liver enzyme that is used to evaluate liver function.

glycogenesis Conversion of glucose into glycogen in the liver and muscles.

glycogenolysis The conversion of glycogen to glucose in the liver.

glycohemoglobin See *glycosylated hemoglobin*.

glyconeogenesis The production of glucose from noncarbohydrates, primarily in the liver.

glycoprotein hormones A family of protein hormones that have identical α subunits but unique β-chains; in humans, these include chorionic gonadotropin, follicle-stimulating hormone, luteinizing hormone, and thyroid-stimulating hormone.

glycoprotein A protein that is composed of a peptide chain with one or more carbohydrate moieties. Glycoproteins are abundant in living organisms and have diverse functions related to their specific structures.

glycosylated hemoglobin Also known as glycohemoglobin; hemoglobin that is bound to glucose; can be measured to quantitate an individual's blood glucose level. See *hemoglobin A$_{1C}$*.

gonadotropin-releasing hormone A hormone secreted by the hypothalamus; stimulates the release of follicle-stimulating hormone and luteinizing hormone from the pituitary.

Goodpasture syndrome A rare pulmonary-renal syndrome in which a type II hypersensitivity reaction creates autoantibodies against collagen type IV in the glomerular basement membrane.

gout An arthritic condition in which monosodium urate monohydrate crystals are deposited in joints.

governing board The body responsible for the financial health of a hospital organization and for setting institutional policies and goals; appoints the medical staff as the party responsible for quality patient care.

grading A system of measuring and identifying tumor size and behavior performed by a pathologist according to medical standards; usually based on a scale from least aggressive (grade I) to most aggressive (grade III or IV). Higher-grade tumors are poorly differentiated, have highly atypical cells, and tend to metastasize early in the disease.

graft-versus-host disease GVHD; occurs when immunoreactive cells of a transplanted organ begin to attack the tissues of the transplant recipient.

gram per deciliter concentration g/dL; the number of grams of a compound dissolved in 100 mL of water.

granuloma A response to chronic inflammation in which macrophages accumulate around a walled-off local infection.

Graves disease Autoimmune disease in which the body produces antibodies to thyroid-stimulating hormone receptors, resulting in overproduction of thyroid hormones; the most common hyperthyroid disease.

growth hormone GH; a peptide hormone produced by the anterior pituitary that promotes growth in infants, children, and adolescents.

Guillain-Barré syndrome GBS; a nervous system disorder that is usually temporary and is caused by the production of an autoantibody against myelin after immunization or an infection; if not treated, it can lead to paralysis of the respiratory muscles.

H

hairy cell leukemia HCL; a type of chronic lymphoid leukemia in which the abnormal B lymphocytes have hairlike cytoplasmic projections on their surface.

half-life The time it takes for the concentration of a drug to fall by half.

Halotron A clean fire-extinguishing agent that is approved for use in handheld extinguishers and larger fire-extinguishing systems for marine and aviation applications. It leaves no residue, is noncorrosive, and will not damage equipment after discharge.

hapten A small molecule that cannot elicit an immune response unless it is attached to a large carrier molecule such as a protein.

haptoglobin A protein that is synthesized in the liver and binds to any free hemoglobin released into the circulation by hemolysis.

Hashimoto thyroiditis A thyroid disease in which autoantibodies cause cell- and antibody-mediated destruction of the thyroid gland, leading to goiter or atrophy; the most common form of primary hypothyroidism.

hazard communication Regulated by the Hazard Communication standard, which is intended to protect workers from illnesses and injuries due to chemical exposure and specifies information and training about chemical hazards and protective measures.

hazardous chemicals Regulated by the Occupational Exposure to Hazardous Chemicals in Laboratories standard, which covers routes of exposure, chemical inventory, storage of chemicals, chemical spills, and compressed gases.

health A state of complete physical, mental, and social well-being and not merely the absence of disease or infirmity.

heart valvular disease A disease in which one or more of the primary valves of the heart (bicuspid, tricuspid, aortic, and pulmonary) has been damaged by infection, medication, or trauma.

heat cramps The mildest form of heat illness; painful muscle cramps that occur when an individual loses water and salt through excessive sweating.

heat exhaustion Heat illness with symptoms that include pale and moist skin, fever, nausea, vomiting, diarrhea, headache, fatigue, weakness, anxiety, and faint feeling; usually diagnosed clinically, but glucose and troponin I and T tests are needed to rule out hypoglycemia and coronary disease.

heat stroke A medical emergency that can lead to death if not treated immediately; heat gain overwhelms the body's ability to lose heat, leading to hyperthermia, neurologic dysfunction, tachycardia, hyperventilation, gastrointestinal hemorrhage, hepatic injury, rhabdomyolysis, and acute kidney injury.

helicase An enzyme that enables DNA and RNA replication by separating the double-stranded nucleic acids.

Helicobacter pylori A species of bacteria, several strains of which are pathogenic and are associated with the formation of ulcers in the stomach and small intestine; can be detected by biopsy and culture or by breath tests for bacteria-secreted urease or stool tests for *H. pylori* antigen.

HELLP syndrome A pregnancy-related condition characterized by hemolysis, elevated liver enzymes, and low platelet counts with preeclampsia; leads to thrombocytopenia and disseminated intravascular coagulation.

hematology The study of blood, blood-forming organs, and blood diseases.

hematopoietic stem cells Multipotent progenitor cells that give rise to all other blood cells; located primarily in the bone marrow and in umbilical cord blood.

hematuria Blood cells in the urine.

hemochromatosis Iron overload.

hemodialysis A method for cleansing the blood of metabolic waste by use of a device that employs semipermeable membranes as filters when the kidneys are unable to function appropriately.

hemoglobin A$_{1c}$ Test that measures the average level of glucose in red blood cells over the last 2 to 4 months; used as an indicator for the adequacy of glucose control in individuals with diabetes mellitus.

hemoglobin C A hemoglobin variant in which a lysine residue is substituted for glutamic acid

at position 6 of the β-globin chain; this mutation reduces the normal plasticity of red blood cells.

hemoglobin E A β-globin chain hemoglobin variant in which a lysine residue replaces glutamic acid at position 26; the substitution may produce a mild anemia.

hemoglobin electrophoresis A technique in which a cellulose acetate medium is used to separate different types of hemoglobin in whole blood samples.

hemoglobin S A form of hemoglobin in which there is a substitution of valine for glutamic acid at position 6 in the α-helix of the β-globin; see *heterozygous hemoglobin S* and *homozygous hemoglobin S*.

hemoglobin SC Refers to the inheritance of one gene for hemoglobin S and one for hemoglobin C. Both β-globin chains have substitutions for the glutamic acid at position 6: a valine in the hemoglobin S and a lysine in the hemoglobin C.

hemoglobin structure The hemoglobin molecule is composed of four globin chains, two α-proteins and two β-proteins, each of which cradles a molecule of heme in its tertiary structure.

hemolysis The rupture or destruction of red blood cells, as when they are mechanically lysed by the phlebotomy needle.

hemolytic disease of the newborn HDN; an autoimmune disease that develops when a fetus's red blood cells (RBCs) contain an antigen that the mother's RBCs lack, usually because of Rh or ABO blood group incompatibility; the mother's immune system produces antibodies against the fetal antigen that pass through the placenta and cause hemolysis and other serious effects in the fetus.

hemopexin A protein that binds heme after breakdown of the hemoglobin molecule.

hemosiderin Iron-storage granules that represent partly degraded, aggregated ferritin molecules whose shells have been digested by lysozymes. Hemosiderin is the end of the intracellular storage iron pathway.

Henderson-Hasselbalch equation Equation that quantitates how carbon dioxide (i.e., the concentration of bicarbonate ion), pH, and the partial pressure of carbon dioxide (pCO_2) in the blood are interrelated: $pH = 6.103 + log[HCO_3^-]/0.306 \times pCO_2$.

Henry's law At a constant temperature, the amount of gas dissolved in a solution is directly proportional to the partial pressure of the gas and the solubility of the gas.

hepatic artery The artery that delivers oxygenated blood to the liver.

hepatic duct The duct that transports bile out of the liver, then joins with the cystic duct from the gallbladder to empty into the small intestine.

hepatic encephalopathy Neurologic condition caused by the deleterious effects of liver failure on the central nervous system; can result in sleep issues, psychiatric changes, tremors, coma, and death.

hepatic portal vein The vein that delivers nutrient-rich but oxygen-poor blood to the liver.

hepatitis Inflammation of the liver caused by chemicals, trauma, drugs, or a virus.

hepatomegaly Enlargement of the liver.

HER2 A gene that is mutated in about 20% of advanced breast cancers and produces the human epidermal growth factor receptor 2

(HER2). *HER2* amplification is a prognostic factor (indicating susceptibility of the tumor to treatment with trastuzumab) and can be used to monitor therapy.

hereditary hemochromatosis An autosomal recessive genetic defect that causes abnormally high absorption of iron from the gastrointestinal tract and iron deposition in the liver and other organs.

heterogeneous immunoassay A type of immunoassay that requires a wash step to separate free labeled antigen from bound labeled antigen in the test solution.

heterozygous hemoglobin S Refers to inheritance of only a single copy of the hemoglobin S gene; the severity of the resulting disease, called sickle cell trait, correlates with the amount of hemoglobin S in red blood cells, but the hemoglobin S also provides some protection against malaria.

hexokinase method A coupled enzyme assay commonly used to measure glucose in body fluids; in the first reaction, hexokinase modifies glucose to glucose-6-phosphate (G6P), and in the second reaction (the indicator reaction), the G6P is acted on by G6P dehydrogenase to form 6-phophogluconate. Reduced nicotinamide adenine dinucleotide (NADH) or the reduced phosphate (NADPH) is produced as part of the indicator reaction in direct proportion to the amount of glucose in the specimen.

high-density lipoprotein HDL; the smallest and densest of the lipoprotein particles; transports cholesterol from the cells to the liver for conversion into bile acids.

high-performance liquid chromatography Modern liquid chromatography that uses very small stationary phase particles and a relatively high performance.

hirsutism A condition, usually caused by increased androgen levels, that in women consists of excessive terminal hair growth in a post-pubertal male pattern.

histamine A chemical mediator of acute inflammation; contracts bronchial smooth muscle, increases vascular permeability, and dilates blood vessels.

HLA typing See *tissue typing* and *human leukocyte antigen*.

Hodgkin lymphoma Abnormal growth of lymphoid tissue in lymph nodes and vessels that originates from abnormal B cells; see also *non-Hodgkin lymphoma*.

homeostasis A balanced or relatively stable state of equilibrium.

homocysteine A protein synthesized in the body from the amino acid cysteine that is a risk factor for development of atherosclerosis; it is toxic to endothelial cells, and elevated blood levels can produce heart attacks and strokes even in teenagers.

homozygous hemoglobin S Refers to the inheritance of two copies of the hemoglobin S gene, resulting in sickle cell disease.

hormone One of many regulatory substances secreted into the blood by endocrine glands to communicate within and among local cells, distant cells, and the nervous system; hormones assist development, enable reproduction, support body processes, and direct responses to stimuli.

human chorionic gonadotropin hCG or β-hCG; a hormone secreted by the placenta that is measured as a reliable indicator of pregnancy; it is also a tumor marker for gonadal (ovary and testicular) choriocarcinoma.

human leukocyte antigen HLA; a protein of the major histocompatibility complex in humans that serves as a marker of self; class I HLAs are present on almost all cells, whereas class II proteins are concentrated on more specialized antigen-presenting cells such as macrophages, dendritic cells, and B cells.

hybridoma A hybrid cell line formed when antibody-producing B cells from mice sensitized to a particular antigen are fused with myeloma cells.

hydrocarbon A compound made of hydrogen and carbon atoms; can be arranged as straight chains, branched chains, or rings.

hydrocephalus A hydrodynamic disorder characterized by disturbance of the flow, formation, or absorption of cerebrospinal fluid (CSF); leads to increased volume occupied by the CSF in the central nervous system and associated neurologic symptoms.

hydrolase An enzyme that catalyzes hydrolysis reactions.

hydrostatic edema Edema that occurs when increased hydrostatic pressure exerted by the intracellular fluid forces water out of the vessels and into the tissue.

hydrostatic pressure Pressure exerted on the outer walls of blood vessels by the intracellular fluid of the cells in the surrounding tissue.

β-hydroxybutyric acid Hydroxybutyrate; an acid that has both hydroxyl and carboxylic acid functional groups; one of three ketone bodies produced in the liver as a result of catabolism of fatty acids.

hyperbilirubinemia A condition in which there is a high level of unconjugated (indirect) bilirubin in the blood, usually with no serious consequences.

hypercalcemia Increased plasma calcium level.

hypercapnia An increased partial pressure of carbon dioxide (pCO_2) in arterial blood.

hyperchloremia An increased level of chloride in plasma.

hyperemesis gravidarum A severe form of nausea and vomiting in pregnancy that is accompanied by ketosis and weight loss.

hyperkalemia An elevated blood potassium level that results when potassium leaves the cells faster than it can be excreted by the kidneys.

hypermagnesemia Rare condition of increased magnesium levels.

hypernatremia An increased sodium level in the blood.

hyperosmolar hyperglycemic nonketotic syndrome HHNKS; a complication of diabetes mellitus (primarily type 2) in which very high glucose levels lead to severe volume depletion, intracellular dehydration, and neurologic changes.

hyperphosphatemia An increased level of phosphate in the blood.

hyperplasia An increase in the number of cells of a specific type in response to injury or stress.

hypersensitivity An exaggerated immune response that leads to tissue damage; signals, cells, or processes of the immune response can become abnormal or impaired due to genetic or environmental influences.

hypertension Abnormally high blood pressure.

hypertensive retinopathy Damage to the retina that is caused by high blood pressure and leads to loss of vision.

hyperthermia Increased body temperature.

hyperthyroidism Increased levels of thyroid hormones.

hypertrophy Increase in cell size in response to injury or stress.

hyperventilation Increased breathing rate.

hypocalcemia Decreased plasma calcium level.

hypocapnia A decreased partial pressure of carbon dioxide (pCO_2) in arterial blood.

hypochloremia A decreased level of chloride in plasma.

hypoglycemia A blood glucose level lower than 55 mg/dL in an adult.

hypokalemia A decreased level of potassium in the blood; can result from low potassium intake over time or from increased loss due to vomiting, diarrhea, gastrointestinal problems, or diuretic use.

hypomagnesemia Common condition of decreased magnesium levels.

hyponatremia A decreased plasma sodium level.

hypoparathyroidism A disease involving caused by low or zero levels of parathyroid hormone that results from an injury to the parathyroid or thyroid gland during neck trauma or surgery.

hypophosphatemia A decreased level of phosphate in the blood.

hypopigmentation A disorder involving loss of pigment in the skin, hair, and/or eyes caused by a mutation in one or more genes responsible for melanin synthesis, distribution of pigment by the melanocyte, and melanosome biogenesis.

hypopituitarism A condition in which the secretion of specific hormones by the pituitary is reduced; may be caused by low or absent hypothalamic tropic hormones, pituitary stalk damage, or a defect in pituitary gland hormone secretion (the most common cause).

hypothalamic-pituitary-adrenal axis HPA axis; system by which the release of inhibitory, releasing, and tropic hormones affects physiologic functions, tying the central nervous system to the endocrine system.

hypothalamus A specific small portion of the brain, located below the thalamus and above the pituitary, that controls hormone release by the pituitary and maintains homeostasis by regulating electrolyte balance, fluid balance, body temperature, blood pressure, and body weight.

hypothermia Reduced body temperature lower than 37° C.

hypothyroidism Underproduction or decreased levels of thyroid hormones.

hypoxemia Decreased arterial oxygen.

hypoxia Oxygen deficiency; refers to decreased partial pressure of oxygen (pO_2) and decreased oxygen saturation (sO_2) resulting from lack of oxygen.

I

idiopathic pulmonary fibrosis A form of chronic, progressive, fibrosing interstitial pneumonia in which the patient's lungs become stiff and inelastic, limiting both the lung expansion volume and the rates of expansion and contraction.

IgA A type of immunoglobulin that exists as a monomer and as a dimer; it makes up about 15% of the immunoglobulins present in the blood.

IgD A type of immunoglobulin that exists as a monomer; its function is unknown, and it makes up only about 1% of the immunoglobulins in the blood.

IgE A type of immunoglobulin that exists as a monomer and is usually found attached to mast cells; there is very little IgE present in the blood.

IgG A type of immunoglobulin that exists as a monomer and is found in the extravascular compartment (65%) and in the blood (35%); it makes up 70% to 75% of the total immunoglobulins in the body.

IgM A type of immunoglobulin that exists as five monomers connected at their bases; it is the largest, least specific, and most abundant immunoglobulin in the blood.

immediate hypersensitivity reaction A hypersensitivity immune reaction that manifests within minutes or hours after exposure to an antigen.

immunity The body's defense against pathogens and toxins; usually involves immune cells that produce antibodies against a foreign invader.

immunodiffusion A laboratory technique that allows antigens and antibodies to diffuse at various rates through agar or agarose; used to determine relative concentrations, compare antigens, or determine the purity of a preparation.

immunoelectrophoresis IEP; a qualitative technique in which charged antigen and antibody particles are moved through a diffusion medium under the influence of an electrical field.

immunofixation Test to determine whether there is abnormal expression of monoclonal immunoglobulins.

immunoglobulin Any of a group of proteins that function as antibodies; there are five types: IgA, IgD, IgE, IgG, and IgM.

immunosuppressant A drug used to prevent transplant rejection.

immunosuppression Suppression of the immune system of an individual; induced to help prevent rejection of a transplanted organ.

incandescent lamp A type of lamp that uses a tungsten filament housed in a fused silica envelope with a low pressure of iodine or bromine vapor within the lamp.

incapacitating agent A chemical that impairs brain function or causes an altered state of consciousness such as disorientation, hallucination, or unconsciousness.

incident management Part of an emergency preparedness plan; defines responsibilities for responder roles and coordination of activities involved in managing a hazardous incident.

induction Activity of a drug or enzyme that leads to an increased amount of one or more metabolic enzymes in the liver; not permanent or instantaneous.

inflammation Reaction in which neutrophils and macrophages as well as chemicals are released into the circulation or tissues to repair an injury or destroy a foreign invader.

inflammatory bowel disease IBD; refers to either ulcerative colitis or Crohn disease; intestinal disease usually associated with abdominal pain, inflammation, destruction of tissue in the gastrointestinal tract, and blood and mucus in the stool.

inhibition Process by which the rate of metabolism of a drug or the activity of a body process is slowed or prevented.

insulin Secreted by the islets of langerhans in the pancreas to help regulate blood glucose levels.

interference filters Filters that have a narrow spectral bandwidth (in the range of 5 to 15 nm); commonly used as monochromators in automated multichannel instruments.

internal audit Systematic assessment of all policies, processes, and procedures in the laboratory conducted by individuals from different departments within the organization.

internal respiration The exchange of oxygen and carbon dioxide between the capillaries and cellular tissue.

international unit IU; a Système Internationale (SI) unit of measurement based on the amount, mass, or volume of a substance required for a specific biological effect, such as the amount of enzyme needed to convert 1 μmol of substrate to product in 1 minute.

interstitial fluid That part of the extracellular fluid that is found between the body's cells.

intracellular Inside the cell.

intracellular fluid Fluid that is contained inside individual cells.

intravascular compartment Refers to the fluids and other constituents inside the lymph and blood vessels.

inventory management Part of a laboratory quality management system; a program of detailed record keeping to manage equipment and ensure that supplies and reagents are available when needed. Efficient inventory management helps prevent waste and maximize cost savings and productivity.

ion exchange chromatography Also known as ion chromatography; uses an ion exchange mechanism to separate analytes based on their charge.

ionic bond An electrovalent bond that is established when one atom transfers its electrons to another atom, completing the valence shells of both.

ion A positively or negatively charged atom or molecule.

ion-selective electrode An electrode in which a membrane selectively interacts with a single ionic species; used for measuring particular electrolytes.

iontophoresis A procedure used to introduce drug-carrying ions through the skin by means of a weak electrical current; also used to perform a sweat chloride test during screening for cystic fibrosis.

iron circulating pool Refers to iron that is present in the blood, primarily bound to transferrin; excludes the iron found in hemoglobin, myoglobin, and tissue iron stores.

iron deficiency anemia A type of anemia that occurs when there is insufficient iron in the body to support healthy red blood cell production. The anemia gradually worsens as iron stores are depleted.

irritable bowel syndrome A disorder of the colon and large intestine that causes cramping, abdominal pain, bloating, discomfort, and chronic diarrhea.

ischemia Lack of oxygen in tissues; caused by decreased blood flow to the cells.

islets of Langerhans Areas within the pancreas containing the beta cells that secrete insulin.

ISO 15189 *Medical Laboratories—Particular Requirements for Quality and Competence*, 2007, a quality standard developed by the International Organization for Standardization (ISO) for industrial manufacturing that applies to the clinical laboratory; requires the engagement of laboratory personnel at all levels in implementing quality indicators to systematically monitor and evaluate the laboratory's contribution to patient care.

ISO/IEC 17025 *General Requirements for the Competence of Testing and Calibration Laboratories,* 2005, a quality standard developed by the International Organization for Standardization (ISO) and the International Electrotechnical Commission (IEC) for industrial manufacturing that applies to the clinical laboratory; covers technical requirements for correctness and reliability of tests and management requirements for the operation and effectiveness of quality management systems within the laboratory.

isocratic procedure In liquid chromatography, a separation technique in which the composition of the mobile phase remains constant throughout the procedure.

isoelectric focusing IEF; in electrophoresis, a technique used to separate proteins based on their migration through a pH gradient under the influence of an electrical field.

isoelectric point The level on the pH scale at which a particular molecule has no electrical charge.

isoenzymes Enzymes that catalyze the same reaction but have different structural and biochemical properties.

isomerase An enzyme that catalyzes the interconversion of isomers.

isotachophoresis A focusing technique based on the migration of sample components between leading and terminating electrolytes; used primarily for sample concentration.

J

jaundice Yellow color in the skin and eyes caused by excess bilirubin.

Joint Commission See *The Joint Commission.*

K

Kallmann syndrome A rare genetic condition that is characterized by a deficiency of gonadotropin-releasing hormone.

Kashin-Beck disease A severe chronic arthritis endemic to certain areas of Asia; one of the suspected causes is selenium deficiency.

kernicterus Type of brain damage that results from hyperbilirubinemia in an infant.

Keshan disease A type of congestive cardiomyopathy related to severe selenium deficiency.

ketone bodies A group of chemicals—acetoacetate, β-hydroxybutyric acid (hydroxybutyrate), and acetone—which are produced by the metabolism of fatty acids; if they accumulate in the blood, they decrease the blood pH, causing a metabolic acidosis.

ketones The ketone functional group consists of an oxygen atom double-bonded to a carbon atom that is bonded to two other carbon atoms; measured in urine as an indication of the use of fat metabolism for energy, as in diabetics.

key quality concept An important aspect of a clinical laboratory that must be considered when developing quality practices; an example is the three-phase workflow concept.

kidney dialysis The artificial process by which blood is filtered and wastes removed; a lifesaving procedure that may be performed frequently in an individual whose kidneys, due to damage or disease, have lost their ability to remove waste.

kidney failure A gradual or sudden decline in the ability of the kidneys to filter blood and remove metabolic wastes.

kidney transplantation A procedure in which a kidney is removed from a donor and surgically implanted into a recipient whose own kidneys have failed.

kinetic or multipoint fixed time method A method used to measure the catalytic activity of enzymes in which reaction progression is monitored continuously as a function of time.

Klinefelter syndrome A common genetic disorder that causes hypogonadism and infertility in men.

koilonychia Also known as spoon nails; a nail disease that can be a sign of anemia, hyperthyroidism, and hemochromatosis.

kwashiorkor A type of malnutrition involving low protein intake associated with famine.

L

label A chemical tag, such as an enzyme, fluorophore, or radioisotope, that is applied to antibodies or antigens; used in immunochemical assays to facilitate detection or quantification of small quantities of clinically important substances.

laboratory information system LIS; a computerized system for receiving, processing, storing, and distributing information generated by medical laboratory testing, such as patient test results and quality control data.

laboratory manager Person responsible for the daily activities of the laboratory; he or she has at least a bachelor's degree and is a clinical laboratory scientist.

laboratory quality manual A regularly updated compilation of a laboratory's policies and procedures related to the quality management system.

Laboratory Response Network LRN; a network of 150 laboratories created in 1999 by the Centers for Disease Control and Prevention that can quickly respond to biological and chemical emergencies or other public health emergencies; includes federal, state, and local public health laboratories as well as veterinary, military, and international laboratories.

lactate dehydrogenase An enzyme that catalyzes the conversion of pyruvate to lactate (and the reverse) in heart and skeletal muscle, facilitating anaerobic (and aerobic) energy production.

lactic acidosis A metabolic disorder caused by low pH due to lactic acid buildup in the bloodstream.

large cell lung cancer A type of cancer that begins in the outer regions of the lungs and is strongly linked to smoking; the rarest of the lung cancers.

Laurell technique Also called rocket electroimmunodiffusion; an adaptation of radial immunodiffusion in which electrophoresis is used to move antigens into an antibody-containing agar medium. The resulting pattern of precipitin lines forms a spike that resembles the shape of a rocket, and the height of the rocket is directly proportional to the amount of antigen in the sample.

LD$_{50}$ See *median lethal dose.*

Lean A process used in the laboratory to optimize space, time, and activity to improve physical paths of workflow.

lecithin/sphingomyelin ratio L/S ratio; a test used to assess fetal lung maturity.

lecithin A major component of airway surfactant.

lectin pathway One of the three activation methods for the complement cascade, using specific bacterial carbohydrates.

left-to-right shunting Occurs when blood from the left atrium or ventricle flows to the right atrium or ventricle and subsequently back to the lungs; may result in heart failure, pulmonary arterial hypertension, and heart rhythm problems.

lethal dose LD; the amount of a chemical or agent that causes death; compare *median lethal dose.*

leukemia Malignant disease in which abnormal, nonfunctional white blood cells are released into peripheral blood instead of mature, normal cells.

leukocyte esterase An enzyme released by white blood cells; when present in the urine, it is an indicator of the presence of white blood cells and other abnormalities associated with infection.

leukotriene Class of eicosanoids that act as chemical mediators of acute and chronic inflammation; they increase vasodilation and vascular permeability.

level 1 laboratories Laboratories capable of the highest level of response to a chemical emergency as part of the Laboratory Response Network; employ high-throughput processes and can detect exposure to cyanide, nerve agents, toxic metals, mustard agents, and toxic industrial chemicals.

level 2 laboratories Laboratories capable of a medium level of response to a chemical emergency as part of the Laboratory Response Network; employ chemists trained to detect agents such as cyanide, nerve agents, and toxic metals.

level 3 laboratories Laboratories capable of the lowest level of response to a chemical emergency as part of the Laboratory Response Network; work with hospitals and first responders to ensure the quality of clinical specimen collection, storage, and shipment.

Levey-Jennings chart A medical laboratory quality control process designed to detect, reduce, and correct errors in a laboratory's analytical processes before release of patient test results.

lewisite An oily, arsenic-containing liquid that is extremely toxic and was developed as a chemical weapon but has not been used in wartime.

ligase Any of a group of enzymes that catalyze the joining of two molecules by formation of a covalent bond accompanied by hydrolysis of adenosine triphosphate (ATP).

linear ion trap A type of trapping mass spectrometry in which a set of quadrupole rods and a static electrical potential are used to confine ions; functions as a selective mass filter or as an actual trap for the ions.

linear regression Statistical technique for comparing the values obtained when two methods are used to examine a set of samples.

linearity Range of values within which a given laboratory procedure, instrument, or reagent provides accurate results.

linoleic acid An ω-6 essential fatty acid found in vegetable oils; it is metabolized in a complex process to arachidonic acid and eicosanoids that increase the inflammatory response.

linolenic acid An ω-3 essential fatty acid found in seed oils; it is metabolized in a complex process to eicosanoids that decrease the inflammatory response.

lipase Any of a group of enzymes that help break down fatty acids and perform essential roles in the digestion and processing of dietary lipids. The serum lipase level is measured to diagnose and monitor acute pancreatitis and other diseases.

lipemia A high concentration of emulsified fat in the blood.

lipids Fat-soluble molecules that are found throughout the body; includes fatty acids, triglycerides, phospholipids, sterols, sphingolipids, and cholesterol.

lipogenesis Fat synthesis.

lipolysis Fat breakdown.

lipoprotein Composed of a mixture of cholesterol triglycerides and phospholipids linked to apolipoproteins.

lipoprotein (a) (Lp(a)) A distinct type of lipoprotein molecules with a structure similar to that of low-density lipoprotein because both contain an apo B-100 particle; Lp(a) also contains a protein, apo(a), that is bound to the apo B-100 particle. Lp(a) is considered an independent risk factor for cardiovascular disease, atherosclerosis, and related disorders.

lipoprotein lipase (LPL) An enzyme found in capillaries and fatty tissues of the body that helps turn fat into triglycerides.

lipoxin A class of eicosanoids produced by leukocytes that act as chemical mediators with immunomodulatory and antiinflammatory actions.

liquid chromatography A separation technique for nonvolatile analytes in which the mobile phase is a liquid.

liquid-phase adsorption A separation technique in which the free antigen is adsorbed onto charcoal particles added to the solution.

lithium Metal element that is chemically similar to sodium and potassium; enhances the reuptake of neurotransmitters, producing a calming effect on the manic symptoms of an affective or bipolar disorder and preventing possible attacks.

liver biopsy Surgical procedure by which a small part of the liver is removed for testing.

liver enzymes Enzymes produced by the liver that are analyzed to assess for liver disease; include bilirubin, alanine transaminase (ALT), aspartate transaminase (AST), alkaline phosphatase (ALP), and γ-glutamyl transferase (GGT).

liver failure Acute or chronic condition in which the liver cannot perform its usual functions.

loading dose An initial dose that is given to achieve the desired blood concentration quickly.

low-density lipoprotein LDL; cholesterol-rich particles that are formed by the removal of triglycerides from very-low-density lipoproteins during catabolism; their major function is to carry cholesterol in the plasma.

lowest observed effect level LOEL; the first dose at which an effect is measured.

luminometer An instrument that measures types of luminescence in which the excitation event is caused by a chemical, biochemical, or electrochemical reaction rather than by photoillumination.

luminophor A chemical group that gives the property of luminescence to a chemical compound; used to label an antibody or antigen of interest in an immunoassay.

luteinizing hormone LH; chemical released from the anterior pituitary gland that stimulates the ovary to produce progesterone; responsible for ovulation in females and for production of testosterone by the testes in males.

lyase Any of a group of enzymes that catalyze the removal of chemical bonds by means other than hydrolysis or oxidation, leaving double bonds, or that add groups to double bonds.

lymphatic system System by which lymph capillaries collect the fluid leaked from blood capillaries and empty it into larger vessels (collecting ducts), which contain valves to prevent backwash; muscle activity helps to move the lymph fluid, which bathes the lymph nodes and eventually empties into the subclavian veins.

lymphedema Edema caused by blockage or damage to lymph vessels, such as after surgery.

lymphoma Malignant tumor of lymphoid tissue; one of the exceptions to the naming conventions for cancer.

lyophilized Freeze-dried.

lysosomal enzymes Enzymes that are synthesized in the endoplasmic reticulum and stored within membrane-bound vesicles (lysosomes); they are involved in many cell signaling and metabolic processes in health and disease and are capable of breaking down materials in the cytoplasm as well as cellular debris and engulfed materials.

M

α₂-macroglobulin A serine protease inhibitor (serpin) that can inhibit many different types of proteinases; a very large protein molecule that contains four identical polypeptide chains linked together.

macronutrient A nutrient that is required by the body in large amounts.

macrophage A immune specialized cell that ingests bacteria and debris.

maintenance dose The amount of drug required to maintain the desired therapeutic level over time.

major histocompatibility complex MHC; part of the adaptive immune system consisting of transmembrane proteins with a peptide-binding fold (i.e., groove) by which class I and class II MHC cells present processed peptide antigens to T lymphocytes to stimulate an immune response (see *human leukocyte antigen*).

malabsorption A general term associated with an inability to absorb one or more nutrients from the gastrointestinal system, most likely due to inefficiencies or pathologies of the pancreas or intestines.

malar rash Butterfly rash; a hallmark of systemic lupus erythematosus; a red rash over the cheeks and nasal bridge that does not extend into the nasolabial folds.

maldigestion An inability to digest one or more nutrients.

malignant cells Cells that are genetically damaged and undergo uncontrollable cell division, creating a malignant tumor as more and more cells are produced.

malignant melanoma A type of cancer caused by the malignant transformation of melanocytes.

malignant tumor A tumor that is invasive, grows rapidly, is not encapsulated, and possesses the microscopic hallmarks of nuclear irregularities and no normal tissue structure.

malnutrition Lack of appropriate nutrients for health.

maple syrup disease Branched-chain ketoacidosis; a genetic disorder that prevents the body from processing certain amino acids properly. The name refers to the sweet odor of the urine produced by affected infants.

marasmus Inadequate intake of both protein and calories; it is characterized by emaciation.

mass spectrometer A detector that provides structural information and positive identification of a wide variety of substances; an analytical instrument that first ionizes a target molecule and then separates and measures the mass of the molecule or its fragments.

mean The average value of a group of results from the same test.

mechanism of action The process that occurs at the target area and produces the pharmacological or other designated effect.

meconium First stool passed in the days immediately after birth; contains a large concentration of bile pigments. Meconium may be passed in utero; if found in the amniotic fluid, it may indicate that the fetus is in distress.

median lethal dose LD_{50}; the acute toxicity of a substance; the amount of a chemical that is capable of killing one half of the members of a tested population.

median The value that appears in the middle of a batch of values (i.e., half of the values are higher and half are lower than the median).

mediator Any biochemical agent that transmits a signal or otherwise plays an intermediary role in a specific response or process in the body.

medical ethics System of moral principles and judgments, as applied to medicine and related situations.

medical laboratory assistant Laboratory personnel who are trained to perform or assist in routine laboratory testing as allowed by law and to perform administrative tasks.

medical staff Health care providers who may or may not be employees of the hospital system; in the traditional structure, the medical staff is granted the right to admit patients and perform procedures in the hospital.

medical technologist (MT (ASCP)) A laboratory professional certified by the ASCP Board of Registry who tests and analyzes body fluids and records the findings. This individual is also called a clinical or medical laboratory scientist and holds a bachelor's degree.

melanocyte Cell that distributes pigment to the skin, hair, or eyes.

melanoma Malignant tumor of melanocytes; one of the exceptions to the naming conventions for tumors.

melatonin A hormone secreted by the pineal gland.

membrane attack complex The end product of the complement cascade; a structure of four complement proteins that attaches to the plasma membrane of an infected or abnormal cell to cause cell lysis and death.

Meniere disease A chronic condition caused by an imbalance of fluid in the inner ear; increased pressure and volume in the area creates symptoms including episodic vertigo, tinnitus, and hearing loss.

meningitis A clinical syndrome involving inflammation of the meninges, usually caused by a bacterial infection.

meningomyelocele A type of spina bifida in which the lower end of the neural tube fails to fuse.

Menkes disease An X-linked, recessive, multi-system disorder of copper metabolism.

menopause Cessation of menses for 12 months or longer in a previously menstruating woman; caused by decreased levels of reproductive hormones and marks the end of reproductive capability.

metabolic acidosis Reduced pH in body fluids or tissues caused by a metabolic problem (i.e., increased production or decreased ability to excrete acids).

metabolic alkalosis Increased pH in body fluids or tissues caused by a metabolic problem (e.g., repeated vomiting, severe dehydration, certain endocrine disorders).

metabolic syndrome The presence of at least three of the following risk factors: (1) abdominal obesity, (2) high triglyceride levels, (3) low levels of high-density lipoprotein, (4) hypertension, and (5) high fasting blood sugar levels; increases the risk for heart disease, stroke, and diabetes.

metalloprotein Generic term for a molecule in which a protein is bound to a metal ion or forms a complex with a metal (e.g., hemeproteins).

metanephrine Intermediate product in the metabolism of epinephrine.

metaplasia The initial abnormal, but reversible, change of a cell from one type to another due to an injury.

metastasize Travel of cells from a malignant tumor to distant parts of the body, where they lodge and form secondary or metastatic tumors.

methemoglobin Molecule that results when hemoglobin reacts with oxidizing agents such as nitrates, quinines, or aniline dyes to produce heme containing Fe^{3+} instead of Fe^{2+}; because oxygen cannot bind to the iron in its oxidized state, methemoglobin is nonfunctional.

methylenedioxymethamphetamine MDMA; member of the class of amphetamine drugs; can induce euphoria, sense of intimacy with others, and diminished anxiety.

Michaelis-Menten kinetics Model that accounts for enzymatic reaction rates based on the concentrations of the enzyme and its substrate.

microalbumin Test that detects tiny amounts of a blood protein (albumin) in urine that are not detectable by conventional methods but provide an early indication of renal damage.

microbiology department Clinical pathology unit that identifies disease-causing microorganisms and determines the most effective antibiotic to destroy them.

micronutrient A nutrient that is needed by the body in very small amounts but is essential for good health and may cause disease if deficient.

microparticle enzyme immunoassay MEIA; a type of immunoassay in which the antibody–antigen complexes are isolated on the surface of small beads called microparticles.

microvilli Microscopic hairlike projections of the cellular membrane, especially on the villi of the small intestine, that further increase the surface area for absorption of nutrients.

mineralocorticoid Aldosterone; a hormone produced by the adrenal cortex that controls the excretion of electrolytes, especially sodium, through the kidneys, colon, stomach, and sweat glands.

mitigate Reduce.

mobile phase A gas or a liquid that flows in a chromatographic system and carries the sample past the stationary phase.

mode Value that occurs most frequently in a batch of test results.

molality A system of expressing concentration that is more accurate but less convenient than molarity and is infrequently used in the clinical laboratory. The molal concentration (mol/kg) of a solution is equal to the number of moles of solute per 1000 g of solvent.

molarity A system of expressing concentration. The molar concentration (mol/L) of a solution is equal to the number of moles of solute per contained in 1 L of the solution. A 1 molar (1 M) solution has 1 mole of solute in each liter of solution.

mole 1 mole of a substance is equal to its equivalent weight in grams (gram molecular weight).

monochromatic Refers to light of a single wavelength.

monochromator A device that can separate light into distinctive wavelengths.

monoclonal antibody An antibody that comes from a single B-cell clone and has activity against one specific epitope of an antigen.

mucoprotein A glycoprotein composed primarily of mucopolysaccharides and protein.

multiple of the median MoM; a statistical tool used to normalize results during test interpretation, especially for screening tests such as α-fetoprotein.

multiple sclerosis An autoimmune disease that destroys the myelin sheaths on motor and sensory nerves in the central nervous system.

mustard-lewisite mixture HL (military designation); a dark, oily liquid that can be distributed by aerial spraying; a blister agent and alkylating agent that damages the DNA of rapidly dividing cells.

myasthenia gravis An autoimmune disease in which impulses from the brain fail to reach skeletal muscles due to the formation of antibodies against acetylcholine nicotinic postsynaptic receptors at the neuromuscular junction.

mycophenolic acid MPA; the active form of the prodrug mycophenolate mofetil; a selective inhibitor of inosine monophosphate dehydrogenase that is found in activated lymphocytes and is necessary for purine synthesis and replication. It is also prescribed as an immunosuppressant with a different mode of action from calcineurin inhibitors and mammalian target of rapamycin (mTOR) inhibitors.

myelodysplastic syndromes A group of malignant hematopoietic stem cell disorders characterized by ineffective blood cell production resulting in a hypercellular or hypocellular marrow and decreased numbers of all blood cells.

myocardial infarction Also known as a heart attack; the irreversible death of cardiac muscle tissue, most often caused by ischemia.

myocarditis Inflammation of the muscle layer of the heart.

myoglobin A small, single-polypeptide protein found in heart and skeletal muscles that stores oxygen molecules and is released into the bloodstream when muscles are damaged.

N

nail clubbing Condition in which the nails are curved and appear to bulge, similar to the bottom of an upside-down spoon; often caused by lung cancer.

Nalgene Company that provides laboratories with high-quality plasticware, made from polystyrene, polypropylene, polycarbonate, Teflon, or nylon, that is biologically inert, chemically resistant, break resistant, and durable.

narcotics Drugs used to treat severe pain; can induce sleep, insensibility, or mental stupor.

narrow-spectrum antibiotics Drugs that are useful in treating only a few types of bacteria.

National Cholesterol Education Program NCEP; established by the National Heart, Lung, and Blood Institute in 1985; educates clinicians, patients, and the public about the role played by elevated cholesterol levels in cardiovascular disease.

National Fire Protection Association (NFPA) label Put on all chemicals in the laboratory that are shipped to others.

national laboratory A federally funded center with unique resources for handling highly infectious agents and identifying specific microbial strains.

natriuretic peptide A small protein that inhibits aldosterone release to help prevent extracellular water accumulation.

necrosis Cell death with the release of intracellular chemicals that damage the living tissue surrounding the necrotic cells.

Needlestick Safety and Prevention Act of 2000 Mandates use of self-sheathing needles and other systems to eliminate or lessen exposure of employees to bloodborne pathogens and training in the proper use of engineering devices, record keeping, and work practice controls to improve employee safety.

negative feedback loop Process by which a change in the normal range of function elicits a response that opposes or resists that change; a method by which the endocrine system controls hormonal responses to stimuli.

neonatal drug testing Applied in cases of suspected maternal drug abuse during pregnancy; a means of preventing low birth weight, premature birth, and impaired neurologic functioning due to drug exposure during gestation.

neoplasia Uncontrolled growth of cells resulting in a benign or malignant tumor.

neoplasm New and abnormal growth of tissue that forms a tumor or mass of cells.

nephelometry Method of measuring light scattered by particles in a solution to determine the amount of a substance in a sample; method of choice for assaying larger particles at lower concentrations.

nephrogenic diabetes insipidus Condition in which the renal collecting tubules are resistant to the effects of antidiuretic hormone.

nephrolithiasis Process of forming a stone in the kidney.

nephrosclerosis Progressive renal disease resulting from hardening of the small blood vessels in the kidneys.

nephrotic syndrome Kidney disease characterized by edema, increased glomerular permeability, proteinuria, hypertension, hyperlipidemia, and hypoalbuminemia.

nerve agent Any highly poisonous chemical that interferes with the conduction of nerve impulses.

neural tube defect Major birth defect caused by abnormal development of the neural tube, the embryonic structure that gives rise to the central nervous system; results in permanent defects of the brain and spinal cord.

neuroblastoma A malignant, catecholamine-secreting tumor made of postganglionic sympathetic neurons; occurs mainly in children.

neurogenic diabetes insipidus Also called central diabetes insipidus; condition caused by deficient production of antidiuretic hormone in the hypothalamus.

neuron-specific enolase Enzyme found in neuronal and neuroendocrine tissues that is used as a tumor marker.

neutralization reaction Reaction in which an acid and a base are combined to produce a salt and water.

next-generation sequencing NGS; a type of high-resolution DNA sequencing.

niacin Also known as nicotinic acid; a water-soluble B vitamin that is converted to niacinamide (nicotinamide).

nitrogen mustards HN (military designation); oily, colorless to yellow liquids with musty, fruity, or bitter almond smells that evaporate slowly and do not dissolve in water; nonspecific DNA alkylating agents used in chemotherapy and potentially in warfare.

no observable effect level NOEL; the highest dose at which no response is measured.

noncompetitive immunoassay A type of immunoassay in which the analyte is bound to a labeled antibody or sandwiched between labeled and unlabeled antibody; the analyte concentration is directly proportional to the measured amount of labeled antibody. These assays have the highest level of sensitivity and specificity and are used to measure cardiac markers and hepatitis markers.

noncompetitive inhibition Reaction in which an inhibitor, rather than competing with the substrate for the active site on an enzyme molecule, binds at a regulatory site (i.e., allosteric site), thus inhibiting enzymatic function.

non-Hodgkin lymphoma Abnormal growth of lymphoid tissue in lymph nodes and vessels that originates from abnormal B or T cells; it is eight times more common than Hodgkin lymphoma.

non–small cell lung cancer Most common type of lung cancer; onset is insidious, and 55% of patients have widespread disease at diagnosis.

norepinephrine Also known as noradrenaline; one of the catecholamine hormones secreted by the adrenal medulla.

normal Refers to a typical finding; objective interpretations of data show that test results fall within the reference range.

normal anion gap acidosis Acidosis that includes a normal anion gap; also known as non–anion gap acidosis.

normal distribution or curve See *Gaussian curve*.

normality A system of expressing concentration; the normal concentration (N) of a solution is the molar concentration divided by the equivalence factor. It is the gram equivalent weight of a compound per liter of solution.

normetanephrine Metabolite of norepinephrine.

nucleic acids Building block of deoxyribonucleic acid (DNA), which forms genes, and ribonucleic acid (RNA), which governs protein synthesis.

nucleoprotein Complex consisting of a nucleic acid (DNA or RNA) bonded to a protein.

nucleotide Compound composed of a sugar, a phosphate group, and a heterocyclic nitrogenous base; the basic structural unit of nucleic acids.

nucleus Central part of the cell that contains genetic material and is enclosed in a membrane.

nutrition Process by which organisms take in and metabolize food for growth and maintenance; also, the branch of science that deals with nutrients and nutrition.

O

obesity Excessive accumulation of body fat that adversely affects health.

Occupational Safety and Health Administration OSHA; agency created within the U.S. Department of Labor by Congress in 1970 to help employers and employees reduce on-the-job injuries, illnesses, and deaths by maintaining a safe and healthy workplace.

occurrence Event with a negative impact on an organization, its personnel, or the organization's product, equipment, or environment.

occurrence management Proactive process by which the laboratory identifies and handles errors and develops changes in policies, procedures, processes, or communication to prevent errors from occurring.

oliguria Production of smaller than normal amounts of urine.

oncofetal antigen Proteins, such as carcinoembryonic antigen and α-fetoprotein, that are produced by some tumors in adults but also are produced normally by a fetus.

oncogenic virus A virus that can induce a tumor by affecting the DNA or RNA of the host.

one-step format Design of a competitive assay that allows labeled antigen and an unlabeled specimen to compete for a limited amount of antibody.

onycholysis Painless separation of the nail from the nail bed caused by local trauma, fungal infection of the nail, or periungual warts.

open neural tube defect Neural tube defect in which the neural tissue is exposed and cerebrospinal fluid leaks out; usually it is apparent at birth and involves the entire central nervous system.

optics Study of the behavior of light or the properties of transmission and deflection of other forms of radiation.

orchitis Inflammation of the testes that is usually caused by the mumps virus but can be caused by other viruses or bacteria.

organ Part of an organism that is typically self-contained and has a specific vital function, such as the heart or liver; tissues group together to form organs.

osmolality Concentration of dissolved substances relative to the mass of the solvent; a 1 molal solution contains 1 osmol of solute per 1 kg of water.

osmotic edema Type of low-protein edema that results from low osmotic pressure.

osmotic pressure Physical force exerted by the movement of solvent molecules from a higher-concentration solution through a semipermeable membrane to a lower-concentration solution to achieve a balanced solution (i.e., osmosis).

osteitis deformans Former name for Paget disease.

osteoarthritis Most common form of arthritis; results from mechanical wear and tear on the joint that leads to degeneration of cartilage and bone.

osteogenesis imperfecta Also called brittle bone disease; genetic disease with an autosomal dominant inheritance pattern that affects collagen throughout the body; characterized by blue sclerae and defective bone development that leads to deafness, abnormal dentition, frequent fractures, and bone deformities.

osteoid Unmineralized organic component of bone.

osteomalacia Softening of the bones due to loss of calcium; typically caused by a deficiency of vitamin D or calcium.

osteoporosis Condition in which bones become brittle and fragile due to loss of tissue; typically caused by hormonal changes or deficiency of calcium or vitamin D.

other potentially infectious materials OPIM; includes semen, vaginal secretions, cerebrospinal fluid, synovial fluid, pleural fluid, pericardial fluid, peritoneal fluid, amniotic fluid, saliva, and any body fluid contaminated with visible blood.

ototoxicity Damage to the hearing or balance functions of the ear caused by a drug or chemical.

Ouchterlony double immunodiffusion A technique in which the antigen and antibody are placed in separate cells and allowed to diffuse toward each other into the gel medium; used to test the similarity between antigens.

out of control Occurs when quality control values are not within the limits established for that control.

outpatient clinic Place where patients receive short-term medical care but are not admitted, as in a hospital, for inpatient service.

ovulation Discharge of a secondary oocyte from the graafian follicle; occurs when follicle-stimulating hormone stimulates the ovary to release an ovum into the peritoneal cavity.

oxidoreductase Enzyme that catalyzes an oxidation-reduction reaction.

oxygen binding The joining of an oxygen molecule (O_2) to one of the four heme groups in a hemoglobin molecule; in the red blood cell, this process continues until all four heme groups are bound.

oxygen saturation sO_2; percentage of hemoglobin bound to oxygen in the blood.

oxytocin A polypeptide hormone that is made in the hypothalamus and stored and released by the posterior pituitary.

P

Paget disease The second most common bone disorder in the elderly; identified by Sir James Paget as osteitis deformans in 1877. It is a chronic disease that typically results in enlarged, deformed bones due to excessive breakdown and formation of bone.

pancreatic amylase Enzyme secreted by the pancreas that helps break down carbohydrates.

pancreatic elastase Enzyme secreted by the pancreas. The test for elastase may be used to detect pancreatic insufficiency.

pancreatic insufficiency Form of maldigestion in which the pancreas fails to produce sufficient digestive enzymes because the enzyme-secreting acinar cells are destroyed; clinical symptoms do not appear until 90% of acinar cells are destroyed.

panhypopituitarism Type of hypopituitarism in which concentrations of all pituitary hormones are low or zero.

pannus Condition in which a highly vascular, inflamed membrane extends over the surface of an organ or other specialized anatomic structure.

parafollicular cells Also called C cells; they are found in the thyroid gland and secrete calcitonin, which lowers blood calcium levels by inhibiting osteoclasts.

paresthesia An abnormal sensation of tingling in the fingertips, toes, or perioral area caused by pressure on or damage to peripheral nerves

Parkinson disease Slow-onset degenerative disease that involves the basal ganglia, leading to a lack of the neurotransmitter dopamine and faulty nerve transmission; characterized by tremor, difficulty walking, muscle rigidity, slurred speech, sleep disturbances, and a wooden, emotionless facial expression.

paroxysmal nocturnal hemoglobinuria A hereditary disease in which red blood cells are lysed by complement, releasing hemoglobin.

partial pressure Amount of pressure contributed by each gas to the total pressure exerted by a mixture of gases.

partition chromatography Analysis of chemical substances based on the differential distribution of solutes between two immiscible liquids, as in liquid chromatography or gas chromatography.

pathologist A medical doctor who examines tissues and oversees the quality of clinical laboratory testing.

pathology Study of the causes and effects of diseases, especially the branch of medicine that deals with the laboratory examination of samples of body tissue for diagnostic or forensic purposes.

pCO₂ Partial pressure of carbon dioxide.

peak level Highest concentration of a drug in the patient's bloodstream.

pepsin An enzyme secreted by the chief cells of the stomach that helps break down protein.

pepsinogen Enzyme precursor that is converted to pepsin by hydrochloric acid in the stomach.

peptidase An enzyme produced in the pancreas that breaks down protein in the small intestine into absorbable oligopeptides and amino acids.

peptide bond Covalent bond formed by joining the amino group of one amino acid to the carboxyl group of a second amino acid.

peptide or polypeptide hormones Water-soluble hormones composed of a few amino acids that circulate freely in the blood and have half-lives of a few minutes; they initiate chemical reactions that change the metabolism of the targeted cell.

pericardial effusion Fluid in the pericardium.

pericarditis Inflammation of the pericardium.

perimenopausal period The years before menopause during which the ovaries have a decreased response to gonadotropins, leading to symptoms such as irregular menses, hot flushes, and weight gain.

peripheral chemoreceptors Specialized cells located in the carotid artery and aorta that involuntarily affect breathing rate and depth and other homeostatic factors.

peripheral neuropathy Malfunction of sensory or motor nerve signals by a disease process; causes weakness, paralysis, numbness, tingling, or pain.

peristaltic pump Type of positive displacement pump in which fluids are forced along by waves of contraction produced mechanically in flexible tubing to separate samples and reagents.

peritoneal dialysis Use of a peritoneal membrane to filter metabolic waste products from blood.

peritubular epithelial cells Epithelial cells that line the kidney tubules.

pernicious anemia An autoimmune macrocytic anemia that leads to gastric atrophy due to reduced vitamin B_{12} absorption caused by lack of intrinsic factor.

personal protective equipment PPE; includes clothing, helmets, goggles, gloves, and other equipment worn to minimize exposure to hazardous materials.

Peyer patches Aggregated lymphoid nodules that are part of the immune system; they are found in the small intestine and provide a setting for the maturation of B cells.

pH An expression of the acidity or alkalinity of a solution on a logarithmic scale (1 to 10) on which 7 is neutral, values lower than 7 are more acid, and values higher than 7 are more alkaline.

pharmacodynamics Study of the biochemical and physiologic effects of drugs and their mechanisms of action.

pharmacokinetics Assesses the rate of absorption, distribution, biotransformation, and excretion of drugs.

phenol Also called carbolic acid; an aromatic organic compound that is highly toxic to most organisms, especially microorganisms, and is used as an ingredient in many antiseptics and disinfectants.

pheochromocytoma Small, vascular tumor of the adrenal medulla that secretes catecholamines.

phlebotomist A technician who draws blood from patients.

phosgene oxime A colorless solid or yellow-brown liquid with a disagreeable, irritating odor that causes erythema and hives on contact with skin but does not produce blistering like other chemicals in its class.

phosphate buffer system System that ensures acid-base balance inside the cell; relies on the equilibrium between dihydrogen phosphate ions ($H_2PO_4^-$) and hydrogen phosphate ions (HPO_4^{2-}).

phospholipid Any of a group of compounds composed mainly of fatty acids, a phosphate group, and a simple organic molecule such as glycerol; cell membrane components that provide structure and protection.

phosphoprotein A conjugated protein in which the protein molecule is bound to phosphate groups.

photodetector A device that converts light into an electrical signal by detecting photons that strike a photosensitive or photoemissive surface; the surface emits electrons in proportion to the number of photons striking it.

photodiode A light-sensing semiconductor device with two terminals that typically allows the flow of current in one direction only; used to measure transmittance in routine chemistry tests. Photodiodes have begun to replace photomultiplier tubes in many clinical laboratory instruments because they are capable of measuring light simultaneously at many wavelengths with speed and accuracy.

photomultiplier tube PMT; an electron tube that contains a cathode, a light-sensitive metal, a series of dynodes in a glass enclosure, and an anode that collects the amplified electrons; a type of photodetector used to amplify and detect very small amounts of light.

photosensitivity Oversensitivity of skin to light that can be a side effect of medications or result from diseases such as lupus erythematosus.

physicians' office laboratories POLs; range from a small laboratories that serve one to five physicians and perform a few tests to large-volume laboratories that serve up to 200 physicians.

pineal gland Small structure located near the center of the brain that secretes melatonin, which maintains the circadian rhythm and regulates levels of luteinizing hormone and follicle-stimulating hormone.

pinocytosis Ingestion of liquid into a cell by budding of small vesicles from the cell membrane.

pipettes Small tubes used to transfer a specific amount of a liquid between containers; classified as manual, semiautomated, and automated.

pitting edema Accumulation of low-protein, watery fluid in the tissues, usually in the extremities.

pituitary gland Endocrine gland located at the base of the brain and attached to the hypothalamus that controls growth, development, and other glands in the endocrine system.

planar chromatography Separation technique in which the stationary phase exists on a plane, as in paper chromatography or thin-layer chromatography.

plaque Accumulation of lipoproteins and inflammatory cells on the walls of arteries.

plasma membrane Selectively permeable membrane that allows specific chemicals to enter and exit the cell under certain conditions; see *cell membrane*.

pleural effusion Accumulation of fluid in the thorax.

pneumatic tubes Cylindrical containers that are propelled through networks of tubes by compressed air or by partial vacuum; used to transport specimens from the collection point to the laboratory.

pneumonia Infection of the lungs that can be caused by viruses, bacteria, or fungi; the sixth leading cause of death in the United States.

pO$_2$ Partial pressure of oxygen.

point-of-care testing POCT; mode of testing performed close to the patient or at the bedside, using portable equipment, for convenience and to obtain rapid results; procedures are usually performed by non-laboratorians.

poison Chemical that can cause illness or death at very low levels when absorbed or introduced into the body.

policy Written statement of intentions and directions defined by a laboratory and endorsed by institutional management.

polyacrylamide Polymer prepared by heating acrylamide with a variety of catalysts; when used in electrophoresis, its advantages include thermostability, transparency, and durability.

polyclonal antibodies Antibodies secreted by different B-cell lineages against a specific antigen, with each antibody identifying a different epitope.

polycystic kidney disease A genetic disorder with an autosomal dominant or autosomal recessive pattern of inheritance in which clusters of cysts develop primarily within the kidneys.

polycystic ovary syndrome Also called Stein-Leventhal syndrome; a hypothalamic-pituitary disorder in which hormonal abnormalities and the development of multiple cysts in the ovaries lead to insulin resistance, excessive production of androgen hormones, high lipid levels, and oligomenorrhea.

polymerase chain reaction PCR; method for exponentially amplifying DNA, creating many copies of a DNA sequence.

polynucleotide Linear arrangement of many nucleotides, constituting a section of a nucleic acid molecule.

polyp Small growth, typically benign and with a stalk, protruding from a mucous membrane; may be associated with an increased incidence of colon cancer.

porphyria Any of a group of clinical syndromes caused by defects in enzymes that catalyze various stages of heme production.

porphyrin Photosensitive pigment consisting of four pyrrole rings that bind to an iron molecule to form heme; important porphyrins in humans are uroporphyrin, protoporphyrin, and coproporphyrin.

porphyrinogen Reduced form of a porphyrin (Fe^{2+}); the functional intermediate in the biosynthesis of heme.

postanalytical phase Laboratory testing phase that includes releasing test results and reporting test results to providers.

posterior pituitary Neurohypophysis; stores antidiuretic hormone and oxytocin; does not synthesize hormones.

postmortem sample Specimen collected after death, as in forensic toxicology.

potentiometric Measurement of an electrical potential difference between two electrodes or half-cells in an electrochemical cell.

potentiometric sensor A type of chemical sensor that measures the electrical potential of an electrode when no voltage is present; used to determine the analytical concentration of components of an analyte gas or solution.

preanalytical phase Phase of laboratory testing that includes all of the tasks that occur before the sample arrives in the laboratory, such as patient preparation, collection and identification of samples, storage, and delivery to the appropriate work unit.

precipitation Process by which a chemical added to a solution causes an insoluble solid (precipitate) to form; in immunologic precipitation, the precipitate is an antigen-antibody complex within a gel or in solution.

precision Reproducibility of results; control values must be within an acceptable range before patient results can be released to the practitioner; precise methods have a coefficient of variation below 5%.

preeclampsia Condition of pregnancy characterized by hypertension and proteinuria that occurs after the 20th week of gestation.

pregnancy Condition of growing a fertilized egg into a fetus within the female uterus; the period from conception to birth.

pressure gradient The difference or change in pressure across a membrane.

preventive maintenance program Schedule of tasks to be performed at daily, weekly, monthly, or yearly intervals. Following the manufacturer's preventive maintenance program allows a laboratory instrument to perform with maximum efficiency, accuracy, and precision and increases its life span.

primary aldosteronism Also called Conn syndrome; uncommon disorder in which the adrenal glands produce excess aldosterone, often associated with an aldosterone-secreting adrenal adenoma; causes hypertension, hypokalemia, renal potassium wasting, and neuromuscular changes.

primary amenorrhea Failure to start menses by 16 years of age.

primary disease Disease that originates in a specific target organ and is not associated with or caused by a previous disease or injury.

primary hyperparathyroidism Common endocrine disorder in which one or more of the parathyroid glands are enlarged and overactive, secreting too much parathyroid hormone; caused by adenoma, hyperplasia, and carcinoma.

primary infertility No successful pregnancies after at least 1 year of having sex without using birth control methods.

primary structure Identity and sequence of amino acids in a polypeptide chain.

primer Short strand of RNA that serves as the starting point for DNA synthesis.

prism Transparent, solid body with a triangular base that separates white light into a continuous spectrum by refraction (i.e., shorter wavelengths are bent more than longer wavelengths as they pass through).

probe assembly Part of a peristaltic pump system; if the instrument accesses capped sample tubes; this assembly includes a cap piercer and liquid sensor.

procainamide A drug used to treat cardiac arrhythmia.

procedure A step-by-step guideline for performing a test.

process A set of interrelated activities that converts inputs (i.e., test requisitions) into outputs (i.e., test results).

product Result produced in a chemical reaction, such as the conversion of a substrate by an enzyme.

product formation The conversion of a substrate by an enzyme; the rate of reaction is affected by enzyme concentration, pH, temperature, cofactors, and inhibitors.

proficiency testing A form of quality control mandated by CLIA 88 for a laboratory to retain accreditation; samples are provided and the results of diagnostic tests are analyzed for accuracy by the accrediting agency.

progesterone receptor A tumor marker that may be overexpressed in breast cancer; the presence of estrogen and progesterone receptors suggests that the cancer is likely to respond to hormonal treatment.

prolactin Hormone secreted by the pituitary gland; it is suppressed by high estrogen levels during pregnancy, increases and stimulates lactation after childbirth, and helps maintain the immune system.

prolactinoma A benign but hormonally active pituitary tumor that secretes prolactin.

prostaglandins Chemical mediators of inflammation that dilate blood vessels; they also control the production of hormones and physiologic functions such as uterine contractions.

prostate-specific antigen Tumor marker used to screen high-risk populations for prostate cancer.

prosthetic group Tightly bound, nonprotein molecules that combine with or form part of a protein and are required for biological function; may be organic (i.e., sugar, vitamin, or lipid) or inorganic (i.e., metal ion).

protease An enzyme that breaks down protein by hydrolysis of the peptide bonds that link amino acids.

protein Molecule made of linear or folded chains of amino acids. Proteins are responsible for structure (e.g., hair, skin, nails), for movement (e.g., actin in muscle), for catalyzing chemical reactions (e.g., enzymes), for transport (e.g., carrier proteins), for defense (e.g., immunoglobulins), and for storage (e.g., iron in the liver by ferritin).

protein buffer system Mechanism for controlling blood hydrogen ion homeostasis; the largest concentration of nonbicarbonate substances in the blood.

proteinuria Abnormal quantities of protein in the urine; may indicate kidney damage.

prothrombin time PT; test that measures the clotting factors in the extrinsic clotting system.

proto-oncogenes Normal genes that become cancer-causing oncogenes when altered by mutations.

pseudohypoparathyroidism An inherited disease in which the parathyroid hormone receptors are unable to produce a response when bound with the hormone.

psychological assessment Examination of a patient that helps to identify psychosocial or psychiatric barriers to a good outcome of a procedure such as transplantation.

pulmonary diffusion Process of gas exchange between the lungs and the red blood cells.

pulmonary edema Accumulation of fluid in the alveoli.

pulmonary embolism Blood clot that has moved from another location in the body to the pulmonary artery.

pulmonary hypertension Elevated pulmonary artery pressure.

pyelonephritis Infection or inflammation of the kidneys that may begin as a lower urinary tract infection such as cystitis or prostatitis.

pyonephrosis Infection of the renal collecting system that produces pus in and around the kidneys.

Pyrex Borosilicate glassware widely used laboratories because of its chemical and thermal stability and good optical clarity. It can be used in high-temperature experiments, and it is resistant to heat shock and acids.

pyrrole ring Heterocyclic compound that is part of a porphyrin molecule and binds to an iron molecule to form heme.

Q

QNB 3-quinuclidinyl benzilate; white, crystalline solid that incapacitates individuals who are exposed through air, water, or food routes by blocking the transmission of nerve signals.

quadrupole mass spectrometer A spectrographic instrument whose quadrupole component (i.e., four parallel metal rods) filter sample ions based on their mass-to-charge ratio and the stability of their trajectories in the oscillating electric fields that are applied to the rods.

quality control chart Essential method for observing the validity of test results from run to run.

quality control chart rules Guidelines for interpretation of control sample results that enable a laboratory to detect an analytical error quickly and maintain a small false-alert rate.

quality control plan A set of written policies and procedures (including corrective actions), instructions for laboratory staff training, documentation, and methods for review and analysis of quality control data. It evaluates the risks of patient harm, applies manufacturers' recommendations for risk mitigation, and considers local health care conditions.

quality improvement Broad-based program designed to evaluate functions of the laboratory or health care system and to improve patient care.

quality improvement plan First step of the continuous quality improvement cycle (followed by corrective actions, monitoring, and further evaluation).

quality management system QMS; overall system that includes the twelve quality system essentials: facilities and safety, customer service, process improvement, documents and records, occurrence management, assessment, purchasing and inventory, process control, information management, equipment, personnel, and organization.

quantitative human chorionic gonadotropin Diagnostic test for ectopic pregnancy that determines whether the hCG levels being produced match the estimated gestational age.

quaternary structure Spatial arrangement of a protein after multiple polypeptide subunits aggregate.

R

radial immunodiffusion RID; technique used to determine the concentration of an antigen in a sample by measuring the diameter of the ring of precipitin formed by the antigen–antibody complex.

radioimmunoassay RIA; technique for determining antibody levels by introducing an antigen labeled with a radioisotope and measuring the resulting radioactivity of the antibody component. In the 1960s, radioisotopes were replaced with enzymes and color generation; this method had faster reaction times and longer shelf lives of components compared with RIA.

random access analyzer Device that allows a laboratory technician to select tests to be performed on each specimen; each specimen and its reagents are independent of other specimens in the analyzer.

random error Unforeseen abnormal test result that is usually due to temperature or technique but may have no apparent cause; the most difficult type of error to detect.

random sampling Ability of the analyzer to run multiple tests on one sample or multiple samples one test at one time.

Raynaud syndrome Disease characterized by vasoconstriction of capillaries in the extremities, especially the fingers.

reactive oxygen species Oxygen molecules that have an unpaired electron, rendering them extremely reactive in enzyme-driven reactions and likely to attack cellular structures.

reagent Chemical solution used in diagnostic tests; usually liquid, lyophilized, or frozen and available in various degrees of purity.

reagent-grade water Type I (highest quality) reagent-grade water is used in tests requiring minimal interference and maximum sensitivity; type II water is used for general laboratory testing; and type III water is used for initial rinsing and washing of glassware.

record Permanent documentation of laboratory information (no revisions are allowed) that can be used for continuous monitoring, sample tracking, evaluation of problems, and management of the laboratory.

redox electrode Inert metal electrode that is immersed in a solution containing redox couples or one in which the metal functions as a member of a redox couple; capable of measuring the potential of an oxidation-reduction reaction.

reference laboratory Large, independent, commercial laboratory that performs routine and specialty testing on samples received from physicians' office laboratories, nursing homes, and hospital laboratories.

reference range Span of normal values determined by analyzing at least 120 specimens obtained from apparently normal individuals and calculating the mean and range (±2 standard deviations from the mean) of those results.

reflectance density Amount of light absorbed by the colored reaction product on the smooth surface.

reflection Occurs when light (i.e., an incident ray) is deflected by the surface of a substance.

refraction Change in direction of light as it passes from one medium to another.

rejection Immune response after transplantation in which the recipient's body produces antibodies to the foreign cells (i.e., antigens) and ultimately destroys the transplanted tissue.

renal calculi Kidney stones.

renal insufficiency Disorder in which the kidneys do not effectively filter waste products from the blood.

renal obstruction Blockage of the flow of urine from the renal pelvis to the ureter, as from kidney stones.

renal threshold Amount of a substance that can be reabsorbed by kidney tubules and returned to the circulation.

renal tubular acidosis Low blood pH level produced by inability of the kidney tubules to secrete hydrogen ions or retain bicarbonate.

renin Proteolytic enzyme that is synthesized and released from specialized renal cells when the pressure in the afferent arterioles and the sodium concentration in the tubules decrease; plays a role in regulating blood pressure.

renin-angiotensin-aldosterone pathway Hormone system that regulates sodium balance, fluid volume, and blood pressure by a negative feedback loop in which renin, secreted in response to reduced renal perfusion, stimulates release of angiotensin release, which in turn stimulates aldosterone secretion; the aldosterone causes sodium retention, water retention, increased blood pressure, and restoration of renal perfusion, shutting off the signal for renin secretion.

resolution Smallest interval measurable by a scientific instrument; affects how well analytes are separated by chromatography.

resorption atelectasis Occurs when a bronchial obstruction blocks air from entering part of the lung and the gas in the alveoli is reabsorbed into the blood, deflating the alveoli.

respiration Process by which oxygen is delivered to tissues and metabolic byproducts such as carbon dioxide are removed from tissues.

respiratory acidosis Reduced pH in body fluids or tissues caused by a respiratory condition (i.e., buildup of carbon dioxide in the blood).

respiratory alkalosis Increased pH in body fluids or tissues caused by a respiratory condition (i.e., loss of carbon dioxide).

respiratory distress syndrome Breathing disorder in newborns caused by fetal lung immaturity usually due to insufficient lung surfactant.

restriction Type of enzyme found in bacteria that cuts human DNA at specific locations.

rhabdomyolysis Rapid destruction of skeletal muscle cells caused by muscle injury and the consequent release of large quantities of myoglobin.

rheumatoid arthritis Chronic, systemic, autoimmune disease that causes inflammation, deformity, and immobility of synovial joints, especially in the fingers, wrists, feet, and ankles; occurs more often in women than in men.

ricin Also called abrin; biological toxin made from castor beans that inhibits protein synthesis in the body.

rickets Bone disease of children and adolescents in which osteoid fails to calcify; caused by deficiency of vitamin D metabolites or dietary deficiency of calcium or phosphorus.

right middle lobe syndrome Usually refers to atelectasis in the right middle lobe of the lung caused by obstruction of the bronchus and partial lung collapse; also found in Sjögren syndrome.

rotor The rotating unit of a centrifuge that creates a centrifugal force.

S

Safety Data Sheets SDS; printed materials used to communicate the properties of a specific product; the physical, health, or environmental hazards it may present; and advice on safety precautions and handling of exposures.

salivary amylase An enzyme secreted by the salivary glands that breaks down carbohydrates.

sarcoidosis Chronic inflammatory disease of unknown cause characterized by the enlargement of lymph nodes in many parts of the body and the widespread appearance of granulomas derived from the reticuloendothelial system.

sarcoma Tumor that originates in connective or other nonepithelial tissue, such as bone, cartilage, fat, muscle, or fibrous tissue.

sarin Nerve agent that is a clear, colorless, odorless, and tasteless liquid.

saturated fatty acids Carboxylic acids with long carbon chains that contain only single bonds between the carbon groups; includes most of the fatty acids from animal sources.

saxitoxin Neurotoxin produced by dinoflagellates of the genus *Gonyaulax* and by the blue-ringed octopus; binds to sodium channels in neuron membranes, blocking transmission of signals to muscles.

scleroderma Systemic autoimmune disease of connective tissue that produces hardening and contraction of the skin as well as blood vessel abnormalities, collagen overproduction, and immune system dysfunction.

secondary aldosteronism Also called secondary hyperaldosteronism; increased aldosterone secretion from a source other than the adrenal glands; most often, angiotensin II is elevated through a renin-dependent mechanism, increasing aldosterone secretion.

secondary amenorrhea Absence of menses in a woman who has been having normal menstrual cycles.

secondary disease An endocrine disease originating in the hypothalamus or pituitary gland.

secondary hyperparathyroidism Occurs when a chronic disease such as kidney failure lowers blood calcium levels, leading to parathyroid hormone resistance and subsequent increased secretion.

secondary hyperthyroidism Increased thyroid hormone levels caused by increased thyroid-stimulating hormone with or without increased thyrotropin-releasing hormone.

secondary hypocortisolism Adrenal insufficiency caused by deficiency of adrenocorticotropic hormone produced by the pituitary gland.

secondary hypothyroidism Underproduction of thyroid hormones caused by failure of the pituitary gland to secrete thyroid-stimulating hormone.

secondary infertility Inability to become pregnant or to carry a pregnancy to term after the birth of one or more biological children.

secondary structure One-dimensional protein assemblies called α-helixes and β-pleated sheets that are created by hydrogen and disulfide covalent bonds.

secondhand smoke The smoke produced from a lit cigarette that is exhaled by a smoker.

secretin A hormone secreted by the S cells of the duodenum that prevents the pH of the small intestine from falling below 4.5; inhibits secretion of hydrochloric acid produced by parietal cells and stimulates the pancreas to secrete bicarbonate.

secretin-cholecystokinin test Combination of two tests that is used to assess the function of both the pancreas and the gallbladder.

secretin test A test used to diagnose pancreatic malfunction.

selectin Type of adhesion molecule.

sensitization Process by which the immune system "learns" from exposure to an antigen such that a subsequent exposure results in an amplified response.

sentinel laboratory First laboratory to learn of a bioterrorism attack and collect patient specimens for testing.

sequelae of diabetes Include renal failure, nontraumatic amputations, blindness, retinopathy, nerve damage, and atherosclerotic disease.

serapin Protein which blocks the enzymatic activity of serine proteases.

serial dilution Stepwise dilution of a substance in solution, producing a series of solutions having equal increments of variation.

serologic glass pipette Glass tube etched with gradations so that different amounts can be delivered with the same pipette.

serologic typing In transplantation medicine, use of a typing tray from a commercial source to identify antigen groups of a donor or recipient.

serotonin Neurotransmitter synthesized from tryptophan and secreted by the gastrointestinal tract; involved in sleep, depression, memory, and smooth muscle contraction.

severe combined immunodeficiency SCID; spectrum of genetic disorders which, in the most severe form (reticular dysgenesis), results in no development of T cells, B cells, or phagocytic cells in the bone marrow.

sharps Anything that can puncture the skin, such as needles, broken glass, glass pipettes, razor blades, and scalpels.

shift Abrupt change in control data with at least six results lying on one side of the mean value.

sirolimus Also known as rapamycin; an inhibitor of the mammalian target of rapamycin (mTOR). Inhibition of mTOR blocks the activation of interleukin-2 and prevents the G- to S-phase transition of T lymphocytes. Like tacrolimus and everolimus, sirolimus has a nephrotoxic effect that is synergistic with calcineurin inhibitors such as cyclosporine.

Six Sigma Laboratory management philosophy that emphasizes setting high objectives, collecting data, and analyzing results to a fine degree as a way to reduce errors in products and services; uses a five-step cycle: Define, Measure, Analyze, Improve, and Control.

size exclusion chromatography Separates molecules according to their size; also known as gel permeation chromatography or gel filtration chromatography.

Sjögren syndrome Autoimmune disease that damages exocrine glands, especially those that produce saliva, tears, and other secretions in the body; associated with dry membranes.

small cell lung cancer The most aggressive form of lung cancer, which can cause death within weeks of diagnosis if not treated.

sodium pump The enzyme, sodium-potassium adenosine triphosphatase (Na^+/K^+-ATPase), that actively transports sodium and potassium across the cell membranes of all animal cells.

solid-phase adsorption Separation technique in which antibody binding to an analyte takes place on the surface of a solid support, such as the inner surface of plastic tubes or microtiter wells or the outer surface of cellulose beads, latex beads, or magnetic particles.

soman Nerve agent; a clear, colorless liquid that smells like camphor or rotting fruit.

somatostatin Peptide hormone produced by the hypothalamus and delta cells of the pancreas that regulates blood glucose, lipids, peptides, vasoactive intestinal peptide, and cholecystokinin.

Southern blot Procedure for identifying specific sequences of DNA, in which fragments separated on a gel are transferred directly to a second medium on which detection by hybridization may be carried out.

specimen processing Samples arriving in the laboratory are checked for proper labeling, sufficient quantity, condition, correct tube, and appropriate and complete paperwork and are then entered into the laboratory system and centrifuged before being delivered to the laboratory department for testing.

spectral bandwidth Width in nanometers of the spectral transmittance curve at a point equal to one half of the peak transmittance.

spectral purity Quantification of the monochromaticity of a given light sample.

spectrophotometry The measurement of light at selected wavelengths.

specular reflectance Analytical technique that measures light reflected from a smooth or mirrorlike surface (in contrast to diffuse reflectance, which occurs when light is reflected from an irregular surface).

sphingolipids Lipid components that occur chiefly in the cell membranes of red blood cells and nerve cells.

sphingomyelin Any of the class of phospholipids that occur in membranes, chiefly in the brain and spinal cord, and that serve as a good internal standard for fetal lung maturity.

spina bifida Closed neural tube defect in which the bottom end of the neural tube fails to fuse; can manifest as a fluid-filled cyst, area of hypopigmentation or hyperpigmentation, capillary telangiectasia or hemangioma, hairy patch, skin appendage, or asymmetric gluteal cleft.

spirometry Measurement of mechanical pulmonary function through lung volumes and capacities.

spondyloarthropathies A group of chronic, systemic, inflammatory conditions that affect the joints and axial skeleton (e.g., ankylosing spondylitis).

spongiform encephalopathy Degenerative disease characterized by the development of porous, spongelike lesions in brain tissue and by deterioration in neurologic functioning.

staging Evaluation of the extent and aggressiveness of a tumor according to its size and spread from the primary location.

standard curve Graph showing properties that are known for multiple samples (standards); used for determining properties of unknown samples by comparison against the curve.

standard deviation Measure of the dispersion of a set of data from the mean.

standard operating procedures SOPs; one way a laboratory can reduce the exposure of workers to hazards; step-by-step instructions for performing tests and operating equipment in the laboratory.

standard precautions Minimum infection control practices recommended by the Centers for Disease Control and Prevention for health care in all settings, regardless of the known or suspected infection status of the patient.

staphylococcal enterotoxin B SEB; one of many toxins produced by *Staphylococcus aureus*; it is toxic to cells and is the primary cause of staphylococcal food poisoning.

stationary phase A solid or a liquid in a chromatographic system that interacts with components of the mobile phase.

status asthmaticus Potentially fatal condition in which asthma attacks follow one another without pause.

steady state Condition in which the amount of drug entering the body is equal to the amount of the drug being eliminated from the body.

steatorrhea Excretion of abnormal quantities of fat in feces.

sterilization Destruction of all microorganisms to create an aseptic environment.

steroid hormone Lipid-soluble hormones that are derived from cholesterol and produced as needed by the gonads, placenta, and adrenal glands; must bind to a carrier protein to move through the blood. Examples include cortisol, aldosterone, testosterone, estrogen, and progesterone.

sterols High-molecular-weight, polycyclic alcohols, also known as steroid alcohols, that are synthesized from acetyl-coenzyme A.

storage iron Iron that is stored in molecules such as ferritin and hemosiderin rather than circulating in the blood.

strychnine A strong poison produced from the plant *Strychnos nux-vomica;* intravenous, gastrointestinal, or respiratory exposure can cause muscle failure and death. It is used as a pesticide and rat poison.

subarachnoid hemorrhage Bleeding into the subarachnoid space of the brain; can be caused by trauma, a ruptured cerebral aneurysm, or an arteriovenous malformation.

subclinical hyperthyroidism Low or undetectable serum thyroid-stimulating hormone levels accompanied by normal thyroid hormone concentrations; hyperthyroidism symptoms are absent, but the condition can cause atrial fibrillation and osteoporosis.

subclinical hypothyroidism Normal thyroid hormone levels with a serum thyroid-stimulating hormone level above the upper limit of normal.

subdural hematoma Bleeding into the space beneath the dura mater and above the arachnoid membrane; the most common type of traumatic lesion to the brain.

Substance Abuse and Mental Health Services Administration SAMSHA; sets federal guidelines for the use of drugs of abuse that apply to employees such as truck drivers in the transportation industry. They must pass a standardized urine drug screen for five categories of drugs of abuse: amphetamines, cannabinoids, opiates, phencyclidine, and cocaine.

substrate Substance on which an enzyme acts.

subtherapeutic dose Concentration of a drug that is below the therapeutic range.

Sudan Stain IV Used in fecal fat test to diagnose malabsorption/maldigestion.

sulfhemoglobin Modified hemoglobin molecule in which sulfur atoms have attached to the hemoglobin, preventing oxygen from attaching to the iron in heme and rendering the hemoglobin molecule nonfunctional.

sulfur mustard A DNA-alkylating agent that damages rapidly growing cells; used in World War I as a chemical warfare agent.

sympathomimetics Drugs that mimic the effects of the sympathetic nervous system; used to treat cardiac arrest and low blood pressure and to delay premature labor.

syndrome of inappropriate antidiuretic hormone secretion SIADH; occurs when the pituitary secretes high levels of ADH without being stimulated to do so. SIADH can be caused by secretion of ADH by ectopic tumors, such as small cell carcinoma of the lung, duodenum, stomach, or pancreas; bladder cancer; prostate cancer; endometrial cancer; lymphomas; and sarcomas.

systematic error Reproducible inaccuracies that are consistently in the same direction and are often due to an equipment failure that persists throughout the experiment; includes trends and shifts.

systemic lupus erythematosus SLE; chronic, inflammatory, autoimmune disease in which the body produces antibodies to nucleic acids, red blood cells, coagulation proteins, phospholipids, lymphocytes, and platelets.

systole Period of contraction of the ventricles during which blood is forced into the aorta and pulmonary artery.

systolic First number of a blood pressure measurement; amount of pressure generated by the heart when it pumps blood into arteries.

T

tabletop exercises Planning scenarios in which participants discuss a plausible incident; consider its impact on buildings, businesses, and customers; and judge the response plan on how well it promotes survivability.

tabun GA (military designation); nerve agent in the form of a clear, colorless to pale or dark amber liquid that smells fruity like bitter almonds.

tachycardia Abnormally rapid heartbeat, usually more than 100 beats per minute.

tacrolimus FK506; immunosuppressive drug used mainly after allogeneic organ transplantation to lower the risk of organ rejection; calcineurin inhibitor that produces less nephrotoxicity than cyclosporine but otherwise has similar long-term side effects.

Tamm-Horsfall protein Also known as uromodulin; a glycoprotein that is synthesized in kidney tubules and excreted in urine; may act as an inhibitor of calcium crystallization to prevent kidney stones and may provide defense against urinary tract infections caused by uropathogenic bacteria.

tandem mass spectrometry Procedure in which two mass spectrometers are used in series and are connected by a chamber known as a collision cell. An ion with a particular mass-to-charge ratio is selected in the first instrument and directed into the collision cell, where it is broken into fragments. The second instrument acquires the mass of the ion fragments.

Tangier disease A disease in which defective catabolism of apolipoprotein A-I causes accumulation of cholesterol esters in tissues.

Terry's nails Condition in which the nail bed is white and opaque, obscuring the lunula; occurs mostly in patients with liver disease, especially cirrhosis, but also in those who are hospitalized for long periods.

tertiary hyperthyroidism Form of hyperthyroidism caused by stimulation of the thyroid gland by increased thyrotropin-releasing hormone levels.

tertiary hypothyroidism Hypothyroidism caused by thyrotropin-releasing hormone deficiency.

tertiary structure Three-dimensional structure resulting from folding and covalent cross-linking of a protein or polynucleotide molecule.

testosterone Steroid hormone derived from cholesterol, produced by the testes, regulated by luteinizing hormone, and bound to sex hormone–binding globulin in the blood; functions in the development and maturation of the male reproductive system.

test profile Array of laboratory tests run on many specimens.

tetraiodothyronine Occurs naturally as L-thyroxine (T_4); a hormone, 3,5,3′5′-tetraiodothyronine, produced by the thyroid gland that contains iodine and is a derivative of the amino acid tyrosine.

tetralogy of Fallot Congenital heart defect caused by failure of the right ventricular tract to form properly in the embryo, causing four congenital heart defects: ventricular septal defect, pulmonic stenosis, malpositioned aorta, and ventricular hypertrophy.

tetrodotoxin Strong neurotoxin secreted by certain fish and bacterial species and by the blue-ringed octopus; causes convulsions and paralysis leading to death.

α-thalassemia Condition caused by the inheritance of genes for Barts hemoglobin, which consists of four γ-globin chains; deletion of all four α-globin genes makes the hemoglobin incapable of effective oxygen delivery to tissues.

β-thalassemia intermedia Type of β-thalassemia that is less severe than β-thalassemia major because patients have some β-chain formation, decreased production of hemoglobin A, and increased production of hemoglobin F.

β-thalassemia major Condition that prevents the formation of β-globin chains; patients have mostly hemoglobin F, have no hemoglobin A, and may have a small amount of hemoglobin A_2. Symptoms include failure to thrive and severe anemia (also called Cooley anemia).

β-thalassemia minor Type of β-thalassemia in which only one of the two β-globin alleles contains a mutation and β-chain production is not intolerably compromised; patients may be relatively asymptomatic.

The Joint Commission Formerly known as the Joint Commission for the Accreditation of Healthcare Organizations (JCAHO); organization that accredits hospitals and other health care institutions such as ambulatory care facilities, stand-alone surgery centers, long-term care facilities, behavioral health centers, and laboratories.

therapeutic index Difference between the dose of a drug that has a lethal effect and the dose that has a therapeutic effect.

therapeutic range Range of concentrations at which a drug effectively treats diseases with minimal toxicity to most patients.

thromboemboli Blood clots that form within blood vessels and circulate through the bloodstream.

thromboxane Any of a group of lipid eicosanoids that function as chemical mediators in hormone production and in physiologic functions such as blood clotting and constriction of blood vessels; an intermediate in the metabolic pathway of arachidonic acid.

throughput Number of tests performed per hour.

thymopoietin TPO; polypeptide hormone secreted by the thymus; induces the proliferation of lymphocyte precursors and their differentiation into T cells.

thymosin TMO; humoral factor secreted by the thymus; promotes maturation of T cells.

thyroglobulin Iodine-containing glycoprotein produced by the follicular cells of the thyroid gland; acts as a substrate for synthesis of the hormones thyroxine and triiodothyronine.

thyroid cancer Disease in which the cells of the thyroid gland become abnormal, grow uncontrollably, and form a mass of cells called a tumor.

thyroid hormone resistance Rare autosomal dominant disorder that is characterized by elevated serum levels of thyroid hormones, inappropriately elevated levels of thyroid-stimulating hormone, and diminished responsiveness of target tissues to the effects of thyroid hormones.

thyroiditis Inflammation of the thyroid gland.

thyroid-stimulating hormone TSH, also called thyrotropin; hormone produced by the pituitary gland; promotes thyroid cell growth and secretion of thyroid hormones.

thyroid storm Exacerbation of symptoms of hyperthyroidism; occurs when uncontrolled thyrotoxicosis follows shock, injury, or thyroidectomy and causes rapid pulse, extreme nervousness, coma, and death.

thyrotoxicosis A hypermetabolic syndrome resulting from serum elevations of the thyroid hormones.

time-of-flight mass spectrometer Device used for the identification of microorganisms. The mass spectra generated are analyzed by dedicated software and compared with stored profiles.

tissue Aggregates of similar cells (e.g., hepatocytes) and their products.

tissue iron Iron found in iron-dependent peroxidases and cytochromes.

tissue typing Histocompatibility matching between a donor and a recipient; a fundamental step in planning organ and tissue transplantation.

tolerance Progressively decreased responsiveness to a drug; necessitates larger doses of the drug to achieve the effect originally obtained by a smaller dose.

total iron-binding capacity TIBC; measures the total amount of iron that can be bound by transferrin.

toxic dose The amount of a chemical that produces a harmful (not lethal) effect.

toxicity Degree to which a substance causes damage in the body.

toxic multinodular goiter Enlargement of the thyroid gland in the setting of low thyroid-stimulating hormone and normal thyroxine levels (i.e., subclinical hyperthyroidism) or clinical hyperthyroidism.

traceability Serial comparisons of measurements that lead to a known NIST reference value; used to ensure reasonable agreement between measurements of routine methods.

transcutaneous Through the skin.

transferase Enzyme that catalyzes the transfer from one molecule to another of a functional group that does not exist in the free state during the transfer.

transferrin Small protein that contains two iron (Fe^{3+}) binding sites; used to transport iron in the body.

transferrin saturation The ratio of serum iron to total iron-binding capacity, multiplied by 100; it is decreased with iron deficiency and increased with iron overload.

transition state An unstable, high-energy configuration assumed by reactants on the way to making products in a chemical reaction; has a much higher level of free energy than the substrate or product.

transplantation Transfer of tissue, an organ, or bone marrow cells from a donor to a recipient.

transposition of the great arteries Congenital disease in which the two major blood vessels that carry blood away from the heart, the aorta and the pulmonary artery, are reversed (transposed).

transthyretin α-globulin secreted by the liver that transports retinol-binding protein and thyroxine through plasma and cerebrospinal fluid.

transudate Fluid that contains low amounts of protein, few cells, and high water content; produced in liver and kidney diseases and by cancerous processes.

trend Drift of laboratory results in an upward or downward direction from the mean; occurs when six consecutive control results gradually move in a positive or negative direction on the control chart.

trichothecene mycotoxins Biological poisons produced by *Fusarium, Myrothecium, Trichoderma, Cephalosporium, Verticimonosporium,* and *Stachybotrys* fungi; thought to have been aerosolized and used as weapons ("yellow rain").

triglycerides Molecules formed from glycerol and three fatty acid groups that serve as the backbone of many lipids; elevated levels in the bloodstream are considered to be a risk factor for atherosclerosis.

triiodothyronine T_3; an iodine-containing hormone produced by the thyroid gland; regulates growth and development, controls metabolism and body temperature, and inhibits the secretion of thyrotropin by the pituitary gland.

triple phosphate crystals Magnesium ammonium phosphate ($MgNH_4PO_4$) crystals, also called struvite crystals; may be normal or may be associated with urinary tract infection or kidney stones.

tropical sprue Rare condition found in tropical regions that is associated with inflammation and malabsorption and is likely caused by an infectious agent.

troponin I and troponin T Regulatory proteins in cardiac cells that are integral to muscle contraction; used as significant biomarkers of heart damage when found in the bloodstream in high amounts.

trough level Lowest concentration of a drug in the patient's bloodstream.

trypsin Digestive enzyme produced in the small intestine that converts procarboxypeptidase and chymotrypsinogen into carboxypeptidase and chymotrypsin and breaks down proteins into oligopeptides.

trypsinogen Released by the pancreas during digestion; converted to trypsin in the small intestine.

tumor markers Substances produced by tumor or other cells that can be measured in blood and used to differentiate malignant from normal tissue.

tumor suppressor genes Type of gene whose products prevent mutation and inhibit damaged cells from proliferating.

turbidimetry Technique that uses spectrophotometers to measure the amount of light transmitted through or absorbed by particles suspended in a solution; values are used to determine the amount of a substance in the sample.

two-step format Design of a competitive assay in which excess antibody is incubated with the sample and binds antigens in the serum (step 1), after which labeled antigen is added to the solution (step 2) and binds with any open antibody binding sites. Less bound labeled antigen indicates that there is a higher amount of antigen in the sample.

type 1 diabetes mellitus Formerly known as juvenile diabetes; destruction of beta cells in the islets of Langerhans in the pancreas leads to absolute insulin deficiency.

type 2 diabetes mellitus Spectrum of disorders ranging from insulin resistance with relative insulin deficiency to a defect of insulin secretion with insulin resistance. Risk factors include increased age, obesity, hypertension, physical inactivity, and family history.

U

ulcer An open sore on an external or internal surface of the body caused by a break in the skin or mucous membrane that fails to heal.

ulcerative colitis Disease in which chronic inflammation affects the large intestine.

unassayed control Control sample for which no assigned analyte value has been provided by the manufacturer; the control value must be determined by the individual laboratory.

uncompetitive inhibition Type of inhibition in which the inhibitor binds to the enzyme-substrate complex, preventing formation of the expected product.

unconjugated bilirubin Indirect bilirubin; fraction of serum bilirubin that has not been conjugated with glucuronic acid in the liver; it is not excreted in urine and circulates with plasma proteins.

universal precautions Set of procedural directives and guidelines by the Centers for Disease Control and Prevention for infection prevention and control that treat all body fluids as if they contained infectious pathogens.

unsaturated fatty acid Molecule with long chains of carbon groups that contain single and double bonds between the carbon atoms; called unsaturated because it is capable of absorbing additional hydrogen atoms.

ureterolithiasis Formation or presence of calculi (stones) in one or both ureters.

uric acid End product of the breakdown of purines; can accumulate in tissues and cause gout.

urinalysis Examination of the physical, chemical, and microscopic properties of urine.

urinary tract infection Infection of the bladder or kidney.

urine Fluid remaining in the collecting ducts after the kidneys filter blood and concentrate waste.

urobilinogen A byproduct of bilirubin metabolism that is analyzed during urinalysis.

urosepsis A blood infection that occurs secondary to a urinary tract infection.

V

valence The number of electrons that can be lost, gained, or shared by an atom when forming a compound.

validation Assessment of results from new reagent kits compared with the results obtained from the old kit; ensures that there will be no clinically significant differences between results obtained with the two sets.

vanillylmandelic acid VMA; primary end product of epinephrine or norepinephrine metabolism; measured in urine to screen patients for neuroblastomas and pheochromocytomas.

vapor pressure The pressure of an evaporated solvent; the value decreases as the concentration of solute particles increases.

vascular permeability Capacity of the walls of small blood vessels to allow small molecules to filter in and out.

vasculitis Inflammation of the blood vessels that can increase wall thickness, weaken the structure, and cause narrowing or scarring.

vasodilation Dilation or widening of blood vessels.

ventricular septal defect Abnormal opening in the septum that divides the two ventricles of the heart.

vertigo Erroneous sensation that the environment is moving (i.e., illusory movement) that can cause balance problems, nausea, and vomiting.

very-low-density lipoprotein Type of cholesterol produced in the liver and released into the bloodstream to supply the body with triglycerides.

vestibular neuronitis Inflammatory condition that results in severe, limited episodes of nausea and vertigo, usually after an infection.

vitamin A A lipid-soluble micronutrient that contains retinol and plays an important role in vision; ingested as dietary β-carotene.

vitamin B$_1$ Thiamine; coenzyme that is required for decarboxylation reactions and has roles in the production of energy from food, synthesis of nucleic acids, and conduction of nerve impulses.

vitamin B$_2$ Riboflavin; an essential part of coenzymes involved in redox reactions, such as flavin adenine dinucleotide (FAD).

vitamin B$_6$ Pyridoxine; used for the synthesis, catabolism, and interconversion of amino acids.

vitamin B$_{12}$ Cyanocobalamin; water-soluble micronutrient produced by gut bacteria; plants do not use or contain this compound.

vitamin C Ascorbic acid; a water-soluble micronutrient that is needed for growth and repair of tissues in all parts of the body.

vitamin D Micronutrient that is necessary for bone health. It is regulated by parathyroid hormone and maintains the concentrations of calcium and phosphate in serum through a feedback mechanism.

vitamin E Complex of ten lipid-soluble micronutrients, with α-tocopherol being the most common form in American diets and the major form found in blood; a potent antioxidant that prevents the production of molecular oxygen and free radicals during fat oxidation.

vitamin H Biotin; a member of the vitamin B complex. It is usually bound to protein and must be released by the action of gastrointestinal hormones to be absorbed from the intestines.

vitamin K Composed of K$_1$ (phylloquinone) and K$_2$ (menaquinone); required for the production of several clotting factors and may be involved in bone metabolism. It is produced in part by gut bacteria.

voltammetry Measurement of current flowing into or out of an electrode in a solution. The study of current as a function of applied potential; used to measure oxygen.

volumetric pipette Long glass tube with a bubble in the middle; allows extremely accurate measurement of a volume of solution.

VX Nerve agent; clear amber, oily, tasteless, and odorless liquid.

W

Waldenström macroglobulinemia A monoclonal gammopathy that is a type of non-Hodgkin lymphoma.

Western blot Technique used to identify specific amino acid sequences in proteins and for quantitation of antigens.

Westgard rules A set of rules used to define calculated control value limits for a particular assay; valuable for detecting random and systematic errors.

Wilson disease Autosomal recessive genetic disease of copper metabolism that leads to copper deposition in body tissues.

Wiskott-Aldrich syndrome Rare X-linked recessive disease in which a protein that is involved in signaling and organizing the cytoskeletal structure in blood cells is mutated; causes thrombocytopenia, immunodeficiency, eczema, and increased susceptibility to tumors and autoimmune disease.

X

xanthomas Small, yellow-red papules deposited on the back of forearms, shins, and pressure points. They erupt when the triglyceride level is greater than 2000 mg/dL.

D-xylose absorption Test used to determine whether malabsorption has a pancreatic or an intestinal origin.

Y

yellow nail syndrome Rare condition producing yellow nails that lack a cuticle, grow slowly, and can be detached (as in onycholysis); usually occurs in people with lung disease or lymphedema.

Youden plot A graphic depiction that is used to analyze data variability from two levels of control materials within a laboratory or between two laboratories. It is used with both normal and abnormal controls and can differentiate between systematic and random errors.

Z

zero-order kinetics Describes a reaction under conditions of substrate excess.

Zollinger-Ellison disease Rare disorder involving benign, non–β-islet cell, gastrin-secreting tumors (i.e., gastrinomas) located in the pancreas or duodenum.

zona fasciculata Middle portion of the adrenal cortex; secretes the glucocorticoids cortisol, cortisone, and corticosterone.

zona glomerulosa Outer portion of the adrenal cortex; produces the mineralocorticoid aldosterone.

zona reticularis Inner portion of the adrenal cortex; secretes mineralocorticoids, sex hormones, and glucocorticoids.

Answer Key

Chapter 1

Practice Problems

1. KBr: The atomic weight of potassium (K) is 39. The atomic weight of bromine (Br) is 80. When they are combined, the molecular weight of potassium bromide (KBr) is 119.

    H_2O: The atomic weight of hydrogen (H) is 1. Because there are two atoms of hydrogen in the compound, the total for hydrogen will be 2. The atomic weight of oxygen (O) is 16. Because there is only one atom oxygen in the compound, the total for oxygen will be 16. Therefore, the molecular weight of water (H_2O) is 2 + 16 = 18.

    $AgNO_3$: The atomic weight of silver (Ag) is 108. There is only one silver atom in the compound, so the total for silver will be 108. The atomic weight of nitrogen (N) is 14. There is only one nitrogen atom in the compound, so the total for nitrogen will be 14. The atomic weight of oxygen (O) is 16. Because there are three atoms of oxygen in the compound, the total for oxygen will be 48. Therefore, the molecular weight of silver nitrate ($AgNO_3$) is 108 + 14 + 48 = 170.

    $Fe_2(SO_4)_3$: The atomic weight of iron (Fe) is 56. Because there are two iron atoms in the compound, the total for iron will be 112. This compound has three molecules of a radical, SO_4, so the final compound will have three sulfur (S) atoms and twelve oxygen (O) atoms. The atomic weight of sulfur is 32. Because there are three atoms of sulfur in the compound, the total for sulfur will be 32 × 3 = 96. The atomic weight of oxygen is 16. Because there are twelve oxygen atoms in the compound, the total for oxygen will be 12 × 16 = 192. Therefore, the molecular weight for ferric sulfate ($Fe_2(SO_4)_3$) is 112 + 96 + 192 = 400. The molecular weight of ferric sulfate is 400.

2. If 1 L of solution contains 5 moles of NaCl, it is a five molar (5 M) solution; 5 moles of NaCl dissolved in 5 L is a 1 M solution because there is 1 mole per liter of solution.

3. The molecular weight of $CaCl_2$ is 40 + 2(35.5) = 111, so 1 L of a 1 M solution would be made by dissolving 111 g of $CaCl_2$ in enough water to make 1 L. Therefore, a 2 M solution would require 2(111) = 222 g of $CaCl_2$ and enough water to make 1 L of solution.

4. The molecular weight of KOH = 39 + 16 + 1 = 56. One liter of 1.5 molar KOH is made by dissolving 1.5(56) = 84 g of KOH in 1 L of solution, so 3.5 liters would be made by dissolving 3.5(84) = 294 g of KOH in 3.5 L of solution.

5. The molecular weight of NaCl is 23 + 35.5 = 58.5, so 58.5 g of NaCl in 1 L is 1 molar solution. We have 9 g in 1 L, so the molarity is 9/58.5 = 0.15 M.

6. The molecular weight of NaCl again is 58.5. Our solution contains 100 g of NaCl in 2 L, so 1 L contains 100/2 = 50 g. Because 1 mole of NaCl is 58.5 g, the molarity of a solution of 50 g in 1 L is 50/58.5 = 0.85 M.

7. a. One liter of 3 M NaOH is made by dissolving 3(23 + 16 +1) = 120 g of NaOH in enough water to make 1 L of solution.

    b. Dissolve 3(39 + 35.5) = 223.5 g of KCl in 3 L of solution.

    c. Dissolve (2.5)(2)(40 +2[35.5]) = 555 g of $CaCl_2$ in 2.5 L of solution.

8. The molecular weight of KCl is 74.5. If there are 200 g of KCl in 900 mL of water, there are x grams in 1000 mL:

    $$200/900 = x/1000$$

    $$900x = 200,000$$

    $$x = 222$$

    The molarity is 222/74.5 = 3.0 M.

9. The atomic weight of Na is 23 and that of Cl is 35.5. The molecular weight of NaCl is 58.5. To make a 3 molal solution, add 3 × 58.5 g of NaCl to 1000 g of solvent (which in the case of water is 1 L).

10. The atomic weight of Li is 7, O is 16, and H is 1. The molecular weight of LiOH is 24. Therefore, 35 g of LiOH is 35/24 = 1.45 moles, and the molality of the solution would be 1.45 moles ÷ 0.75 kg = 1.94 mol/kg.

11. The atomic weight of Na is 23 and that of Cl is 35.5, making the molecular weight of NaCl 58.5.

Therefore, 44 g of NaCl is 44/58.5 = 0.75 mole. A 2.75 molal solution would contain 2.75 moles in 1 kg of solvent:

$$0.75/x = 2.75/1000$$

$$x = 0.75/2.75$$

$$x = 273$$

The required amount of solvent is 273 g.

12. The atomic weight of Ca is 40, and the atomic weight of Cl is 35.5. The molecular weight of $CaCl_2$ is 40 + 2(35.5) = 110, so 110 g equals 1 mole. To make a 1.4 molal solution would require 1.4 × 110 = 154 g of $CaCl_2$ for every 1000 g of solvent. However, we have only 475 g of solvent, so only 154 × (475/1000) = 73.15 g of $CaCl_2$ is required. Put another way, we need only 1.4 × (475/1000) or .665 moles, and 110 × .665 = 73.15 g of $CaCl_2$.

13.

Element	Electrons in Outer Orbit	Valence
K	1	+1
Ca	2	+2
Br	7	−1
Fe	3	+3
O	6	−2

14. a. Molecular weight of NAOH is 40 g. The total valence is 1. Find the number of moles of NaOH: 10 g/40 g/mol. There are 0.25 moles. Divide by valence of 1 to get the gram equivalent weight = 0.25. 0.25 gram equivalent weight of NaOH divided by total liters of solution (0.5 L) = 0.5 N solution.

b. The gram molecule weight of $MgCl_2$ is 95 g (24 + 71). The total valence for this compound is 2. The gram equivalent weight for this compound is 95 g/2 = 47.5. We will divide 90 g by the gram equivalent weight (47.5 g) to find out we have 1.89 gram equivalent weights of $MgCl_2$. This is dissolved in 1.5 L of water, which produces a 1.26 N solution: 1.89 gram equivalent weights/1.5 liters of solution.

15. a. To make 1 L of 3 N KOH, dissolve 168.3 g of KOH in enough water to make 1 L of solution.

b. To make 5 L of 1 N $CaCl_2$, dissolve 277.5 g of $CaCl_2$ in enough water to make 5 L of solution.

16. a. To make 3 L of 1.5 g/dL KOH, dissolve 45 g of KOH in 3 L of water.

b. To make 600 mL of 4 g/dL $MgCl_2$, dissolve 24 g of $MgCl_2$ in 600 mL of water.

c. To make 50 mL of 10% NaOH, dissolve 5 g of NaOH in 50 mL of water.

17. a. A 10% NaOH contains 100 g or 2.5 moles per liter of solution; therefore, the molarity is 2.5 M.

b. To prepare 20 L of 0.9% NaCl, dissolve 180 g of NaCl in 20 L of water.

c. A 0.1 N KOH solution would have a concentration of 560 mg/dL.

18. It takes 277.8 mL of concentrated (36 N) H_2SO_4 to make 5 liters of 2 N H_2SO_4.

19. It takes 65 L of 1 M NaCl diluted to 10 L to make a 0.9% NaCl solution. Convert 1 M solution of NaCl to %: 1 M = 58.5 g/mol/1 liter of solution or 5.85 g per 100 mL solution = 5.85%

Ratio: 0.9%/10 L = 5.85% (x)

$$0.9\%(x) = (10)(5.85\%)$$

$$x = (10 L)(5.85\%)/0.9\%$$

$$x = 65 L$$

20. 1000 mL; 21. 20,000 mL; 22. 30 mg; 23. 100 mL; 24. 1000 g; 25. 0.001 kg; 26. 0.001 L; 27. 10 mg; 28. 0.01 g; 29. 4° C; 30. 122° F; 31. 19° C; 32. 91° F; 33. 37° C; 34. 113° F; 35. 12° C; 36. 326° K; 37. 273° K; 38. 319° K

39. $C_{unknown} = A_{unknown} \times C_{standard}/A_{standard}$
     = .16/.14 × 100
     = 114.3 mg %

Review Questions

1. a; 2. c; 3. c; 4. d; 5. c

6. a. Add 98 g of H_2SO_4 to enough water to make 1 L of solution.

b. Add 24.5 g $Cu(NO_3)_2$ to enough water to make 300 mL of solution.

c. Add 2.83 g of KBr to enough water to make 250 mL of solution.

d. Add 490 g of $CaCO_3$ to enough water to make 700 mL of solution.

e. Add 54.4 g of H_2O_2 to enough water to make 500 mL of solution.

f. Add 339 g of NaBr to enough water to make 3 L of solution.

g. Add 820 g of Na_3PO_4 to enough water to make 2.5 L of solution.

h. Add 122.9 g of $NaC_2H_3O_2$ to enough water to make 450 mL of solution.

i. Add 363.2 g of $Ni_2(S_2O_3)_3$ to enough water to make 200 mL of solution.

7. a. 0.4 M; b. 11.76 M; c. 17.0 M; d. 1.2 M; e. 0.18 M; f. 0.18 M; g. 0.94 M; h. 3.6 M; i. 0.03 M; j. 1.81 M; k. 0.095 M

8. a. 0.56 N; b. 9.9 N; c. 0.017 N; d. 7.2 N; e. 1.46 N; f. 0.0146 N; g. 1.21 N; h. 163.7 N; i. 0.0798 N; j. 11.5 N; k. 9.1 N

9. a. 0.19 N; b. 0.0008 M; c. 0.001 N; d. 0.16 M; e. 0.0042 N; f. 0.0088 M; g. 0.00177 N; h. 0.00478 M; i. 0.0055 N; j. 0.00506 M

10. a. 1000 mg%; b. 314,000 mg%; c. 4170 mg%; d. 3465 mg%; e. 10,500 mg %; f. 2550 mg%; g. 32,520 mg%; h. 6450 mg%; i. 16,250 mg%; j. 33,210 mg%

11. a. 73.3 mg%; b. 120 mg%; c. 634.9 mg/dL; d. 238.6 mg/dL; e. 2.7 mg/dL; f. 568 mg/dL; g. 16.8 mg/dL; h. 2.34 mg/dL

Chapter 2

Case in Point

The worker should use a dustpan and a brush to pick up the pieces of the glass. Personal protective equipment, including gloves, should be worn to pick up the glass fragments. The worker should not use her hands to pick up the glass because the sharp pieces can easily cut her hands. A cut can allow bloodborne and other pathogens to infect the worker.

Review Questions

1. a; 2. c; 3. d; 4. c; 5. d; 6. a; 7. a; 8. b; 9. a; 10. a

Critical Thinking Questions

1. The laboratory safety program helps employers and employees reduce on-the-job injuries, illnesses, and deaths by maintaining a safe and healthy workplace. It also leads to lower workers' compensation insurance costs and medical expenses for employers and greater productivity from healthier workers. The goal of any laboratory safety program is to minimize the risk of injury or illness to employees by ensuring that they have the training, information, support, and equipment needed to work safely in the laboratory.
2. One piece of personal protective equipment (PPE) is a face shield. The face shield helps protect the eyes and mucous membranes from blood and body fluid splatter by providing a physical barrier that does not allow liquid to pass through. Gloves, another piece of PPE, are worn on the hands to prevent blood and body fluids from entering cuts or sores. The physical barrier prevents liquid from reaching the skin. An N-95 respirator is a third piece of PPE that protects individuals from inhaling airborne pathogens. The physical barrier blocks infectious agents from entering the body through the nose and mouth.
3. The acronyms RACE (Rescue, Alarm, Contain, Evacuate) and PASS (Pull, Aim, Squeeze, Sweep) provide emergency instructions. RACE indicates the responses to encountering a fire. If it is safe, rescue (R) individuals who need help to get away; pull the fire alarm (A) to bring the fire department to the site of the fire; if possible, contain (C) the fire by moving other debris or flammable materials far away from the burning fire; and evacuate (E) yourself and others to a safe place. When using a fire extinguisher, the PASS acronym indicates the sequence of actions needed by the user: pull (P) the pin on the fire extinguisher so it can be used; aim (A) the nozzle of the extinguisher to the base of the fire; squeeze (S) the handle to activate the extinguisher; and sweep (S) the fire to ensure it is covered to put it out.

Case Study

A specific protocol to be used when handling gas cylinders. The maintenance worker should have brought the cylinder into the department, secured the new cylinder near the incubator, and then taken away the used cylinder. Eddie did not have the correct hand truck to transport cylinders, and he should not have tried to move the cylinder himself.

Chapter 3

Review Questions

1. a; 2. c; 3. b; 4. a; 5. d; 6. b; 7. c; 8. c; 9. d; 10. a

Critical Thinking Questions

1. See Figure 3-3.
2. See Figure 3-36.
3. Electrophoresis separates molecules according to their electrical charges in a medium. Most often, it is used to separate proteins using agarose as a medium. Cellulose acetate is the medium of choice for separating hemoglobin. Equipment used in this technique includes a power supply, a chamber, and a cover. To perform electrophoresis, the chamber is filled with a specific buffer at a specific pH, and the medium is placed in the chamber, ensuring contact with the buffer. The cover is applied, and the power supply is connected. A timer is set, and the power is turned on to allow electricity to flow through the medium. The medium is removed from the chamber at the end of the time frame. The medium is stained and dried, and it is read on a densitometer for protein quantitation.

Chapter 4

Case in Point

The consistently high values can be explained by poor washing. All extraneous materials were not removed.

Review Questions

1. b; 2. d; 3. b; 4. b; 5. d; 6. a; 7. b; 8. d; 9. c; 10. c

Critical Thinking Questions

1. The antigen of interest is prepared, and then it is purified so that only antibodies to the targeted antigen are produced. The purified antigen is injected into a rabbit to produce a population of antibodies to the antigen. This population consists of heterogeneous subpopulations of antibodies directed at individual epitopes on the antigens. After a specified time, the animal is checked for antibodies in its blood against the injected antigen. After antibodies are detected, the animal is bled. The serum is separated from the cells, and the generated antiserum is stored. The antiserum varies from bleeding to bleeding and from

animal to animal because the immune response in a particular animal at a particular time can modify the concentration, affinity, or specificity of the antibodies (see Fig. 4-6).

2. The high-dose hook effect is usually seen when performing sandwich immunoassays. Very high antigen concentrations in the sample bind to all available antibody binding sites in the antibody–solid phase and to the antibody-labeled conjugate, preventing formation of the sandwich and falsely decreasing the test result.

Case Study

The sandwich method is modified by the high-dose hook effect when the sample values are very high. This occurs when the large amount of antigen in the sample binds to all antibodies, producing a lower sample value. The diluted sample does not contain as much antigen, and it is therefore not subject to the high-dose hook effect and provides a more accurate result.

Chapter 5

Review Questions

1. a; 2. b; 3. c; 4. d; 5. c; 6. a; 7. d; 8. c; 9. d; 10. b

Critical Thinking Questions

1. To draw a diagram that describes the complex steps in replication, see Figures 5-10, 5-11, and 5-12.
2. To discuss the bonding structure in DNA and draw diagrams to illustrate the bonds, see Figures 5-4 and 5-5.
3. RNA and DNA are similar or different as follows:
   - The sugar is deoxyribose in DNA and ribose in RNA.
   - The five nucleotides found in DNA and RNA are adenine, guanine, thymine, cytosine, and uracil. Adenine and guanine are classified as purines, and thymine, cytosine, and uracil are classified as pyrimidines.
   - In DNA, the bases adenine and thymine bind together and guanine and cytosine bind together. Adenine and thymine do not form bonds with guanine or cytosine.
   - RNA plays an important role in biological functions and has three forms: ribosomal RNA (rRNA), messenger RNA (mRNA), and transfer RNA (tRNA). RNA has a chemical makeup similar to that of DNA, consisting of a heterocyclic base, ribose sugar, and phosphate. Similar to DNA, the sugar forms the backbone of the molecule, with phosphodiester bonds occurring between the 3′ and 5′ carbons. The bases found in RNA are adenine, guanine, cytosine, and uracil.
   - rRNA is an integral part of the ribosome, the site where protein synthesis occurs. A cell contains approximately 80% rRNA, 5% mRNA, and 15% tRNA.
   - mRNA is transcribed from DNA, and the molecule then migrates from the nucleus to the ribosome in the cytoplasm, where it serves as the template for synthesizing a specific protein.
   - tRNA transports amino acids to the ribosome, where proteins are synthesized.

Chapter 6

Review Questions

1. d; 2. a; 3. c; 4. c; 5. a; 6. b; 7. d; 8. d; 9. c; 10. a

Critical Thinking Questions

1. In discrete analyzers, each specimen is contained in a separate reaction vessel, and the analyzer can run multiple tests on one sample or multiple samples one test at a time. A continuous flow analyzer uses large amounts of tubing to move reagents and samples to a reaction chamber. The samples and reagents are separated by bubbles as they move through the tubing.
2. Batch analyzers perform one test on a number of specimens. It is difficult to interrupt a run and insert a stat (i.e., needed immediately) specimen. Sometimes, all specimens have all tests performed on them, whether the test was ordered or not.
3. Reagent storage, reagent aspiration, and reagent delivery are important. Reagents must be prepared and handled according to manufacturer's instructions. If the instructions are not followed, tests will not produce correct results for quality controls and patient specimens. Attention to detail in this area is important for valid and accurate test results.

Chapter 7

Case in Point

Incomplete centrifugation results in inadequate coverage of the red blood cells (RBCs) so that serum sits directly on the RBCs. As we know, RBCs continue to live and metabolize glucose while they are in a tube. Acids are produced as the end product of glucose metabolism, and this causes the blood in the tube to become more acidic. It also lowers the glucose level of the serum in the tube. Sodium from the RBCs leaks into the serum and increases the potassium level. If the specimen was drawn less than 1 hour ago, the technician should recentrifuge the specimen to ensure that the gel at the bottom of the tube covers the cells completely. If the specimen was collected more than 1 hour ago, the technician should contact the physician's office, explain the situation, and ask for the specimen to be redrawn.

Review Questions

1. a; 2. c; 3. a; 4. c; 5. d; 6. a; 7. c; 8. b; 9. b; 10. d

Critical Thinking Questions

1. The quality management system (QMS) helps to reduce the level of inaccuracy as much as possible and alerts technicians when systems are not functioning properly. Patients' health outcomes depend on the accuracy of the laboratory test results. Inaccurate results can cause

unnecessary treatment, treatment complications, failure to provide the proper treatment, delay in correct diagnosis, and additional and unnecessary laboratory testing. The QMS examines all the processes, procedures, and components that lead to quality, reliable, and accurate laboratory results and includes troubleshooting and adjusting components to guide necessary improvements.

2. Westgard established quality control (QC) interpretive rules that have been adopted by clinical laboratories to determine when a method is out of control. Safeguards and practices based on this system help to demonstrate quality of results, prevent errors, and identify potential problem areas before test results are distributed to the offices of medical practitioners and to medical records. Statistical process control verifies that test results are producing the expected variability from a properly calibrated and stable operating system. A laboratory chooses rules to detect calibration and precision anomalies that require corrective action before patient results can be reported. The most common Westgard rules used in clinical laboratories are the following:
   - 1_{2s} A control value that exceeds the established mean by ±2 SD is considered a warning to carefully inspect the control data.
   - 1_{3s} When a control exceeds the established mean by ±3 SD, a random error is suspected.
   - 2_{2s} When two control values on two consecutive runs exceed the same mean +2 SD or mean −2 SD limit, a systematic error is probable.
   - R_{4s} When one control measurement exceeds the mean +2 SD limit and another exceeds the mean −2 SD limit, a random error is indicated.
   - 4_{1s} When four consecutive control values exceed the same mean +1 SD (or mean −1 SD) limit, a systematic error is indicated.
   - 10_x When ten consecutive control values fall on the upper or lower side of the mean (without regard to distance from the mean), a systematic error is indicated.

3. Continuous monitoring is the key to a successful continuous quality improvement (CQI) cycle. It starts with a quality improvement plan, carries through with corrective actions, and finally examines the result through monitoring and evaluation. Audits can help a laboratory monitor and evaluate policies, procedures, and processes. Proficiency testing is an external quality assessment method used by laboratories to determine the accuracy of test results.

Case Studies

1. Rule 1_{3s} is the rule that is broken. This indicates a random error, so the control specimen should be repeated.

2. The rule that is broken is 2_{2s}. This is no longer an isolated incident and a random error; it may be a systematic error. The control specimen should be repeated. The lot number of the control should be checked to make sure it is correct. A new aliquot of control should be run to determine

whether the control value is within limits. If not, preventive maintenance should be performed, and the controls should be repeated along with the run. If the control value is still out, the technician should consult the laboratory supervisor or the technical service representative, or both, according to the laboratory's procedures.

Chapter 8

Case in Point

Acute pancreatitis should be considered as the cause for this man's discomfort due to his symptoms: abdominal pain located in the epigastric area and radiating to the back. Amylase and lipase assays can help diagnose this condition.

Review Questions

1. c; 2. b; 3. d; 4. d; 5. a; 6. c; 7. b; 8. c; 9. b; 10. c

Critical Thinking Questions

1. The number of substrate binding sites (active sites) on enzymes is limited. Competitive inhibition describes the binding of an inhibitor to the active site of an enzyme. This prevents the substrate from binding to the enzyme and consequently inhibits the enzymatic function. Competitive inhibitions are reversible, and their effect can be decreased by increasing the substrate concentration. The affinity of the enzyme to the substrate (K_m) increases, but the rate of substrate formation (V_{max}) remains the same, as shown in Table 8-2.

   In noncompetitive inhibition, the inhibitor binds at a regulatory site (allosteric site) on the enzyme molecule instead of competing with the substrate for the active site (see Fig. 8-5). The regulatory site of an enzyme determines the conformation and activity of the enzyme. Therefore, this type of inhibition cannot be reversed by an increase in substrate concentration. The K_m remains unaffected because there is no competition for the substrate binding site, but the rate of product formation is reduced, resulting in a decreased V_{max}.

   Uncompetitive inhibition occurs when the inhibitor binds to the enzyme–substrate complex, preventing the formation of product. This type of inhibition is not reversible by adding substrate, so both K_m and V_{max} are negatively affected.

2. The clinical applications of aminotransferases are exclusively related to the evaluation of liver disease. Alanine aminotransferase (ALT) activity is higher than aspartate aminotransferase (AST) activity in most forms of liver disease except for alcoholic hepatitis, hepatic cirrhosis, and hepatocellular carcinoma.

   Liver disorders associated with destruction of hepatic tissue (necrosis), including viral hepatitis, display elevated AST and ALT activity before the appearance of clinical signs and symptoms. AST and ALT values are elevated usually 10 to 40 times and can be as high as 100 times the upper limit of the reference interval.

Nonalcoholic fatty liver disease is another common cause of aminotransferase activity increases.

An important characteristic of ALT activity elevation is its increased specificity for the liver, compared with AST. Elevations in ALT activity are very rare in nonliver disorders. In addition, ALT activity elevations persist longer than those of AST due to the longer half-life of ALT in serum.

Increases in γ-glutamyl transferase (GGT) are not specific and are seen in the majority of individuals with liver disease, although the highest increases are seen in hepatobiliary disorders. In addition, patients with primary and metastatic hepatocellular carcinoma display unusually high GGT activity. Another subset of patients with elevated GGT activity includes those with alcoholic hepatitis and chronic alcohol drinkers.

Determination of GGT activity can be useful in the context of elevated alkaline phosphatase (ALP) activity. GGT activity is normal during pregnancy and in the presence of bone disorders, conditions that exhibit elevated ALP activity.

Case Study

The diagnosis of hepatitis, probably hepatitis A, should be considered. Travel to other countries where water purification procedures are not as strict as those in the United States can result in infection with the hepatitis A virus. The ALT level is higher than the AST level, indicating a liver disease. Remember that although ALP is mostly associated with bone, some ALP is present in the liver, and ALP can be elevated in hepatobiliary disease. The GGT level is within normal limits, so this condition is probably not caused by alcoholic hepatitis. The elevated bilirubin level points to a liver disease. To definitively diagnose this patient, a hepatitis panel should be ordered.

Chapter 9

Case in Point

It is likely that Laurie's metabolic test results would be normal. Even though her tests were normal, it would not mean that she was not sick. The terms "health" and "disease" qualitatively describe the condition of an individual. "Normal" and "abnormal" refer to the objective interpretations of data used to determine whether an individual has a disease.

Review Questions

1. c; 2. a; 3. b; 4. c; 5. d; 6. d; 7. a; 8. c; 9. a; 10. d

Critical Thinking Questions

1. No, healthy does not mean normal, and diseased does not mean abnormal. "Health" and "disease" qualitatively

describe the condition of an individual. "Normal" and "abnormal" refer to the objective interpretations of data used to determine whether an individual has a disease.

2. Clinical chemistry tests are ordered based on a medical history, symptoms, and physical examination. Health care providers will perform the most sensitive test first, then follow up with more specific tests, as necessary. By performing a highly sensitive test, providers will not miss many people who have the disease. Based on the positivity of the sensitive test, the provider will order a highly specific test to identify those who actually have the disease (true positives) and the false positives. Usually, no single test is 100% accurate in diagnosing disease. This is why the objective test results must be combined with the medical history and the physical examination findings. This process resembles putting together a puzzle—several pieces must come together to reveal the whole picture. Many diseases and conditions share similar symptoms, and this makes it extremely hard to correctly diagnose a person without knowing all the pieces.

3. As the name implies, a false-positive test result occurs when an individual does not have a condition but the laboratory test result indicates that the condition is present. The other type of error, false negative, occurs when an individual does have a condition but the test indicates that he or she does not have the condition. There are also tests results that are considered true positives and true negatives. In the case of a true positive, the test results are positive and the individual indeed has the condition. With a true negative, the test results are negative and the individual in fact does not have the condition.

Technicians need to understand the concepts of false-positive and false-negative tests, because physicians will take this into consideration when trying to diagnose an individual.

Case Study

The first test was a highly sensitive test; such a test will be abnormal in many people, especially those with the disease in question. The second test was a highly specific test that actually identifies people who have the particular disease. The first test result for this woman had a false-positive result.

Chapter 10

Case in Point

Alcohol is a toxic substance the directly injures the liver cells. Damage to cells can occur through direct chemical injury after exposure to alcohol. The two laboratory tests that would indicate whether liver damage has occurred are aspartate aminotransferase and alanine aminotransferase.

Review Questions

1. a; 2. d; 3. c; 4. b; 5. a; 6. a; 7. c; 8. c; 9. d; 10. b

Critical Thinking Questions

1. Mountain climbers may experience the following types of stress:
   a. Hypoxia—due to the high altitude, there is little oxygen available. Low oxygen can lead to a pH imbalance in the body, and this leads to cellular injury.
   b. Cold injury—prolonged exposure to below-freezing temperatures can allow water in the blood to freeze, causing frostbite and tissue necrosis.
   c. Radiation—Mt. Everest is 29,029 feet tall. The higher you go above the earth, the thinner the atmosphere. The atmosphere protects us from much of the ionizing radiation that bombards the earth in space, so at an elevation of 5+ miles, you will be bombarded by much ionizing radiation.
2. Ionizing radiation is the stress that the workers at this plant endured. The reaction vessels in the main reactor portion of the plant contain radioactive elements that emit gamma rays. Gamma rays penetrate deep into the body and disrupt cells in tissues. Gamma rays affect fast-growing cells more than other tissue cells. As a result, red and white blood cells and intestinal lining cells are dramatically affected. After exposure to gamma rays, an individual's red and white blood cell counts drop precipitously, and the intestinal lining sloughs off. All of these occurrences make the individual extremely susceptible to infection.
3. A myocardial infarction occurs when a coronary artery is blocked. The blockage causes the tissue receiving nutrients and expressing waste through that artery to die. The tissue builds up metabolic wastes and does not receive oxygen, so it dies. Creatine kinase isoenzymes (especially the MB fraction) are useful for determining whether an acute myocardial infarction has occurred.

Case Study

In phenylketonuria and hypothyroidism, enzymes and hormone products are not being produced by the newborn. This results in a buildup of metabolic byproducts, which are toxic to a newborn's brain. The result is brain damage later in life.

Chapter 11

Case in Point

Inflammation is the body's response to injury. It is a protective response used to rid the body of invaders. In this case, the stick broke the man's defenses—his skin. The body is undergoing acute inflammation to rid itself of the microorganisms present on the stick. This is causing the red, warm, swollen area of his face around the injury. The inflammatory response also signaled for leukocytes to help in the effort and can be seen in the pus that is found at that site. This man is experiencing the hallmarks of inflammation: edema (swelling), redness, warmth, and pus.

Review Questions

1. c; 2. c; 3. c; 4. b; 5. c; 6. a; 7. d; 8. b; 9. a; 10. c

Critical Thinking Questions

1. The complement cascade is one of the body's nonspecific defense systems. It can be activated by antibody–antigen complexes, properdin, C-reactive protein, and bacterial and fungal cell walls. Some components of the complement system (i.e., C3b) help leukocytes phagocytize bacteria, viruses, and other invaders. The result of activating the complement system is lysis of the bacteria, fungus, or invader.
2. Cells involved in inflammation include segmented neutrophils, bands, eosinophils, basophils, monocytes, macrophages, B and T lymphocytes, and plasma cells.
   Neutrophils and bands—play a role in migration, infiltration, and phagocytosis
   Eosinophils—release chemicals to enhance migration of white blood cells
   Basophils—play a role with allergies and asthma (inflammatory reactions)
   Monocytes—are immature macrophages
   Macrophages—are active in phagocytosis and in tissue destruction and repair; produce reactive oxygen species
   B lymphocytes and plasma cells—carry out the specific immune response by producing antibodies to specific invaders
   T lymphocytes—destroy infected cells
3. C-reactive protein (CRP) is measured qualitatively by mixing a drop of serum and a drop of latex-coated antibody reagent onto a slide, rotating the slide for a period of time, and observing the mixture for a precipitate. It can also be measured quantitatively with the use of ELISA, particle-enhanced immunoturbidimetry, nephelometry, immunofluorescence, immunoprecipitation, or immunochemiluminescence.
   Cytokines can be measured with bioassays, immunoassays, and flow cytometry.

Case Study

Chronic inflammation produces a dense infiltration of an area with lymphocytes and macrophages. Sometimes the body walls off an area with an excessive migration of macrophages to protect the rest of the body. The accumulation of macrophages around a walled-off infection is called a granuloma. The wall of the tuberculosis bacterium is resistant to all other body defenses.

Chapter 12

Case in Point

In this type of a condition, the man's serum and urine osmolality results would be abnormal. He would have an elevated blood glucose level. Because he is also dehydrated, he would have an elevated sodium level.

Review Questions

1. b; 2. c; 3. a; 4. a; 5. d; 6. b; 7. c; 8. c; 9. a; 10. a

Critical Thinking Questions

1. Dehydration occurs when there is too little intravascular water. The blood thickens and becomes more difficult to pump throughout the body. If the dehydration is severe enough, it can also lead to hypernatremia.
2. Sodium functions to help transmit nerve impulses, maintain osmotic pressure of extracellular fluid and retain water, contract muscles, maintain the acid-base balance, and maintain blood viscosity. Disease states include hypernatremia and hyponatremia.

   Potassium is found at high concentrations in intracellular fluid and at lower concentrations in extracellular fluids. Potassium helps control muscle activity in the body. High potassium levels can paralyze muscles and cause the heart to stop beating. Low potassium levels lead to irregular heartbeats and abnormal electrocardiograms.

   Chloride is the most important extracellular enzyme and has the highest concentration of any extracellular anion. The major function of chloride is to maintain electrical neutrality. When blood is oxygenated, chloride participates in the "chloride shift": chloride shifts from the red blood cell into the plasma, causing bicarbonate to leave the plasma and enter the red blood cell. When blood contains carbon dioxide, bicarbonate exits the red blood cells and enters the plasma, while chloride shifts from the plasma and enters the red blood cells.

   Bicarbonate is an electrolyte that plays a major role in maintaining the body's acid-base balance.

   Lithium is a small ion that is used to treat manic depression.
3. The term "anion gap" is a misnomer, but it is used to determine whether the body's electrolytes are in balance: the total positive charges should equal the total negative charges. The anion gap is calculated by the following formula: Anion Gap = $[Na^+ + K^+] - [Cl^- + HCO_3^-]$. Abnormal anion gaps may indicate a significant medical problem, such as renal failure or diabetic ketoacidosis.

   For the data given—Na, 145 mmol/L; K, 4.2 mmol/L; Cl, 100 mEq/L; and HCO₃, 28 mEq/L—the anion gap would be (145 + 4.2) – (100 + 28) = 21. This anion gap is abnormally high.

Case Study

Potassium is one of the electrolytes that is involved in muscle function. It is especially active in cardiac muscle. Hypokalemia increases the irritability or contractions of the heart muscle, leading to irregular heartbeats and abnormal findings on electrocardiography.

The patient's potassium level was so low because she had experienced diarrhea for 2 months. Diarrhea causes large amounts of potassium to be excreted through the intestines because it is not reabsorbed into the blood.

Chapter 13

Case in Point

The blood gas results indicate the following: pH, alkalosis; pCO₂, decreased; and pO₂, decreased. This individual appears to be in respiratory alkalosis. Hyperventilation is a state in which a person breathes extremely fast, like a dog panting. Hyperventilation produces a respiratory alkalosis because the individual is blowing off much carbon dioxide, causing the blood to become more alkalotic. This is why the amount of carbon dioxide in the blood is decreased. Hypoxia and ventilation are not synonyms. Hypoxia refers to a low blood oxygen level, whereas ventilation refers to the mechanical process of bringing air into the lungs and breathing it back into the environment. Panic attacks can cause respiratory alkalosis. The man's other symptoms are nonconsequential. He is feeling ill because he is in respiratory alkalosis. Panic attacks are treated with several types of tranquilizers or tricyclic antidepressants.

Review Questions

1. a; 2. b; 3. a; 4. d; 5. b; 6. d; 7. a; 8. c; 9. b; 10. c

Critical Thinking Questions

1. The human body maintains a very narrow range for its blood pH. This range produces optimal functioning of organs and tissues. If conditions such as hyperventilation cause the pH to increase, the body will stimulate the kidneys to retain more hydrogen ions to try to restore the pH to its narrow range. Systemic conditions that disturb this delicate balance can produce serious diseases.
2. Normal values are as follows: pH, 7.35-7.45; pO₂, 83-108 mm Hg; pCO₂, 35-48 mm Hg; and bicarbonate (also called total carbon dioxide, or tCO₂), 23-30 mEq/L.
3. A person is in *acidosis* if the blood pH is lower than 7.35. If the blood pH is higher than 7.45, the person is in *alkalosis*. Respiratory acidosis describes an acidosis that is caused by a respiratory condition. If the condition is caused by a metabolic problem, it is called metabolic acidosis. Likewise, respiratory alkalosis is caused by respiratory conditions, and metabolic alkalosis is caused by metabolic conditions. Respiratory acidosis is caused by any condition that results in retention of carbon dioxide in the lungs (e.g., chronic obstructive pulmonary disease). Respiratory alkalosis is caused by any condition that results in quick elimination of carbon dioxide from the blood, such as hyperventilation. Metabolic acidosis is caused by any condition that produces large quantities of organic acids, such that the kidneys cannot excrete enough hydrogen ions to maintain the acid-base balance. An example is diabetic ketoacidosis. Finally, metabolic alkalosis is caused by any condition that

produces a primary bicarbonate excess, such as ingesting large amounts of antacids.

Case Study

The patients' glucose level is very elevated, carbon dioxide is very decreased, sodium is decreased, potassium is very elevated, chloride is low normal, pH is low (acidotic), pCO_2 is low, bicarbonate is low, and pO_2 is low normal.

Drinking large amounts of water after vomiting can dilute the electrolytes in the blood. The sodium level is especially susceptible to large influxes of plain water. This is why athletes who sweat out a large amount of fluid during the course of a workout replenish their electrolytes by drinking an electrolyte-balanced drink as opposed to plain water.

A high blood sugar level will increase urinary output of water, thus making the blood even more viscous.

The low pCO_2 is caused by the body's attempt to compensate for the acidosis by breathing fast and shallow.

This patient is in diabetic ketoacidosis.

Chapter 14

Case in Point

She has iron deficiency anemia. In addition to the complete blood count that was already completed, her doctor should order testing for total iron, total iron-binding capacity (TIBC), and ferritin to confirm this diagnosis.

Review Questions

1. b; 2. a; 3. d; 4. a; 5. c; 6. c; 7. d; 8. b; 9. b; 10. See Table 14-4

Critical Thinking Questions

1. Iron deficiency anemias are microcytic (mean corpuscular volume [MCV] <83 fL) and hypochromic, whereas anemia of chronic disease produces decreased iron in the blood, decreased erythropoietin, and a decreased red blood cell life span; it is normochromic and normocytic.
2. Common hemoglobinopathies include sickle cell disease (homozygous for hemoglobin S), which is diagnosed using a hemoglobin S screen and electrophoresis. In this disorder, valine is substituted for glutamic acid in the β-globin. Hemoglobin E is a β-globin chain variant in which a lysine residue replaces a glutamic acid; it produces a mild anemia. In hemoglobin C, another hemoglobinopathy, a lysine is substituted for glutamic acid in the β-globin chain. This condition can also be found in α- and β-thalassemia. There are individuals who can have one copy of the S gene and one copy of the C gene; have hemoglobin SC. This hemoglobinopathy produces fewer sickle cells and fewer acute vaso-occlusive events than homozygous hemoglobin S does.

    Thalassemias result when globin chains are missing from the hemoglobin molecule. There are α-thalassemias and β-thalassemias. These conditions involve a defective hemoglobin molecule, and some are very severe, leading to death immediately after birth. Others are mild and may be asymptomatic.

Case Study

For sickle cell disease to be transmitted, the individual must inherit the gene from both parents, so they must be homozygous for hemoglobin S. At low oxygen levels, the hemoglobin S precipitates into long thin crystals with pointed ends. The red blood cells in sickle cell crisis lose their characteristic biconcave shape and resemble the shape of a crescent; the pointed ends of the hemoglobin S crystal tear blood vessels and tissue and cause much pain. This can be diagnosed with the use of a sickle screening test and hemoglobin electrophoresis. If an individual has sickle cell trait, he or she is heterozygous for hemoglobin S and has a milder disease. It is diagnosed the same way as sickle cell anemia in the laboratory.

Chapter 15

Case in Point

The abnormal results are hemoglobin (decreased) and total protein (elevated).

The probable diagnosis is multiple myeloma. High total protein and bone pain with low hemoglobin indicates that other cells are probably crowding out the red blood cell precursors.

The predominant cell would be plasma cells.

Review Questions

1. d; 2. a; 3. a; 4. c; 5. d; 6. d; 7. a; 8. b; 9. c; 10. c

Critical Thinking Questions

1. Proteins separate on agarose gel in the following order: prealbumin, albumin, α_1 proteins, α_2 proteins, β proteins, and γ-proteins. If the patient had an inflammatory condition, one would expect the α regions to be increased because of the increased production of acute phase reactants. In liver disease, all serum proteins will be decreased because the liver is unable to synthesis them at a healthy level.
2. The five classes of immunoglobulins are as follows:

    IgG—monomer, most abundant immunoglobulin in blood
    IgM—nonspecific, pentamer, largest of immunoglobulins; capable of activating complement
    IgA—dimer, secreted in tears
    IgD—monomer, function unknown
    IgE—monomer, binds with mast cells and is responsible for histamine release; functions in allergic reactions and parasitic infections

3. Monoclonal antibodies are made from one clone and are very specific. Polyclonal antibodies are made from several clones and are lower in specificity than monoclonal antibodies.

Case Study

The probable diagnosis is agammaglobulinemia because the γ region on serum protein electrophoresis shows no γ-globulins. Confirmatory tests would include individual levels for all immunoglobulins.

Chapter 16

Case in Point

The result is abnormal. The next step would be a prostate biopsy to determine whether the enlarged prostate is caused by a benign or a malignant tumor. PSA tests are used to screen only men who are at high risk for prostate cancer, because PSA can be elevated in other conditions that are not cancer.

Review Questions

1. a; 2. d; 3. c; 4. b; 5. a; 6. a; 7. c; 8. c; 9. d; 10. b

Critical Thinking Questions

1. Genetic mutations disrupt the normal cellular division cycle and allow the cells to continue to divide and proliferate. In addition, tumor suppression genes are inactivated, and this also allows the cells to continue to proliferate.
2. Tumor markers are not used to screen the general population for cancer because these substances can be elevated in benign conditions as well.
3. Markers used to guide therapy include estrogen receptors (ERs), progesterone receptors (PRs), and the human epidermal growth factor receptor 2 gene (HER2). The density of ERs and PRs indicates whether a tumor is likely to respond to hormone therapy. Receptor-positive patients have a better prognosis; receptor-negative patients need alternative treatments such as chemotherapy. Amplification of the HER2 gene indicates that the tumor may be successfully treated with trastuzumab (Herceptin). CA 15-3 and CA 27.29 are used together to monitor therapy for breast cancer. Increased CA 15-3 and CA 27.29 levels indicate disease progression. For best results, CA 15-3 and CA 27.29 are measured before each course of chemotherapy and every 3 months after beginning hormone therapy.

Case Study

The patient likely has colon cancer. The best screening procedure for this type of cancer is the colonoscopy. Carcinoembryonic antigen (CEA) is the tumor marker for this cancer, and it is usually used for monitoring therapy and recurrence.

Chapter 17

Case in Point

Diabetics have a lipoprotein lipase deficiency, which causes a buildup of chylomicrons. The presence of elevated glucose in the blood promotes synthesis of VLDL molecules that are high in triglycerides. This means that the triglyceride and total cholesterol values will be elevated. (Total cholesterol is elevated because the VLDL, which contains cholesterol, is elevated.) This specimen would be considered type V in Fredrickson's classification.

Review Questions

1. c; 2. c; 3. b; 4. c; 5. c; 6. a; 7. b; 8. c; 9. a; 10. d

Critical Thinking Questions

1. Friedewald formula is used to estimate LDL: LDL = Total cholesterol − (HDL − Triglycerides/5). This formula is not valid when the triglyceride level is greater than 400 mg/dL.
2. Triglycerides are usually determined by the enzymatic method:

$$\text{Triglycerides} \xrightarrow{\text{(Lipase)}} \text{Glycerol} + \text{Fatty Acids}$$

$$\text{Glycerol} + \text{APT} \xrightarrow{\text{(GK)}} \text{Glycerol-1-phosphate} + \text{ADP}$$

$$\text{Glycerol-1-phosphate} + O_2 \xrightarrow{\text{(GPO)}} \text{DAP} + H_2O_2$$

$$H_2O_2 + \text{4-AA} + \text{4-Chlorophenol} \xrightarrow{\text{(POD)}}$$

$$\text{Quinoneimine dye} + \text{HCL} + 2H_2O$$

3. Type V

Case Study

The most likely diagnosis is Tangier disease (the patient's HDL level is abnormally low). Because this condition is inherited in an autosomal dominant pattern, genetic testing would be appropriate as well as a measurement of total cholesterol.

Chapter 18

Case in Point

The likely diagnosis is myocardial infarction. No other tests need to be ordered because the most specific test for detecting a myocardial infarction is the troponin I, which has already been done. An acute myocardial infarction occurs when a coronary artery to the heart is occluded. This occlusion stops blood flow (including oxygen flow) to the heart tissue, and the tissue dies from lack of oxygen. The blood levels of these analytes are elevated, indicating tissue damage in the heart.

Review Questions

1. c; 2. b; 3. a; 4. b; 5. c; 6. b; 7. d; 8. a; 9. b; 10. b

Critical Thinking Questions

1. Environmental and genetic risk factors include age, gender, heredity, lipid metabolism, diabetes mellitus, hypertension, clotting factors, smoking, and behavior. The risk factors that can be changed by individuals include lipid metabolism, diabetes mellitus, hypertension, clotting factors, smoking, and behavior. There is no additional laboratory test that can predict someone's risk for developing atherosclerosis or coronary heart disease.
2. Myocarditis and pericarditis are diagnosed with the use of blood cultures, echocardiography, electrocardiography, radiography, magnetic resonance imaging, angiography, and cardiac biopsies. Because myocarditis can also be caused by infectious agents (e.g., virus, bacteria, parasite), antibody levels are also used to help diagnose the condition. IgM levels are used for recent or current infections, and IgG antibodies are used to detect past exposure to infectious agents.

Case Study

The most probable condition is congestive heart failure. Rheumatic heart disease causes damage to the heart, and heart damage is a prerequisite for congestive heart failure to occur. B-type natriuretic peptide (BNP) is the best test to order to detect both ventricle damage and swelling in and around her heart.

Chapter 19

Case in Point

The probable diagnosis is emphysema because his α_1-antitrypsin level is 8 mmol/L. Any value less than 11 mmol/L leads to lung tissue destruction and emphysema.

Review Questions

1. a; 2. c; 3. b; 4. d; 5. d; 6. b; 7. a; 8. c; 9. c; 10. b

Critical Thinking Questions

1. Cystic fibrosis (CF) is an autosomal recessive genetic disease. CF is distinguished by abnormal secretions that block the respiratory, digestive, and reproductive systems (Fig. 19-7). The fundamental abnormality is in transport of the chloride ion (Fig. 19-8). Over time, the hypoxic state causes the alveolar arteries to form new branches in an effort to oxygenate more red blood cells (Fig. 19-9). Individuals with CF produce more mucus than normal and are unable to adequately clear mucus from the lungs. In addition, the mucus they produce is abnormally thick.

This thick mucus retains bacteria, which form biofilms that can be hard to treat with antibiotics.
2. A pulmonary embolism is considered a medical emergency because larger thromboemboli that travel into the lungs can completely obstruct the pulmonary artery bifurcation, causing immediate death.
3. Blood gas values in emphysema, chronic bronchitis, cystic fibrosis, and asthma differ from normal values because of the pathology of each disease.

    Emphysema: The alveoli are destroyed to the point that the air spaces in the lung enlarge. The destruction of the alveoli also leads to loss of elasticity and poor gas exchange. The low blood oxygen results in lowered cardiac output and hyperventilation, leading to tissue hypoxia throughout the body. These patients suffer from wasting and weight loss and are called "pink puffers."

    Chronic bronchitis: Chronic bronchitis is characterized by enlargement of mucous cells as well as inflammation and neutrophil infiltrations. Chronic bronchitis is considered to be an obstructive disease because the large amounts of mucus in the bronchi, inflammation of the bronchi and alveoli, and neutrophil infiltration in the airways all lead to obstruction of air flow in and out of the lungs.

    Cystic fibrosis: CF is distinguished by abnormal secretions that block the respiratory, digestive, and reproductive systems. The lungs are the main organs affected, and respiratory failure is the usual cause of death in people diagnosed with CF. Over time, the hypoxic state causes the alveolar arteries to form new branches in an effort to oxygenate more red blood cells. Individuals with CF produce more mucus than normal and are unable to adequately clear mucus from the lungs. In addition, the mucus they produce is abnormally thick. This thick mucus retains bacteria, which form biofilms that can be hard to treat with antibiotics.

    Asthma: The bronchial tree constricts especially during exhalation, causing obstruction of air flow. Chronic inflammation is responsible for constriction of the bronchial tree. The bronchi in chronic asthma are different from normal bronchi. The bronchial lumen is narrow and contains a lot of mucus and inflammatory cells, fluid from edema, and hypertrophied smooth muscle.

Case Study

This woman has a pleural effusion that is causing her dyspnea that may be due to compression atelectasis. This pleural effusion is caused by cirrhosis of the liver and decreased total plasma protein concentration.

Chapter 20

Case in Point

The urease test methodology is as follows:

$$CO(NH_2)_2 + 2H_2O \xrightarrow[\text{(Urease)}]{} H_2O + CO_2 + 2NH_3$$

The causative agent is *Helicobacter pylori*. *H. pylori* stimulates inflammation and causes erosion of the stomach lining (gastric ulcers) and the small intestine (duodenal ulcers).

Review Questions

1. d; 2. d; 3. b; 4. d; 5. b; 6. b; 7. b; 8. b; 9. b; 10. a

Critical Thinking Questions

1. The primary organs of the gastrointestinal (GI) tract are the mouth, esophagus, stomach, small intestine, and large intestine. Accessory GI organs, which aid in digestion, include the liver, gallbladder, and pancreas. The functions of the GI tract include the ingestion of food, digestion of food, absorption of nutrients from food, and waste elimination. Accessory organs are probably called that because they supply necessary enzymes and hormones to allow the primary organs to digest the food.

2. Diarrhea is characterized by loose, watery, and frequent stools. Diarrhea is considered chronic when frequent stools are present for longer than 4 weeks. Diarrhea may be accompanied by abdominal pain, cramping, nausea, blood, or mucus. Usually, acute diarrhea is short lived and self-limited. However, when diarrhea is severe or persistent (chronic), it can lead to dehydration due to large water loss and dangerously low potassium levels, resulting in serious complications or even death. Some patients affected by diarrhea require hospitalization. In infants, significant dehydration can occur within hours. The causes of acute diarrhea are divided into bacterial, viral, or parasitic causes. Table 20-1 lists some etiologic agents of acute diarrhea. Acute diarrhea can also be caused by the effects of antimicrobial use. Broad-spectrum antimicrobials can destroy the normal gut bacteria and allow opportunistic bacteria to multiply, causing diarrhea. *Clostridium difficile* is an example of such an opportunistic infectious agent. The primary causes of chronic diarrhea are ulcerative colitis and Crohn disease, irritable bowel syndrome, celiac disease, malabsorption, food intolerances, and chemotherapy or radiation. In addition, parasitic infection, colon cancer, polyps, and excessive laxative use can cause chronic diarrhea.

   Stool cultures, immunoassays, ova and parasites, fecal fat, and antibody assays are used for diagnosis. In a stool culture, stool bacteria in are grown on selective and differential media to identify an infectious agent. For some infectious agents, such as *C. difficile*, rotavirus, and *Escherichia coli* O1:57, enzyme-linked immunoassays (ELISAs) can detect the presence of the infectious agent without culturing. The ova and parasites test detects the presence of parasites in stool.

3. Malabsorption is defective absorption of nutrients by the GI tract. The absorption defects can be associated with a single nutrient or all nutrients. Most patients with malabsorption conditions experience diarrhea, abdominal discomfort, and weight loss. Treatment depends on the underlying etiology. Maldigestion occurs when the small intestine or pancreas do not produce appropriate levels of digestive hormones. This leads to incomplete digestion of food. Only way to differentiate is to assay digestive enzyme levels.

   Diagnostic laboratory tests for malabsorption may include a CBC, a chemistry screen, prothrombin time, and vitamin or mineral assays. Other tests, such as pancreatic elastase, celiac antibodies, fecal fat, a stool culture, or ova and parasites, are also used to diagnose these conditions.

   A CBC is used to detect anemia. Anemia can be present in malabsorption due to lower amounts of iron, vitamin B_{12}, and folate. Malabsorption can also cause a vitamin K deficiency, which can be detected by the prothrombin time. Various vitamins and minerals, such as iron, folate, vitamin B_{12}, magnesium, calcium, vitamin D, and vitamin A, are measured to detect malabsorption and are usually decreased. Other useful chemistry tests include albumin, triglycerides, cholesterol, sodium, and potassium.

   Serologic tests are needed to detect celiac disease. Tests such as anti-AGA, anti-TTG, anti-DGP, or anti-EMA may help rule out celiac disease as a cause of malabsorption. Pancreatic elastase 1 is an enzyme detected in stool that can help providers understand a patient's exocrine pancreatic status to differentiate between maldigestion and malabsorption.

Case Study

Diagnostic tests for inflammatory bowel disease (IBD) include a complete blood count (CBC) showing anemia or an increased white blood cell count. Fecal examinations will reveal red and white blood cells; white blood cells can signify infection or inflammation, whereas red blood cells are indicative of bleeding. Blood can also be detected by occult blood tests. Imaging and endoscopy are also used to diagnose these conditions.

IBD includes ulcerative colitis and Crohn disease. Ulcerative colitis produces inflammation of the colon, whereas Crohn disease produces inflammation primarily in the small intestines, although it can also affect any part of the gastrointestinal tract. The characteristics of both diseases are summarized in Table 20-3. Their pathology and appearance are shown in Figures 20-5 and 20-6. Both ulcerative colitis and Crohn disease exhibit bouts of remission and bouts of exacerbation or "flare-ups." The causes of ulcerative colitis and Crohn disease are not known. Both appear to have autoimmune components; the body attacks its own tissue or fails to stop the inflammatory process once it has begun. There appears to be a genetic link or susceptibility in both diseases. Environmental factors such as infectious agents, food antigens, or medications also appear to play a role. Both ulcerative colitis and Crohn disease are associated with abdominal pain, cramping, anorexia, bloody diarrhea, and anemia.

Chapter 21

Case in Point

The elevated bilirubin and liver enzyme levels indicate that this individual has hepatitis. The next tests to order would be a hepatitis panel so that the provider can determine which hepatitis virus is causing the inflammation. If the hepatitis panel comes back negative, then the provider should look for other causes of the inflammation, such as parasites, chemicals, drugs, or alcohol.

Review Questions

1. a; 2. c; 3. c; 4. a; 5. b; 6. b; 7. b; 8. b; 9. b; 10. c

Critical Thinking Questions

1. Many tests can be performed to appropriately diagnose and monitor HBV infection, including hepatitis B surface antigen (HB_sAg), antibody against the hepatitis B surface antigen (anti-HB_s), anti-hepatitis core antigen (anti-HB_c), and anti-hepatitis core antigen IgM (anti-HB_c IgM).

Hepatitis Disease	Presentation	Progression	Laboratory Results
Hepatitis A	Sudden symptoms: lethargy, jaundice, fever, chills, weight loss, myalgia	Self-limited: resolves about 8-9 weeks after infection	Elevated AST, ALT, total bilirubin; anti-HAV IgM increases when symptoms appear; anti-HAV IgG appears during recovery
Hepatitis B	Gradual onset of symptoms: tea-colored urine, fatigue, myalgia, jaundice	Recovery in 6 months; 15-25% develop chronic liver disease	Elevated AST, ALT, total bilirubin; hepatitis B surface antigen present with symptoms, hepatitis B core antigen, then anti-hepatitis surface and core antigens

2. Functions of the liver include metabolism of carbohydrates, lipids, and proteins; production of bile; chemical detoxification; porphyrin catabolism; bilirubin metabolism; and protein synthesis. The liver also forms waste products (urea) from toxic metabolites such as ammonia.

Cirrhosis of the liver is end-stage liver disease characterized by scarring of the liver and decreasing ability of the liver to function. Liver failure occurs when large parts of the liver become damaged and are unlikely to be repaired and the liver is no longer able to function. In both liver failure and cirrhosis, the liver is unable to function well. Carbohydrate and lipid metabolism will be affected, as will protein synthesis. The liver will be unable to conjugate toxic substances, and as a result, the toxic substances will build up in the blood. The liver will no longer manufacturer clotting factors, so individuals with liver failure or cirrhosis will experience abnormal bleeding due to lack of coagulation factors. In liver failure, ALT, AST, bilirubin, and GGT would all be elevated. ALP would be normal.

Case Study

This patient probably has Wilson disease. Serum copper and ceruloplasmin can be normal in this disease, but the urinary copper level is always elevated.

Chapter 22

Case in Point

The patient's glucose level is extremely elevated (800 mg/dL), electrolytes are decreased, and acetone is very high. This individual is experiencing diabetic ketoacidosis produced by diabetes mellitus. In an individual with insulin deficiency, lipolysis is increased, so more fatty acids are transported to the liver. The liver uses the fatty acids for glyconeogenesis, which produces more glucose for the body. Without insulin, the adipocytes (i.e., fat cells) release free fatty acids, stimulating the liver to produce more ketone bodies (i.e., acetoacetate, hydroxybutyrate, and acetone) than the body can use. The ketone bodies accumulate in the blood, decreasing the blood pH and causing metabolic acidosis. This type of metabolic acidosis is called diabetic ketoacidosis (DKA). In DKA, acetone is exhaled, giving the breath an acetone smell or a fruity odor. In severe cases of DKA, brown crystals of acetone can form on the lips.

Review Questions

1. b; 2. d; 3. a; 4. b; 5. c; 6. d; 7. a; 8. d; 9. b; 10. a

Critical Thinking Questions

1. Insulin stimulates lipogenesis (i.e., fat synthesis) and inhibits lipolysis (i.e., fat breakdown). Insulin removes the glucose from the blood and uses it to synthesize fats.

2. Pancreatic secretion of insulin and glucagon helps to regulate blood glucose levels and the amount of glucose stored in the liver in the form of glycogen.

3. Starches are metabolized starting in the mouth. Salivary amylase is mixed with food during chewing. The amylase metabolizes the starch as the food makes its way down to the stomach. The acid in the stomach further metabolizes the starch, breaking it into monosaccharides, disaccharides, and polysaccharides. The monosaccharides and disaccharides are absorbed into the blood, and the polysaccharides are excreted.

Case Study

A Sudan stain would reveal that this man is experiencing fat in his stool (steatorrhea) as a result of chronic pancreatitis. In chronic pancreatitis, digestion of the organ causes fibrosis and scarring. The pancreas progressively loses function over time and is slowly destroyed. The loss of function leads to diabetes and pancreatic insufficiency, a form of maldigestion.

Chapter 23

Case in Point

The probable diagnosis is Cushing syndrome. Symptoms of Cushing syndrome include central obesity, thin limbs, and a round, moon-shaped face. She also has hypertension and hyperglycemia. Her cortisol levels are abnormal because the morning level is higher than the afternoon level.

Review Questions

1. c; 2. d; 3. c; 4. b; 5. c; 6. a; 7. d; 8. c; 9. b; 10. a

Critical Thinking Questions

1. The adrenal glands are composed of the adrenal cortex (i.e., outer portion) and the adrenal medulla (i.e., inner portion). The adrenal cortex is composed of the zona glomerulosa (an outer layer that secretes mineralocorticoids), the zona fasciculata (a middle layer that secretes glucocorticoids), and the zona reticularis (an inner layer that secretes androgens). The adrenal medulla secretes the catecholamines epinephrine and norepinephrine.

2. The parathyroid glands produce PTH (i.e., parathormone), which interacts with vitamin D to increase blood calcium levels. Calcium binds to receptors on the parathyroid chief cells, generating a signal that increases PTH secretion when calcium levels rise and decreases PTH secretion when calcium levels decline. Increased phosphate levels lead to decreased calcium levels and increased PTH secretion.

3. Most often, the angiotensin II level is elevated through a renin-dependent mechanism that causes increased aldosterone secretion. Increased angiotensin II levels can be caused by dehydration, shock, hypoalbuminemia,

renal artery stenosis, heart failure, or hepatic cirrhosis. Increased angiotensin II levels lead to increased aldosterone levels, which lead to increased sodium and water reabsorption by nephron collecting duct.

Case Study

The abnormal test results include bicarbonate, calcium, chloride, free T_3, free T_4, glucose, magnesium, phosphorus, potassium, sodium, thyroid peroxidase antibodies, thyroxine-binding globulin, total T_3, total T_4, and tyrosine. The preliminary diagnosis would be hyperthyroidism.

Thyroid-stimulating hormone (TSH) stimulates the thyroid gland to produce T_3 and T_4. T_3 and T_4 exert effects on cellular metabolism. Thyroglobulin is the binding protein that transport T_3 and T_4 in the blood. The final differential diagnosis would be thyroid hormone resistance because TSH is normal while T_3 and T_4 are elevated. Additional tests would include a thyroid biopsy.

Chapter 24

Case in Point

The diabetic man is experiencing diabetic nephropathy. His high blood sugar levels are damaging the kidneys and allowing protein to be excreted in the urine. If the urine protein level were 3 g or greater in 24 hours, the likely diagnosis would be nephrotic syndrome.

Review Questions

1. a; 2. c; 3. a; 4. a; 5. a; 6. b; 7. b; 8. d; 9. b; 10. c

Critical Thinking Questions

1. The three parts of a urinalysis are the physical, chemical, and microscopic examinations. The physical examination detects the color and clarity of the urine, and unusual odors noticed during the physical examination may indicate a particular condition. Color usually ranges from pale yellow to deep amber. The sample may be clear to very cloudy.

The chemistry examination includes specific gravity, pH, protein, glucose, ketones, blood, leukocyte esterase, nitrites, bilirubin, and urobilinogen. It is usually performed with the use of a dipstick test kit (Fig. 24-10).

The microscopic examination looks for cells (i.e., epithelial cells, bacteria, yeast, white blood cells, and red blood cells), casts, and crystals (Fig. 24-11). Casts are formed from Tamm-Horsfall proteins in the distal convoluted tubules and collecting ducts of the nephron. Casts can be hyaline, cellular (i.e., red cells, white cells, or epithelial cells), granular, or waxy. Waxy and finely granular casts indicate profound stasis of urine in the kidney tubules or collecting ducts. Included are calcium oxalate crystals, triple phosphate crystals, hippurate crystals, uric acid crystals, cysteine crystals, and tyrosine crystals. Most crystals are considered nonpathogenic, but some, such as cysteine and tyrosine, are considered pathogenic.

Aromas detected in the physical examination can lead to diagnosis of aminoacidurias or infections. The chemical examination can diagnoses diabetes and diabetic ketoacidosis. The microscopic examination can diagnosis renal failure and renal tubular acidosis.

2. The primary function of the renal system is to maintain homeostasis in the body. The kidneys maintain homeostasis by removing metabolic waste and organic substances from the plasma and by regulating plasma volume, electrolytes, and the hydrogen ion concentration. They also maintain homeostasis by regulating erythropoietin, renin, and vitamin D production.

Hypoxemia and anemia stimulate the peritubular epithelial cells of the renal cortex to synthesize erythropoietin. Renin is a proteolytic enzyme that is released from specialized cells when the pressure in the afferent arteriole and sodium concentration in the tubule decrease. The proximal tubule of the kidney secretes 1α-hydroxylase, which converts 25-hydroxyvitamin D to biologically active 1,25-dihydroxyvitamin D_3 (i.e., calcitriol).

3. Cystitis and pyelonephritis are both urinary tract infections. Cystitis occurs in the bladder, whereas pyelonephritis occurs in the kidney. If left untreated, cystitis can progress into pyelonephritis. If left untreated, severe pyelonephritis can result and can lead to pyonephrosis (i.e., pus around the kidney), urosepsis (i.e., systemic infection), kidney failure, and death.

Case Study

Polycystic kidney disease (PKD) is a genetic disorder with an autosomal dominant or autosomal recessive pattern of inheritance. PKD is characterized by cysts in the kidneys. The cysts are often filled with fluid and can be few or numerous. The cysts replace functioning nephrons with nonfunctioning space. They increase the size of the kidney and decrease kidney function.

PKD is common in the United States and is a leading cause of kidney transplantation (Fig. 24-8). Performing genetic testing for the PKD gene in affected persons or in family members is expensive but can yield a diagnosis. There is no cure for PKD. Individuals with the disease are treated with medication for various symptoms such as hypertension.

Chapter 25
Case in Point

Many female marathon runners experience amenorrhea due to a syndrome known as female athletic triad. Women with athletic triad syndrome exercise vigorously and may have amenorrhea, disordered eating, and osteoporosis. Ovarian tumors, ovarian failure, polycystic ovary syndrome (PCOS), and Cushing syndrome can also cause secondary amenorrhea. Evidence demonstrates that a critical body fat level is necessary for the female reproductive system to function normally.

Other hormone tests may be helpful in ruling out other conditions that could cause amenorrhea, especially primary ovarian failure. Other tests that need to be ordered are tests to rule out male infertility. Although this woman may have some issues, it may actually be the male who is infertile.

Review Questions

1. c; 2. b; 3. a; 4. a; 5. d; 6. d; 7. b; 8. c; 9. c; 10. a

Critical Thinking Questions

1. Because the hypothalamic-pituitary-gonadal axis produces the gonadotropin that controls the rest of the reproductive hormones, it would make sense that any dysfunction in this system would cause infertility and other issues.
2. Menopause is the cessation of menstruation and reproductive capabilities in women. This only affects women because men do not menstruate.

Case Study

The significant event is menopause. Levels of estrogen in the blood decline, and this leads to bone resorption and dysfunctional rebuilding of bones. The resulting bones are porous and very brittle.

Most women go through menopause at age 50 or 51. Reaching menopause does not automatically create brittle bones. Reaching menopause is when the bone changes begin. It takes time for a woman to develop osteoporosis.

Any condition that decreases the amount of estrogen in a woman's system, such as primary or secondary ovarian failure, may justify doing a bone density scan on a woman before age 60.

Chapter 26
Case in Point

A high fasting glucose level indicates that this woman may have gestational diabetes. The provider should order the oral glucose tolerance test to confirm gestational diabetes. This should be done to protect both the mother and the child during the remainder of the pregnancy.

Review Questions

1. b; 2. b; 3. b; 4. a; 5. a; 6. a; 7. a; 8. a; 9. a; 10. a

Critical Thinking Questions

1. Ectopic pregnancies can be medical emergencies if the fertilized egg continues to grow and ruptures the fallopian tube; the resulting hemorrhage releases a large volume of blood into the abdominal cavity. The following symptoms suggest a medical emergency: abdominal

rigidity, severe tenderness, and evidence of hypovolemic shock (orthostatic blood changes due to hemorrhage).

2. Preeclampsia is characterized by hypertension (blood pressure >140/90 mm Hg on two separate occasions) and proteinuria (protein in the urine) after the 20th week of pregnancy. The exact cause of preeclampsia is unknown, but risk factors for this condition include age greater than 40 years, black race, family history of preeclampsia, chronic renal disease, chronic hypertension, diabetes mellitus, twin gestation, and a high body mass index (>31). Severe preeclampsia is defined as the presence of at least one of the following symptoms in addition to hypertension and proteinuria: blood pressure 160/110 mm Hg or higher, proteinuria (>5 g in 24-hour collection, or >3+ on two random specimens), pulmonary edema, cyanosis, oliguria (<400 mL in 24 hours), persistent headaches, epigastric pain, impaired liver function, thrombocytopenia (platelet count <100,000/mm^3), and decreased fetal growth or placental abruption (placenta breaking away from uterus). The only treatment for preeclampsia is delivery.

3. A life-threatening manifestation of preeclampsia is eclampsia, in which a mother experiences grand mal seizures or falls into a coma. This is important because eclampsia can lead to intracranial hemorrhage.

Case Study

Ms. D has preeclampsia. This is considered a serious situation because the only treatment for preeclampsia is delivery. Individuals who have mild preeclampsia can have labor induced after 37 weeks' gestation. Because the fetus must survive after birth, it can be treated with corticosteroids to speed fetal lung maturity. If a woman develops preeclampsia before 34 weeks' gestation, the severity of the disease and its effect on the mother and child must be weighed against the risks of infant prematurity.

Possible complications include going from a mild preeclampsia condition to a severe preeclampsia condition that could harm both the mother and the baby. Severe preeclampsia is defined as the presence of at least one of the following symptoms in addition to hypertension and proteinuria: blood pressure 160/110 mm Hg or higher, proteinuria (>5 g in 24-hour collection, or >3+ on two random specimens), pulmonary edema, cyanosis, oliguria (<400 mL in 24 hours), persistent headaches, epigastric pain, impaired liver function, thrombocytopenia (platelet count <100,000/mm^3), and decreased fetal growth or placental abruption (placenta breaking away from uterus).

Chapter 27

Case in Point

Rhabdomyolysis causes rapid destruction of skeletal muscle cells. It often results from muscle injury and the consequent release of large quantities of myoglobin, which can be toxic. Symptoms include muscle weakness, muscle pain, and dark urine caused by excreted myoglobin. Life-threatening complications include renal failure and disseminated intravascular coagulation (DIC). Other complications include electrolyte abnormalities and hypoalbuminemia.

Review Questions

1. b; 2. a; 3. a; 4. b; 5. c; 6. d; 7. d; 8. a; 9. c; 10. b

Critical Thinking Questions

1. There are three different types of calcium in the body—ionized calcium, calcium bound to albumin, and calcium bound to diffusible ions such as phosphate or citrate. Ionized calcium is the biologically active form of calcium. About 50% of the calcium in the body is in the free or ionized form, 40% is bound to plasma proteins, and 10% bound to diffusible anions. The calcium cation (Ca^{2+}) binds to negatively charged sites on the albumin molecule. As the pH of the blood increases, more calcium binds to albumin, and there is a smaller amount of free calcium in the blood. As the pH of the blood decreases, less calcium binds to albumin, and there is a larger amount of free calcium in the blood. Calcium plays an important role in many body processes. For example, extracellular calcium serves as an intracellular messenger by binding and releasing cellular proteins. The proteins change their structure and function on binding to calcium. Calcium as an intracellular messenger helps regulate muscle contraction, hormone and fluid secretion, mitosis, and ion transfer across cell membranes. Bones are dynamic systems that constantly absorb, reabsorb, and release calcium, and bones serve as a storehouse for calcium. The dynamic balance of calcium in the body is controlled by hormones.

2. Diagnostic laboratory tests for rheumatoid arthritis (RA) include C-reactive protein (CRP), complete blood count (CBC), rheumatoid factor (RF), erythrocyte sedimentation rate (ESR), anti–cyclic citrullinated peptide (anti-CCP), and anti–mutated citrullinated vimentin (anti-MCV) assays. The ESR and CRP levels are elevated in this disease, and the CRP level increases as the disease progresses. Many people with RA also have anemia from the disease process or from the medications used to treat it. Disease activity corresponds to the severity of anemia, which can be reversed with therapy. The most specific tests for RA are the autoantibody tests. The RF test is not specific for RA because RF is also elevated in connective tissue diseases, infections, and other autoimmune disorders. RF levels can fluctuate with disease activity, but they tend to remain high even during drug-induced remissions. RF levels predict progression of bone erosions. Anti-CCP and anti-MCV

levels are used to diagnose RA. Elevated anti-CCP levels in conjunction with an elevated RF level are specific for RA. If both antibodies are present, a worse prognosis is indicated. RF is detected by latex agglutination or immunoturbidimetric tests. Anti-CCP and anti-MCV are measured by enzyme-linked immunoassay (ELISA) methods.

3. The weakness associated with Duchenne muscular dystrophy occurs mainly in the pelvic and shoulder muscles. Infants with Duchenne muscular dystrophy appear to be normal and may not be suspected of having the disease unless a sibling was previously diagnosed with it. Muscle weakness is not apparent until the child begins to walk. Children with this disease may delay walking due to muscle weakness, and they may also have intellectual impairment that can affect the ability to walk. At age 5 years, children struggle with school-related activities such as climbing stairs and playing at recess. As the disease progresses, children fall often and have a hard time getting up from a sitting or lying posture. Some children become wheelchair bound by 6 years of age, after which the disease progresses more rapidly. Duchenne muscular dystrophy is a terminal disease, and death usually occurs before the age of 30.

Case Study

Myasthenia gravis is an autoimmune disease caused by the formation of antibodies against acetylcholine nicotinic post-synaptic receptors at the neuromuscular junction of skeletal muscles. This prohibits impulses from the brain from reaching muscles, causing the muscles to cease functioning. Symptoms include specific muscle weakness and extra-ocular muscle weakness. Muscle weakness tends to grow worse throughout the day. The weakness is progressive, and approximately 13 months after onset the disease becomes generalized. Symptoms are exacerbated by bright sunlight, surgery, immunization, emotional stress, menstruation, and medications. The anti-acetylcholine receptor test is used for diagnosing the disease. The test is 100% specific, and the result is positive for approximately 90% of individuals with the disease.

Chapter 28

Case in Point

The provider is probably looking for signs of multiple sclerosis. Multiple sclerosis is a chronic disease that is caused by demyelination of the neurons. When nerves lose their coverings, they short-circuit and do not carry nerve impulses well. The disease increases in severity as years go by and more and more myelin is removed from the nerves.

Review Questions

1. b; 2. a; 3. b; 4. c; 5. d; 6. b; 7. a; 8. c; 9. d; 10. d

Critical Thinking Questions

1. Routine tests performed on a CSF sample include a Gram stain and culture, protein, glucose, and cell count. Normally, there are no microorganisms in a CSF sample, so the Gram stain and culture should be negative. A positive finding would be identification of a microorganism in the CSF. The reference range for CSF glucose is 75% of plasma glucose, which is approximately 45 to 75 mg/dL. A positive finding would be an elevated or decreased glucose level. A decreased glucose level would indicate an infection.

   The reference range for CSF protein is 15 to 45 mg/dL. An elevated or decreased protein level would be considered abnormal. An elevated level may indicate an infection.

   There are normally five or fewer red or white blood cells in CSF. An abnormal result would be finding more than five red or white blood cells in CSF. Increased cells in the CSF indicate a traumatic tap, a subarachnoid hemorrhage, or an infection.

2. Test methods for CSF protein include sulfosalicylic acid, pyrogallol red, and Coomassie blue. The reference range for CSF protein is 15 to 45 mg/dL, whereas the reference range for total protein in serum is 6.4 to 8.3 g/dL. The biuret test method is very accurate for specimens with high protein concentrations, but CSF has very low protein levels (measured in milligrams, not grams).

3. Closed neural tube defects are confined to one area and usually involve only the spine. Spinal presentations include spina bifida. Closed neural tube defects commonly manifest as an abnormality along the spine, such as a fluid-filled cyst, an area of hypopigmentation or hyperpigmentation, capillary telangiectasia or hemangioma, a hairy patch, a skin appendage, or an asymmetric gluteal cleft (Fig. 28-4). The neural tube is not visible at birth. An α-fetoprotein measurement is performed at 15 to 20 weeks' gestation to detect neural tube defects. The procedure and the interpretation of the test results are discussed in Chapter 25.

Case Study

This man was just immunized for the flu. An overreaction of the body to an immunization can cause Guillian-Barré syndrome (GBS). GBS is an acute autoimmune disorder that involves an anti-myelin antibody. It represents an excessive immune response to immunization or an infection. If the syndrome is not treated, it can be fatal because it can lead to respiratory muscle paralysis. The motor nerve dysfunction causes weakness that begins in the legs and arms and then moves upward to the respiratory muscles in a few days to a few weeks. No laboratory tests are used for the diagnosis.

Chapter 29

Case in Point

The woman had albinism, which is caused by a genetic mutation.

Review Questions

1. c; 2. d; 3. b; 4. b; 5. a; 6. d; 7. a; 8. b; 9. c; 10. b

Critical Thinking Questions

1. *Candida* thrives in warm, moist, dark places such as skin folds. The fungal infection commonly occurs on the genitals or in skin folds around the genitals or buttocks. The high blood sugar level of diabetics provides a steady source of carbohydrates for the fungi to live on. Diabetic ulcers usually occur on the foot and are caused by decreased circulation and neuropathy, which together promote skin breakdown rather than healing after an injury.

2. Also called *systemic sclerosis,* scleroderma is an autoimmune disease of connective tissue that can produce thick, leather-like skin. The progressive disease that affects many other systems in addition to the skin. Different forms of the disease are characterized by limited skin involvement, diffuse skin sclerosis, severe and progressive organ involvement, or fulminant systemic sclerosis. The form with limited skin involvement affects areas above the elbows and knees, the face, and the neck. The diffuse cutaneous form causes skin thickening of the trunk and areas below the elbows and knees; the face is also involved. Involvement of the heart, lungs, or kidneys can be life-threatening. Systemic sclerosis is most obvious in the skin and in the gastrointestinal, respiratory, renal, cardiovascular, musculoskeletal, endocrine, and genitourinary tracts. Loss of range of joint motion is caused by skin tightening. Thickening of the skin is caused by chronic inflammation leading to fibrosis of tissue. The trigger for this autoimmune reaction is unknown.

3. Albinism is a group of disorders caused by mutations in genes responsible for melanin synthesis, distribution of pigment by melanocytes, and melanosome biogenesis. Symptoms are complete or partial loss of pigment in the skin, hair, and eyes. With complete pigment loss, the hair is white, and the eyes appear pink because light is reflected from the back of the eye.

Case Study

Diabetic foot ulcers are caused by poor perfusion of blood in the extremities and exacerbated by diabetic neuropathy that compromises feeling in the extremities, especially the feet. The two conditions work in tandem to allow skin breakdown initiated by pressure or an injury to progress to an ulcer. Proper healing requires a supply of nutrients and structural materials for repair. However, the diabetic's blood is thicker than normal because of increased glucose levels, and it moves slowly through the small capillaries in the skin, impeding the rate of healing.

Chapter 30

Case in Point

The condition is vertigo, and it cannot be detected through laboratory tests. Vertigo causes a temporary change in laboratory tests results, especially electrolytes and glucose, due to vomiting.

Review Questions

1. a; 2. c; 3. d; 4. a; 5. b; 6. b; 7. a; 8. d; 9. c; 10. d

Critical Thinking Questions

1. Chronically high blood sugar levels cause hypertension, increasing the microaneurysms and oxidative damage in retinal arteries. Microaneurysms burst, leaking plasma or blood and causing hemorrhages and retinal exudates in the early phase of the disease. Later phases of diabetic retinopathy often involve proliferative vascular changes, including growth of new blood vessels in the retina that are delicate, bleed easily, and hinder vision. Scarring can occur, eventually leading to blindness.

2. Hypertensive individuals have high blood pressure in all arteries, including those of the eye. Atherosclerosis (i.e., hardening of the arteries) also involves the eye arteries, causing small aneurysms (i.e., blood-filled bulges) in the arterial walls that can rupture if the hypertension remains untreated, similar to a cerebrovascular accident involving a small artery. The damaged retina and reduction in blood supply impair eyesight. Atherosclerosis also causes the arteries to become less flexible, reducing their ability to deliver oxygenated blood to the eye. This further damages the retina and leads to impaired vision.

3. Ototoxic drugs such as aminoglycosides (e.g., streptomycin, gentamicin), vancomycin, furosemide, quinine, and related compounds can damage the auditory nerve. Large doses of aspirin can cause tinnitus (i.e., ringing in the ears) and temporary hearing loss.

Case Study

Younger people with genetic conditions that cause abnormally high lipid levels can produce a lipid arc around the cornea. The triglyceride levels usually exceed 4000 mg/dL, and cholesterol levels exceed 1200 mg/dL. Tangier disease, an inherited disorder characterized by abnormally low blood levels of high-density lipoprotein (HDL) cholesterol (<5 mg/dL), results in diffuse opacity of the cornea due to deposition of cholesterol.

Chapter 31

Case in Point

The physician would order a vitamin D measurement to find out why the calcium level is low. Because the patient lives in the Pacific Northwest, where it rains often, she does not have much exposure to the sun to help increase her vitamin D level, which is probably low. The woman should be treated with vitamin D supplements.

Review Questions

1. b; 2. b; 3. c; 4. a; 5. a; 6. d; 7. c; 8. c; 9. d; 10. d

Critical Thinking Questions

1. In addition to macronutrients, many micronutrients play a large part in keeping the human body healthy. Micronutrients are needed in very small amounts but are essential for good health and may cause disease if deficient. Vitamins and trace metals are micronutrients that are important reactants in many physiologic reactions.

2. The metabolism of fatty acids leads to the production of eicosanoids, including prostaglandins, thromboxanes, and lipoxins. Eicosanoids control the production of hormones and many physiologic functions. Prostaglandins and thromboxanes, also called *prostanoids,* are made from dihomo-γ-linolenic acid (DGLA) by an alternative pathway. They inhibit gastric acid secretion, increase vasodilation, decrease the inflammatory response, and inhibit platelet aggregation and thrombosis. Lipoxins are potent antiinflammatory molecules that are created through lipoxygenase interactions.

3. All newborns in the United States are tested for phenylketonuria (PKU). In the original test developed by Guthrie in the 1960s, a sample of blood from a newborn was collected on filter paper and transferred to a bacterial culture to determine whether it contained high levels of phenylalanine. Most states now use tandem mass spectrometry (MS/MS) to test for more than 30 substances. All infants are tested for PKU because it causes microcephaly and severe mental retardation, which can be avoided by eliminating foods containing phenylalanine from the diet of the affected infant.

Case Study

The physician should order a mercury level test because the patient's symptoms indicate mercury poisoning. He eats a lot of fish, and fish caught in some areas contain high levels of mercury. Mercury attacks the insulating myelin sheaths surrounding some nerves and can disturb vision and hearing.

Chapter 32

Case in Point

Abnormal laboratory results include the white blood cell count and 1+ level of ketones in the urine. The child has an immunodeficiency disease, and follow-up tests should include total and individual immunoglobulin levels. The probable diagnosis is Wiskott-Aldrich disease.

Review Questions

1. c; 2. d; 3. b; 4. b; 5. b; 6. b; 7. b; 8. a; 9. d; 10. b

Critical Thinking Questions

1. Cell-mediated immunity is controlled by T cells and involves activation of phagocytes and antigen-specific T lymphocytes in response to antigens. The immune response generates cytotoxic T cells that destroy pathogen-infected cells and cancer cells. The humoral and cell-mediated components are controlled by helper T cells through the secretion of chemical messengers called *cytokines.* The cell-mediated component also regulates immune reactions so that they do not become excessive and harm normal tissues. The normal immune response mounts an acute defense against pathogens and then returns the system to homeostasis.

   Type IV hypersensitivity is also called delayed hypersensitivity because it can take 48 to 72 hours before symptoms appear. It differs from other hypersensitivity reactions in that it is mediated by T lymphocytes instead of antibodies (see Fig. 32-11). The natural killer (NK) cells target and destroy aberrant cells by using cytotoxic molecules stored in secretory lysosomes. Examples of type IV hypersensitivity include contact dermatitis associated with sensitivity to jewelry, allergy to poison oak or ivy, and graft rejection. Type IV hypersensitivity mechanisms may play a part in autoimmune conditions. T cells destroy collagen and joints in rheumatoid arthritis, attack thyroid tissue in Hashimoto disease (i.e., autoimmune thyroiditis), and kill beta cells in the islets of Langerhans of the pancreas in type 1 diabetes.

   Helper T cells are the most important cells in the immune system because they secrete the cytokines necessary for stimulating antibody production by B cells, killing infected cells, monitoring and killing cancer cells, and controlling the immune system. When the population of helper T cells is low or nonexistent, all phases of the immune response are compromised. Persons infected with the human immunodeficiency virus (HIV) have increased numbers and severity of infections by bacteria, viruses, fungi, and parasites. Many of these can be life-threatening in the setting of HIV infection. Because cancer surveillance is compromised, the incidence of certain cancers increases. The lack of immune regulation in individuals with advanced HIV infection increases the likelihood of autoimmune conditions.

2. Hypersensitivity reactions are categorized by the antigen that is attacked by the immune system (i.e., allergy, autoimmunity, or alloimmunity) or by the mechanism of the attack (i.e., type I, II, III, or IV). Type I hypersensitivity reactions are immunoglobulin E mediated and responsible for most allergies. Hypersensitivity type II reactions

are tissue specific, and type III reactions are immune complex mediated. Types I, III, and III are immediate reactions. All four types of hypersensitivity reactions are seen in autoimmune diseases (see Table 32-2).

The cell-mediated type IV reaction is also called *delayed hypersensitivity* because the response can take 48 to 72 hours. It differs from other hypersensitivity reactions in that it is mediated by T lymphocytes instead of antibodies (see Fig. 32-11). Natural killer cells target and destroy aberrant cells by using cytotoxic molecules stored in secretory lysosomes. Examples of type IV hypersensitivity include contact dermatitis associated with sensitivity to jewelry, allergy to poison oak or ivy, and graft rejection. T cells destroy collagen and joints in rheumatoid arthritis, attack thyroid tissue in Hashimoto disease, and kill beta cells in the islets of Langerhans of the pancreas in type 1 diabetes.

3. In rheumatoid arthritis, the immune system produces antibodies against the synovial lining of the joints, resulting in a chronic, systemic, autoimmune inflammatory disease. Inflammation causes joint pain, swelling, and stiffness and eventually destroys the joints. During the course of the disease, damage spreads from the synovial to the articular cartilage, the fibrous joint capsule, and surrounding ligaments and tendons.

Case Study

HIV infection causes a long-term immunodeficiency disease that progresses to acquired immunodeficiency syndrome (AIDS) when the total T-cell count falls to 200 cells/mm^3 or less. Tests used for diagnosing HIV include the Western blot assay, and the viral load test is used to track disease progression.

Chapter 33

Case in Point

The patient is suffering from theophylline toxicity. Symptoms of theophylline overdose include seizures, arrhythmias, and gastrointestinal disturbances. Theophylline (proprietary name: Theo-Dur) is used to treat moderate or severe asthma.

Review Questions

1. a; 2. c; 3. b; 4. d; 5. b; 6. a; 7. d; 8. b; 9. c; 10. a

Critical Thinking Questions

1. Therapeutic drug monitoring (TDM) is used to measure medication levels in the blood and maintain the right amount of drug in a patient's system. Too little drug in the blood may not effectively treat the disease or symptoms, and too much may cause toxic side effects.
2. Drugs that are administered orally are absorbed through the gastrointestinal tract. They are then carried through the hepatic portal vein into the liver, where they are extensively metabolized (first-pass effect) before entering the systemic circulation. The absorption rate is influenced by the drug formulation and is affected by abnormal gastrointestinal motility, diseases or infections of the gastrointestinal tract, irradiation, and interactions with food and other substances. These variables should be taken into consideration when performing TDM and management.
3. The aim of TDM is to inform the provider about drug levels in a patient to ensure that they do not reach toxic levels (i.e., concentrations above the upper end of the therapeutic range). For some drugs, the difference between a functional dose and a lethal dose is very small; these drugs are said to have a low therapeutic index, and their levels must be monitored closely. Symptoms of toxicity vary depending on the drug and may affect the gastrointestinal tract, the cardiovascular system, and the central nervous system, as well as kidney and liver function.

Case Study

Therapeutic range for gentamicin is 1 to 5 mg/dL. The peak and trough levels in this case are not accurate. For antibiotics administered intravenously, specimens are drawn 30 minutes before the dose to measure the trough level and 30 minutes after completion of the infusion to measure the peak level. To determine true peak and trough levels, the samples will have to be redrawn following these guidelines. The values are not within acceptable trough and peak levels because they were drawn at the wrong time intervals.

Chapter 34

Case in Point

Normal circulating levels of carbon monoxide (CO) in blood are between 0% and 3%. The patient has CO poisoning; it is cold outside, so he could have been using a space heater that gives off CO. Space heaters should be used only in well-ventilated rooms. CO is called the silent killer because it is odorless, tasteless, and colorless. It has more affinity for hemoglobin than oxygen does, and after it binds to hemoglobin, it cannot be removed easily. Because oxygen cannot bind to the CO-bound hemoglobin, it cannot be delivered to nourish organs, and the body dies.

Review Questions

1. a; 2. d; 3. b; 4. b; 5. c; 6. a; 7. c; 8. a; 9. b; 10. c

Critical Thinking Questions

1. Each drug or toxin produces a specific toxic syndrome (i.e., toxidrome) when a large amount of the chemical is

introduced into the body. Most exhibit a dose-response curve: Low doses may produce no observable effect, but the effects increase as the dose increases. This curve is different for each drug or toxin and may vary according to the exposure time and exposure route.

2. Blood or urine samples are used to detect ethanol. Enzymatic methods are used for ethanol analysis. Ethanol is oxidized to acetaldehyde by alcohol dehydrogenase, and NAD+ is converted to NADH; the amount of NADH produced is directly proportional to the amount of ethanol in the sample.

Devices that detect the amount of alcohol in a person's breath (breathalyzers) have been developed for determining the blood alcohol level of an impaired driver. The device is based on the principle that the ratio of alcohol in capillary blood to that in alveolar (exhaled) air is about 2100:1.

An alcohol test has been developed in which saliva is absorbed by a swab, which is inserted into a test cartridge. The test is based on an alcohol dehydrogenase method coupled with a chromophore to produce a visual end point. This method is also used on card or strip tests.

When blood is drawn to determine the blood alcohol level, the individual must give consent. The blood alcohol kit should include betadine or another disinfectant to prepare the site (rather than alcohol) and a sticky label for the tube of blood that must be completed. The phlebotomist may be subpoenaed to testify about the collection of the specimen. A chain of custody form must be completed when a blood alcohol specimen is drawn for legal purposes.

3. Most opiates are μ opioid receptor agonists. They affect numerous regions of the central nervous system, and their effects include reduced pain transmission and activation of the reward system. Opiates (i.e., morphine and heroin) have a high potential for addiction and tolerance and can produce severe withdrawal symptoms on cessation, ranging from dysphoria to stroke, heart attack, and death.

Case Study

The anion gap for this patient is 140 – (100 + 15) = 25. The is an abnormal value, because the normal anion gap is 8 to 16. The measured osmolality is 230 mOsm/kg, whereas the calculated osmolality is higher, at 294 mOsm/kg. The two values are different because of the presence of volatile chemicals in the patient's urine. A methanol level test should be ordered, because illegally altered alcohol drinks can contain significant amounts of methanol. The most probable diagnosis is methanol intoxication.

Chapter 35

Case in Point

Numerous criteria are used to determine whether an individual with organ failure can be considered a candidate for transplantation. Indications include (1) a condition for which transplantation is considered effective treatment, (2) severe and progressive disease that no longer responds to medical treatment and may be fatal, (3) willingness to accept the risks of surgery and subsequent medical treatment, and (4) being physically and emotionally capable of tolerating surgery and subsequent medical treatment. A family profile and thorough psychological assessment of the patient help to identify psychosocial or psychiatric barriers to a good outcome. Laboratory medicine also plays a central role in the success of solid organ and hematopoietic stem cell transplantation (HSCT). Responsibilities include testing the donor for infectious disease, pretransplantation testing for immunologic compatibility of donor and recipient, and posttransplantation monitoring of organ function, immunosuppressant therapy, and adverse effects of immunosuppression.

Review Questions

1. c; 2. b; 3. d; 4. c; 5. b; 6. d; 7. b; 8. b; 9. a; 10. d

Critical Thinking Questions

1. Graft-versus-host disease (GVHD) is a potentially fatal condition that occurs when the immunoreactive cells of a transplant attack the tissues of the transplant recipient. It is a likely complication of hematopoietic stem cell transplantation (HSCT) because the graft replaces major components of the recipient's immune system and because the recipient's bone marrow is depleted to allow acceptance of the donor marrow. The immune reaction initiated by T cells of the graft can destroy liver, skin, and gastrointestinal tissues. GVHD can also affect the transplantation of organs rich in lymphocytes, such as the liver. The risk of developing GVHD is minimized by HLA matching, but it is not completely eliminated due to intact donor T cells in some grafts.

2. Transplant rejection is based on incompatibility of major histocompatibility complex proteins (i.e., HLAs). Humoral or cellular mechanisms can be responsible. Hyperacute rejection can occur almost immediately and is caused by preformed antibodies to donor HLAs or ABO blood type incompatibility. Acute rejection occurs over a longer period and is caused by T-cell recognition of donor organ HLAs (i.e., acute cellular rejection) or by formation of antibodies to donor organ HLAs. Immunosuppressant drugs block these responses. The primary drugs prescribed are corticosteroids such as prednisolone, calcineurin inhibitors (CNIs) such as cyclosporine and tacrolimus, mammalian target of rapamycin (mTOR) inhibitors such as sirolimus and everolimus, and mycophenolic acid (MPA).

Prednisolone stimulates promoter-enhanced transcription of genes (e.g., interleukin-1 receptor) that are involved in antiinflammatory responses and blocks the function of other factors that are required for transcription of proinflammatory mediators. Corticosteroids suppress antiinflammatory responses by macrophages and monocytes.

Cyclosporine binds to the cytoplasmic protein cyclophilin, and the resulting complex binds to and inhibits calcineurin, a regulated serine/threonine protein phosphatase that normally activates transcription factors necessary to produce the cytokines that are essential for lymphocyte proliferation. Tacrolimus, which is commonly used for maintenance of immunosuppression, binds first to FK506 binding protein 12 in the cytoplasm and then to calcineurin. The long-term side effects of tacrolimus are similar to those of cyclosporine but less nephrotoxic.

Sirolimus binds to an FK protein, and the complex then binds to mTOR. Inhibition of mTOR blocks the activation of interleukin-2 and prevents the G- to S-phase transition of T lymphocytes. Side effects of sirolimus and everolimus (a derivative of sirolimus with different pharmacokinetics) include hyperlipidemia, anemia, edema, proteinuria, thrombosis, hyperlipidemia, and decreased glucose tolerance due to insulin resistance. They are also nephrotoxic in a way that is synergistic with CNIs.

MPA is the active form of the prodrug mycophenolate mofetil. Because its mode of action is different from those of CNIs and mTOR inhibitors, it can be prescribed in addition to them. MPA is an antimetabolite and a selective inhibitor of inosine monophosphate dehydrogenase, which is found in activated lymphocytes and is necessary for purine synthesis and replication. MPA is regarded as safe for long-term immunosuppression, but it can cause abdominal pain, nausea, diarrhea, anemia, and leukopenia.

Case Study

Cyclosporine, tacrolimus, and mycophenolic acid are likely to be prescribed for the patient. After liver transplantation, liver function tests will be used for monitoring, as well as kidney function tests to check for nephrotoxicity due to cyclosporine. The induction phase of drug therapy lasts for at least 2 to 4 weeks after transplantation, after which the maintenance phase continues as a lower-intensity, long-term, stable regimen. If acute rejection occurs, immediate intensification of therapy with high-dose corticosteroids is required. Long-term use of immunosuppressant drugs can lead to problems such as atherosclerosis, diabetes, and renal insufficiency, for which patients must be monitored throughout their lives.

The exact regimen and combinations of immunosuppressants for different transplant types remains an active area of research. Each drug has a mechanism of action that interferes with the proliferation of lymphocytes and suppresses the immune response. In the future, expert systems will allow all variables for a patient to be analyzed to develop an individualized treatment plan.

Chapter 36

Case in Point

Because there is no confirmation of the type of chemical agent, both urine and blood specimens would need to be collected, according to the Centers for Disease Control and Prevention (CDC) and hospital guidelines. For example, the laboratory technician may collect 12 mL of blood in four 3-mL or three 4-mL EDTA tubes (marking the tubes with the order of draw), at least 3 mL of blood in one gray or green top tube, and 25 to 50 mL of urine. A label should be attached to each specimen and positioned so that the barcode resembles a ladder. Three empty 4-mL EDTA tubes and one empty gray top tube should be included in the shipment.

The specimens should be prepared for shipment as mandated by the CDC:

- Use a gridded-type box lined with an absorbent pad, and arrange the tubes by patient number. Place the gridded box into a secondary container, then place a plastic bag around the secondary container.
- Encircle the width of the box with one continuous piece of evidence tape (which cannot be moved once placed). The individual making the seal must write his or her initials half on the tape and half on the plastic bag.
- Wrap the gridded box and secondary container in an absorbent pad and seal it with regular tape. Place this wrapped container in a Saf-T-Pak clear inner, leakproof polybag or something similar.
- Place the Saf-T-Pak package into a white Tyvek (or equivalent) outer envelope.
- Seal the envelope all around with one continuous piece of evidence tape. Again, initial half on the evidence tape and half on the envelope.
- Next, place absorbent pads in the bottom of a polystyrene, foam-insulated, cardboard box.
- Place approximately four reusable ice packs in a single layer on top of the absorbent material.
- Place the wrapped package of specimens on top of the reusable ice packs. Then add additional packing material to cushion the specimens from all sides and additional ice packs on top.
- Place the shipping manifest (obtained on CDC website) in a sealed plastic bag on top of the samples. Place the lid on the box, and secure it with shipping tape.

Because these specimens may become part of legal evidence, it is imperative that the CDC instructions be followed to the letter. The chain-of-custody documents should be kept in the laboratory's files. The box is then shipped to the CDC as follows:

- Address the box top with the return address of the laboratory facility. The receiving address of the CDC Laboratory is listed on the website that describes the shipping requirements (http://emergency.cdc.gov/labissues/specimens_shipping_instructions.asp).

- On the same side with the addresses, add the "UN 3373" label and the words "Biological Substance, Category B."
- Send the box via FedEx (or an equivalent service) to the address listed on the CDC instructions for shipping specimens.

Review Questions

1. a; 2. d; 3. b; 4. b; 5. e; 6. c; 7. a; 8. d; 9. b; 10. a

Critical Thinking Questions

1. Terrorist groups are not opposed to killing people but rely more on the resulting chaos and psychological effects of an attack to make an impact. They are usually politically motivated to gain some type of an advantage by using chemical weapons as an offensive weapon. A government may think that using chemical agents as an offensive weapon will give them an edge over an opponent in a warlike situation.
2. As of 2010, fifty-three laboratories are part of the Laboratory Response Network (LRN) (see Fig. 36-13). All of them have level 3 capacity and can work with hospitals and first responders to ensure the quality of clinical specimen collection, storage, and shipment. The thirty-four level 2 laboratories in the LRN employ chemists who are trained to detect agents such as cyanide, nerve agents, and toxic metals. The ten level 1 laboratories in the LRN are top-level laboratories that aid the CDC in a chemical emergency response. They have high-throughput analysis capabilities and can detect exposure to cyanide, nerve agents, toxic metals, mustard agents, and toxic industrial chemicals.
3. Briefly, the groups and characteristics of chemical agents are the following:
   - Blister agents are chemicals that produce blisters when they come in contact with the eyes, skin, or respiratory tract. They include the nitrogen mustards and other mustard agents, lewisite, and phosgene oxime.
   - Blood agents are chemicals that become poisonous after they are absorbed into the blood. They include arsine and cyanogen chloride.
   - Caustics are acids that produce chemical burns on the skin, eyes, and mucous membranes on contact. An example is hydrofluoric acid.

- Pulmonary agents are chemicals that cause severe irritation or swelling of the respiratory tract. Chemicals in this group include ammonia, chlorine, mercury, diphosgene, phosgene, and phosphorus.
- Incapacitating agents are chemicals that impair brain function or cause an altered state of consciousness (e.g., unconsciousness). This group includes benzene (BZ), fentanyl, and 3-quinuclidinyl benzilate (QNB).
- Heavy metals usually act as poisons after being absorbed into the body by interfering with the production of hemoglobin. The metallic poison group includes arsenic, barium, mercury, and thallium.
- Organic solvents dissolve fats and oils, including cell membranes and other organs made with fat and oils. An example is benzene.
- Nerve agents are highly poisonous. After they enter the body, they interfere with the conduction of nerve impulses and can lead to death. Nerve agents are classified as G agents, including sarin (GB), soman (GD), and tabun (GA), or V agents such as VX.
- Riot control agents cause irritation to the eyes and mucous membranes on contact. This group of chemicals includes bromobenzyl cyanide (military designation: CA), chloroacetophenone (CN), chlorobenzylidenemalononitrile (CS), chloropicrin (PS), and dibenzoxazepine (CR).
- Alcohols produce toxic effects on the heart, kidney, and nervous system. The most common example is blindness caused by ethylene glycol.
- Adamsite is the only chemical classified as a vomiting agent. Exposure to it causes nausea and vomiting.

Case Study

It is likely that the chemical is some sort of blister agent. The blisters are the result of second- and third-degree burns. Individuals can also experience runny nose, sneezing, bloody nose, sinus pain, shortness of breath, and cough. When treating or drawing blood from these patients, it is important to wear the correct protective equipment to avoid worker exposure to the same agents. The patient must also be decontaminated as soon as possible after exposure. Many times, this means removing clothing immediately after exposure.

Index

Note: Page numbers followed by "*b*", "*t*", and "*f*" refer to boxes, tables, and figures respectively.